Volume two

ALIMENTARY TRACT ROENTGENOLOGY

Volume two

ALIMENTARY
TRACT ROENTGENOLOGY

Edited by

Alexander R. Margulis, M.D.

Professor and Chairman, Department of Radiology,
University of California School of Medicine,
San Francisco, California

and

H. Joachim Burhenne, M.D.

Clinical Professor of Radiology,
University of California School of Medicine, San Francisco;
Chairman, Department of Radiology,
Children's Hospital and Adult Medical Center,
San Francisco, California

with 2949 illustrations, including 16 in full color in Chapter 55

SECOND EDITION

The C. V. Mosby Company

SAINT LOUIS   1973

SECOND EDITION

Copyright © 1973 by The C. V. Mosby Company

All rights reserved. No part of this book may be reproduced in any manner without written permission of the publisher.

Previous edition copyrighted 1967

Printed in the United States of America

Distributed in Great Britain by Henry Kimpton, London

Library of Congress Cataloging in Publication Data

Margulis, Alexander R
 Alimentary tract roentgenology.

 Includes bibliographies.
 1. Alimentary canal—Radiography. I. Burhenne,
Hans Joachim, joint author. II. Title. [DNLM:
1. Gastrointestinal system—Radiography. WI 141 M331a
1973]
RC804.R6M3   1973   616.3'07'57   72-14444
ISBN 0-8016-3131-9

Contributors

John R. Amberg, M.D.

Professor and Chairman, Department of
Radiology, Vanderbilt University School of
Medicine, Nashville, Tennessee

Marcel Brombart, M.D.

Maître de Stage à l'Université Libre de Bruxelles;
former Chief of the X-ray Department
of the C. dePaepe Clinic, Brussels;
Honorary President, Belgian Society
of Gastro-Enterology, Avenue L. Lepoutre,
Brussels, Belgium

H. Joachim Burhenne, M.D.

Clinical Professor of Radiology,
University of California School of Medicine, San
Francisco; Chairman, Department of Radiology,
Children's Hospital and Adult Medical Center,
San Francisco, California

John V. Carbone, M.D.

Professor of Medicine,
University of California School of Medicine,
San Francisco, California

Harley C. Carlson, M.D.

Consultant,
Department of Diagnostic Roentgenology,
The Mayo Clinic,
Rochester, Minnesota

Arthur R. Clemett, M.D.

Clinical Professor of Radiology,
New York University School of Medicine;
Chief, Gastrointestinal Radiology Section,
St. Vincent's Hospital and Medical Center,
New York, New York

Wylie J. Dodds, M.D.

Associate Professor of Radiology,
Department of Radiology,
The Medical College of Wisconsin;
Chief of G. I. Radiology Section,
Milwaukee County General Hospital,
Milwaukee, Wisconsin

J. Scott Dunbar, M.D.

Professor and Head,
Department of Diagnostic Radiology,
The University of British Columbia Faculty
of Medicine, Vancouver, B. C., Canada

S. Boyd Eaton, Jr., M.D.

Clinical Assistant Professor of Radiology,
Emory University School of Medicine, Atlanta;
Radiologist, West Paces Ferry Hospital,
Atlanta, Georgia

John A. Evans, M.D.

Professor and Chairman, Department of
Radiology, The New York Hospital–Cornell
Medical Center, New York, New York

Joseph T. Ferrucci, Jr., M.D.

Assistant Professor in Radiology,
Harvard Medical School, Boston;
Associate Radiologist,
Massachusetts General Hospital,
Boston, Massachusetts

†Felix G. Fleischner, M.D.

Clinical Professor of Radiology (Emeritus),
Harvard Medical School;
Radiologist-in-Chief (Emeritus),
Beth Israel Hospital,
Boston, Massachusetts

†Deceased.

Barry D. Fletcher, M.D.

Assistant Professor of Diagnostic Radiology
and Lecturer in Pediatrics,
McGill University Faculty of Medicine,
Montreal, Quebec, Canada

Wolfgang Frik, M.D.

Professor of Radiology, Director,
Department of Radiology,
Faculty of Medicine,
Techn. University, Aachen, Germany

J. Frimann-Dahl, M.D.

Professor of Radiology, University of Oslo;
Head, Roentgen Department, Ullevål Hospital,
Oslo, Norway

Hermann Frommhold, M.D.

Scientific Assistant, Department of Radiology,
University Hospital, University of Bonn,
Bonn, Germany

Walter Frommhold, M.D.

Professor of Radiology and Director of Radiology,
University of Tübingen Institute,
Tübingen, Germany

Henry I. Goldberg, M.D.

Associate Professor of Radiology,
Department of Radiology,
University of California School of Medicine,
San Francisco, California

C. Allen Good, M.D.

Professor of Radiology,
Mayo Graduate School of Medicine,
Section of Diagnostic Roentgenology,
The Mayo Clinic, Rochester, Minnesota;
Secretary, The American Board of Radiology

Mordecai Halpern, M.D.

Professor of Radiology,
University of Southern California
School of Medicine; Attending Radiologist,
Los Angeles County–University
of Southern California Medical Center,
Los Angeles, California

George S. Harell, M.D.

Assistant Professor of Radiology,
Stanford University School of Medicine,
Stanford, California

J. N. Hunt, M.D., D.Sc.

Chairman of Physiology Department,
Guy's Hospital Medical School,
London, England

Makoto Ishikawa, M.D.

Associate Professor of Medicine,
Tohoku University School of Medicine,
Sendai, Japan

Leonard R. Johnson, Ph.D.

Professor, Program in Physiology,
University of Texas Medical School,
Houston, Texas

Mansho T. Khilnani, M.D.

Professor of Radiology,
Mount Sinai School of Medicine;
Attending Radiologist, Mount Sinai Hospital,
New York, New York

M. T. Knox, B.Sc., Ph.D.

Research Associate, Department of Physiology,
Guy's Hospital Medical School, London, England

Elliott C. Lasser, M.D.

Professor and Chairman, Department of
Radiology, University of California School of
Medicine, San Diego, California

Arthur E. Lindner, M.D.

Associate Professor of Medicine,
New York University School of Medicine,
New York, New York

James J. McCort, M.D.

Chairman, Division of Radiology,
Santa Clara Valley Medical Center,
San Jose, California;
Clinical Professor of Radiology,
Stanford University School of Medicine,
Stanford, California

Alexander R. Margulis, M.D.

Professor and Chairman,
Department of Radiology,
University of California School of Medicine,
San Francisco, California

Richard H. Marshak, M.D.

Clinical Professor of Radiology,
Mount Sinai School of Medicine
of The City University of New York;
Attending Radiologist,
Mount Sinai Hospital,
New York, New York

Harry Z. Mellins, M.D.

Professor of Radiology, Harvard Medical School;
Director, Division of Diagnostic Radiology,
Peter Bent Brigham Hospital,
Boston, Massachusetts

J. Howard Middlemiss,
C.M.G., M.D., F.R.C.P., F.F.R.

Department of Radiodiagnosis,
The Medical School;
Director of Radiology, Bristol Royal Infirmary,
Bristol, England

Earl R. Miller, M.D.

Professor of Radiology, Director,
Radiological Research Laboratory,
Department of Radiology,
University of California School of Medicine,
San Francisco, California

Roscoe E. Miller, M.D.

Professor of Radiology,
Indiana University Medical Center,
Indianapolis, Indiana

Ian W. Monie, M.B., Ch.B., M.D.

Professor of Anatomy and Embryology,
University of California School of Medicine,
San Francisco, California

Antonio Navarrete, M.D.

Assistant Professor of Pathology,
Baylor College of Medicine; Surgical Pathologist,
Ben Taub General Hospital, Houston, Texas

Walter L. Palmer, M.D., Ph.D.

Richard T. Crane Professor of Medicine
(Emeritus), University of Chicago;
Active Attending Staff, Woodlawn Hospital,
Chicago, Illinois

Robert Prévôt, M.D.

Professor and Ordinarius of Radiology
(Emeritus), University of Hamburg; Director,
Department of Radiology (Emeritus), University
Hospital, Hamburg-Eppendorf, Germany

Maurice M. Reeder, M.D.

Chief, Radiology Department,
Walter Reed General Hospital;
Consultant in Radiology
to Surgeon-General, U. S. Army,
Washington, D. C.

Leo G. Rigler, M.D.

Professor of Radiology,
University of California School of Medicine,
Los Angeles, California

Francis F. Ruzicka, Jr., M.D.

Professor of Radiology,
University of Wisconsin,
Madison, Wisconsin

Ralph Schlaeger, M.D.

Professor of Clinical Radiology,
Columbia University College of Physicians and
Surgeons; Attending Radiologist, Presbyterian
Hospital, Columbia-Presbyterian Medical
Center, New York, New York

William B. Seaman, M.D.

Professor and Chairman, Department of
Radiology, Columbia University
College of Physicians and Surgeons;
Chief of Radiology Service,
Columbia-Presbyterian Medical Center,
New York, New York

Edward B. Singleton, M.D.

Clinical Professor of Radiology,
Baylor College of Medicine, Texas Medical
Center; Director of Radiology,
St. Luke's Episcopal and Texas Children's
Hospital and the Texas Heart Institute,
Houston, Texas

Harlan J. Spjut, M.D.

Professor of Pathology,
Baylor College of Medicine;
Attending in Pathology, St. Luke's Hospital,
Houston, Texas

Hooshang Taybi, M.D., M.Sc.

Clinical Professor of Radiology,
University of California School of Medicine,
San Francisco, California;
Chief, Department of Radiology,
Children's Hospital Medical Center,
Oakland, California

Frederic E. Templeton, M.D.

Professor of Radiology,
University of Washington School of Medicine,
Seattle, Washington

Jack A. Vennes, M.D.

Associate Professor of Medicine,
University of Minnesota, School of Medicine;
Chief, Endoscopic Unit,
Veterans Administration Hospital,
Minneapolis, Minnesota

Marvin Weiner, M.D.

Associate Professor of Radiology,
University of California School of Medicine,
Los Angeles, California

Sölve Welin, M.D.

Professor of Radiology (Emeritus),
University of Lund;
Director and Chairman (Emeritus),
University X-ray Department,
Malmö General Hospital, Malmö, Sweden

Walter M. Whitehouse, M.D.

Professor and Chairman, Department of
Radiology, The University of Michigan Medical
School, Ann Arbor, Michigan

Ifor Williams, M.R.C.P., D.M.R.D.

Radiologist, Northwick Park Hospital
and Clinical Research Centre,
Harrow, London, England

Robert E. Wise, M.D.

Clinical Professor of Radiology,
Boston University School of Medicine;
Chairman, Department of Diagnostic Radiology,
Lahey Clinic Foundation, Boston;
Chairman, Department of Radiology,
New England Baptist Hospital,
Boston, Massachusetts

Bernard S. Wolf, M.D.

Professor and Chairman, Department of
Radiology, Mount Sinai School of Medicine
of The City University of New York;
Director, Department of Radiology,
Mount Sinai Hospital,
New York, New York

Shoichi Yamagata, M.D.

Professor of Medicine,
Tohoku University School of Medicine,
Sendai, Japan

James E. Youker, M.D.

Professor and Chairman, Department of
Radiology, The Medical College of Wisconsin;
Director, Department of Radiology,
Milwaukee County General Hospital,
Milwaukee, Wisconsin

F. Frank Zboralske, M.D.

Professor of Radiology, Director,
Division of Diagnostic Radiology,
Stanford University School of Medicine,
Stanford, California

Preface

The second edition of *Alimentary Tract Roentgenology* follows the first edition by 6 years. The field of gastrointestinal radiology is progressing at a steady pace and reference books must be kept up to date. The reader who compares the second edition to our first effort will notice that almost every chapter has been changed and that a number of new chapters have been added. Although the first edition had forty-nine chapters, the second edition has grown to sixty-four. This increase includes corrections for some omissions and attempts a more logical sequence of chapters. It also reflects the growth in the field. The number of illustrations has been doubled.

As before, there is a certain overlap of material in the chapters, since we have encouraged the expression of different views on controversial subjects. Some of these views are in direct opposition to each other and are included for the sake of completeness in areas where proof is still not available.

The international character of the contributors to the book has been jealously maintained and expanded. We are extremely grateful to all coauthors of both editions for their diligent work and excellent contributions. We sincerely hope that many of them will join us again when the time comes to revise this work.

We would also like to express our appreciation to Miss Hildegarde Braun, Mrs. Rae Saxon, Mrs. Livia De Wath, and Mrs. Jane Reille for their help in preparing this book.

A. R. M.
H. J. B.

Contents

xi

Volume two

PART V   THE SMALL BOWEL

PART VI   THE COLON

PART VII   THE PANCREAS AND THE LESSER SAC

PART VIII   THE LIVER AND THE BILIARY TRACT

PART IX   SPECIAL PROCEDURES

PART X   PEDIATRIC ROENTGENOLOGY

Part V

The small bowel

Pathology of the small bowel | 30

Harlan J. Spjut
Antonio Navarrete

SMALL BOWEL
Malformations
Atresias

Atresias of the small intestine may occur in the jejunum or ileum or in both. Occasionally the colon is affected when the small intestine is involved with atresia. There may be multiple sites of atresia. One case report describes atresia of the small intestine and part of the colon from the jejunum to the transverse colon.[35] The segment proximal to the area of an atresia is often greatly dilated, whereas the segment distal to the atresia is very tiny, sometimes measuring as little as 4 mm. in diameter. The atretic segment may be represented only as a fibrous strand (Fig. 30-1). Some atresias are associated with a mucosal diaphragm that effectively blocks the passage of the intestinal content; in others there is complete separation of the bowel segments. Other anomalies of the intestinal tract or other viscera may be associated with the atresias. These include intestinal malrotations, hypoplasia of the kidney, clubfoot, and Meckel's diverticulum.

The pathogenesis of the lesion has been suggested in the section on the esophagus. A number of the atresias have been thought to be caused by mechanical obstruction in utero such as volvulus and intussusception, resulting in strangulation of the intestine with compromise of the blood supply. This perhaps is not the only etiologic factor but seems at the moment to be a major consideration.[19,28]

In addition to atresia two other lesions must be considered in the infant with clinical evidence of intestinal obstruction. Rare examples of segmental absence of the musculature of the small intestine have been reported. A second cause is aganglionosis of the small bowel. The colon has always been involved in the cases reported thus far. The aganglionosis may involve the entire small intestine and even the duodenum, but most commonly affects the terminal ileum.[49,51]

Meckel's diverticulum

Meckel's diverticulum is said to be the most frequent anomaly of the gastrointestinal tract, occurring in approximately 3% of patients. Generally speaking, it is not of great importance unless a complication develops. The Meckel's diverticulum is the result of a persistence of the omphalomesenteric duct, which should be obliterated and detached from the embryo by the fifth week. The diverticulum may occur anywhere within the terminal 6 feet of the ileum and is almost invariably on the antimesenteric border (about 6% occur on the mesenteric border).

The major complications of Meckel's diverticulum are ulcer, inflammation, and obstruction, which includes obstruction caused by intussusception, fibrous bands, and volvulus and occasionally the occurrence of tumors. Among the tumors that have been reported in Meckel's diverticulum (about 60) are carcinomas, sarcomas, and carcinoids.[24]

Microscopically, the Meckel's diverticulum consists of the full thickness of the wall of the small intestine. Heterotopic tissue (12% to

787

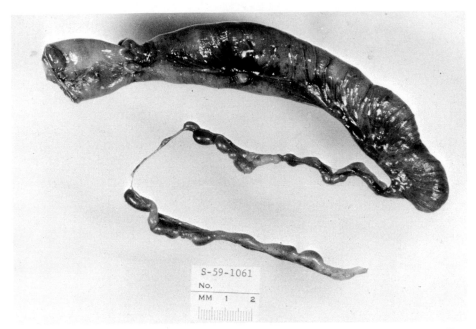

Fig. 30-1. Jejunal atresia with an extremely narrow segment that becomes a fibrous cord. (Courtesy Dr. Harvey Rosenberg.)

16%) is most likely to be found in symptomatic diverticula in the following order of frequency: gastric, pancreatic, and colonic.[3,23]

Diverticula

The jejunum is the most common site of diverticula, with the ileum alone the next most common, and both simultaneously involved the least common.[29] A solitary diverticulum is most likely to be noted in the ileum and multiple diverticula in the jejunum. Diverticula usually have a wide mouth and are composed of mucosa, submucosa, and muscularis mucosae, the muscularis propria not being a portion of the wall. Most are located on the mesenteric border of the bowel. The majority of diverticula of the small intestine do not produce symptoms. Occasionally complications occur such as volvulus, obstruction, inflammation, perforation, and bleeding.[33] An interesting association of multiple diverticula of the jejunum with steatorrhea, macrocytic anemia, and glossitis has been noted.[9]

Intussusception

Intussusception is the invagination of one portion of the intestine into another (Fig. 30-2). It is most frequently encountered in infants and children and is uncommon after the age of 5. Most of the episodes of intussusception occur within the first 2 years of life. In childhood the cause is usually inapparent whereas after the age of 4 years and into adulthood the etiologic factor leading to intussusception usually can be found. Ileoileal and ileocolic types of intussusception are the most frequent, with the latter comprising the majority. A rare form of intussusception is that of the appendix into itself or into the cecum or colon.

When a cause is demonstrated in intussusception in children it includes Meckel's diverticulum, polyps, duplication, and lymphoid hyperplasia. The latter is especially important in recurrent intussusception. The causes in adults also include Meckel's diverticulum, polyps, lipomas, carcinomas, lymphomas, and other tumors.[4,37,41]

Ulcer

Aside from the gastrojejunal ulcer, which is ordinarily a complication of surgical therapy for peptic ulcer, the nonspecific ulcer of the jejunum and ileum has recently received a great deal of attention in the literature. The fre-

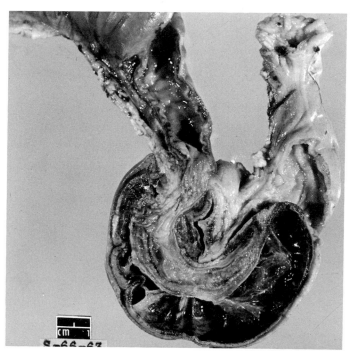

Fig. 30-2. Ileoilial intussusception. The intussusceptum is the dark, dilated portion. Histologically, it was necrotic. BTGH #66012.

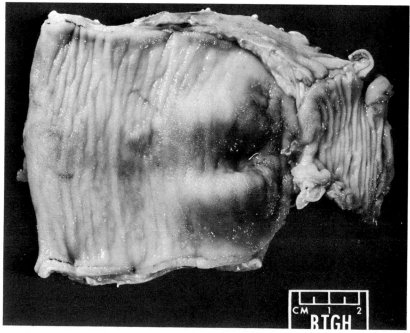

Fig. 30-3. The dilated and narrow portions of the ileum are separated by a narrow circumferential ulcer. There was no history of drug intake. BTGH #64158.

quency of the location as to jejunum or ileum varies with different reports. It has been demonstrated that a number of the ulcers formerly considered nonspecific have been related to the ingestion of enteric-coated potassium chloride tablets with or without accompanying thiazides. Recently the vascular and ischemic origin of some of the nonspecific ulcers of the small bowel has been reconsidered. Also, one must consider the Zollinger-Ellison syndrome in the case of jejunal ulcers.[57]

The ulcers of the small intestine are often annular and may be as long as 4 cm. and as narrow as 0.5 cm.; others are punched out having the same appearance as gastric or duodenal ulcers (Fig. 30-3). They may be multiple and rarely perforate. Histologically, the ulcers are similar to those described in the duodenum and stomach.[15,52]

Enteropathies

A number of diseases of the small bowel result in malabsorption or loss of proteins. Among them are nontropical sprue, lymphoid hyperplasia, Whipple's disease, lymphangiectasis, and allergic gastroenteropathies.[10,21] Among the more common, nontropical sprue is a disease characterized by steatorrhea, which is caused by poor absorption of fats. The jejunum is most commonly involved, but the ileum may be. Grossly, there is flattening of the plicae circulares. The histologic alterations seen in nontropical sprue have been greatly advanced by the use of peroral biopsies. Three major changes are seen; these consist of shortening of the villi, elongation of the crypts, and an associated chronic inflammation. In addition, the basement membrane may be focally thickened. Schenk and associates noted that lipid droplets are situated supranuclearly in celiac disease, whereas in tropical sprue lipid droplets are found in the basement membrane.[42] By electron microscopy additional findings have been eluciated; these include a shortening of the microvilli, resulting in decrease of the absorptive surfaces. Mucosal biopsies from patients with nontropical sprue who have been treated with a gluten-free diet have shown a reversion of the mucosal epithelium to normal by light and electron microscopy. However, this is not a constant finding.[42,45,50]

Whipple's disease

Whipple's disease occurs predominantly in middle-aged men and is associated with steatorrhea and migratory arthritis among other symptoms. Rather than being confined to the bowel, Whipple's disease is now considered to be a systemic disorder. For example, histologic evidence of it may be found in the myocardium lymph nodes, adrenal glands, and subcutaneous fat. With involvement of the intestine the gross appearance is that of a shaggy and velvety mucosa apparently caused by thickening of the villi by the accumulation of large numbers of foamy macrophages. The plicae circulares also appear to be enlarged. Histologically, numerous macrophages are found in the mucosa; in other tissues that are involved, similar macrophages are found. It has been demonstrated that the material in these macrophages is PAS positive (periodic acid, Schiff) and considered by some to be a glycoprotein. Others have considered that the material represents alterations induced by organisms that have been identified within these cells by electron microscopy. In addition to the electron microscopic identification of organisms. *Hemophilus*-like rods and *Corynebacteria* have been isolated in cultures of jejunum obtained by peroral biopsies.[11,25] These organisms have not been proved to be the etiologic agent in Whipple's disease.

Enteritis

Although regional enteritis is one of the most important inflammatory lesions, clinically, tuberculosis must still be considered in the differential diagnosis of inflammatory lesions of the small bowel. Tuberculosis is usually associated with pulmonary tuberculosis, and there is an increased incidence of small-bowel involvement related to the severity of the pulmonary lesion. The ileocecal area is the most common site in tuberculous involvement of the small bowel. The other areas of the gastrointestinal tract that are involved by tuberculosis, listed in descending order of frequency, include the ascending colon, jejunum, appendix, duodenum, stomach, sigmoid, and rectum. Actually, the cecal area accounts for 85% to 90% of the tuberculosis involvement of the gastrointestinal tract. Grossly, the tuberculous lesions in the bowel may be present as ulcerative areas, hypertrophic areas, or combinations of the two. The ulcerative form is the most frequently seen. The ulcers have their long axis perpendicular to the axis of the intestine. However, the ulcers are rarely circumferential. They may be associated with undermining and pseudopolyps. The hypertrophic variation of tuberculous involvement may actually be difficult to distinguish from regional enteritis because of the thickening of the bowel wall. Histologically, the tuberculous lesions appear as does tuberculosis elsewhere.[1]

Eosinophilic granuloma and eosinophilic gastroenteritis may involve the small bowel as part of a diffuse gastrointestinal process or as a solitary lesion. The lesion may present as a narrowing of the bowel lumen because of mural involvement or as a polypoid mass that may be single. The latter may be dominantly fibrous. Other solitary lesions are plaque-like and often ulcerated.

Necrotizing enterocolitis in infancy may perforate in 50% of patients. The terminal ileum is often involved in combination with the colon. Occasionally the small bowel alone is the site of the necrotizing process. Histologically there is acute inflammation, ulceration, and widespread necrosis. Pneumatosis intestinalis may complicate the process.[55]

Regional enteritis (Crohn's disease)

Regional enteritis, of unknown cause, is an inflammatory lesion of the bowel that occurs predominantly in young adults but may be encountered in children and older persons. In fact, 60% of the patients have indication of the disease before the age of 40. Regional enteritis occurs with nearly equal frequency in males and females.[30] The ileum is the most common single site of regional enteritis; however, all areas of the gastrointestinal tract have been involved. The ileum alone or in combination with some other portion of the gastrointestinal tract accounts for approximately 95% of the cases. Colonic involvement, usually combined with ileal involvement, has been reported as occurring in 22% to 55% of cases. Skip areas have been described as occurring in roughly 14% of patients. The length of the segment involved in the small bowel has been as great as 76 cm., with an average of about 20 cm. Grossly, the bowel wall is diffusely thickened, and the serosa appears thickened and hyperemic. Sometimes a fibrinous or even a purulent exudate may be

seen on the serosa. Adhesions may cause a matting of loops of the ileum. A reasonably characteristic finding in regional enteritis is a thickening of the mesentery with finger-like projections of the mesenteric fat onto the bowel serosa. The demarcation between the involved and uninvolved portions of bowel is usually quite abrupt. The mucosa may appear to be hypertrophic; it may actually be nodular and in some instances atrophic. Nearly always the mucosa is ulcerated and edematous, to produce a cobblestone effect (Fig. 30-4). Many of the ulcers are superficial. Others may be very deep, producing sinuses and fistulas.[38] As a matter of fact, sinuses and fistulas are common complications of regional enteritis. For example, rectal abscesses and fistulas have been described as occurring as frequently as in 26% of the patients studied.[26] Krause and his colleagues reported no difference in the chance of an anal fistula in relation to whether the colon was or was not involved.[26]

Jejunal involvement has often been described as being less severe than ileal. Also, it is much less likely to result in fistula formation. However, stenosis has been described as being more likely to occur.

Williams has noted three patterns of the inflammatory involvement of regional enteritis: (1) diffuse inflammatory, (2) diffuse granulomatous, and (3) focal granulomatous.[53] The latter is seen in 50% of the specimens. However, whichever pattern is observed microscopically, the full thickness of the bowel wall from mucosa to serosa is involved. The mucosa is ulcerated very commonly, and occasionally one may find crypt abscesses as are seen in ulcerative colitis. Occasionally pseudopolyps are seen. Submucosal lymphoid aggregates and lymphatic channel dilatation are a frequent accompaniment of regional enteritis. The inflammatory cells may involve the muscularis, which is often hypertrophied; lymphoid aggregates may be actually seen in the muscularis. Lymphoid aggregates and nodules are noted in the serosa along with other inflammatory cells. Granulomas may be seen in all layers and in the mesenteric lymph nodes.

Ulcerative colitis may involve the ileum (55% in one series)[38] and generally maintains a recognizable gross and microscopic pattern of that disease. The lesion is dominantly a mucosal and submucosal one rather than involving the full

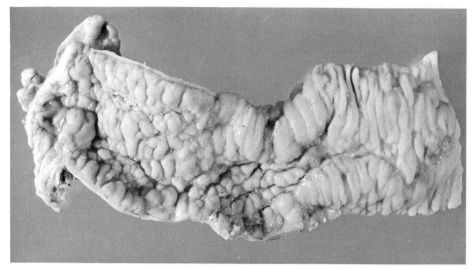

Fig. 30-4. Cobblestone effect of regional enteritis. Narrow ulcers and loss of the plicae circulares are noted. BUCM #17414.

thickness of the bowel wall as seen in regional enteritis. With ileal involvement, the histologic features of ulcerative colitis are maintained.

Crohn's disease has a high recurrence rate, as high as 39% in some series. The chance of recurrence after a second resection is even higher. The mortality of this disease is estimated at 7% at 5 years and 12% at 10 years after the first resection.[26,27]

Irradiation

Irradiation injuries should be entertained in the differential diagnosis of patients who have signs and symptoms of small-bowel obstruction and a history of irradiation to the abdomen or pelvis. Small-bowel epithelium has been shown to be extremely radiosensitive. Early findings of irradiation include edema and hyperemia, which eventually may lead to ulceration and necrosis. The ulcerated areas are well demarcated, with the intact surrounding mucosa being edematous. The muscularis propria is remarkably resistant to irradiation, but with intense irradiation severe damage may occur with necrosis. Vascular changes may be seen: they inuclude endothelial proliferation and even more severe alterations such as necrosis and thrombosis. The vascular changes may aggravate the mucosal and submucosal lesions to induce further necrosis. Healing is effected by scarring and may result in stenosis. Animal experiments indicate that when

ulcers and particularly stenotic areas are encountered after irradiation the ulcers and stenoses are the result of a previously more extensive segmental involvement. Known lengths of small bowel in dogs have been irradiated, replaced into the abdominal cavity, and studied at various intervals of time. It has been demonstrated that long segments have undergone essential autoanastomosis; that is, the stenosis becomes a very narrow circumscribed ulcer, hardly more than 0.5 cm. in length.[48]

Mechanical and vascular lesions

Infarction of the small bowel may be of two varieties, venous or arterial, with the former occurring in younger patients and often following abdominal surgical procedures. The latter is usually a complication of arteriosclerosis. Grossly, both may be similar, the bowel wall being thickened, dark red, and edematous. Usually the infarction following arterial complications is better demarcated than venous infarction. Necrosis of the bowel may also follow incarceration in a hernia, volvulus, constriction by adhesive bands, endotoxic shock (gastroenteritis in children), disseminated intravascular coagulation, and intussusception.[20,47]

Hemorrhagic infarction of the small bowel may also be seen in patients who have severe cardiac disease, with the infarction occurring without demonstrable occlusion of the arterial or venous supply. These infarcts have been considered to be caused by reduced blood flow associated with poor cardiac function.

Rare lesions

Recurrent edema of the small intestine, possibly of an allergic background, has been described. Grossly, the small bowel is greatly thickened and has clubbing of the plicae circulares. Microscopically, there is marked submucosal edema.[39]

Pneumatosis cystoides intestinalis, a collection of gas in the submucosa and serosa of the bowel, may involve the stomach, small bowel, and large bowel. Grossly, there are gas-filled cysts that may be seen through the serosa. The submucosal cysts tend to broaden the mucosal folds, and the bowel wall is thickened. The cause of this disease is not known, but it is thought that it may be on either a mechanical, a bacterial, or a chemical basis.[36]

Benign tumors

The frequency of benign tumors of the small intestine is demonstrated by the compilation of three series. These include leiomyoma, 180; hemangioma, 60; adenomatous polyp, 56; lipoma, 52; lymphangioma, 17; and neurogenic tumors, 5. The lesions are fairly equally distributed between the jejunum and ileum with minor variation. Most of them are present as mucosa-covered protuberances in the bowel lumen. An occasional lesion, other than the adenomatous polyps, may be pedunculated. A leiomyoma may be ulcerated and may be the source of gastrointestinal bleeding. Any part of the lesion may serve as a leading point for intussusception.[5,13,32]

Many of the epithelial polyps of the small bowel are associated with hereditable disorders, for example, Peutz-Jeghers syndrome. The latter is associated with pigmentation in the oral area, which may also be seen in the toes and fingers. About 90% of the polyps in this disorder occur in the small bowel and have been seen in the stomach and colon. They are nearly always multiple (Fig. 30-5, *A*). Histologically, the polyps in this disorder are considered to be hamartomatous, that is, a mixture of mucosa and the muscularis mucosae maintaining to some degree a recognizable pattern (Fig. 30-5, *B*). Except in rare instances the polyps in this syndrome have been benign.[7,12,16,31] Most of the carcinomas reported in the Peutz-Jeghers syndrome have arisen in mucosa not involved by the Peutz-Jeghers hamartomatous polyps.[12]

Endometriosis

Although endometriosis is not a true neoplasm it may present in such a fashion as to mimic a neoplasm of the large or small bowel. Although it is much more common in the large bowel, it may cause obstructive signs and symptoms of the small bowel. When of clinical consequence it will present as a constricting mass that is covered by mucosa. Histologically, endometrial glands often associated with an endometrial stroma may be found in all areas of the bowel but are most frequent in the submucosa and the muscularis. The constriction caused by endometriosis is the result of hypertrophy of the muscularis propria.[40]

Malignant tumors

Primary malignant tumors of the small intestine occur in adults and rarely in children, although leiomyosarcoma and angiosarcomas have been reported in the neonate.[44] A compilation of several series of malignant tumors of the small bowel reveal the following occurrence rate: carcinoid, 177; adenocarcinoma, 92; lymphoma, 59; leiomyosarcoma, 33; vascular malignancies, 3; and fibrosarcoma, 1.[5,13,32] Except for adenocarcinoma the malignant neoplasms dominate in the ileum; this is especially true of the carcinoid.

Adenocarcinomas usually encircle the bowel to produce obstructive signs and symptoms. The lesions are frequently ulcerated. Histologically, the tumors are fairly well-differentiated adenocarcinomas. Carcinoids, on the other hand, rarely encircle the bowel, are usually present as mucosa-covered lesions, and are comparatively small. They may become large enough, however, to kink the bowel and thus, produce symptoms. Approximately 30% of carcinoids are multiple. The carcinoids are included among the malignant tumors because of the frequency of metastases to regional lymph nodes; the metastatic rate is related to the size of the tumor. The relationship of carcinoids to the carcinoid syndrome (approximately 7% of small-bowel carcinoids) is well recognized. A second primary malignant neoplasm occurs in a high percentage (17% surgical, 36% necropsy) of patients with

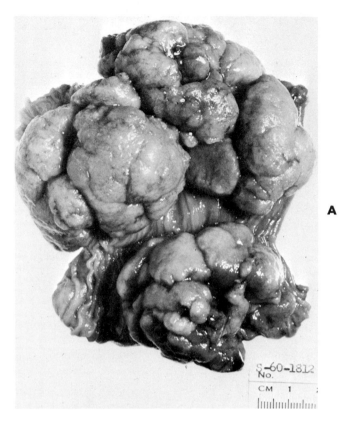

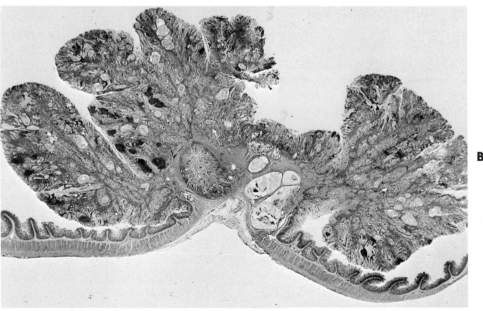

Fig. 30-5. A, Two large hamartomatous polyps from the small intestine of a 6-year-old girl with Peutz-Jeghers syndrome. **B,** Photomicrograph of one of the polyps. Strands of smooth muscle extend into the mucosal component of the polyp. (×1.5.) (Courtesy Dr. Harvey Rosenberg.)

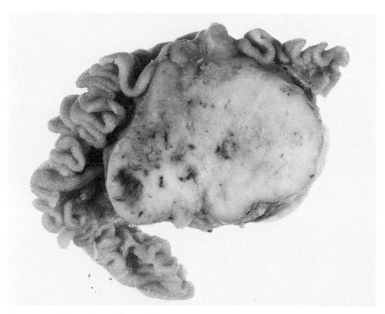

Fig. 30-6. Cross section through a leiomyosarcoma of the jejunum, demonstrating the large extraluminal component and the ulceration of the mucosal attachment. The tumor measured 4.5 cm. in greatest dimension and had metastasized to the liver. SLEH #710600.

carcinoids. The second lesion is found commonly in the alimentary tract.[32]

Leiomyosarcomas tend to grow outside of the bowel, for example, into the mesentery, having therefore, a relatively small mucosal and luminal component. The lesions may be ulcerated and result in gastrointestinal bleeding (Fig. 30-6). Histologically, the features are similar to those described under diseases of the stomach.

Of the primary lymphomas involving the small bowel, lymphosarcoma and reticulum cell sarcoma are the most common; Hodgkin's disease is relatively rare. Grossly, lymphomas are frequently present as polypoid lesions; they may be annular or they may show diffuse thickening of the bowel to give it a hoselike appearance. Not frequently recognized but of some importance is the fact that they might present ulcerative lesions, which at times are complicated by perforation. There may be multiple sites of involvement. The lesions are often well demarcated, particularly those of the ulcerative and the diffuse variety. Perforation following the treatment of lymphomas of the small bowel by chemotherapeutic or radiotherapeutic methods has been described. Plasmacytoma, a related disease, has also been described as involving the small bowel.[8,22,46]

The survival after treatment for primary malignant tumors of the small intestine depends upon the type; for example, the 5-year survival for carcinoid is 68% whereas for carcinoma it is 32%. Less optimistic figures of an overall 5-year survival of 20% have been reported.[43]

The small bowel is a fairly common site for secondary involvement by malignant tumors (Fig. 30-7), particularly in peritoneal seeding by carcinomas. Secondary involvement may result in a constriction of a portion of the small bowel. Lymphatic permeation of the small bowel has also been described as being secondary in occurrence to linitis plastica of the stomach. The bowel wall becomes diffusely thickened and less pliable as the tumor permeates it. This is thought to be the result of the milking effect of peristalsis. Metastases from distant sites to the bowel, apparently blood borne, occur in the following descending order of frequency: (1) melanoma, (2) lung, (3) breast, (4) choriocarcinoma, (5) kidney, and (6) stomach.[17,54]

Secondary involvement of the gastrointestinal tract by malignant lymphoma is common, being found in 63% of patients with disseminated disease. The small intestine is less frequently involved than are other sites (19%). Reticulum cell sarcoma is more likely to involve the gastro-

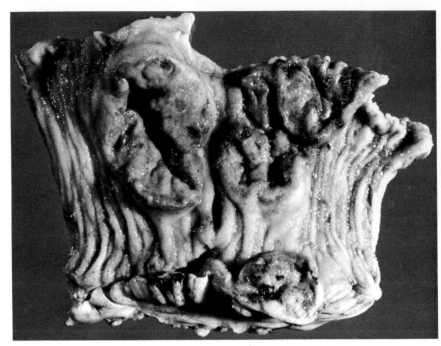

Fig. 30-7. Metastatic reticulum cell sarcoma of the small bowel. Ulcerated protuberant masses are present. One ulcerated lesion had perforated. BTGH #64469.

intestinal tract than are the other histologic types.[14]

DISEASES OF THE MESENTERY

Metastatic carcinoma is the most common neoplasm of the mesentery. Primary mesenteric neoplasms are infrequent, and benign tumors are more common than the malignant. The frequency of cystic mesenteric tumors is greater than that of the solid type. Lymphatic cysts are the cost common of the cystic group of tumors. Lipomas, xanthogranulomas, fibromatoses, hemangiomas, neurofibromas, mesenchymomas, and smooth muscle tumors are some examples of primary solid mesenteric neoplasms, among which the fibromatoses are the most common. In some reports mesenteric fibromatosis has been described as associated with familial polyposis and considered as a manifestation of Gardner's syndrome. As in the omentum, mesenteric smooth muscle tumors are among the more common, but in the mesentery, leiomyosarcomas are more frequent then leiomyomas.[6,56]

Mesenteric panniculitis, a nonspecific chronic inflammatory process restricted to the adipose tissue of the mesentery, often presents clinically as an intra-abdominal tumor commonly associated with gastrointestinal symptoms.[34] Roentgenograms are helpful in diagnosis only in patients in whom the mesenteric masses displace viscera or cause partial intestinal obstruction. This condition involves the root of the mesentery more frequently than other portions of it. The mesentery becomes markedly thickened, forming a mass that is most frequently single. The peritoneal surface of the mesenteric mass may be puckered or elevated and presents reddish brown to white-yellowish plaques. Some authors have expressed the belief that this entity is related to some or to all of the following entities: isolated lipodystrophy of the mesentery, lipogranuloma of the mesentery, retractile mesenteritis, Weber-Christian disease, systemic nodular panniculitis, and febrile mesenteric panniculitis.[18]

REFERENCES

1. Abrams, J. S., and Holden, W. D.: Tuberculosis of the gastrointestinal tract, Arch. Surg. (Chicago) **89:** 282, 1964.
2. Appleman, R. M., and Jackman, R. J.: Regional enteritis; proctoscopic clues in diagnosis, Dis. Colon Rectum 5:361, 1962.

3. Aubrey, D. A.: Meckel's diverticulum, Arch Surg. (Chicago) **100**:144, 1970.

4. Bond, M. R., and Roberts. J. B. M.: Intussusception in the adult, Brit. J. Surg. **51**:818, 1964.

5. Braasch, J. W., and Denbo, H. E.: Tumors of the small intestine, Surg. Clin. N. Amer. **44**:791, 1964.

6. Burnett, W. E., Rosemond, G. P., and Bucher, R. M.: Mesenteric cysts, Arch. Surg. (Chicago) **60**:699, 1960.

7. Calabro, J. J.: Hereditable multiple polyposis syndromes of the gastrointestinal tract, Amer. J. Med. **33**:276, 1962.

8. Christensen, H. E.: Polypous reticulum cell sarcoma of the gastrointestinal tract, Acta Path. Microbiol. Scand. **45**:53, 1959.

9. Dick, A. P.: Association of jejunal diverticulosis and steatorrhea, Brit. Med. J. **1**:145, 1955.

10. Dobbins, W. O.: Diseases associated with protein losing enteropathy; electron microscopic studies of the intestinal mucosa, Southern Med. J. **60**:1077, 1967.

11. Dobbins, W. O., and Ruffin, J. M.: A light and electron microscopic study of bacterial invasion in Whipple's disease, Amer. J. Path. **51**:225, 1967.

12. Dozois, R. R., Judd, E. S., Dahlin, D. C., and Bartholomew, L. G.: The Peutz-Jeghers syndrome: is there a predisposition to the development of intestinal malignancy? Arch. Surg. (Chicago) **98**:509, 1969.

13. Ebert, P. A., and Zuidema, G. D.: Primary tumors of the small intestine, Arch. Surg. (Chicago) **91**:452, 1965.

14. Ehrlich, A. N., Stalder, G., Geller, W., and Sherlock, P.: Gastrointestinal manifestations of malignant lymphoma, Gastroenterology **54**:1115, 1968.

15. Ellis, K.: Gastrojejunal ulcer, Radiology **71**:187, 1958.

16. Falkinburg, L. W., and Kay, M. N.: Intestinal polyposis with oral pigmentation (Peutz-Jeghers syndrome), J. Pediat. **54**:162, 1959.

17. Fernet, P., Azar, H. A., and Stout, A. P.: Intramural (tubal) spread of linitis plastica along the alimentary tract, Gastroenterology **48**:419, 1965.

18. Graciansky, P., Paraf, A., and Timsit, E.: Le problieme de la maladie de Weber-Christian panniculite nodulaise aigui fibrike recidivante au cervis diem cuuch acineaux du pancreas, Ann. Derm. Syph. **93**:503, 1966.

19. Grosfeld, J. L., and Clatworthy, H. W., Jr.: The nature of ileal atresia due to intrauterine intussusception, Arch. Surg. (Chicago) **100**:714, 1970.

20. Grosh, J. L., Mann, R. H., and O'Donnell, W. M.: Nonthrombotic intestinal infarction in heart disease, Amer. J. Med. Sci. **250**:613, 1965.

21. Hodgson, J. R., Hoffman, H. N., and Huizenga, K. A.: Roentgenologic features of lymphoid hyperplasia of the small intestine associated with dysgammaglobulinemia, Radiology **88**:883, 1967.

22. Irvine, W. T., and Johnstone, J. M.: Lymphosarcoma of the small intestine, Brit. J. Surg. **42**:611, 1955.

23. Johns, T. N. P., Wheeler, J. R., and Johns, F. S.: Meckel's diverticulum and Meckel's diverticulum disease, Ann. Surg. **150**:241, 1959.

24. Johnston, R. H., Jr., Hall, R. A., and Erickson, E. E.: Argentaffin cell tumor of Meckel's diverticulum, Arch. Surg. (Chicago) **90**:172, 1965.

25. Kleyn, K. A., Mandell, G. H., Sakwa, S., and Kobernick, S. D.: Glomus tumor of the stomach, Arch. Surg. (Chicago) **97**:111, 1968.

26. Krause, U., Bergman, L., and Norlen, B. J.: Crohn's disease, Scand. J. Gastroent. **6**:97, 1971.

27. Lennard-Jones, J. E., and Stalder, G. A.: Prognosis after resection of chronic regional ileitis, Gut **8**:332, 1967.

28. Louw, J. H.: Investigations into the etiology of congenital atresia of the colon, Dis. Colon Rectum **7**:471, 1964.

29. Macbeth, W. A. A.: Jejunal diverticula, Brit. J. Surg. **51**:580, 1964.

30. Mendeloff, A. J., Monk, M., Siegel, C. D., and Lilienfeld, A.: Some epidemiological features of ulcerative colitis and regional enteritis, Gastroenterology **51**:748, 1966.

31. Michalany, J., and Ferraz, M. D.: Peutz syndrome in a mulatto family; with special reference to the histological structure of the intestinal polyps, Gastroenterologia (Basel) **97**:119, 1962.

32. Moertel, C. G., Sauer, W. G., Dockerty, M. B., and Baggenstoss, A. H.: Life history of the carcinoid tumor of the small intestine, Cancer **14**:901, 1961.

33. Nobles, E. R., Jr.: Jejunal diverticula, Arch. Surg. (Chicago) **102**:172, 1971.

34. Ogden, W. W., Bradburn, D. M., and Rives, J. D.: Mesenteric panniculitis, Ann. Surg. (Chicago) **161**:864, 1965.

35. Okmian, L. G., and Kövamees, A.: Jejunal atresia with intestinal aplasia; strangulation of the intestine in the extraembryonic coelum of the belly stalk, Acta Paediat. (Stockholm) **53**:65, 1964.

36. Paris, L.: Pneumatosis cystoides intestinalis in infancy, J. Pediat. **46**:1, 1955.

37. Ponka, J. L.: Intussusception in infants and adults, Surg. Gynec. Obstet. **124**:99, 1967.

38. Rappaport, H., Burgoyne, F. H., and Smetana, H. F.: The pathology of regional enteritis, Mil. Surgeon **109**:463, 1951.

39. Renton, C. J.: Recurrent oedema of the small intestine, Brit. J. Surg. **52**:536, 1965.

40. Rio, F. W., Edwards, D. L., Regan, J. F., and Schmutzer, K. J.: Endometriosis of the small bowel, Arch. Surg. (Chicago) **101**:403, 1970.

41. Sarason, E. L., Prior, J. T., and Prowda, R. L.: Recurrent intussusception associated with hypertrophy of Peyer's patches, New Eng. J. Med. **253**:905, 1955.

42. Schenk, E. A., Samloff, I. M., and Klipstein, F. A.: Morphologic characteristics of jejunal biopsy in celiac disease and tropical sprue, Amer. J. Path. **47**:765, 1965.

43. Sethi, G., and Hardin, C. A.: Primary malignant tumors of the small bowel, Arch. Surg. (Chicago) **98**:659, 1969.

44. Shafie, M. E., Spitz, L., and Ikeda, S.: Malignant tumors of the small bowel in neonates presenting with perforation, J. Pediat. Surg. **6**:62, 1971.

45. Shearman, D. J., Girdwood, R. H., Williams, A. W., and Delamore, I. W.: A study with the electron microscope of the jejunal epithelium in primary malabsorptive disease, Gut **3**:16, 1962.
46. Sherlock, P., and Oropeza, R.: Jejunal perforations in lymphoma after chemotherapy, Arch. Intern. Med. (Chicago) **110**:102, 1962.
47. Shor-Pinsker, E., and Hernandez, O. A.: Intestinal infarction, Arch. Surg. (Chicago) **102**:187, 1971.
48. Spratt, J. S., Jr., Heinbecker, P., and Saltzstein, S. L.: The influence of succinylsulfathiazole (Sulfasuxidine) upon the response of canine small intestine to irradiation, Cancer **14**:862, 1961.
49. Steiner, D. H., Maxwell, J. G., Rasmussen, B. L., and Jones, R.: Segmental absence of intestinal musculature, Amer. J. Surg. **118**:964, 1969.
50. Thurlbeck, W. M., Benson, J. A., Jr., and Dudley, H. R., Jr.: The histopathologic changes of sprue and their significance, Amer. J. Clin. Path. **34**:108, 1960.
51. Walker, A. W., Kempson, R. L., and Turnberg, J. L.: Aganglionosis of the small intestine, Surgery **60**:449, 1966.
52. Wayte, D. M., and Helwig, E. B.: Small-bowel ulceration—iatrogenic or multifactorial origin? Amer. J. Clin. Path. **49**:26, 1968.
53. Williams, W. J.: Histology of Crohn's disease, Gut **5**:510, 1964.
54. Willis, R. A.: The spread of tumours in the human body, ed. 2, London, 1952, Butterworth & Co., Ltd.
55. Wilson, S. E., and Woolley, M. M.: Primary necrotizing enterocolitis in infants, Arch. Surg. (Chicago) **99**:563, 1969.
56. Yannopoulos, K., and Stout, A. P.: Primary solid tumors of the mesentery, Cancer **16**:914, 1963.
57. Zollinger, R. M., and Grant, G. N.: Ulcerogenic tumor of the pancreas, J.A.M.A. **190**:181, 1964.

Examination of the small bowel | 31

Ralph Schlaeger

Evaluation of the mesenteric small bowel by roentgenologic methods is based upon sequential film documentation after the administration of a nonabsorbable contrast agent. Modifications of this technique, including pharmacologic acceleration of transport, have gained acceptance. In an effort to localize lesions more precisely, intubation as well as retrograde techniques have been employed.

During the past 40 years, Golden's radiologic contributions[28,29] have served to alter the concept of the relative diagnostic inaccessibility of the small bowel and to establish the small-bowel study as a frequently employed routine procedure. It is to him that we radiologists owe much of our understanding of the radiology of this area in both health and disease. Incorporated into his classic work, *Radiological Examination of the Small Intestine*,[29] is a wealth of information representing a summation of his research and experience in context of the investigation of others.

Marshak's contributions in the past 20 years have shed new radiologic light on various established entities, placing them into the perspective of the modern era of gastroenterology. Gleaned from a vast clinical experience and supportd by an avid interest, his observations are detailed in many publications.[58-61]

The inherent features of the small bowel account for the challenge to any form of radiologic investigation. While the mesenteric small intestine is the longest portion of the alimentary canal, its surface length is augmented by the folds forming the valvulae conniventes and by the mucosa formed as villi that project into the lumen. Even though the villi do not enter into the scope of radiologic investigation, one should be aware that the difficulty in evaluating this vast morphologic unit, the small bowel, is compounded by the superimposition of loops and the constant changes caused by pendular and peristaltic movements. Even when the patient has been fasting, secretions are constantly present within the lumen. Other factors compli-

INDICATIONS FOR SMALL-BOWEL EXAMINATION

EVOLUTION OF CONCEPTS IN ROENTGENOLOGIC EXAMINATION

SUSPENDING AGENTS AND PARTICLE SIZE OF THE CONTRAST MEDIUM

INTERVALS BETWEEN ROENTGENOGRAPHS

PHARMACODYNAMIC TECHNIQUES

THE EXAMINATION

Examination of the patient after operation
Antegrade intubation techniques
Examination with the Miller-Abbott tube
Examination in the presence of obstruction
The case against water-soluble media
Complete reflux examination
New methods of examination

cating evaluation include the effects of drugs, neurogenic stimuli, and psychic responses such as fear and rage. These conditions, coupled with a relatively low incidence of organic disease and the subtle changes produced by disease, have provided sufficient reason for dissatisfaction with the techniques for examination and have prompted the various modifications.

There is now no universal technique of examination that is suited to all radiologic equipment and that conforms to the philosophy of examination of all radiologists. The mode of investigation frequently is conditioned by the interests of the radiologist and his clinical colleagues. Therefore, in practice the small-bowel examination varies appreciably. The method employed seems unimportant if, indeed, the necessary information is obtained. Golden, in a discussion of one of the modifications of procedure, commented on personal preference as a determinant in selection of such a technique, "What we like sometimes depends on what we are used to. To me, it seems more important for each of us to use a technique the results of which we understand than for all of us to use exactly the same procedure.[96]

INDICATIONS FOR SMALL-BOWEL EXAMINATION

Awareness of the possibility of organic disease of the small bowel in a specific clinical problem is the prime consideration in the evaluation of this portion of the bowel. The indications proposed by Golden[29] many years ago continue to be the basis for roentgenographic examination of the small bowel. These include: (1) gastrointestinal blood loss, either occult or manifest, which cannot be localized to the esophagus, stomach, duodenum, or colon; (2) unexplained abdominal pain, particularly when it is periumbilical or in the right lower quadrant; (3) change in the frequency or character of the stool, notably diarrhea or steatorrhea.

From this broad basis the indications have been extended to include specific problems, particularly as investigation with other modalities has demonstrated various alterations in absorption. Unexplained anemia, even though gastrointestinal blood loss cannot be documented at the time stool guaiac testing is done, deserves critical appraisal after the other portions of the bowel have been exonerated as sites of organic disease. Nonaddisonian macrocytic anemia, which may be of intestinal origin, caused by faulty B^{12} absorption in the ileum as a result of stasis proximal to a stricture, or a blind pouch equivalent, occasioned by a side-to-side anastomosis, other surgery, or small-bowel diverticulosis. In the presence of crampy abdominal pain with nausea and intermittent vomiting, when the colon has been cleared as a site of organic stenosis, contrast examination is indicated even though small-bowel obstruction is a major consideration. Anomalies of midgut rotation are investigated in this manner, and in young patients unexplained growth retardation is an indication for small-bowel study to detect asymptomatic regional enteritis as the cause. A host of conditions is included in the category of the so-called malabsorption syndrome. It should be stressed that even in the absence of diarrhea or characteristic stools the possibility of steatorrhea cannot be excluded when fat absorption is impaired. Although the radiologic findings may not be diagnostic of a specific malabsorption problem, examination is nevertheless indicated as a base line with which comparison is made after therapy. A report of a normally appearing small-bowel pattern does not invalidate evidence of malabsorption established by more precise techniques.

Because signs and symptoms of disease in the small intestine are frequently nonspecific, clinical appraisal frequently fails to focus attention on this portion of the bowel. It is therefore not surprising that localized lesions are entirely overlooked when the small intestine has not been examined radiologically. In addition, such common lesions as hiatal hernia, duodenal ulcer, colonic diverticulosis and gallstones may be suggested by nonspecific clinical findings, when in reality the underlying disease is a small-bowel tumor. The difficulty in establishing a sound, accurate diagnosis is compounded when diagnoses such as antral gastritis and duodenitis, reached by some physicians on nebulous radiologic grounds, are used as comfortable simplifications to explain poorly defined or inadequately investigated symptoms. The radiologist will do well to avoid the pitfalls of such vague diagnostic categories.

EVOLUTION OF CONCEPTS IN ROENTGENOLOGIC EXAMINATION

The information to be obtained from a small-bowel study is based on critical assessment of the caliber of the lumen, the relief contours of the mucosal surface, and the thickness of the wall as inferred from the appearance of juxtaposed loops. From a practical standpoint, motility as measured by the transit time is of little diagnostic value except in the context of change in the caliber of the lumen or in the mucosal pattern.

Kim analyzed the marked variation in transit time in 315 normal small-bowel examinations performed in adults.[42] The normal range, from 15 minutes to 5 hours, did not vary significantly between males and females or between younger and older groups. Goldstein and associates obtained comparable transit time values in twenty male volunteers studied by conventional means and also by various accelerated techniques.[33] The examinations in the control group, in which the barium mixture differed from that of Kim's, had a normal range of from 15 minutes to 3 hours with an average of 58 minutes. Localized displacement of a loop takes on importance especially in the presence of alteration in the wall or in the adjacent mucosal pattern. It is in an effort to obtain such information that various modifications in the small-bowel study have evolved.

Over the years, the barium meal has been the single most important variable in the small-bowel examination. The nature of the barium meal has been altered simply because radiologists have realized that the pattern of the small bowel is in part dependent upon the composition of the material introduced into the bowel. Pendergrass and his associates early established the validity of this concept and in addition pointed out that the consistency of the meal, its size, the gastric emptying time, and the tonicity of the gastrointestinal tract were factors in the radiologic appearance of the mucosal pattern.[81]

The early investigators were concerned with the purity of the barium sulfate and the water, and, at one time, Pendergrass proposed that distilled water be used as a vehicle to avoid the possible effects of chlorine.[79] Physiologic saline for a period replaced water as the suspending agent. Other workers varied the consistency of the barium suspension from the ratio of 1 part of water to 1 part of barium by volume; Akerlund[4] advocated a 3:4 ratio by volume. The voume of the meal was varied as well; ultimately an 8-ounce mixture, consisting of equal parts of barium and water by volume was widely used.

SUSPENDING AGENTS AND PARTICLE SIZE OF THE CONTRAST MEDIUM

There was no significant advance in the diagnostic medium until 1949, when Frazier, French and Thompson showed that flocculation of the barium occurred in the presence of mucus and that in normal individuals this accounted for changes indistinguishable from the deficiency pattern.[19] That this phenomenon was not a function of neurogenic activity was documented in isolated small-bowel segments removed from the body. Zimmer[98] established that pure barium, both in vivo and in vitro, produced a coarsened mucosal pattern as well as segmentation and that the addition of protective colloids prevented the appearance of such spurious changes in the absence of disease.[98] Ardran, French, and Mucklow demonstrated that barium suspended with a protective colloid maintained

a continuous column in dilated small bowel and that the valvulae conniventes were clearly delineated in such loops.[5] Their impression that motility was more rapid was confirmed by Kirsh, who compared separate examinations in the same patients, using pure barium and nonflocculating suspensions.[44] Accordingly, the concept of the deficiency pattern lost its validity on the basis of these studies and subsequent use of barium protected by colloids.

Although suspending agents influence the appearance of the small bowel roentgenographically, barium particle size is also a factor. As early as 1936, Pendergrass compared standard barium with a finely divided preparation and noted differences in the small-bowel pattern as well as in motility.[80] Adolph and Taplin found that micropulverization of barium to less than 1μ in diameter was of help in preventing flocculation.[3] Recently, an effort to determine the nature of the numerous barium preparations was reported by Miller.[62]

INTERVALS BETWEEN ROENTGENOGRAPHS

Another variable in performing the examination has been the interval between films during the course of transit of the meal. In addition, the role of fluoroscopy has held varying degrees of importance among the examiners. Golden advocated films at one-half hour intervals with two or three fluoroscopic examinations and spot films to define areas suspected of disease.[28] An effort at reducing the patient's exposure to radiation included films at 1, 2½, and 5 hours after ingestion of the opaque meal.[38] While the radiation exposure was reduced, it was at the expense of the critical evaluation of the small bowel. Fluoroscope examinations with spot films, rather than being performed at specified intervals, have been reserved for evaluation of those areas which, at the time each interval film is seen, are suspected of containing organic disease. In addition, the terminal ileum, ileocecal valve, and cecum are evaluated in this manner near the completion of the examination.

PHARMACODYNAMIC TECHNIQUES

Dissatisfaction with the time consumed by the procedure has motivated continuing attempts at accelerating the transit of the contrast medium through the small bowel. Many of the techniques for doing so antedated the use of nonflocculating barium. Thirty years ago Weber and Kirklin gave a food stimulus to increase peristalsis and accelerate transit at a time in the examination when the stomach had been empty.[94] Weintraub and Williams' rapid technique made use of a barium-saline meal followed by ice cold saline at the completion of the upper gastrointestinal examination and again 5 minutes later.[96] Others have used ice cold carbonated water to achieve the same end. An increase in the volume of contrast material introduced into the small bowel also has been employed to accelerate transit. Marshak routinely has employed large volumes, 20 ounces or more, in the examination of the small bowel.[59] The proponents of Golden's 8-ounce technique have pointed out that the problem of overlapping loops outweighs the advantages of distention and rapid transit. Those who insist on large volumes use external compression to resolve this problem. Caldwell and Floch, who compared Golden's use of 8 ounces of barium with Marshak's use of larger volumes, concluded that an increased quantity of barium provided a more satisfactory examination of the small bowel.[11]

An accelerated technique evolved by Nice includes preliminary preparation of the colon with castor oil, placement of the patient in the right lateral recumbent position, a 10-ounce barium and water suspension, and 10 ounces of water 30 minutes later.[73,74] This technique produced rapid, uniform filling of the small intestine as well as a diagnostically excellent roentgenographic pattern. However, the use of castor oil adds an additional variable because of its effect on the small intestine. In patients suspected of small-bowel disease, some of whom have diarrhea, the routine use of castor oil is open to question. Golden[29] has stated that the transit time is not influenced by the rate of emptying of the stomach, an observation made by Lönnerblad[61] in normal persons and by Weigen and co-workers[95] in dogs.

Use of neostigmine

Pharmacologic methods have been employed to accelerate transit of barium through the small intestine. Neostigmine (Prostigmin) methylsulfate inhibits the enzymatic destruction of acetylcholine by cholinesterase; the resultant sustained action of acetylcholine is comparable to simulation of the parasympathetic nervous system. The effect on the bowel is an increase in the amplitude and frequency of propulsive waves and a resultant acceleration of intestinal transport. Margulis and Mandelstam employed neostigmine in physiologic doses as a survey procedure of the small bowel on all patients undergoing gastrointestinal examination.[55] If disease was suspected or discovered, a more detailed examination was performed.

More recently Margulis summarized his thoughts on the augmented examination with neostigmine and stressed that the drug was effective only when neuromotor function of the small intestine was intact.[56] The disturbance in the neuromotor mechanism in sprue precludes neostigmine acceleration of transport. He noted that the tone of the small bowel was increased, with resultant narrowing of the lumen and reduction in the overlapping of loops. The details of the valvulae conniventes were more apparent and fistulas, sinuses, and kinks were more readily demonstrable.

Friedenberg and co-workers compared the use of neostigmine, iced saline, and iced water in improving the speed of small-bowel transport and the quality of the examinations.[20] The results for neostigmine and iced saline were the same, with approximately 72% of the patients in each group having a transit time of 1 hour; however, neostigmine provided some improvement in quality of the small-bowel examination. In the group of patients receiving iced water, the results were inferior to either neostigmine or ice cold saline. Twenty ounces of barium suspension was used in each of the examinations by these workers; after fluoroscopy of the upper gastrointestinal tract 0.5 mg. of neostigmine was injected subcutaneously in adults who weighed less than 190 pounds, and 0.75 mg. was used for those who weighed more.

Marshak, in conjunction with large volume barium meals, routinely employs neostigmine in 0.5 mg. doses, which he repeats when indicated to obtain the necessary effect.[61] Neostigmine does not alter significantly the small-bowel pattern, although "intestinal hurry" may result in confusing spurious areas of narrowing. No side effects were encountered in Marshak's large series of patients; he does not use neostigmine in anyone over the age of 55 or in patients who have hypertension or angina. Atropine should be readily available as an antidote for untoward reactions. Margulis cautions that patients with low blood pressure of long duration should remain recumbent during the examination to avoid syncope.[56] In the series of 10,000 roentgenographic examinations reported by Friedenberg and co-workers, essentially no untoward reactions were encountered.[20] They did not give the drug to patients suspected of having intussusception, volvulus, complete intestinal obstruction, perforation, or peritonitis; in addition, it was not used in those with a history of recent myocardial infarction.

Use of cholecystokinin

Highly potent, physiologically active decapeptides, notably caerulein and cholecystokinin, stimulate propulsive muscular activity in the mesenteric small intestine and therefore have been used to accelerate transit. Cholecystokinin in this role has been investigated by Monod,[67] Morin and co-workers,[68] Backlund,[6] and Parker and Beneventano.[78] Since these hormones produce inhibition of muscular activity of the proximal half of the duodenum and stimulation of the distal duodenum and mesenteric small bowel, a sufficient quantity of contrast material first must be presented to the intestine distal to the ligament of Trietz before the drug is administered. This requires a period of approximately 30 minutes after ingestion of a barium suspension. Forty units of cholecystokinin are given intravenously, and abdominal roentgenograms are made at 1, 3, 5, 7, and 10 minutes after drug administration. Some of the investigators have documented the appearance of the small intestine by cineradiographic techniques. In 129 of 186 patients Backlund found a normal small-bowel transit time of less than 10 minutes.[6] Parker and Beneventano observed transit times of less than 15 minutes in 21 of 26 subjects (Fig. 31-1).[78] They noted that in celiac sprue, granulomatous enteritis, and enterocolitis the small bowel was as responsive to cholecystokinin as the normal bowel. However, the drug was ineffectual in accelerating transit in progressive systemic sclerosis with intestinal involvement. Transient untoward effects included nausea and abdominal cramps; no late sequellae were observed. The side effects of caerulein were similar to those noted with cholecystokinin.

Use of metoclopramide

Metoclopramide hydrochloride, an antiemetic agent, increases gastric emptying, produces dilatation of the pylorus and duodenum, and results in rapid propulsive movements of the jejunum. James and Hume investigated the effects of a 20 mg. intravenous dose of metoclopramide on gastric clearance of a barium meal and on transit through the small bowel.[41] The effect on small-bowel motility was not nearly as striking as with cholecystokinin, and the incidence of untoward reactions was greater. Dystonic movements have been reported in children after the therapeutic use of metoclopramide. Thus far the use of the drug in gastrointestinal roentgenology has been limited to investigation outside the United States.

Use of sorbitol

Another pharmacologic method of accelerating transit is the use of sorbitol, which is incorporated into the barium suspension and which provides satisfactory documentation of the small intestinal status in 40 to 60 minutes. Sovenyi and Varro employed 30 gm. of sorbitol in a cold suspension of barium and water and observed an increased amount of fluid in the small bowel. This fluid produced lack of sharpness of the mucosal pattern as seen on the roentgenogram but did not interfere with interpretation.[93] However, they commented that sprue could not be diagnosed. On the other hand, it is of interest that Ingelfinger and Moss reported that the motility of the small bowel in sprue was not influenced by neostigmine.[40]

Use of anticholinergic agents

Anticholinergic induction of small-bowel hypotonia is the basis for several roentgenologic techniques of investigation. Linevsky and Pavlova employed 1 ml. of 0.1% atropine sulfate in 10 ml. of 10% calcium chloride and filled the small bowel in a retrograde manner with a barium suspension introduced via a tube positioned in the distal small bowel and gradually withdrawn.[48] Pajewski and co-workers have evolved a double-contrast examination that makes use of a barium suspension containing sorbitol and sodium citrate, depression of motility with an anticholinergic agent (propantheline [Pro-Banthine] bromide) after filling of the small intestine with barium, and insufflation of

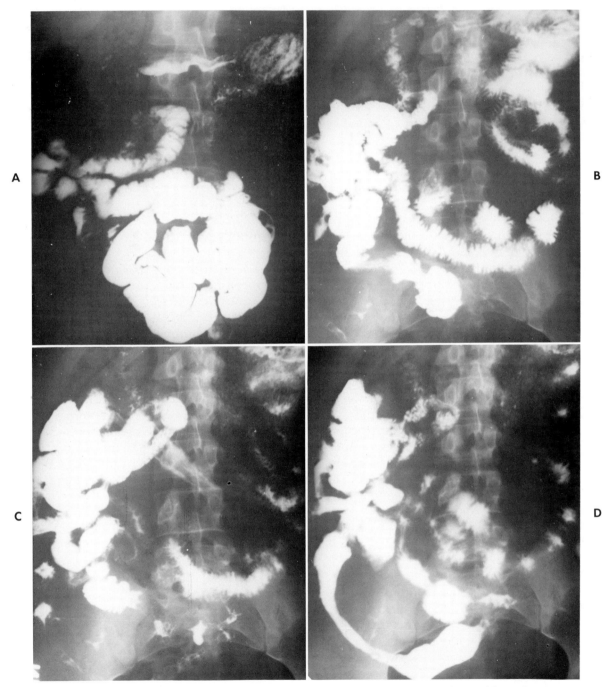

Fig. 31-1. Accelerated small-bowel transit by cholecystokinin in a patient with regional enteritis. **A,** Baseline conventional examination, 3½-hour film showing barium in proximal portion of the small bowel. **B,** 3 minutes, **C,** 5 minutes, and **D,** 7 minutes after cholecystokinin, showing progressive filling of distal small intestine and passage into the colon. (Courtesy Dr. Thomas Beneventano.)

the stomach with air means of a nasogastric tube.[76] Following gastric distention, air enters the small intestine, producing an appearance of ileus with the mucosal surface of the atonic loops coated by barium. Ferrucci and Benedict have obtained excellent mucosal detail by passing a tube to the duodenojejunal junction and instilling 8 to 12 ounces of barium.[17] When the barium reaches the area of interest propantheline is administered and air is insufflated through the tube. Side effects of propantheline have been encountered, and such examinations are not employed if there are contraindications to anticholinergic agents.

Use of glucagon

The use of glucagon for duodenal hypotonia has been recently reported.[13a] By injecting 2 mg. of glucagon intravenously or intramuscularly even better results in obtaining relaxation of the duodenum have been achieved than with propantheline bromide. The use of glucagon was virtually free of side effects.

Use of methylglucamine diatrizoate

Goldstein and associates employed methylglucamine diatrizoate (Gastrografin) as a barium suspension additive to accelerate transit during small-bowel examinations.[33] This technique is an extension of that used by Bradfield and Chrispin to expedite studies in children.[8] Goldstein and associates found that the best method for accelerating small-bowel transit was the addition of 10 ml. of methylglucamine diatrizoate to the barium mixture. In a series of normal volunteers studied by different techniques, 10 ml. of methylglucamine diatrizoate was superior to 30 ml. added to the barium not only in rapidity of transit but also without producing the effects of hyperosomolarity. Also, the transit time was significantly shortened when compared to controls receiving only barium, to examinations with the patients lying in the right lateral decubitus position, and to those performed following a 0.5 mg. dose of neostigmine.

Techniques in perspective and drug interference

In attempting to evaluate the various techniques and place them in perspective, it must be reiterated that there is no ideal or universal method that will meet the requirements of all examiners. There are, nevertheless, certain values that are not predicated on mere preference and that are accepted rather widely. A barium suspension that does not respond to the mucus content of the small-bowel fluid should be used; each examiner or group of examiners should accept one medium as standard, evolve base line values concerning the normal and abnormal small bowel though constant use of that medium, and avoid resorting to multiple preparations. Suitably spaced interval films are necessary to document the appearance of the small bowel, notably each segment, on more than one film. If accelerated techniques are employed, it is well to heed Golden's admonition that shortening the time of the examination is desirable provided that speed in itself does not become the ultimate objective and certain observations bearing on disease are not obscured.[29] It is a dictum that, when a question is raised as to the validity of a finding and it cannot be resolved even on a creditable examination, the examination must be repeated.

When reliance is placed on the transport function of the small bowel, as in all antegrade nonintubation techniques, drugs affecting motility should be discontinued well in advance of the examination. Twenty-four hours should elapse after the last dose of anticholinergic drugs, such as propantheline, and ganglionic blocking agents, such as tetraethylammonium chloride. Lumsden and Truelove have shown that the alteration in motility produced by propantheline is accompanied by some dilatation of the loops, with little change in the feathery pattern created by the valvulae conniventes.[52] Tetraethylammonium chloride, according to Holt and coworkers, cases a marked inhibition of propulsive movements; coarsening of the mucosal markings, which are fixed in one position; and generalized dilatation of the small bowel.[39] Because of impairment of motility, dilatation, coarsening of the valvulae, and increase in the fluid within the lumen of the small bowel, diphenoxylate (Lomotil) hydrochloride with atropine sulfate also should be discontinued for 24 hours prior to the examination (Fig. 31-2). Other drugs that produce relative atony of the small intestine are morphine, dihydromorphinone hydrochloride (Dilaudid), pantopium (Pantopon), codeine, and atropine; a period of approximately 6 hours after discontinuation is sufficient to obtain re-

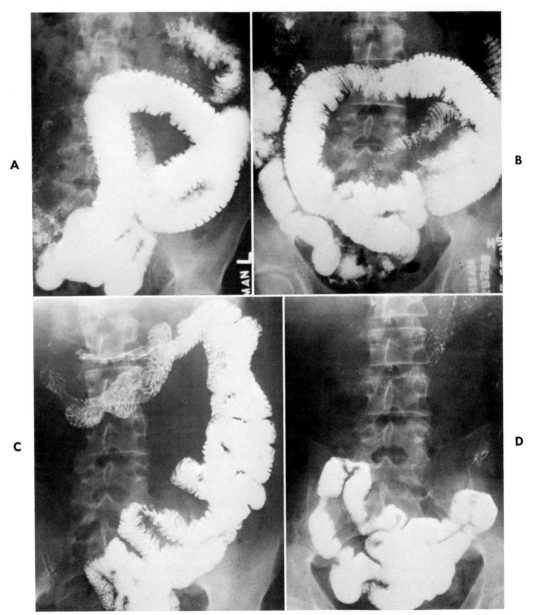

Fig. 31-2. Transitory effect of diphenoxylate hydrochloride with atropine sulfate (Lomotil) on the pattern and transit of the normal small intestine. **A** and **B,** Interval films at 3 and 5½ hours showing changes related to atropine ingested on the day prior to examination. The caliber of the loops is widened grossly, the folds are prominent, the volume of secretions is increased, and transport is impaired. **C** and **D,** Interval films at 30 minutes and 2½ hours on reexamination 9 days later, following discontinuation of the medication. The loop caliber, the fold pattern, the volume of secretions, and transit time have returned to normal. The total transit time reverted to 3 hours as compared to 5½ during the sustained effect of atropine.

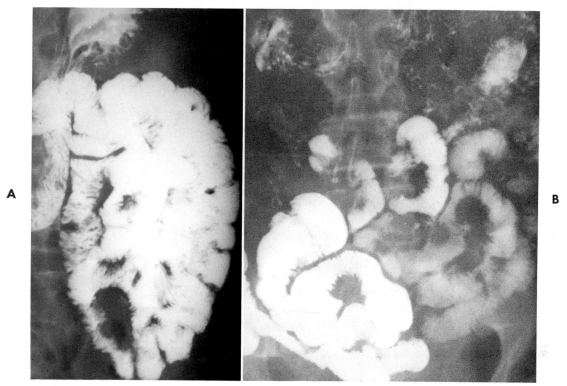

Fig. 31-3. Serosal implants and submucosal metastases from a primary carcinoma of the stomach. **A,** Two-hour interval film showing submucosal nodules in the distal duodenum and subserosal implants producing separation of adjacent jejunal loops and encroachment on the lumen. **B,** Five hours later, after the barium column has passed distally, the constancy of the subserosal alterations has been documented, the fold preservation has been established, and other lesions previously obscured by barium in the jejunum have become apparent. Still other similar lesions are apparent in the ileum.

lease from the effects of these drugs. If, indeed, base-line values without extraneous effects are to be obtained, then oral cholecystography should not be performed concurrent with or immediately prior to a small intestinal examination. It will be recalled that iopanoic acid (Telapaque) effect on the small bowel results in diarrhea in a large percentage of patients.

THE EXAMINATION

After an overnight period of fasting, patients requiring small-bowel study are examined as early as possible in the morning so that studies involving prolonged transit may be completed at a reasonable hour. So that residual barium in the colon does not interfere with interpretation of the films, patients who have had recent contrast studies are given preliminary cleansing enemas.

As a matter of personal preference, I have employed a 12-ounce nonflocculating barium meal (Figs. 31-3 and 31-4) that provides for filling of longer segments than do smaller volumes and that seemingly avoids the problems incident to flooding of ileal loops in the pelvis. The contrast material, administered under fluoroscopic control, is used for examination of the upper gastrointestinal tract to the level of the proximal jejunum. This phase of the examination is completed with erect films in the frontal and left lateral projections, and a prone film at that time serves to document the status of the proximal jejunum.

Sequential films generally are made at half hour intervals unless, at the time of the initial fluoroscopy, the radiologist gains the impression that transit is extremely rapid. Such a timing sequence would not apply to an accelerated tech-

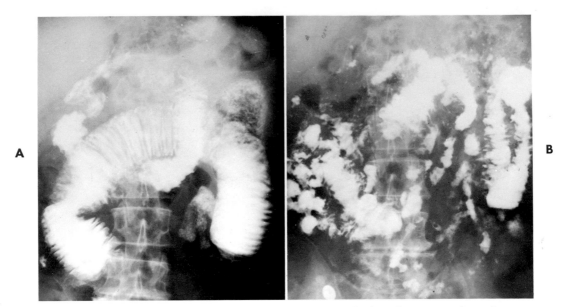

Fig. 31-4. Primary adenocarcinoma of the jejunum, producing almost complete obstruction and a spuriously abnormal small-bowel pattern that may be confused with sprue. **A,** Jejunal obstruction with proximal dilatation and a small amount of barium distal to the obstruction site on a 3½-hour film. **B,** At 5 hours the major portion of the contrast material has passed the obstruction, after having first mixed with a large volume of secretions. The segmentation of the column is a function of the intermittent passage through the high-grade obstruction; the peculiar pattern, in spite of nonflocculating barium having been employed, reflects the effect of the increased volume of secretions.

nique such as that using neostigmine. Each film is immediately reviewed for progress of the meal and for evidences of abnormality that might be evaluated further with fluoroscopy and spot films (Fig. 31-5). Iced water or food stimulation is employed when the stomach is empty in those patients who do not have problems of malabsorption. For patients who do have such conditions, base line values are desired without the additional variable of food stimulation. The time and nature of the food stimulus is recorded for use during evaluation of the completed examination. With patients who have markedly delayed transit, as those with amyloidosis, scleroderma (Fig. 31-6), and occasionally sprue, the interval between films may be extended to 1 hour.

While the study may be completed when contrast material enters the cecum, it often is necessary to continue the examination in order to facilitate the delineation of ileal loops with extrinsic pressure during fluoroscopy. At this time pressure spot films are taken of the terminal ileum, the ileocecal valve, and the cecum. Unless specifically indicated, a 24-hour film is not obtained. The ultimate evaluation of the completed examination requires a rather time-consuming, careful scrutiny and critical appraisal of each segment in continuity from the ligament of Treitz to the cecum.

Examination in disaccharidase deficiency

Laws and Neale[45,46] have evolved a roentgenologic technique for assessment of disaccharidase deficiency, which also has been employed by Haemmerli and Kistler[36] and extended in range by Preger and Amberg.[83] Of the disaccharidase deficiency states, hypolactasia is sufficiently common to justify roentgenologic attempts at diagnosis. Laws and Neale employed a 25 gm. challenging dose of lactose incorporated into the barium suspension administered for small-bowel examination. In patients with lactase deficiency the osmotic effect is similar to that produced by a saline cathartic such as magnesium sulfate. Small-bowel transit is accelerated, the caliber of the intestine increases, the contrast material is diluted, and it literally "hurries" into the colon.

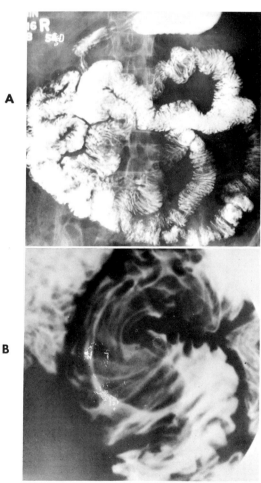

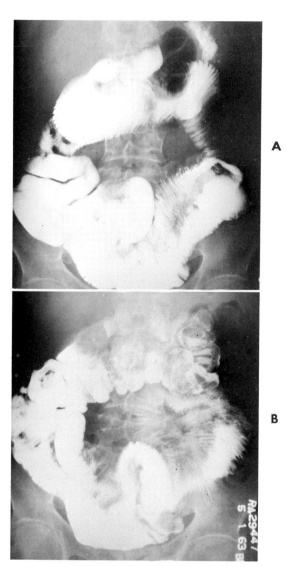

Fig. 31-5. Small-bowel filling defects resulting from multiple lipomas. **A,** Thirty-minute interval film demonstrating the lesions at the duodenojejunal junctional region and distally. **B,** Pressure spot film made during fluoroscopy, documenting the importance of this technique in establishing the nature of abnormalities observed or suspected on immediate review of each film by the examiner. The larger lipoma is sharply delimited and is attached by a long pedicle in an area where the mucosal pattern is preserved.

Fig. 31-6. Small-bowel changes in progressive systemic sclerosis (scleroderma). **A,** Interval film at 3 hours showing dilatation of the small intestine and residual barium in a hypotonic megaduodenum. **B,** At 6½ hours the contrast material has passed into the colon, and the dilated small bowel is delineated by valvulae conniventes that are not thickened but are stretched. Slow transit as such, unless accompanied by alterations in the caliber of the lumen or in the valvulae, generally is not an indicator of organic disease.

Similar changes have been observed following a challenging dose of sucrose in patients with sucrase deficiency.

For critical evaluation of such enzymatic deficiencies, a base line, conventional, small-bowel examination is performed. On a subsequent day, examination with the challenging dose of disaccharide provides the changes from the base line findings, which often are diagnostic. Preger and Amberg showed that in some of their control patients who were given 100 gm. of lactose, the roentgenographic findings were similar to those in documented lactase deficiency.[83] In patients with primary gastrointestinal disorders, such as regional enteritis or previous gastrectomy, challenging doses produced positive roentgenographic alterations that may be accounted for on the basis of secondary deficiency states.

Examination of the patient after operation

Certain modifications of radiographic procedure are important in the successful examination of patients after surgery. For patients who have had a gastrectomy or a gastroenterostomy, in whom gastric emptying is independent of a functioning pylorus, films are made at 15-minute intervals during the first hour and thereafter at 30-minute intervals until the study is completed. Schlaeger has shown that, while the total transit time in these patients is within the range of normal variation, the transit through the proximal small intestine is accelerated; this decreased transport time is thereafter compensated for by prolonged transport in the distal small bowel.[89]

Following ileostomy, interval films are dependent on a knowledge of the length of the remaining small bowel and upon the rapidity of transit as documented on the early roentgenograms. Attention is focused especially on the prestomal portion of the distal small bowel. This segment is evaluated with spot films during fluoroscopy with the patient turned in varying degrees of obliquity until he has almost reached a true lateral position. In examining the transmural portion of the small bowel, one must wait for a wave to propel the bolus through the stoma; it is during the passage of a wave that distention of the terminal segment is achieved. Alterations in the transmural portion of the distal bowel are obscured by the introduction of a tube into the stoma and, accordingly, retrograde

contrast studies would appear to have no place in evaluation of the postileostomy state.

After partial enterectomy, unless there is narrowing, end-to-end anastomotic sites are difficult to locate even with painstaking pressure techniques. Meckel's diverticula and postsurgical blind pouches may often be demonstrated only on delayed films after the mainstream of barium has passed into the colon.

Antegrade intubation techniques

Various antegrade intubation techniques have been developed for examination of the small intestine. These have involved the administration of barium through short tubes positioned in the duodenum in order to render filling of the distal portion of bowel independent of pyloric function. As initial diagnostic procedures, these methods have had sporadic vogue among only a few proponents. Pesquera's description[82] of such a method in 1929 was followed 9 years later by Ghelew and Mengis' report on the use of both barium and air to evaluate the small intestine.[26] Barium enteroclysis, a method used by Gershon-Cohen and Shay in 1939, was based on gravity flow of a diluted barium suspension through a tube with the tip in the third portion of the duodenum.[25] This was also an effort at delineating the entire small bowel by single- and double-contrast techniques. Subsequently, Wissenberg[97] applied the technique of Gershon-Cohen and Shay in twenty-one cases but succeeded in demonstrating few abnormalities. In 1943 Schatzki popularized the small-bowel enema, which was a gravity technique similar to that reported by Pesquera.[82] Lura has used the short tube technique to investigate the proximal small bowel.[53] On the day following the initial examination, after the colon has been cleansed, he studies the distal small intestine by retrograde filling through the ileocecal value. Scott-Harden in 1960 reawakened interest in the short tube examination with his modification.[91,92] This technique involves the use of a Ryle tube positioned with its tip in the region of the duodenojejunal junction. The rapid injection of 60 to 90 ml. of a nonflocculating barium suspension is immediately followed by water containing magnesium sulfate. Successive injections of barium and water provide limited obscuring loops by total barium filling. Pygott and co-workers have used the Scott-Harden technique of small-bowel intubation and stress that it is not to be undertaken as a routine procedure but rather in the demonstration of obstructive and infiltrative lesions and in problems of occult bleeding.[84] At the present time there are few advocates of the short tube contrast examination in the United States.

Examination with the Miller-Abbott tube

Contrast studies through double lumen intestinal tubes are predicated on the fundamental investigations of Miller and Abbott and their co-workers. As early as 1938 Abbott and Johnston pointed out the usefulness of this technique in establishing the location and nature of small bowel obstructions.[1] They also recommended aspiration of intestinal contents to determine the source of bleeding. Leigh and co-workers subsequently championed the cause of the Miller-Abbott tube as a tool useful in reaching a definitive diagnosis of both obstruction and bleeding.[48] A method of evaluating an isolated segment of bowel suspected of organic disease was evolved by Friedman and Rigler, who used a triple-lumen double-balloon tube.[22] Lofstrom and Noer's early observations, among others, stressed the diagnostic superiority of the highest viscosity barium suspension that could be passed without difficulty through the tube.[49,50] In one of their techniques they sealed off the end lumen of the tube distal to the balloon, in order to perform a segmental survey of the small bowel. Twenty years later the same tube modification and method were used by Greenspon and Lentino in a technique termed "retrograde enterography."[34] This involved incremental filling and interval films until overlapping of loops established the end point at the lesion. Not only are Miller-Abbott tube studies of practical value in diagnosing small-bowel obstruction and in establishing the site and possible cause of bleeding but they also extend the usefulness of the conventional small intestinal examination by resolving indeterminate findings.

Variations in procedure

Variations in the examination with the Miller-Abbott tube are dependent upon the problem to be investigated. In bleeding, intermittent aspirations are made during the course of passage of the tube distally. When guaiac-

positive material is identified the tube is secured at that point and the patient is transported to the radiology department. In an attempt at definitive evaluation of the suspected lesion, the tip of the tube is positioned at the approximate level of the alterations observed on the conventional small-bowel study. Generally, repositioning of the tube is necessary during fluoroscopy when barium is introduced.

In small-bowel obstruction, the progress of the tube and the effectiveness of decompression are documented on interval films of the abdomen. When the distended loops are decompressed and the tip of the tube has remained stationary, the diagnostic procedure should be undertaken. The air-containing balloon is deflated in the fluoroscopic room, and under fluoroscopic guidance a nonflocculating barium suspension is manually injected through the tube. Although examinations have been performed with relatively small quantities, approximately 150 ml. of barium is required to complete such a study satisfactorily. The need for such a volume is accounted for by the following factors: (1) following deflation of the baloon, the tip of the tube usually is well proximal to the obstruction site; (2) there frequently is residual dilatation of the bowel, and the secretions cause dilution of the barium; and (3) the openings in the tube proximal to the balloon, together with retrograde peristalsis, permit much of the bolus to pass proximally rather than beyond the end of the tube. Spot films with compression and variation in the position of the patient are invaluable in demonstrating the obstructing lesion (Figs. 31-7 and 31-8); frequently, the examination may be completed during the initial fluoroscopic session. However, when proximal passage of the contrast material prevents documentation of the lesion the tube is withdrawn slightly, so that there is a column of barium distal to the tip of the tube, and the balloon is reinflated. This reinflation frequently stimulates peristalsis, and the contrast material may pass to or beyond the point of narrowing. Depending on the information obtained, the examination is discontinued or continued with additional interval fluoroscopy and films. If a need for more barium is indicated it is introduced after the balloon has been deflated. The contrast material is withdrawn through the indwelling tube by continuous suction when the ex-

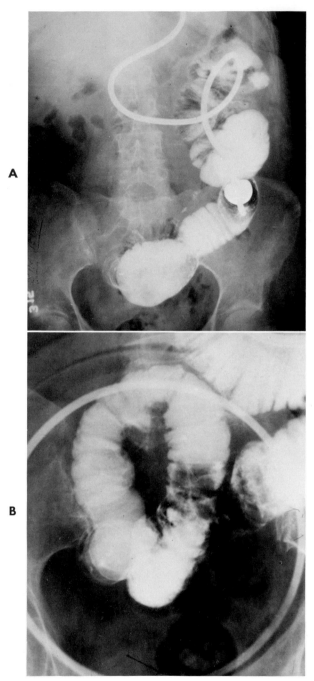

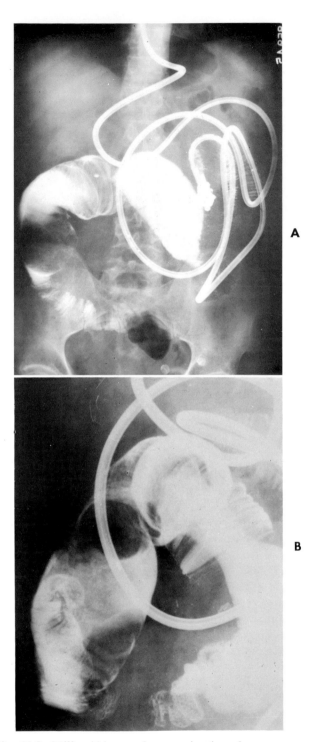

Fig. 31-7. Miller-Abbott tube examination demonstrating gallstone obstruction of the small intestine. **A,** Following attempted decompression, a nonflocculating barium suspension was introduced through the tube in spite of residual dilatation of the small bowel. The tip of the tube generally moves somewhat proximally following deflation of the balloon in the presence of obstruction; the balloon has been reinflated to maintain a continuous contrast column between it and the obstruction site. **B,** A spot film made during fluoroscopy with extrinsic pressure separating the superimposed loops more clearly delineates the large calculus with an opaque periphery.

Fig. 31-8. Miller-Abbott tube examination demonstrating an intussuscepting leiomyoma of the small intestine. **A,** Intussusceptum, intussuscipiens, and large leading mass outlined by nonflocculating barium administered as a suspension through an intestinal tube following decompression. **B,** A spot film made during fluoroscopy further documents the characteristic coil-spring appearance, the mass producing the intussusception, and the short segment of normal small intestine distally.

amination has been completed. There are no inherent dangers to the use of barium in this procedure.

Examination in the presence of obstruction
Oral barium

Oral barium, without preliminary intestinal intubation, has been used in suspected small-bowel obstruction, but in the United States it has had few if any outspoken advocates. Schwarz in 1911, after having recognized the significance of fluid- and gas-filled loops, administered a thin barium mixture to facilitate further delineation.[90] Frimann-Dahl during the past two decades has advocated the use of oral barium when acute small-bowel obstruction is suspected but cannot be confirmed with certainty on abdominal films.[23,24] While the barium reaches the obstruction site after varying periods, recumbent patients should be maintained in the right lateral position to ensure prompt and continuous gastric emptying. With the patient in the supine position the barium gravitates to the dependent fundus and gastric emptying is significantly delayed. This factor does not pertain in patients who are able to sit or stand. Frimann-Dahl employs a 50 ml. suspension consisting of 2 parts of barium to 3 parts of water. When there is no free perforation into the peritoneal cavity and no stenotic lesion in the colon, the use of barium, in itself, provides no hazard to the patient (Fig. 31-9).

Nelson and Christoforidis have advocated a more aggressive approach in patients clinically suspect of intestinal obstruction whose abdominal roentgenograms are normal or equivocal.[72] After ingestion of 300 to 400 ml. of a barium suspension, interval abdominal films generally are made in the prone position. Usually they are done at hourly intervals; however, the time period may vary from 15 minutes to 3 hours and the examination is terminated when the lesion is found or the barium passes into the cecum.

There is no evidence to substantiate the widely held beliefs that barium will convert an incomplete obstruction into a complete one or that it will inspissate in the small intestine proximal to an area of stenosis. Donato, Mayo, and Barr approached this problem experimentally by producing high-grade distal small-bowel obstruction in dogs and then introducing a bar-

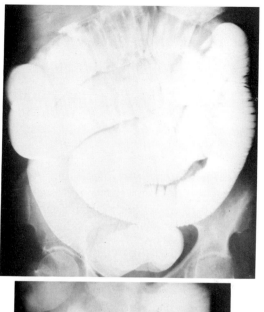

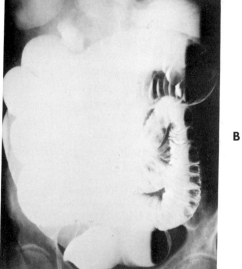

Fig. 31-9. Small-bowel obstruction resulting from an incarcerated right femoral hernia as demonstrated by barium administered orally. Because of the suspicion of a gastric carcinoma, upper gastrointestinal tract contrast studies were performed elsewhere and the patient was referred to the hospital. Roentgenograms of the abdomen were made 24 hours after the first studies, shortly after her arrival. **A,** The supine film shows marked small-bowel dilatation. **B,** Lateral decubitus–horizontal beam film, demonstrating the beaked end of the obstructed small bowel at the site of the femoral hernia. There were no untoward effects incidental to the oral administration of barium in the presence of a complete obstruction.

ium suspension by intubation techniques.[15] At autopsy, there were no instances of barium having produced a complete obstruction by inspissation. Rather, the barium was more liquid than usual in the area of stasis proximal to the stenosis.

The case against water-soluble media

The accumulated experimental evidence has served to dispel the unfounded fears of the dangers of barium in small-bowel obstruction and to place the use of water-soluble iodinated contrast media into its proper perspective. Nelson has summarized these data in an editorial appropriately entitled "Facts versus Folklore."[69a] The experimental studies reported by Nelson and co-workers in 1963 compared water-soluble iodinated contrast media with barium in surgically produced proximal and distal complete nonstrangulating small-bowel obstructions in two groups of dogs.[69b] The results indicated that barium was tolerated better by the animals, that it did not produce impaction at or proximal to the obstruction site, and that the studies using barium were invariably more diagnostic from the roentgenographic standpoint. Neuhauser and his colleagues tested in dogs his belief that infants undergoing examination with water-soluble contrast media may succumb to a severe state of hypovolemia.[37] They showed that the decrease in opacity of the iodinated material was correlated with a progressive fall in circulating plasma volume which ranged from 15% to 30%. When iodinated material was injected into closed loops of small animals there was a marked plasma loss from the circulating volume, and shock ensued. Therefore, in small patients with an initially depressed circulating volume, the hypovolemia occasioned by iodinated contrast media presents a potential as well as a real hazard. Nelson and co-workers also showed that the decrease in plasma volume, resulting from fluid shift into the bowel because of hyperosmolarity of the medium, is aggravated by additional fluid and electrolyte loss caused by the vomiting evoked by the water-soluble contrast medium.[70] Accordingly, the evidence indicates that barium is preferable as a contrast agent in any type of obstruction, especially when the alternative is a hypertonic, pharmacologically active iodinated compound that becomes so diluted as to preclude its use in definitive diagnostic techniques.

Barium is a more desirable contrast agent than is iodinated material when injected through a Miller-Abbott tube following decompression. Dilution is not nearly as critical a problem, especially when delayed interval films are necessary in order to document transit. Epstein pointed out that in the postoperative state, after contrast material had reached the colon, water-soluble media were not impressive in their ability to differentiate ileus from partial mechanical small bowel obstruction.[16] When lesions became suspected with this technique, they required subsequent documentation with barium. Rubin and his co-workers also found that an unequivocal distinction between adynamic ileus and partial mechanical obstruction was not possible with water-soluble media.[86] Even in the absence of obstruction or ileus the secretions and increased fluid caused by the hyperosmolarity of the medium result in dilution, which precludes definitive evaluation distal to the duodenum. (See also Chapter 12.)

Complete reflux examination

Complete reflux examination represents an attempt to overcome the limitations imposed by physiologic transit of barium in conventional antegrade studies.[63] Miller's method of rapid total filling of the small bowel by way of the colon represents an extension of Cherigie's technique of retrograde delination of the ileum.[13] This method employed intravenous atropine and calcium gluconate for an alleged effect on the ileocecal valve and was used to complete the examination of the small bowel after the proximal portion had been investigated in an antegrade fashion on the preceding day. Lura[53] used a similar method to shorten the time of the examination, decrease the radiation to the patient, and lessen the cost of the procedure. For the most part, retrograde studies have been limited to the delineation of the terminal ileum in the course of examination of the colon; Figiel and Figiel have demonstrated tumors of the terminal ileum in this manner.[18]

Miller continues to be the major proponent of complete reflux examination of the small bowel.[66] The details of Miller's technique have been described in his reports on inflammatory lesions and obstructions diagnosed by this method.[63,65] He does not propose the examination as a substitute for antegrade small-bowel evaluation and does not believe that it should be used routinely. All patients, except those with acute obstructions, are investigated first by antegrade techniques. Patients are prepared with castor oil and enemas as for a routine barium enema; however, in suspected bowel obstruction, no preparation is employed. A recent addition to premedication with meperidine (Demerol) hydrochloride and atropine is intravenous diazepam (Valium). Miller now uses a 15% weight-to-volume suspension of barium, which is administered through a large bore retention catheter until the duodenal bulb is filled or until 4,000 to 5,000 ml. have been introduced. After a prone film of the abdomen, the colon is drained and fluoroscopy of the filled small bowel is followed by high kilovoltage films. These often are repeated after further attempts at spontaneous evacuation. In spite of patient discomfort, the procedure has the merit of brevity.

In Miller's series, there have been no complications. However, the examination is not done when mesenteric infarction or gangrene as a result of other causes is suspected. Myocardial infarction is a contraindication, and relative contraindications include congestive heart failure and pulmonary insufficiency.

Castellino and co-workers reported aspiration of barium into the lungs of an infant several hours after retrograde small-bowel examination was performed.[10] Miller previously had cautioned against this hazard from the use of too much barium.[64]

New methods of examination

Cinefluoroscopy has in the past provided little practical information when used for the examination of the small intestine. As an investigative tool it has potential value in documenting alterations of motility produced by various drugs or in studying a limited number of disease states. The use of a so-called physiologic contrast meal, consisting of small food particles mixed with barium, offers little in the practical examination of the small intestine.[10] The extended use of selective arteriography may provide additional insight into organic disease of the small bowel.

The new frontiers in study of the small intestine probably are in the area of opacification by intravenously administered contrast material. Salzman and McClintock have shown that high doses of diatrizoate sodium or diprotrizoate sodium, when injected intravenously in cats, results in visualization of the small intestine and gallbladder by appearance of the material in the wall of the bowel as well as in the lumen.[87] Opacification is more striking in nephrectomized cats, where the prolonged blood level elevation of contrast material makes larger amounts available for excretion by the bowel wall. With high dose diatrizoate radiography, visualization of the small bowel has been observed in infants and also in patients with renal insufficiency. If in adults without renal damage the dose is sufficiently high, the small intestinal wall will be delineated by the contrast material in the course of opacification of the kidneys and extrarenal organs such as the liver, spleen, and gallbladder.

REFERENCES

1. Abbott, W. O.: Intubation studies of the human small intestine. XII, The treatment of intestinal obstruction and a procedure for identifying the lesion, Arch. Intern. Med. **63**:453, 1939.
2. Abbott, W. O., and Johnston, C. G.: Intubation studies of the human small intestine. X, A nonsurgical method of treating, localizing and diagnosing the nature of the obstructive lesions, Surg. Gynec. Obstet. **66**:691, 1938.
3. Adolph, W., and Taplin, G. V.: Micropulverized barium sulfate in x-ray diagnosis, Radiology **54**:878, 1950.
4. Akerlund, A.: Zur direkten Röntgendiagnostik der Dünndarmtumoren, Acta Chir. Scand. **71**:1, 1932.
5. Ardran, C. M., French, J. M., and Mucklow, M. B.: Relationship of the nature of the opaque medium to the small intestine radiographic pattern, Brit. J. Radiol. **23**:267, 1950.
6. Backlund, V.: The use of cholecystokinin in radiology, Radiology **10**:36-39, 1970.
7. Bertaccini, G., and Agosti, A.: Action of caerulein on intestinal motility in man, Gastroenterology **60**:55-63, 1971.
8. Bradfield, G. P., and Chrispin, A. R.: The 90 minute follow through; a simple technique for examination of the small intestine, Brit. J. Radiol. **38**:691-693, 1965.
9. Brown, F. O.: On routine barium examination of the small bowel, Lancet **2**:530, 1959.
10. Burhenne, H. J.: Roentgenologic approach to a physiologic examination of the alimentary tract. In Gamble, J. R., and Wilbur, D. L., editors: Current concepts of clinical gastroenterology, Boston, 1965, Little, Brown and Co.
11. Caldwell, W. L., and Floch, M. H.: Evaluation of the small bowel barium motor meal with emphasis on the effect of volume of barium suspension ingested, Radiology **80**:383, 1963.
12. Castellino, R. A., Verby, H. D., Friedland, G. W.,

and Northway, W. H., Jr.: Delayed barium aspiration following complete reflux small bowel enema, Brit. J. Radiol. 41:937-939, 1968.

13. Cherigie, E.: Radiologie de l'intestin grele normal, Arch. Mal. Appar. Dig. 38:523, 1949.

13a. Chernish, S. M., Miller, R. E., Rosenak, B. D., and Scholz, N. E.: Hypotonic duodenography with the use of glucagon, Gastroenterology 63:392, 1972.

14. Dedick, A. P., and Collins, L.: The roentgen diagnosis of bleeding lesions of the small intestine, Amer. J. Roentgen. 69:926, 1953.

15. Donato, H., Mayo, H. W., Jr., and Barr, L. H.: The effect of peroral barium in partial obstruction of the small bowel; an experimental study, Surgery 35:719, 1954.

16. Epstein, B. S.: Nonabsorbable water-soluble contrast mediums, their use in diagnosis of intestinal obstruction, J.A.M.A. 165:44, 1957.

17. Ferrucci, J. T., Jr., and Benedict, K. T., Jr.: Anticholinergic-aided study of the gastrointestinal tract, Radiol. Clin. N. Amer. 9:23-39, 1971.

18. Figiel, L. S., and Figiel, S. J.: Tumors of the terminal ileum; diagnosis by retrograde filling during barium enema study, Amer. J. Roentgen 91:816, 1964.

19. Frazier, A. C., French, J. M., and Thompson, M.D.: Radiographic studies showing the induction of a segmentation pattern in the small intestine in normal human subjects, Brit. J. Radiol. 22:123, 1949.

20. Friedenberg, M. J., McAlister, W. H., and Margulis, A. R.: Roentgen study of the small bowel in adults and children with neostigmine, Amer. J. Roentgen. 88:693, 1962.

21. Friedman, J.: Roentgen studies of the effects on the small intestine from emotional disturbances, Amer. J. Roentgen. 72:367, 1954.

22. Friedman, J., and Rigler, L. G.: A method of double-contrast roentgen examination of the small intestine, Radiology 54:365, 1950.

23. Frimann-Dahl, J.: The administration of barium orally in acute obstruction; advantages and results, Acta Radiol. 42:285, 1954.

24. Frimann-Dahl, J.: Roentgen examinations in acute abdominal diseases, ed. 2, Springfield, Ill., 1960. Charles C Thomas, Publisher.

25. Gershon-Cohen, J., and Shay, H.: Barium enteroclysis; a method for the direct immediate examination of the small intestine by single and double contrast techniques, Amer. J. Roentgen. 42:456, 1939.

26. Ghelew, B., and Mengis, O.: Mise en evidence de l'intestin grele par une nouvelle technique radiologique, Presse Med. 46:444, 1938.

27. Goin, L. S.: Some obscure factors in production of unusual small bowel patterns, Radiology 59:177, 1952.

28. Golden, R.: Radiologic examination of the small intestine, Philadelphia, 1945, J. B. Lippincott Co.

29. Golden, R.: Radiologic examination of the small intestine, ed. 2, Springfield, Ill., 1959, Charles C Thomas, Publisher.

30. Golden, R.: Technical factors in the roentgen examination of the small intestine, Amer. J. Roentgen. 82:965, 1959.

31. Golden, R., Leigh, O. C., and Swenson, P. C.: Roentgen-ray examination with the Miller-Abbot tube, Radiology 35:521, 1940.

32. Golden, R., and Morales, P. L.: Radiological examination in organic diseases of small intestine, J.A.M.A. 153:1431, 1953.

33. Goldstein, H. M., Poole, G. J., Rosenquist, C. J., Friedland, G. W., and Zboralske, F. F.: Comparison of methods for acceleration of small intestinal radiographic examination, Radiology 98:519-523, 1971.

34. Greenspon, E. A., and Lentino, W.: Retrograde enterography; a new method for roentgenologic study of the small bowel, Amer. J. Roentgen. 83:909, 1960.

35. Grivaux, M., Cornet, A., and Wattez, E.: Metoclopramide in digestive radiology, Sem. Hop. Paris 40:23382345, 1964.

36. Haemmerli, U. P., and Kistler, H.: Disaccharide malabsorption, D.M., Chicago, 1966, Yearbook Medical Publishers, Inc., pp. 1-51.

37. Harris, P. D., Neuhauser, E. B. D., and Gerth, R.: The osmotic effect of water-soluble contrast media on circulating plasma volume, Amer. J. Roentgen. 91:694, 1964.

38. Hodges, F. J., Rundles, R. W., and Hanelin, J.: Roentgenologic study of the small intestine, I. Neoplastic and inflammatory disease, Radiology 49:587, 1947.

39. Holt, J. F., Lyons, R. H., Neligh, R. B., Moe, G. K., and Hodges, F. J.: X-ray signs of altered alimentary function following autonomic blockade with tetraethylammonium, Radiology 49:603, 1947.

40. Ingelfinger, F. J., and Moss, R. E.: Motility of small intestine in sprue, J. Clin. Invest. 22:345, 1943.

41. James, W. B., and Hume, R.: Action of metoclopramide on gastric emptying and small bowel transit time, Gut 9:205, 1968.

42. Kim, S. K.: Small intestine transit time in the normal small bowel study, Amer. J. Roentgen. 104:522-524, 1968.

43. Kirsh, I. E., and Spellberg, M. A.: Examination of small intestine with carboxymethylcellulose, Radiology 60:701, 1953.

44. Kirsh, I. E.: Motility of the small intestine with non-flocculating medium; a review of 173 roentgen examinations, Gastroenterology 31:251, 1956.

45. Laws, J. W., and Neale, G.: Radiological diagnosis of disaccharidase deficiency, Lancet 2:139-143, 1966.

46. Laws, J. W., Spencer, J., and Neale, G.: Radiology in the diagnosis of disaccharidase deficiency, Brit. J. Radiol. 40:594-603, 1967.

47. Leigh, O. C., Jr., Nelson, J. A., and Swenson, P. C.: The Miller-Abbott tube as an adjunct to surgery of small intestinal obstructions, Ann. Surg. 111:186, 1940.

48. Linevsky, Y. V., and Pavlova, I. S.: The value of radiological examination of the artificially hypotensive small intestine for the diagnosis of chronic enteritis, Vetn. Roentgen. Radiol. 43:34-37, 1968.

49. Lofstrom, J. E., and Noer, R. J.: The role of intestinal intubation in the diagnosis and localization of intestinal obstruction, Radiology 35:546, 1940.

50. Lofstrom, J. E., and Noer, R. J.: The use of intestinal intubation in localization of lesions of the gastrointestinal tract, Amer. J. Roentgen. 42:321, 1939.

51. Lonnerblad, L.: Transit time through the small intestine; a roentgenologic study on normal variability, Acta Radiol. 88 (Supp.):1, 1951.

52. Lumsden, K., and Truelove, S. C.: Intravenous probathine in diagnostic radiology of the gastrointestinal tract with special reference to colonic disease, Brit. J. Radiol. 32:517, 1959.

53. Lura, A.: Radiology of the small intestine, IV, Enema of the small intestine with special emphasis on the diagnosis of tumours, Brit. J. Radiol. 24:264, 1951.

54. McAlister, W. H., and Margulis, A. R.: Small bowel transit time of barium sulfate preparations and iodine contrast media in dogs, Amer. J. Roentgen. 91:814, 1964.

55. Margulis, A. R., and Mandelstam, P.: The use of parenteral neostigmine in the roentgen study of the small bowel, Radiology 76:223, 1961.

56. Margulis, A. R.: Some new approaches to the examination of the gastrointestinal tract, Amer. J. Roentgen. 101:265-286, 1967.

57. Marks, M. M.: Barium modification with Methocel in diagnosis of bowel lesions, J. Int. Coll. Surg. 15:143, 1951.

58. Marshak, R. H.: Roentgen findings in lesions of the small bowel, Amer. J. Dig. Dis. 6:1084, 1961.

59. Marshak, R. H., and Lindner, A. E.: Malabsorption syndrome, Seminars Roentgen. 1:138, 1966.

60. Marshak, R. H., Wolf, B. S., and Adlersberg, D.: Roentgen studies of the small intestine in sprue, Amer. J. Roentgen. 72:380, 1954.

61. Marshak, R. H., and Lindner, A. E.: Radiology of the small intestine, Philadelphia, 1970, W. B. Saunders Co.

62. Miller, R. E.: Barium sulfate suspensions, Radiology 84:241, 1965.

63. Miller, R. E.: Complete reflux small bowel examination, Radiology 84:457, 1965.

64. Miller, R. E., and Miller, W. J.: Inflammatory lesions of the small bowel: complete reflux small bowel examination, Amer. J. Gastroent. 45:40, 1966.

65. Miller, R. E., and Miller, W. J.: Small bowel obstruction; complete reflux small bowel examination, Amer. J. Surg. 109:572, 1965.

66. Miller, R. E.: Reflux examination of the small bowel, Radiol. Clin. N. Amer. 7:175-184, 1969.

67. Monod, E.: Action enter-kinetique de la cecekin, Arch. Mal. Appar. Dig. 53:607-608, 1964.

68. Morin, G., Fescancon, F., Grall, A., Jouve, R., and Debray, C. R.: Technique d'accélération due grèle, Arch. Mal. Appar. Dig. 54:1285-1290, 1965.

69a. Nelson, S. W.: facts versus folklore, Amer. J. Surg. 109:543, 1965.

69b. Nelson, S. W., Christoforidis, A. J., and Roenigk, W. J.: Barium suspensions versus water-soluble iodine compounds in the study of obstruction of the small bowel; an experimental study of physiologic characteristics and radiographic value, Radiology 80:252, 1963.

70. Nelson, S. W., Christoforidis, A. J., and Roenigk, W. J.: Dangers and fallibilities of iodinated radiopaque media in obstruction of the small bowel, Amer. J. Surg. 109:546, 1965.

71. Nelson, S. W., and Christoforidis, A. J.: The use of barium sulfate suspensions in the study of suspected mechanical obstruction of the small intestine, Amer. J. Roentgen. 101:367-378, 1967.

72. Nelson, S. W., and Christoforidis, A. J.: The use of barium sulfate suspensions in the diagnosis of acute disease of the small intestine, Amer. J. Roentgen. 104:505-519, 1968.

73. Nice, C. M., Jr.: Roentgenographic pattern and motility in small bowel studies, Radiology 80:39, 1963.

74. Nice, C. M., Jr.: A simple experiment in small bowel motility, Indian J. Radiol. 14:149, 1960.

75. Osgood, E. C.: The role of the radiologist in the management of patients with intestinal obstruction, with special reference to the use of the Miller-Abbott tube, Radiology 49:529, 1947.

76. Pajewski, M., Itzchak, Y., and Profis, A.: The double contrast examination of the small intestine: preliminary communication of a new technique, Clin. Radiol. 21:83-86, 1970.

77. Pansdorf, H.: Die fraktionierte Dünndarmfüllung und ihre klinische Bedeutung. Fortschr. Geb. Röntgenstr. 56:627, 1937.

78. Parker, J. G., and Beneventano, T. C.: Acceleration of small bowel contrast study by cholecystokinin, Gastroenterology 58:679-684, 1970.

79. Pendergrass, E. P.: Roentgen diagnosis of small intestinal lesions, Texas J. Med. 35:528, 1939.

80. Pendergrass, E. P.: The small intestine, J.A.M.A. 107:1859, 1936.

81. Pendergrass, E. P., Ravdin, I. S., Johnston, C. G., and Hodes, P. J.: Studies of the small intestine. II, Effects of food and pathological states on gastric emptying and small intestinal pattern, Radiology 26:651, 1936.

82. Pesquera, G. S.: Method for direct visualization of lesions in small intestines, Amer. J. Roentgen. 22:254, 1929.

83. Preger, L., and Amberg, J. R.: Sweet diarrhea: roentgen diagnosis of disacharidase deficiency, Amer. J. Roentgen. 101:287-295, 1967.

84. Pygott, F., Street, D. F., Shellshear, M.F., and Rhodes, C. J.: Radiological investigation of the small intestine by small bowel enema technique, Gut 1:366, 1960.

85. Ravdin, I. S., Pendergrass, E. P., Johnston, C. G., and Hodes, P. J.: The effect of foodstuffs on emptying of the normal and operated stomach and the small intestinal pattern, Amer. J. Roentgen. 35:306, 1936.

86. Rubin, R. J., Ostrum, B. J., and Dex, W. J.: Water-soluble contrast media; their use in the diagnosis of obstructive gastrointestinal disease, Arch. Surg. 80:495, 1960.

87. Salzman, E., and McClintock, J. T.: Opacification of the small bowel with intravenously administered contrast medium, Radiology **80**:748, 1963.

88. Schatzki, R.: Small intestinal enema, Amer. J. Roentgen. **50**:743, 1943.

89. Schlaeger, R.: Radiologic observations with barium and food in the postgastrectomy state, New York J. Med. **60**:1780, 1960.

90. Schwarz, G.: Die Erkennung der tieferen Dünndarmstenosen mittels des Röntgenverfahrens, Wien. Klin. Wchschr. **24**:1386, 1911.

91. Scott-Harden, W. G.: Examination of the small bowel. In McLaren, J. W., editor: Modern trends in diagnostic radiology, New York, 1960, Harper & Row, Publishers.

92. Scott-Harden, W. G., Hamilton, H. A. R., and McCall-Smith, S.: Radiological investigation of the small intestine, Gut **2**:316, 1961.

93. Sovenyi, E., and Varro, V.: Über eine neue Methode zur Röntgenuntersuchung des Dünndarms, Fortschr. Rontgenstr. **91**:269, 1959.

94. Weber, H. M., and Kirklin, B. R.: Roentgenologic investigation of the small intestine, Med. Clin. N. Amer. **22**:1059, 1938.

95. Weigen, J. F., Pendergrass, E. P., Ravdin, I. S., and Machella, T. F.: A roentgen study of the effect of total pancreatectomy on the stomach and small intestine of dogs, Radiology **59**:92, 1952.

96. Weintraub, S., and Williams, R. G.: A rapid method of roentgenologic examination of the small intestine, Amer. J. Roentgen. **61**:45, 1949.

97. Wissenberg, P.: Roentgen examination of small intestine following introduction of contrast substance by means of duodenal tube, Nord. Med. **16**:3422, 1942.

98. Zimmer, E. A.: Radiology of the small intestine, I. Studies on contrast media for the x-ray examination of the gastrointestinal tract, Brit. J. Radiol. **24**:245, 1951.

Regional enteritis 32

Richard H. Marshak
Arthur E. Lindner

Regional enteritis is a chronic, nonspecific, granulomatous, inflammatory disease of the small bowel. The cause of the illness is not known.[7] It was first described in 1932 by Crohn, Ginzburg, and Oppenheimer, who reported 14 patients with an obstructing inflammatory lesion of the terminal ileum.[2] Such lesions in the past had been considered to be intestinal tuberculosis; but Crohn and his associates demonstrated the absence of tuberculous infection and called the disease "terminal ileitis," since inflammation was confined to the terminal ileum in all their cases. Subsequently the name was changed to "regional enteritis" or "regional ileitis," and it became apparent that although the disease usually does involve the terminal ileum, any part of the gastrointestinal tract from the esophagus to the anus can be affected. British authors call the illness *"Crohn's disease"* wherever it occurs in the intestine, but American authors, who tend to avoid eponyms, have used a variety of terms: "granulomatous gastritis," for stomach involvement; "regional enteritis," for small-bowel disease; "granulomatous colitis," for disease of the colon; and "granulomatous ileocolitis," for involvement of both small bowel and colon. Granulomatous colitis and ileocolitis, which pose a problem in differentiation from ulcerative colitis, are discussed in Chapter 37. The pathology of the granulomatous disease process is the same at all levels of the gastrointestinal tract.

PATHOLOGY

The wall of the bowel involved with regional enteritis is thick and rigid, and the segment of diseased bowel is often sharply delimited from normal contiguous intestine. The mesentery is thick and swollen, and mesenteric lymph nodes are enlarged. When the bowel is opened, the lumen is found to be narrowed, sometimes to a stricture. The mucosa is red and swollen and often has an appearance that has been lickened to a cobblestone road. Such an appearance re-

PATHOLOGY

CLINICAL FEATURES

ROENTGENOGRAPHIC FINDINGS
Nonstenotic phase
Stenotic phase

SITE OF INVOLVEMENT
Ileitis
Jejunoileitis
Jejunitis
Duodenitis
Gastritis

RECURRENT REGIONAL ENTERITIS
Healing in regional enteritis
Regional enteritis in children
Carcinoma with regional enteritis

LYMPHOID HYPERPLASIA

DIFFERENTIAL DIAGNOSIS

sults from the intersection of rather regular longitudinal and transverse ulcers, with swollen intervening mucosa. Sinus tracts and abscesses may be present, and fistulas may extend from the diseased segment to adjacent viscera or to the body wall. Two or more areas of disease ("skip lesions") may be identified in the bowel, separated by lengths of normal-appearing intestine.

On histologic examination regional enteritis proves to be a transmural disease, with a chronic granulomatous inflammatory reaction marked by edema and fibrosis involving all layers of the intestinal wall.[4,13] Changes are most prominent in the submucosa. Ulcers are often present in the mucosa and may extend deep into the submucosa and muscularis as fissures. The most useful diagnostic feature is the presence of noncaseating granulomas containing multinucleated giant cells and epithelioid and mononuclear cells. Granulomas may also be found in regional lymph nodes. It is possible to identify granulomas in approximately three fourths of surgical specimens that otherwise meet clinical, roentgenographic, and pathologic criteria for regional enteritis, but their presence is not essential for diagnosis. Jones Williams found nonspecific inflammation as the only finding in 25% of cases studied, a diffuse granulomatous inflammation in another 25%, and focal granulomatous inflammation with sarcoid-like granulomas in 50%.[6]

CLINICAL FEATURES

The clinical course of regional enteritis usually begins with diarrhea, abdominal cramps, fever, anemia, anorexia, and weight loss.[3,12] Often the onset is insidious, especially in children, and in the early stages symptoms may increase only gradually in severity. At times the symptoms are so low grade or so intermittent that the patient does not seek medical attention for a long time or appropriate diagnostic studies are delayed for months or years; in these cases the true onset of the disease is recognized only in retrospect. Sometimes the onset is sudden and the patient has apparent acute appendicitis. At laparotomy on these occasions, however, the small bowel usually appears to be chronically inflamed, so it is likely that "acute ileitis" is really an acute exacerbation of a previously quiescent chronic disease.

A characteristic finding on physical examination is the presence of a tender abdominal mass, usually in the right lower quadrant. The mass represents chronically thickened bowel and mesentery, enlarged lymph nodes, and sometimes and intra-abdominal abscess.

Stricture formation and partial small-bowel obstruction are common in regional enteritis, but complete obstruction is unusual even in severe disease. For this reason obstruction rarely requires emergency surgical intervention. Spasm and edema contribute to the obstruction and relief may be obtained by small-bowel intubation and medical supportive measures.

Free perforation of the small bowel is rare, but small sealed-off perforations are not only common but are also quite characteristic of the disease. These small perforations represent extensions of inflammatory disease through the bowel wall to the serosa and into the mesentery. The perforations are small, the inflammatory reaction is intense, and the leak becomes sealed off. Such small sealed-off perforations are the genesis of the fistulas that are so common in regional enteritis. Fistulas may extend from one loop of small bowel to another, from small bowel to colon, or from small bowel to vagina, bladder, or abdominal wall. Perianal fistulas and abscesses are frequent features of the illness; indeed they may be the first clinical finding in regional enteritis and may antedate the other clinical features by many months or even years.

Gross blood in the stools is unusual; when it occurs it is usually only an occasional episode and not a regular feature of the clinical course. Occult bleeding is common, however, and iron deficiency is a principal cause of the anemia that occurs in the disease.

Extraintestinal manifestations, such as peripheral arthritis, ankylosing spondylitis, iritis, erythema nodosum, and pyoderma gangrenosum, occur in patients with regional enteritis but are less frequent than in ulcerative colitis.

Regional enteritis does not usually spread anatomically, either proximally or distally, in the absence of surgery. When patients are followed with serial small-bowel examinations year after year on medical programs, the disease may become more severe within a given area, and abscesses, strictures, or fistulas may develop; however, the linear extent of the disease throughout followup usually appears to be the same as on the initial examination. The failure of the disease to extend during medical treatment is remarkable, for the disease is notorious for its tendency to recur and to spread after surgery. Disease recurs in at least half the patients who are operated upon, usually within the first 2 years after operation but sometimes many years later. As a rule the disease recurs just proximal to the old diseased area, at the site of anastomosis, but sometimes the recurrence is quite distant and skip lesions may develop. A "cure" of regional enteritis by either medical or surgical means is unusual, but prolonged remissions of many years' duration may occur.

ROENTGENOGRAPHIC FINDINGS

Several investigators divide the roentgenographic findings in this disease into acute, subacute, and chronic stages. Since the classic form of regional enteritis is that of a low-grade inflammatory process with episodes of acute

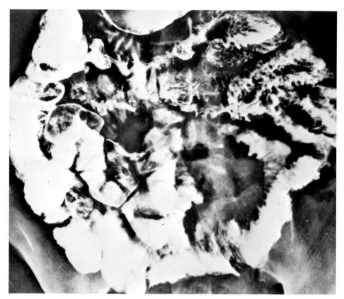

Fig. 32-1. Nonstenotic regional enteritis. There is involvement of the distal jejunum and the proximal ileum with thickening and blunting of the folds, rigidity, and separation of the loops of intestine.

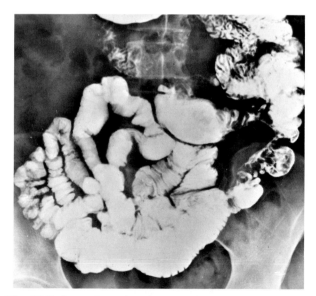

Fig. 32-2. Stenotic regional enteritis, same patient as in Fig. 32-1 6 years later. There is more extensive narrowing of the lumen, with alternating areas of constriction and dilatation, but there has been no longitudinal spread of the inflammatory process. Resection was carried out at this time because of repeated intestinal hemorrhages.

exacerbation, we find it difficult to identify such clear-cut patterns indicative of the stage of the disease. It is possible that acute granulomatous regional enteritis does occur, but the determination of the precise onset of regional enteritis is almost impossible; what is described as acute regional enteritis may be a more active phase of the chronic illness.

Proximal and distal extension of the disease process, despite repeated roentgenographic examinations over a period of many years, is rarely seen. The maximum length of the involved area is determined by the initial studies (Figs. 32-1 and 32-2). This is not true after exclusion operations or resections when longitudinal spread is frequent.

One of the prominent features of this disease is the development of stenosis with obstruction. Roentgenologically, cases may conveniently be classified as stenotic or nonstenotic.[8] The majority of patients may continue without stenosis for many years. Again division into active and inactive phases seems inappropriate, for a patient with long segments of stenotic and probably fibrotic intestine may have chronic bouts of fever, abdominal pain, or leukocytosis.

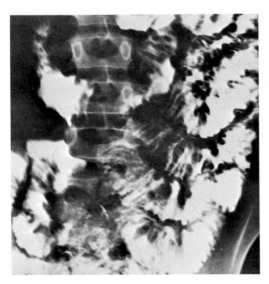

Fig. 32-3. Nonstenotic type of regional enteritis. There is thickening and blunting of the folds and moderate irregularity of the contour of the bowel. Numerous small defects are noted, which in some areas appear to be submucosal.

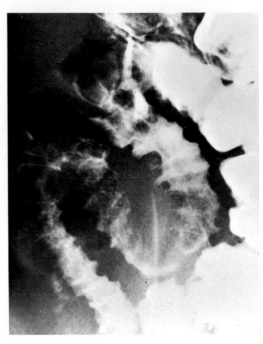

Fig. 32-4. Nonstenotic type of regional enteritis in a young male with a 10-day history of illness. The folds are thickened and blunted in the distal ileum with evidence of an inflammatory edema. There is moderate separation of the loops of bowel associated with narrowing and rigidity.

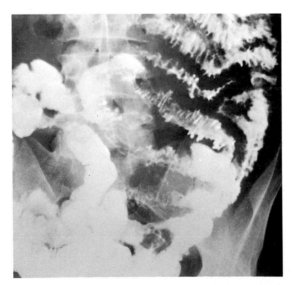

Fig. 32-5. Nonstenotic type of regional enteritis. The mucosal folds are thickened, blunted, and in some areas fused. The contour of the bowel is irregular with moderate narrowing of the lumen. There is rigidity and separation of the intestinal loops, which appear straight.

Nonstenotic phase

The roentgenographic findings closely parallel the pathologic features. Early changes are blunting, flattening, thickening, distortion, or straightening of the valvulae conniventes. The folds may be quite distorted or may be arranged in a fairly regular, symmetrical, parallel fashion. They may appear rigid and are perpendicular to the long axis of the intestine. The folds become thicker, irregular, indistinct, and partially fused (Figs. 32-3 to 32-5). The lumen and contour become irregular. Occasionally the irregularity of contour and of the valvulae conniventes is seen without distinct blunting or thickening of the folds (Fig. 32-6). These early changes are caused by the inflammatory submucosal and mucosal thickening. When ulceration occurs, a more characteristic pattern is produced. Longitudinal streaks of barium, which are recognizable as ulcerations, appear (Fig. 32-7) and are usually associated with transverse ulcerations producing, in some cases, a cobblestone pattern (Fig. 32-8).

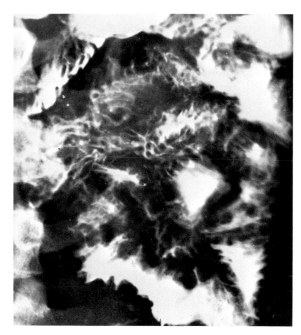

Fig. 32-6. Nonstenotic regional enteritis. There is spasm and irritability of the proximal jejunal loops, associated with thickening of the folds and irregularity of the contour.

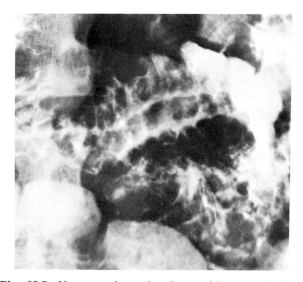

Fig. 32-7. Nonstenotic regional enteritis. Longitudinal and transverse ulcerations are noted with intervening mucosal edema.

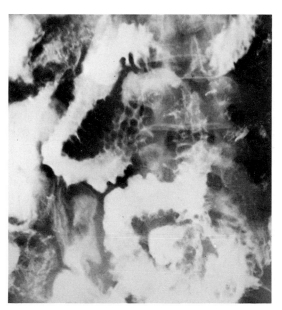

Fig. 32-8. Nonstenotic regional enteritis. Longitudinal and transverse ulcerations produce a characteristic cobblestone pattern. In other areas the folds are thickened and blunted with moderate irregularity of the contour of bowel.

This specific pattern is more common in the jejunum, probably because of the thicker valvulae conniventes in this region. Ulceration continues at the expense of the intervening island of mucosa, replacing the cobblestone pattern by an irregular network of interlacing streaks of barium. At this stage the ulceration is neither uniform nor symmetric but appears hazy and reticulated (Fig. 32-9). Denudation of the mucosa is usually incomplete, leaving behind islands of inflamed mucosa (inflammatory polyps) that produce multiple smooth defects of varying size (Figs. 32-10 to 32-12.) Their prominence is increased by the narrowing of the bowel lumen, resulting from the beginning of cicatrical contraction that occurs at this stage. Finally, one may see the roentgenologic image of a uniform, rigid, castlike tube filled with barium and presenting no mucous membrane pattern. This roentgenologic image is similar to that of ulcerative colitis and represents the stage when scarring and regeneration of an atrophic mucosa is progressing (Fig. 32-11). As scarring proceeds, the transition to the stenotic phase occurs.

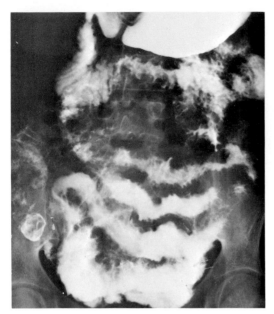

Fig. 32-9. Nonstenotic regional enteritis. Virtually the entire small bowel is involved with regional enteritis. There is almost complete ulceration of the mucosa, which appears hazy and reticulated. The granular appearance of the barium is caused by the inflammatory edema.

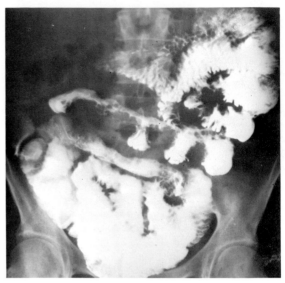

Fig. 32-10. Nonstenotic regional enteritis. There is rigidity and separation of the loops of intestine with numerous small filling defects caused by inflammatory polyps. Eccentric skip areas are also noted.

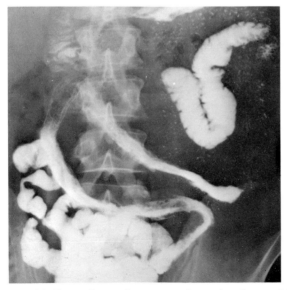

Fig. 32-11. Late phase of nonstenotic regional enteritis. The distal jejunum and proximal ileum are involved. The mucosal pattern appears castlike, with no evidence of a normal mucous membrane pattern. The loops of bowel are moderately rigid, narrowed, and separated.

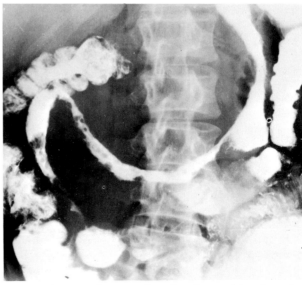

Fig. 32-12. Stenotic type of regional enteritis of moderate severity. The mucosa is extensively ulcerated, and small inflammatory polyps are present. The loops are rigid and narrowed, with slight proximal dilatation. The loops of bowel appear to surround a mass that is the result of the inflamed indurated mesentery.

Coincident with changes in the mucosa, other characteristic roentgenographic features appear. The bowel lumen reveals varying degrees of narrowing. In the early stages submucosal thickening and spasm, secondary to the inflammatory process, are responsible for the narrowing of the lumen. Later, as fibrosis occurs, the narrowing is more complete and leads finally to the stenotic stage. In the early stages, rigidity of the countour and mucosal pattern is incomplete. Some flexibility or dynamic activity becomes evident during successive roentgenograms. Later, the roentgenologic appearance is fixed and unvarying. Pliability is also lost. Furthermore, early in the disease the normal serpentine or coiled pattern of the loops of small intestine disappears. The diseased segments seem to be straightened and rigid. This is probably a result of loss of flexibility in the intestinal wall and mesentery as well as longitudinal shortening caused by spasm.

At times the loops of intestine appear to surround a mass (Fig. 32-12). Although this may be caused by an abscess resulting from perforation, more often it is secondary to the indurated mesentery associated with the marked increase in the mesenteric fat and the enlarged lymph nodes. The silhouette of the intestine may be hazy. This is because the intestine is diffusely ulcerated; it contains exudate and excessive secretions, and the barium does not adhere to the walls. Despite the increase in intestinal content, the barium mixture remains fluid and homogeneous. Neither agglutination, clumping, nor formation of masses of barium is found in regional enteritis as contrasted with the findings in the sprue pattern. Segmentation, such as is characteristic of sprue, is not observed. When unequivocal segmentation occurs, the diagnosis of regional enteritis should be suspect. Skip areas (Fig. 32-10), that is, segments of normal intestine intervening between diseased segments, represent another charcteristic feature. The length of the skip area may vary from a few inches to several feet. In most cases the extent of involvement may be quite accurately determined on a roentgenogram since the transition from the diseased to the normal intestine is fairly abrupt. In some instances, spasm and irritability may be seen in intrinsically normal small bowel because of their proximity to diseased segments. Several examinations may be

necessary before it can be accurately determined that these spastic and irritable loops of bowel are not involved with regional enteritis. This is important for both the surgeon and the radiologist in planning a resection in these cases.

An outpouching of the mucosa between the thickened folds (Fig. 32-13) occurs in some cases, creating an appearance much like diverticula. Pseudodiverticula are probably caused by eccentric skip areas affecting one side of the bowel wall and not the other.

Stenotic phase

In the stenotic stage many of the rigid loops previously described become constricted to a remarkable degree. These stenotic segments resemble rigid pipestems (Figs. 32-14 to 32-18). This appearance is caused by a marked thickening and contraction of the wall of the small intestine. The stenosis may extend 1 or 2 cm. or over long segments. With severe narrowing, dilatation of the proximal intestine may be pronounced. In many instances it is difficult to state whether or not intrinsic disease is present in a dilated area. Very often disease is present when a loop of dilated intestine exists between two points of constriction. On the other hand, when there is a single area of constriction with proxi-

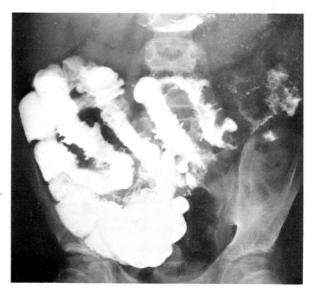

Fig. 32-13. Nonstenotic type of regional enteritis. Normal bowel protrudes between thickened, blunted folds, producing multiple pseudodiverticula. These represent eccentric skip areas.

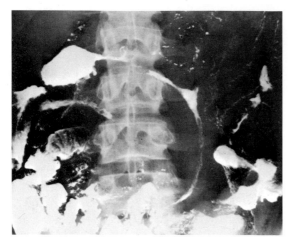

Fig. 32-14. Stenotic type of regional enteritis. Long segments of constricted bowel alternate with small areas of dilatation. The loops of bowel are unduly separated because of the thickening of the mesentery.

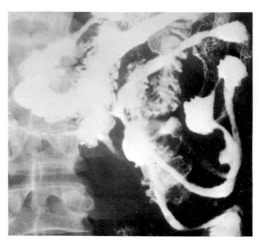

Fig. 32-15. Stenotic type of regional enteritis. There are multiple areas of constriction and dilatation. In the constricted segments the mucosa is ulcerated. This patient died of an exsanguinating hemorrhage.

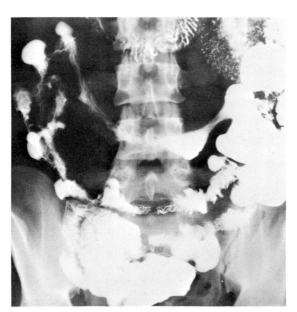

Fig. 32-16. Stenotic type of regional enteritis. There are multiple areas of constriction associated with pseudo-diverticula and proximal dilatation of the bowel.

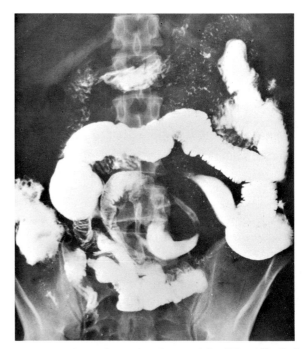

Fig. 32-17. Stenotic regional enteritis. The distal jejunum and proximal ileum are involved with the stenotic form of regional enteritis. The proximal small bowel is moderately dilated.

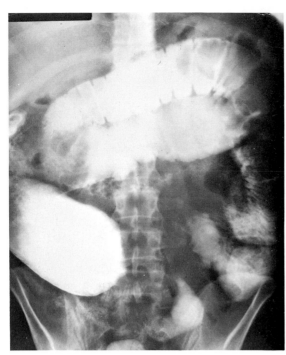

Fig. 32-18. Stenotic regional enteritis. Same patient as in Fig. 32-17 9 years later. There is tremendous dilatation of the jejunum associated with a large amount of secretions. The stenotic segments are difficult to identify.

mal dilatation, regional enteritis may not be present in the dilated segment. However, because of retained secretions, secondary inflammatory changes, tension ulcers, and muscular hypertrophy, the appearance of the dilated loops may be confused with the alterations seen in regional enteritis. This distinction is of great importance when surgery is considered. Many patients have not undergone operative intervention because the surgeon believed that the entire intestine was involved. Extreme dilatation of long segments of the intestine is rarely associated with intrinsic granulomatous disease.

Many of the roentgenologic phenomena observed in the nonstenotic phase of the disease are again noted in the stenotic phase. The mucosal pattern is usually reticulated or castlike. Small filling defects and inflammatory polyps, irregularly distributed throughout the diseased segments, are noted. Skip areas and wide spacing between the segments of intestine are more striking than in the nonstenotic phase. The loops are rigid and maintain a constant

position from film to film. The diseased segments of intestine seem to encircle an inflammatory mass. Fistulas, usually involving the distal ileum and adjacent loops of intestine, may be seen. Occasionally these are difficult to demonstrate, especially when dilated loops of intestine produced overlapping. The fistulas may extend to and penetrate the abdominal wall.

In general, the roentgenographic findings in regional enteritis are as described; however, certain characteristics are peculiar to the area of involvement.

SITE OF INVOLVEMENT
Ileitis

The most frequent site of involvement of the small bowel with regional enteritis is the terminal ileum. Depending on the degree of involvement, this segment exhibits varying roentgenographic alterations. The early cases may be difficult to detect. There may be only slight disturbance in peristaltic activity, manifested by minimal flattening of the contours or irregular pseudodiverticular contractions, and minimal limitation in distensibility. Spasm and irritability are common and may be so pronounced that the involved segment is difficult to see. Slight spiculation of the contours may be identified with minimal thickening and irregularity of the mucosal folds (Figs. 32-19 and 32-20). Repeat studies are important with patients who have minimal symptoms. If the findings disappear, the diagnosis of regional enteritis should be questioned. As ulceration proceeds, there is more spasm and irritability, more coarsening and thickening of the folds, and, finally, the string sign may be seen.

The string sign has come to be identified as a pathognomonic roentgenographic manifestation of regional enteritis and is most frequently noted in this region. It has been described as a thin, linear shadow, suggesting the appearance of a frayed cotton string (Fig. 32-21). The string sign is caused by incomplete filling resulting from irritability and spasm associated with extensive ulceration. It may be seen in both the nonstenotic and stenotic phases of this disease. Repeated spot films will demonstrate that some distensibility is present in this segment (Fig. 32-22). The bowel proximal to the string sign may or may not be dilated, depending on the stage of the disease. In the nonstenotic phase,

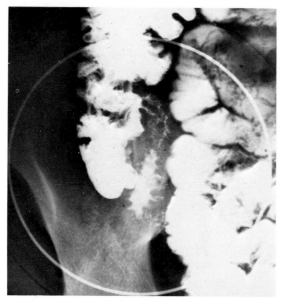

Fig. 32-19. Early regional enteritis. Minimal changes involving the terminal ileum are noted, characterized by spasm, irritability, and slight thickening and irregularity of the mucosal folds.

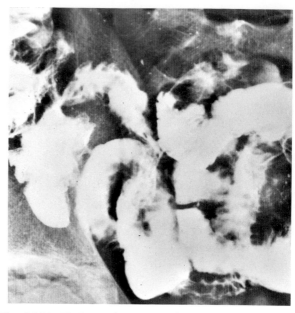

Fig. 32-20. Early regional enteritis. In comparison to Fig. 32-19 there is identifiable a slightly greater involvement of the distal 2 feet of ileum. The patient is a 15-year-old boy. There is ulceration of the mucosa, which produces a cobblestone pattern of a loop of ileum above the symphysis pubis. Moderate thickening and blunting of the folds are seen.

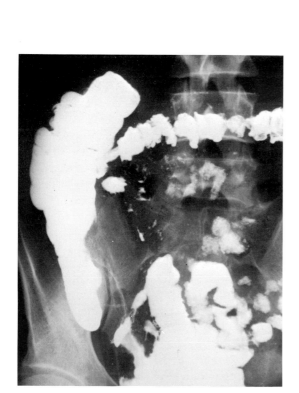

Fig. 32-21. String sign in regional enteritis.

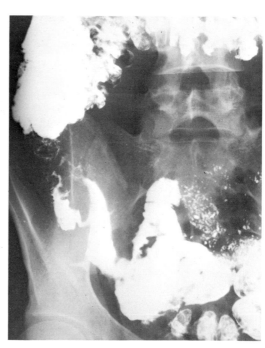

Fig. 32-22. Same patient as in Fig. 32-21 a few moments later. There is more distensibility of the distal ileum. The findings in the ileum are caused by pronounced ulceration and secondary spasm. Several intramural sinus tracts and fistulas extending from the distal ileum into the narrowed cecum are noted. The proximal bowel is not dilated.

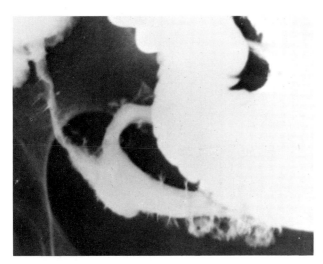

Fig. 32-23. Regional enteritis. Numerous fistulas extend from the terminal ileum into the mesentery.

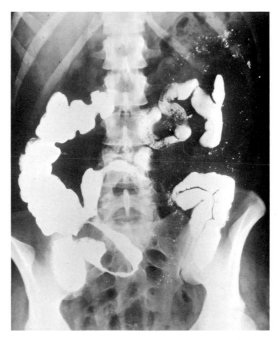

Fig. 32-24. Regional enteritis. There is a fistulous communication extending from the terminal ileum into the medial aspect of the ascending colon.

the proximal intestinal lumen is generally not dilated, despite the narrowing associated with the string sign, which indicates the importance of spasm in producing this characteristic appearance. This spasm is usually inconstant. When the spasm is persistent, however, temporary proximal dilatation may occur with symptoms of obstruction. In the stenotic phase there is constant proximal dilatation that may be accentuated by spasm secondary to ulceration. Despite the narrowing, complete intestinal obstruction is rare. Recognizing that the string sign does not always indicate significant fibrosis and stenosis is important, since operations during the stage of ulceration and activity are often followed by a high degree of recurrence.

Fistulas and perforation (Figs. 32-23 and 32-24), thickening of the mesentery, and separation of the loops of bowel are more frequent in the distal ileum than in the remainder of the small bowel because of the ulceration. A possible explanation of extensive ulceration in the distal ileum may be the higher bacterial content in this area.

Deformities of the cecum and ascending colon are not unusual with involvement of the terminal ileum. This may vary from a gentle concavity in the mesial aspect of the cecum at the ileocecal region (Figs. 32-21 and 32-22) to pronounced narrowing of the cecum. This is an important sign, particularly if at the time of the first examination by barium enema the terminal ileum cannot be filled with barium because of undue spasm and irritability. The presence of this sign is strongly suggestive of regional enteritis, and reexamination for filling of the terminal ileum is important. This deformity of the mesial aspect of the cecocolic region is most often the result of the pressure on the colon from the thickened terminal ileum with its inflamed mesentery and from the heavy pad of mesenteric fat. In some cases it is caused by fistulas or intramural sinus tracts arising from the terminal ileum and extending into the right side of the colon.

Jejunoileitis

Characteristically, the distal half of jejunum and proximal half of ileum are involved in jejunoileitis (Figs. 32-16 and 32-17).[9] Skip areas are frequent and large inflammatory polyps may be noted. Ulceration is not as marked as in the terminal ileum, and fistula formation is less frequent. Because of the extent of involvement, operative intervention until recently has been rare, and long follow-up of the natural course of the disease has been possible. The transition from the nonstenotic to the stenotic stage can be observed, and in the average case the interval varies from 4 to 16 years (Figs. 32-1 and 32-2).

It is of interest that many of these patients with such extensive involvement of the intestinal tract, despite numerous episodes of partial intestinal obstruction, can maintain an adequate nutritional status. This is observed most often in patients without fistulas.

Jejunitis

Regional jejunitis is that variety of regional enteritis in which the initial manifestations are mainly or exclusively in the jejunum. The roentgenographic pattern of regional jejunitis differs somewhat from that of disease localized in the ileum. The most common site of granulomatous involvement is the distal portion of the ileum, and the frequency of involvement progressively diminishes in the more proximal and distal portions of the gastrointestinal tract. Practically all patients we have seen with jejunitis appeared to have long-standing disease. However, early cases of jejunitis are being recognized with increasing frequency. Most of these proceed to the more chronic form. On the other hand, there have been reports of isolated instances of acute regional jejunitis that have healed completely without sequelae. In these instances, the diagnosis has arisen from observations made during a laparotomy, not necessarily with pathologic or roentgenographic confirmation.

Roentgenographically, the prestenotic phase of the disease has been demonstrated on a number of occasions and is similar to the changes previously described. Some of these cases have been followed up until the actual development of stenosis. However, since none of the patients we have seen have been operated upon in the prestenotic period we have not observed the pathologic signs of that phase. It would seem that this stage of the disease would be encountered when log segments of jejunum are resected because of involvement in multiple areas. However, our experience has revealed that such resected specimens show all the involved areas to be in the cicatrizing stenotic phase. This observation suggests that the disease appears in different segments at approximately the same time and progresses in them at the same rate.

In distal ileitis the roentgenographic picture

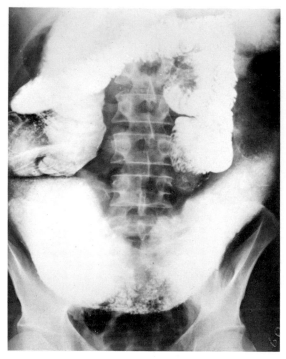

Fig. 32-25. Stenotic regional enteritis. There is undue dilatation of the midjejunal loops and a considerable amount of secretions. The stenotic segments are obscured by the dilated loops of bowel.

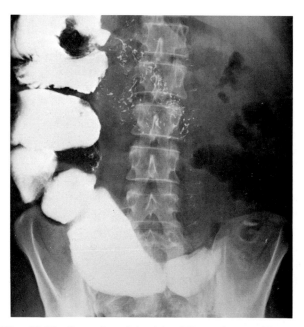

Fig. 32-26. Stenosing jejunitis. There is considerable dilatation of the jejunal loops. Multiple dilated sacs are identified obscuring the stenotic segments. Additional stenotic segments in the distal jejunum were visualized on later films.

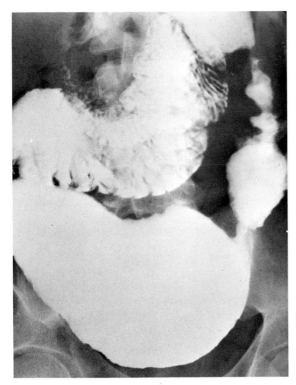

Fig. 32-27. Stenosing jejunitis. There is an immensely dilated loop of jejunum between two short strictured segments. Additional narrowed segments are also identified.

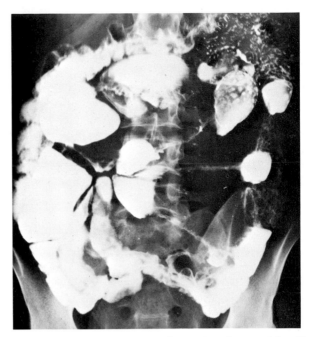

Fig. 32-28. Recurrent stenotic regional enteritis. Six years after surgery for a localized jejunitis, multiple stenotic segments alternating with areas of dilatation developed.

is dominated by the appearance of diseased segments of bowel per se. In regional jejunitis, on the other hand, the sequelae of the diseased stenotic segments, that is, the dilated, chronically obstructed loops, are the striking findings (Figs. 32-25 and 32-26). The retention of food and secretions, and the inflammatory reaction that frequently develops in these chronically obstructed loops, produce roentgenographic features that are characteristic of prolonged obstruction. It is often impossible in this situation to determine roentgenologically whether there is intrinsic involvement or whether changes are produced by the long-standing obstruction. The diameter of the doubly obstructed loops may attain the proportions of a significantly distended colon (Fig. 32-27).

In most instances, the stenotic segments are easily visualized (Fig. 32-28). However, when numerous overlapping and dilated intestinal loops are present, a single short stricture may be difficult to delineate (Fig. 32-29).

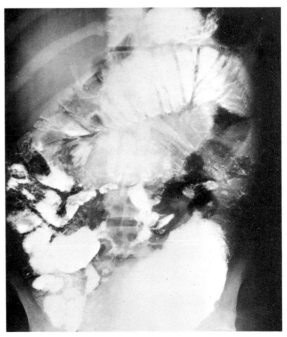

Fig. 32-29. Stenotic regional enteritis. Immensely dilated loops of small bowel in a patient with extensive regional enteritis are shown.

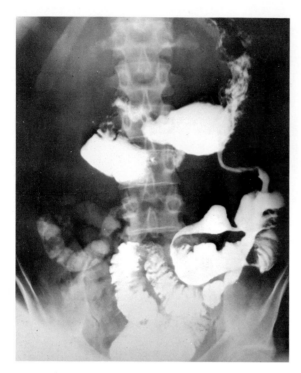

Fig. 32-30. Stenosing jejunitis. Starting at the ligament of Treitz, alternating areas of constriction and dilatation of the proximal jejunum are seen. The duodenum is dilated. There is rigidity and narrowing of the bowel loops with effacement of the mucosal folds.

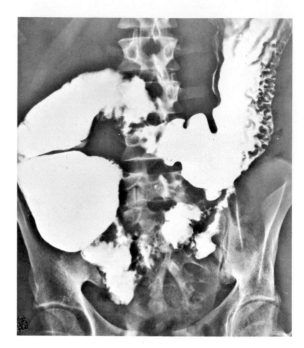

Fig. 32-31. Stenosing jejunitis. There is marked dilatation of the second and third portions of the duodenum caused by stenosing jejunitis of the proximal jejunum.

Although the stenotic segments indicate a considerable degree of fibrosis, the narrowing may be further enhanced by superimposed edema and spasm resulting from the inflammation. The contours of the narrowed segments generally are smooth. The lumen is concentrically located. The mucosa may be castlike or may reveal numerous pseudopolyps and ulcerations. The stenotic segments are rigid. They may be single or multiple and may vary in length (Fig. 32-30). If there is only a single area of constriction, a more or less uniform dilatation of the proximal bowel may be seen. The presence of skip lesions may result in a "hammock type" or "sausage-link" type of deformity. When obstruction occurs near the fossa of Treitz, duodenal and even gastric dilatation may be evident (Fig. 32-31). Ulceration, perforation, and their sequelae are much less common in regional jejunitis than in ileitis.

Duodenitis

Duodenitis is uncommon, but the roentgenographic findings are similar to those seen in the jejunum. Moderate stenosis is present and ulceration is difficult to identify. Most patients have involvement of other portions of the small bowel. The diagnosis of duodenitis should be made with circumspection, because spasm and irritability of the doudenum in patients with extensive ileojejunitis is not uncommon. Some cases reported in the literature are without any or with only meager pathologic confirmation. A diagnosis of regional enteritis of the duodenum when there is no involvement of other segments of the small bowel is extremely difficult. It should be considered in the differential diagnosis of stenotic lesions in this region if there is no destruction of the mucosa (Fig. 32-32).

Gastritis

Gastric involvement with granulomatous disease is uncommon. Usually in granulomatous gastritis the antrum of the stomach is involved there is a narrow lesion with fairly smooth margins and no evidence of discrete ulceration. The finding of a solitary ulcer militates against the

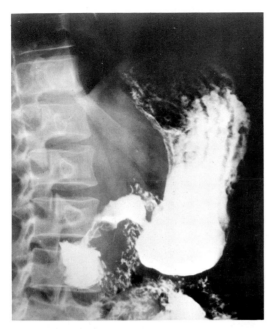

Fig. 32-32. Regional enteritis involving the second portion of the duodenum. Other loops of the small bowel are also involved.

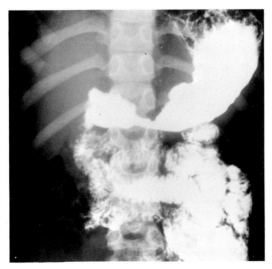

Fig. 32-33. Regional enteritis involving the stomach. The distal loops of ileum are also involved.

diagnosis of granulomatous gastritis. When there is no involvement of other portions of the gastrointestinal tract, the diagnosis of granulomatous disease of the stomach is difficult. Granulomatous gastritis apparently unrelated to regional enteritis also occurs and usually involves the entire stomach rather than the antrum alone.[11]

Granulomatous disease of the esophagus has rarely been observed.

RECURRENT REGIONAL ENTERITIS

Following operation for regional enteritis, recurrence of the disease is common. It recurs most frequently during the first 2 years after the operation, but many years may elapse before new involvement is seen. Many patients with early recurrent lesions may be asymptomatic for long periods of time. Recurrences appear more frequently in those patients in whom the original disease is most active, and sinus tracts and fistulas are found. If operation is performed in the more chronic and stenotic phase of the disease and in the absence of fistulas, the recurrence rate is less.

In general, the recurrent lesions are similar to the original process. The earliest roentgenographic findings are thickening and blunting of the folds progressing through the nonstenotic to the stenotic phase. Fistula formation appears less frequently. The length of the original lesion has no effect on the recurrence rate. A remarkable feature of regional enteritis is that the recurrences are almost always at the site of the new terminal ileum (Figs. 32-34 and 32-35). Extension into the colon has also been seen (Figs. 32-36 and 32-37).

Healing in regional enteritis

Roentgenologic demonstrations of improvement in regional enteritis without operation are rare. However, cases have been observed where remarkable changes indicating healing have occurred (Figs. 32-38 and 32-39). Despite these instances of improvement, the large majority of cases demonstrate the disease to be continuous (Figs. 32-1 and 32-2). Many years may elapse, however, before stenosis supervenes. It should be pointed out that, in patients who are clinically improved, secondary changes may occur, notably stenosing lesions and permanent loss of the normal small-bowel structure. These changes are caused by healing with scar formation.

Regional enteritis in children

The roentgenographic findings of regional enteritis in children are essentially the same as those described for adults (Figs. 32-20 and 32-40). Of twenty-eight cases of regional enteritis studied in children ranging in age from 2 to 15

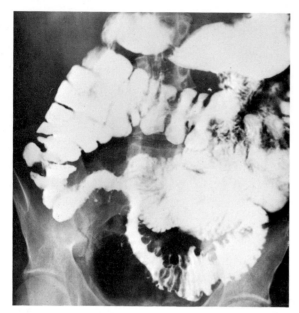

Fig. 32-34. Recurrent regional enteritis. This patient had two resections of the terminal ileum with an anastomosis of the new terminal ileum to the ascending colon. Following each resection there was a recurrence of the disease. This roentgenogram of the third recurrence reveals the characteristic involvement of the small bowel adjacent to the stoma.

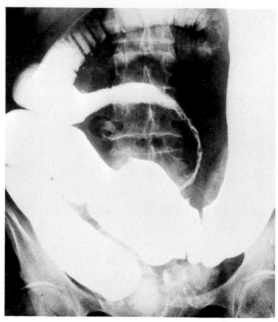

Fig. 32-35. Recurrent regional enteritis following an ileosigmoidostomy. Recurrent disease adjacent to the stoma is identified.

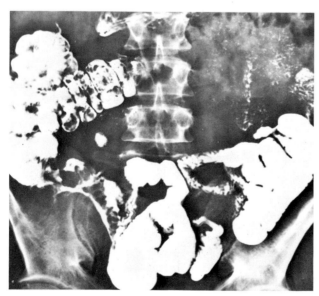

Fig. 32-36. Regional enteritis. The inflammatory process involves the terminal ileum, with multiple sinus tracts into the mesentery.

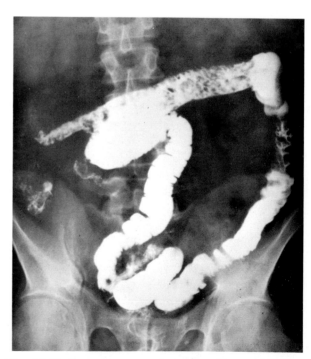

Fig. 32-37. Recurrent granulomatous disease. Same patient as in Fig. 32-36. Six months after ileotransverse colostomy and resection of the involved ileum there is a recurrence of the inflammatory process in the transverse colon (recurrent granulomatous disease).

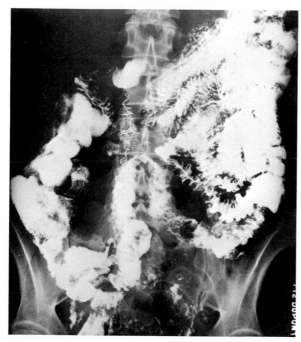

Fig. 32-38. Regional enteritis. The distal jejunum and entire ileum are involved with an inflammatory process, characterized by acute spasm, irritability, narrowing, rigidity, thickening of the folds, and ulceration of the mucosa.

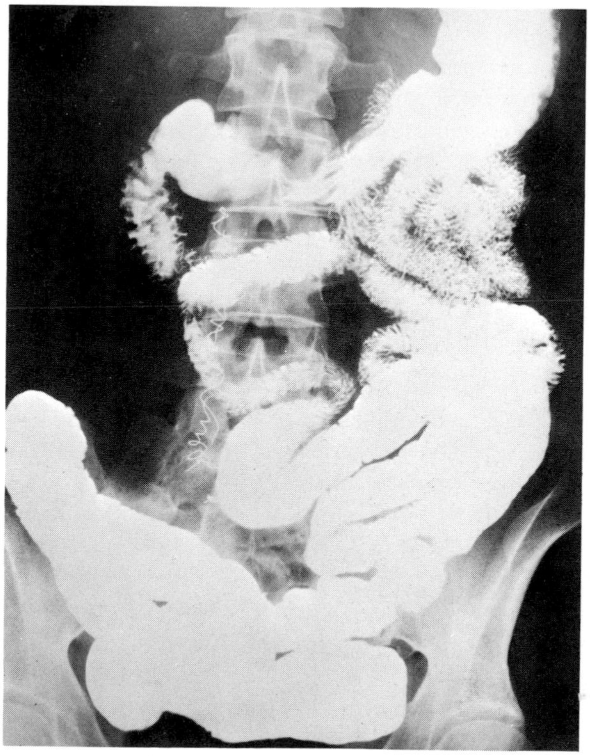

Fig. 32-39. Regional enteritis. Same patient as in Fig. 32-38 2 years later. There is significant improvement in the appearance of the small bowel. However, there is a minimal area of narrowing in the ileum that is obscured by the overlying loops of bowel in this region. The healing in this case is unusual and remarkable.

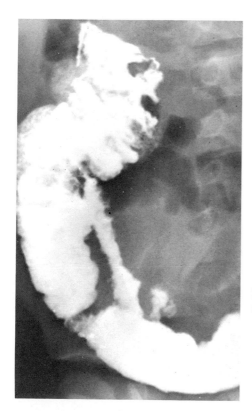

Fig. 32-40. Typical regional enteritis in a 2-year-old infant.

years, the distal ileum was involved in twenty, the jejunoileum in four, and four were examples of ileocolitis. Twenty-three of the twenty-eight cases were of the nonstenotic variety, reflecting the relatively short duration of the disease, which had not been present long enough for stenosis to develop. In five of the twenty-eight cases, fistulas of the distal ileum were observed. None of the children with involvement of the proxical ileum and the jejunum showed roentgenologic evidence of fistula formation.

In recent years there has been an increasing number of reports of so-called acute ileitis occurring in children.[10] The condition is clinically indistinguishable from acute appendicitis. At operation the terminal ileum is found to be congested, thickened, and possibly rigid, and in most cases there is an associated mesenteric adenitis. The majority of such patients recover spontaneously, and there is no progression to the chronic stage. The condition is considered by some clinicians to be a distinct nonrecurring, nonsclerosing form of acute ileitis, which is essentially unrelated to chronic cicatrizing granulomatous enteritis. A number of such cases, however, apparently develop into regional enteritis, and a clear distinction between the two forms of the acute disease has not been satisfactorily established in the current literature. The roentgenographic findings in so-called acute ileitis are similar to the early changes of regional enteritis and consist of slight spiculation of the contours of the bowel with minimal thickening and irregularity of the mucosal folds. The roentgenographic alterations in the few cases of acute ileitis that were studied did not persist and disappeared in a few weeks (Fig. 32-41).

Carcinoma with regional enteritis

Primary carcinoma of the small bowel is an uncommon lesion. In recent years a number of cases of adenocarcinoma of the small bowel have been reported in association with long-standing regional enteritis or in surgically excluded loops.[1] The diagnosis is very difficult to establish preoperatively because the presence of multiple strictures with intervening segments of dilated bowel obscures the associated malignancy on small-bowel examination (Fig. 32-42) and the clinical features of the carcinoma mimic those of the obstructing inflammatory disease.

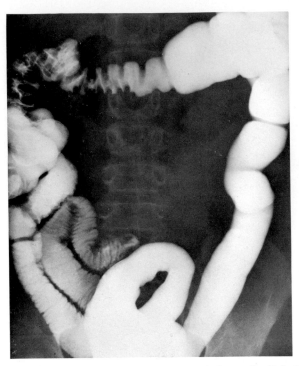

Fig. 32-41. Acute ileitis. The terminal ileum is slightly dilated, with a moderate irregularity of the contour. There is thickening of the folds and increased secretions. The alterations in the terminal ileum completely disappeared in 1 month. The relationship of this entity to regional enteritis has not been established.

LYMPHOID HYPERPLASIA

The normal terminal ileum in children contains sufficient lymphoid tissue to produce small filling defects within the lumen. These are usually symmetric and fairly sharply demarcated, with no evidence of an inflammatory process. This appears to be a normal finding in adolescents, since follow-up examinations have invariably shown the disappearance of these small defects (Fig. 32-43).

Diffuse nodular lymphoid hyperplasia occurs throughout the small intestine, the colon, or both. The process should be considered pathologic when it extends beyond the confines of the terminal ileum. A number of patients with nodular lymphoid hyperplasia have been found to have an associated dysgammaglobulinemia.[5] The absence of inflammatory changes permits differentiation from regional enteritis.

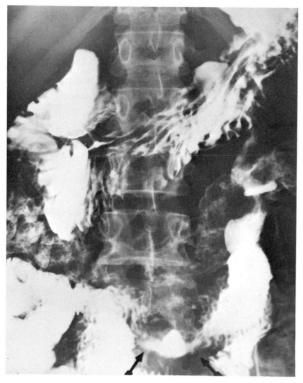

Fig. 32-42. Regional enteritis with an associated carcinoma. There are alternating areas of narrowing and dilatation involving the jejunum. An associated carcinoma of the jejunum indicated by the arrow can be seen. This was not diagnosed prior to surgery.

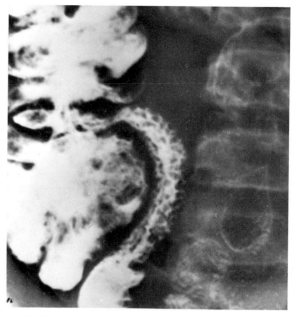

Fig. 32-43. Numerous small, fairly sharply demarcated radiolucent filling defects in an asymptomatic young woman. This is a normal finding and is presumably secondary to lymphoid tissue.

DIFFERENTIAL DIAGNOSIS

In most instances the roentgenographic alterations in regional enteritis are sufficiently characteristic that differential diagnosis is not difficult. The following diseases may, on occasion, simulate the roentgenographic findings previously described.

Lymphosarcoma can simulate the nonstenotic phase of regional enteritis. Thickening and blunting of the folds, irregularity of the contour, ulceration, and intraluminal nodules and fistulas are features that are common to both diseases (Fig. 32-44 to 32-46). In regional enteritis there is more inflammation, producing spasm and narrowing of the bowel lumen. Irregular nodules that can be identified as tumors are an uncommon feature of regional enteritis but are a frequent finding in lymphosarcoma. Although, owing to tumor encroachment, narrowing of the bowel lumen can be seen in lymphosarcoma, as a rule the bowel is of normal caliber or slightly dilated. Ulcerations in lymphosarcoma are usually discrete or multiple and do not have the linear configuration seen in regional enteritis. Separation of the loops of bowel in regional enteritis is more pronounced than in lymphosarcoma.

Hodgkin's disease can produce all the roentgenographic alterations described in lymphosarcoma. In addition, however, marked fibrosis of the bowel can be seen with constriction of the lumen (Fig. 32-47). The features that distinguish this disease from a single stenotic lesion of regional enteritis are the eccentric lumen, the presence of a tumor nodule, and the absence of chronic intestinal obstruction. In regional enteritis, multiple areas of stenosis are more frequent, and the proximal dilated loops of bowel are usually longer, with evidence of considerable secretion and chronic obstruction.

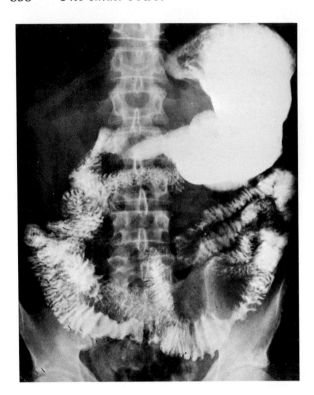

Fig. 32-44. Lymphosarcoma of the jejunum simulating regional enteritis. The recognition of nodular defects along the contours helps in differentiating the two lesions. However, this is not always possible.

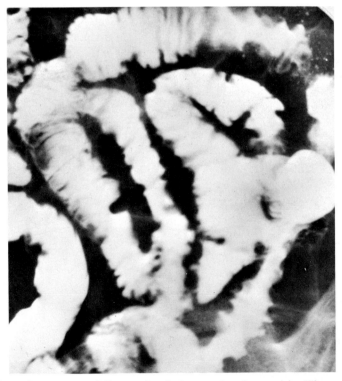

Fig. 32-45. Lymphosarcoma of ileum simulating regional enteritis. There is thickening of the folds, narrowing of the bowel lumen, slight separation of the loops of bowel, and small tumor nodules. Differentiation from regional enteritis in this case depends on the detection of the small tumor nodules.

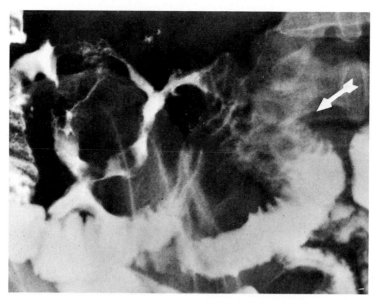

Fig. 32-46. Endo-exoenteric lymphosarcoma of the distal ileum. The normal bowel lumen is replaced by many intercommunicating tortuous tracts through the tumor. The arrow points to the nodular mucosal pattern proximal to the mass. The lumen in this segment is not narrowed. A mass developed in the neck of this patient and on biopsy was diagnosed as lymphosarcoma.

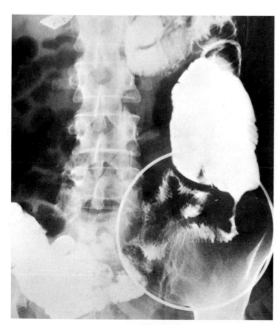

Fig. 32-47. Hodgkin's disease of the jejunum. There is a narrowed rigid segment producing obstruction to the barium column and proximal dilatation. The contours are slightly scalloped, and no overhanging margins are seen. The lumen is eccentric, with a gradual transition between normal and abnormal bowel. A single stenotic segment in regional enteritis occurs but is unusual.

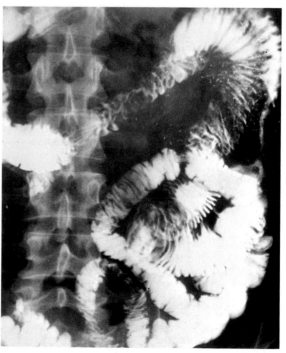

Fig. 32-48. Segmental infarction of the jejunum. There is a segment of stenosis with smooth contours in the proximal jejunum. Earlier films (taken 4 weeks previously) on this patient revealed ulceration of the mucosa and a normal lumen. The rapid progression to stenosis is more characteristic of infarction than of regional enteritis.

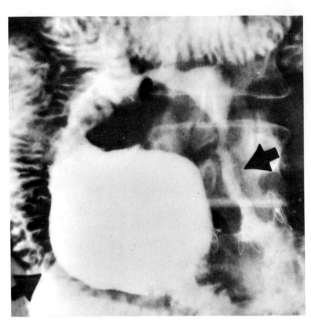

Fig. 32-49. Infarction of the small bowel secondary to a strangulating incisional hernia. Again note the resemblance to regional enteritis.

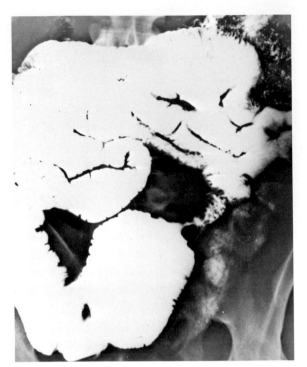

Fig. 32-50. Tuberculosis of the small intestine. Note the resemblance to Fig. 32-47. A single diagnosis in this type of case is impossible.

Segmental infarction of the small intestine may show fairly rapid progressive changes leading to stricture formation. An individual segment may completely mimic a stenotic segment in regional enteritis, but again the evidence of chronic proximal intestinal obstruction is less pronounced and the patient's history is usually characteristic (Figs. 32-48 and 32-49).

Carcinoma of the intestine produces lesions that are usually short with an eccentric rigid lumen. The mucosa shows destruction and occasionally ulceration. Proximal dilatation and overhanging edges are frequent roentgenographic findings.

Malabsorption syndromes and regional enteritis may show similar clinical features, but the roentgenographic features are quite different. In the spruelike states there is no stenosis. Evidence of an inflammatory process is either minimal or completely absent. Dilatation, segmentation, and increased secretions are the prominent roentgenographic features in the spruelike states.

Tuberculosis can completely mimic the find-ings associated with regional enteritis. With tuberculosis, however, there is generally greater involvement of the colon than of the terminal ileum. The lesion has a tendency to be associated with more irregular contours, and the mucosal markings are coarser than in regional enteritis. This results from the large irregular ulcerations frequently seen in tuberculosis. When tuberculosis of the small intestine is not associated with involvement of the lungs, the problem of differential diagnosis may be extremely difficult (Fig. 32-50).

Amebiasis involving the small bowel has been observed rarely in the United States. A cone-shaped appearance of the cecum is frequently mentioned as a pathognomonic feature of ameboma, but we have seen this configuration much more often with regional enteritis, appendicitis, and ulcerative colitis.

Carcinoid tumors may involve long segments of the small bowel with muscle hypertrophy and fibrosis. These changes resemble those of regional enteritis. Usually tumor nodules can be identified and permit differentiation from in-

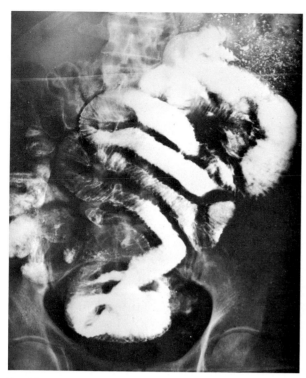

Fig. 32-51. Radiation ileitis. Following irradiation, various degrees of necrosis of the small bowel may occur, producing changes that are indistinguishable from regional enteritis.

flammatory disease, but sometimes the distinction cannot be made roentgenologically and the tumor is an unexpected finding at laparotomy or in the pathology laboratory.

Radiation ileitis may occur following irradiation treatment. Various degrees of necrosis of the small intestine may occur, producing changes of that area that are indistinguishable from regional enteritis (Fig. 32-51).

REFERENCES

1. Ben-Asher, H.: Adenocarcinoma of the ileum complicating regional enteritis, Amer. J. Gastroent. **55:** 391, 1971.
2. Crohn, B. B., Ginzburg, L., and Oppenheimer, G. D.: Regional ileitis, J.A.M.A. **99:**1323, 1932.
3. Crohn, B. B., and Yarnis, H.: Regional ileitis, ed. 2, New York, 1958, Grune & Stratton, Inc.
4. Hadfield, G.: Primary histological lesion of regional ileitis, Lancet **2:**773, 1939.
5. Hermans, P. E., Huizenga, K. A., Hoffman, H. N., Brown, A. L., and Markowitz, H.: Dysgammaglobulinemia associated with nodular lymphoid hyperplasia of the small intestine, Amer. J. Med. **40:**78, 1966.
6. Jones Williams, W.: Histology of Crohn's syndrome, Gut 5:510, 1964.
7. Leading article: Etiology of Crohn's disease, Lancet 2:193, 1970.
8. Marshak, R. H., and Wolf, B. S.: Roentgen findings in regional enteritis, Amer. J. Roentgen. **74:**1000, 1955.
9. Marshak, R. H., and Wolf, B. S.: Chronic ulcerative granulomatous jejunitis and ileojejunitis, Amer. J. Roentgen. **70:**93, 1953.
10. Moseley, J. E., Marshak, R. H., and Wolf, B. S.: Regional enteritis in children, Amer. J. Roentgen. **84:**532, 1960.
11. Present, D. H., Lindner, A. E., and Janowitz, H. D.: Granulomatous diseases of the intestinal tract, Ann. Rev. Med. 17:243, 1966.
12. Van Patter, W. N., Bargan, J. A., Dockerty, M. B., Feldman, W. H., Mayo, C. W., and Waugh, J. M.: Regional enteritis, Gastroenterology **26:**347, 1954.
13. Warren, S., and Sommers, S. C.: Cicatrizing enteritis (regional ileitis) as a pathologic entity, Amer. J. Path. 24:475, 1948.

33 | Malabsorption

Richard H. Marshak
Arthur E. Lindner

The term "malabsorption refers to the defective absorption from the small intestine of the main foodstuffs—carbohydrate, protein, and fat. Often this defect results in the so-called malabsorption syndrome, which is characterized by steatorrhea, the passage of stools that are bulky, fatty, and foul smelling. In addition, as part of the malabsorption syndrome there may occur such clinical features as diarrhea, weight loss, abdominal distention, skin pigmentation, retarded growth and development, and various nutritional deficiency states, including lack of folic acid, vitamin B[12] and other B-complex vitamins, vitamin K, iron, calcium, or magnesium.

Before discussing in detail diseases associated with the malabsorption syndrome, we will consider briefly the mechanisms and processes involved in normal absorption.

PHYSIOLOGY OF ABSORPTION

The small intestine is remarkably adapted to its function of absorption by means of several features that serve to increase the surface area of its mucosa. There are the mucosal folds, or valvulae conniventes; the villi, finger-like mucosal processes about a millimeter in length that project into the lumen; and the microvilli, structures similar to the villi, but about a micron in length and visible only through an electron microscope, which form the luminal border of the columnar absorbing cell. Wilson has estimated that these features may increase the small bowel surface area for absorption to some six hundred times what it would be if the small bowel were a simple tube.[29]

The villi are lined by columnar absorbing cells and mucus-producing goblet cells and contain smooth muscle fibers, blood capillaries, and lymphocytes. Substances absorbed through the villi by way of the blood capillaries ultimately enter the portal vein; those absorbed by way of the lymph vessels enter the thoracic duct. Between the bases of the villi are the glandlike crypts of Lieberkühn from which the cells lining the villi are generated. Radioautographic studies have demonstrated that intestinal epithelial cells originate in the crypts of Lieberkühn and, as sheets of cells, migrate upward along each villus to its apex where they are extruded into the lumen. The intestinal epithelium is completely renewed within 2 or 3 days. As the epithelial cells move upward, they become more differentiated for absorptive functions. These functions are at their peak at the tip of the villus where the most mature cells are located just prior to their extrusion.[17]

At least four processes of general physiology—passive diffusion, active transport, facilitated diffusion, and pinocytosis—are thought to be involved in absorption from the small intestine. *Passive diffusion* is the movement of a substance across a membrane in accordance with a concentration gradient and in electrical charge. *Active transport* is the movement of a substance across a membrane against an electrochemical gradient. Such a process requires energy, which is supplied by cellular metabolism. *Facilitated diffusion* is the movement of a substance across a membrane without direct expenditure of energy but at a rate greater than would be expected by simple diffusion. A carrier mechanism has been postulated to account for this phenomenon. Unlike active transport, facilitated diffusion is not against a concentration gradient. *Pinocytosis* is the process of engulfing particles or materials by vesiculation, as happens in the ameba. Fat droplets, for example, have appeared to invaginate the cell membrane and become pinched off to enter the cell.

Carbohydrates are broken down into the monosaccharides glucose, galactose, and fructose by intestinal enzymes. These monosaccharides are absorbed, largely in the proximal jejunum, by mechanisms of active transport. Protein is hydrolyzed to amino acids that are also absorbed largely in the proximal jejunum by active transport. Fats are hydrolyzed by action of pancreatic lipase and bile salts; most fat is absorbed in the upper jejunum also. There is controversy whether fat droplets may enter the absorbing cell by pinocytosis or by diffusion through the lipid membrane of the cell. Fatty acids, glycerol, and some monoglycerides and diglycerides are believed to be the end products absorbed after the hydrolysis of fats. Normally almost all the dietary fat is absorbed; about 5 gm. of fat is excreted in the stool each day, but this is derived largely from bacterial bodies and desquamated intestinal cells. In man most fluid and electrolytes are absorbed from the jejunum. Relatively little net fluid absorption occurs in the duodenum where the intestinal contents are made isotonic.

DISEASES ASSOCIATED WITH MALABSORPTION
Sprue

The name "sprue" is given to a group of three diseases of the small bowel, which have a close clinical relationship. This group comprises celiac disease of children, nontropical sprue or idiopathic steatorrhea of adults, and tropical sprue. All available evidence now indicates that celiac disease and nontropical sprue are the same entity, occurring at different times of life. Whether tropical sprue is a distinct disease or a variant of nontropical sprue is not yet established.

All three members of the sprue group demonstrate similar lesions upon small-bowel biopsy. There is flattening, broadening, coalescence, and sometimes complete loss of villi. The crypts of Lieberkühn become elongated, so that the overall thickness of the mucosa may not be much different from the normal thickness. The lamina propria is infiltrated with lymphocytes, plasma cells, and occasionally eosinophils. The epithelial cells of the villi are flattened and cuboidal,

and the nuclei of these cells, instead of maintaining a regular basal orientation, appear at irregular levels. These mucosal abnormalities associated with sprue tend to be more pronounced in the jejunum than in the ileum. Histochemical evidence suggests that when sprue is present, the tip of the villus, physiologically the most active site of absorption, is not formed but instead is replaced by an abnormal epithelium that has both morphologic and chemical defects.[17] Patients with sprue present the classic clinical expressions of malabsorption, which were mentioned previously.

Celiac disease and nontropical sprue have in common a peculiar relationship to diet—a feature that distinguishes them from tropical sprue. In 1950 in Holland, Dicke demonstrated that in children with celiac disease, removal of wheat from the diet caused the signs and symptoms of the disease to disappear and that reintroduction of wheat caused their recurrence.[5] Subsequently the list of offending cereals was extended to include wheat, rye, oats, and barley, and it was shown that a rigorous diet avoiding these grains brought dramatic remissions to children with celiac disease and to adults with nontropical sprue.

The toxicity of the cereal grains to the sprue patient lies in the water-insoluble protein fraction of the grain, which is called gluten, but the specific cause of the toxicity of gluten remains elusive.[2] It has been suggested that patients with sprue may, as an inborn or acquired error of metabolism, lack an enzyme in the small-bowel mucosa that can inactivate the deleterious agent in gluten.

The nature of the relationship between gluten and the intestinal lesion is obscure. The lesion may improve or disappear within 3 months to a year in young patients with celiac disease who are on a gluten-free diet. In adults some improvement as a result of diet may be noted but in the great majority of cases the lesion persists. The fact that complete clinical remission may occur, although the small-bowel mucosal lesion persists without change, suggests that the morphologic changes are a secondary effect rather than the cause of sprue. Moreover, the severity of the histologic lesion does not correlate with the clinical state or with the degree of absorptive impairment.

When a patient on a gluten-free diet is in

clinical remission, reintroduction of gluten into the diet will increase the fecal fat excretion to abnormal levels and cause a clinical exacerbation. The time that it takes for this change to occur varies from several days to several weeks.

Tropical sprue is probably distinct from non-tropical sprue and celiac disease, although the clinical manifestations of all three are similar and the intestinal mucosal lesions appear to be the same. The principal differences seem to lie in their responses to clinical treatment. Tropical sprue often responds dramatically to folic acid or antibiotic therapy, or both, while celiac disease and nontropical sprue do not. (Severe deficiency of folic acid and of vitamin B_{12} occurs frequently in tropical sprue but is uncommon in nontropical sprue.) On the other hand, celiac disease and nontropical sprue usually respond to a gluten-free diet, which is ineffective in the treatment of tropical sprue. Nontropical sprue appears to be widespread in its geographic incidence, but tropical sprue is remarkably localized. It occurs, for example, in India and the Far East but not in Africa; it is common in Puerto Rico but not in Jamaica.

Although folic acid rapidly improves the clinical status in tropical sprue, it fails to improve intestinal function or heal the mucosal lesion so quickly. In one study about half the patients with the disease eventually recovered from the initial episode with healing of the mucosal lesion and return of biochemical tests to normal. Those who failed to enter a full remission remained relatively asymptomatic but showed persistent biochemical and histologic evidence of disease.[22]

The sprue pattern

The roentgenographic findings to be described in tropical sprue, celiac disease, and nontropical sprue are identical. They are present in virtually all patients in the active phase of these diseases, and in addition may be found in many patients suffering from other diseases associated with malabsorption. This is the reason for the use of the term "sprue pattern" later in the text to refer to roentgenographic findings in these other diseases.

Inflammatory changes are not seen in sprue. However, practically every patient with sprue exhibits in the small intestine changes in the form of varying degrees of dilatation and hyper-

secretion, and of segmentation, fragmentation, and scattering of the barium column.[11,15] Thickening or thinning of the fold pattern of the small intestine, which depends on the degree of dilatation and the amount of secretion, may also be present. In clinical remissions, the roentgenographic findings, corresponding to severity of the small bowel lesion, may show improvement toward normal or may not change.

Dilatation. Dilatation of the lumen of the small intestine is one of the most important and constant findings in sprue. Some of the individual features of the sprue pattern are seen in other disorders, but in none is dilatation more striking or constant than it is in sprue (Figs. 33-1 to 33-4). The exact cause of dilatation remains unknown. At autopsy, the only gross finding may be a thinning of the small-bowel wall. Whether this is the cause of the dilatation or its sequela has been subject to speculation.

Dilatation is the most frequent of the roentgenographic findings in sprue. It is usually best visualized in the mid- and distal jejunum. Dilatation is not as common in the distal ileum as it is elsewhere in the small intestine, but it may occur diffusely throughout the small intestine. The large intestine may also show dilatation. The dilated intestinal loops are generally long and tortuous and have pliable walls. The degree of dilatation is exceedingly variable; often a single intestinal segment may manifest varying degrees of dilatation during the course of a single roentgenographic study. In general, dilatation appears to be related to the severity of the disease and is most pronounced in advanced cases of sprue.

Fluoroscopic observations of the altered contractility of the dilated small-bowel loop are of some interest. In many patients the barium column flows more freely than usual through the dilated intestinal loops, apparently unhindered by the tone of the contracted segment that is normally found ahead of it. When secretions are encountered, progress is slowed and the barium column becomes segmented. In other patients with severe dilatation, there is prolonged transit time, which appears to be the result of ineffective peristaltic activity. These fluoroscopic findings suggest that in sprue the tonicity of the small intestine is altered, offering little resistance to dilatation by ingested substances, possibly even by secretions, and that,

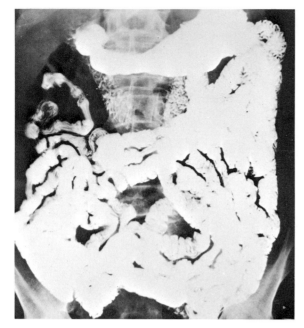

Fig. 33-1. Normal small bowel. A half hour after the ingestion of barium the column has reached the mid-ileum. Ingestion of a large quantity of barium permits demonstration of a continuous column and the study of the relationship of one intestinal loop to the other.

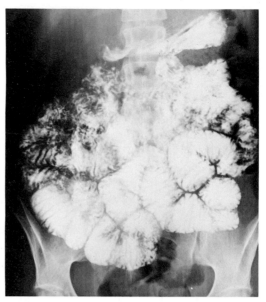

Fig. 33-2. Sprue. There is moderate dilatation of the mid and distal jejunum, and the intestinal loops are pliable and flaccid.

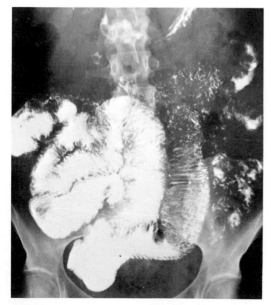

Fig. 33-3. Sprue. There is moderate dilatation of the entire jejunum, associated with thinning of the valvulae conniventes, minimal fragmentation, and increased secretions. Minimal intussusception, which has occurred here in the distal jejunum, is frequently seen in sprue.

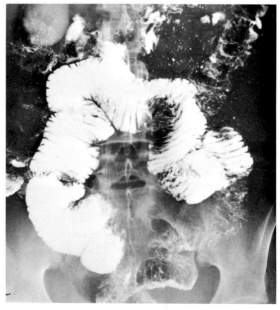

Fig. 33-4. Sprue. There is considerable dilatation of the midjejunum, associated with thinning of the valvulae conniventes, and the intestinal loops are again flaccid. Thinning of the valvulae is probably a mechanical phenomenon related to the dilatation of the bowel.

once dilated, peristalsis becomes disordered and ineffective. Secretions in themselves, however, do not appear to be a factor in the production of dilatation. Dilatation is generally greatest in the jejunum where secretions are minimal, and least pronounced in the ileum, where excessive secretions are most often found. In severe cases of sprue with extensive prolonged small-bowel dilatation and subsequent ineffective peristalsis, decompensation of the bowel wall may occur.

Intussusceptions may be demonstrated in sprue (Fig. 33-3). They are characteristically nonobstructive, with a typical coiled-spring appearance, and they usually are transient and extend over a short distance.[20]

Hypersecretion. An excessive amount of fluid in the intestinal tract is a constant phenomenon in most patients manifesting sprue symptoms and especially in those whose roentgenograms show marked segmentation of barium within the small intestine.[1,6] Such fluid is as likely to represent a defect in absorption of water by the deranged mucosa as it is to represent the excessive movement of water into the lumen, but the common roentgenologic term for the phenomenon is "hypersecretion." As a result of hypersecretion air-fluid levels may occasionally be seen in the small intestine during the course of a contrast study. In addition, instead of the homogenous appearance that indicates the normal small intestine, the barium has a coarse granular appearance, with areas of flocculation dispersed irregularly in the intestinal loops. Flocculation is best visualized at the periphery of the intestinal segment.

Segmentation. We restrict the term "segmentation" to refer to those masses of barium that are moderately large, definitely separated from adjacent clumps, usually in dilated segments that contain excessive secretions. The small, contracted, barium-filled segments of small intestine that are connected by strands of barium and seen in association with spasm are not included in this definition.

Segmentation, most pronounced in the ileum and best seen in more advanced cases of sprue, occurs in two forms—immediate, and delayed. The more common form is delayed segmentation, that is, segmentation that occurs in those intestinal segments that are in the process of evacuation. The less common immediate segmentation is noted as soon as barium enters the

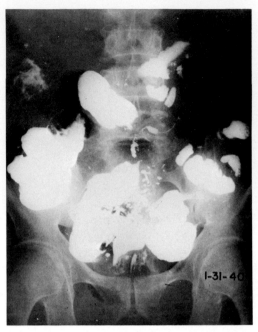

Fig. 33-5. Sprue. There is immediate, persistent, and marked segmentation. The segmented loops are moderately dilated and contain a considerable amount of fluid.

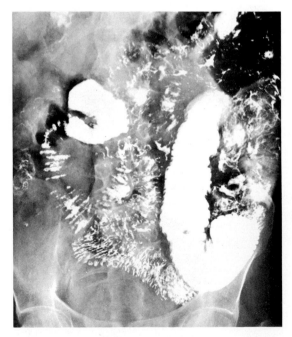

Fig. 33-6. Sprue. There is delayed segmentation best visualized in the distal jejunum and proximal ileum; marked fragmentation has also taken place.

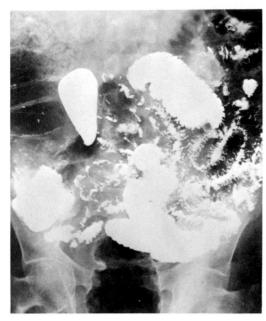

Fig. 33-7. Sprue. There is marked segmentation with stringlike strands of barium appearing between the barium clumps. The absence of folds in the segmented loops has been referred to as the moulage phenomenon. The contracted loops of bowel probably represent barium within a fluid-filled intestinal loop.

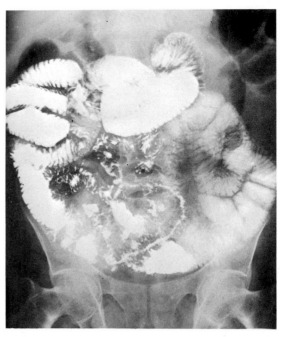

Fig. 33-8. Sprue. In the same patient as in Fig. 33-7, after the administration of a special collodial barium segmentation has almost completely disappeared, and instead, there is a continuous dilated column of barium. The administration of this type of barium mixture permits better visualization of the intestinal wall, but the segmentation characteristic of sprue is not seen.

small intestine, and it persists throughout the contrast study (Fig. 33-5). In a mild or moderately severe case of sprue, diffuse dilatation of the jejunum and proximal ileum is noted, followed by delayed segmentation of the barium column in the distal ileum (Fig. 33-6). In more severe cases, segmentation may be accounted for by the amount of secretions within the intestinal tract. In patients with markedly increased secretions, segmentation appears to be immediate.

Segmentation is probably a physical response of barium to the excessive fluid within the bowel lumen in sprue. When micropulverized barium preparations containing suspending agents are employed, segmentation is greatly reduced (Figs. 33-7 and 33-8).

Between the segmented clumps of barium, worm- or stringlike barium strands are often noted, apparently indicating seemingly collapsed intestinal loops. These strands are inconstant and vary from film to film, possibly because of altered motor activity of the bowel segment, or incomplete filling and emptying. Since they occur only in the presence of segmentation (which is always associated with hypersecretion), they may actually only represent the barium stream as it passes through a secretion-filled loop (Figs. 33-7 and 33-8).

As the barium leaves the small intestine, a faint, irregular stippling of residual barium may be seen along the course of the jejunum. This is a normal finding; however, in sprue the stippling is coarser, more amorphous, and resembles snow flakes. This phenomenon is called "scattering" or "fragmentation" and is usually associated with segmentation and increased secretion (Figs. 33-9 and 33-10).

Fold pattern. When dilatation of the jejunum occurs, whether as a result of mechanical or functional changes, the mucosal folds appear thin, straightened, and less prominent. The apparent mucosal thickening previously reported in some cases was thought to be caused by edema.[15] Postmortem examination of one of

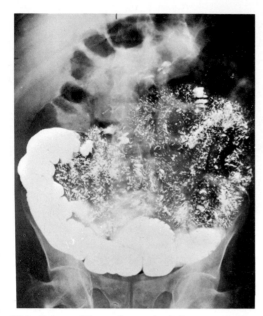

Fig. 33-9. Sprue. There is marked fragmentation, associated with slight dilatation and segmentation.

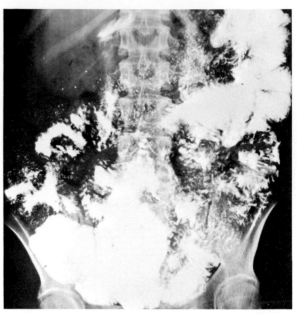

Fig. 33-10. Sprue. There is marked fragmentation, giving a disorganized appearance to the entire small bowel.

these patients, however, showed atrophy of the intestinal wall. Actual thickening of the folds, such as seen in lymphosarcoma and Whipple's disease, is not present. An abnormal fold pattern, then, is not an important factor in recognizing the presence of sprue, but appearance of such a pattern on the x-ray film which probably represents a functional phenomenon, may be misleading.

Transit time. Transit time refers to the time period during which the barium traverses the small intestine and enters the cecum. The average transit time in adults has been found to be approximately 3 hours; however, there is a wide range of variation. In most patients with sprue, transit time varies from 3 to 5 hours. In a few it is less, diminishing to as little as 30 minutes. In occasional patients, it is as long as 6 or 7 hours. Rarely is there undue prolongation of transit time when larger quantities of barium (20 fluid ounces) than usual are used to overcome the effect of puddling in a single dilated segment.

Moulage sign. This term—derived from the French *moulage,* which means "moulding" or "casting"—has been utilized to describe the roentgenographic appearance of the jejunum in sprue. The mucosal folds appear to be com-

pletely effaced and the barium-filled lumen resembles a tube into which "wax has been poured and allowed to harden" (Fig. 33-7). The moulage sign is most frequently noted in association with hypersecretion and segmentation. In these cases secretions probably obscure the mucosal markings. In a few cases, no mucosal markings are seen even when there is no dilatation and no hypersecretion. The bowel wall appears flaccid. In these cases the cause of the moulage sign is not clear.

Constitutional diseases
Whipple's disease

In 1907 G. H. Whipple reported the first case of the disease that now bears his name. He described a clinical picture of weight loss, steatorrhea, abdominal signs, and arthritis. At autopsy he found deposits of fat and fatty acids in the intestinal wall and the mesenteric lymph nodes. Large pale macrophages that gave a negative reaction to stains for fat were present in those areas. The next case of the disease was not reported until 1923, and it was not until 1949 that the material within the macrophages of the lamina propria of the small bowel and lymph nodes was discovered to be a glycoprotein that reacts positively to periodic acid-Schiff (PAS) stain. In recent years, especially since the advent of small-bowel biopsy techniques, more cases of Whipple's disease have been reported, and although its cause remains obscure, much has been learned about its pathology and treatment.

Characteristically, Whipple's disease causes a syndrome of intermittent arthralgia or arthritis, abdominal pain, diarrhea, steatorrhea, and weight loss. Physical findings include, besides evidence of dehydration and weight loss, lymphadenopathy, distention and diffuse tenderness of the abdomen, and abnormal skin pigmentation. Biochemical, radiologic, and hematologic findings resemble those of sprue. Pathologic examination shows polyserositis and generalized lymphadenopathy. In addition the lumen of the small bowel is dilated and the small-bowel wall and mesentery are thickened.

The hallmark of Whipple's disease is the presence in the lamina propria and in the lymph nodes of macrophages that are Sudan-negative and PAS-positive. The diagnosis of Whipple's disease can be established by demonstrating macrophages exhibiting these reactions in material obtained from small-bowel biopsy, from abdominal lymph nodes during laparotomy, or from peripheral nodes.

The nature and significance of the PAS-positive material are of great interest. Light and electron microscopic studies in Whipple's disease utilizing small-bowel biopsy specimens obtained during the active phase of the disease and during remission have been reported.[26] When the disease is active, biopsy specimens show abundant PAS-positive and gram-positive granules within the macrophages and extracellularly in the lamina propria. During treatment there is a decrease in both extracellular and intracellular granules. Electron microscopy and histochemical studies show that the PAS- and gram-positive rods and granules seen under the light microscope are bacteria and bacterial substances. The significance of the bacteria found in the mucosa of patients with Whipple's disease is difficult to evaluate. These organisms may be the cause of the disease, or they may be secondary invaders through a damaged epithelium. Whether their role is primary or secondary, the organisms, although they do tend to disappear or be modified by antibiotic treatment, disappear very slowly, suggesting that prolonged treatment may

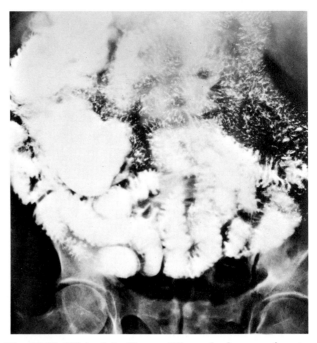

Fig. 33-11. Whipple's disease. The valvulae conniventes are thickened and slightly redundant. Several of the loops of bowel are dilated, and there is minimal fragmentation.

be required to effect remission or cure.[4] However, patients have now been reported with complete clinical, biochemical, radiologic, and histologic recovery.

Although a large series of cases of Whipple's disease is difficult to accumulate, enough individual cases have appeared in the literature so that a roentgenographic pattern has emerged. The most prominent single roentgenographic finding of Whipple's disease is the alteration in the appearance of the mucosal fold pattern. The valvulae conniventes are thickened and sometimes appear slightly nodular (Fig. 33-11). The mucosal folds may appear to be wild and redundant and to lack a homogeneous configuration (Fig. 33-12). The lumen of the bowel may be normal or slightly dilated. A slight amount of secretion, segmentation, and fragmentation may be identified (Fig. 33-13). Rigidity and inflammatory change or ulceration of the bowel wall, such as are noted in regional enteritis, are not seen. The transit time of barium is within normal limits. Two diseases—sprue and intestinal lymphangiectasia—exhibit radiographic signs similar to those of Whipple's disease and make

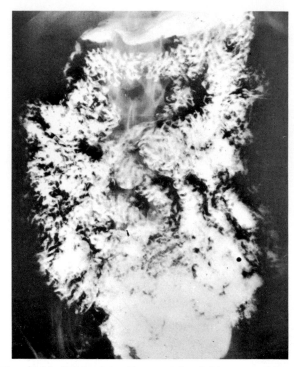

Fig. 33-12. Whipple's disease. The folds are wild, redundant, thickened, slightly nodular, and sharply delineated. Minimal dilatation, fragmentation, and segmentation are seen. This patient demonstrates the typical roentgenographic features in Whipple's disease.

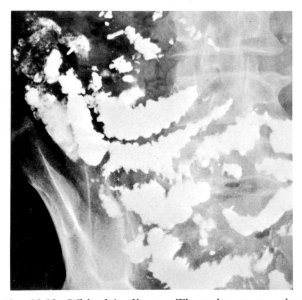

Fig. 33-13. Whipple's disease. There is segmentation, fragmentation, increased secretions, and thickening of the folds, but no evidence of any dilatation. The lack of dilatation differentiates the roentgenographic signs of Whipple's disease from the sprue pattern.

differential diagnosis difficult. Of the two, sprue is the more difficult to distinguish from Whipple's disease, but the less marked dilatation and characteristic thickening of the mucosal folds together with only minimal evidence of segmentation and fragmentation in the latter should enable a distinction to be made. Intestinal lymphangiectasia may completely simulate the roentgenographic findings in Whipple's disease, except for the distribution of the thickened mucosal folds. In Whipple's disease thickened folds are usually confined to the jejunum, whereas in intestinal lymphangiectasia they may be found throughout the small bowel. In some cases the nodularity of the mucosal contour is so extensive that its appearance suggests lymphosarcoma.

Scleroderma

Scleroderma is a systemic disease that may involve the small bowel and be associated with the malabsorption syndrome.[13] Although the small intestine may become involved at any time in the course of the disease, its involvement is usually preceded by skin changes, Raynaud's phenomenon, or symptoms of joint involvement. When the small intestine is affected, pathologic examination shows atrophy of the muscular layers and their replacement by collagen tissue. Both the mucosa and submucosa are atrophic. The villi are atrophic and round cell infiltration of the submucosa may also occur. Mesenteric vascular arteritis has been noted, and in a recent report biopsy of the mucosa of the duodenum demonstrated considerable fibrosis of the submucosal tissue and fibrosis of tissue around Brunner's glands.[19] The mucosa itself was normal. Up to the present time there have been no extensive studies of the mucosa by small-bowel biopsy.

Although the cause of the malabsorption associated with scleroderma is speculative, several possible explanations exist. Replacement of the muscular layers with fibrous tissue may alter peristaltic activity. Arteritis may contribute to alterations in small-bowel absorptive capacity. Changes in bacterial flora as a result of changes in motility may be a cause of malabsorption. Long-term administration of broad-spectrum antibiotics may improve absorption from the small bowel.

The roentgenographic findings in the esophagus in scleroderma are atony, hypomotility or absent peristaltic activity, shortening, sliding hiatus hernia, regurgitation, esophagitis, and stricture. The inability of the esophagus to empty with the patient in the prone position is a characteristic finding.

The roentgenographic findings in the remainder of the intestinal tract are similar to those described in the esophagus but occur less frequently. A considerable delay in peristaltic activity associated with dilatation is the most conspicuous roentgenographic feature of scleroderma. In the stomach and the duodenal bulb this is usually minimal. The second portion of the duodenum demonstrates varying changes in its caliber, characterized by dilatation and delayed emptying. This dilatation may be pronounced, suggesting an obstruction at the ligament of Treitz from metastasis, from extension from carcinoma of the pancreas, from regional enteritis, or from adhesions (Fig. 33-14). In one of our cases, the dilatation of the duodenum was so pronounced that it filled the proximal two thirds of the abdomen.

In the jejunum and ileum roentgenographic findings show that the most striking alteration is hypomotility with varying degrees of dilatation. Segmentation, fragmentation, and increased secretions are usually not present. There is no roentgenographic evidence of an inflammatory process. The mucosal fold pattern is normal and there is no evidence of any disturbance of the normal architecture of the small bowel. When the hypomotility is significant, a small-bowel obstruction may be simulated; several patients have been operated upon to exclude this possibility. Several patients have also had exploratory surgery with removal of the dilated loops in an effort to relieve the severe stasis that was present. When the hypomotility is especially pronounced, sacculation with the formation of pseudodiverticula may occur (Fig. 33-15). This finding is more frequently seen in the colon in association with fecaliths (Fig. 33-16).

The colon in addition exhibits other changes similar to those in the small bowel. The degree of dilatation may be enormous and occasionally may simulate Hirschsprung's disease occurring in adults. Stercoral ulceration caused by retained fecal material may be seen pathologically, but it is difficult to identify in a roentgenographic examination.

As a rule differential diagnosis from sprue

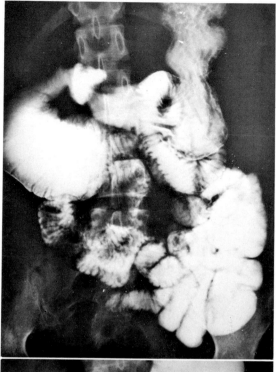

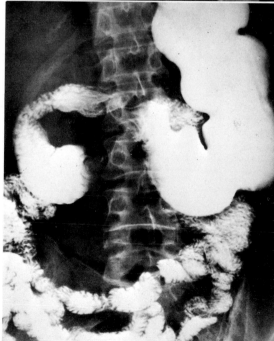

Fig. 33-14. Scleroderma. **A,** Marked dilatation of the duodenal loop, unassociated with obstruction at the ligament of Treitz, is evident on this film. There is also considerable hypomotility of the barium through the small bowel. **B,** Metastasis at ligament of Treitz, producing obstruction and dilatation of the duodenal loop, simulates scleroderma.

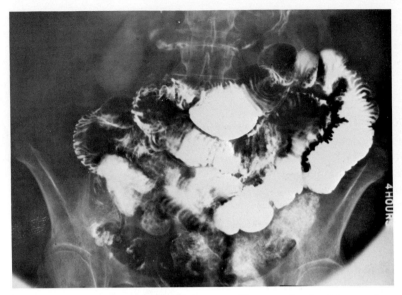

Fig. 33-15. Scleroderma. There is marked hypomotility associated with pseudosacculation and minimal dilatation. The valvulae conniventes are closer together than usual, presumably as a result of intramural fibrosis.

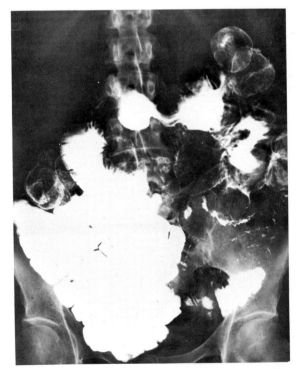

Fig. 33-16. Scleroderma. There is dilatation of the duodenal loop, and marked hypomotility in the small bowel associated with numerous fecaliths in the colon.

is not difficult because the lack of increased secretions, segmentation, and fragmentation in scleroderma make a distinction possible. Moreover, the dilatation of sprue is most significant in the midjejunum and is usually associated with normal motility while the dilatation in scleroderma is more diffuse. The presence of sacculation should also suggest a diagnosis of scleroderma.

Dilatation of the bowel secondary to obstruction from adhesions may simulate the dilatation and hypomotility of scleroderma; but the history, lack of esophageal changes, and absence of pseudodiverticula help rule out scleroderma.

Idiopathic intestinal pseudo-obstruction is a poorly understood condition that simulates mechanical obstruction in appearance and symptoms. At laparotomy no cause is found, and histologic examination is negative. The condition usually occurs in young patients. The three young patients recently reported by Moss and his co-workers were clinically suspected to have scleroderma.[15a]

Lymphosarcoma

When lymphosarcoma of the small bowel occurs with malabsorption and steatorrhea, differentiation from sprue can be very difficult.[25] If there is enlargement of extra-abdominal lymph nodes or if abdominal masses are palpable, a diagnosis of lymphosarcoma may be suspected and confirmed on biopsy. In the absence of such findings, differentiation from sprue rests largely on the shorter and more fulminant course of lymphosarcoma, on bowel complications such as perforation and ulceration in lymphosarcoma, and on failure of the patient to respond completely to a gluten-free diet, folic acid, or antibiotics.

The distinction between the two diseases is further confused by reported cases of the development of lymphosarcoma in patients with sprue. It is more likely that in these cases lymphosarcoma develops as a complication of long-standing sprue than that it had been responsible for the entire course of the disease. The complication of lymphosarcoma should be considered when a patient with sprue develops fever, bowel perforation, or hemorrhage, or shows exacerbation of sprue symptoms despite maintenance treatment.

Along with the clinical and laboratory findings of sprue that can occur in lymphosarcoma of the small bowel and mesentery, roentgenographic alterations simulating sprue may also be found. In some cases of lymphosarcoma dilatation of small intestinal loops, hypersection, and segmentation of the barium column are seen. Often the dilatation is less extensive than it would be in sprue alone, and the intestinal folds appear to be coarsened, thickened, and sometimes nodular (Figs. 33-17 to 33-20). At times there may be obvious evidences of lymphosarcoma with evidence of extraluminal masses, thickening of the bowel wall, and displacement and invasion of the small-bowel loops, superimposed upon the sprue pattern.

It must be remembered that extensive involvement of the small bowel with lymphosarcoma may occur with little evidence of malabsorption.

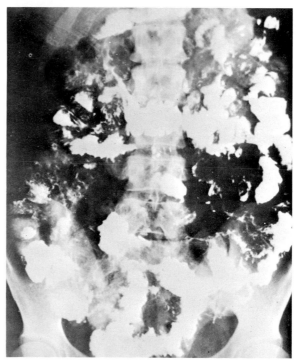

Fig. 33-17. Lymphosarcoma. Diffuse lymphosarcoma of the mesentery and retroperitoneum, mimicking the sprue pattern, is manifested by segmentation, hypersecretion, and flocculation of the barium column. No dilated flaccid loops, such as those seen in sprue, are identified.

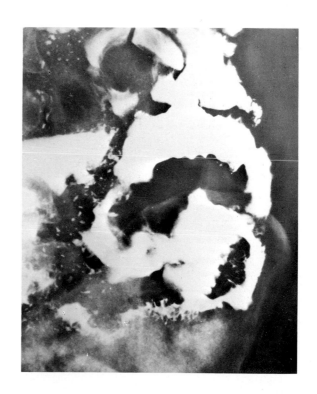

Fig. 33-18. Lymphosarcoma. There is segmentation, fragmentation, and increased secretions. The irregularity of the bowel contour is the result of infiltration of the wall by lymphosarcoma.

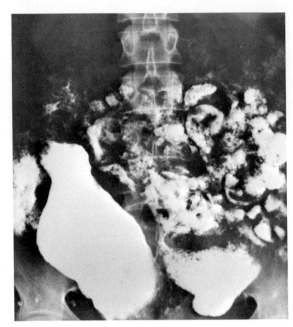

Fig. 33-19. Lymphosarcoma. The increased thickness of the bowel wall is indicated by the increase in the soft tissues intervening between the dilated segments (aneurysmal dilatation) and adjacent small-bowel loops. The proximal portion of the bowel shows minimal evidence of the sprue pattern.

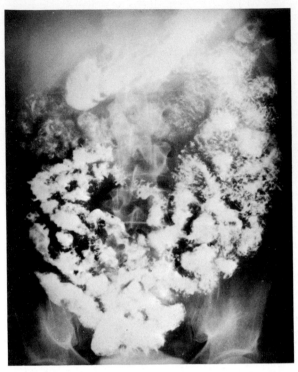

Fig. 33-20. Lymphosarcoma. A diffuse involvement of the small bowel with lymphosarcoma is shown on this film. The mucosal folds are thickened with numerous intraluminal and contour defects. This pattern may be confused with some of the features seen in Whipple's disease or in intestinal lymphangiectasia, but the presence of tumor nodules indicates lymphosarcoma.

Amyloidosis

The small bowel may be involved in both primary and secondary amyloidosis, but development of malabsorption and steatorrhea is uncommon. The diagnosis of small-bowel amyloidosis can be made by oral biopsy. Histologically, the deposits of amyloid are heaviest in the mucosa and in the submucosal arterioles. The epithelial cells may be intact in cases of amyloid involvement, but with more extensive deposits the villi are flattened and in some areas may be destroyed and replaced by amyloid bands.

Recent studies have tended to blur the distinction between primary and secondary amyloidosis and have suggested that most, if not all, cases of amyloidosis represent a neoplasm or a dyscrasia, or plasma cells that elaborate the abnormal proteins that are incorporated into amyloid.

The conspicuous roentgenographic finding in primary amyloidosis is thickening of the valvulae conniventes. This may be symmetrical, producing a striking uniform appearance throughout the entire intestinal tract of large folds unassociated with ulceration, tumor nodules, or significant dilatation (Fig. 33-21). When the thickening of the folds is patchy and uneven, the differential diagnosis from Whipple's disease, intestinal lymphangiectasia, and lymphosarcoma is difficult. The diagnosis in these instances can be made only by process of elimination. In secondary amyloidosis, with large amyloid deposits distributed throughout the intestinal tract, tumor-like defects may be seen, but again unless the primary cause of the condition is established, it is impossible to make a definite diagnosis.

Amyloidosis has been reported in association with intestinal pseudo-obstruction,[12] an entity

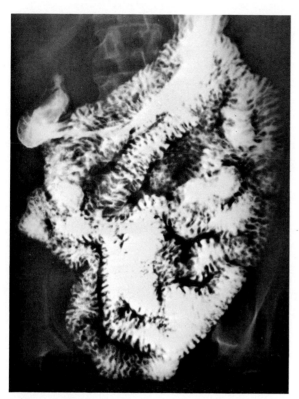

Fig. 33-21. Amyloidosis. There is a striking symmetrical, diffuse, sharply demarcated thickening of the valvulae conniventes, associated with minimal dilatation. No segmentation, fragmentation, or any evidence of an inflammatory lesion appears.

in which clinical manifestations of mechanical small-bowel obstruction occur in the absence of organic occlusion of the lumen. The findings are presumed to be secondary to infiltration of the bowel wall by deposits of amyloid. If the diagnosis can be established by small-bowel or rectal biopsy, the patient can be managed conservatively and be spared laparotomy. The prognosis of systemic amyloidosis is extremely poor.

Immunoglobulin disorders

The relation of the serum immunoglobulins to malabsorption syndrome is a subject of current active investigation.[7] The immunoglobulins, or antibodies, have been classified into a number of groups, of which the three most important have been named IgG, IgM, and IgA.

IgG globulin comprises most of the serum antibodies, including those against bacteria and viruses. IgM globulins are large molecules that make up the macroglobulins of serum. IgA globulins have a special relationship to the intestine. It is believed that the plasma cells of the lamina propria of the bowel locally synthesize IgA globulin, which is found in the serum and is also taken up by the intestinal epithelial cells. Within these cells two molecules combine with a nonimmunoglobulin glycoprotein called the "secretory piece," which is synthesized within the cell, to form secretory IgA, which is secreted into the lumen. It is likely that IgA provides a line of defense for the intestinal epithelium and may help regulate the normal bacterial and viral flora of the bowel.

Most patients with congenital or acquired hypogammaglobulinemia are deficient in all three serum immunoglobulin fractions. Clinical manifestations may include a variety of gastrointestinal features, including diarrhea and malabsorption syndrome. Jejunal biopsy in hypogammaglobulinemia has usually been reported to be normal, but a spruelike lesion has been described in a few cases.

Insufficient numbers of cases of hypogammaglobulinemia have been studied to warrant a roentgenographic description. Of the several cases that we have studied, some have had minimal changes of the sprue pattern and others had thickening and slight rigidity of the folds (Fig. 33-22). The cause of the thickening has not been determined, but the possibility should be considered that it is the consequence of a secondary infection of the intestine, such as giardiasis. *Giardia lamblia* infection is a common accompaniment of hypogammaglobulinemia.

Certain patients with hypogammaglobulinemia, however, (so-called dysgammaglobulinemia, type I) who have very low levels of IgA and IgM but borderline normal levels of IgG,[7] display a pattern of nodular lymphoid hyperplasia on small-bowel biopsy. This feature can be recognized on roentgenographic examination as well. Many of these patients have also been found to have intestinal giardiasis.

Although lymph follicles large enough to be visible on roentgenograms of the small bowel may be found in the terminal ileum of normal persons, a pathologic process must be suspected when this finding extends into the proximal small bowel. It is in this group of patients with diffuse nodular lymphoid hyperplasia that a

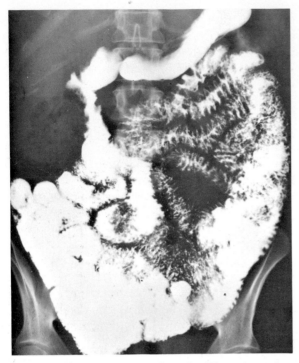

Fig. 33-22. Hypogammaglobulinemia. There is moderate thickening of the valvulae conniventes in the jejunum, associated with slight rigidity and narrowing of the lumen, and increased secretions. The exact cause of these changes in hypogammaglobulinemia is unknown, but it is thought that they may be secondary to an inflammatory process.

clinical syndrome has recently been described,[8] consisting of hypogammaglobulinemia with predominant depression of IgA and IgM concentrations, diarrhea, malabsorption syndrome, and *Giardia lamblia* infection. The significance and the interrelationships of the components of the syndrome remain uncertain at present.

A new immunoglobulin abnormality associated with malabsorption syndrome, termed "alpha-chain disease," has been described by Seligmann[21] and his colleagues. The patient studied had clinical characteristics of a previously described "Arabian lymphoma" found in young Arabs and non-European Jews, with diffuse plasma call infiltration of the entire small bowel, resembling a lymphoma, and profound malabsorption. In the patient's serum and urine were found alpha chains, which are the heavy-chain components of IgA. The levels of serum

immunoglobulins were low. It seems possible that less severe variants of alpha-chain disease may occur, with infiltration of the small bowel by plasma cells and variable alterations in the serum immunoglobulins and in small-bowel absorptive function. We have seen one such case.

Abnormalities of IgM globulins may also be associated occasionally with malabsorption syndrome. Primary (Waldenstrom's) macroglobulinemia is a plasma cell dyscrasia involving those cells that synthesize macroglobulins (IgM). Large amounts of IgM are found in the serum. Manifestations of the disease include anemia, lymphadenopathy, and hepatosplenomegaly. Gastrointestinal symptoms are not usually conspicuous, but a few patients have now been reported with malabsorption syndrome.[10] Small-bowel examination in patients with macroglobulinemia and malabsorption has shown dilatation of the bowel and thickening of the mucosal folds. The roentgenographic features are nonspecific, but they do suggest involvement of the small bowel in this systemic disease process.

Diabetes

Severe diarrhea occasionally occurs in patients with diabetes mellitus who have normal exocrine pancreatic function. This diarrhea has been attributed to visceral neuropathy. In some patients with diarrhea, steatorrhea has been reported. Such evidences of malabsorption may in part reflect a rapid transit time, but recent small-bowel biopsy studies have suggested that malabsorption may be the result of concomitant sprue.[27] Alternatively, secondary spruelike changes in the small-bowel mucosa may be induced by the diabetes itself, but thus far there has been no direct evidence to support this. However, in some cases diabetic patients with diarrhea and malabsorption have displayed a sprue pattern in a small-bowel roentgenographic examination.

Carcinoid

A rare cause of diarrhea and malabsorption is metastatic carcinoid. Presumably the diarrhea is secondary to increased levels of circulating serotonin. The cause of the malabsorption, however, remains uncertain. When malabsorption is present there are no roentgenographic changes superimposed on those caused by carcinoid.

Primary small-bowel diseases
Intestinal lymphangiectasia

Intestinal lymphangiectasia, first defined by Waldmann in 1961, is a distinctive cause of protein loss into the gastrointestinal tract, of hypoproteinemia, and in some patients, of malabsorption and steatorrhea.[28]

Clinically, the condition is manifested by edema, serous effusions, and diarrhea. Laboratory studies demonstrate hypoalbuminemia and hypogammaglobulinemia, increased protein catabolism, and loss of albumin into the gastrointestinal tract.

The pathologic findings in the small bowel are characteristic.[16] The bowel appears edematous, and the serosal surface is dark and congested. The lumen is only slightly dilated and the valvulae conniventes are swollen and broad. The tips of the villi are enlarged and bleblike. Histologically, the hallmark is dilatation of the lymph vessels in the mucosa and submucosa. Within the mucosa are abundant foamy macrophages that stain for fat and are negative to PAS stain.

In some patients with onset of symptoms in infancy, intestinal lymphangiectasia appears to be congenital; in others onset of symptoms takes place late in life and the condition is probably an acquired abnormality. Multiple abnormalities of the systemic lymph vessels may be present.

It is not clear how protein is lost through the bowel wall in intestinal lymphangiectasia. Waldmann has suggested that dilated lymphatic vessels may rupture and discharge their contents into the lumen of the intestine.[28] Alternatively, lymphatic blockage may result in leakage of protein from an intact epithelium.

Steatorrhea, which sometimes occurs in intestinal lymphangiectasia, may be the result of obstruction of intestinal lymph vessels, damage to the mucosal epithelial cells, or chronic leakage of fat-containing lymph into the lumen.

Efforts to treat intestinal lymphangiectasia with steroids, gluten-free diet, and segmental small-bowel resection have proved unsuccessful. Treatment of patients with a low-fat diet, however, results in increase in serum proteins, decrease in albumin catabolism, and decrease in intestinal protein loss. It has been suggested that the low-fat diet may decrease pressure in obstructed intestinal lymph vessels by a decrease in

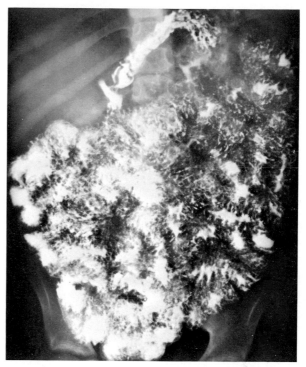

Fig. 33-23. Intestinal lymphangiectasia. There is symmetrical thickening of the valvulae conniventes throughout the entire small bowel, associated with increased secretions. The mucosal folds are somewhat redundant and excessive with no evidence of nodularity. Minimal fragmentation of the folds is seen.

lymph production and consequent decrease in lymph leakage. Availability of synthetic medium-chain triglycerides, which are absorbed by way of the intestinal capillaries and portal blood rather than by the lymph vessels, provides another possible means of treating intestinal lymphangiectasia.

Thickening of the mucosal folds is an outstanding feature in all cases, and it is usually diffuse. The fold pattern is symmetrical, but the folds appear to be redundant and excessive. Nodular defects, especially of varying size, are unusual. Increased secretions are invariably present (Fig. 33-23). The combination of edema and secretion may produce blunting and fragmentation of the folds (Fig. 33-24). Segmentation is usually minimal. Dilatation is minimal or absent, with slight evidence of rigidity of the folds, ulceration, or separation of the loops of bowel (Fig. 33-25). Differential diagnosis from other lesions producing thickening of the folds can be difficult: In Whipple's disease there is

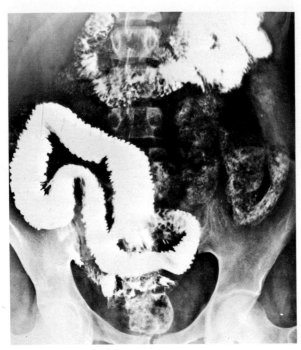

Fig. 33-24. Intestinal lymphangiectasia. There is thickening and blunting of the folds, associated with slight rigidity and moderately increased secretions.

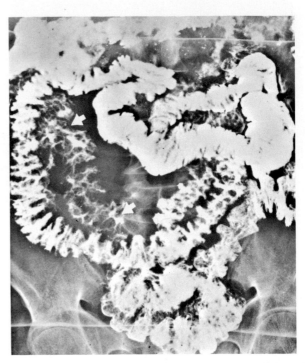

Fig. 33-25. Intestinal lymphangiectasia. The small bowel shows thick folds that in places are coarsely nodular. The caliber of the bowel is slightly increased. The lack of homogeneity of the barium appears to be the result of punctate mucosal prominences rather than excessive secretions.

usually more segmentation and fragmentation, and the fold appearance is usually wild, less symmetrical, and not as diffuse. In amyloidosis, edema and secretions are usually absent. In patients with hypoalbuminemic states, such as nephrosis or cirrhosis, a symmetrical diffuse thickening of the folds of the small intestine may be demonstrated, but the thickening is usually less pronounced and the secretions less prominent than in patients with intestinal lymphangiectasia.

In an occasional patient with intestinal lymphangiectasia, tiny punctate lucencies can be demonstrated on roentgenograms of the small intestine (Fig. 33-25). Whether these are caused by droplets of secretion or the tiny, pebble-like prominences seen pathologically is difficult to determine. When ascites is present, bulging of the flanks with a central configuration of the small-bowel loops is seen.

Hypoproteinemia, which affects the gastrointestinal tract in the same way as it does other areolar tissues, deserves some special comments. A collection of fluid that can be detected by barium meal examination occurs in the peritoneum and the wall of the gastrointestinal tract. Hypoproteinemia may be the result of malfunctioning kidneys, liver, or intestinal tract. The roentgenographic changes that have been observed include the widening and redundancy of the mucosal folds, together with minimal dilatation and multiple contractions of the small bowel that make it appear shirred or seem overactive. In most cases the folds are distinct, but as a result of active peristalsis may be blurred and uneven. Segmentation and fragmentation of barium during an examination may be present, but they are not conspicuous features. When ascites occurs, the small bowel assumes a central configuration like that seen with an internal hernia. When the albumin level is sufficiently diminished and edema is present in varying degrees throughout the body, the changes described above have been noted in many patients with nephrosis, cirrhosis of the liver, and congestive heart failure (Fig. 33-26).

How much a role the changes of hypopro-

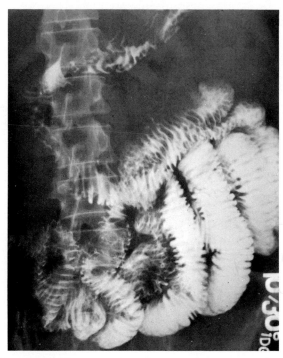

Fig. 33-26. Hypoproteinemia secondary to nephrosis (albumin content = 1.5 gm./100 ml.). There is a diffuse prominence of the valvulae conniventes of the jejunum associated with dilatation. Active contraction of the bowel loops is also seen. There is no evidence of increased secretions.

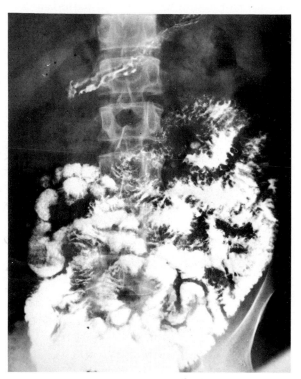

Fig. 33-27. Giardiasis. There is marked spasm and irritability of the jejunum, associated with slight narrowing of the bowel lumen. The valvulae conniventes are distorted, thickened, and fragmented. The marked spasm and irritability of the bowel associated with disorientation of the folds are distinguishing features of giardiasis. The findings are usually limited to the jejunum.

teinemia play in the roentgenographic appearance of disorders such as sprue, Whipple's disease, or intestinal lymphangiectasia is not known. In intestinal lymphangiectasia thickening of the folds associated with edema is certainly closely correlated with the degree of protein loss.

Parasitic infections

The incidence of malabsorption in parasitic infection is difficult to assess because nutritional deficiencies and dietary inadequacy are common in those geographic areas where these diseases are endemic. Most authorities agree that hookworm, *Strongyloides,* and *Giardia,* however, may produce malabsorption when infection is severe.[3,23]

The roentgenographic findings in giardiasis are more striking than in hookworm infestation and are limited to the duodenum and jejunum.[14] The mucosal folds of the intestine appear thickened, blunted, and in many areas distorted and fragmented. Associated with the mucosal changes is a significant degree of spasm and irritability of the bowel that produces a rapid change in the direction and configuration of the valvulae conniventes (Figs. 33-27 and 33-28). The lumen of the bowel is frequently narrowed because of spasm. Dilatation, when present, is minimal. Increased secretions are frequent and cause blurring and indistinctness in the appearance of the folds, which on occasion is accompanied by fragmentation and slight segmentation (Fig. 33-29). Motility through the jejunum may be so rapid that multiple filming with considerable amounts of barium is necessary to study roentgenographic alterations. The ileum is within normal limits. In several cases complete return to normal has been observed in the fold pattern following treatment (Fig. 33-28). Roentgenographic changes similar to these have been noted with *Strongyloides.*

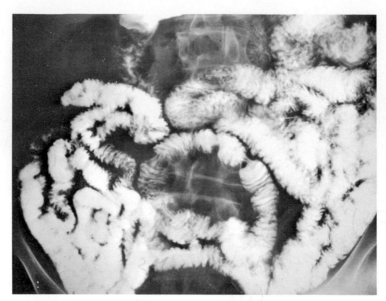

Fig. 33-28. Giardiasis. After a course of quinacrine hydrochloride (Atabrine) medication, there has been a return to normal in the appearance of the small bowel.

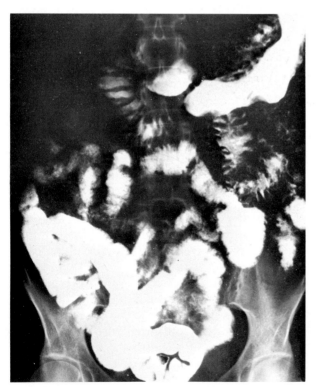

Fig. 33-29. Giardiasis. There is marked spasm and irritability of the jejunum associated with narrowing of the lumen. The thickening of the folds is associated with increased secretions secondary to inflammatory edema.

The roentgenographic findings associated with parasitic diseases have been incorrectly ascribed to the accompanying malabsorption. The changes that are observed are primarily the result of an inflammatory reaction and do not have the usual appearance associated with malabsorption. Although malabsorption may exist clinically, the roentgenographic findings in parasitic diseases are the result of inflammation rather than of a sprue pattern.

Diverticula, blind loops, and strictures

Malabsorption syndrome may develop in patients with spontaneously occurring or surgically created small-bowel diverticula, blind loops, or strictures. The significant features common to these anatomic abnormalities are local hypomotility, stasis, and overgrowth of intestinal bacteria. A macrocytic anemia may also develop because the bacteria compete with the mucosal absorbing cells for supplies of intraluminal vitamin B^{12}. Both the macrocytic anemia and the malabsorption syndrome can be corrected by the administration of systemic antibiotics or by surgical correction of the anatomic anomaly. The mechanism by which bacterial overgrowth may induce malabsorption is not clear. It has been suggested that bacteria may deconjugate

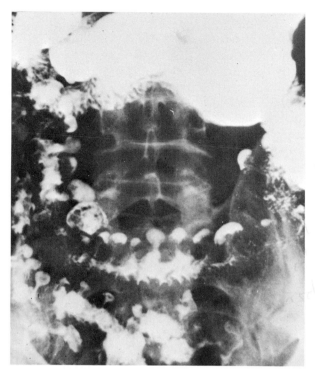

Fig. 33-30. Diverticulosis of the small bowel associated with malabsorption. Multiple diverticula are distributed throughout the small bowel.

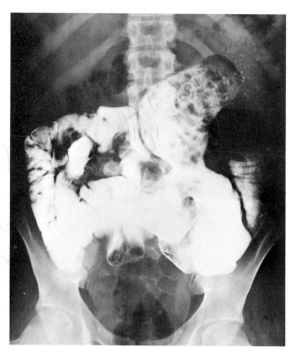

Fig. 33-31. Regional enteritis. Two large blind loops secondary to side-to-side anastomosis performed for stenotic regional enteritis.

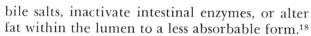

bile salts, inactivate intestinal enzymes, or alter fat within the lumen to a less absorbable form.[18]

The roentgenographic diagnosis of diverticulosis depends on the visualization of the multiple sacs that may appear as oval, circular, or flask-shaped projections from the bowel lumen (Fig. 33-30). They can be tiny or large and are usually smooth in outline with no distinct mucosal folds. Because of the motility of the intestinal loops, these sacs may change in position rapidly. When large and numerous, they may stimulate the segmentation seen in sprue. Enteroliths are also occasionally noted in connection with diverticulosis. A lateral projection or a film taken while the small bowel is emptying is useful in differentiating diverticulosis and sprue.

Blind loops are frequently associated with an intestinal side-to-side anastomosis (Fig. 33-31), but a blind loop effect may be produced when there are two segments of constricted bowel with an intervening area of dilatation, as is seen in the stenotic phase of regional enteritis (Fig. 33-32). Bleeding from an erosion in a blind loop occurs more frequently than from diverticula.

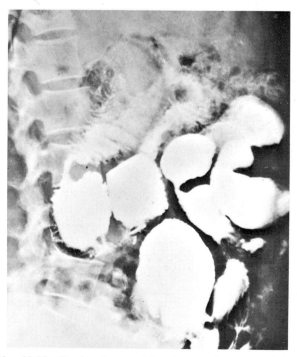

Fig. 33-32. Regional enteritis. Areas of stenosis intervene between markedly dilated loops. In this patient there was associated malabsorption and macrocytic anemia.

Regional enteritis and tuberculosis

In many patients with regional enteritis malabsorption can be demonstrated by specific tests of absorption, but only occasionally is malabsorption a feature of major clinical significance in the disease. When the regional enteritis is extensive and involves the jejunum as well as the ileum, appreciable malabsorption is a likely finding. For the most part, the malabsorption of regional enteritis is probably caused by mechanical obstruction of intestinal lymph vessels by the inflammatory process, but it can also be the result of secondary changes induced in the mucosal absorbing cells or disruption of the enterohepatic circulation of bile salts. Atrophic changes have been demonstrated in small bowel mucosal biopsy specimens proximal to the principal areas of inflammatory disease.

There is no relationship between the type of roentgenographic findings in regional enteritis and the degree of malabsorption present. Malabsorption appears to be more severe in those cases with the more extensive involvement of the intestine or those with jejunal involvement.

The roentgenographic findings in tuberculosis are extremely difficult to differentiate from those of regional enteritis. In general, there is more angulation of the loops of bowel, more irregularity of the bowel contour, and deeper, larger ulcerations. Irregular involvement of the cecum and ascending colon is frequent.

Mesenteric vascular insufficiency

Malabsorption may result from the acute or chronic occlusion of the superior mesenteric artery which results in vascular insufficiency of the small bowel. The clinical picture in mesenteric vascular insufficiency is one of postprandial abdominal cramps, and progressive diarrhea, steatorrhea, and weight loss. A diagnosis may be established by the aortographic demonstration of occlusion of the superior mesenteric artery or by the roentgenographic demonstration of alterations in the small bowel pattern. Successful treatment, involving endarterectomy and vascular grafts, has been reported.

Eosinophilic gastroenteritis

Eosinophilic gastroenteritis is a rare disease of unknown cause in which there is a diffuse infiltration of eosinophils in the wall of the bowel.[2a] The bowel wall is thickened by muscle hypertrophy and by edema and infiltration with chronic inflammatory cells and eosinophils. Peripheral eosinophilia is usually present. Clinically the patients have bouts of abdominal pain, vomiting, and diarrhea. The course is usually benign, and corticosteroids have provided effective treatment. Malabsorption syndrome has been documented,[9] but the mechanism is unknown. Presumably the infiltration of inflammatory cells and the edema are responsible for derangement of absorptive functions. The roentgenographic alterations are nonspecific. Both stomach and small bowel may be involved. Changes simulate those of regional enteritis or lymphoma, and without clinical or pathologic data a specific diagnosis is impossible.

Postoperative conditions

Roentgenographic examination may contribute to a diagnosis of malabsorption syndrome by demonstrating a surgical reconstruction of the gastrointestinal tract. Partial resection of the small bowel reduces the principal areas for absorption in the duodenum and jejunum; inadvertent gastroileostomy bypasses them. The ileum appears able to undertake some of the absorptive function of the jejunum when this has been lost. The prognosis for a child who has had a small bowel resection is probably better than it is for an adult since growth, with increased length and greater adaptability of the remaining gut, may still occur. It has been shown that absorption of fat is less impaired after gastroduodenostomy (Billroth I) than after gastrojejunostomy (Billroth II).

Following both total and subtotal gastrectomy there is a decrease in absorption of protein and fat. One of the major complications of gastric resection is failure to gain or maintain weight. After gastrectomy malabsorption may be caused by loss of the reservoir function of the stomach, by rapid small-bowel motility and decreased transit time, by decreased stimulation of bile and pancreatic secretions and consequent poor mixing of digestive enzymes and food within the gut, or by alterations in small-bowel bacterial flora.

In most patients with a partial gastric resection the appearance of the small bowel is normal. Slight dilatation of the jejunum is frequently identified because of overfilling of its loops, especially when large quantities of barium are employed in an examination. The interpretation of minimal degrees of segmentation, hypersecretion, and fragmentation is difficult, especially in a patient with diarrhea. In these patients laboratory tests are of much greater significance for diagnosis. When anatomic and functional changes in the small bowel are greatest, patients usually have an associated spruelike disorder.

Faulty digestion
Diseases of the liver and biliary tract

Diseases of the liver and biliary tract that exclude bile from the small bowel may be associated with malabsorption. Absence of bile salts from the intestine results in impaired digestion and absorption of fat. Steatorrhea is therefore a feature of primary and secondary biliary cirrhosis. Absorption of fat returns to normal if liver function improves or biliary obstruction can be relieved. In a limited number of cases some of the roentgenographic features associated with sprue may be found.

Zollinger-Ellison syndrome

As it is usually defined, the Zollinger-Ellison syndrome consists of gastric acid hypersecretion and severe peptic ulceration in association with noninsulin-producing islet cell tumors of the pancreas. Diarrhea is also frequently reported.

Recent studies have suggested that patients with diarrhea and islet cell tumors may be divided into two distinct categories.[24] In one group the diarrhea is associated with classic Zollinger-Ellison findings of peptic ulceration and gastric hypersecretion, and it is often accompanied by steatorrhea. Serum electrolyte levels tend to be normal. The steatorrhea in these patients appears to be directly related to the large volumes of highly acid gastric juice entering the small bowel. The precise mechanism of the malabsorption is unknown, but it may result from inactivation of intestinal enzymes by the abnormal acidity of the upper small bowel or from the irritant and inflammatory effects of acid on the small bowel mucosa. Small bowel biopsies in the patients in this group have indicated no abnormalities or have shown only mild inflammatory changes.

Another group of patients with islet cell tumors and diarrhea displays hypokalemia and electrolyte abnormalities but no steatorrhea. In this group gastric hypersecretion and peptic ulceration are uncommon and in some cases anacidity has been reported. In these patients diarrhea seems unlikely to be related to the presence of acid in the small bowel, and it has been suggested that some substance is elaborated by the pancreatic tumors which directly stimulates small bowel motility. Whether this postulated substance might be related to the gastrin identified in some islet tumors of patients with classic Zollinger-Ellison syndrome has not yet been established.

There are six roentgenographic findings associated with classic Zollinger-Ellison syndrome: (1) large mucosal folds (hyperrugosity); (2) single or multiple ulcerations situated in the stomach, duodenal bulb, duodenal loop, or proximal small bowel; (3) dilatation of the second portion of the duodenum; (4) thickening of the folds in some areas of the duodenal loop, simulating the haustral pattern of the colon; (5) severe hypersecretion; and (6) a lacelike or reticulated pattern of the small intestine, probably secondary to gastric hypersecretion.

Pancreatic insufficiency

Malabsorption may occur in patients with pancreatic disease that involves obstruction to the duct system or destruction of acinar tissue. Thus malabsorption may be a manifestation of chronic pancreatitis, carcinoma of the pancreas, or fibrocystic disease. Malabsorption in this type of pancreatic disease is actually maldigestion, the principal defect being absence of pancreatic lipase from the intestine. The stool contains neutral fat, and absorption of radioactive oleic acid is normal. Tests of carbohydrate absorption are normal. Treatment of pancreatic steatorrhea consists of the oral administration of large amounts of commercial pancreatic extracts at mealtime.

The roentgenographic examination of a patient with pancreatic insufficiency usually indicates no abnormalities. In an occasional patient with severe chronic pancreatitis, segmentation of the barium column and increased secretions may be seen within the small bowel. Dilatation such as occurs in sprue is absent. A normal x-ray film of patients with severe steatorrhea immediately suggests that underlying chronic pancreatitis may be present.

REFERENCES

1. Ardran, G. M., French, J. M., and Mucklow, M. B.: Relationship of the nature of the opaque medium to the small intestine radiographic pattern, Brit. J. Radiol. 23:697, 1950.
2. Benson, G. D., Kowlessar, O. D., and Sleisenger, M. H.: Adult celiac disease with emphasis upon response to the glutten-free diet, Medicine (Balt.) 43:1, 1964.
2a. Burhenne, H. J., and Carbone, J. V.: Eosinophilic (allergic) gastroenteritis, Amer. J. Roentgen. 96:332, 1966.
3. Cortner, J. A.: Giardiasis, a cause of celiac syndrome, Amer. J. Dis. Child. 98:311, 1959.
4. Davis, T. D., McBee, J. W., Borland, J. L., Jr., Kurtz, S. M., and Ruffin, J. M.: The effect of antibiotics and steroid therapy in Whipple's disease, Gastroenterology 44:112, 1963.
5. Dicke, W. K., Weijers, H. A., and van de Kramer, J. H.: Coeliac disease; presence in wheat of factor having a deleterious effect in cases of coeliac disease, Acta Paediat. 42:34, 1953.
6. Frazer, A. C., French, J. M., and Thompson, M. D.: Radiographic studies showing the induction of a segmentation pattern in the small intestine in normal human subjects, Brit. J. Radiol. 22:123, 1949.
7. Hobbs, J. R.: Immunoglobulins and malabsorption, Proc. Roy. Soc. Med. 62:982, 1969.
8. Hodgson, J. R., Hoffman, H. N., and Huizenga, K. A.: Roentgenologic features of lymphoid hyperplasia of the small intestine associated with dysgammaglobulinemia, Radiology 88:883, 1967.
9. Kaplan, S. M., Goldstein, F., and Kowlessar, O. D.: Eosinophilic gastroenteritis; report of a case with malabsorption and protein-losing enteropathy, Gastroenterology 58:540, 1970.
10. Khilnani, M. T., Keller, R. J., and Cuttner, J.: Macroglobulinemia and steatorrhea: roentgen and pathological findings in the intestinal tract, Radiol. Clin. N. Amer. 7:43, 1969.
11. Laws, J. W., Booth, C. C., Shawdon, H., and Stewart, J. S.: Correlation of radiological and histological findings in idiopathic steatorrhea, Brit. Med. J. 5341:1311, 1963.
12. Legge, D. A., Wollaeger, E. E., and Carlson, H. C.: Intestinal pseudo-obstruction in systemic amyloidosis, Gut 11:764, 1970.
13. Leneman, F., Fierst, S., Gabriel, J. B., and Ingegno, A. P.: Progressive systemic sclerosis of the intestine presenting as malabsorption syndrome, Gastroenterology 42:175, 1962.
14. Marshak, R. H., Ruoff, M., and Lindner, A. E.: Roentgen manifestations of giardiasis, Amer. J. Roentgen. 104:557, 1968.
15. Marshak, R. H., Wolf, B. S., and Adlersberg, D.: Roentgen studies of the small intestine in sprue, Amer. J. Roentgen. 72:380, 1954.
15a. Moss, A. A., Goldberg, H. I., and Brotman, M.: Idiopathic intestinal pseudoobstruction, Amer. J. Roentgen. 115:312, 1972.
16. Nugent, F. W., Ross, J. R., and Hurxthal, L. M.: Intestinal lymphangiectasia, Gastroenterology 47:536, 1964.
17. Padykula, H. A.: Recent functional interpretations of intestinal morphology, Fed. Proc. 21:873, 1962.
18. Panish, J. F.: Experimental blind loop steatorrhea, Gastroenterology 45:394, 1963.
19. Rosson, R. S., and Yesner, R.: Peroral duodenal biopsy in progressive systemic sclerosis, New Eng. J. Med. 272:391, 1965.
20. Ruoff, M., Lindner, A. E., and Marshak, R. H.: Intussusception in sprue, Amer. J. Roentgen. 104:525, 1968.
21. Seligmann, M., Danon, F., Hurez, D., Mihaesco, E., and Preud'homme, J-L.: Alpha-chain disease; a new immunoglobulin abnormality, Science 20:1396, 1968.
22. Sheehy, T. W., Baggs, B., Perez-Santiago, E., and Floch, M. H.: Prognosis of tropical sprue; a study of the effect of folic acid on the intestinal aspect of acute and chronic sprue, Ann. Intern. Med. 57:892, 1962.
23. Sheehy, T. W., Meroney, W. H., Cox, R. S., Jr., and Soler, J. E.: Hookworm disease and malabsorption, Gastroenterology 42:148, 1962.
24. Singleton, J. W., Kern, F., Jr., and Waddell, W. R.: Diarrhea and pancreatic islet cell tumor, Gastroenterology 49:197, 1965.
25. Sleisenger, M. D., Almy, T. P., and Barr, D. P.: The sprue syndrome secondary to lymphoma of the small bowel, Amer. J. Med. 15:666, 1953.
26. Trier, J. S., Phelps, P. C., Eidelman, S., and Rubin, C. E.: Whipple's disease: light and electron microscope correlation of jejunal mucosal histology with antibiotic treatment and clinical status, Gastroenterology 48:684, 1965.
27. Vinnik, I. E., Kern, F., Jr., and Struthers, J. E., Jr.: Malabsorption and the diarrhea of diabetes mellitus, Gastroenterology 43:507, 1962.
28. Waldmann, T. A., Steinfeld, J. L., Dutcher, T. F., Davidson, J. D., and Gordon, R. S., Jr.: The role of the gastrointestinal system in "idiopathic hypoproteinemia," Gastroenterology 41:197, 1961.
29. Wilson, T. H.: Intestinal absorption, Philadelphia, 1962, W. B. Saunders Co.

Neoplasms of the small bowel | 34

Harley C. Carlson
C. Allen Good

Benign neoplasms

It has been said that one of the most important aspects of accurate roentgenology is the correct psychologic state of the roentgenologist conducting the examination. If this is true, there are numerous reasons why the psyche of the roentgenologist may be at low ebb while he is examining the small intestine for benign neoplasms. He is called on to do relatively few of these examinations, since they usually constitute only about 3% to 4% of all gastrointestinal work. The number of neoplasms of the small bowel found during such examination is similarly small, averaging between 1.5% and 6% of all neoplasms found in the gastrointestinal tract.[15,25] In addition, the reliability of an examination of the small bowel in the detection of neoplasms is decidedly less than that of an examination of the colon and stomach. Accuracy rates as low as 40% have been reported. Of the errors that do occur, however, about 40% are caused either by the inattention or by the ignorance of the roentgenologist, for accuracy rates in the detection of neoplasms of the small bowel as high as 90% have been reported from institutions where the examination is carried out with enthusiasm and skill.[9,16]

The roentgenologist should be stimulated by the realization that benign tumors of the small intestine can cause profound morbidity and even mortality. Armed with knowledge of the pathologic forms taken by benign neoplasms as well as with some enthusiasm and persistence in obtaining the fullest possible visualization of all loops of the small intestine, the roentgenologist can perform the examination with acceptable accuracy.

INCIDENCE

As already mentioned, all neoplasms of the small intestine constitute somewhere between 1.5% and 6% of all neoplasms in the gastroin-

testinal tract. This proportion is probably a correct approximation for benign tumors in the small intestine as well. Although malignant tumors are more common than benign tumors in the stomach, and benign tumors are more common than malignant tumors in the colon, in the small intestine the total incidence of benign and malignant tumors is about equal. About a third of benign neoplasms are discovered during operation and about two thirds during autopsy, whereas, in the case of malignant neoplasms, the reverse is true (Table 34-1).[15]

CLINICAL FEATURES

The vast majority of benign neoplasms (about 80%) cause no symptoms, and even when discovered during operation, they are incidental to some more pressing abdominal disease. The commonest symptoms are melena, pain, and weakness. These symptoms arise from two underlying mechanisms: ulceration with hemorrhage and obstruction. Lesions with heavy surface vascularity, such as leiomyomas and hemangiomas, bleed most frequently, but almost every histologic variety of lesion bleeds with some frequency. Obstruction is most commonly caused by intussusception, which may occur anywhere except in that portion of the duodenum that is not freely suspended by mesentery. Complete obstruction resulting from narrowing of the lu-

men by a benign neoplasm itself is almost unknown.

Physical signs of benign neoplasms include pallor, loss of weight, and a palpable abdominal mass. The pallor and loss of weight result from recurrent bleeding, obstruction, and occasional anorexia that may be present even though the patient has no obvious history of bleeding or obstruction. A palpable abdominal mass occurs with surprising frequency (about one of five cases) and may be caused by a large tumor, which is itself palpable; or the mass may be a loop of intussuscepted bowel. It is most uncommon for a benign neoplasm of the duodenum to be palpable. This is true probably because intussusception cannot occur in most of the duodenum and because a lesion in this segment often is not only symptomatic when quite small but is also discoverable by the radiologist with a relatively high rate of accuracy (Table 34-2).*

PATHOLOGIC TYPES

The form taken by any neoplasm in the gastrointestinal tract is dependent on: (1) the degree of invasiveness of the neoplasm, (2) the consistency of neoplastic tissue, and (3) the layer of origin of the neoplasm in the intestinal wall. Since benign neoplasms usually do not invade adjacent tissue, but rather push it aside, they commonly form a somewhat spherical mass. One notable exception is angioma, which may be plaquelike and may infiltrate the entire intestinal wall. The consistency of the neoplastic tissue is important in determining its gross form. Leiomyoma, for example, is usually rather firm and often forms almost perfect spherical masses, whereas hemangioma is almost completely compressible and, therefore, difficult to identify by palpation either at the time of physical examination or at the time of contrast roentgenologic examination. Glandular and lipomatous neoplasms, on the other hand, are firm enough for ready identification at the time of roentgenologic examination but are pliable enough so that they often form ovoid masses that conform to the intestinal lumen.

The layer of origin in the intestinal wall is probably one of the most important factors in

Table 34-1. Benign neoplasms of the small intestine seen at the Mayo Clinic (1938-1958)

Histologic type of neoplasm	Discovery		Total
	At autopsy	At operation	
Leiomyoma	63	56	119
Adenoma	40	27	67
Lipoma	34	19	53
Hemangioma	33	10	43
Other	30	16	46
Total	200	128	328

Table 34-2. Clinical features encountered at the Mayo Clinic in patients with benign tumors of the small intestine

Histologic type of neoplasm	No. cases	Pain, obstruction, or both	Loss of blood	Palpable mass	Loss of weight
Leiomyoma	29	17	23	7	11
Adenoma	11	7	7	2	..
Lipoma	15	13	6	4	3
Hemangioma	10	..	10	..	..
Total	65	37	46	13	14

*See references 1, 4, 6, 7, 9, 11, 12, 15, 16, 17, 23, 25-29, and 36.

determining the gross form taken by benign neoplasms. Mucosal growths always project into the lumen and usually are pedunculated, although the pedicle may be broad and short. On the opposite side of the intestinal wall, lesions arising near the serosa grow into the peritoneal cavity and also may become pedunculated. These serosal projections do not deform the intestinal lumen. Thus, both pedunculated intraluminal and pedunculated and sessile intraperitoneal growths occur, as well as all intermediate forms. Although no classification of these intermediate forms is completely satisfactory, they may be reasonably divided into the following groups: (1) sessile intraluminal tumors, (2) mostly intramural or extramural tu-

mors with only a relatively small portion of the mass projecting into the lumen, and (3) combinations of these forms in lobulated tumors (Fig. 34-1). Of course the determination of the relationship of the neoplastic mass to the lumen and wall of the intestine does not identify its histologic type. However, a determination of this relationship plus the determination of the presence or absence of ulceration, consistency of the mass, and general gross form (lobulated, oval, spherical, and so forth) will constitute a large step toward classification and differential diagnosis.

With the exception of the peritoneum, all varieties of tissues making up the intestinal wall form benign growths. About half of all sympto-

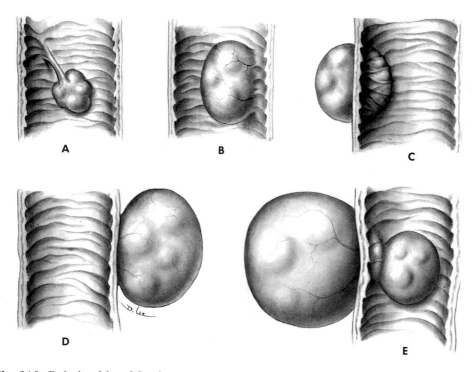

Fig. 34-1. Relationship of benign tumors of the small intestine to the lumen and wall of the intestine. **A,** Pedunculated intraluminal tumor. The mass is movable, and its surface may be smooth or irregular with no visible mucosal pattern. **B,** Sessile intraluminal tumor. The mass is relatively fixed with a broad base of attachment to the wall. The length of this attachment, however, is less than the diameter of the mass. Its surface may be smooth or irregular, and usually no recognizable mucosal pattern is present. **C,** Chiefly intramural or extramural tumor. A relatively small portion of the mass projects into the lumen. Mucosal pattern usually is recognizable over the surface. **D,** Serosal tumor. None of the mass projects into the lumen. The mucosa is not deformed by the mass; it may become pedunculated in the peritoneal cavity. **E,** Combined forms of tumors. Here the large lobule is chiefly extramural and the small lobule, sessile intraluminal.

matic tumors and about a third of all benign tumors of the small intestine arise from smooth muscle. Other tumors less common than leiomyoma and of about equal frequency with one another are tumors of glandular origin (adenomas), lipomas, and hemangiomas. Much less common are lymphangiomas, fibromas, and neurofibromas. In rare instances, osteomas, teratomas, and tumors of mixed cell types occur (Table 34-1).

A most remarkable feature of the distribution of histologic types of benign neoplasms of the small intestine is the low incidence of mucosal tumors, since the small intestine possesses about 90% of the mucosal surface of the alimentary canal. In addition, among this small number it is uncommon to find neoplasms resulting from proliferation of a single cell type. Most of them are of the multiple cell, hamartomatous variety found in Peutz-Jeghers syndrome.*

ROENTGENOLOGIC MANIFESTATIONS
Plain roentgenogram

Evidence of abnormality resulting from high-grade, persistent mechanical obstruction by neoplasm of the small intestine is apparent on the ordinary roentgenogram in about 95% of the instances in which it occurs. An unequivocal diagnosis of high-grade obstruction can be made in 80% of these cases. This type of obstruction of the small intestine, however, is rare, since the most common obstructing mechanism, intussusception, is often transient, and high-grade obstruction by the benign tumor itself is almost unknown. If intussusception persists, however, the tissues become edematous, and high-grade obstruction results. Rarely, a serosal tumor becomes adherent to the wall of the peritoneal cavity, and volvulus can occur around this point of fixation. In extremely rare instances necrosis and perforation of a tumor may occur, resulting in free gas in the peritoneal cavity that is demonstrable on the plain film.

Intussusception

If the use of plain roentgenograms is equivocal for diagnosis of obstruction in symptomatic patients and if there is an absence of clinical evidence of necrosis of the intestinal wall, it may

*See references 1, 11, 13-15, 26, 29, and 36.

be an opportune time for contrast study. Intussusception may be developing but may not be established well enough to cause positive roentgenologic signs on the plain film; the use of contrast study may lead to detection of a lesion that might escape direct visualization in the absence of evidence of intussusception.

Intussusception occurs when the motor action of the intestine propels the tumor forward, and the attached bowel is pulled along (intussusceptum) and enfolded into the receiving loop (the intussuscepiens). This phenomenon usually is associated with pedunculated, intraluminal lesions, but it can also occur with relatively sessile lesions. It is usually a dynamic process and may appear and disappear while the patient is under fluoroscopic observation. The roentgenologic picture that results depends on whether or not the contrast medium passes through an established intussusception, or the intussusception develops after the bowel is filled with contrast medium. When contrast medium passes through an established intussusception, the somewhat dilated lumen narrows abrupty, and the mucosal pattern assumes a longitudinal orientation. At the distal end of the involved segment, the lumen and mucosal pattern assume a normal configuration except for the filling defect caused by the tumor and the intussusceptum. If barium refluxes into the space between the intussusceptum and the intussuscepiens, a so-called coil-spring pattern can be seen in the mucosa of the intussuscepiens distended by the sausage-like filling defect, the intussusceptum (Fig. 34-2, *A*). When intussusception occurs in a segment of intestine already filled with contrast medium, all channels and reflections can be seen clearly. The coil-spring pattern then dominates the picture, and the compressed central channel often is barely evident and occasionally cannot be seen at all (Fig. 34-2, *B*). Intussusception in an adult is presumptive evidence of an intraluminal, usually pedunculated mass, which is often a benign neoplasm.

Contrast medium

Contrast media used in examining the small intestine are either suspensions of barium sulfate or water solutions of iodine-containing organic compounds. A nonflocculating suspension of barium sulfate is probably the most satisfactory. It has the advantages of being dense, resulting

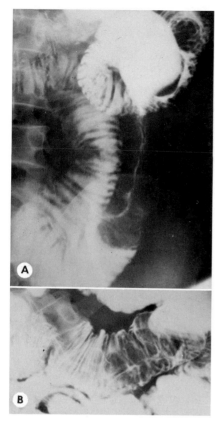

Fig. 34-2. A, Barium passing an established intussusception. The lumen narrows, and the mucosa assumes longitudinal orientation. A filling defect and coil-spring pattern are at the distal end. **B,** Intussusception after barium filling. All reflections are clearly shown, with the coil-spring pattern predominant.

counted for by hypermotility induced by the hypertonic solution and by physical diffusion of the solute. When a contrast medium such as barium sulfate is used, mechanical propulsion is necessary, since diffusion of a suspension does not occur.

In most instances, the patient is simply asked to drink the contrast medium, which is usually about 16 ounces of barium suspension. Mechanical expression of the contrast medium from the stomach into the duodenum often will result in the opportunity to visualize the entire duodenal loop and a large portion of the jejunum in the distended state at the beginning of the examination. From this point on, however, control of the barium column is rather variable and has led some roentgenologists to advocate the use of the so-called small-bowel enema. A tube is passed through the pylorus, and the entire small bowel is distended and visualized as a relatively continuous column. This tube also can be advanced to points of interest, such as obstruction, and contrast medium can be injected into the specific region to opacify it more precisely without its being obscured by adjacent barium-filled loops. The entire small bowel may also be opacified via the colon if the ileocecal valve is patent. This procedure is especially useful in the presence of obstruction of the small intestine, since almost all of the contrast medium will be distal to the point of obstruction and the patient can be expected to pass it spontaneously.

Tumor outline

Deformities of the barium column caused by the tumor itself reflect the gross pathologic forms already described. In general, it is wise to remember that the contrast material makes possible the visualization of the lumen of the intestine and that the lumen must be deformed by the tumor in order for detection and localization of the tumor to be possible. In addition, it must be recalled that the gross form assumed by the tumor does not identify the tissue of origin, that intermediate or combined forms are encountered that are sometimes difficult to classify, and that forms assumed by benign lesions are often identical to those assumed by malignant ones.

Roentgenologic deformities can be divided into the following five groups depending on the relationship of the neoplasm to the lumen and

in clear visualization of the lumen; it has little osmotic activity and therefore does not become diluted by stimulation of the mucosa of the small bowel; and it coats the mucosa intimately. A water-soluble medium has the disadvantage of being hypertonic in concentrations that result in adequate roentgenologic density; therefore, it is rapidly diluted to isotonicity by the secretory activity of the small-bowel mucosa, reducing radiodensity to the point of only faint visualization. However, with the ordinary roentgenogram, which is equivocal for small-bowel obstruction, ingestion of water-soluble medium will enable the roentgenologist to distinguish between complete and incomplete obstruction. Rapid appearance of the medium in the cecum in the presence of incomplete mechanical obstruction or an adynamic ileus is probably ac-

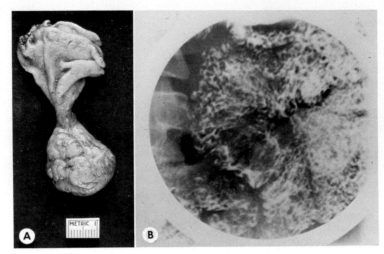

Fig. 34-3. Pedunculated intraluminal adenomatous polyp. **A,** Polyp, pedicle, and adjacent bowel wall. The surface is irregular with no mucosal pattern. **B,** Filling defect of polyp.

wall of the intestine: (1) pedunculated intraluminal, (2) sessile intraluminal, (3) mostly intramural or extramural with only a relatively small portion of the mass projecting into the lumen, (4) chiefly intraperitoneal, and (5) combined forms (Fig. 34-1).

Pedunculated intraluminal tumors

Roentgenologically, a pedunculated intraluminal neoplasm appears as a lucent mass that is completely surrounded by contrast medium with the exception of its attachment to the bowel wall by a stalk that is often invisible (Fig. 34-3). This filling defect remains the same regardless of the plane of visualization, but it can be moved up and down the lumen for a distance approximately double the length of the pedicle. Most benign tumors originating from the mucosa, and some originating from tissues outside the mucosa, have this form. The mass may be spherical and, if large enough, may distend the lumen of the bowel, or it may be relatively oval and conform to the shape of the lumen. The surface of the mass may be smooth or irregular, and a small-bowel mucosal pattern is never recognizable overlying this surface. Ulceration may occur, and if the crater is deep enough or large enough to affect the contour of the mass or to retain contrast material, it can be recognized roentgenologically.

Sessile intraluminal tumors

In the sessile intraluminal variety of tumors most of the mass appears to project within the lumen when viewed in profile, but there is no stalk. The lesion cannot be moved up and down the lumen, and the diameter of the intraluminal projection is greater than the length of the attachment (Fig. 34-4). Face-on views of this type of tumor give the same appearance as the pedunculated variety. In rare instances, benign mucosal tumors may assume this form, but it is usually caused by masses arising from tissues outside the mucosa. The surface may be smooth or irregular, and no mucosal pattern is visible on the surface of those tumors of mucosal origin or over the surface of most of those tumors of submucosal origin. Ulceration is recognized in the same manner as in the case of the pedunculated lesion (Fig. 34-5).

Tumors mostly intramural or extramural

If the mass is mostly intramural or extramural a curved filling defect is seen when the lumen filled with contrast medium is viewed in profile. The base of the tumor is greater than the diameter of any part projecting into the lumen. All of such masses arise from tissue outside the mucosa, and, therefore, it is common to see a small-bowel mucosal pattern overlying the mass. As the mass enlarges, the mucosa assumes a stretched appearance and may ultimately become completely effaced (Fig. 34-6). By far the most common histologic type of tumor causing this defect is the leiomyoma. With this variety central necrosis is likely to develop. A subsequent development is deep ulceration that can frequently be recognized roentgenologically as

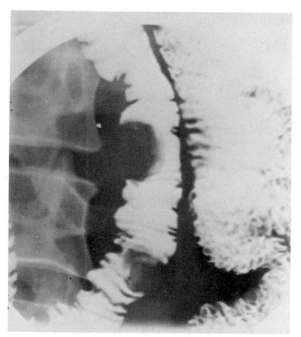

Fig. 34-4. Profile of filling defects caused by two sessile intraluminal leiomyomas.

a relatively large collection of barium extending beyond the anticipated limit of the bowel lumen.

Tumors chiefly serosal

If the mass projects chiefly from the serosal surface and is, therefore, in large part, intraperitoneal, no deformity of the barium column is seen until the mass assumes generous proportions. At that time its presence may be implied by the displacement of adjacent opacified loops, as a blank space on the roentgenogram (Fig. 34-7). Most of these lesions are leiomyomas and often undergo central necrosis. This necrotis material may enter the lumen of the bowel through a small ulceration in the overlying mucosa, forming a huge crater that may be recognized when filled with barium suspension and gas during the roentgenologic examination. Rarely, a fistula may be identified between adjacent portions of the bowel or between its lumen and the peritoneal cavity.

Combined form tumors

Gross lobulation occurs in neoplasms of the small bowel, especially those of smooth muscle origin. When this happens, combinations of previously mentioned forms may be visualized. For example, one lobule may be sessile intraluminal, and another larger lobule, chiefly intraperitoneal, or, in much of the duodenum,

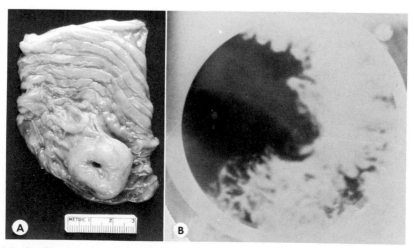

Fig. 34-5. Sessile intraluminal leiomyoma. **A,** Specimen with no mucosal pattern on surface and a rather deep crater. **B,** Profile of filling defect with barium extending into crater.

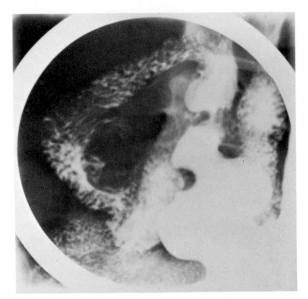

Fig. 34-6. Profile of broad filling defect caused by leiomyoma, chiefly intramural and extramural. The surface of the lesion does not show a mucosal pattern, but that of the overlying bowel can be seen.

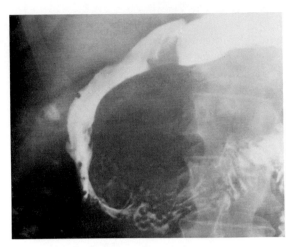

Fig. 34-8. Lobulated smooth muscle tumor. The large lobule located between the duodenum and the pancreas showed considerable mitotic activity and was considered to be a sarcoma. A smaller lobule caused the smooth sessile intraluminal filling defect.

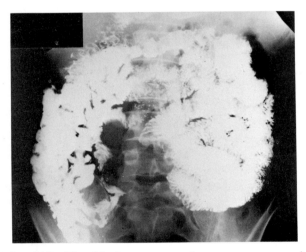

Fig. 34-7. The blank space on the roentgenogram is caused by a smooth muscle tumor projecting almost entirely from the serosa, although to the right a short segment of intestinal wall is fixed to the mass and is deformed.

located between the intestinal wall and the adjacent organs. These are sometimes called "dumbbell tumors," and the roentgenologic examination may conspicuously reveal only the intraluminal portion of the tumor (Fig. 34-8).

It should be emphasized that the chief responsibility of the roentgenologist is the detec-

tion and localization of the neoplasm. Its specific histologic identity is commonly not apparent, although its general layer of origin can usually be identified. Although it is often possible to make a definite diagnosis of malignant neoplasm of the small intestine, it usually is impossible to make a diagnosis of benign neoplasm with complete assurance, since the gross form assumed by many malignant neoplasms is identical to that assumed by benign varieties.*

HISTOLOGIC TYPES
Leiomyoma
Incidence and location

Leiomyoma is the most common benign neoplasm of the small bowel, constituting about a third of all benign lesions and about a half of all symptomatic benign lesions. Approximately equal numbers of cases are found during operation and during autopsy. Lesions are usually single (about 97% of cases), and the total number of lesions is about evenly distributed in the three segments of the small intestine (Fig. 34-9; Table 34-3). However, if one considers the rela-

*See references 2, 9, 15-18, 23, 29, 33, 34, 36, and 37.

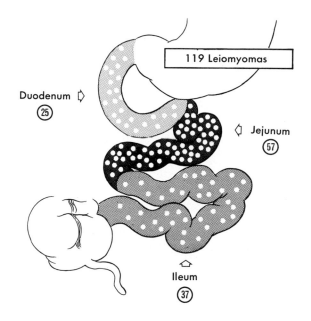

Fig. 34-9. Distribution of 119 leiomyomas found among 328 benign neoplasms in the small intestine.

Table 34-3. Site of benign tumors of the small intestine

Histologic type	Duode-num	Jejunum	Ileum	Total cases
Leiomyoma	25	57	37	119
Adenoma	14	24	29	67
Lipoma	17	9	27	53
Hemangioma	1	24	18	43
Other	11	14	21	46
Total	68	128	130	328

tively short length of the duodenum and calculates the occurrence rate on the basis of unit length, leiomyomas occur seven times more frequently in the duodenum than in the jejunum or ileum.

Pathologic findings

Microscopically, leiomyomas consist of spindle-shaped smooth muscle cells, the nuclei of which are often palisaded. Tumors projecting chiefly on the serosal surface generally attain a larger size than those projecting intraluminally. Of all benign smooth-muscle tumors occurring in the small intestine, about half are smaller than 5 cm., about a fourth range from 5 to 10 cm., and about a fourth are larger than 10 cm. Their distribution with respect to location in the intestinal wall is rather unfortunate for the roentgenologist, since about half project chiefly from the serosal surface and may actually be pedunculated. Only about a fifth project chiefly into the lumen, and these may also be pedunculated.

Pedunculated leiomyomas occur intraluminally and intraperitoneally with approximately equal frequency. About a tenth of the growths are chiefly intramural, and slightly more than a tenth are lobulated, giving rise to combined forms. The surface often exhibits a rich blood supply, visible grossly, and the central portion of the tumor is often virtually avascular. This undoubtedly accounts for their tendency to become necrotic and form craters that are much larger deep within the tumor than they are on the surface. The rich surface vascularity also accounts for their tendency to be associated with rather massive hemorrhage.

The intraluminal lesions usually give rise to intussusception if located in the jejunum or ileum, but almost never do so when located in the duodenum. The vast majority of patients who have symptoms show evidence of tumor ulceration. The intramural and serosal forms are larger and tend to be necrotic, to ulcerate on the mucosal surface, to form cavities and fistulas, and to cause secondary infection.

Clinical features

Combined surgical and autopsy series showed that tumors give rise to intestinal symptoms or physical signs in only about a fourth of all cases. Most lesions are found incidentally at operation or at autopsy. A palpable mass is present in about a fifth of symptomatic patients, a finding that is dependent on the size of the tumor itself as well as on the presence of intussusception. Leiomyomas in the duodenum are almost never palpable (about 2%), probably because intussusception is not possible except in the most proximal portion of the duodenum. In addition these lesions in the duodenum tend to ulcerate and bleed when relatively small, and the patients are, therefore, symptomatic when the lesion is much smaller. Finally, roentgenologic examination of the duodenum is more accurate than that of the jejunum and ileum, since filling is under better control and palpation of the duodenal loop by the roentgenologist is possible, leading to the early detection of these growths.

About half of the patients who have symptoms experience pain that may be caused by the inflammatory reaction accompanying gross ulceration and necrosis or that may be secondary to intussusception and obstruction. Hemorrhage occurs in slightly more than half of them. It is usually massive and intermittent, especially when associated with smaller intramural or intraluminal forms. Larger intramural and serosal lesions that cavitate, communicate with the intestinal lumen, and bleed, tend to continue toward exsanguination. The patient has a history either of melena or of grossly bloody stools but rarely of hemoptysis. Loss of weight and nausea occur somewhat less commonly (Table 34-2).

Roentgenologic manifestations

The roentgenologic manifestations of leiomyomas reflect the gross pathologic forms and changes already described. Roentgenologic examination is moderately effective in detecting these lesions. Of all patients who have both malignant and benign smooth muscle tumors of the small intestine, the diagnosis of neoplasm can be made in about two thirds by means of conventional barium examination of the small intestine. In about one fifth, the histologic type of neoplasm can be suggested. Undoubtedly the accuracy rate for benign neoplasms alone would be somewhat lower, since they are smaller and subject to less extensive secondary pathologic change.

Most leiomyomas project chiefly from the serosal surface and cause roentgenologically detectable change only when they are large enough to cause displacement of adjacent barium-filled loops of small intestine, which appear as blank spaces on the roentgenogram (Fig. 34-7). Since these lesions are subject to necrosis and communication with the lumen through relatively small ulcers on the mucosal surface, a large cavity filled with barium and gas may appear as a small deformity of the adjacent bowel on examination with contrast medium. Those lesions that project into the lumen but are intramural, appear as round, filling defects when viewed face-on, but appear as curved indentations into the lumen when viewed in profile. If the mass is largely intramural and extramural, the base

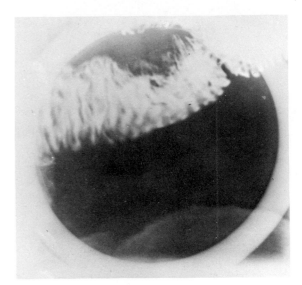

Fig. 34-10. Profile of broad filling defect caused by chiefly intramural and extramural leiomyoma with mucosal pattern visible on the surface of the mass.

of the indentation into the lumen is wider than the projection into the lumen. If the mass is only slightly intramural, its center may be seen within the lumen with a sessile attachment, which is shorter than the diameter of the mass, projecting into the lumen (Fig. 34-4). Intestinal mucosal folds may be visible over the filling defect, especially in forms that are chiefly intramural and extramural (Fig. 34-10). In forms that are largely intraluminal, the mucosal folds become almost completely effaced and the pattern unrecognizable.

Contrast medium is commonly retained in a relatively small portion of mucosal ulceration communicating with a relatively deep pit, a situation that is characteristic of leiomyoma. This pit may become a large cavity and may communicate with a second mucosal ulceration or with the peritoneal cavity forming a fistulous tract. These fistulous tracts associated with benign lesions are usually less than 1.5 cm. in length. Sarcomatous change cannot be excluded from diagnostic considerations by means of x-ray examination alone. In somewhat less than one tenth of cases the leiomyoma may become pedunculated within the lumen. Its outline may be irregular, and mucosal folds are not recognizable on the surface (Fig. 34-11). Ulcer pits develop rather frequently, and occasionally they can be recognized by their retention of barium

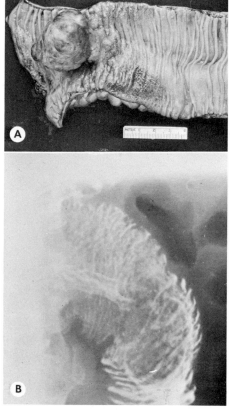

Fig. 34-11. Pedunculated intraluminal leiomyoma. **A,** Polyp, pedicle, and adjacent intestinal bowel wall. Note the irregular surface with no visible mucosal pattern. **B,** Intussuscepting leiomyoma.

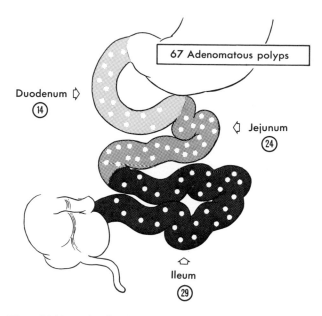

Fig. 34-12. Distribution of sixty-seven adenomatous polyps found among 328 benign neoplasms in the small intestine.

near the surface of the lesion. Those that occur in the jejunum and ileum usually cause intussusception; those in the duodenum almost never do so. These pedunculated lesions are indistinguishable from pedunculated intraluminal lesions of other histologic types.*

Glandular tumors
Incidence and location

Benign glandular tumors are about half as common as smooth-muscle tumors (Table 34-1). They are found in approximately equal numbers in each of the three segments of the small intestine (Fig. 34-12; Table 34-3). However, when the relative lengths of the segments of small intestine are considered, the incidence is

_____
*See references 2, 15, 26, 28, 32-34, 36, and 37.

several times higher in the duodenum than in the jejunum and ileum. This is especially true if discrete, dominantly polypoid lesions composed of Brunner's glands are included in this category, since all of these lesions occur in the duodenum.

Pathologic findings

Some understanding of the microscopic anatomy of the glandular tumors is extremely important in appreciating their significance. Gannon and associates carried out a notable pathologic study of polypoid glandular lesions of the small intestine in sixty cases.[13] In forty-six cases the lesions were of the hamartomatous variety seen in Peutz-Jeghers syndrome; in only eight were the lesions adenomatous polyps composed of a single cell type, and in six the lesions were polypoid gastric heterotopic tumors.

Of the hamartomatous polyps in forty-six cases in the same study, those in twenty-seven were found during operation and those in nineteen were found during autopsy. Characteristics noted on microscopic examination were the presence of all three types of epithelial cells of the small bowel (vacuolated goblet cells, columnar absorptive cells, and dark granular Paneth's cells) and mimicry of intestinal villi, as well as inter-

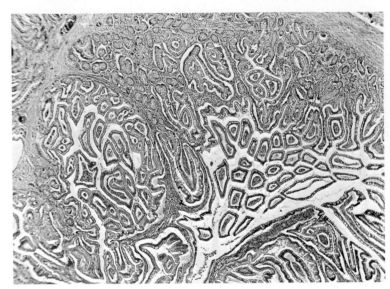

Fig. 34-13. Section of hamartomatous polyp from small intestine showing formation of villi, interspersed smooth muscle, and all three epithelial cell types (goblet cell, absorptive cell, Paneth's cell). (Hematoxylin and eosin; ×35.)

spersed smooth muscle and connective tissue (Fig. 34-13). In addition, the muscularis propria at the base of the lesion was often interspersed with islands of intestinal glands that had sometimes been interpreted as evidence of invasion and, hence, of malignancy. However, in no case was there gross tumefaction in the wall at the base of the lesions, and there was no instance of distant spread. These growths are best considered developmental anomalies with only slight malignant potential. Almost half of the group with hamartomatous polyps had multiple gastrointestinal polyps (twenty-one patients); about half of these had hamartomatous growths in the stomach, and about three fourths had hamartomatous colonic lesions. In eight of the twenty-one patients, diffuse involvement with innumerable polypoid lesions of varying sizes in a limited segment of intestine was found, and in seven of the eight, characteristic pigmentation of the skin and oral mucosa associated with Peutz-Jeghers syndrome was observed. Scattered multiple lesions were present in thirteen patients, and only two of these had characteristic Peutz-Jeghers pigmentation. Of nine patients having this interesting syndrome, three reported that other members of their families had characteristic "freckles." None of the twenty-five patients who had only a single hamartomatous polyp in the small intestine had characteristic oral or mucosal pigmentation.

Of the eight patients in Gannon's material who had a single, true adenomatous polyp composed of a single cell type, similar to that which is so common in the colon, one had cellular atypia and one had adenocarcinoma in situ. These lesions, then, may be regarded as having some malignant potential, but the potential seems small and the lesions are extremely rare.

The polypoid gastric heterotopic tumors in the small intestine of six patients contained mucous, chief, and parietal cells and were ectopic hamartomatous lesions. The growths were in the duodenum in two patients, in the jejunum in two, and in the ileum in two, and they were as large as 5 cm. in diameter.

Over a 20-year period at the Mayo Clinic, five pedunculated polypoid lesions consisting of a collection of Brunner's glands, which emptied into the normal overlying duodenal mucosa covering the glandular mass, were found in the duodenum. The largest was 6 cm. in diameter.[15]

Clinical features

Clinically, there is little to distinguish these lesions from other benign tumors of the small bowel (Table 34-2). Since most of these glandular lesions are pedunculated and intraluminal, intussusception is common when they are located in the jejunum and ileum. About two thirds of the symptomatic patients experience pain or obstruction, about two thirds have a history or laboratory evidence of loss of blood, and about one fifth have a palpable mass. Those patients with multiple hamartomatous polyps in the small intestine often have characteristic skin and mucosal pigmentation, especially if the lesions are of the diffuse form involving a segment

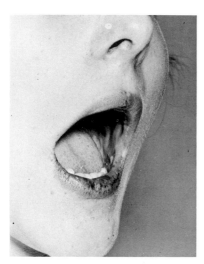

Fig. 34-14. Pigmentation of facial skin and oral mucosa of a patient with multiple hamartomatous polyps in the small intestine and colon.

of small intestine. This pigmentation may occur on the mucous membrane of the lips, cheeks, gums, or palate, or on the skin of the lips, of the nose, around the eyes, on the fingers, and on the toes (Fig. 34-14). It appears as dark brown or black specks, which represent deposits of melanin. These patients often have a history of multiple bowel resections, which often have been undertaken because of the mistaken notion that these lesions are malignant or have malignant potential, and a history or roentgenologic evidence of polyps in the stomach and colon.

Roentgenologic manifestations

Most benign glandular neoplasms in the small intestine manifest themselves roentgenologically as intraluminal pedunculated masses. They are most easily, and therefore most frequently, found in the duodenum, the proximal portion of the jejunum, and the terminal part of the ileum, since in these regions the loops are more easily separable, distensible, and available for manual palpation by the roentgenologist. Intussusception may be observed, and if it is reduced, the lesion may be visualized and identified as an intraluminal mass. If there are multiple lesions in the small intestine or if the patient is known to have polyps in the colon or stomach, the radiologist would do well to personally inspect the

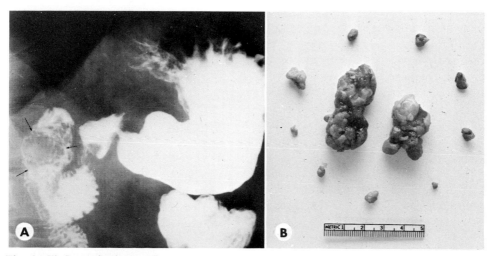

Fig. 34-15. Peutz-Jeghers polyps. **A,** Intraluminal filling defect in duodenum. **B,** During operation two large polypoid growths and a number of smaller ones were removed. Innumerable smaller lesions were left.

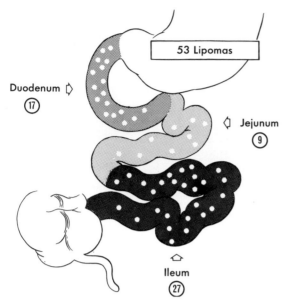

Fig. 34-16. Distribution of fifty-three lipomas found among 328 benign neoplasms in the small intestine.

appropriate areas of skin and mucous membrane for evidence of characteristic Peutz-Jeghers pigmentation. The diffuse type of polypoid involvement of a segment of small intestine is usually appreciable only by visualization of the larger polypoid lesions, since most of the small lesions escape detection (Fig. 34-15). A specific diagnosis of this syndrome and a knowledge of the hamartomatous, relatively nonmalignant nature of the so-called neoplasms by the radiologist may save the patient nutritionally crippling resection of the bowel, since only local excision is usually necessary to prevent intussusception and hemorrhage. Hamartomatous polyps can only be suspected on the basis of roentgenologic examination, however, and the diagnosis must be confirmed by finding the characteristic pigmented spots on the skin and mucous membrane.*

Lipoma
Incidence and location

Lipomas occur only slightly less frequently than glandular tumors and are found more frequently in the ileum (one half) and duodenum (one third) than in the jejunum (Fig. 34-16 and Table 34-3). The lesions are found during operation in about one fourth of the cases and during

*See references 8, 13, 15, 18, 30, and 31.

autopsy in about three fourths. Of those tumors found surgically, about a third are incidental findings. In symptomatic patients lipomas are found in the small intestine only about a fifth as frequently as in the colon.

Pathologic findings

Microscopically, lipomas in the small bowel appear similar to those in other locations, consisting of large cells filled with fat and supported by a framework of fibrous septa. The growths arise in the submucosa, and, as they protrude into the lumen, they are covered with intestinal epithelium. The surface usually becomes extremely smooth as the growth enlarges. Although they are usually relatively small, they may measure up to 6 cm. in diameter. The mass usually projects into the lumen and has a sessile attachment to the bowel wall, although occasionally it may become pedunculated and cause intussusception. Ulceration of the overlying mucosa occurs in about two thirds of the symptomatic patients and slightly more than two thirds of these patients experience intussusception.

Clinical features

Only about a sixth of the small intestinal lipomas that are found are associated with intestinal symptoms. Pain, characteristic of intermittent obstruction of the small bowel, occurs in about three fourths of symptomatic patients and almost always is associated with intussusception, although a rare instance of a tumor becoming detached and impacted in the ileum has been reported. About a third of symptomatic patients have a history or laboratory evidence of loss of blood, but ulceration of the lesion occurs in almost twice this number, reflecting the relative avascularity of the tumor. About a fourth have a palpable mass, and usually it is associated with intussusception (Table 34-2).

Roentgenologic manifestations

Lipomas of the small bowel are discovered rather infrequently by the radiologist, probably because the lesions are of relatively small size and their consistency is such that the mass itself is rather easily deformed even when palpated with contrast medium overlying it. Those that are discovered are almost all in the duodenum and terminal part of the ileum for reasons al-

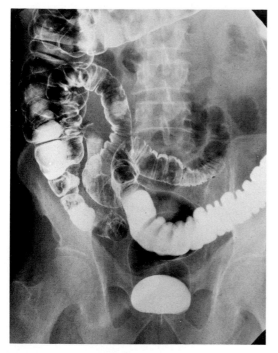

Fig. 34-17. Lipoma in the terminal portion of the ileum demonstrated by a double-contrast medium during a barium enema. Note the smooth outline and lack of mucosal pattern on the surface.

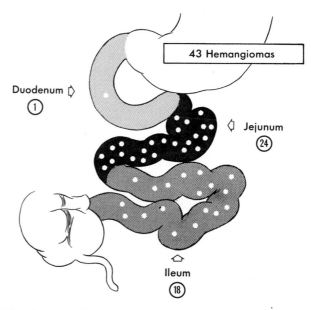

Fig. 34-18. Distribution of forty-three hemangiomas found among 328 benign neoplasms in the small intestine.

ready mentioned. The mass is usually seen as an intraluminal filling defect with a smooth surface and a broad base of attachment indicating likely intramural origin (Fig. 34-17). Those that become pedunculated may be associated with intussusception in the jejunum and ileum.*

Hemangioma
Incidence and location

Hemangiomas occur somewhat less frequently than do grandular and lipomatous tumors (Table 34-1). Unlike almost all other histologic varieties, however, hemangiomas develop more often in the small intestine than in the stomach or the colon; about two thirds of all gastrointestinal vascular lesions are found in the small bowel. They are rare in the duodenum (about 2%) and most common in the jejunum (about 55%) and ileum (42%) (Fig. 34-18; Table 34-3).

---

*See references 15, 22, 26, 35, and 36.

Pathologic findings

Microscopically, hemangiomas appear as cavernous, blood-filled, endothelial-lined spaces or as masses of capillaries or mixtures of these two. The vascular mass may be covered by mucosal epithelium or serosa, or it may be interspersed throughout the muscular wall of the bowel. In about two thirds of cases, multiple, small (less than 1 cm. in diameter), cavernous hemangiomas are located on either serosal or mucosal surface or both. Rarely, these are mixed cavernous and capillary types. In about a seventh of the cases, single polypoid growths, usually of the cavernous variety, are found on the mucosal surface. They are often larger than the multiple lesions and are associated with a high incidence (80%) of hemorrhage, or, less commonly, with obstruction associated with intussusception. More unusual (about 3%) is the diffuse, expansive type involving a segment or segments of the intestine. The Rendu-Osler-Weber syndrome is a rare complex characterized by (1) repeated hemorrhage from the nose or mouth, (2) telangiectatic lesions of the mucosa of the nasal or oral cavities, and (3) familial occurrence. Two varieties of intestinal lesions develop in this complex: spider telangiectasia and multiple nodular angiomas measuring about 1 to 3 mm. in diameter. By 1961, twenty-eight cases with visceral lesions had been reported in the literature.[14]

Clinical features

Surprisingly, five sixths of the patients with intestinal hemangiomas are asymptomatic, and the lesions arc found incidentally during autopsy or operation. One would think that these multiple cavernous vascular lesions with thin walls would be rather subject to physical and chemical trauma and subsequent hemorrhage. Perhaps their compressibility and rarity in the duodenum, with its wide fluctuations in tonicity and pH, explain this failure to cause more symptoms. Hemorrhage, usually, recurrent and unexplained by clinical, laboratory, and roentgenographic investigation and even by laparotomy, occurs in almost all symptomatic patients (Table 34-2). Symptoms of obstruction occasionally occur, usually in association with the larger, single polypoid variety of hemangioma. A palpable mass is reported with variable frequency, occurring in as high as 25% in one series and in none of the symptomatic patients in another. Some patients who have unexplained gastrointestinal hemorrhage exhibit dermal hemangiomas that may suggest the nature of the intestinal lesion. At least one case has been reported in which small intestinal hemangiomas were associated with the freckle pigmentation of Peutz-Jeghers syndrome.[3]

Roentgenologic manifestations

Roentgenologic examination of the small intestine rarely shows evidence of hemangioma, probably because of the consistency of the lesion, which is almost completely compressible and easily obliterated by palpation. The masses are usually relatively small and do not cause rigid deformity of the intestinal wall or mucosa. This failure of roentgenologic detection is not too surprising in view of the fact that they are sometimes missed at the time of surgical exploration. When they are visualized roentgenologically, they may be seen as (1) multiple, sessile, compressible intraluminal filling defects (Fig. 34-19) (2) nodular-appearing, segmental mucosal ab-

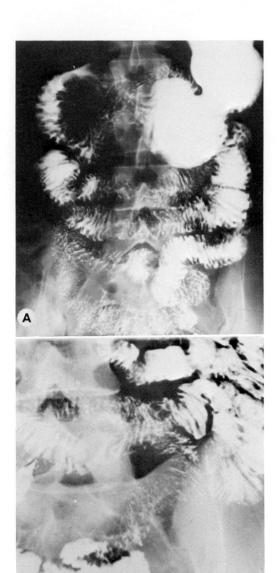

Fig. 34-19. A and **B,** Multiple smooth, sessile filling defects caused by hemangiomas in the duodenum and jejunum.

normalities, or (3) phleboliths occurring in the wall of an involved segment, which may have the nodular abnormal mucosal pattern.*

Other benign neoplasms

Since all types of tissue found in the wall of the small intestine, with the exception of peri-

---

*See references 3, 6, 10, 14, 15, 19, 24, 26, and 38.

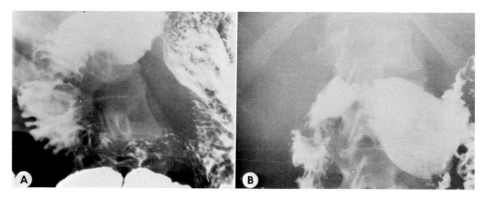

Fig. 34-20. Filling defects from sessile neurofibroma, **A,** and from pedunculated intraluminal ganglioneuroma in the second portion of the duodenum, **B.**

toneum, form neoplasms, several smaller but significant groups of tumors may be encountered, such as those made up of lymphatic vessels, neural elements, and connective tissue (fibroma, osteoma). In one series of 328 cases of benign small intestinal neoplasm, sixteen lymphangiomas, eleven fibromas, and five tumors made up of nerve tissue were reported. Various lesions derived from epithelial and connective tissue elements and mixtures thereof were exhibited in nine cases.[15]

The clinical manifestations of these lesions depend mainly on their gross form. Those that project into the lumen may ulcerate and bleed. If the lesion becomes pedunculated, intussusception often occurs, leading to obstruction and a palpable mass.

The roentgenologic manifestations are similar to those described for other neoplasms and are dependent on the gross form of the neoplasm.

Neurogenic tumors

Neurofibromas may be single or multiple and may occur as pedunculated or sessile filling defects in the barium column (Fig. 34-20). About a third are symptomatic, and symptoms are usually associated with intussusception. Some disagreement persists regarding the histologic classification of these lesions containing neural elements, and it is almost certain that many lesions considered by some pathologists to be primarily of nerve tissue origin are considered by others to be primarily of smooth muscle origin and vice versa.*

---

*See references 5, 15, 20, 26, and 27.

Lymphangioma

Lymphangioma of the small intestine is about half as common as hemangioma. About half are symptomatic and are associated with pain and obstruction, a palpable mass, and, rarely, hemorrhage. No characteristic roentgenologic picture has been reported.[11,15,26,27]

PSEUDOTUMORS

A number of pathologic processes result in nonneoplastic masses in the small intestine. Roentgenologically, they may not be distinguishable from neoplasms, but the patient's history may help in the differentiation. Endometrioma occurs in women during the age span of fertility and may be suspected on the basis of physical findings on pelvic examination. Cysts may be lined with endothelium (Fig. 34-21, *A*) or may represent duplication of the intestine; they are usually indistinguishable from intramural neoplasms. Occasionally, a duplication communicates with the principal lumen and may fill with contrast medium. Aberrant pancreatic tissue may be seen as a sessile or even as a pedunculated intraluminal filling defect and cannot be distinguished from other similar lesions, unless one is able to recognize a "dimple" of retained barium in the duct, in which case the histologic nature of the mass can be stated with a high degree of confidence (Fig. 34-21, *B*). Rarely, a Meckel diverticulum may become inverted and may result in a filling defect in the lumen of the small intestine or lead to intussusception. Hyperplasia of Brunner's glands usually occurs in a diffuse form involving the proximal portion of the duodenum and results in a

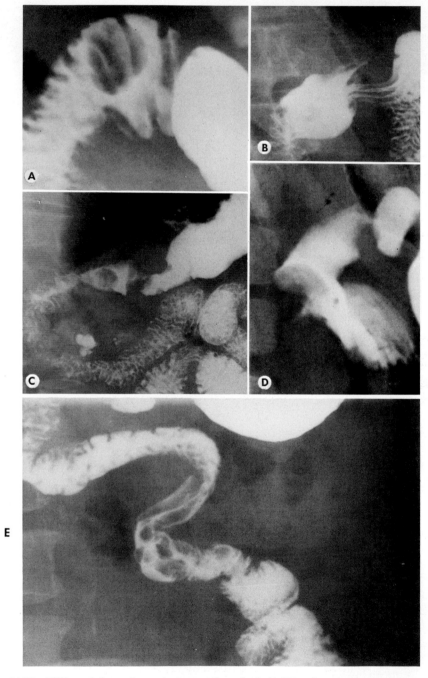

Fig. 34-21. Filling defects from intramural endothelial-lined cyst, **A,** aberrant pancreatic tissue, **B,** adenoma of Brunner's gland, **C,** hematoma in the wall of the duodenum in a child who had been run over by a tractor, **D,** and focal varices, **E,** in the jejunum of a man with unexplained loss of blood.

rather nodular appearance of the duodenal mucosa. Occasionally, however, focal hyperplasia, which results in a sessile or even pedunculated intraluminal filling defect, can be recognized roentgenologically. Whether these lesions should be considered as adenomas or focal hyperplasia is a matter of preference (Fig. 34-21, *C*). Hematoma of the small intestine gives the appearance of an intramural tumor with intact overlying mucosa, but it is seen only in patients on anticoagulant therapy or in patients who have experienced recent abdominal trauma (Fig. 34-21, *D*). Focal varices in the submucosa may protrude into the lumen and resemble a lobulated neoplasm (Fig. 34-21, *E*).[15,21,22]

COMMENT ON DIAGNOSIS AND TECHNIQUE

The major role of the radiologist in the study of benign neoplasms of the small intestine is to detect the presence of such abnormalities and to determine their location. In this effort the same diagnostic criteria must be applied as are applied in the study of any segment of the intestine, that is, the determination of (1) the size and distensibility of the lumen, (2) the gross mobility of the organ, (3) the presence of filling defects projecting into the lumen, and (4) the presence or absence of persistent collections of contrast medium representing ulceration and necrosis.

To this end, segments of small intestine must be visualized separately and compressed manually in as complete a manner as possible. In most instances this requires fluoroscopic examination, vigorous manual manipulation of the loops of bowel, and frequent evaluation of the patient, probably at least every 15 minutes early in the examination. This is especially true with the use of a finely divided barium suspension, when it is not uncommon to visualize the cecum within 30 minutes after oral ingestion in normal persons. Most important for the radiologist are high degrees of interest and concentration on the conduct of the examination.

The actual identification of the lesion is usually a somewhat secondary function. Although it is often impossible, occasionally it can be accomplished with disarming ease. To identify the lesion, the roentgenologist must determine: the location of the mass with respect to the intestinal wall and mucosa; whether or not the lesion is solitary or multiple; and the shape (spherical, oval), surface form (smooth, irregular), and consistency of the mass, as well as the presence and form of ulceration. If this essential information is combined with knowledge of the incidence and occurrence of neoplastic lesions of the small intestine, of the pathologic findings and clinical implications of the lesions, and of a reasonable amount of clinical information, a likely diagnosis and useful suggestions for management of the case will result.

Malignant neoplasms

INCIDENCE

If one considers all neoplasms of the small intestine discovered at surgical intervention and at autopsy, malignant neoplasms are almost as common as benign tumors. More than two thirds of all malignant neoplasms, however, are discovered at operation, and approximately a third are found at autopsy. In the case of benign neoplasms, the reverse is true. If one considers only those neoplasms that result in clinical manifestations, malignant neoplasms of the small bowel are three times as common as benign neoplasms. Since roentgenologic examination of the small intestine is usually undertaken only in circumstances that are rather suggestive of disease, it follows that the overwhelming majority of neoplasms discovered at examination will be malignant (Table 34-4).[52]

CLINICAL FEATURES

About two thirds of all malignant neoplasms produce clinical manifestations as compared to

Table 34-4. Malignant neoplasms of the small intestine seen at the Mayo Clinic (1938-1958)

Histologic type of neoplasm	*Discovery*		*Total*
	At autopsy	*At operation*	
Carcinoid tumor	85	67	152
Adenocarcinoma	8	77	85
Malignant lymphoma	8	47	55
Leiomyosarcoma	1	34	35
Other	2	2	4
Total	104	227	331

about a fifth of the benign neoplasms. If one excludes carcinoid tumors, which are a rather special type of malignant neoplasm and which are symptomatic in less than a third of cases, more than 90% of the remaining malignant neoplasms exhibit clinical manifestations prior to discovery. However, since carcinoid tumors usually should be considered malignant, they are included in this study.

In patients with intestinal malignant disease, pain or other evidence of obstruction is present in about four out of five, loss of weight in more than two out of three, evidence of loss of blood in about half, and a palpable abdominal mass in about half of the patients.

Pain is usually the result of obstruction, which is caused most commonly by narrowing of the lumen as a result of infiltration of the tumor and, frequently, by the fibrotic response of the intestinal wall to this infiltrating tumor. If the gross form of the neoplasm is polypoid or pedunculated, this can lead to intussusception, just as in the case of benign tumors, which are found in these forms somewhat more frequently than are malignant tumors. Ulceration is common in all forms of malignant tumors, except for carcinoid, and this leads to loss of blood especially in adenocarcinoma, leiomyosarcoma, and somewhat less frequently in lymphoma. Evidence of loss of blood is almost never found in patients with carcinoid tumors.

Loss of weight is attributed both to obstruction of the small intestine and to ulceration; this manifestation, therefore, is also common in malignant tumors.

A palpable mass may be caused by intussusception of a small intraluminal tumor, as is true with benign neoplasms; more often, however, it is the result of an accumulation of the abnormal tumor tissue itself. The tissue may be the primary growth, as in leiomyosarcoma, or it may result chiefly from metastasis of the primary growth, as in carcinoids. In some cases the mass is a combination of these two features, a typical example being lymphoma of the small intestine (Table 34-5).[44,52]

PATHOLOGIC TYPES

Although benign tumors enlarge and merely displace adjacent normal tissues and organs, most malignant neoplasms are characterized by infiltration and invasion of adjoining normal tissue. Thus, the form taken by a malignant tumor is determined less by its layer of origin in the intestinal wall and more by its invasiveness together with the response of the intestinal wall to this invasion. Since the invasiveness of different neoplasms is widely variable, as is response of normal tissue to neoplasms, the result is a spectrum of gross forms, which range from those that may appear clearly benign and seem to be characterized simply by displacement of adjacent tissue to those that are extensively invasive.

Of the tumors that are invasive, some, such as adenocarcinoma, incite a rather vigorous fibrotic response in the intestinal wall resulting in rather rapid narrowing of the lumen of the bowel before the tumor becomes extensive (Fig. 34-22). Other infiltrating neoplasms, such as lymphoma, are extremely cellular and do not incite a fibrotic response; as a result, the lumen is usually not compromised until the growth is extremely extensive. This bulky cellular growth tends to undergo necrosis, resulting in ulceration and actual widening of the lumen, which gives the lesion a rather characteristic gross appearance (Fig. 34-23). Although all malignant

Table 34-5. Clinical features encountered at the Mayo Clinic in patients with malignant tumors of the small intestine

Histologic type of neoplasm	Number of cases	Pain, obstruction, or both	Loss of blood	Palpable mass	Loss of weight
Carcinoid tumor	49	28	——	21	29
Adenocarcinoma	77	69	54	25	66
Malignant lymphoma	54	51	19	30	36
Leiomyosarcoma	34	17	28	19	22
Total	214	165	101	95	153

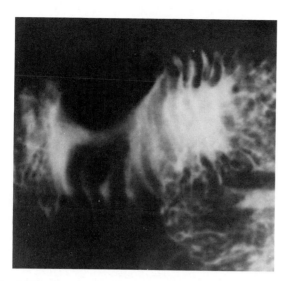

Fig. 34-22. Almost annular, short adenocarcinoma of the proximal portion of the jejunum, with ulcerated surface and considerable narrowing of the lumen.

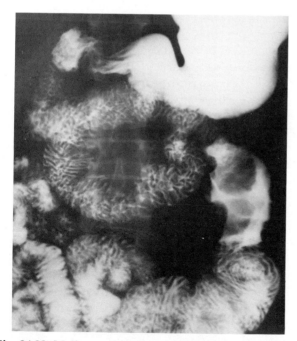

Fig. 34-23. Malignant lymphoma of the proximal portion of jejunum, which is long, is extensively ulcerated, and has a rather nodular surface resulting in a widened lumen.

tumors of the small bowel are inclined to invade and metastasize, the form of metastasis varies and in many cases determines the actual clinical manifestations of the neoplasm. For example, leiomyosarcomas almost never metastasize to lymph nodes and the blood-borne metastasis usually deposits outside of the abdominal cavity. At the other end of the spectrum, carcinoid tumors almost never invade and destroy the overlying mucosa of the small intestine but do invade the intestinal wall and extend into the mesentery. They metastasize to regional nodes, and it is this extension and local metastasis that incites an almost violent fibrotic reaction in the mesentery and brings about the symptoms and signs of bowel obstruction (Fig. 34-24). Malignant lymphomas form large bulky lymph node metastases in many instances, resulting in a rather high frequency of palpable abdominal masses. Adenocarcinomas, on the other hand, metastasize in a large proportion of cases to regional lymph nodes, but more frequently they spread early to more distant organs, such as the liver, and later in some cases to the lungs. The region of the primary growth is not usually palpable.

Most malignant tumors of the small intestine originate from tissues located in the mucosa and submucosa, whereas the most common benign tumor of the small intestine arises from the muscularis propria.*

ROENTGENOLOGIC MANIFESTATIONS
Plain roentgenogram

If high-grade obstruction occurs, as it occasionally does in malignant neoplasms of the small intestine, a plain roentgenogram will lead to a diagnosis of mechanical obstruction in approximately 80% of such cases. This situation is most commonly encountered in cases of adenocarcinoma. Complete obstruction is uncommon in any form of neoplasm of the small bowel. If obstruction occurs, especially if unheralded by any forerunning symptoms, it usually indicates that the mechanism of obstruction is either intussusception or volvulus.

Contrast medium

Since complete obstruction is relatively uncommon, one has the opportunity to study most

---

*See references 40, 41, 43, 45, 52, 59, 60, 62, and 64.

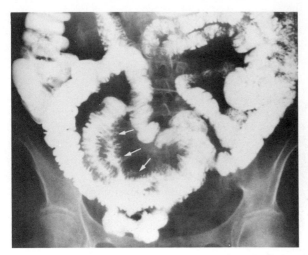

Fig. 34-24. Extensive abdominal carcinoid with primary tumor in the distal portion of the ileum (not demonstrated) and mesenteric mass and kinked loop of bowel (arrows) in the right lower quadrant.

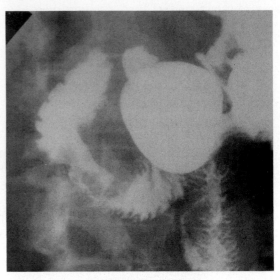

Fig. 34-25. Ulcerating, almost annular adenocarcinoma of the descending portion of the duodenum, resulting in low-grade obstruction.

patients with contrast medium. About the only contraindications to contrast study are (1) roentgenographic evidence of such high-grade obstruction that surgical intervention is clearly and immediately indicated, and (2) clinical or roentgenographic evidence of perforation of the bowel. The best and virtually the only satisfactory contrast medium for examination of the small bowel is a nonflocculating suspension of barium sulfate. The examination should be conducted as outlined earlier in this chapter.

Tumor outline

Deformity of the intraluminal barium reflects the gross form of the tumor and its manner of spread. Tumors that are more expansive and less invasive have the same forms and cause the same roentgenologic picture as benign neoplasms. Tumors that are primarily invasive cause a wide variety of roentgenologic abnormalities. Some forms, adenocarcinoma in particular, invade circumferentially rather than longitudinally. If the narrowing caused by the vigorous fibrotic response is sufficient, some dilatation of the bowel usually develops just proximal to the lesion; this feature attracts the roentgenologist's attention when he is examining the bowel fluoroscopically. The narrowed segment may show evidence of polypoid projections into the normally distensible portion. This narrowed portion is usually devoid of normal mucosal pattern, either because of ulceration or infiltration of the surface by neoplasm (Fig. 34-25).

Other forms of malignant neoplasm, such as lymphoma, invade along the longitudinal axis rather than circumferentially and heavily infiltrate the submucosa and muscularis, forming plaques of tumor in the wall of the bowel. Early in this infiltrative process there is usually preservation of the mucosal layer (Fig. 34-26, *A*), but the pattern is abnormal with thickening of the folds, which in profile appear rather corrugated. As the growth enlarges, necrosis often occurs in its central portion (Fig. 34-26, *B*), leading to mucosal ulceration that may become rather extensive. This results roentgenologically in a rigid segment of bowel with a rather wide lumen, often without recognizable mucosal pattern within the widely ulcerated lumen (Fig. 34-23). One is usually attracted by the rigidity of this bowel segment, by its resistance to compression, and, especially on roentgenograms, by the abnormality or absence of mucosal pattern in and adjacent to the rigid segment.

Another variation of growth results in deformity of the lumen primarily because of mesenteric invasion and fibrosis. In this situation the lumen seems to be stretched transversely, which results in a rather sharp, cleanly delineated mucosal pattern, often combined with

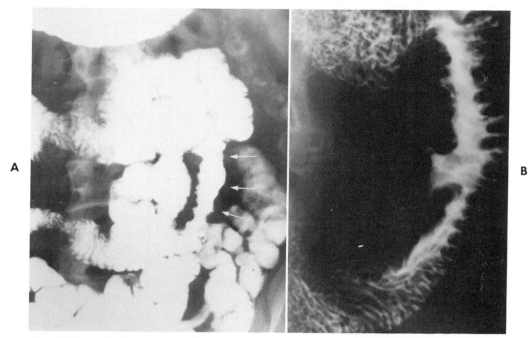

Fig. 34-26. A, Rigid segment of jejunum with malignant lymphoma. The scalloped border is caused by thickening of mucosal folds medially and complete effacement of folds laterally. **B,** Somewhat similar lesion with ulceration near the midportion.

knuckling of the longitudinal axis of the bowel (Fig. 34-24). Rather frequently, the primary mass is overlooked because of its relatively small size or because of the associated deformity caused by the mesenteric involvement.

Naturally, combinations of these gross forms and roentgenologic patterns occur so that one must think in terms of a wide spectrum of pathologic change as one seeks to translate roentgenologic findings into terms of pathologic anatomy.*

HISTOLOGIC TYPES
Carcinoid tumor
Incidence and location

Carcinoid is the most common neoplasm of the small intestine, and, if all carcinoids are considered to have malignant potential, it is overwhelmingly the most common malignant tumor. Unlike most malignant growths, however, about two thirds of the carcinoids are not symptomatic and, consequently, are found chiefly at autopsy.

When considering the entire gastrointestinal

*See references 39, 41, 43-45, 48, 52-54, 59, 66, and 69.

tract, more than half of all carcinoids are found in the region of the appendix. However, these tumors rarely metastasize. Excluding the appendix, about 80% of gastrointestinal carcinoids are found in the small bowel and the remainder are divided about evenly between the stomach and the rectum. Of those found in the small bowel, 90% are located in the ileum, and of these, 80% are situated in the distal third (Fig. 34-27). The tumor occurs in males about twice as frequently as in females.

Pathologic findings

The cells of carcinoid tumors have an affinity for silver stain much like the silver-staining cells at the base of the crypts of Lieberkühn in normal mucosa of the small intestine. It seems reasonable, then, that such tumors arise from these cells, proliferate, and form a mass in the submucosa. They are covered with normal intestinal mucosa. Most of these lesions have neither invaded nor metastasized when they are identified at autopsy. Those that are invasive extend into the submucosa, muscularis, and serosa or mesentery. Here they incite an intense fibrotic reaction, first causing local deformity of the in-

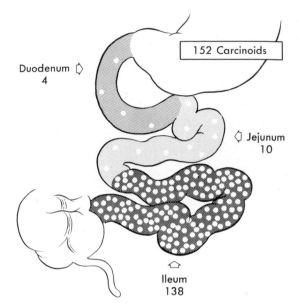

Duodenum ◁
4

152 Carcinoids

◁ Jejunum
10

⇧
Ileum
138

Fig. 34-27. Distribution of 152 carcinoids found among 331 malignant neoplasms in the small intestine.

testinal wall and then causing kinking of a longer segment comparable to the kinking of a sharply flexed garden hose. Massive metastasis to the lymph nodes, as well as to the liver, may occur, but rarely does the tumor leave the abdominal cavity. The frequency of metastasis is clearly related to the size of the primary lesion; those less than 1 cm. in diameter almost never metastasize, and those more than 2 cm. in diameter metastasize in about 80% of such cases. The submucosal primary tumor is multicenteric in almost a third of all cases; when this is true, there are usually three or more independent primary masses. About a third of the carcinoids, especially those found at autopsy, are associated with malignant tumors arising in other locations. Obstruction occurs in more than half of the patients with symptomatic lesions, kinking being the mechanism in most instances, and narrowing of the lumen caused by local invasion or by intussusception being the cause in a much smaller proportion.

Clinical features

About a third of all carcinoids are manifest clinically, and when they are, symptoms and signs are almost invariably caused by metastasis to the lymph nodes or to the liver. Metastasis to the lymph nodes frequently results in partial mechanical obstruction often accompanied by loss of weight; a palpable mass is present only slightly less frequently. In some patients a systemic effect also occurs, as a result of the elaboration by the tumor of 5-hydroxytryptamine, also called "serotonin." In excess, this substance can produce diarrhea, wheezing, and flushing of the skin. In addition, fibrotic changes in the valves of the right side of the heart can occur, resulting in pulmonary stenosis and tricuspid insufficiency and, ultimately, right heart failure with ascites. Liver and lung tissue inactivate normal amounts of 5-hydroxytryptamine by converting it to 5-hydroxyindoleacetic acid, which is physiologically inert and excreted by the kidneys. When this substance is excreted in excess in the urine, carcinoid can be diagnosed confidently. Virtually all such systemic manifestations result from extensive metastasis to the liver. The serotonin, which causes changes in the right side of the heart, overwhelms the "neutralizing" capacity of the lung tissue and then enters the systemic circulation. Not all elements of this so-called carcinoid syndrome are always present—diarrhea being common and flushing being rare. Attacks of the syndrome are often precipitated by the ingestion of food or alcohol (Table 34-5).

Roentgenologic manifestations

On barium examination the demonstration of a small intraluminal mass together with obstruction caused by a fixed, kinked loop of bowel is virtually diagnostic of carcinoid tumor (Figs. 34-28 to 34-32). Unfortunately, few such masses have been identified before operation, although the number seems to be increasing somewhat.

Since most carcinoids occur in the terminal portion of the ileum, they can be demonstrated either by the oral administration of barium or by reflux filling of the terminal portion of the ileum at the time of barium enema (Fig. 34-33). Regardless of the route of administration of contrast medium, in about half of such examinations carried out on patients with clinically manifest carcinoids of the small intestine no abnormality has been reported. Of the examinations reported as showing an abnormality, carcinoid tumor has been recognized in a few, but the changes are most commonly attributed to other pathologic processes, such as regional en-

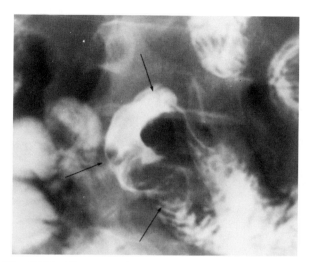

Fig. 34-28. Three centimeter polypoid carcinoid with a fixed kinked loop of jejunum and multiple metastatically involved regional nodes.

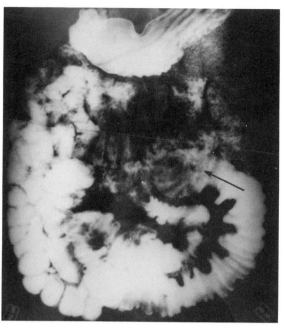

Fig. 34-29. Multiple (thirty-seven) carcinoids of ileum causing partial obstruction as a result of kinking and a polypoid mass (arrow). Note extension to lymph nodes and liver.

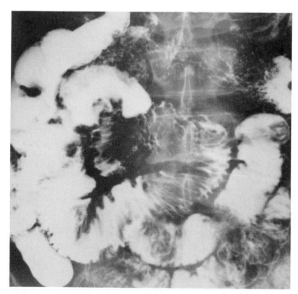

Fig. 34-30. Multiple (eight) carcinoids of distal ileum (not demonstrated). Severe kinking of the lumen and thickening of mucosal folds results in obstruction. Patient had carcinoid syndrome.

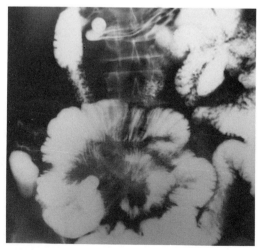

Fig. 34-31. Carcinoid of ileum with evidence of mesenteric involvement, including obstruction caused by kinking of the lumen and thickening and transverse elongation of mucosal folds.

teritis or other more commonly recognized polypoid neoplasms.

Many of the primary growths themselves are overlooked either because of their small size or because they are obscured by the deformity brought about by extension of the tumor to the mesentery. Nevertheless, a significant portion of the overall error is attributable to failure by the radiologist to translate the roentgenologic findings into correct terms of pathologic change as well as failure to recognize this change as characteristic of carcinoid. Such a characteristic combination of roentgenologic signs, especially when they occur in the right lower quadrant of the abdomen, should not be missed so frequently.

Selective mesenteric arteriography may lead to more accurate identification. In the presence of a carcinoid tumor there is narrowing of the arteries in the mesentery and a mass of stellate, abnormal vessels in the region of the involved mesentery. Unlike other neoplasms, accumulation of contrast medium within the tumor is minimal; and unlike regional enteritis, usually no veins are visualized. The role of angiography in the detection of carcinoids that have eluded discovery in the barium examination is not clear at this time.*

Adenocarcinoma
Incidence and location

Although not as common as carcinoids, adenocarcinomas more often cause symptoms and because of this, are almost always identified at operation rather than at autopsy. They comprise about a fourth of all malignant lesions of the small bowel, and about a third of all those causing clinical manifestations. About 90% are lo-

*See references 50, 52, 55, 58-61, 63, and 67.

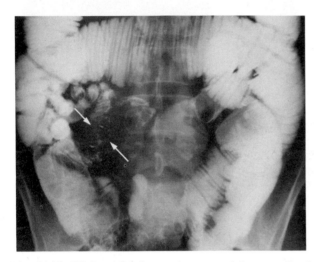

Fig. 34-32. High-grade obstruction caused by very localized kinking of ileum (arrow) as a result of metastasis from a 2 cm. polypoid carcinoid (arrow).

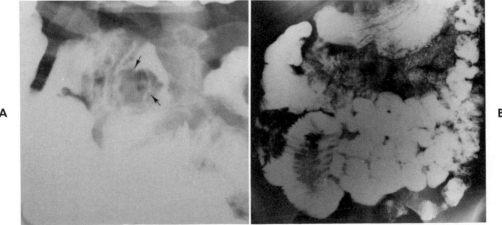

Fig. 34-33. A, Polypoid carcinoid in the terminal portion of the ileum seen on barium enema examination. **B,** Mesenteric involvement in the small intestine as evidenced by kinking as well as thickening and transverse elongation of mucosal folds, seen by oral ingestion of barium.

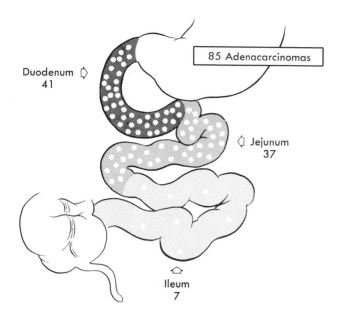

85 Adenacarcinomas

Duodenum
41

Jejunum
37

Ileum
7

Fig. 34-34. Distribution of eighty-five adenocarcinomas found among 331 malignant neoplasms in the small intestine.

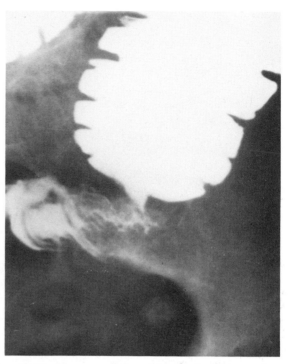

Fig. 34-35. Short, annular, ulcerated adenocarcinoma with intense scirrhous reaction in wall and mesentery.

cated in the duodenum and jejunum, with almost the same number in each segment (Fig. 34-34).

Pathologic findings

Most adenocarcinomas are rather aggressively infiltrative. A small proportion form broad-based polypoid masses and, although extremely rare, they may take the form of a pedunculated polyp.

The common, infiltrative form usually extends rapidly around the circumference of the bowel, inciting a fibrotic reaction and a narrowing of the lumen that soon cause obstruction. The mucosa in the narrowed segment is replaced by tumor, which may undergo necrosis, forming a somewhat irregular channel. It has been suggested recently that the presence of regional enteritis predisposes to the development of adenocarcinoma, with most of these lesions being found in the ileum.

Clinical features

About 90% of adenocarcinomas are clinically manifest, with pain and obstruction occurring in 70% of the patients, blood loss in about half, loss of weight in about half, and a palpable mass in about a third (Table 34-5).

Roentgenologic manifestations

A small proportion of patients are operated on because of high-grade obstruction and never have barium examinations of the small bowel. Of those who do have such contrast examinations, a positive result should be forthcoming in about 90%. Since most of the growths are located in the proximal portion of the bowel, the segment usually can be well filled with contrast medium and the bowel manipulated manually, all of which undoubtedly explains the high diagnostic accuracy. Tumors located in the ileum, where they may be within the bony pelvis and difficult to palpate and separate from adjacent loops, are overlooked much more frequently than those in other portions of the bowel.

The most common and most characteristic finding is a short, sharply demarcated, often annular filling defect. If the lumen is rather narrow, the bowel is usually somewhat dilated proximally. If the tumor is infiltrative, there may not be any polypoid projection into the dilated lumen, and the lesion may appear deceptively similar to an inflammatory stricture (Fig. 34-35). If surface proliferation is more promi-

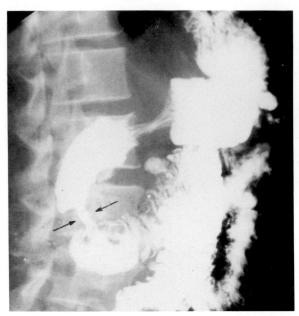

Fig. 34-36. Annular, ulcerated adenocarcinoma of the duodenum with polypoid growth at each edge (arrows) of lesion.

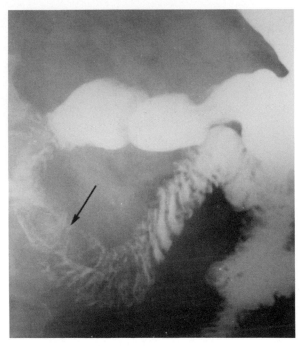

Fig. 34-38. Lobulated, polypoid, high-grade adenocarcinoma of the midduodenum.

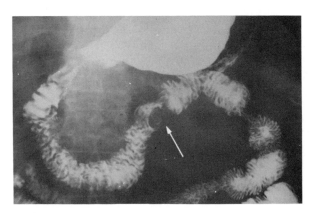

Fig. 34-37. Sessile, polypoid, low-grade adenocarcinoma of the distal duodenum.

nent than infiltration, such polypoid projections are present. When the surface of the narrowed segment becomes necrotic, it forms an irregular channel and the lesion may resemble the common form taken by annular carcinoma of the colon (Fig. 34-36). An oval or lobulated sessile polypoid filling defect can be detected much less commonly, especially early in the course of low-grade tumors (Figs. 34-37 and 34-38). The surface may become necrotic, forming a rather flat ulcer, which, in the stomach, might be thought to be benign (Fig. 34-39). Finally, a rare adenocarcinoma may be suspended within the lumen by a pedicle and may not be distinguishable roentgenologically from most other slightly irregular intraluminal neoplasms (Fig. 34-40). If the adenocarcinoma can be detected and localized, histologic identification usually can be made by roentgenologic examination.*

Malignant lymphoma
Incidence and location

Primary malignant lymphoma of the small intestine is somewhat less common than adenocarcinoma, comprising a little less than a fifth of all malignant growths. Unlike adenocarcinoma, about half of the lesions are found in the ileum and half in the jejunum. They are rarely found in the duodenum (Fig. 34-41).

Pathologic findings

Almost any gross form is possible with lymphoma. Most commonly it forms a cellular infiltrate beginning in the submucosa and usu-

*See references 40, 44, 48, 52-54, 62, 65, 66, and 69.

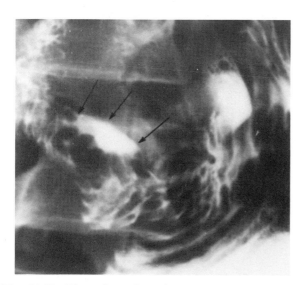

Fig. 34-39. Ulceration of a plaquelike adenocarcinoma of the duodenum, resembling a benign ulcer of the stomach.

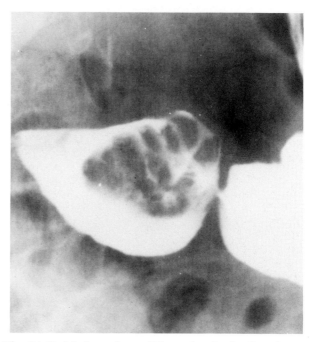

Fig. 34-40. Moderately undifferentiated adenocarcinoma presenting as a pedunculated polyp in the duodenal bulb.

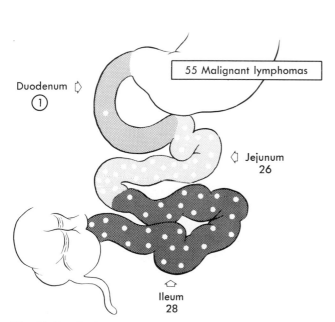

Fig. 34-41. Distribution of fifty-five malignant lymphomas found among 331 malignant neoplasms in the small intestine.

ally extending longitudinally to form a plaque of tumor. More than 80% of growths are longer than 5 cm, and 20% are longer than 10 cm. The infiltrate does not stimulate the formation of fibrous tissue. The mucosal folds become thickened and in profile may have a corrugated appearance that becomes more and more effaced as the mass grows (Fig. 34-42). The growth gradually encircles the bowel, but before obstruction occurs, extensive necrosis often takes place on the luminal surface, which has the effect of widening the lumen. This presents a distinctive appearance in about a third of all cases (Figs. 34-23 and 34-43). However, a wide variety of forms exist, including a single polypoid mass, multiple small nodular or small polypoid masses, short extramucosal annular growths, short ulcerated annular lesions that may look identical to adenocarcinomas, and, finally, chiefly transmural and extraluminal growths, which may undergo necrosis and cavitation. Since multiple sites of involvement are present in about a fifth of cases, any combination of these forms may exist in one patient. If one considers all lymphomatous involvement of the small intestine, those patients

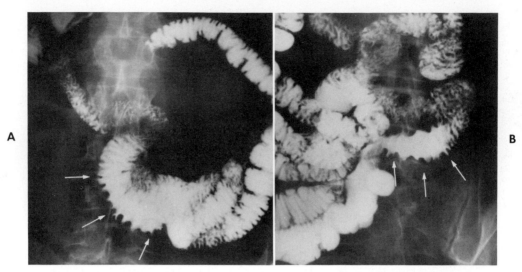

Fig. 34-42. A, Segment of malignant lymphoma of jejunum exhibiting "corrugated" (arrows) mucosal pattern. **B,** The same segment 7 months later, with effacement of the folds caused by growth of neoplastic infiltrate.

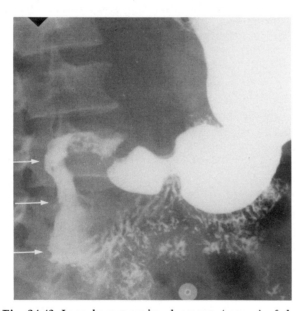

Fig. 34-43. Lymphomatous involvement (arrows) of duodenum, with widened lumen without mucosal pattern.

who have multiple sites of involvement have widely disseminated lymphomatous disease much more frequently than those patients with a single lesion in the bowel.

Several histologic types are found, including the chiefly lymphocytic variety, reticulum cell sarcoma, giant follicular lymphosarcoma, and Hodgkin's disease. These cannot be distinguished by gross forms.

Clinical features

Clinical manifestations occur in almost all patients with malignant lymphoma. Pain or obstruction is present in about 90%, a palpable mass in about two thirds, loss of weight in about two thirds, and evidence of blood loss in about one third (Table 34-5).

Roentgenologic manifestations

Since a wide variety of gross pathologic forms exists, there are many roentgenologic manifestations. The single most common gross form is that of a long growth encircling the lumen, which is extensively smoothly ulcerated and hence is widened, thereby providing a striking roentgenologic picture that portrays exactly these changes and leads to a histologic diagnosis (Figs. 34-23 and 34-43). The plaque-like infiltrating form that is seen before necrosis and ulceration occur also has a distinctive appearance. The segment is stiff on manipulation, does not empty itself of barium, and its mucosal surface has a rather distinctive corrugated appearance caused by the cellular infiltration of the folds (Fig. 34-42). This form, too, allows a histologic diagnosis roentgenologically. In many cases, however, malignant lymphomas assume forms resembling other neoplasms, and precise identification is often impossible. The diffuse form may resemble regional enteritis if the lesions are relatively flat and nodular (Fig. 34-44), or the lesions may present as multiple, small, peduncu-

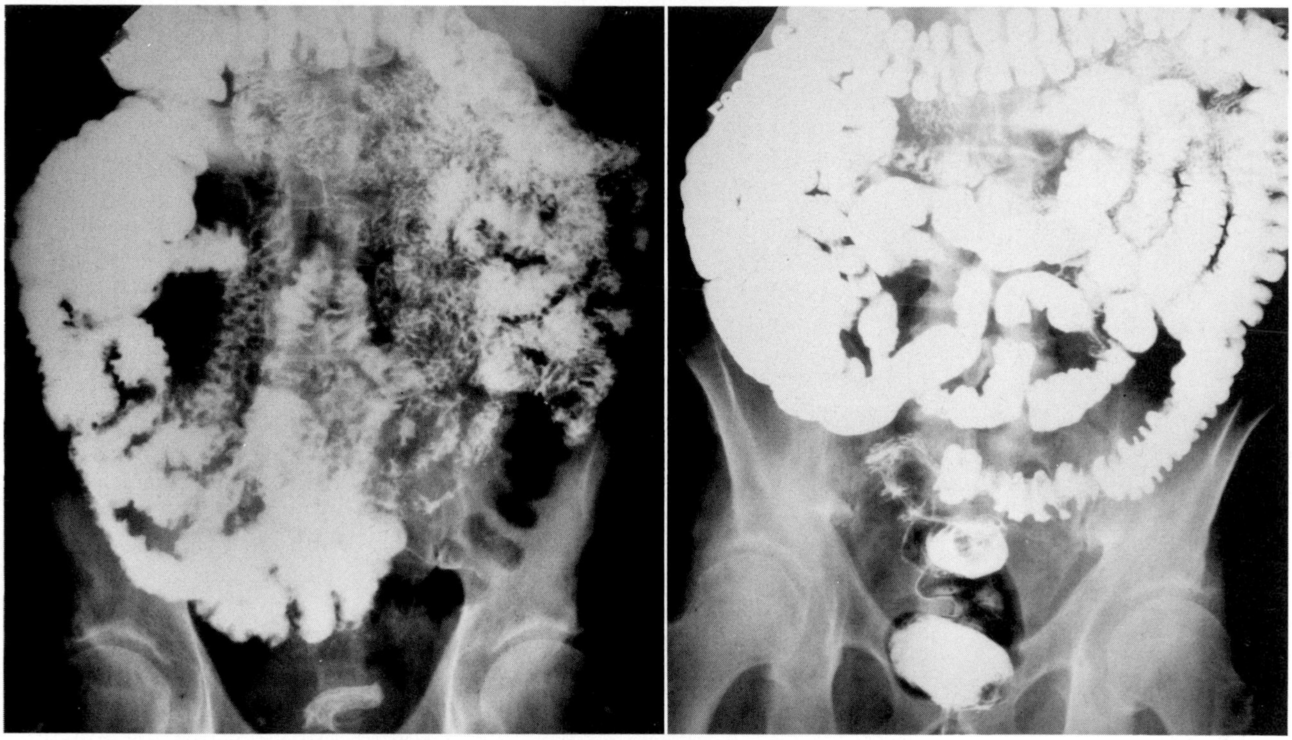

Fig. 34-44. A, Multiple nodules of lymphoma involving the distal portion of the ileum and ascending colon. **B,** Normal appearance on examination 9 months after irradiation.

lated polyps. In either case, involvement of the colon is frequently present and the process may be identified by a proctoscopic biopsy. Multiple sites of involvement with varying gross forms are suggestive of lymphoma but must be distinguished from metastasis (Fig. 34-45). Finally, the accumulation of barium in a large irregular cavity, which occurs sometimes with lymphomatous involvement, resembles rather closely the cavities occurring in smooth-muscle neoplasms as well as those occurring with abscess formation associated with regional enteritis (Fig. 34-46). Thus a histologic diagnosis can be strongly suggested from the roentgenologic examination in about half of the cases in malignant lymphoma of the small intestine.*

Leiomyosarcoma
Incidence and location

Leiomyosarcoma comprises about 10% of all malignant neoplasms of the small intestine and about 16% of all of those that cause symptoms and signs. The lesions are found in almost equal numbers in each of the three segments of the

---

*See references 40-43, 45, 47, 51, 52, 54, 57, 66, and 69.

small bowel. Considering all cases of smooth-muscle tumors identified at autopsy and operation, benign tumors are about three times as common as malignant. However, of those smooth-muscle lesions identified in the small bowel at operation, about half are malignant and half are benign (Table 34-4 and Fig. 34-47).

Pathologic findings

Malignant smooth-muscle tumors assume exactly the same forms and combination of forms as the benign variety and cannot be distinguished from them grossly with any accuracy. In fact, differentiation by the histologist is often difficult, and, in some cases, lesions that exhibit no cellular signs of malignancy invade and metastasize.

About 10% project chiefly into the lumen and a few of these are pedunculated; about two thirds project chiefly into the peritoneal cavity and a few of these are pedunculated as well; about 15% are chiefly intramural and about 10% are multilobulated with a portion projecting into the lumen and a second lobule projecting chiefly into the abdominal cavity. Like the benign variety, the surface vascularity is rich

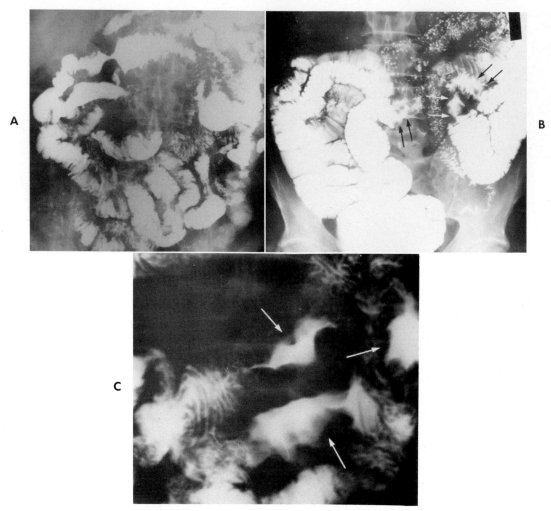

Fig. 34-45. Multiple sites of involvement in three patients with malignant lymphoma of the small intestine. **A,** Lymphosarcoma with disease in testicle and abdominal wall. **B,** Three sites of involvement, with Hodgkin's disease limited to small intestine (arrows). **C,** Multiple sites of reticulum cell sarcoma of jejunum with disease in the neck as well.

and the central portion of the mass is poorly vascularized and often necrotic. If surface ulceration occurs, which happens in about half of the cases, deep craters may form. The mass may become huge, and although malignant specimens are, on the average, somewhat larger than the benign lesions, the range of diameters is almost identical. It is probably best to regard all large smooth-muscle tumors as malignant. Metastasis occurs almost always via the vascular route.

Clinical features

Blood loss, pain, and a palpable mass are the most common manifestations, and each occurs in about two thirds of the cases. Blood loss, because of the rich surface vascularity of the mass, is often massive and intermittent. Intervals between such episodes may be long, sometimes extending to years. Obstruction occurs much less commonly than in most other types of small-bowel malignancy, being present in only about a fourth of cases. About half of the obstructions are associated with intussusception. Occasionally, the peritoneal surface of the lesion may become necrotic and cause symptoms and signs of peritonitis. In rare instances this may be associated with a so-called ulcer cavity in the mass and may allow leakage of the intestinal content into the peritoneal cavity (Table 34-5).

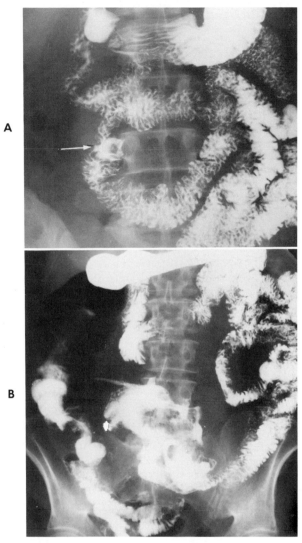

Fig. 34-46. Small, **A,** and large, **B,** cavitating reticulum cell sarcomas of the jejunum.

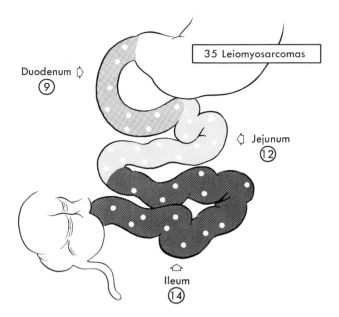

Fig. 34-47. Distribution of thirty-five leiomyosarcomas found among 331 malignant neoplasms in the small intestine.

Roentgenologic manifestations

As one might expect, the roentgenologic manifestations are exactly the same as those described for the benign varieties of smooth-muscle neoplasms, since their gross forms are almost indistinguishable. Since more than two thirds of these lesions project chiefly into the peritoneal cavity, their chief manifestation on x-ray examination is displacement of adjacent loops of bowel. Of all cases of smooth-muscle tumor having barium examination, positive results are forthcoming in about two thirds and a diagnosis of smooth-muscle tumor can be made in about a fifth of such cases. Those that deform

the lumen exhibit a wide spectrum of size and projection from the mucosal surface. A small proportion of these (less than 5%) present as intraluminal pedunculated masses (these often result in intussusception); more frequently, the mass is broad based with or without mucosal pattern on its surface depending on how much the growth has effaced the mucosal folds (Fig. 34-48). Ulceration of the mucosa covering these lesions occurs in about half of the cases. The ulcers appear as small deep pits in the smaller masses and may communicate with a large necrotic cavity in the large, chiefly extramural forms (Fig. 34-49). Fistulas may form through the mass and, if identified roentgenologically, these provide a characteristic sign (Fig. 34-50). The craters are usually larger and the fistulous tracts are longer in malignant than in benign myomas, but this is seldom of importance in management of the patient. As noted, it is best to regard all smooth-muscle tumors as *potentially* malignant, and all large tumors as *actually* malignant, regardless of histology. As in the case of the benign variety, if the growth is multilobulated a portion may manifest itself as a sessile, submucosal mass and a second or third portion may take the form of a largely extramural tumor with displacement of adjacent loops of bowel (Fig. 34-51).*

*See references 39, 40, 52, 62, and 64.

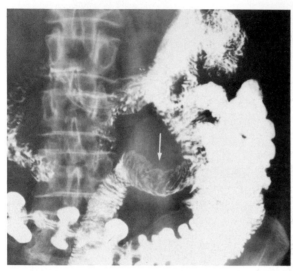

Fig. 34-48. Large intramural leiomyosarcoma with only about a fourth of its profile circumference projecting into the jejunal lumen. There is no ulceration. Mucosa, probably on the opposite wall, is "stretched" transversely. (From Good, C. A.: Tumors of the small intestine, Caldwell lecture, 1962, Amer. J. Roentgen. **89:** 685, 1963.)

Metastatic neoplasms
Incidence and location

Although overlooked for some time, it has become apparent within the past decade that lesions demonstrated to involve the small intestine may be the first detected evidence of metastasis from a variety of primary neoplasms, including those from the uterine cervix, skin, ovary, kidney, lungs, stomach, colon, breast, and pancreas. Only those patients who do not have obvious evidence of abdominal carcinomatosis or evidence of generalized widespread metastasis should be considered in this category. Extension from an adjacent neoplasm also represents a separate and distinct situation. Such metastatic deposits may occur anywhere in the small bowel, and their frequency in patients seen at the Mayo Clinic is only somewhat less than that of primary leiomyosarcoma of the small bowel.

Pathologic findings

Most commonly, most of the mass is located in the mesentery adjacent to the bowel wall. Here it incites a fibrotic response and causes kinking of the bowel much like that caused by carcinoid tumor. Metastatic deposit also may grow intramurally and project into the lumen as a sessile mass. Another common form is an annular infiltrating process resembling adenocarcinoma. Finally, submucosal deposits may result in largely intraluminal lesions, which may become pedunculated and rather frequently ex-

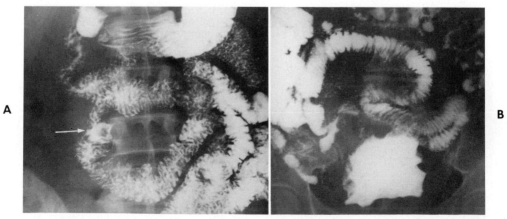

Fig. 34-49. A, Small, partially necrotic leiomyosarcoma of the jejunum (arrow). **B,** Large, necrotic leiomyosarcoma of the ileum.

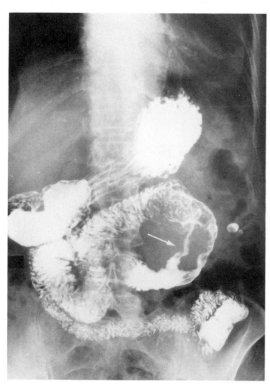

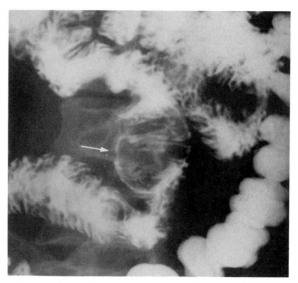

Fig. 34-50. Fistula (arrow) through dumbbell-shaped leiomyosarcoma of jejunum. (From Good, C. A.: Tumors of the small intestine, Caldwell lecture, 1962, Amer. J. Roentgen. **89:**685, 1963.)

Fig. 34-51. Dumbbell-shaped leiomyosarcoma of jejunum. Arrow indicates one 3 cm. pedunculated lesion within the lumen connected to a second 3 cm. pedunculated subserous mass (undetectable roentgenologically).

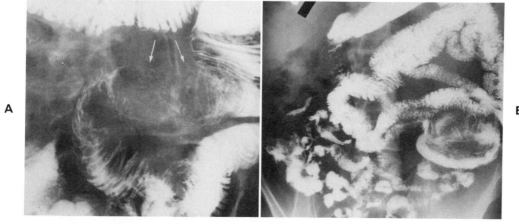

Fig. 34-52. A, Metastasis from carcinoma of rectum, largely mesenteric but with an intraluminal component (arrow). **B,** Metastatic carcinoma of appendix, largely mesenteric.

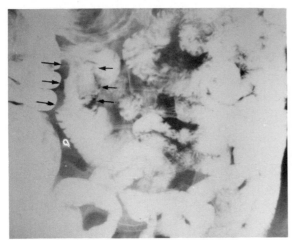

Fig. 34-53. Single metastasis from malignant melanoma resembling primary adenocarcinoma.

tensively ulcerated on the surface opposite the short pedicle, with the result that the name "buttercup" has been applied to them by surgical pathologists.

About half of all metastatic growths in the small intestine are multiple. In the case of malignant melanoma, multiple lesions, some of which are usually extensively pedunculated and ulcerated, are exhibited in almost 100% of the patients.

Clinical features

All patients must have a demonstrable primary growth. Most patients have evidence of intestinal obstruction, and this usually is the indication for roentgenologic examination.

Roentgenologic manifestations

A wide spectrum of roentgenologic change reflects the wide variety of gross forms taken by these tumors. The most common signs are those of mesenteric and peritoneal infiltration and fixation. These may result in a fixation and "tenting up" of the wall and mucosa of the small bowel with transverse stretching of the mucosal folds (Fig. 34-52). A mass may protrude into the lumen, usually in association with mesenteric disease. The mass may undergo extensive ulceration and may resemble annular carcinoma (Fig. 34-53). Finally, polypoid masses may form, even with short pedicles and surface ulceration. These "buttercups" of the pathologists have become "bull's-eyes" of the roentgenologist because of the sizable ulcer craters surrounded by an equal size rim of neoplasm, giving the ap-

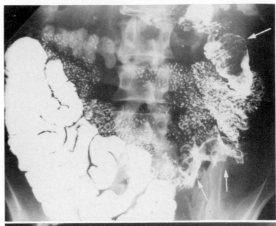

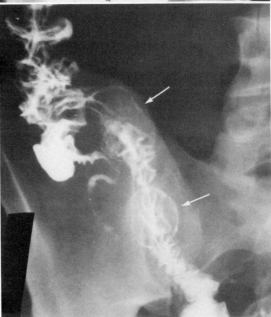

Fig. 34-54. Four polypoid masses from malignant melanoma. **A,** One mass in the jejunum has caused intussusception (arrow) and a second is extensively ulcerated (two arrows). **B,** Two smooth polypoid masses in ileum in same case as **A.**

pearance of a target. If one encounters neoplasms of the small bowel roentgenologically in a patient with a history of a primary malignant neoplasm capable of metastasis, this possibility should be considered. This is especially true if there are multiple sites of involvement with varying forms (Figs. 34-54 and 34-55). Metastatic disease of the small bowel may strongly resemble lymphomas with multiple sites or carcinoid tumors with both mesenteric and luminal signs. The history of malignant melanoma together with the finding of multiple polypoid and ul-

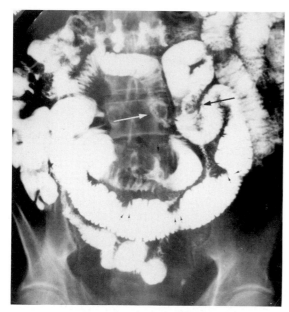

Fig. 34-55. Multiple sites and forms (polypoid annular, eccentric, infiltrate) of metastatic carcinoma from the appendix.

cerated lesions in the small intestine is virtually diagnostic of metastasis.*

REFERENCES
Benign neoplasms

1. Alrich, E. M., Blank, R. H., and Fomon, J. J.: Primary tumors of the small intestine, Amer. J. Surg. 99:33, 1960.
2. Baker, H. L., Jr., and Good, C. A.: Smooth-muscle tumors of the alimentary tract: their roentgen manifestations, Amer. J. Roentgen. 74:246, 1955.
3. Bandler, M.: Hemangiomas of the small intestine associated with mucocutaneous pigmentation, Gastroenterology 38:641, 1960.
4. Bernstein, J. S., and Chey, W. Y.: Small bowel tumors: a clinical study of 109 cases, J. Mount Sinai Hosp. N. Y. 25:1, 1958.
5. Biese, L., and Wade, W.: Solitary schwannoma of the small intestine, Amer. J. Surg. 101:184, 1961.
6. Botsford, T. W., Crowe, P., and Crocker, D. W.: Tumors of the small intestine: a review of experience with 115 cases including a report of a rare case of malignant hemangio-endothelioma, Amer. J. Surg. 103:358, 1962.
7. Broders, A. C., Jr., Hightower, N. C., Jr., Hunt, W. H., III, Stinson, J. C., White, R. R., and Laurens, H., Jr.: Primary neoplasms of the small bowel: analysis of one hundred two cases, Arch. Surg. 79: 753, 1959.
8. Bruwer, A., Bargen, J. A., and Kierland, R. R.: Surface pigmentation and generalized intestinal polyposis (Peutz-Jeghers Snydrome), Proc. Staff Meet., Mayo Clin. 29:168, 1954.
9. Cooley, R. N.: The diagnostic accuracy of radiologic studies of the biliary tract, small intestine and colon, Amer. J. Med. Sci. 246:610, 1963.
10. Copple, P. J., and Kingsbury, R. A.: Hemangiomas of the small bowel in children: report of a case and review of the literature, J. Pediat. 59:243, 1961.
11. Darling, R. C., and Welch, C. E.: Tumors of small intestine, New Eng. J. Med. 260:397, 1959.
12. Deshpandle, D. H., and Purandare, N. M.: Clinicopathologic study of 45 cases of tumors of the small intestine, J. Postgrad. Med. 10:114, 1964.
13. Gannon, P. G., Dahlin, D. C., Bartholomew, L. G., and Beahrs, O. H.: Polypoid glandular tumors of the small intestine, Surg. Gynec. Obstet. 114:666, 1962.
14. Gentry, R. W., Dockerty, M. B., and Clagett, O. T.: Collective review: vascular malformations and vascular tumors of gastrointestinal tract, Int. Abstr. Surg. 88:281, 1949.
15. Good, C. A.: Tumors of the small intestine: Caldwell lecture, 1962, Amer. J. Roentgen. 89:685, 1963.
16. Keats, T. E., and Sakai, H. Q.: An evaluation of the sources of error in the roentgenologic diagnosis of neoplasms of the small intestine, Gastroenterology 29:554, 1955.
17. Krouse, J. M., Eyerly, R. C., and Babcock, J. R.: Tumors of the small bowel, Amer. J. Surg. 101:121, 1961.
18. Lillie, R. H., and Bares, G. C.: Multiple polyposis of the small intestine, Ann. Surg. 154:133, 1961.
19. Madell, S. H.: A case of hemangioma (angiomatosis) of the small intestine and mesentery: a radiographic clue to diagnosis, Radiology 69:564, 1957.
20. Marshak, R. H., Freund, S., and Maklansky, D.: Neurofibromatosis of the small bowel, Amer. J. Dig. Dis. 8:478, 1963.
21. Martel, W., Whitehouse, W. M., and Hodges, F. J.: Small-bowel tumors, Radiology 75:368, 1960.
22. Muratore, R., and Gambarelli, J.: Endométriose et lipome de l'intestin grêle, Arch. Anat. Path. (Paris) 10:125, 1962.
23. Patterson, J. F., Callow, A. D., and Ettinger, A.: The clinical patterns of small-bowel tumors: a study of 32 cases, Ann. Intern. Med. 48:123, 1958.
24. Polak, M.: Benign tumors of small intestine, Clin. Sympos. 13:27, 1961.
25. Raiford, T. S.: Tumors of the small intestine: their diagnosis, with special reference to the x-ray appearance, Radiology 16:253, 1931.
26. River, L., Silverstein, J., and Tope, J. W.: Collective review: benign neoplasms of small intestine; a critical comprehensive review with reports of 20 new cases, Int. Abstr. Surg. 102:1, 1956.
27. Roddy, S. R.: Small-bowel tumors: clinical review of thitry-four cases, Arch. Surg. 75:847, 1957.
28. Sawyer, R. B., Sawyer, K. C., Jr., Sawyer, K. C., and Larsen, R. R.: Benign and malignant tumors of the small intestine, Amer. Surg. 29:268, 1963.
29. Schmutzer, K. J., Holleran, W. M., and Regan, J. F.: Tumors of the small bowel, Amer. J. Surg. 108: 270, 1964.

---

*See references 46, 49, 56, 68, and 70.

30. Sheward, J. D.: Peutz-Jeghers syndrome in childhood: unusual radiological features, Brit. Med. J. 1:921, 1962.

31. Silverman, L., Waugh, J. M., Huizenga, K. A., and Harrison, E. G., Jr.: Large adenomatous polyp of Brunner's glands, Amer. J. Clin. Path. 36:438, 1961.

32. Silverton, R.: Smooth muscle tumours of the small intestine, Med. J. Aust. 2:745, 1964.

33. Skandalakis, J. E., Gray, S. W., and Shepard, D.: Smooth muscle tumors of the small intestine, Amer. J. Gastroent. 42:172, 1964.

34. Skandalakis, J. E., Gray, S. W., Shepard, D., and Bourne, G. H.: Smooth muscle tumors of the alimentary tract: leiomyomas and leiomyosarcomas—a review of 2,525 cases, Springfield, Ill., 1962, Charles C Thomas, Publisher.

35. Smith, F. R., and Mayo, C. W.: Submucous lipomas of the small intestine, Amer. J. Surg. 80:922, 1950.

36. Southam, J. A.: Benign tumors of the small intestine, Surg. Gynec. Obstet. 117:473, 1963.

37. Starr, G. F., and Dockerty, M. B.: Leiomyomas and leiomyosarcomas of the small intestine, Cancer 8:101, 1955.

38. Wimer, B. M., and Hijaz, I.: Simple polypoid cavernous hemangioma of the small intestine: case report and review, Guthrie Clin. Bull. 30:34, 1961.

Malignant neoplasms

39. Baker, H. L., Jr., and Good, C. A.: Smooth-muscle tumors of the alimentary tract: their roentgen manifestations, Amer. J. Roentgen. 74:246, 1955.

40. Brookes, V. S., Waterhouse, J. A. H., and Powell, D. J.: Malignant lesions of the small intestine: a ten-year survey, Brit. J. Surg. 55:405, 1968.

41. Burman, S. O., and van Wyk, F. A. K.: Lymphomas of the small intestine and cecum, Ann. Surg. 143:349, 1956.

42. Cornes, J. S.: Multiple lymphomatous polyposis of the gastrointestinal tract, Cancer 14:249, 1961.

43. Cupps, R. E., Hodgson, J. R., Dockerty, M. B, and Adson, M. A.: Primary lymphoma in the small intestine: problems of roentgenologic diagnosis, Radiology 92:1355, 1969.

44. Darling, R. C., and Welch, C. E.: Tumors of the small intestine, New Engl. J. Med. 260:397, 1959.

45. Dawson, I. M. P., Cornes, J. S., and Morson, B. C.: Primary malignant lymphoid tumours of the intestinal tract: report of 37 cases with a study of factors influencing prognosis, Brit. J. Surg. 49:80, 1961.

46. De Castro, C. A., Dockerty, M. B., and Mayo, C. W.: Metastatic tumors of the small intestines, Surg. Gynec. Obstet. 105:159, 1957.

47. Deeb, P. H., and Stilson, W. L.: Roentgenologic manifestations of lymphosarcoma of the small bowel, Radiology 63:235, 1954.

48. Doub, H. P.: Malignant tumors of the small intestine, Radiology 49:441, 1947.

49. Farmer, R. G., and Hawk, W. A.: Metastatic tumors of the small bowel, Gastroenterology 47:496, 1964.

50. Foreman, R. C.: Carcinoid tumors: a report of 38 cases, Ann. Surg. 136:838, 1952.

51. Frazer, J. W., Jr.: Malignant lymphomas of the gastrointestinal tract, Surg. Gynec. Obstet. 108:182, 1959.

52. Good, C. A.: Tumors of the small intestine: Caldwell lecture, 1962, Amer. J. Roentgen. 89:685, 1963.

53. Keats, T. E., and Sakai, H. Q.: An evaluation of the sources of error in the roentgenologic diagnosis of neoplasms of the small intestine, Gastroenterology 29:554, 1955.

54. Kohler, R.: Primary malignant tumors in the small intestine with special reference to their roentgen diagnosis, Acta Radiol. 30:217, 1948.

55. MacDonald, R. A.: A study of 356 carcinoids of the gastrointestinal tract: report of four new cases of the carcinoid syndrome, Amer. J. Med. 21:867, 1956.

56. Marshak, R. H., Khilnani, M. T., Eliasoph, J., and Wolf, B. S.: Metastatic carcinoma of the small bowel, Amer. J. Roentgen. 94:385, 1965.

57. Marshak, R. H., Wolf, B. S., and Eliasoph, J.: The roentgen findings in lymphosarcoma of the small intestine, Amer. J. Roentgen. 86:682, 1961.

58. Masson, P.: Carcinoids (argentaffin-cell tumors) and nerve hyperplasia of the appendicular mucosa, Amer. J. Path. 4:181, 1928.

59. Miller, E. R., and Herrmann, W. W.: Argentaffin tumors of the small bowel: a roentgen sign of malignant change, Radiology 39:214, 1942.

60. Moertel, C. G., Sauer, W. G., Dockerty, M. B., and Baggenstoss, A. H.: Life history of the carcinoid tumor of the small intestine, Cancer 14:901, 1961.

61. Reuter, S. R., and Boijsen, E.: Angiographic findings in two ileal carcinoid tumors, Radiology 87:836, 1966.

62. Sethi, G., and Hardin, C. A.: Primary malignant tumors of the small bowel, Arch. Surg. 98:659, 1969.

63. Stark, S., Bluth, I., and Rubinstein, S.: Carcinoid tumor of the ileum resembling regional ileitis clinically and roentgenologically, Gastroenterology 40:813, 1961.

64. Starr, G. F., and Dockerty, M. B.: Leiomyomas and leiomyosarcomas of the small intestine, Cancer 8:101, 1955.

65. Steiger, E., and Dudrick, S. J.: Adenocarcinoma with regional enteritis, New Eng. J. Med. 283:875, 1970.

66. Swenson, P. C.: X-ray diagnosis of the primary malignant tumors of the small intestine, Rev. Gastroent. 10:77, 1943.

67. Thorson, A., Biörck, G., Björkman, G., and Waldenström, J.: Malignant carcinoid of the small intestine with metastases to the liver, valvular disease of the right side of the heart (pulmonary stenosis and tricuspid regurgitation without septal defects), peripheral vasomotor symptoms, bronchoconstriction, and unusual type of cyanosis: a clinical and pathologic syndrome, Amer. Heart J. 47:795, 1954.

68. Tillotson, P. M., and Douglas, R. G., Jr.: Metastatic tumor of the small intestine: three cases presenting unusual clinical and roentgenographic findings, Amer. J. Roentgen. 88:702, 1962.

69. Weber, H. M., and Kirklin, B. R.: Roentgenologic manifestations of tumors of the small intestine, Amer. J. Roentgen. 47:243, 1942.

70. Zboralske, F. F., and Bessolo, R. J.: Metastatic carcinoma to the mesentery and gut, Radiology 88:302, 1967.

Part VI

The colon

Pathology of the colon | 35

Harlan J. Spjut
Antonio Navarrete

MALFORMATIONS

Imperforate rectum is often considered in discussions of imperforate anus, but the two have been separated by some authors. The middle rectal segment is most often involved; this involvement is caused by a failure of division of the cloaca. Thus the rectum may end blindly, or there may be formation of rectovesical or rectourethral fistulas. In the female, rectovaginal fistulas involving the posterior vagina may be present. The imperforate rectum is frequently accompanied by severe sacral and genitourinary deformities.[69,70]

Other major deformities of the large bowel may occur such as malrotations, duplications, and atresias.[21,71] Atresias are fewer in number than in the small bowel. Etiologically, atresias of the colon are considered the result of interruption of the blood supply to a segment of colon in utero. Three types of atresias have been described to involve the colon: (1) a diaphragm that occludes the lumen, (2) proximal and distal blind ends that are connected by a cord-like remnant of large bowel, and (3) complete separation of the proximal and distal blind ends. Type 1 is more commonly found on the left side of the large bowel, and types 2 and 3 are more common on the right. The importance of the early diagnosis of this disease lies in the fact that very few of these patients have been saved by surgical intervention.[35,71]

Hirschsprung's disease represents another congenital malformation in the large bowel and is more accurately referred to as an aganglionic megacolon. It occurs in 1:5,000 births and there is a male sex preponderance.[61] The main defect lies in the absence of Meissner's and Auerbach's plexi. The nerve defect is seen in the narrowed segment and not in the dilated portion of the large bowel. The rectum is almost invariably involved in an aganglionic megacolon; this is evidenced by the successful use of rectal biopsies in

the delineation of this disease. At times the whole colon and a portion of the terminal ileum may be aganglionic. Of equal importance, in order to avoid unnecessary surgical procedures, is the recognition of functional and acquired megacolon. In the functional form there are no abnormalities of the ganglion cells, and the disease is usually noted in patients who are mentally retarded, in cretins, or in patients who have anal obstruction. The acquired form of megacolon is most often seen in adults and, in one series, was associated with degenerative changes in myenteric plexus, which were thought to be secondary to nutritional deficiencies. Another form of acquired megacolon or megasigmoid has been described as occurring in patients in neuropsychiatric hospitals.[30,31,49,72]

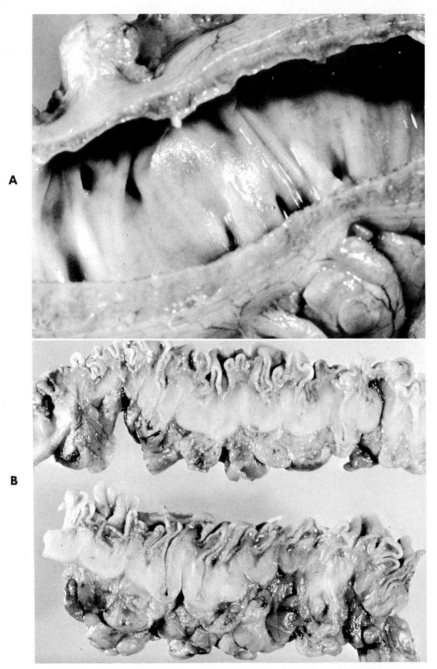

Fig. 35-1. A, Mouths of several diverticula of the sigmoid colon. BUCM #18446. **B,** Longitudinal section through a sigmoid colon with diverticulosis. Note the penetration of the diverticula into the muscularis and the hypertrophy of the muscularis. BUCM #18446.

Diverticula

Diverticula are a common finding, which occur in approximately 5% to 10% of the autopsies studied. Even though the lesion is common, complications of diverticula are relatively rare. Approximately 80% of the diverticula are found in the sigmoid portion of the colon; they are otherwise fairly uniformly distributed. They tend to line up along the taenia of the colon, apparently at the point of penetration of the nutrient arteries, which represents a weakness in the muscular wall (Fig. 35-1). Recent studies suggest that diverticulosis of the colon is a muscle abnormality as evidenced by the frequency of thickening of the muscle layers of the colonic segments resected for diverticulitis (Fig. 35-1, B). At times the diverticula dissect into the appendices epiploicae. Histologically, the wall of the diverticulum is composed of mucosa, submucosa, and the muscularis mucosae. The complications of the diverticula are well known and include inflammation, perforation, and hemorrhage.[40,60]

VASCULAR LESIONS

Infarction of the large intestine is uncommon when compared to the occurrence of this lesion in the small bowel. Ischemic necrosis has been reported following ligation of the inferior mesenteric artery and as spontaneous thrombosis. The latter condition is rare and occurs in patients who have severe cardiovascular disease. Infarction may follow mechanical insults to the bowel, such as volvulus.[28] The lesions of ischemic colitis have recently been divided into three types: (1) ischemic infarction, (2) ischemic stricture, and (3) a transient form that is considered to be reversible. In addition to the etiologic factors listed above, hypotension and bacterial pathogens are to be considered.[38,42]

ULCER

Idiopathic ulcers occur in any segment of the large intestine but are more common in the cecum and rectum. The next most common site is the sigmoid. They are rarely diagnosed, clinically or radiologically. Grossly, most of the ulcers are round to ovoid and fairly well circumscribed and vary in size from a few millimeters to 4 cm. The ulcers are usually solitary. A few have been described as linear or annular. Histologically, the changes are nonspecific, and heal-ing may lead to stenosis of the bowel. These ulcers are frequently found without any associated lesion. Ulcers (stercoral) may be found in the proximal portion of a segment of bowel that is the site of an obstructive lesion such as carcinoma or functional obstruction such as Hirschsprung's disease (Fig. 35-2). These ulcers may be multiple and are often ragged in outline. Similar ulcers and inflammations of the colon have been produced experimentally in dogs by surgically created obstruction.[4,16,17]

INFLAMMATORY LESIONS

A number of inflammatory lesions involve the colon; among them are the granulomatous diseases such as tuberculosis, histoplasmosis, and lymphogranuloma venereum. The most frequent site of gastrointestinal tract involvement by tuberculosis is the ileocecal region. As far as the large bowel itself is concerned, it is less frequently involved than other parts of the gastrointestinal tract. Histoplasmosis may involve the gastrointestinal tract, including any portion of the colon. It is often present as an ulcerative or a nodular thickening of the colonic wall and at times may be polypoid. Gastrointestinal histoplasmosis usually indicates disseminated disease.[1,45]

Ulceration in the large bowel may be caused by *Entamoeba histolytica*. This disease may occur in any portion of the large bowel, but the likeliest sites are the cecum, then the rectum, then sigmoid, and then transverse colon. At times the inflammatory reactions of the *Entamoeba histolytica* may produce a mass termed ameboma. It occurs in ulcerative sites and may be present as a nodular or polypoid mass. Histologically, there are necrosis, granulation tissue, and fibrosis. The lesion may be large enough to partially obstruct the large bowel. Other complications include perforation, stenosis, volvulus, and intussusception (Fig. 35-3).[52]

A number of colonic complications have been described among patients on immunosuppressive therapy as homotransplant recipients. Perforated diverticulitis, enterocolitis, ulceration, and fecal impaction have occurred in a group of more than 200 patients described by Penn and associates.[44]

CHRONIC ULCERATIVE COLITIS

Chronic ulcerative colitis is a disease that usually involves the entire colon and occurs

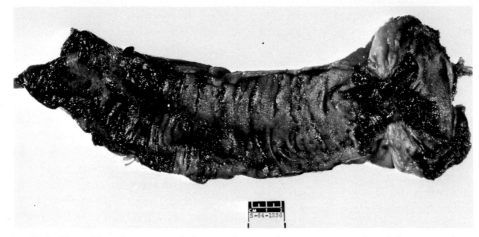

Fig. 35-2. Sigmoid colon resected for carcinoma that is seen at the right extremity of the specimen. Near the left margin is an irregularly shaped, large, stercoral ulcer. BTGH #64111.

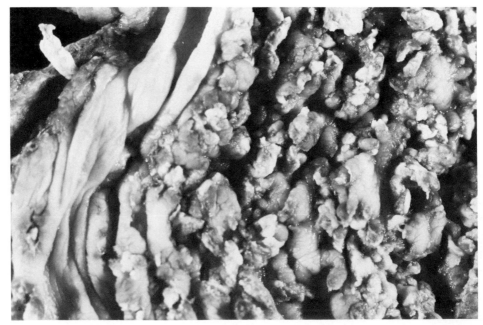

Fig. 35-3. Amebic colitis. The mucosa exhibits numerous exudate-covered ulcers and pseudopolyps. The colon has perforated. BTGH #27268.

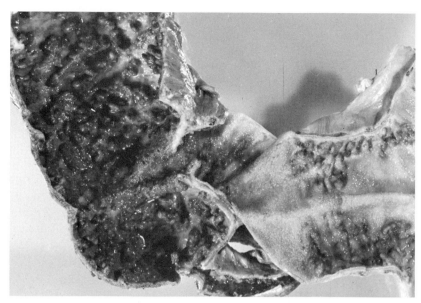

Fig. 35-4. Chronic ulcerative colitis with involvement of the appendix (bottom) and the terminal ileum (right). Numerous pseudopolyps are seen in each of the sites along with ulceration. MH #66-1162.

about equally in men and women. It is most frequently seen in the third to the fifth decades but does occur in childhood and even infancy. It is often clinically associated with periods of activity and remission, and this same variation of activity is grossly apparent in resected specimens. Basically, chronic ulcerative colitis is a mucosal and submucosal lesion, but in advanced disease the entire bowel wall may be involved. The earliest lesions begin as hyperemic foci that in reality are small abscesses. The abscesses occur in the crypts and result in ulceration. These unite to form larger and more extensive ulcers. Isolated islands of mucosa occur, and these are referred to as pseudopolyps (Fig. 35-4). There may be bridging of mucosal remnants; remnants of mucosa are undermined. In severe disease and in the late stage there may be actual narrowing and shortening of the colon. Stenosis is uncommon. Histologically, the ulcers are nonspecific with a granulation base that is richly vascular. Healing of the denuded areas is effected by reepithelialization with varied states of proliferation. The areas that have healed may appear atrophic.

One of the numerous complications of chronic ulcerative colitis is extreme dilatation of the colon. This massive dilatation of the colon usu-

ally occurs during an acute fulminating episode of ulcerative colitis and histologically shows damage to the entire wall of the colon. Other complications include malnutrition, perforation, and bleeding. Perforation and bleeding have been reported as more common in patients who have been treated with steroids, yet others report no such increased incidence. Another major complication that has been of great interest is the association of carcinomas and chronic ulcerative colitis. It has been demonstrated that carcinomas are related in general to the duration of the disease, the age of the patient at onset, and to some extent the severity of the disease. In collected groups of patients with chronic ulcerative colitis the percentage of patients having a carcinoma varies from less than 1% to 16%. The risk of developing carcinoma for a patient with chronic ulcerative colitis of over 10 years' duration is 4% per year for the colon and rectum combined. Grossly, the carcinomas have a variable appearance. Some are flat and difficult to detect grossly; others are annular, polypoid, or ulcerative. Histologically, they are adenocarcinomas, with mucinous carcinoma being fairly frequent. The distribution of carcinomas complicating chronic ulcerative colitis is more uniform throughout the colon than is ordinary carcinoma. For example, ordinary carcinoma is found most frequently in the rectum and sigmoidal areas. Multiple tumors are fairly common in this complication of chronic ulcerative colitis.*

An entity that is being increasingly discussed in the literature is Crohn's disease of the colon. The exact histologic definition of this lesion in the colon remains somewhat obscure. However, clinically, the lesion is associated with regional enteritis in about one fourth of the cases of the latter disease. There are instances in which the lesion has been confined to the colon and may involve it diffusely, be segmental, or have skip areas. It is most commonly diagnosed in the second and third decades of life but may be seen in older persons or in children. An unusual feature of the disease is that the rectum is often spared. The lesion has been described under a number of different names including segmental colitis, granulomatous colitis, ileocolitis, and regional colitis. Grossly and histologically, the lesion differs from chronic ulcerative colitis. Grossly, the mucosa is given a cobblestone pattern by numerous small intercommunicating ulcers. Long linear ulcers have also been described with this lesion. The whole bowel wall is involved, and fissures may be seen leading from the mucosa to the serosa. Another common accompaniment has been anal fistulas; on biopsy a granulomatous change may be present in the anus in 80% to 85% of patients with Crohn's disease of the large intestine and in 100% when the rectum is involved.[3] Histologically, the appearance of Crohn's disease of the colon is similar to that in the small intestine.[33,34,54,57,83]

Ulcerative proctitis is considered a mild form of ulcerative colitis, which tends to remain localized to the rectum. Roentgenographically, narrowing of the rectum and irregularity of the mucosa may be seen.[62] The earliest signs are edema and thickening of the rectal valves.

CHRONIC RADIATION EFFECT

Most frequent sites of involvement are the rectum and sigmoid and generally follow irradiation for pelvic carcinomas. The lesion is important, since it may, clinically and radiologically, pose as a carcinoma, either new, persis-

tent, or invasive. Grossly and histologically, the findings are not necessarily related to the interval between resection and radiotherapy. Grossly, ulceration and stenosis are common. The ulcer usually circumscribes the diseased area and is sharply outlined, but at either side there is edema of the mucosa. (Fig. 35-5). The wall of the bowel is thickened, with the major portion of the thickening being caused by fibrosis and edema. Histologically, the ulcers and the other findings are not specific effects of irradiation but when combined they are strongly suggestive of it; there may be peculiar alterations (loss of distinctness) of the collagen tissue indicative of radiation effect. Necrosis of smooth muscle and vascular alterations are suggestive of radiation effect.[46]

UNUSUAL DISEASES

Pneumatosis cystoides intestinalis may be confined to the colon and misinterpreted radiologically as polyposis. The gross and microscopic findings have been previously described[51] (Fig. 35-6).

Whipple's disease may involve the colon and may actually be diagnosed by rectal biopsies. Histiocytosis of the colon has been found in children, and it is similar to Whipple's disease. It is known that Whipple's disease is ordinarily detected in middle-aged and older men. The histiocytosis in children in an asymptomatic phase may represent the beginning of Whipple's disease to be manifested in adult life.[6,53]

Malakoplakia, usually considered to be a disease of the urinary tract, has been described as involving the colon and presents as a polypoid mass in the cecum. Histologically, it is a granulomatous lesion with numerous histiocytes and the diagnostic siderocalcific bodies (Michaelis-Gutmann bodies).[73]

Gallstones may be found in the intestine and have been referred to as secondary enteroliths. Primary enteroliths are rare in the colon and are said to be related to diseases that result in stasis of the bowel contents. Calcium accumulation in the enteroliths makes them radiopaque.[22]

A lesion that may be inflammatory in origin is colitis cystica profunda. It may occur either as a diffuse form or the more common localized form. The diffuse form presents a nodular mucosal thickening with submucosal cysts. Localized colitis cystica is nearly always found in the

---

*See references 11, 15, 18, 19, 24, 36, and 37.

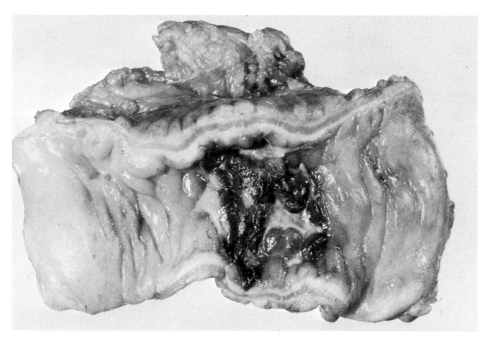

Fig. 35-5. Ulcer and stenosis of the sigmoid colon 9 months after irradiation for carcinoma of the vagina. The ulcer is sharply demarcated; the adjacent mucosa is edematous. Submucosal fibrosis is prominent. (From Moss. W. T., and Brand, W. N.: Therapeutic radiology, ed. 3, St. Louis, 1969, The C. V. Mosby Co.)

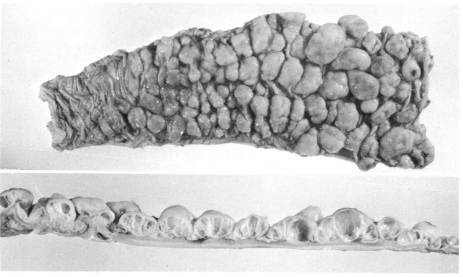

Fig. 35-6. Pneumatosis cystoides intestinalis. The mucosa is distorted by the submucosal collections of gas seen in the longitudinal section. (From Ackerman, L. V., and Rosai, J.: Surgical pathology, ed. 5, St. Louis, 1973, The C. V. Mosby Co.)

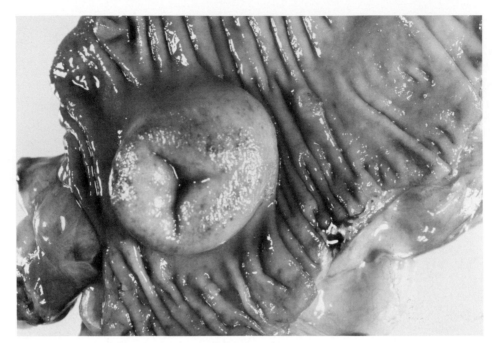

Fig. 35-7. Lipoma of the ileocecal valve. The mucosa is intact over the mass, which resulted in a filling defect by barium enema. SLEH #710536.

rectum and is a polypoid or nodular mass. Histologically, submucosal cysts with an associated chronic inflammation are seen. The cysts are frequently filled with mucin and because of their submucosal location have been diagnosed mistakenly as mucinous adenocarcinoma.

TUMORS

Benign tumors other than adenomatous polyps of the large intestine are relatively uncommon. Most of those that do occur are covered by mucosa, and are present as protuberances into the lumen of the bowel, which are sometimes pedunculated. Hemangiomas are common in the distal colon and rectum but may occur at any site and be the cause of rectal bleeding. Leiomyomas may be present as polypoid or sessile masses and occur in the submucosa. Lipomas are said to be one of the most common of the benign tumors other than adenomatous polyps and are usually found in the submucosa (Fig. 35-7). Occasionally subserosal lipomas have been described. The most common location for lipomas is the cecum,[20,48] becoming progressively less frequent in the distal segments of the colon.

Neurofibromas, often associated with neurofibromatosis, may affect the large bowel. Another rare lesion is a dermoid cyst, which has been described as occurring in the cecum.[43,78]

A reasonably common benign tumor of the large bowel is the lymphoid pseudotumor sometimes inappropriately referred to as benign lymphoma. These are most common in the lower one third of the rectum and may vary in size from 3 mm. to 3 cm. They may be the source of rectal bleeding. Grossly, they are rounded, smooth, mucosa-covered nodules that may occasionally have a broad stalk. Microscopically the lesion is composed of lymphoid aggregates with germinal centers. There has been no recorded instance of transformation of this lesion into a lymphosarcoma.[8]

Endometriosis of the large intestine may be mistaken, both clinically and radiologically, for benign and malignant tumors. It is most commonly found in the rectum and sigmoid and should be considered in women who have rectal pain or tenesmus associated with menses. Only rarely is there rectal bleeding associated with the menses. The lesion is covered by mucosa, is smooth, and at times, is multiple (Fig. 35-8).

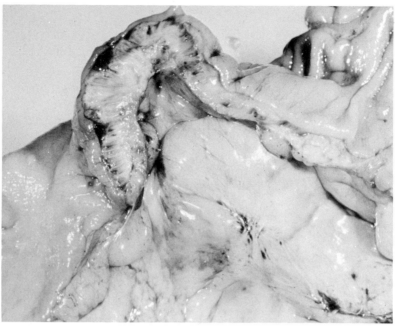

Fig. 35-8. Submucosal nodule of the sigmoid colon resulting from endometriosis. The bulk is caused by hypertrophy of the muscularis. The small dark spots are hemorrhagic foci. BUCM #18446.

Much of the deformity in the contour of the bowel is caused by hypertrophy of the muscularis.[64]

Polyps

Polyps of the large bowel signify a gross configuration of a lesion protruding into the lumen. Therefore many lesions may appear grossly and radiographically as polyps including those previously described and malignant tumors, for example, carcinoids, carcinomas, and metastatic lesions. The most common of the polyps, however, are the epithelial polyps of which there are several histologic types; juvenile or retention polyps, inflammatory polyps, adenomatous polyps, hyperplastic polyps, the mixed villous and adenomatous polyps, and the villous tumors.

Juvenile polyps are probably inflammatory in origin and tend to occur in children. They are a common cause of rectal bleeding in children. Often the lesion may be passed spontaneously and by radiographic examination has been observed to regress spontaneously. There is no relationship between these lesions and malignancy. Inflammatory polyps may occur as isolated lesions or with ulcerative colitis. Pseudopolyps of ulcerative colitis have not been associated with the formation of carcinoma.[2,25]

Hyperplastic polyps are small, usually less than 5 mm. in diameter. They have a distinctive microscopic appearance that sets them off from other epithelial polyps. There is an infolding of the epithelium into the grandular lumen giving a somewhat serrated appearance. These may or may not represent a stage in the development of adenomatous polyps. This point has not yet been settled.[32]

The controversial lesion among the polyps of the large bowel is the adenomatous polyp. The controversy revolves around its relationship to carcinoma. Does transformation from polyp to carcinoma occur rarely, never, or invariably? Histologically, the adenomatous polyp is composed of glands that simulate in structure the normal colonic glands. They are crowded and have nuclear and cytoplasmic alterations. The nuclear alterations consist of nuclear stratification with increased numbers of mitotic figures. Cytoplasmic alterations consist of increased density of the cytoplasm and decreased numbers of goblet cells. They usually have a stalk but may be sessile (Fig. 35-9). Most adenomatous

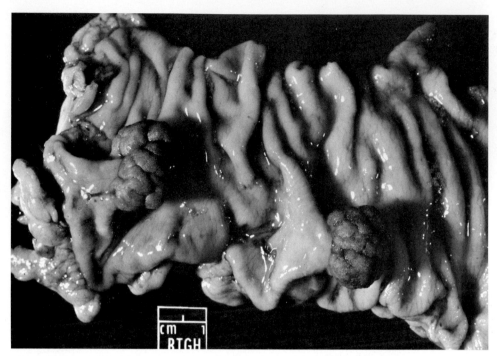

Fig. 35-9. Two adenomatous polyps of the sigmoid colon. Both have a diameter greater than 1 cm. and are on stalks. BTGH #64104.

polyps are in the neighborhood of 1 cm. in greatest dimension but may measure up to 3 or 4 cm. Histologically, there may be foci of carcinoma in situ in the adenomatous polyps, or there may even be invasion of the stalk. The evidence in the literature, which in recent years has been voluminous, seems to support a negative relationship between adenomatous polyps and carcinoma.[7,26,29,67] An occasional patient with a pedunculated polyp with carcinoma in the polyp and metastasis to regional lymph nodes has been reported.[32] However, a number of these polyps have been of the mixed variety although designated as adenomatous. The chance of a polypoid lesion being malignant increases with the size of the lesion. Therefore, high quality roentgenographic studies are needed in order to delineate these lesions Demonstration of a stalk is extremely important in the polypoid masses, since it has been demonstrated that polypoid lesions, such as adenomatous polyps on stalks in which there is a histological focus of carcinoma, are of no consequence as far as endangering the life of the patient is concerned. Serial studies to evaluate possible enlargement are, however, necessary.

Familial polyposis is a genetic disease in which the patients have a high risk of dying of carcinoma of the large bowel. This is estimated at about 40%. There are other familial diseases associated with multiple polyps of the large bowel. One of these is Gardner's syndrome, consisting of multiple adenomatous polyps, osteomas, and soft tissue tumors. The polyps may occur anywhere in the gastrointestinal tract. In the large bowel, the polyps are not as numerous as those seen in familial polyposis; that is, they do not for all practical purposes appear to cover the entire large-bowel surface. The risk of malignant neoplasm is similar to that of familial polyposis. The second noteworthy lesion is Peutz-Jeghers syndrome, a familial intestinal polyposis associated with pigmentation of the oral mucosa, lips, hands, or feet.[5,80]

In addition to the entities listed above the following categories of polyposis have been described[55,76,82]:

1. Turcot syndrome (polyposis with brain tumor)
2. Cronkhite-Canada syndrome (polyposis with ectodermal changes)
3. Multiple glandular adenomatosis with polyposis
4. Multiple polyps of the colon or rectum

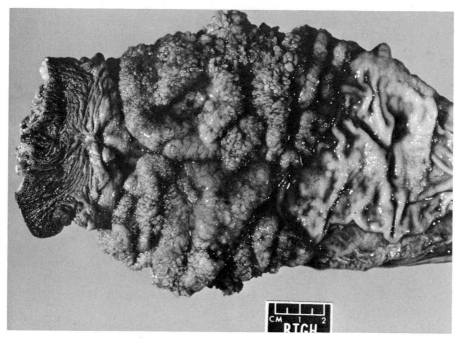

Fig. 35-10. Circumferential villous tumor of the rectum. The lesion has folds, is nonulcerated, and presents innumerable villous projections. Histologically, an invasive carcinoma was found. BTGH #65198.

5. Polyposis of the entire gastrointestinal tract
6. Gastrointestinal juvenile polyposis
7. Juvenile polyposis coli

A histologic variant of the adenomatous polyp is the mixed or villoglandular polyp. As the name suggests, the lesion is composed of an adenomatous component with numerous villous projections. These lesions tend to be larger than the adenomatous polyps; their importance, however, is unknown at the moment. Growth rates as studied by serial roentgenograms indicate that these lesions have a growth rate similar to that of the villous tumors.[77]

Villous tumors most commonly occur in the rectum and sigmoid of the large intestine but may be seen in other portions and even in the small bowel. Seventy-five percent or more are found in the rectum or sigmoid. They vary in size, but many are over 3 cm. in greatest dimension. They usually are broad based and papillary; an occasional villous tumor may have a stalk. It is generally accepted that between 35% and 50% of the lesions contain a histologic focus of carcinoma. This correlates positively with the size of the tumor. Grossly, when the lesion is in reach of the palpating finger, car-

cinoma can be suspected when there is evidence of ulceration, when the villous tumor seems to be fixed, or when firm areas are palpated (Fig. 35-10). Of clinical interest is the association of electrolyte loss with the villous tumor, that is, a loss of sodium, potassium, or chloride. This loss correlates roughly with the size of the lesion; the larger the lesion the more likely this complication is to occur.[50] Another interesting feature, observed by Kaye and Bragg, is the association of other gastrointestinal tumors with villous tumors.[27] About one fourth of their patients with villous tumors had such lesions.

Carcinoids

In the colon the rectum is the most common site of carcinoid tumors, although they may be seen in any portion of the large bowel. Grossly, carcinoid ordinarily is present as a submucosal nodule that may be ulcerated, polypoid, or even annular. On occasions carcinoids may be multiple. Characteristically the lesions are yellowish on their cut surface. Histologically, they are composed of nests of neatly arranged rather uniformly shaped and sized cells, often surrounded by a dense fibrous stroma.

In the rectum a glandular pattern is often

seen and confused with adenocarcinoma. Invasion of the muscularis may be seen. The incidence of metastases from carcinoids is generally related to the size, that is, those lesions over 2 cm. are considered to have the highest chance of metastases. This is of considerable significance in the treatment of these tumors.

Even with widespread metastases the carcinoid syndrome is rare with carcinoids of the colon and rectum. Saegesser and Gross have reported one case—a woman with a rectal carcinoid, liver metastases, and elevated urine levels of 5-HIAA.[56]

Carcinoma

In both men and women carcinoma of the large bowel represents the second most common cause of death caused by carcinoma in the United States. In men it is second to carcinoma of the lung and in women second to carcinoma of the breast. The cause is unknown, but several epidemiologic factors may contribute to the genesis of carcinoma of the large intestine: socioeconomic status, diet, obesity (in men), possible bacterial flora of the large intestine, occupation (asbestos workers), increased risk for Jews (cecum to sigmoid), and the well-known risk for patients with chronic ulcerative colitis of some duration.[58,81]

The majority of carcinomas of the large bowel occur in the rectum and sigmoid, with the cecum representing the third most common site. Grossly, the pattern varies a great deal. Many are ulcerated with raised borders; others are polypoid or annular, and occasionally they may be flat with diffuse infiltration, having somewhat the appearance of linitis plastica (Fig. 35-11). The areas of the tumor are usually sharply demarcated. The majority of the carcinomas are invasive of the wall of the bowel and may extend into the mesenteric fat or serosa. Some may have a bulky extraluminal component. Approximately 15% of carcinomas of the large bowel are associated with a second lesion in the large bowel, as a second carcinoma or adenomatous polyp.

As many as 5% of persons with one malignant tumor of the large bowel will have a second malignancy of the colon or rectum. These are not necessarily synchronous. Diamante and

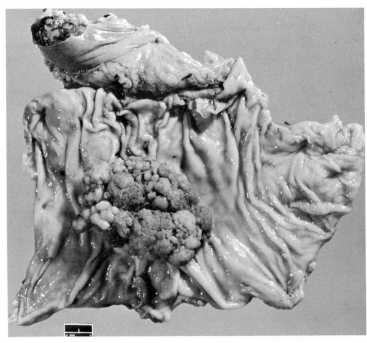

Fig. 35-11. A polypoid carcinoma of the colon that invaded the bowel wall. BTGH #66128.

Bacon also reported that 3.8% of patients with a malignancy of the colorectum have an extracolonic malignancy.[10]

The growth rate of carcinomas of the large bowel has been shown to be slow, indicating that when they are detectable radiologically, it is relatively late in the life of the tumor. Serial measurement of carcinoma by roentgenographic means indicates that most of the lesions have been present for years. It has also been demonstrated that small carcinomas of the large bowel, those 2 cm. or less in greatest dimensions, may have histologically verified metastases.[65,66,77]

Histologically, the majority of carcinomas of the large bowel are adenocarcinomas of varied degrees of differentiation. Most are moderately well differentiated. Recent studies have indicated that a reasonably high percentage of poorly differentiated or undifferentiated carcinomas are located in the right colon as compared to the left. Mucinous carcinomas are relatively uncommon; an occasional one may be of the signet ring cell variety. Mucinous components in ordinary carcinomas, however, are fairly frequent. Mucinous carcinomas comprise a high percentage of the carcinomas of the large bowel in young adults and children. Rare squamous cell carcinomas and adenoacanthomas have been found in the rectum and cecum. Histologically, ossification and calcification occur in a few carcinomas of the colon and these may be detected roentgenographically.[23,59,75,84]

There are many features of carcinomas of the colon that correlate with prognostic values. The most common one used is Duke's classification, which relates to depth of invasion into the bowel wall by the carcinoma. Duke's classification A means the tumor is confined to the bowel wall; Duke's B, the tumor has invaded through the muscularis into the serosa or into the mesenteric fat; and Duke's C means that there is a tumor distant from the bowel. Another feature of importance in relation to prognosis is nerve and vascular invasion, which is generally associated with a poor prognosis. Pushing margins (rounded) when seen histologically indicate a good prognosis. Heavy infiltration of the tumor margins by inflammatory cells or associated abscess formation usually indicates a good prognosis. Of interest is the fact that free perforation of the carcinoma into the peritoneal cavity does not alter the prognosis appreciably.[63,68]

A point of interest in the follow-up of patients having been treated for carcinoma of the large bowel is the relatively high recurrence rate at the line of anastomosis in those patients who have had anterior resection. This percentage is in the neighborhood of 11%. Patients having recurrence at the line of anastomosis usually do poorly, and it has been pointed out that approximately 80% of the recurrences occur within 3 years of the initial treatment. Of equal importance is the fact that patients surviving carcinoma of the colon beyond 5 years have a high risk of developing a second colonic carcinoma or an extracolonic carcinoma. Such a lesion is found in about one third of these patients.[47,74]

Other tumors

Primary lymphomas of the large bowel involve the cecum most frequently, representing 85% of these lesions. Grossly, the lesion may be diffuse, polypoid, or ulcerative. The wall is usually thickened and the lesion may be multiple. Histologically, lymphosarcoma of various degrees of differentiation is the most common type, followed by reticulum cell sarcoma, mixed lymphosarcoma or reticulum cell sarcoma, and Hodgkin's disease.[9,14]

Carcinomas metastatic to the large bowel are most frequently associated with intra-abdominal carcinomas. These may be the result of vascular dissemination, direct extension, or drop metastases. Many are multiple. They present, grossly, a variety of patterns such as ulcers, extrinsic pressure, polypoid lesions, and intramural lesions, but they usually do not have the raised borders seen around primary carcinomas of the colon.[79]

Leiomyosarcomas of the large bowel have somewhat the same gross characteristics as do the leiomyomas; they occur intramurally and are often covered by mucosa. Of the few cases reported only about one half have survived beyond 5 years after treatment.[44]

DISEASES OF THE APPENDIX
Calculi

Lithiasis of the appendix is a condition that occurs more frequently than other well-established appendiceal entities such as mucocele and carcinoid tumors. For many years the roentgenographic finding of a calculus in the appendix has been considered as a rare and unimportant phenomenon. Accumulated evidence indicates now that this condition is of clinical importance, and that it is not as rare as customarily assumed. The clinical importance of this condition lies mainly in the fact that usually such calculi result in acute appendicitis and are associated with a high incidence of acute complications, mainly perforation. The occurrence rates given in the literature vary considerably. When radiologists have become coprolith-conscious, the diagnostic incidence has increased.

Roentgenographic examination of normal appendixes has shown calculi in 0 to 25% of the cases.[12] When acutely inflamed appendices have been examined roentgenographically after surgical removal, the presence of calculi has varied from 33% to 44%. Appendiceal calculi have been demonstrated on abdominal roentgenograms obtained on patients with suspected appendicitis in 3.8% to 33% of the instances, with an average of about 10%. In some series, calculi have occurred predominantly in males; in other series no sex difference has been observed. Although the condition has been reported in patients of all ages, most of the calculi occur within the first three decades of life. The average size of the calculi is 1 cm. Although more often single, multiple calculi are not uncommon (Fig. 35-12).

The clinical diagnosis of this condition depends entirely on the roentgenologic findings. A laminated calculus in the right lower quadrant of a patient with acute abdominal symptoms will almost invariably prove to be an appendiceal calculus.[13]

Mucocele and myxoglobulosis

Myxoglobulosis is a rare type of mucocele of the appendix, characterized by clusters of pearly white mucous balls that resemble frog or fish

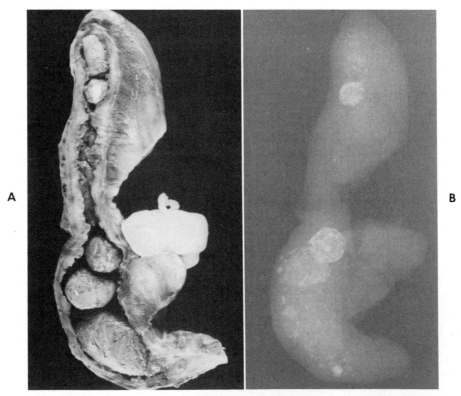

Fig. 35-12. A, An appendix opened longitudinally, revealing five coproliths. There is associated appendicitis. **B,** Roentgenogram of the appendix in **A,** illustrating calcific densities in each of the coproliths. These were noticed in retrospect on the flat film of the abdomen of this patient.

eggs intermixed with mucus. Like simple mucocele of the appendix, myxoglobulosis is usually asymptomatic and is found incidentally at operation or postmortem examination. Occasionally, both lesions can appear clinically as acute appendicitis and result in pseudomyxoma peritonei. The prevalence of myxoglobulosis is much lower than that of mucocele. Mucocele has been reported in 0.07% to 0.24% of appendectomy specimens and in 0.2% of appendixes examined at autopsy, whereas myxoglobulosis is said to comprise only 0.35% to 7.8% of mucoceles.

If judged by the sparsity of reported cases, the incidence of calcification of simple mucocele seems to be uncommon. When calcification occurs, it is usually the wall of the appendix that becomes calcified and appears on roentgenograms as a slender, curvilinear shadow of increased density. Occasionally the contents of myxoglobulosis become calcified, and when this happens the radiologic appearance is pathognomonic. A round, sharply outlined, soft-tissue shadow, attached to the cecum and freely mobile with it, with or without marginal calcifications, with absence of contrast media filling the appendix, with small 1 to 10 mm. rounded calcifications is pathognomonic of myxoglobulosis (Figs. 35-13 and 35-14).[41]

Tumors

Carcinomas of the appendix are classified as carcinoid tumors, malignant mucoceles, and adenocarcinomas of colonic type. Carcinoid tumors are by far the most frequent. Yet the surgical incidence of appendiceal carcinoid tumors ranges from 0.03% to 0.69%. As with carcinoid tumors originating in other parts of the gastrointestinal tract, the size of the appendiceal lesion and the incidence of metastasis to

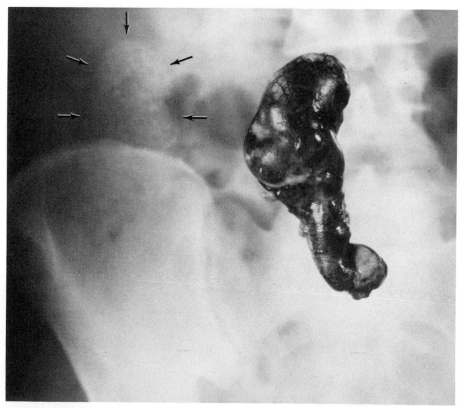

Fig. 35-13. The arrows outline a mass in which numerous punctate densities are seen. The surgically removed appendix is superimposed to the right. (From Navarrete-Reyna, A., Stewart, C. V., and Collins, L. C.: Myxoglobulosis, Texas Med. **65:**52, 1969.)

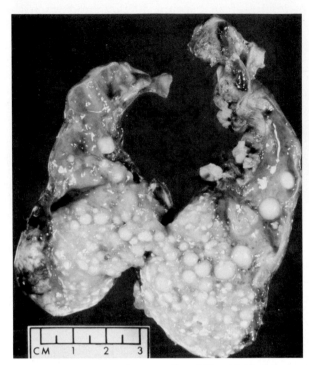

Fig. 35-14. The opened appendix of Fig. 35-13 shows numerous pearly white mucous balls admixed with mucus.

regional lymph nodes are directly related. About 90% of carcinoid tumors of the appendix measure 1.5 cm. or less in diameter, and a carcinoid larger than 2 cm. is rare.[39]

Most of the appendiceal mucosal polyps are of the adenomatous type. Villous or papillary polyps, indistinguishable from those originating in the colon, small intestine, and stomach, have occasionally been reported in the appendix.

REFERENCES

1. Abrams, J. S., and Holden, W. D.: Tuberculosis of the gastrointestinal tract, Arch. Surg. (Chicago) **89:** 282, 1964.
2. Andrén, L., and Frieberg, S.: Spontaneous regression of polyps of the colon in children, Acta Radiol. (Stockholm) **46:**507, 1956.
3. Boggs, H. W., Jr.: Anal lesions of granulomatous (Crohn's) disease of the bowel, Southern Med. J. **63:**1265, 1970.
4. Butsch, J. L., Dockerty, M. B., McGill, D. B., and Judd, E. S.: "Solitary" nonspecific ulcers of the colon, Arch. Surg. (Chicago) **98:**171, 1969.
5. Calabro, J. J.: Hereditable multiple polyposis syndromes of the gastrointestinal tract, Amer. J. Med. **33:**276, 1962.
6. Caravati, C. M., Litch, M., Weisiger, B. B., Rag-
land, S., and Berlinger, H.: Diagnosis of Whipple's disease by rectal biopsy, Ann. Intern. Med. **58:** 166, 1963.
7. Castleman, B., and Krickstein, H. I.: Do adenomatous polyps of the colon become malignant? New Eng. J. Med. **267:**469, 1962.
8. Cornes, J. S., Wallace, M. H., and Morson, B. C.: Benign lymphomas of the rectum and anal canal, J. Path. Bact. **82:**371, 1961.
9. Culp, C. E., and Hill, J. R.: Malignant lymphoma involving the rectum, Dis. Colon Rectum **5:**426, 1962.
10. Diamante, M., and Bacon, H. E.: Primary multiple malignancy of colon and rectum, Dis. Colon Rectum **9:**441, 1966.
11. Edling, N. P., and Eklöf, O.: A roentgenologic study of the course of ulcerative colitis, Acta Radiol. (Stockholm) **54:**397, 1960.
12. Felson, B.: Appendical calculi; incidence and clinical significance, Surgery **25:**734, 1949.
13. Forbes, G. B., and Lloyd-Davies, R. W.: Calculous disease of the vermiform appendix, Gut **7:**583, 1966.
14. Glick, D. D., and Soule, E. H.: Primary malignant lymphoma of colon or appendix, Arch. Surg. (Chicago) **92:**144, 1966.
15. Glotzer, D. J., Gardner, R. C., Goldman, H., Hinrichs, H. R., Rosen, H., and Zetzel, L.: Comparative features and cause of ulcerative and granulomatous colitis, New Eng. J. Med. **282:**582, 1970.
16. Glotzer, D. J., and Pihl, B. G.: Experimental obstructive colitis, Arch. Surg. (Chicago) **92:**1, 1966.
17. Glotzer, D. J., Roth, S. I., and Welch, C. E.: Colonic ulceration proximal to obstructing carcinoma, Surgery **56:**950, 1964.
18. Goldgraber, M. B., and Kirsner, J. B.: Carcinoma of the colon in ulcerative colitis, Cancer **17:**657, 1964.
19. Goldgraber, M. B., Kirsner, J. B., and Palmer, W. L.: The role of ACTH and adrenal steroids in perforation of the colon in ulcerative colitis, Gastroenterology **33:**434, 1957.
20. Haller, J. D., and Roberts, T. W.: Lipomas of the colon; a clinicopathologic study of 20 cases, Surgery **55:**773, 1964.
21. Harbour, M. J., Altman, D. H., and Gilbert, M.: Congenital atresia of the colon, Radiology **84:**19, 1965.
22. Harland, D.: A case of multiple calculi in the large intestine with a review of the subject of intestinal calcula, Brit. J. Surg. **41:**209, 1953.
23. Hermann, G., and Rozin, R.: Calcification in gastro-intestinal carcinomata, Clin. Radiol. **15:**139, 1964.
24. Hijmans, J. C., and Enzer, N. B.: Ulcerative colitis in childhood, Pediatrics **29:**389, 1962.
25. Horrilleno, E. G., Eckert, C., and Ackerman, L. V.: Polyps of the rectum and colon in children, Cancer **10:**1210, 1957.
26. Hughes, L. E.: The incidence of benign and malignant neoplasms of the colon and rectum; a postmortem study, Aust. New. Zeal. J. Surg. **38:**30, 1968.
27. Kaye, J. J., and Bragg, D. G.: Unusual roentgeno-

logic and clinicopathologic features of villous adenomas of the colon, Radiology 91:799, 1968.

28. Kerry, R. L., and Ransom, H. K.: Volvulus of the colon, Arch. Surg. (Chicago) 99:215, 1969.
29. Koppel, M., Bailar, J. C., Weakley, F. L., and Shimkin, M. B.: Incidence of cancer in the colon and rectum among polyp-free patients, Dis. Colon Rectum 5:349, 1962.
30. Kottmeier, P. K., and Clatworthy, H. W., Jr.: Aganglionic and functional megacolon in children—a diagnostic dilemma, Pediatrics 36:572, 1965.
31. Kraft, E., Finby, N., Egidio, P. T., and Glenn, J. S.: The megasigmoid syndrome in psychotic patients, J.A.M.A. 195:1099, 1966.
32. Lane, N., and Lev, R.: Observations on the origin of adenomatous epithelium of the colon, Cancer 16:751, 1963.
33. Lindner, A. E., Marshak, R. H., Wolf, B. S., and Janowitz, H. D.: Granulomatous colitis, New Eng. J. Med. 269:379, 1963.
34. Lockhart-Mummery, H. E., and Morson, B. C.: Crohn's disease of the large intestine, Gut 5:493, 1964.
35. Louw, J. H.: Investigations into the etiology of congenital atresia of the colon, Dis. Colon Rectum 7:471, 1964.
36. Lumb, G., and Protheroe, R. H. B.: Ulcerative colitis, Gastroenterology 34:381, 1958.
37. Lumb, G., Protheroe, R. H. B., and Ramsay, G. S.: Ulcerative colitis with dilatation of the colon, Brit. J. Surg. 43:182, 1955.
38. Marston, A., Pheils, M. T., Thomas, M. L., and Morson, B. C.: Ischaemic colitis, Gut 7:1, 1966.
39. Moertel, C. G., Dockerty, M. B., and Judd, E. S.: Carcinoid tumors of the vermiform appendix, Cancer 21:270, 1968.
40. Morson, B. C.: The muscle abnormality in diverticular disease of the sigmoid colon, Brit. J. Radiol. 36:385, 1963.
41. Navarrete-Reyna, A., Stewart, C. V., and Collins, L. C.: Myxoglobulosis, Texas Med. 65:52, 1969.
42. Payan, H., Levine, S., Bronstein, L., and King, E.: Subtotal ischemic infarction of the colon simulating ulcerative colitis, Arch. Path. (Chicago) 80:530, 1965.
43. Pear, B. L., and Wolff, J. N.: Epidermoid cyst of the cecum, J.A.M.A. 207:1516, 1969.
44. Penn, I., Brettschneider, L., Simpson, K., Martin, A., and Starzl, K. E.: Major colonic problems in human homotransplant recipients, Arch. Surg. (Chicago) 100:61, 1971.
45. Perez, C. A., Sturim, H. S., Kouchoukos, N. T., and Kamberg, S.: Some clinical and radiographic features of gastrointestinal histoplasmosis, Radiology 86:482, 1966.
46. Perkins, D. E., and Spjut, H. J.: Intestinal stenosis following radiation therapy, Amer. J. Roentgen. 88:953, 1962.
47. Polk, H. C., Jr., Spratt, J. S., Jr., and Butcher, H. R., Jr.: Frequency of multiple primary malignant neoplasms associated with colorectal carcinoma, Amer. J. Surg. 109:71, 1965.
48. Quan, S. H. Q., and Berg, J. W.: Leiomyoma and

leiomyosarcoma of the rectum, Dis. Colon Rectum 5:415, 1962.
49. Raia, A.: Pathogenesis and treatment of acquired megacolon, Surg. Gynec. Obstet. 101:69, 1955.
50. Ramirez, R. F., Culp, C. E., Jackman, R. J., and Dockerty, M. B.: Villous tumors of the lower part of the large bowel, J.A.M.A. 194:863, 1965.
51. Ramos, A. J., and Powers, W. E.: Pneumatosis cystoides intestinalis, Amer. J. Roentgen. 77:678, 1957.
52. Recio, P. M.: Ameboma of the colon, Philipp. J. Surg. Spec. 20:61, 1965.
53. Rowlands, D. T., Jr., and Landing, B. H.: Colonic histiocytosis in children, Amer. J. Path. 36:201, 1960.
54. Rudhe, U., and Keats, T. E.: Granulomatous colitis in children, Radiology 84:24, 1965.
55. Sachatello, C. R., Pickren, J. W., and Grace, J. T., Jr.: Generalized juvenile gastrointestinal polyposis, Gastroenterology 58:699, 1970.
56. Saegesser, F., and Gross, M.: Carcinoid syndrome and carcinoid tumors, Amer. J. Proctol. 20:27, 1969.
57. Saltzstein, S. L., and Rosenberg, B. F.: Ulcerative colitis of the ileum and regional enteritis of the colon, Amer. J. Clin. Path. 40:610, 1963.
58. Selikoff, I. J., Churg, J., and Hammond, E. C.: Relation between exposure to asbestos and mesothelioma, New Eng. J. Med. 272:560, 1965.
59. Sessions, R. T., Riddell, D. H., Kaplan, H. J., and Foster, J. H.: Carcinoma of the colon in the first two decades of life, Ann. Surg. 162:279, 1965.
60. Soger, K., and Wacks, M. R.: Exsanguinating arterial bleeding associated with diverticulating disease of the colon, Arch. Surg. (Chicago) 102:9, 1971.
61. Soper, R. T., and Miller, F. E.: Congenital aganglionic megacolon (Hirschsprung's disease), Arch. Surg. (Chicago) 96:554, 1968.
62. Sparberg, M.: Ulcerative proctitis, Texas Med. 64: 52, 1968.
63. Sperling, D., Spratt, J. S., Jr., and Carnes, V. M.: Adenocarcinoma of the large intestine with perforation, Missouri Med. 60:1104, 1963.
64. Spjut, H. J., and Perkins, D. E.: Endometriosis of the sigmoid colon and rectum, Amer. J. Roentgen. 82:1070, 1959.
65. Spratt, J. S., Jr., and Ackerman, L. V.: The growth of a colonic adenocarcinoma, Amer. Surg. 27:23, 1961.
66. Spratt, J. S., Jr., and Ackerman, L. V.: Small primary adenocarcinomas of the colon and rectum, J.A.M.A. 179:337, 1962.
67. Spratt, J. S., Jr., Ackerman, L. V., and Moyer, C. A.: Relationship of polyps of the colon to colonic cancer, Ann. Surg. 148:682, 1958.
68. Spratt, J. S., Jr., and Spjut, H. J.: Prevalence and prognosis of individual clinical and pathologic variables associated with colorectal carcinoma, Cancer 20:1976, 1967.
69. Stephens, F. D.: Congenital imperforate rectum, recto-urethral and recto-vaginal fistulae, Aust. New Zeal. J. Surg. 22:161, 1953.
70. Stephens, F. D.: Malformations of the anus, Aust. New Zeal. J. Surg. 23:9, 1953.

71. Sturim, H. S., and Ternberg, J. L.: Congenital atresia of the colon, Surgery 59:458, 1966.

72. Swenson, O.: Hirschsprung's disease (aganglionic megacolon), New Eng. J. Med. **260**:972, 1959.

73. Terner, J. Y., and Lattes, R.: Malakoplakia of colon and retroperitoneum, Amer. J. Clin. Path. **44**:20, 1965.

74. Vandertoll, D. J., and Beahrs, O. H.: Carcinoma of rectum and low sigmoid, Arch. Surg. (Chicago) **90**:793, 1965.

75. VanPatter, H. T., and Whittick, J. W.: Heterotopic ossification in intestinal neoplasms, Amer. J. Path. **31**:73, 1955.

76. Veale, A. M. D., McColl, I., Bussey, H. J. R., and Morson, B. C.: Juvenile polyposis coli, J. Med. Genet. **3**:5, 1966.

77. Welin, S., Youker, J., and Spratt, J. S., Jr.: The rates and patterns of growth of 375 tumors of the large intestine and rectum observed serially by double contrast enema studies (Malmö technique), Amer. J. Roentgen. **90**:673, 1963.

78. Weston, S. D., Marren, M., Cohan, M. H., and Schlachter, I. S.: Neurofibroma of the rectum and colon, J. Int. Coll. Surg. (Bull.) **40**:285, 1963.

79. Wigh, R., and Tapley, N. DuV.: Metastatic lesions to the large intestine, Radiology **70**:222, 1958.

80. Woolf, C. M.: Mutation and cancer of the colon. In Burdett, W. J., editor: Carcinoma of the alimentary tract, Salt Lake City, 1965, University of Utah Press.

81. Wynder, E. L., and Shigematsu, T.: Environmental factors of cancer of the colon and rectum, Cancer **20**:1520, 1967.

82. Yanemoto, R. H., Slayback, J. B., Byron, R. L., Jr., and Rosen, R. B.: Familial polyposis of the entire gastrointestinal tract, Arch. Surg. (Chicago) **99**:427, 1969.

83. Yarnis, H., Marshak, R. H., and Crohn, B. B.: Ileocolitis, J.A.M.A. **164**:7, 1957.

84. Zirkin, R. M., and McCord, D. L.: Squamous cell carcinoma of the rectum, Dis. Colon Rectum **6**:370, 1963.

Examination of the colon | 36

Alexander R. Margulis

The colon is one of the organs that lends itself well to a precise and reliable roentgenologic procedure. It is the organ that in its entirety is examined best by roentgenology.

A multitude of approaches to roentgenologic examination of the colon is available. Considerable information about the colon is often obtainable from plain films of the abdomen. More precise methods for evaluating the state of the colon and for discovering lesions within it employ the use of contrast agents. Of these, the method most preferred is that of introduction of barium sulfate suspensions by enema. A modification of this method of examination of the colon is the insufflation of air after the barium sulfate has coated the mucosa. This modified method is employed with great frequency and is held in high regard by most radiologists.

These two methods are the present standard roentgenologic approaches to the examination of the colon, but other special techniques have been developed for examination of specific areas. These techniques include the silicone foam enema for study of the sigmoid and the descending colon, the shaving foam enema for examination of the rectum, and the peroral barium sulfate examination for the right colon and the ileocecal valve. The radiologist's armamentarium also includes the water enema to establish the specific diagnosis of lipoma of the colon and selective arteriography for locating the site of bleeding in the colon.

These special examinations are performed rarely and only in a few centers; however, the conventional barium sulfate enema examination of the colon is one of the most frequent examinations performed in departments of radiology throughout the world. Thomas estimated that in 1963 2,550,000 such examinations were performed in the United States.[111] When properly performed and individualized to meet the particular problem, a barium enema is a highly accurate examination. The radiologist and the staff must give a great deal of care to the prepa-

ration of the patient and to the technique of the examination. The many aspects involved in each examination must be carefully considered in order to achieve the high accuracy that the method offers. A barium enema is no more routine than is a physical examination or a laboratory work-up. Standardization and observance of meticulous care are only the bases on which individualization of each case is built in order to render a satisfactory result.

PRELIMINARY PLAIN ROENTGENOGRAMS OF THE ABDOMEN

The preliminary plain roentgenogram of the abdomen is an indispensable part of the examination of the colon. It is part of the complete record of the examination, bearing the same relationship and importance that roentgenograms of the spine or chest bear to the myelogram or bronchogram. Calcifications, unusual air or fat collections, bone abnormalities, intraperitoneal and retroperitoneal tissues, and organ changes observed on plain films are of great importance in the final evaluation of the colon by contrast medium examination. Any barium sulfate or iopanoic acid (Telepaque) remaining in the bowel or stomach from a previous examination may be recorded on the plain roentgenogram. Foreknowledge of the presence of either will relieve the anxiety and doubts that arise when they are observed during fluoroscopy as the barium sulfate enema centers the colon, or when they are seen on the edge of spot films or the large films of the barium examination. A scout film of the abdomen also permits a much more reliable evaluation of the air in the small bowel as well as the appearance of the bowel loops than do films exposed when the colon is filled with contrast medium. In addition, careful fluoroscopic scanning of the abdomen before barium sulfate starts to flow is an indispensable part of examination of the colon. Spot radiographs made with the modern intensifying systems, with or without television, are utilized because of their excellent detail and clarity. The advantages of a permanent record over the memorized impressions of even an expert fluoroscopist are so obvious that they need no further discussion.

Ideally, in the examination of the abdomen preliminary to roentgenography of the colon, the same projections that constitute the routine plain roentgenographic examination of the abdomen should be used (see Chapter 10). Rays parallel to air-fluid levels should be applied to at least one film of the abdomen in which the pelvis as well as the diaphragm is shown. The roentgenograms should be exposed with conventional technique in the 60 to 80 kv range, with the shortest possible exposure time.

In many medical centers the barium enema examination is performed after extensive radiographic examination, including radiography of the abdomen and excretory pyelograms. If this is the routine practice, in order to limit radiographic exposure another plain film examination may be omitted, provided that these roentgenograms are studied before the colon examination. Any roentgenographic and fluoroscopic disparity apparent on these films should be recorded immediately on new films of the abdomen. In any event, the use of preliminary roentgenograms may prove in the long run to be the most economical approach in an examination of the colon. This is especially true when some form of contrast material has been ingested by the patient preceding colon examination.

A survey was made of the value of routine plain roentgenograms of the abdomen, obtained consecutively on admission to the hospital of 500 patients more than 40 years of age.[91] These routine films suggested ninety-six previously unsuspected clinical conditions, which were present in 17.4% of the 500 patients. Another survey of some of the leading centers in the United States, Canada, and Europe disclosed surprising results.[63] Fewer than one third of the centers included preliminary plain films of the abdomen as part of their routine barium enema examinations.

In a survey of techniques employed by 224 radiologists in Australia and New Zealand, only 7% obtained routine preliminary roentgenograms of the abdomen, according to a report in 1971.[66]

CONTRAST-MEDIUM EXAMINATIONS OF THE ENTIRE COLON

The historic aspects of the barium enema and other examinations of the colon are dealt with in greater detail in Chapter 1. As far back as 1904 Schüle performed an enema examination of the colon using radiopaque material.[93] In 1911 Haenisch described a fluoroscopic method of examination in which bismuth subcarbonate suspension was used as the contrast medium, and the examination was performed on a table equipped with a horizontal fluoroscope.[43] More advances followed the subsequent substitution of bismuth by barium, with Fischer describing the double-contrast (barium and air) enema examination.[35] Later, with improvements, this procedure gained wide favor.[5,105-107,113-116] With increasing use the conventional barium enema examination came to be more heavily relied on and advances were made in specific aspects of the technique. Recent years have seen emphasis placed on preparation of the colon,[5,106,107,114] the addition of tannic acid to the suspension,[22,44,81] and the use of supplementary spot films, compression during screening and exposure,[33] special roentgenographic views to resolve the tortuous sigmoid colon, high kilovoltage technique for radiography,[38] and thinner suspensions of barium sulfate to enhance the penetration. A further advancement in specific conditions is the addition of cineradiography.[17]

Conventional examination with the barium sulfate enema

Equipment for roentgenography

The subject of roentgenographic equipment is discussed in greater detail in Chapter 2. It should be pointed out that in the United States and in most of Europe image-intensified fluoroscopy with or without television is rapidly replacing the conventional fluoroscopic screen technique. This development is most significant, since it permits brilliant visualization with excellent detail and individual adaption of the examination as it is being performed. Additional subtler benefits have also been derived from the decrease of radiation exposure and the advantage of working in a lighted room. The latter improves the patient-radiologist relationship during the examination and eases the apprehension of the patient. It also creates smoother cooperation between the radiologist and his assistant and enhances the appearance of the examination room. Most importantly, it provides a safe examination for the patient because the examining team is able to observe simultaneously the patient and any tubes attached to him. Television systems usually offer less resolution than mirror viewing, but they have the advantage of permitting the patient to view the screen, thus further allaying his apprehension and improving his cooperation.

The fluoroscopic table should be capable of being tilted into both the upright and Trendelenburg positions. The latter position need not exceed 45 degrees. Foam-rubber-padded shoulder holders like those used in myelography should be available for use in the Trendelenburg position. Every fluoroscopic room should be equipped with overhead tubes, preferably suspended from the ceiling. Cable pulleys that retract cable slack are also advisable for maximum maneuverability in the fluoroscopic room. The fluoroscopic unit should be equipped

with a spot device having a stationary or an oscillating fine grid, and for economy and quality of detail a selection of multiple exposure on one film should be available. The unit generator should be capable of delivering exposures in at least the 130 kv and, preferably, the 150 kv range. For optimum detail the time of exposure must be short, which necessitates equipment capable of high milliampere output. Although adept and experienced radiologists are able to select the time of exposure for each spot film, a device for phototiming spot films is recommended, especially for large departments.

Compression devices. The use of the gloved hand or fingers for palpation of the colon in the direct x-ray beam, as is practiced by many radiologists, is to be discouraged. Many devices, from wooden spoons to more elaborate plastic paddles with inflatable rubber balloons and cones, which are attached to the fluoroscopic screen, are available.[33,34] Almost every inventive radiologist has developed a compression device that has advantages in his own hands. One simple self-made device is a wooden stick 50 cm. long, with its distal end wrapped in multiple layers of rolled elastic bandage. An inconspicuous metallic marker should be incorporated into any compression device to identify the spot films in which it was used. With such a marker, the suspicion that extrinsic but intracorporeal masses produce the compression defect is eliminated.

Equipment for administration of the enema

The large metallic can with rubber tubing and sterilized or disposable rectal tips is no longer the mainstay in most departments of radiology. It has been abandoned in favor of a disposable plastic bag, tubing, and tip (Fig. 36-1). Bacterial contamination from retrograde fecal flow into the enema apparatus has been demonstrated.[69,103] Sterilization of the metallic cans and tubing before each examination is expensive and impractical, and a disposable valve preventing reflux from the rectum is not available. Disposable plastic bags, tubing, and tips are therefore preferable for the administration of the barium enema.

The bag should hold at least 2,000 ml. and should be translucent. The internal diameter of most tubes in use is 1/4 inch.[101] An internal

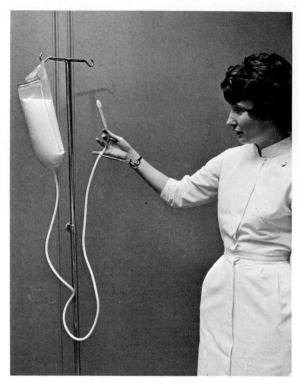

Fig. 36-1. The disposable enema apparatus consisting of a plastic bag, tube, and tip, which is used for cleansing enemas and the administration of the barium suspension. The bag holds 2,300 ml.

diameter of ⅜ inch, which permits greater choice of speed of administration of even viscous suspensions, is being advocated.[70] Plastic disposable enema tips should always be used and usually are part of the disposable plastic bag and tubing sets. If nondisposable sterilizable metal cans and rubber tubing are employed, the rectal tips should still be disposable. Most patients experience no difficulty in holding the enema and need no devices for retention. If the examination is performed in a lighted room, cooperation may be further encouraged when the patient is able to observe the examination on the television screen.

Patients who are uncooperative, senile, mentally deranged or retarded, unconscious, severely debilitated, paraplegic, or who have an incompetent anal sphincter, may require a retaining balloon. The most common balloon used for this purpose in the United States is the Foley type (Fig. 36-2). Since fatalities after improper insertion have been reported, great caution must be exerted in the insertion and inflation of such balloons. Fatalities have occurred from rupture of the large bowel when insertion was above the peritoneal reflection in the rectosigmoid, in the

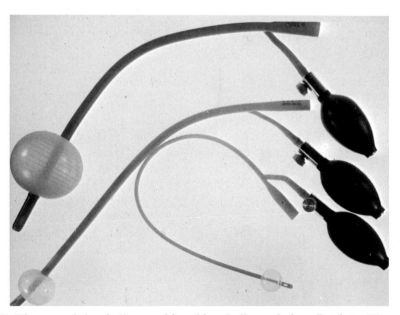

Fig. 36-2. Three retaining balloons with rubber bulbs and shutoff valves. The volumes of the balloons vary. The bottom balloon for the catheter used in small children has a volume of 15 ml.; the middle one, used in average adults, 30 ml.; and the top one, for use in adults who are incontinent, 140 ml.

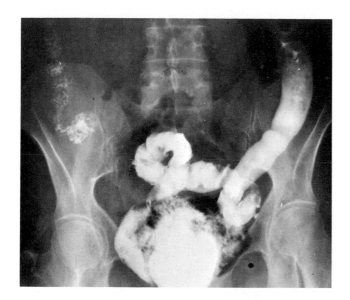

Fig. 36-3. Perforation of the rectum as a result of over-inflation of the retaining balloon. There was extraperitoneal leakage of barium and rectal contents into the pelvis. The patient died of septicemia.

middle of a rectal annular carcinoma, or in a scarred, fibrotic, or weakened rectum with ulcerative colitis.* Rupture of the rectum with leakage of bowel content and barium (Fig. 36-3) into the peritoneal cavity or extraperitoneal tissues frequently results in death. Alertness to this complication and immediate laparotomy, peritoneal lavage, and administration of antibiotics may save the patient's life. The barium may then remain in the peritoneal cavity for life (Fig. 36-4).

In order to safeguard the patient, the following precautionary measures should be taken with the use of a retaining balloon:

1. The radiologist should introduce the catheter and balloon into the rectum of the patient in the presence of a female assistant or nurse. The radiologist should wear rubber gloves and should perform a rectal examination before introducing the balloon except when hospital records indicate that a rectal examination or a sigmoidoscopic examination has been performed and the findings are normal. A low rectal neoplasm may rupture under the pressure of the distending balloon (Fig. 36-5).

2. The bulb for the insufflation must be of

low capacity and be equipped with a valve for release of air.

3. The job of inflating the balloon should not be delegated. The examining radiologist should pump the air into the balloon, while watching it on the fluoroscopic screen. If a trained assistant is permitted to inflate the balloon, the radiologist must direct the operation, again observing the balloon on the screen.

4. The barium suspension should be introduced into the rectum before any inflation of the balloon is attempted. This measure locates the balloon in relation to the rectal ampulla and gives an idea of the distensibility of the distal colon. If there is no difficulty with the retention of barium, this may encourage the radiologist and the patient to proceed with the examination without any inflation of the balloon.

5. The radiologist should be familiar with the shape and volume of the balloon he uses (Fig. 36-2). The fully inflated balloon of the usual design is perfectly spherical and appears round on the screen. Should the shape of the balloon become elliptical, asymmetric, or irregular, inflation should be discontinued immediately. After the air is released from the balloon, the rectum should then be

_____

*See references 20, 46, 75, 78, 79, 94, 124, and 199.

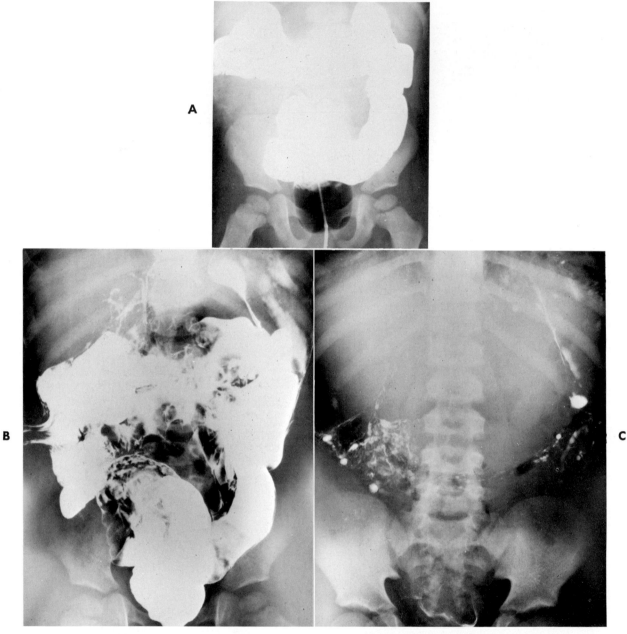

Fig. 36-4. Perforation of the rectum above the peritoneal reflection in a 22-month-old child after overinflation of a retaining balloon. A colostomy of the ascending colon had been performed in infancy at another hospital. **A,** The rectal balloon is seen inflated. Minimal irregularity of the barium contour is seen along the posterior upper border of the balloon; this was the site of perforation. **B,** During the same examination, a massive extravasation of barium throughout the peritoneal cavity takes place. Barium outlines the external wall of the stomach and the inferior border of the liver. **C,** The child survived the laparotomy and peritoneal lavage. Four years later barium is still seen in the peritoneal cavity, outlining the external wall of the stomach and inferior wall of the liver, and deposited around the porta hepatis.

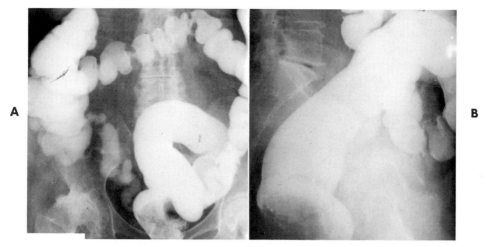

Fig. 36-5. Preevacuation roentgenograms of a barium enema examination. **A,** Frontal projection; **B,** lateral projection. A large villous adenoma is present in the lower rectum. Blind inflation of retaining balloon in the rectum in similar circumstances may cause serious complications.

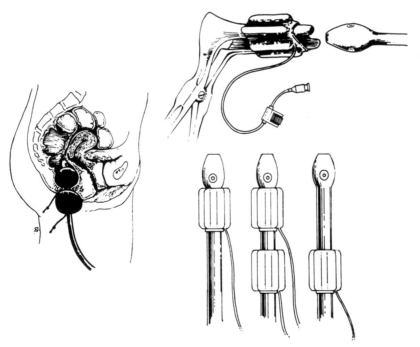

Fig. 36-6. The double-cuff enema apparatus. The schematic drawing on the left shows one cuff inflated inside the anal canal, the other inflated externally. The drawing on the upper right shows the method of placing the cuff on the enema tip. The drawing on the lower right shows three different methods of using the enema cuff with a conventional enema tip. (From Miller, R. E.: Radiology **87:**756, 1966.)

carefully examined by digital palpation.

6. A new double-cuff apparatus, that is, inflatable rubber cuffs applied on the plastic enema tip, has recently been described.[40,72] With this system, the balloons can be inflated either inside or outside the anal canal, or in both locations simultaneously (Fig. 36-6). The use of this device prevents insertion of the balloon too far cephalad, beyond the rectal ampulla where the colon is narrower and ruptures more easily. Inflation of the external as well as the internal balloon permits less distention of the retrorectal balloon.

7. If there is continuous leakage of barium while the balloon is being inflated, a mild pull maintained on the balloon by the assistant will bring it against the anal opening. Thus, a safe seal may result without further inflation.

8. Another maneuver that may combat incontinence without jeopardizing safety is to perform the examination with the patient prone, in a slight head down, feet up (prone Trendelenburg) position.

9. It must be emphasized that the use of rectal balloons should be an exception. Their use is not a routine procedure, as is frequently advocated by assistants who wish to eliminate the cleansing of the room, the equipment, and the patient.

10. Balloons should never be inflated within the bowel of a patient with a colostomy stoma. If a balloon is used in such an instance, it should be inflated externally and held against the stoma. Discussion of this procedure will be amplified in the statements about examination through a colostomy.

11. In a few conditions inflation of a balloon is absolutely contraindicated. These include, among others, a low rectal carcinoma and acute ulcerative colitis.

An interesting approach to prevent leakage of barium from the anus during barium enema was described by Clark.[23] He uses a cannula that has electrodes powered by a transistorized generator with batteries, stimulating the anal sphincter at the rate of 20 pulses per second. Clark reports excellent success in obtaining anal sphincteric competence during the examination.

Drainage of colon during examination. Drainage of barium suspension from the filled colon may be desirable for better cleansing of the colon. The study of a lesion may be more satisfactory with less barium or with drainage of some of the barium before the introduction of air. When a patient is sent to the toilet for evacuation, the examiner cannot control the drainage, and the resultant delay and inconvenience are costly. Instead, a combination suction and drainage system may be used, which is combined with the table and connected with the hospital plumbing system.[110] In departments without this convenience, a second plastic bag, connected to the rectal tube through a Y connector, can be part of the enema injection apparatus (Fig. 36-7). Removing the clamp that connects the second bag to the system and clamping off the barium bag enables gravity to suction off the colon content into the second bag.

Ancillary facilities. In the design of a modern diagnostic roentgenology department several aspects must be taken into account. For the barium enema examination, facilities should be such that it can be performed safely and smoothly, with minimum discomfort to the patient.

A sufficient number of fluoroscopic rooms must be available so that the patient with the filled colon need not be moved to another room for overhead exposure of films. An adequate number of toilets—a minimum of two or three toilets per fluoroscopic unit—should be available. A survey of centers disclosed that more than half provided only one toilet per room.[63] One of the reasons for the success of Welin's method of examination of the colon is the accessibility to eight toilets from one fluoroscopic room and five toilets from a second. The availability of one or several rooms in the department where cleansing enemas may be administered is also a most important and almost hidden factor in successful preparation of the colon. Finally, strongly recommended in a department of radiology in which cleansing and barium enemas are done, are one or more rooms for respite of patients. Here they may rest between the various steps of the examination, and during the time the radiologist is checking the films.

Ancillary personnel. The current problem of shortage of radiologists makes ancillary person-

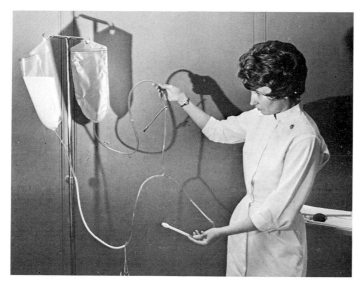

Fig. 36-7. Double enema bag that is used simultaneously for administration of barium sulfate and drainage of the colon. Clamps are used to direct the flow of barium during administration of the enema and to prevent its mixing with contents of the large bowel during drainage.

nel necessary to safeguard the quality of the roentgenologic examination. Besides the radiologic team, there must be receptionists, darkroom technicians, and circulating nursing personnel to check on ill patients. The team performing the barium enema examination must consist of at least a radiologist, a fluoroscopic aide, and an x-ray technologist. In less busy departments the technologist may administer the barium enema, clean the room and equipment between examinations, administer the cleansing enema that is given in the department, and assist and supervise the patient in going to the toilet. The more economic arrangement, however, is to assign an aide to the fluoroscopy room, one technologist to two fluoroscopic rooms, and a nurse or trained aide to administer cleansing enemas for two busy fluoroscopic rooms.

Preparation of the patient for the examination

To achieve maximum accuracy in the barium sulfate enema examination, the colon must be free of fecal material and cathartic oil droplets, and mucous secretions must be diminished or absent. In order to accomplish this goal a rigor-

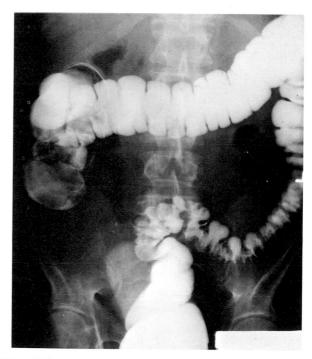

Fig. 36-8. Example of a poorly cleansed right colon containing large amounts of fecal material, which masked a polypoid carcinoma of the cecum, 2 cm. in diameter. Unless the colon is properly cleansed before the barium enema is administered, the examination must be repeated if it is to be worthwhile.

ous preparation, consisting of alterations in diet, use of cathartics, and administration of preparatory cleansing enemas is necessary (Fig. 36-8). Patients who are not ill or debilitated usually complain only that this preparation has been fairly uncomfortable and exhausting. Elderly or debilitated patients, or those suffering from heart disease, severe diabetes, adrenal disease, or other severe illnesses may be severely taxed by the rigors of this preparation.[10] The examination, therefore, must be performed with the utmost care so that the added trauma of a repetitive preparation is not necessary.

In a small number of institutions the radiologist himself issues the orders for the preparation. This practice requires a working rapport with the referring physician, which enables the radiologist to see the patient 24 to 48 hours before the examination. A more workable system is the issuing of standing orders for ward patients and outpatients who are to have a roentgenologic examination. The patient's physician must understand this routine, be educated and convinced of its value, and be able to substitute when these orders might endanger the health of the patient. Coronary artery occlusion, cerebrovascular accidents, or severe electrolyte imbalance in patients being prepared for or having a barium enema occur.

Diet. In almost one fourth of the centers surveyed, a normal diet was permitted up to the time of barium enema examination.[63] In the rest of the centers a low-residue diet or clear liquid diet was prescribed. The former was used by a few more centers than the latter. We at the University of California Medical Center (San Francisco) prescribe a 24-hour clear liquid diet consisting of broth, Coca-Cola, black coffee, ginger ale, gelatin, syrup from canned fruit, and tea with sugar only. A typical low-residue diet consists of tender meats, eggs, bread and cereals without roughage or bulk, clear soups, pureed bland vegetables and fruits limited to two servings of each, soft desserts, boiled milk, and potatoes limited to one serving. Such a diet for 2 to 3 days is easier for the patient and produces satisfactory results.

Laxatives. Castor oil is still the predominant laxative used throughout the world to prepare patients for a barium enema. The survey, frequently referred to in this chapter, of eighty medical centers in the United States, Canada, and Europe, showed that most radiologists have their patients prepared with 1 to 3 ounces of castor oil 10 to 20 hours before the examination.[63] The preferred dose appeared to be 2 ounces; it is the one we use at the University of California Medical Center (San Francisco). Whether patients took the castor oil before or after meals seemed to make no difference. Castor oil is a dependable laxative of the irritant type.[43] Its activity depends on the hydrolysis of the oil into ricinoleic acid, an irritant to the small bowel that causes massive peristalsis that the patient experiences as cramps.

Purified preparations of castor oil prepared as emulsions with additives to improve their taste are not as effective as castor oil used alone. One such preparation is Neoloid, which is used in many centers in the United States, but even a 4 ounce dose does not produce the same results as 2 ounces of castor oil. Other laxatives, such as bisacodyl (Dulcolax) suppositories and tablets and anthraquinoidal glycosides (X-prep), although effective in many patients, are not as reliable as castor oil. A castor oil laxative that may be indispensable in the preparation of the colon of most patients, however, may be contraindicated in patients with active ulcerative colitis, colostomy, or other conditions. Milder laxatives than castor oil may be required for patients with coronary insufficiency, adrenal cortical insufficiency, severe diabetes, or other serious illnesses.

A new approach to the preparation of the colon was used by five of the institutions that participated in the survey of radiologic techniques.[7,15] We frequently use this technique now at the University of California Medical Center (San Francisco), particularly on outpatients. It has the advantage of eliminating preparatory enemas and the use of castor oil. The preparation consists of a diet of a low-residue lunch, clear liquid dinner, and multiple glasses of water throughout the day and evening. The laxatives consist of 11 ounces of liquid magnesium citrate and three or four bisacodyl tablets taken in the evening. In the morning the patient is given one bisacodyl suppository. The patient is given no breakfast.

Cooperation of the referring physician for the proper preparation is mandatory for the safety of patients. The preparation for a barium enema as well as the performance of the examination itself is an exhausting experience for any patient, and in elderly patients electrocardiographic changes have been recorded during the examination.

Preparatory enemas. Many radiologists order one enema on the evening before, and one on the morning of a barium enema examination. Most radiologists use water, soap suds, or saline solutions for these enemas. Often enemas are given by ward personnel until reflux is clear; the usual limit is three such enemas.

The administration of a cleansing enema requires skill and patience in order that at least 1,000 ml. of solution may be instilled. Ward personnel often do not possess the latter virtue, so whenever possible the last enema should be given in the radiology department by a nurse or an aide trained in the procedure.

The last enema, whether administered on the ward or in the department of radiology, can be made more effective by the use of tannic acid.[83] The Food and Drug Administration has recently approved the re-release of tannic acid and bisacodyl (Clysodrast) provided that a concentration of 0.25% is not exceeded. Good results have been obtained with this enema, particularly in our older inpatients. Tannic acid is an astringent that precipitates mucus and produces evacuation and spasm of the large bowel.[57] To obtain the best results from the tannic acid dosage, an aide should encourage the patient to wait 2 to 3 minutes before evacuation of the cleansing enema. To reduce spasm of the right colon and facilitate the examination, the barium enema should be delayed about one-half hour after the cleansing enema.

If water or saline enemas are administered immediately before the roentgenographic examination, considerable retention of the enema may dilute the contrast medium. Even with tannic acid and bisacodyl it is possible that up to 40% of the cleansing enema may be retained; however, most of the patients in actuality retain very little.[122] In trials at the University of California Medical Center preparatory enemas with oxyphenosatin (Lavema) were not as satisfactory as those with tannic acid and bisacodyl because of adverse side reactions and considerable spasm of the colon.[101] However, Barnhard and Crow reported satisfactory results with oxyphenosatin dissolved in distilled water, although they advised against its routine use and stressed the

poor mucosal detail on the postevacuation roentgenograms.[8]

The tannic acid controversy. The use of tannic acid became part of the roentgenologic examination of the colon in 1946, and since then it has been used in millions of patients throughout the world.[44,51,119] Thomas estimated in 1963 that, as of that time, about 600,000 patients were receiving tannic acid enemas annually for colonic cleansing and mucosal delineation.[111]

Fatalities from liver necrosis were reported in 1942 after topical administration of tannic acid for massive burns.[117] Another group of workers in 1943 reproduced liver necrosis in animals after intravenous use or application of tannic acid to artificial burns.[6] Steinbach and Burhenne commented in 1962 that they had found no report of serious complications to the use of tannic acid administered by enema. Only by personal communication with one radiologist did they learn of "episodes of syncope, marked tetanic contractions of the colon, and occasional true temporary shock."[101] No adverse reactions from tannic acid administered by enema were reported until 1963, when McAlister and his colleagues reported the deaths of three children, occurring after the repeated use of 0.75% tannic acid enemas.[68] Later in 1963, Lucke and his colleagues reported on the deaths of five patients, all of whom had received enemas containing 2% tannic acid.[61] The livers of the patients reported on by McAlister and others showed centrolobular necrosis similar to the type described by Wells and others.[67,117] In one patient a positive reaction in the liver was obtained when Nessler's reagent was used in a nonspecific test for tannic acid and similar compounds. Apparently, radiologists have been using tannic acid in enemas with great confidence as to its safety, and paying little attention to dosage or to differences in concentration when identical volumes of fluffy (crystalline), or amorphous tannic acid were used. Despite the abandon with which tannic acid was used—with concentrations in the enema of up to 3% reported by those who measured the dosage—extremely few complications apparently occurred.

A team of investigators at the University of California Medical Center (San Francisco) consisting of radiologists, a pathologist, and pharmaceutical chemists, reported the results when tannic acid was administered by enema to rats.[45,85,122] The dose at which hepatotoxicity would develop and the conditions under which this hepatotoxic dose would vary were studied. Rats were selected as the experimental animals because of their proved susceptibility to hepatotoxic agents.

The histologic evidence of hepatotoxicity showed that lower concentrations of tannic acid administered by enema produced liver damage if forcibly retained for 1 hour (2.5% concentration of tannic acid) more often than when the enema was forcibly retained for only 1 minute (16%). Colon damage (ulceration and hemorrhage) was also produced by lower concentrations when the enema was forcibly retained for 1 hour. Liver damage depended on the concentration of tannic acid in the enema and the length of time it was retained. Severe colonic injury was almost always associated with hepatic damage. By applying histologic criteria, an enema containing a concentration of 3% of tannic acid forcibly retained for 1 hour produced hepatotoxic changes in all animals. In about 50% of the animals, the hepatotoxic dose was a 2.5% concentration; a concentration of 2% was considered safe under the experimental conditions present. Administering tannic acid intraperitoneally and thus simulating total absorption, the hepatotoxic dose for all animals was 60 to 80 mg./kg. of body weight, whereas the dose causing no hepatotoxic damage was 40 mg./kg.

Minor inflammatory changes and edema of the colon were seen even after the use of isotonic saline enemas and were more frequent after three repetitions of such enemas. Damaged colonic mucosa appears to be a prerequisite for absorption of tannic acid and its detection in the portal venous blood. In clinical situations, therefore, rigorous cleansing of the colon with repeated saline enemas may permit the absorption of a lower concentration of tannic acid, thus reducing the margin of safety relative to which tannic acid can be used. Repetition of the tannic acid enemas and their retention for prolonged periods, ulcerative disease of the colon, and preexisting parenchymal disease of the liver further reduced the margin of safety. The investigators concluded, however, that no proof exists that a tannic acid enema in concentrations of from 0.25% to 0.5% ever produced hepatotoxicity.

Welin had the necropsy slides of livers of all patients who had received tannic acid enemas since 1957 at the Malmö University Hospital reviewed. Not a single case of liver changes was found as the result of tannic acid administration. The liver function in forty-five patients who received cleansing and barium enemas containing tannic acid were studied by Burhenne and his colleagues.[19] From the results of five highly sophisticated tests, they concluded that a cleansing enema with 0.25% tannic acid with subsequent enema of 0.5% tannic acid in the barium enema examination is safe. A double-blind efficacy study showed no conclusive effect of the 0.25% tannic acid on cleansing the colon, or on enhancing the mucosal detail.[58] It did show that tannic acid promotes more complete contraction of the colon than a placebo preparation. These results differ from those of a double-blind study by Wyatt and others.[120] These authors observed that 0.75% tannic acid, as well as 1% ammonium alum produced better colonic contraction and coating of the mucosa than did the barium sulfate alone that was used in controls.

Drug additives in the preparation of the colon. In most centers in the United States and Europe the preparation of the colon for the performance of the conventional barium enema does not include the use of drugs.[63] Their use, however, is on the rise. Thirty to 60 mg. of propantheline bromide (pro-Banthine) is given with increasing frequency[32] before examining an irritable colon (Fig. 36-9) and dihydroxyanthraquinone (Dorbane), which is a smooth-muscle relaxant, is sometimes used in a dose of 75 mg. A significant number of radiologists prescribe 1 mg. of atropine sulfate for reduction of spasm and mucous secretion. These drugs, however, detract from the value of the postevacuation film. Generally they should be reserved for the performance of the double-contrast barium-air study.

Barium sulfate. The characteristics of the available suspensions of barium sulfate and the desirable features of such suspensions are discussed extensively in Chapter 7. Barium sulfate with a suspending agent is in almost general use in the United States and Europe, and only a few centers use USP barium.[63] The advantages of nonprecipitating barium sulfate and the dangers of missing a lesion located in the part of the lumen filled with supernatant water have been sufficiently emphasized (Fig. 36-10).[101] Because of water density, lesions of the bowel can be de-

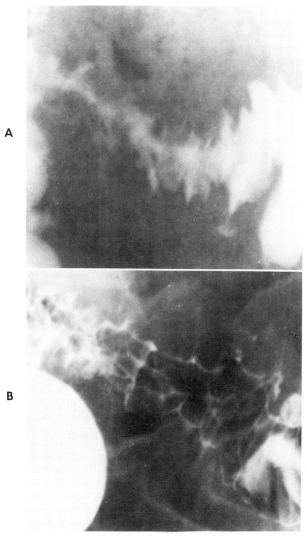

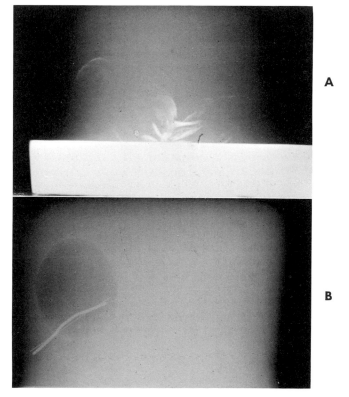

Fig. 36-9. Two spot films showing the sigmoid colon, obtained during the barium enema examination of a patient with proved diverticulitis of the sigmoid colon. **A,** Spot film obtained before administration of propantheline (Pro-Banthine) bromide. **B,** Spot film obtained after intramuscular administration of 30 mg. of propantheline and instillation of air. The spasm of the sigmoid colon has relaxed. The colon did not attain a normal lumen since it was surrounded by an inflammatory mass. We now use glucagon to relax the intestine.

Fig. 36-10. Roentgenograms of two paper cups filled with barium and containing a suspended small plastic balloon filled with water and marked with a metallic wire. The barium in the cups was allowed to settle for 1 hour. **A,** The cup is filled with USP barium sulfate that has largely settled on the bottom. The water-filled balloon is of the same density as the supernatant. A lesion of water-density on the colonic wall, in contact with the supernatant of the barium suspension, would not be visible if USP barium were used in the examination. **B,** With a suspension of barium sulfate with suspending agent (Barotrast) settling after 1 hour is only minimal. If kilovoltage is sufficient to penetrate the barium column, a lesion of water-density is plainly visible during examination.

tected roentgenographically only when immersed in barium. USP barium will precipitate within minutes, while most barium sulfate with a suspending agent that is commercially available will remain in suspension for hours.

The suspending agents used by the manufacturers of the various barium sulfate preparations are also discussed in Chapter 7. They include acacia, honey proteins, pectins, bentonite, methylcellulose, tragacanth, mucilage, monooleate of sorbitan, polyethylene glycol, aluminum hydroxide gel, starches, and ingredients that the manufacturers did not specify. The terms "thick" and "thin" barium depend more on the nature of the suspending agent than on the amount of barium sulfate. A thick barium suspension may appear so because of the great viscosity contributed by the suspending agent, yet it may be relatively radiolucent because it contains little barium sulfate. Barium is best suspended by mixing it with water for 30 seconds with a high-speed electric blender. I use it at approximately room temperature. Miller recommended mixing according to weight per volume, or weight per weight formulas, rather than by hygrometer readings, since viscosity and barium settling can affect the hygrometer readings.[71]

After using many commercially available mixtures of barium sulfate we at the University of California Medical Center (San Francisco) have settled on a mixture recommended by Roscoe Miller. For double-contrast medium examination we use a mixture consisting of 4 volume units of Barosperse to 6 of Intropaque to 16 of water. For a conventional barium enema this stock mixture is diluted with water—5 volume units of the stock mixture to 8 of water. Our results, as those of others who use the same mixture, have been gratifying.

Since barium sulfate suspensions mixed in large amounts and stored for more than 24 hours have been contaminated bacterially,[4] we mix our stock solutions daily. For emergency use, when individual doses are required, we employ a commercially available sterilized suspension in cans.[4]

Additives to the barium sulfate suspension. The addition of tannic acid to an enema in order to cleanse the colon was discussed previously. The controversy regarding its safety and the present knowledge about the hepatotoxic dose were also discussed.

When added to the barium sulfate suspension in an enema, tannic acid precipitated mucus, stimulated evacuation, and produced cantraction of the colon. Most likely because of the latter two actions, an excellent mucosal pattern was obtained in postevacuation films (Fig. 36-11). Polyps larger than 1 cm. are best seen on the postevacuation film, provided tannic acid has been added to the barium sulfate suspension.[22] When tannic acid was used, the postevacuation film of the barium enema examination was so satisfactory that one of the leading centers in the United States used it routinely as the only roentgenogram of the examination.

We have recently started to add two drops of Simethicone per 100 ml. of the barium sulfate suspension in an attempt to break up the gas bubbles.

Oxyphenosatin as an additive produces excellent evacuation of the colon, but frequently no barium is left in the colon, and visualization of the mucosal pattern is generally poor.[8]

Time of performance of the conventional barium enema

Whether the barium enema examination is performed in the morning or afternoon seems to be a matter of convenience for the department, if not for the patient, who is permitted clear liquids for breakfast when the examination is scheduled for afternoon. Many departments use their fluoroscopic suites and personnel for examinations of the upper gastrointestinal tract in the morning. The same facilities and personnel are then used for barium enemas in the afternoon.

The order in which the examinations of the gastrointestinal tract are performed is more controversial. If there is the possibility that an obstruction of the colon exists, the barium enema must be performed first. In this case, to prevent inspissation of barium in the colon proximal to the obstruction, examination of the upper gastrointestinal tract with barium is usually canceled. Most of the centers surveyed avoid this complication by routinely performing the barium enema examination first, but many radiologists do examine the upper gastrointestinal tract first unless obstruction of the colon is suspected.

From the point of view of the patient's welfare the latter procedure is preferable, since the examination of the upper gastrointestinal tract

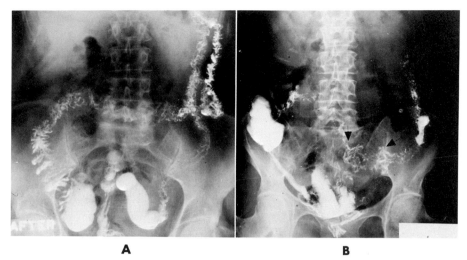

A   **B**

Fig. 36-11. Postevacuation roentgenograms obtained after 0.25% tannic acid (Clyso-drast) had been added to the barium sulfate suspension (Barotrast). **A,** The roentgenogram of one patient shows a normal colon. **B,** In another patient a large villous adenoma of transverse colon (arrows) is shown.

needs no preparation other than overnight fasting. Thus, one whole day is gained for observing a special diet in the preparation of the colon. The film of the abdomen preliminary to examination of the colon will show whether any barium remains in the colon from the previous day's examination of the upper gastrointestinal tract. From this observation the examiner receives reliable and quick information as to whether or not the patient is adequately prepared for the examination. The two examinations done in this order involve rigorous cleansing of the colon only once and the order is therefore easier on the patient.

In some centers the barium enema examination and the upper gastrointestinal examinations are performed, in that order, on the same day. This routine has advantages in speed and convenience to the patient, but it imposes difficulties in the operation of a busy department, and study of the small bowel simultaneously with the upper gastrointestinal examination is almost impossible. In addition it may prove to be an exhausting experience for the ill patient.

The excretory pyelogram frequently precedes the barium enema examination and both are given on the same day. Repetition of preparation is not necessary for the barium enema, and the opacification of the urinary bladder, renal calices, pelvis, and ureters during the pyelogram helps greatly in locating the abdominal masses in the second examination. This is especially true if lateral views are obtained.

Most radiologists refuse to perform barium enemas on the same day that the sigmoidoscopic examination is performed. The introduction of air during sigmoidoscopy, the secretion of mucus, and the increased spasm of the colon result in a difficult and an often unsatisfactory barium enema examination. A 24-hour delay usually effects an adequate examination. If a biopsy was performed at the sigmoidoscopic examination, there should be a delay of at least 7 days, although some centers delay for 2 months.[63] The caution with which barium enema examination is approached after biopsy is justified by the possibility of perforation at the site of biopsy.[94]

Exceptions to this policy are allowed if the radiologist is informed by an experienced colleague that a surface biopsy was performed on a fungating lesion or that a mucosal biopsy was taken from a rectal valve. General knowledge of this policy in the hospital and uniform adherence to it by the radiology staff is recommended.

Performance of the examination

Spot films in cassettes with intensifying screens are generally employed in the barium enema examination; few radiologists use 70 mm. roll film. The reason for preferring the spot films is that with present-day rapid developing, they may be viewed almost instantly. Refilling of the colon with barium or with air is then immediately possible.

Probably no two radiologists perform the barium enema examination in exactly the same way. Opinion and practice on most of the important steps of the examination are amazingly uniform, however. The examiner carefully follows the head of the advancing column of barium and turns the patient to the left to unravel the tortuous sigmoid and the rectosigmoid. One or more spot films of this area are obtained, with compression if possible. The patient is then turned to the right side for a view of the sigmoid at right angles to the previous view. A spot film in this projection is obtained routinely by many examiners. If any positive changes are noted, the examination concentrates on them: more spot films are made, with varied degrees of compression if possible. On occasion, to distend the sigmoid colon, the flow of barium is restarted in spurts. The head of the barium column, however, should be observed by moving the screen rapidly back and forth. The flow of barium must always be stopped when a spot film is obtained.

After examination of the sigmoid colon, the technicians in some institutions obtain overhead films of the rectum and sigmoid colon. These views are usually taken with the patient prone or supine. Often both views are obtained in order to shift any air bubbles or oil droplets that may be present. A lateral view of the rectum is usually obtained, as well as a Chassard-Lapine or an angled view of the sigmoid colon. The value of these views is discussed later. The interruption of the fluoroscopic examination to obtain overhead films has the advantage that no confusing cecal, appendiceal, or ileal structures filled with barium cover the sigmoid. Many examiners are of the opinion that disadvantages—discomfort to the patient, lack of control over proximal flow of barium, and interrupted logistics, requiring more technicians and rooms—outweigh the advantages. Second generation remote control equipment (Chapter 2) using overhead tubes for spot filming permits the exposure of angled and angled oblique views of the sigmoid colon during any desired stage of filling.

Most radiologists proceed with the examination without an interruption to obtain overhead films, and carefully palpate the descending colon as it is being filled. Compression spot films of any possible lesion are obtained. Routine spot films of the splenic and hepatic flexure, opened by placing the patient at an angle, are frequently obtained, especially if residents in training are performing the examination. The two flexures can often be palpated and compressed as they descend on deep inspiration. The examination continues with palpation of the transverse and ascending colon and of the cecum as they fill gradually. A low-lying cecum may be best seen by rotating the patient to the right or left. Similar maneuvers may be necessary to show the cecum well if partial malrotation with a preserved mesentery of the ascending colon exists. Spot films of the cecum with compression are an essential part of the barium enema examination. Malignant lesions of the cecum are frequently missed unless it is examined with meticulous care.[27,33,59]

Before stopping the examination, the radiologist must be sure that the cecum is indeed filled. This end point is reached if the appendix is filled, if the terminal ileum is filled, or if the ileocecal valve is well demonstrated. The knowledge of whether the patient has had an appendectomy or another surgical procedure is imperative. At the University of California (San Francisco), the patient's chart is available to the radiologist at the time of examination, along with a request for radiologic consultation, which contains pertinent history.

Opinion as to whether or not the terminal ileum should be filled during a routine barium enema examination is varied. A filled terminal ileum may result in difficult or impossible evaluation of the sigmoid colon on the overhead films. The course of the colon loops may be confusing and sometimes even difficult to distinguish from a distended ileum. Opinion is unanimous, however, that filling of the small bowel must be attempted when patients have chronic ulcerative colitis, granulomatous colitis, and carcinoma of the cecum or ileocecal valve, and when a Meckel's diverticulum is suspected.

In many Scandinavian departments, in order to ensure better evaluation of the sigmoid colon the patient is encouraged to drink $\frac{1}{2}$ to 1 liter of water an hour before the examination, and he is

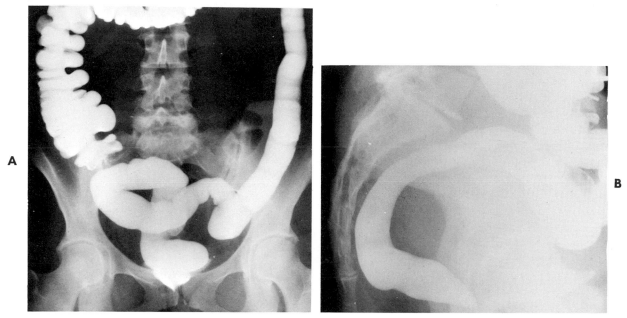

Fig. 36-12. Illustration of the valve of a lateral roentgenogram of the rectum in demonstrating a low pelvic mass (ectopic pregnancy). **A,** The preevacuation frontal roentgenogram is not particularly suggestive of abnormality. **B,** The lateral roentgenogram outlines the pelvic mass.

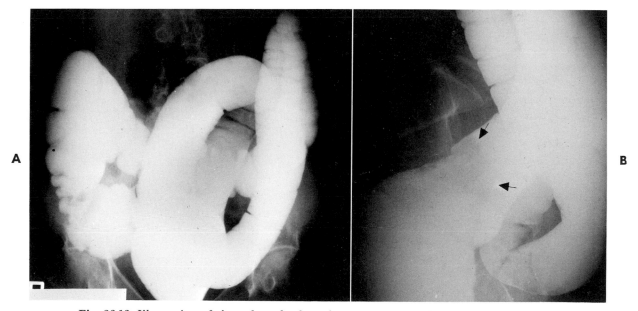

Fig. 36-13. Illustration of the value of a lateral roentgenogram of the rectum in demonstrating adenocarcinoma of the rectum. **A,** A preevacuation roentgenogram, frontal view, shows no evidence of abnormality from superimposition. **B,** A lateral roentgenogram shows a large, irregular polypoid carcinoma (arrows) arising from the posterior wall of the rectum.

instructed not to void until the examination has been concluded. The distended bladder lifts the sigmoid out of the pelvis and helps to unravel its redundant loops. A greatly distended bladder, however, adds to the patient's distress in trying to retain the enema. After exposure of the overhead films the patient is allowed to go to the toilet, at which time the colon and bladder are usually emptied. The dropping of the sigmoid into the pelvis after the bladder is emptied adds important information about the mobility of this part of the colon.

Overhead films. Opinion varies greatly about the number and required projections of pre-evacuation overhead films. A tendency prevalent among many radiologists is to continue adding views as their personal experience increases. One must remember, however, that a routine set of films is meant to be a survey unless circumstances require the addition of special views in a particular patient.

At the University of California (San Francisco) the routine preevacuation views by most of the examiners include prone, supine, and left posterior oblique views of the abdomen, and a left lateral view of the rectum (Figs. 36-12 and 36-13). The first three views are obtained

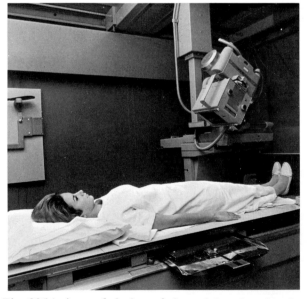

Fig. 36-14. An angled view of the pelvic colon showing the relationship of the roentgenogram in the Bucky tray to the patient and tube. The tube is angled 30 degrees cephalad.

on large (14 by 17 inch) films, the last on a 10 by 12 inch or 11 by 13 inch film. Whenever the sigmoid colon is redundant, which is true in most instances, a view, with the patient lying supine and the x-ray tube angled 30 to 35 degrees (Fig. 36-14), or a Chassard-Lapine view (Fig. 36-15) is obtained. Views with the patient lying oblique or prone and the x-ray tube at an angle (Fig. 36-16) are rarely obtained.[30] The advantages of the angled and Chassard-Lapine views have been well discussed by Ettinger and Elkin, and others.[13,21,25,31] The Chassard-Lapine view will frequently show sigmoid lesions that are missed on routine films (Fig. 36-17). However, it does not give much information about the rectum, which is seen lumen-on, and the required position may be difficult to maintain for a debilitated or an obese patient, or one who has great difficulty in holding the enema. An additional drawback is that an inordinately large dose of radiation is administered to the pelvic organs; therefore, it should not be used in patients of reproductive age. The angled view (Figs. 36-18 and 36-19) is technically easier, is not as taxing on the patient or technician, and gives approximately the same information.

An added view, if mobility of the transverse colon, the flexures, the cecum, and the sigmoid is to be tested, is an upright view of the abdomen. This view may give information about the presence of adhesions and invasion, and is particularly valuable in the diagnosis of a hernia at the foramen of Morgagni. The transverse colon remains fixed at an angle close to or above the diaphragm, depending on whether the hernia includes only the omentum or both the omentum and the colon. With high kilovoltage technique, sufficient penetration of barium in the colon is obtained so that polypoid lesions can be seen as filling defects (Figs. 36-20 and 36-21).[39] The common use of 120 to 150 kv exposures is the single greatest advance in the technique of exposure of preevacuation films.

Postevacuation views. Postevacuation films are generally obtained with kilovoltage of 70 to 100 kv, but many centers insist on higher kilovoltage. A single 14 by 17 inch film with the patient prone is usually obtained. In special circumstances a left posterior oblique, Chassard-Lapine, and lateral films of the rectum, as well as upright films and spot films of any suspicious area may be obtained. The patient must

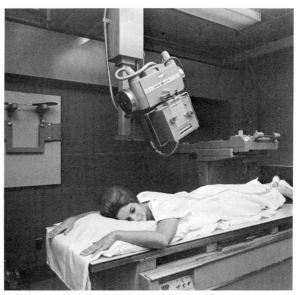

Fig. 36-16. Prone, angled view of pelvic colon. The tube is angled 30 degrees caudad.

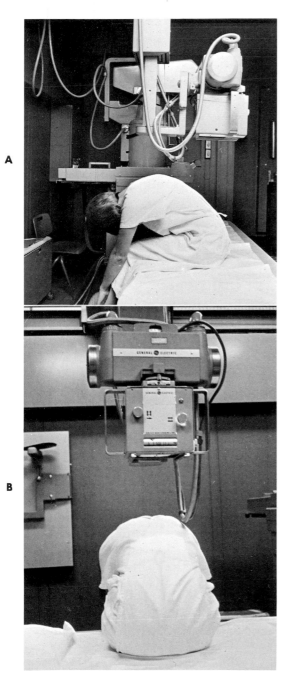

Fig. 36-15. Positioning for the Chassard-Lapiné view. **A,** Note the relationship of the patient to the table and tube. **B,** The localizing light from the collimator shining on the patient's back shows the orientation of the tube to the patient.

not be released from the radiology department until the roentgenograms have been checked and found satisfactory. Beginning residents should have the results of their examinations checked by a more experienced radiologist.

Examination of the colon through a colostomy. The examination of the colon after an abdominoperineal resection through a colostomy is often a difficult and unsatisfactory procedure.[12] The preparation usually omits castor oil since the patient's bowel habits may become disrupted for weeks. A diet of clear liquid for a day and a more vigorous irrigation of the large intestine than usual is generally all that is needed. Never should a balloon be inflated inside the bowel. Perforation may result when the large bowel detaches itself from the site of anastomosis to the skin. Frequently, perforation may cause death, as a result of intraperitoneal spillage of bowel content.[94,99,124] Extraperitoneal spillage of bowel contents and barium following perforation is not always fatal (Fig. 36-22).

In administering the barium enema a large Foley catheter with a long front section (Fig. 36-23) is used to prevent spillage of barium on the skin. The front section of the catheter is introduced into the bowel, preferably by the patient, and the balloon is inflated and kept on the outside. The patient presses the balloon against the

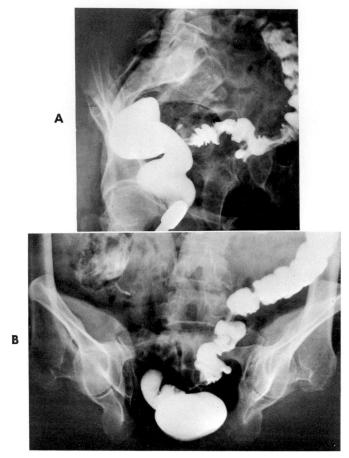

Fig. 36-17. Illustration of the value of the Chassard-Lapiné view for the demonstration of carcinoma of the sigmoid colon. **A,** An oblique view fails to show the lesion. **B,** With the Chassard-Lapiné view an annular carcinoma of the sigmoid is well demonstrated. (Courtesy Dr. Alice Ettinger.)

colostomy opening with his own hand. Types of external devices other than balloons are also used; some have external suction cups and others have the appearance of large pacifiers with an enlarged hole in the rubber part. Packing of towels or bandages around a soft rubber catheter is successfully used by some radiologists. In this case a plastic shield is held outside. An alternative safe approach to the performance of barium enema through a colostomy stoma utilizes the patient's own irrigation device. The patient is instructed to bring the device along for the examination.[18]

Once started, the technique of the examination does not differ significantly from the conventional barium enema. Attention must be given to the most distal portion of the colon leading into the colostomy stoma, which is best seen in steep oblique spot films. When a double-barrel colostomy has been performed, the examination is again usually directed to the distal portion of the colon. Knowledge of the patient's history is of great importance when he has had a colostomy. If the operation was performed because of perforation, a water-soluble contrast medium, such as diatrizoate sodium (Hypaque) should be used. Under these conditions barium can be used only after films obtained with diatrizoate show no leak.

Ileostomy enema. Ileostomy is performed either after total colectomy or as a bypass procedure when the diseased colon is to rest for a

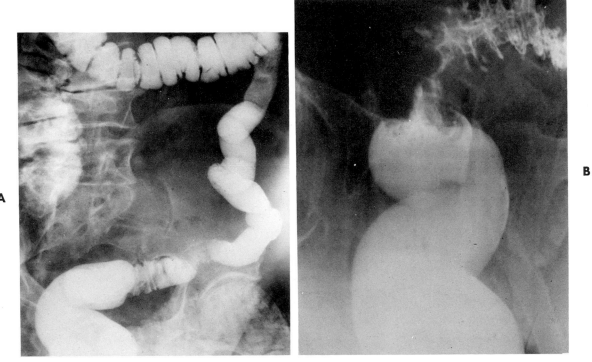

Fig. 36-18. An illustration of the value of the angled view in demonstrating carcinoma of the distal sigmoid colon. **A,** An oblique view fails to show the carcinoma. **B,** In the angled view the annular lesion in the distal sigmoid colon is plainly demonstrated. (Courtesy Dr. Alice Ettinger.)

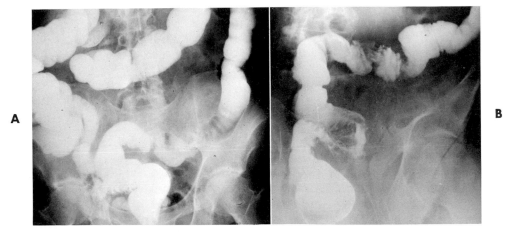

Fig. 36-19. An illustration of the value of the oblique, angled view in demonstrating carcinoma of the sigmoid colon. **A,** A preevacuation roentgenogram with the patient prone fails to show the lesion to best advantage. **B,** The ulcerated carcinoma of the sigmoid colon is plainly shown on the oblique angled view. (Courtesy Dr. Alice Ettinger.)

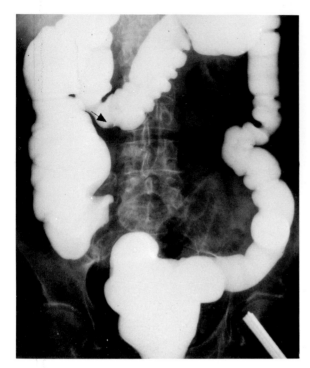

Fig. 36-20. Demonstration of the value of high kilovoltage technique. A preevacuation roentgenogram of the barium-filled colon, with the patient in the prone position, shows a small polyp in the transverse colon (arrow). The colon was well prepared and a filling defect demonstrated repeatedly in various positions can be diagnosed as a polyp.

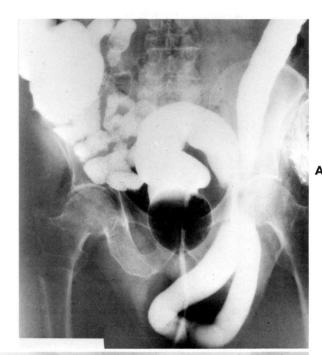

A

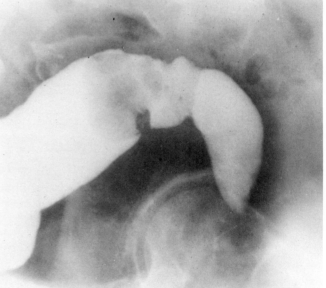

B

period. A permanent ileostomy after total colectomy is most commonly performed in patients with chronic ulcerative colitis, granulomatous colitis, and familial multiple polyposis. In patients with normally functioning ileostomy, the distal prestomal ileum does not distend.[37] Ileostomy dysfunction, resulting in copious uncontrolled discharge from the ileostomy, is a frequent complication in patients who have undergone this operation.[36] The state of the ileostomy stoma and the distal loop should be examined perorally as well as by barium enema.

In the performance of the enema through the ileal stoma, the same precautions must be observed as advocated for the examination through a colostomy stoma. A Foley balloon should never be inserted into the bowel. The method of instilling barium into the stoma can be left to the discretion of the examiner, but all the approaches recommended in performing the ex-

Fig. 36-21. Illustration of the value of high kilovoltage technique for demonstration of intracolonic tumors. **A,** An underexposed roentgenogram of the colon shows a left inguinal colon-containing hernia. No filling defect is seen. **B,** A properly exposed spot film obtained at 120 kv shows a polypoid carcinoma of the sigmoid colon, distal to the neck of the inguinal hernia.

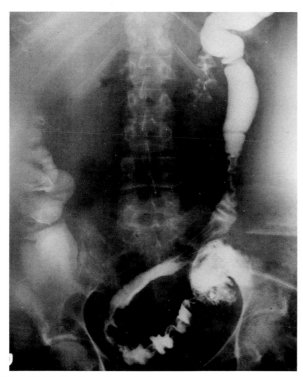

Fig. 36-22. Perforation of the colon at the site of colostomy stoma. A retaining balloon is seen within the stoma. The perforation and the extravasation of barium were extraperitoneal.

amination through a colostomy stoma also hold true for the ileostomy enema. The examiner can insert a soft catheter and surround the stoma with towels. A balloon can be held externally by the patient, with a soft catheter inside the stoma.

In the examination of the postoperative ileostomy by enema, roentgenograms must show the stoma in profile and good detail of the terminal loop should be obtained (Fig. 36-24). Fleischner and Mandelstam have stressed the point that in most patients with ileostomy dysfunction, the terminal loop of the ileum is distended because of partial stomal obstruction.[36]

In addition to roentgenograms of the prestomal ileum before evacuation, I recommend strongly that roentgenograms after evacuation also be obtained. In a patient with a well-functioning ileostomy the terminal loop empties readily and the ileum reduces its diameter. In patients with obstruction the diameter of the ileum reduces little, if any (Fig. 36-24). A cineradiographic examination of the ileostomy stoma and terminal ileum during evacuation can also be helpful in establishing the presence and cause of the dysfunction.

Cineradiography of the colon. As remembered fluoroscopy the value of cineradiography

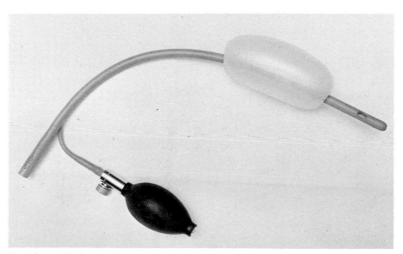

Fig. 36-23. A large Foley catheter used for external occlusion of a colostomy stoma. The patient inserts the catheter tip and holds the inflated balloon outside the stoma, pressing it against the opening.

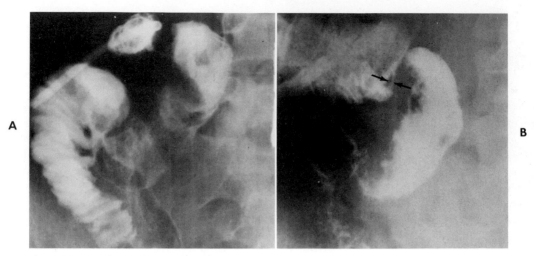

Fig. 36-24. Barium enema examination through an ileostomy stoma in a patient who underwent total colectomy and resection of terminal ileum for Crohn's disease. Patient is suffering from ileostomy dysfunction. **A,** Preevacuation spot film of terminal ileum and stoma. **B,** Postevacuation film of same area. There is a prestomal stricture present (arrows), with the terminal ileum involved with recurrence of regional enteritis.

is to record motion. It often fails to offer good detail. During introduction of barium or a water-soluble medium into the colon, it is of value only in demonstrating leaks not well seen on films, patency of anastomosis, and direction of flow in particularly complicated anastomoses. It must be stressed again that 40% diatrizoate or a similar water-soluble contrast medium must be used if a leak is present. Cineradiography of a barium enema examination may also be the method of choice for the demonstration of fistulous communications between the small bowel and the colon or between the stomach and the colon. These fistulas are usually better shown on barium enema studies than on peroral barium studies, since the greater pressure under which the barium suspension is introduced dislodges the fecal ball valves. When such fistulas are present, cineradiography supplemented by spot films is of value especially during the filling phase.

The greatest advantage that barium enema cineradiography offers is the recording of evacuation.[14,17] When evacuation films are recorded the table is slightly inclined and the patient lies on and evacuates into a plastic bedpan. The main indications are Hirschsprung's disease and other types of megacolon, evacuation of colostomy and ileostomy, and the behavior of the colon after vascular accidents.

The role of double-contrast enema examination

The double-contrast enema examination of the colon is frequently performed by many radiologists.[116] When the colon is properly prepared, this technique permits excellent delineation of minute lesions. For optimum visualization, the colon must be free of fecal material and debris. The colonic mucosa must be evenly coated with a thin film of adherent barium and the colon distended with air. By obtaining films in multiple projections, the bowel loops are separated and the bowel walls can be observed. Observation through the loops is not prevented by their overlapping, and by means of multiple views lesions can be seen from different angles and associated with the proper loops.

Radiologists are not in complete agreement whether the double-contrast enema examination should be performed as the only radiologic examination of the colon, or whether it should be a regularly performed second examination after the conventional barium enema examination. Some radiologists have expressed the belief that the double-contrast enema examination of the colon has no place in modern radiology. They state that it has no advantages over a properly performed conventional examination in which adequate preparation, the use of high kilovoltage, and thin nonflocculating barium sulfate

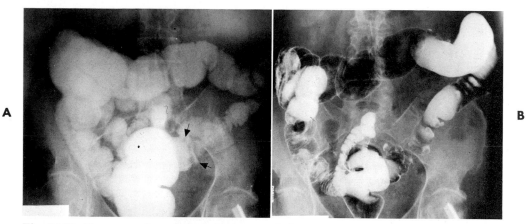

Fig. 36-25. Demonstration of the advantages of the conventional barium enema examination over the double-contrast examination in demonstrating annular neoplasms. **A,** On a conventional preevacuation roentgenogram, frontal view, the annular lesion is seen as an overhanging edge (arrows). **B,** The double-contrast frontal view fails to show the lesion.

suspensions are included. Welin and his associates advocate using only the double-contrast examination,[114,115] but they are in a decided minority as are the radiologists who insist that there is no place at all for this examination. A survey of current practices in centers in the United States, Canada, and Europe disclosed that the performance of the double-contrast study as the only examination is uncommon (nine of 79).[63]

One reason for the lack of reliance on this examination as the only approach is undoubtedly the great effort spent in preparing the colon adequately and the rather narrow margin of deviation from the optimum that can be permitted in preparation and performance of the examination if it is to be worthwhile. The other and more significant objection is that with the high concentration of barium needed for adequate uniform coating of the colon, fluoroscopy is less reliable. Fluoroscopy is also difficult once air is introduced. Furthermore, although polyps can be best seen and evaluated by double-contrast enema examination,* some sessile lesions, particularly annular lesions, might be missed easily were only the double-contrast examination performed (Figs. 36-25 and 36-26).[47]

Most radiologists prefer to perform the double-contrast enema examination if the con-

ventional study leads them to suspect polyps, or if polyps were found on sigmoidoscopy or were present in the past. A double-contrast enema examination is also indicated when a patient has rectal bleeding without hemorrhoids but the conventional barium enema examination is negative, or when there is a single polypoid lesion or any demonstrable lesion on the conventional examination. The double-contrast enema examination is also the method of choice in the follow-up of small polyps and the evaluation of their growth.[116]

Some radiologists introduce air into the colon after they have completed the conventional examination. This maneuver has the advantage that after the barium enema no further preparation is needed, but the lack of a uniform barium coating on the colonic mucosa is a drawback.

Preparation of the patient

Preparation for the double-contrast enema examination should be as vigorous and meticulous as that for the conventional barium enema examination. The preparation observed by Welin is described in detail in Chapter 39.

Most radiologists agree that, as is the case with the conventional examination, a 24-hour clear liquid diet or a 2-day low residue diet should precede the double-contrast examination. The two types of diets were described in the preced-

---

*See references 5, 74, 107, 108, and 114-116.

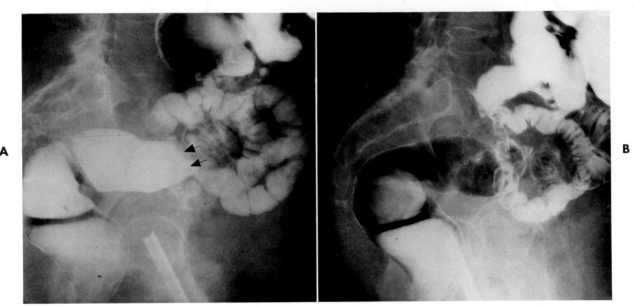

Fig. 36-26. Lateral views of the same patient as in Fig. 36-25. **A,** Lateral preevacuation roentgenogram taken during the conventional barium enema examination again shows the overhanging edge of the tumor (arrows). **B,** A similar air-contrast view fails to show the lesion.

ing section on preparation for the conventional barium enema examination. The laxative of choice for the double-contrast examination is also castor oil. The dose for adults is generally 2 ounces. On the evening preceding the examination enemas should be administered until a clear reflux is obtained, but their number should not exceed three. The "hydration technique" of preparation, which consists of magnesium citrate, biscodyl tablets and suppository as laxatives, clear liquid diet, and the forcing of fluids, can be used instead of the castor oil preparation. On the day of the examination, breakfast is usually withheld. In many centers, following Welin's recommendation, oral atropine sulfate (1 mg. for adults, 0.75 mg. for adolescents, and 0.25 to 0.5 mg. for children) is administered a half hour before the cleansing enema. Most radiologists use water, soap suds, or saline solutions in the cleansing enema. Clysodrast enemas (0.25%) may also be used. In a specially equipped room, the nurse who gives the enema rotates the patient from left to right and from the supine to the prone position until he has received 1 liter of the solution. The patient is encouraged to retain the enema for 5 minutes and is then allowed to empty the colon.

Barium suspension

Many types of barium are used for the double-contrast enema examination of the colon. All of them have in common the presence of a suspending agent. Except for Barosperse, all of the suspensions are rather thick and flow into the colon with difficulty. The use of disposable plastic bags allows the barium flow to be speeded by twisting of the plastic bag. Other systems employ the pumping of barium directly into the colon, under increased pressure. With the plastic bag additional pumping is unnecessary. At the University of California in San Francisco we now use the barium mixture described earlier in this chapter, consisting of 4 volume units of Barosperse, 6 of Intropaque, and 16 of water.

Performing the examination

In performing the double-contrast enema examination, it is important that the entire colon not be filled with barium. Most radiologists agree that the colon should be filled just beyond the splenic flexure. The excess barium is then drained away, either by use of gravity drainage,[101] by a drainage system incorporated in the examination table, or by sending the patient to the toilet to evacuate the excess barium.[110] If the latter method is chosen, the patient must return as soon as possible to the examining room for insufflation, before the barium precipitates. Air is then introduced. Miller and Brahme recommend barium instillation with the patient in the prone position.[73] This they claim prevents barium from entering the ileum. Barium flows more readily from the rectum into the sigmoid when the patient is in the prone position.

If the barium has not filled the entire colon, air must not pass beyond the barium column, since this will produce what is in effect an air block. Such an air block can be avoided by carefully observing the air and barium on the fluoroscope and by positioning of the patient so that air is at all times above the barium column, pushes the barium ahead. In practice this is accomplished by starting the introduction of air with the patient lying on his right side until the barium column has reached the hepatic flexure and ascending colon. He is then turned to the supine position, and gradually assumes an upright or partially upright position so that the ascending colon and cecum are filled. The air is introduced slowly and is stopped when the patient complains of major discomfort.

I prefer, after complete filling of the colon with air, to roll the patient on the table from left to right two or three times. These maneuvers ensure an adequate coating of the bowel walls before spot filming is begun. During the maneuvers particular attention is directed to the flexures. For best distention of the various loops of the colon the oblique, the Trendelenburg, and the partially upright positions are advantageous. The cecum, the sigmoid, and the rectal area are best seen in the Trendelenburg position, while the splenic and hepatic flexures are best distended and filled with air in upright or semi-upright positions.

Should air advance ahead of the barium column, owing to some technical mistake, coating of the right colon with barium may be difficult. Attempts should then be made to break the air-lock by rotating the patient so that the barium slides along the bowel walls. If this is impossible, the examination should be discontinued and the patient be sent to the toilet for evacuation. The administration of barium is then restarted and the entire procedure is again attempted. Usually the examination is salvageable by combining these two steps.

Overhead films

Because of the thickness of the barium introduced, the fluoroscopic examination of the colon in the double-contrast enema examination is not nearly as contributory and productive as it is in the conventional barium enema examination. Fluoroscopy is also of less value during the introduction of air. The most important information in the double-contrast enema examination, therefore, is obtained from spot films and overhead films. The number of overhead films obtained in a double-contrast enema examination considerably exceeds the number obtained in a conventional barium enema examination.

Very few centers or radiologists obtain exactly the same projections. Most radiologists, however, agree that numerous films in various projections are necessary to unravel all the air-distended and barium-coated loops of the large bowel. At the University of California Medical Center (San Francisco) the following projections are employed: left posterior oblique, right posterior oblique, prone, supine, left lateral decubitus, right lateral decubitus, and upright. The angled view of the sigmoid and lateral films of the rectum are also frequently obtained. All except the latter two are taken on 14 by 17 inch films. Welin obtains four oblique views of the rectum and sigmoid, and one frontal, two profile, two lateral decubitus, and three upright views of the colon.

Although the number and the type of projection vary somewhat in different centers, the guiding principles behind any individual's choice in this matter are the same. These are the use of many varied positions of the patient, the employment of parallel rays through any possible fluid levels, and the exposure of multiple oblique roentgenograms. Films are exposed with lower kilovoltage than are those of the conventional barium enema examination. Overpenetration is not necessary, provided that the examination is performed correctly and there are no large amounts of excess barium in the colon.

Contraindications

A double-contrast enema examination of the colon should not be performed for at least 24 hours after a sigmoidoscopy. After a rectal or sigmoid biopsy, it should not be performed for at least 14 days or even longer.[63] The examination is also contraindicated if definite diverticulitis is present. A perforation or a suspected perforation of the colon is a contraindication to both double-contrast barium enema examination and the conventional barium enema examination. Welin and Brahme recommend a double-contrast enema examination in ulcerative colitis.[115] This is a matter of opinion, but fulminating ulcerative colitis (toxic megacolon) contraindicates both the conventional barium enema and the double-contrast enema examinations in this condition. The latter examination, with strain of increased intracolonic pressure, is particularly dangerous.

Water-soluble contrast media for examination of the colon

Water-soluble contrast media should not be used in routine examination of the colon for several reasons. They are expensive, they do not coat the colonic mucosa well, they are hypertonic and irritating, and they may produce fluid and electrolyte imbalance. The postevacuation films obtained after introduction of water-soluble, iodine-containing contrast media are of inferior quality.

Water-soluble contrast media are indicated only if definite perforation is suspected and the demonstration of its exact site is considered important. In the presence of fistulas between the large and small bowel, barium sulfate is the contrast medium of choice. If a vesicocolonic fistula is suspected, however, water-soluble contrast media are preferred.

Water-soluble contrast media should also be used if a sinus tract is reinjected from the skin and collections in soft tissues are to be outlined. The injection should always be performed under fluoroscopy, with introduction of a soft rubber catheter. Sterile technique is practiced by most radiologists to avoid the introduction of additional infectious agents into the sinus tract.

SPECIAL EXAMINATIONS FOR VISUALIZATION OF PARTICULAR AREAS OF THE COLON
Peroral double-contrast enema examination of the right colon

Heitzman and Berne described the introduction of barium orally and air rectally during the

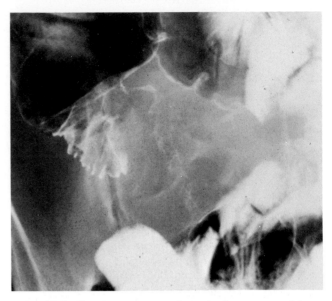

Fig. 36-27. Roentgenogram taken during a peroral barium, double-contrast examination of the right colon and terminal ileum. Granulomatous colitis and terminal ileitis were present; the lesions are well demonstrated.

same examination for visualization of lesions in the right colon and ileocecal valve.[48] This examination is performed at the University of California Medical Center (San Francisco) routinely when a lesion exists or its presence is suspected in the cecum or in the ileocecal valve[123] (Figs. 36-27 and 36-28). The advantage of this type of examination is that the right colon can be visualized without interfering with the barium-filled loops of the sigmoid. The patient is prepared in the same manner as for a double-contrast enema examination of the colon, with a clear liquid diet, preparatory enemas, and a castor oil laxative. Six ounces of barium sulfate with a suspending agent are given by mouth and the progress of the barium column is observed fluoroscopically. When the head of the barium column reaches the transverse colon and both the jejunum and proximal ileum are empty of barium, air is introduced rectally. Multiple spot films are then obtained. Overhead films should include supine, prone, and two lateral decubitus projections. This examination is especially useful for visualizing lesions of the ileocecal valve, cecal polyps, granulomatous colitis, regional enteritis, and simultaneous involvement of the terminal ileum and cecum in enteritis.

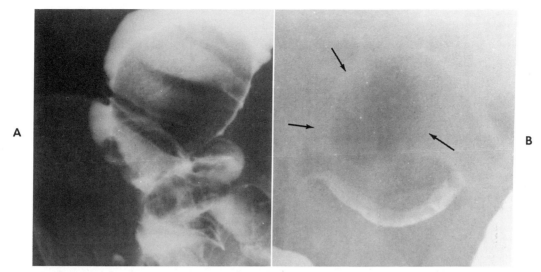

Fig. 36-33. Excellent demonstration of a lipoma of the cecum by water enema and 60 kv exposures. **A,** The smooth polypoid lesion is seen to be surrounded by barium on this spot film of the cecum obtained during a barium enema examination. **B,** The large radiolucency (arrows) is in the same area on a spot film obtained during a water enema. Residual barium is seen in the appendix. The metallic densities in the two lower corners are the edges of the examiner's glove.

the lower kilovoltage range.[98] Furthermore, in roentgenograms obtained in the lower range of radiographic kilovoltage, fatty lesions surrounded by water density can be delineated. The water enema is a supplementary technique; it is performed only when a definite lesion suspected of being a lipoma is identified by the conventional barium enema examinations.[65]

Water is introduced into the colon and spot films and roentgenograms are obtained in exactly the same projections as were the roentgenograms that showed the lesion on barium enema examination. The recommended kilovoltage is between 40 and 70 kv.[98] Demonstration of fat in smooth colonic lesions by the water enema is definite evidence of the presence of a lipoma. All other lesions are of water density and will not be visible on the roentgenograms of the water-filled colon (Figs. 36-32 and 36-33).

To displace air bubbles, both prone and supine positions are advisable when roentgenograms and spot films are obtained. Since not all lipomas are radiolucent, these examinations are of diagnostic value in only about 50% of proved lipomas. Barium in the appendix or diverticula is helpful, since the distention of the colon is difficult to follow by water fluoroscopically.

Water-contrast-barium enema technique using methylcellulose

Sinclair and Buist claim that water can be used instead of air for the double-contrast effect.[95] The use of methylcellulose with water minimizes removal of the barium that coats the bowel wall. This technique helps in the visualization of the cecum and in demonstrating small lesions of the sigmoid colon, such as polyps and carcinoma. It facilitates examination and is reportedly more satisfactory than the usual air-contrast examination. I have had no experience with this examination.

Arteriography

Arteriography is a method that is used to demonstrate bleeding into the colon.[9,52,64,86] The site of bleeding can be demonstrated by catheterization of a vessel at operation, by catheterization of the aorta, or by selected catheterization of the superior mesenteric or inferior mesenteric arteries. Jaffe, Youker, and Margulis have shown in experiments that for aortographic visualization of bleeding into the small bowel, the bleeding rate must be close to 6 ml. per minute.[50] When it is less than 3 ml. per minute, selective arteriography is necessary.[80] Nusbaum and Baum have shown experimentally that bleeding into

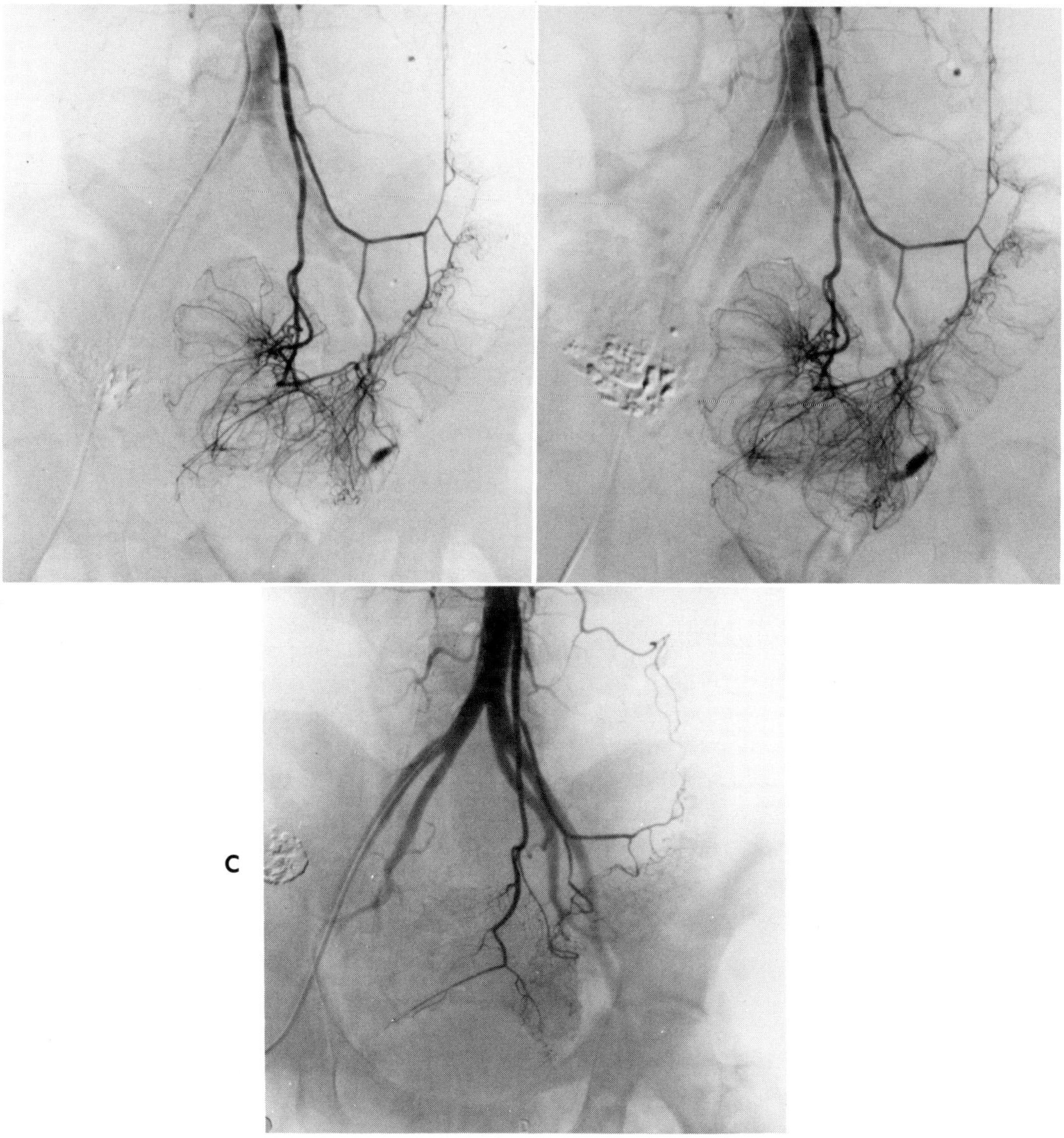

Fig. 36-34. Inferior mesenteric arteriogram in a 53-year-old woman who was bleeding profusely by rectum. The patient had hyperparathyroidism and therefore was a poor operative risk. Subtraction technique was used: **A,** arteriogram in early phase shows bleeding into the lumen of the distal descending colon; **B,** a later film shows the intraluminal accumulation of leaked contrast material to be greater; **C,** following intravenous infusion of .2 unit of vasopressin (Pitressin) per minute for 40 minutes the bleeding stopped. The patient did not require surgery at this time. Elective laparotomy demonstrated an ulcer. (Courtesy Dr. Kent Pearson.)

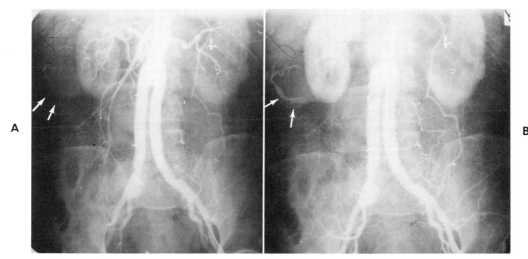

Fig. 36-35. Midstream aortogram injection in a patient with massive rectal bleeding. **A,** Contrast material is leaking from the ileocecal branch of the superior mesenteric artery into the cecum. Contrast medium has accumulated in the lumen (arrows). **B,** A later aortogram shows massive accumulation of contrast medium in the cecum (arrows). The patient was operated on minutes after the aortographic study, and an ischemic ulcer of the cecum was found. The bleeding came from an exposed artery.

the bowel can be demonstrated by selective arteriography if the bleeding rate exceeds 0.5 ml. per minute.[81] The bleeding site is visualized as leakage of contrast material into the bowel lumen (Figs. 36-34 and 36-35).

Arteriography has also been used to demonstrate and study colonic tumors. These studies were directed predominantly at learning more about the vascularity of tumors.[62,68,108,109] Some tumors of the colon are highly vascular, whereas, in others vascularity is only sparse and the diagnosis of tumor is possible only by identification of the individual vessels.[62] Arteriography will probably never be a diagnostic method for locating tumors in the large bowel. It is, however, a method for finding the site of bleeding if this is impossible by more conventional means. Arteriography is also promising in the study of vascular abnormalities, such as arteriovenous communications or hemangiomas, as well as in the study of inflammatory disease.

BARIUM ENEMA AS A THERAPEUTIC TOOL
Reduction of intussusception

The use of the barium enema in the reduction of intussusception was reported almost simultaneously from France, Denmark, and the United States.[11,77,87] The method and its advantages are discussed in Chapter 56. The value of reduction of intussusception by barium enema in children was extensively reported by Nordentoft and Hansen.[77] Of importance is the fact that in three of the patients, perforation occurred in the colon. In all three, symptoms of intussusception had persisted for more than 48 hours.

Berman and Kimble pointed out some contraindications and objections to reduction of intussusception by barium enema.[11] A Meckel's diverticulum may be overlooked, polyps or other lesions may be missed, and incomplete reduction may be unsuspected. In addition, use of the barium enema can result in intestinal perforation when, occasionally, gangrenous bowel may be reduced. It must be emphasized that the height of the barium level in the bag during the enema should never exceed 3 feet above the table, and that the attempt at reduction of the intussusception by barium enema should be abandoned if it is not easily successful.

Should the patient be too ill, the barium enema should not be performed. When leakage of barium from the colon is noted, immediate surgical intervention is mandatory. Intussusception in adults is almost always associated with lesions that require surgical treatment.

Reduction of volvulus

This subject was covered in Chapter 10. Reduction of volvulus by barium enema is only transitory. Although frequently successful, the use of the barium enema, is a method that should follow the attempts at reduction with a sigmoidoscope or a rectal tube, or both. A surgical procedure will frequently be necessary, despite the transient reduction by barium enema.

Barium enema for bleeding from colonic diverticulum

The use of barium enema to stop bleeding from colonic diverticula has been reported in the surgical literature.[2] Barium sulfate in the form of enema is introduced by hydrostatic pressure. No experimental evidence is available, but in my experience this method has been successful. The barium sulfate particles probably serve as a nucleus for clot formation. Adams has reported successful arrest of acute diverticular bleeding in twenty-six of twenty-eight patients by the use of barium enema.[1]

Selective arterial drug infusions in the treatment of acute colonic bleeding

Rösch and his co-workers have described successful control of bleeding from the colon in four patients by means of selective intra-arterial infusions of propranolol hydrochloride followed by infusions of epinephrine.[89] Baum and Nusbaum advocate the use of vasopressin injected through the intra-arterial catheter. They recommend a dose of 0.2 pressor units/ml./minute. The effect after a 20-minute infusion can be observed by subsequent arteriography. The dose can be adjusted upward to 0.3 units/ml./minute if necessary. At the University of California in San Francisco we start the control of arterial bleeding with the infusion of vasopressin as recommended by Baum and Nusbaum.[9a] If that is unsuccessful we follow the program outlined by Rösch and co-workers.[89a] They use a preinjection of propranolol (3 to 5 mg. in 2 minutes) followed by 10 to 20 μg./minute of epinephrine into one of the mesenteric arteries. For superselective injections into the branches of the superior or inferior mesenteric arteries we use a dose of 6 to 8 μg./minute of epinephrine. The injection of the drugs followed the localization of the site of bleeding and was effected through the same catheter. This type of interventional, therapeutic radiodiagnosis may eliminate the necessity of surgical intervention.

We will have to await controlled studies to assess the degree of therapeutic success of drug infusion for intestinal bleeding. Most patients stop bleeding without any medical help.

COMPLICATIONS OF BARIUM ENEMA

Although the barium enema is one of the safer examinations, and a large number of them is performed throughout the world every day, certain complications, which have been alluded to throughout the chapter, may occur. The radiologist must be familiar with the ways to prevent them, and also must be able to recognize them quickly in order to take immediate countermeasures.

Perforation

Perforations of the colon have various causes. Perforation as a result of overinflation of balloons in the rectum, inflation of balloons inside the stoma after a colostomy, and perforation of the colon in a patient with acute fulminating ulcerative colitis, or after biopsy, or as a result of perforation of a colonic carcinoma, have been discussed. Perforations produced in the course of reduction of intussusception were also discussed. Perforations of the colon during enemas can occur without demonstrable underlying disease.[94]

Perforation can be intraperitoneal. In such a case, during fluoroscopy barium can be seen flowing rather freely and outlining the bowel loops and organs surrounding the site of perforation (Fig. 31-5, *B*).[49] Extraperitoneal perforations may occur into the pelvis below the rectoperitoneal reflection (Fig. 36-3), with perforation at the site of colostomy (Fig. 36-2), or more rarely, with posterior perforations into the retroperitoneal tissues in the region of the descending or ascending colon or cecum. Retroperitoneal emphysema after double-contrast enema or barium enema has been reported. Retroperitoneal perforations have a better prognosis than have intraperitoneal perforations.[16,41,83,94]

Perforation may also occur into the venous

system. Perforation into submucosal veins is usually fatal.[90,92,101,121] All perforations, whether into the peritoneal cavity, the extraperitoneal tissues, or other organs, are surgical emergencies and must be recognized as quickly as possible by the radiologist. Familiarity with them will permit immediate stoppage of the examination procedure, thus reducing the amount of barium leaving the colon through the perforation.

Water intoxication

The dangers of instilling large amounts of barium into children with Hirschsprung's disease are well known and have been described.[102] Water intoxication has presumably caused the death of several patients. In preparing a barium suspension for children, lactated Ringer's solution or other physiologic solutions should be used instead of water. An overdilated colon full of fecal material should not be completely filled, whether in a child with Hirschsprung's disease, or in a patient with longstanding carcinoma of the colon producing significant, antegrade obstruction. Once the lesion underlying dilatation is well demonstrated, the radiologist must decide whether the examination should be stopped or should proceed. He can make this decision wisely if he is familiar with possible complications.

REFERENCES

1. Adams, J. T.: Therapeutic barium enema for massive diverticular bleeding, Arch. Surg. **101**:457-460, 1970.
2. Albo, R. J., Grimes, O. F., and Dunphy, J. E.: Management of massive lower gastrointestinal hemorrhage, Amer. J. Surg. **112**:264, 1966.
3. Amberg, J. R.: A hazard of silicone foam enema, Amer. J. Roentgen. **99**:96, 1967.
4. Amberg, J. R., and Unger, J. DeB.: Contamination of barium sulfate suspension, Radiology **97**:182-183, 1970.
5. Andren, L., Frieberg, S., and Welin, S.: Roentgen diagnosis of small polyps in colon and rectum, Acta Radiol. (Stockholm) **43**:201, 1955.
6. Barnes, J. M., and Rossiter, R. J.: Toxicity of tannic acid, Lancet **2**:218, 1943.
7. Barnes, M. R.: How to get a clean colon—with less effort, Radiology **91**:948-949, 1968.
8. Barnhard, H. J., and Crow, N. E.: Evaluation of new colon evacuant: dihydroxyphenylisatin, Amer. J. Roentgen. **79**:876, 1958.
9. Baum, S., Stein, G. N. Nusbaum M. and Chait, A.: Selective arteriography in the diagnosis of hemorrhage in the gastrointestinal tract, Radiol. Clin. N. Amer. **7**:131-145, 1969.
9a. Baum, S., and Nusbaum, M.: The control of gastrointestinal hemorrhage by selective mesenteric arterial infusion of vasopressin, Radiology **98**:497, 1971.
10. Berman, C. Z., Jacobs, M. G., and Bernstein, A.: Hazards of the barium enema examination as studied by electrocardiographic telemetry: preliminary report, J. Amer. Geriat. Soc. **13**:672, 1965.
11. Berman, E. J., and Kimble, J. W.: Barium enema for intussusception in infants and children, Arch. Surg. **92**:508, 1966.
12. Bettman, R. B., Richter, H. M., Jr., and Drugas, T.: Perforation of colostomy loop by soft rubber catheter, J.A.M.A. **151**:206, 1953.
13. Billing, L.: Zur Technik der Kontrastuntersuchung des Colon sigmoideum, Acta Radiol. **25**:418, 1944.
14. Brown, B. S.: Defecography or anorectal studies in children including cinefluorographic observations, J. Canad. Ass. Radiol. **16**:66, 1965.
15. Brown, G. R.: A new approach to colon preparation for barium enema; preliminary report, Univ. Mich. Med. Bull. **27**:225-230, 1961.
16. Brunton, F. S.: Retroperitoneal emphysema as a complication of barium enema, Clin. Radiol. **11**:197, 1960.
17. Burhenne, H. J.: Intestinal evacuation study: a new roentgenologic technique, Radiol. Clin. (Basel) **33**:79, 1964.
18. Burhenne, H. J.: Technique of colostomy examination, Radiology **97**:183-185, 1970.
19. Burhenne, H. J., Vogelaar, P., and Arkoff, R. S.: Liver function studies in patients receiving enemas containing tannic acid, Amer. J. Roentgen. **96**:510, 1966.
20. Burt, C. A. V.: Pneumatic rupture of intestinal canal with experimental data showing mechanism of perforation and pressure required, Arch. Surg. **22**:875, 1931.
21. Chassard and Lapine, M. M.: Etude radiographique de l'arcade pubienne chez la femme enciente; une nouvelle méthod d'appreciation du diàmetre bi-ischiatique, J. Radiol Electr. **7**:113, 1923.
22. Christie, A. C., Coe, F. O., Hampton, A. O., and Wyatt, G. M.: Value of tannic acid enema and post-evacuation roentgenograms in examination of the colon, Amer. J. Roentgen. **63**:657, 1950.
23. Clark, K.: Barium enema examination using an electronic technique—a preliminary report, Brit. J. Radiol. **44**:970-972, 1971.
24. Cook, G. B., and Margulis, A. R.: Detecting small sessile colon cancers with silicone foam, J.A.M.A. **183**:66, 1963.
25. Cook, G. B., and Margulis, A. R.: The silicone-foam diagnostic enema, Surg. Forum **12**:309, 1961.
26. Cook, G. B., and Margulis, A. R.: Use of silicone foam for examining the human sigmoid colon, Amer. J. Roentgen. **87**:633, 1962.
27. Cooley, R. N., Agnew, C. H., and Rios, G.: Diagnostic accuracy of barium enema study in car-

cinoma of colon and rectum, Amer. J. Roentgen. **84**:316, 1960.

28. DeCarlo, J., Jr.: Complications associated with diagnostic barium enema, Surgery **47**:965, 1960.

29. Dietrich, D. C.: Bowel preparation for outpatient radiography, Radiology **86**:488, 1966.

30. Dysart, D. N., and Stewart, H. R.: Special angled roentgenography for lesions of the rectosigmoid: five year survey, Amer. J. Roentgen. **96**:285, 1966.

31. Ettinger, A., and Elkin, M.: Study of the sigmoid by special roentgenographic views, Amer. J. Roentgen. **72**:199, 1954.

32. Ferrucci, J. T., Jr., and Benedict, K. T., Jr.: Anticholinergic-aided study of the gastrointestinal tract, Radiol. Clin. N. Amer. **9**:23-39, 1971.

33. Figiel, L. S., Figiel, S. J., and Hennessey, A.: Carcinoma of the colon; incidence of error in the roentgen diagnosis, Amer. J. Gastroent. **40**:487, 1963.

34. Figiel, S. J., Figiel, L. S., and Rush, D. K.: High-kilovoltage, spot-compression studies: a new approach to colonic polyp detection, Med. Radiogr. Photogr. **34**:34, 1958.

35. Fischer, A. W.: A roentgenologic method for examination of the large intestine: combination of the contrast material enema with insufflation with air, Klin. Wschr. **2**:1595, 1923.

36. Fleischner, F. G., and Mandelstam, P.: Roentgen observations of the ileostomy in patients with idiopathic ulcerative colitis; ileostomy dysfunction, Radiology **70**:469-480, 1958.

37. Fleischner, F. G., Mandelstam, P., and Banks, B. M.: Roentgen observations of the ileostomy in patients with idiopathic ulcerative colitis; the well functioning ileostomy, Radiology **63**:74-80, 1954.

38. Gianturco, C., and Miller, G. A.: Program for detection of colonic and rectal polyps, J.A.M.A. **153**:1429, 1953.

39. Gianturco, C., and Miller, G. A.: Routine search for colonic polyps by high-voltage radiography, Radiology **60**:496, 1953.

40. Gianturco, C., Miller, G. A., and Neucks, H. C.: A modified bardex enema tube. In Selected papers of the Carle Hospital Clinic and Carle Foundation (Urbana, Ill.) **15**:37, 1962.

41. Goldberg, L.: Surgical emphysema following double contrast enema, Treat. Serv. Bull. **6**:25, 1951.

42. Goodman, L. S., and Gilman, A.: Pharmacological Basis of Therapeutics ed. 3, New York, 1965, The Macmillan Co.

43. Haenisch, F.: Value of the roentgen ray in the early diagnosis of carcinoma of the bowel, Amer. Quart. Roentgen. **3**:175, 1911.

44. Hamilton, J. B.: Use of tannic acid in barium enemas, Amer. J. Roentgen. **56**:101, 1946.

45. Harris, P. A., Zboralske, F. F., Rambo, O. N., Margulis, A. R., and Riegelman, S.: Toxicity studies on tannic acid administered by enema, II. The colonic absorption and intraperitoneal toxicity of tannic acid and its hydrolytic products in rats, Amer. J. Roentgen. **96**:498, February 1966.

46. Hartman, A. W., and Hills, W. J.: Rupture of colon in infants during barium enema: report of two cases, Ann. Surg. **145**:712, 1957.

47. Hartzell, H. V.: To err with air, J.A.M.A. **187**:455, 1964.

48. Heitzman, E. R., and Berne, A. S.: Roentgen examination of the cecum and proximal ascending colon with ingested barium, Radiology **76**:415, 1961.

49. Isaacs, I.: Intraperitoneal escape of barium enema fluid perforation of sigmoid colon, J.A.M.A. **150**:645, 1952.

50. Jaffe, B. F., Youker, J. E., and Margulis, A. R.: Aortographic localization of controlled gastrointestinal hemorrhage in dogs, Surgery **58**:984, 1965.

51. Janower, M. I., Robbins, L. L., Tomchik, F. S., and Weylman, W. T.: Tannic acid and the barium enema, Radiology **85**:887, 1965.

52. Kanter, I. E., Schwartz, A. J., and Fleming, R. J.: Localization of bleeding point in chronic and acute gastrointestinal hemorrhage by means of selective visceral arteriography, Amer. J. Roentgen. **103**:386-399, 1968.

53. Kaufman, S. A.: Retrograde vaginal filling during barium enema, Amer. J. Dig. Dis. **10**:732, 1965.

54. Kaye, J., and Solomon, A.: Use of Dulcolax in propylene glycol in the radiological investigation of the colon, Brit. J. Radiol. **37**:913, 1964.

55. Killingback, M.: Acute large bowel obstruction precipitated by barium x-ray examination, Med. J. Aust. **2**:503, 1964.

56. Köhler, R., and Tähti, E.: Cleansing of large bowel before roentgenologic examination of abdomen, Acta Radiol. (Stockholm) **55**:129, 1961.

57. Krezanoski, J. Z.: Tannic acid: chemistry, analysis and toxicology, Radiology **87**:655, 1966.

58. Lasser, E. C., and Gerende, L. J.: An efficacy study of clysodrast, Radiology **87**:649, 1966.

59. Lauer, J. D., Carlson, H. C., and Wollaeger, E. E.: Accuracy of roentgenologic examination in detecting carcinoma of colon, Dis. Colon Rectum **8**:190, 1965.

60. Levene, G.: Low temperature barium water suspensions for roentgenologic examination of colon, Radiology **77**:117, 1961.

61. Lucke, H. H., Hodge, K. E., and Patt, N. L.: Fatal liver damage after barium enemas containing tanic acid, Canad. Med. Ass. J. **89**:1111, 1963.

62. Margulis, A. R.: Arteriography of tumors; difficulties in interpretations and the need for magnification, Radiol. Clin. N. Amer. **2**:543, 1964.

63. Margulis, A. R., and Goldberg, H. I.: The current state of radiologic technique in the examination of the colon: a survey, Radiol. Clin. N. Amer. **7**:27-42, 1969.

64. Margulis, A. R., Heinbecker, P., and Bernard, H. R.: Operative mesenteric arteriography in the search for the site of bleeding in unexplained gastrointestinal hemorrhage; a preliminary report, Surgery **48**:534, 1960.

65. Margulis, A. R., and Jovanovich, A.: Roentgen diagnosis of submucous lipomas of colon, Amer. J. Roentgen. **84**:1114, 1960.

66. Masel, H., Masel, J. P., and Casey, K. V.: A survey of colon examination techniques in Australia and New Zealand, with a review of complications, Aust. Radiol. **15**:140-147, 1971.

67. McAlister, W. H., Anderson, M. S., Bloomberg, G. R., and Margulis, A. R.: Lethal effects of tannic acid in barium enema; report of three fatalities and experimental studies, Radiology **80**:765, 1963.

68. McAlister, W. H., Margulis, A. R., Heinbecker, P., and Spjut, H.: Arteriography and microangiography of gastric and colonic lesions, Radiology **79**: 769, 1962.

69. Meyers, P. H.: Contamination of barium enema apparatus during its use, J.A.M.A. **173**:1589, 1960.

70. Miller, R. E.: Barium enema examination with large bore tubing and drainage, Radiology **82**:905, 1964.

71. Miller, R. E.: Barium sulfate suspensions, Radiology **84**:241, 1965.

72. Miller, R. E.: Enema control for difficult patients, Radiology **87**:756, 1966.

73. Miller, R. E., and Brahme, F.: The clarity of good technic, Amer. J. Dig. Dis. **12**:418-420, 1967.

74. Moreton, R. D.: Double-contrast examination of colon with special emphasis on studies of sigmoid, Radiology **60**:510, 1953.

75. Nathan, M. H., and Kohen, R.: The bardex tube in performing barium enemas, Amer. J. Roentgen. **84**:1121, 1960.

76. Neaman, M. P.: Comparative evaluation of adjuvants to barium enema examinations: use of oxyphenisatin and tannic acid, J. Canad. Ass. Radiol. **16**:17, 1965.

77. Nordentoft, J. M., and Hansen, H.: Treatment of intussusception in children; brief survey based on 1,838 Danish cases (I, 1,042 cases 1928-1935. II. 796 cases 1944-1949), Surgery **38**:311, 1955.

78. Noveroske, R. J.: Intracolonic pressures during barium enema examination, Amer. J. Roentgen. **91**:852, 1964.

79. Noveroske, R. J.: Perforation of the rectosigmoid by a bardex balloon catheter, Amer. J. Roentgen. **96**:326, 1966.

80. Nusbaum, M., and Baum, S.: Radiographic demonstration of unknown sites of gastrointestinal bleeding, Surg. Forum **14**:374, 1963.

81. Pointet, C.: Addition of tannin to barium enemas for the study of the colonic mucosa, Gaz. Med. France **58**:771, 1951.

82. Pratt, J. H., and Jackman, R. J.: Perforation of rectal wall by enema tip, Proc. Staff Meet. Mayo Clin. **20**:277, 1945.

83. Pyle, R., and Samuel, E.: Evaluation of hazards of barium enema examination, Clin. Radiol. **11**:192, 1960.

84. Raap, G.: Position of value in studying pelvis and its contents, Southern Med. J. **44**:95, 1951.

85. Rambo, O. N., Zboralske, F. F., Harris, P. A., Riegelman, S., and Margulis, A. R.: Toxicity studies on tannic acid administered by enema, I. Effects of enema-administered tannic acid on the colon and liver of rats, Amer. J. Roentgen. **96**:488, 1966.

86. Rastelli, G. C., Magnani, L., and Bocchia, C.: L'impiego dell'arteriografia nella diagnostica delle emorragie del tubo digerente, Minerva Chir. **14**: 1188-1194, 1959.

87. Ravitch, M. M.: Intussusception in infancy and childhood; an analysis of seventy-seven cases treated by barium enema, New Eng. J. Med. **259**:1058, 1958.

88. Robinson, J. M.: Polyps of the colon: how to find them, Amer. J. Roentgen. **77**:700, 1957.

89. Rösch, J., Gray, R. K., Grollman, J. H., Jr., Ross, G., Steckel, R. J., and Weiner, M.: Selective arterial drug infusions in the treatment of acute gastrointestinal bleeding; a preliminary report, Gastroenterology **59**:341-349, 1970.

89a. Rösch, J., Dotter, C. T., and Rose, R. W.: Selective arterial infusions of vasoconstrictors in acute gastrointestinal bleeding, Radiology **99**:27, 1971.

90. Roman, P. W., Wagner, J. H., and Steinbach, S. H.: Massive fatal embolism during barium enema study, Radiology **59**:190, 1952.

91. Rosenbaum, H. D.: Lieber, A., Hanson, D. J., and Pellegrino, E. D.: Routine survey roentgenogram of the abdomen on 500 consecutive patients over 40 years of age, Amer. J. Roentgen. **91**:903, 1964.

92. Rosenberg, I. S., and Finc, A. V.: Fatal venous intravasation of barium during a barium enema, Radiology **73**:771, 1959.

93. Schüle, A.: Ueber die Sondierung und Radiographie des Dickdarms, Arch. f. Verdauungskr. **10**: 111, 1904.

94. Seaman, W. B., and Wells, J.: Complications of the barium enema, Gastroenterology **48**:728, 1965.

95. Sinclair, D. J., and Buist, T. A. S.: Instrumental and technical notes; water contrast barium enema technique using methyl cellulose, Brit. J. Radiol. **39**:228, 1966.

96. Slanina, J.: Value of hydrogenperoxide and tannic acid in cleansing enema, Radiol. Clin. (Basel) **27**: 197, 1958.

97. Soila, P., and Wegelius, U.: Comparative study of different methods of evacuation of the large bowel for roentgen examination, Acta Radiol. [Diagn.] (Stockholm) **1**:1105, 1963.

98. Spiers, F. W.: Effective atomic number and energy absorption in tissues, Brit. J. Radiol. **19**:52, 1946.

99. Spiro, R. H., and Hertz, R. E.: Colostomy perforation, Surgery **60**:590-597, 1966.

100. Spjut, H. J., Margulis, A. R., and Cook, G. B.: The silicone-foam enema: a source for exfoliative cytological specimens, Acta Cytol. **7**:79, 1963.

101. Steinbach, H. L., and Burhenne, H. J.: Performing the barium enema: equipment, preparation, and contrast medium, Amer. J. Roentgen. **87**:644, 1962.

102. Steinbach, H. L., Rosenberg, R. H., Grossman, M., and Nelson, T. L.: Potential hazard of enemas in patients with Hirschsprung's disease, Radiology **64**:45, 1955.

103. Steinbach, H. L., Rousseau, R., McCormack, K. R.,

and Jawetz, E.: Transmission of enteric pathogens by barium enemas, J.A.M.A. **174**:1207, 1960.

104. Stevens, G. M.: Use of a water enema in the verification of lipoma of the colon, Amer. J. Roentgen. **96**:292, 1966.

105. Stevenson, C. A.: Clinical roentgenology of the colon, Amer. J. Roentgen. **96**:275, 1966.

106. Stevenson, C. A.: Development of colon examination (Hickey memorial lecture), Amer. J. Roentgen **71**:385, 1954.

107. Stevenson, C. A.: Symposium on gastrointestinal surgery; technic of double contrast examination of colon, Surg. Clin. N. Amer. **32**:1531, 1952.

108. Stewart, W. H., and Illick, H. E.: Method of more clearly visualizing lesions of sigmoid, Amer. J. Roentgen. **28**:379, 1932.

109. Ström, B. G., and Winberg, T.: Percutaneous selective angiography of the inferior mesenteric artery, Acta Radiol. (Stockholm) **57**:401, 1962.

110. Templeton, F. E., and Addington, E. A.: Roentgenologic examination of the colon using drainage and negative pressure: with special reference to the early diagnosis of neoplasm, J.A.M.A. **145**:702, 1951.

111. Thomas, S. F.: All speed and no control, Amer. J. Roentgen. **89**:889, 1963.

112. Truemner, K. M., White, S., and Vanlandingham, H.: Fatal embolization of pulmonary capillaries, J.A.M.A. **173**:1089, 1960.

113. Weber, H. M.: Roentgenologic demonstration of polypoid lesions and polyposis of large intestine, Amer. J. Roentgen. **25**:577, 1931.

114. Welin, S.: Modern trends in diagnostic roentgenology of colon (Mackenzie Davidson memorial lecture), Brit. J. Radiol. **31**:453, 1958.

115. Welin, S., and Brahme, F.: Double contrast method in ulcerative colitis, Acta Radiol. (Stockholm) **55**:257, 1961.

116. Welin, S., Youker, J., and Spratt, J. S., Jr.: The rates and patterns of growth of 375 tumors of the large intestine and rectum observed serially by double contrast enema study (Malmö technique), Amer. J. Roentgen. **90**:673, 1963.

117. Wells, D. B., Humphrey, H. D., and Coll, J. J.: Relation of tannic acid to liver necrosis occurring in burns, New Eng. J. Med. **226**:629, 1942.

118. Wittenborg, M. H.: Aerosol-foam, double-contrast enema for examination of the sigmoid and descending colon. Unpublished data.

119. Wyatt, G. M.: Survey examination of colon with barium and tannic acid. Society proceedings, Scientific exhibit, Fifty-second Annual Meeting of American Roentgen Ray Society, Washington, D. C., Amer. J. Roentgen. **66**:820, 1951.

120. Wyatt, G. M., Thornbury, J. R., Fischer, H. W., and Hierschbiel, E. A.: Comparison of ammonium alum and tannic acid as barium enema additives, J.A.M.A. **195**:537, 1966.

121. Zatzkin, H. R., and Irwin, G. A.: Nonfatal intravasation of barium, Amer. J. Roentgen. **92**:1169, 1964.

122. Zboralske, F. F., Harris, P. A., Riegelman, S., Rambo, O. N., and Margulis, A. R.: Toxicity studies on tannic acid administered by enema. III, Studies on the retention of enemas in humans; IV. Review and conclusions, Amer. J. Roentgen. **96**:505, 1966.

123. Zboralske, F. F., Margulis, A. R., and Sizeler, S.: Peroral right pneumocolon examination. To be published.

124. Zheutlin, N., Lasser, E. C., and Rigler, L. G.: Clinical studies on effect of barium in peritoneal cavity following rupture of colon, Surgery **32**:967, 1952.

Ulcerative and granulomatous colitis | 37

Richard H. Marshak

Arthur E. Lindner

For many years the finding of nonspecific inflammatory disease of the large bowel was equivalent to a diagnosis of ulcerative colitis. In recent years it has become apparent that the granulomatous process, which in the small bowel is known as regional enteritis,* can also involve the colon.[1,29] Therefore the differential diagnosis of nonspecific inflammation of the colon rests between ulcerative and granulomatous colitis. The cause of both diseases remains unknown. As a rule it is possible to distinguish the two entities on the basis of their clinical, roentgenologic and pathologic characteristics, but at times features are mixed or intermediate and it is not possible to make a clear-cut distinction by present criteria. In such cases further observation will usually clarify this diagnosis. When a definite diagnosis cannot be made, we prefer to classify the case for the time being, "colitis, type unknown," with a description of the salient features rather than to force the case into either category or to add intermediate classifications. Although some common cause may in time become apparent, it seems that ulcerative and granulomatous disease represent distinct entities and that subsequent investigation will more likely be advanced by keeping the two groups separate than by trying to unify them.

ULCERATIVE COLITIS

Characteristic findings in patients with ulcerative colitis are fever, abdominal cramps, and diarrhea with blood in the stool. At times constipation rather than diarrhea may occur. In many patients the onset is insidious, with vague abdominal complaints and gradual change in the frequency and character of stools. In others the onset is abrupt, with fever, abdominal pain, and bloody diarrhea becoming rapidly more severe over a period of days or weeks. In a few patients the inception is explosive, with high fever, systemic toxicity, severe diarrhea, and

*See references 2-5, 8, 26-28, and 31.

electrolyte depletion or hemorrhage. Gross blood in the stool is characteristic and may precede the onset of diarrhea. Perianal fistulas and anorectal disease occur in some patients with ulcerative colitis, but they are not characteristic findings. Extracolonic manifestations, including arthritis, uveitis, and such skin changes as erythema nodosum or pyoderma gangrenosum may occur. Ulcerative colitis as a rule involves the rectum, even when the rest of the colon is spared; therefore sigmoidoscopy can be expected to provide positive diagnostic findings of granularity, friability, and ulceration, with blood and exudate in the lumen. Toxic dilatation of the colon and free perforation into the peritoneal cavity are dread complications of ulcerative colitis. Carcinoma of the colon is sometimes a sequel to chronic ulcerative colitis.

The course of ulcerative colitis is variable. In some patients with mild disease the clinical and sigmoidoscopic findings subside. In most patients, however, the disease becomes chronic with periodic clinical exacerbations and remissions. Medical treatment includes dietary manipulations, antispasmodics, antidiarrheal agents, blood transfusions, insoluble sulfa drugs, salicylazosulfapyridine (Azulfidine) and corticosteroids. All of these are useful in managing symptoms and perhaps in inducing remissions, but there is no convincing evidence yet that medical treatment alters the natural history of the disease. About 20% to 30% of the patients sick enough to be hospitalized are ultimately treated surgically with colectomy and either ileostomy or ileoproctostomy. In those not operated upon, the disease may become quiescent or burnt out after years of intermittent activity.

On pathologic examination the colon displays features of an exudative inflammation, which involves primarily the mucosa, secondarily the submucosa, and only occasionally the muscularis. The bowel wall is thin or of normal thickness; however, edema, accumulation of fat, and hypertrophy of muscle caused by inflammation may create the impression of a thickened bowel. Ulcerations are shallow and coalesce, leaving islands of mucosa as irregular tags called pseudopolyps. The classic form of ulcerative colitis involves the entire colon. Often, however, the process is segmental. In such cases the rectum alone is usually involved, or the entire left side of the bowel is diseased. Segmental forms of ulcerative colitis without disease of the rectum are uncommon. The diseased areas of bowel are continuous without intervening areas of normal bowel, and involvement of the gut wall is circumferential and symmetrical. In some cases of universal ulcerative colitis the terminal ileum displays a superficial mucosal inflammation called "backwash ileitis."

Histologic examination of the colon confirms the exudative nature of the disease, with exudate and edema as prominent features that involve especially the mucosa. Occasional foreign body giant cells are noted, but granuloma systems are not identified. With time fibrosis occurs within the bowel wall, and the colon becomes distorted, rigid, and shortened. The lumen narrows and strictures may form. Regional lymph nodes may be enlarged and on section show nonspecific inflammation.

Roentgenologic features
Acute stage

In the acute stage the roentgenologic findings are caused by three factors: edema, ulceration, and alterations in the motility of the bowel.

There is a variable roentgenologic pattern, depending on whether the disease process is mild, moderate, or fulminant in character. Inflammation produces motility changes characterized by spasm and irritability (Figs. 37-1 to 37-4). Because of this spasm, narrowing and incomplete filling are frequent, and in some areas the bowel is so attenuated that a string sign is simulated (Figs. 37-1 and 37-5). Considerable secretions are present within the bowel lumen as a consequence of the edema, mucus, blood, and exudate. The usual homogeneous-appearing barium mixture therefore has a granular, flocculant quality (Fig. 37-6). Ulcerations are tiny and difficult to identify and are recognized either as serrations along the contour of the filled bowel (Fig. 37-7) or, after evacuation, as small spicules extending from the mucosa (Fig. 37-8). It should be noted, however, that serrations along

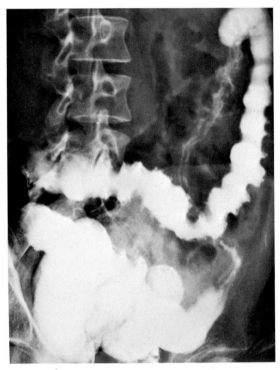

Fig. 37-1. Universal ulcerative colitis. The entire colon is spastic and irritable. The contour of the bowel is hazy because of an inflammatory exudate. Small indistinct ulcers extend from the contour of the transverse colon. The left side is incompletely filled (simulating a string sign) because of marked spasm accompanying the inflammatory process.

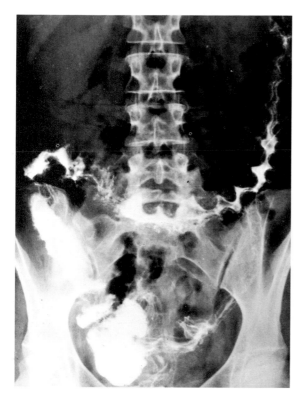

Fig. 37-2. Same case as in Fig. 37-1, after evacuation. The mucosal folds are hazy and thickened in a symmetrical fashion. In contrast to granulomatous colitis there is no evidence of nodularity or irregularity of the contour.

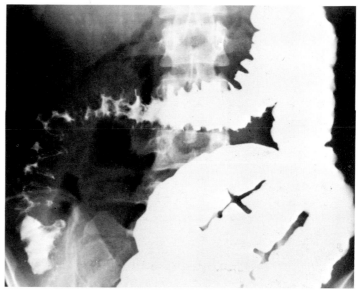

Fig 37-3. Universal ulcerative colitis. The right side of the colon is so spastic and irritable that complete filling was not obtained. The folds are thickened, with tiny ulcerations extending from the contour. Because of overfilling of the left side of the colon, the inflammatory process in this region can easily be missed.

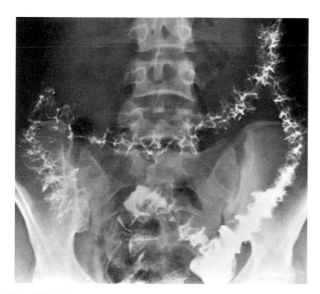

Fig. 37-4. Same case as in Fig. 37-3, after evacuation. The involvement of the entire colon is now better visualized. The folds are thickened throughout and maintain a symmetrical pattern. The extent of involvement in inflammatory disease is often best determined by study of the evacuation film.

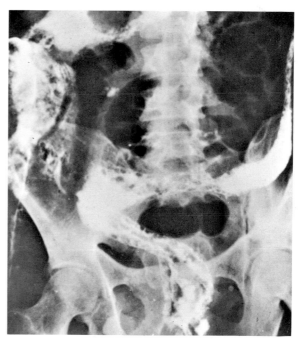

Fig. 37-5. Universal ulcerative colitis. The changes are most marked in the rectum and sigmoid. There is a moderate degree of narrowing and rigidity associated with numerous inflammatory polyps and severe ulceration. Through the entire examination the left side of the colon was impossible to distend because of marked spasm simulating a string sign.

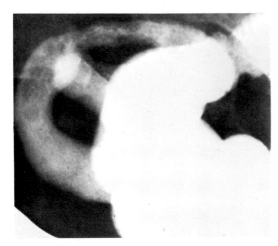

Fig. 37-6. Universal ulcerative colitis; spot film of the sigmoid. The sigmoid is moderately narrowed and rigid. The barium has a granular, flocculant appearance caused by admixture of barium with the blood, pus, and mucus.

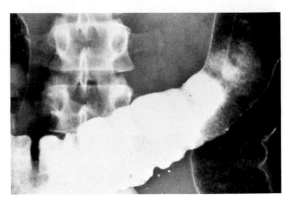

Fig. 37-7. Universal ulcerative colitis; spot film of the distal transverse colon. There are numerous tiny, hazy, indistinct ulcerations along the contour of the bowel. Similar tiny flecks of barium are identified within the lumen of the colon.

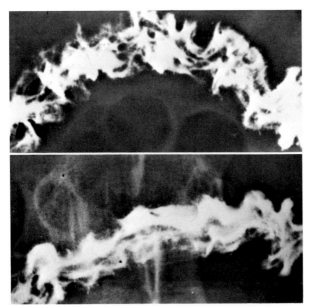

Fig. 37-8. Universal ulcerative colitis; spot film of the transverse colon after evacuation. Thickening, distortion, haziness of the mucosal folds, and numerous tiny ulcerations are seen. This type of ulceration is typical of ulcerative colitis.

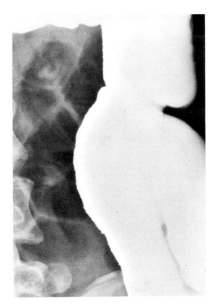

Fig. 37-9. Spicules in a normal bowel. In an occasional normal patient tiny spicules, mimicking ulcerations, are identified. Normal spicules are more symmetric and sharply defined than ulcerations.

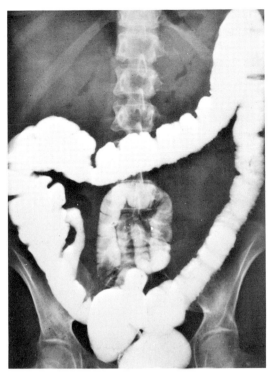

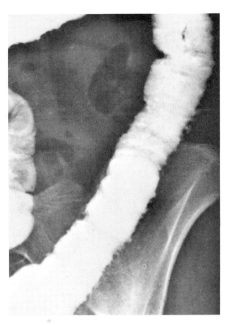

Fig. 37-11. Same case as in Fig. 37-10; spot film of descending colon. The fuzziness of the contour of the bowel is again seen. Some of the ulcerations appear as collar-button projections.

Fig. 37-10. Universal ulcerative colitis with backwash ileitis. There is a minimal degree of narrowing and rigidity of the entire large bowel, associated with absent and irregular haustral markings. There is a fuzziness along the contours of the descending colon and transverse colon because of numerous tiny ulcerations. The terminal ileum is slightly narrowed and rigid, secondary to backwash ileitis.

the contour of the bowel may at times be seen normally perhaps caused by barium penetration of colonic glands. These are sharply defined and have a symmetric, regular, uniform appearance (Fig. 37-9). Ulcerations, in contrast, are hazy, less symmetric, and less uniform.

In the more acute or fulminant phase of this disease, the bowel contour appears obviously hazy. This fuzziness is caused by excessive mucus and ulcerations. When the ulcerations are more pronounced (Figs. 37-10 to 37-13), the fuzziness is replaced by an irregular, serrated border, sometimes appearing as collar-button-like projections as the ulcerations penetrate and become confluent. In some cases the contours are grossly ragged and irregular. As ulceration proceeds, the edematous mucosa produces an appearance that has been called pseudopolyposis

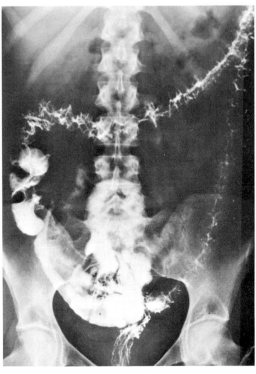

Fig. 37-12. Same case as Figs. 37-10 and 37-11; post-evacuation study. The mucosa throughout the bowel is thickened. There is more narrowing and rigidity of the terminal ileum than is usually seen in backwash ileitis.

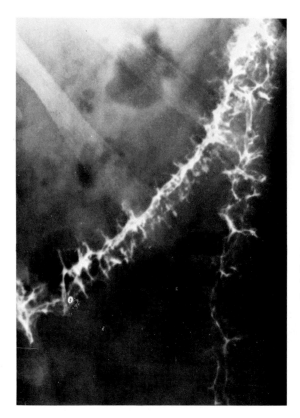

Fig. 37-13. Spot film of the splenic flexure; same case as in Fig. 37-12. The film demonstrates the symmetric thickening of the mucosal folds, associated with numerous tiny ulcerations.

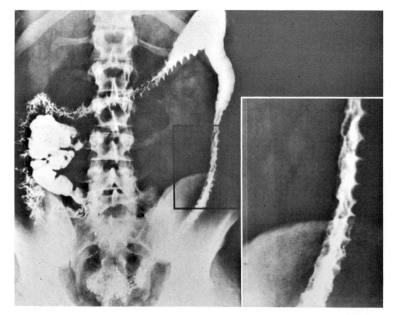

Fig. 37-14. Universal ulcerative colitis; evacuation film. There is symmetric thickening of the folds, with multiple indentations along the contours. These indentations have been referred to as thumb-printing. The granular quality of the barium is caused by an admixture of blood, pus, and mucus.

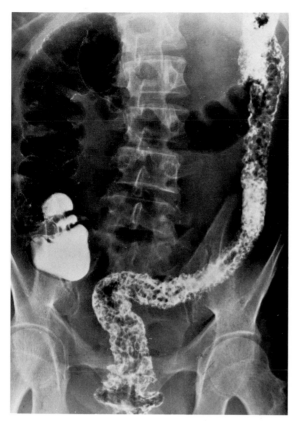

Fig. 37-15. Segmental subacute ulcerative colitis. The left side of the colon is involved with ulcerative colitis, characterized by a moderate degree of narrowing, rigidity, and numerous small inflammatory polyps. The symmetric involvement of the contours is seen. Despite repeated examinations over a period of many years there has been no extension of the inflammatory process in this patient.

(Fig. 37-5). Rarely, localized pneumatosis coli may be recognized in an area of intense ulceration.

The mucosal pattern is best recognized on the evacuation film. The folds are thickened, hazy, and associated with increased secretions. The pattern is regular and symmetric and appears coarsely reticular (Figs. 37-2, 37-4, 37-8, 37-12, and 37-13). Frequently numerous tiny, indistinct ulcerations projecting from the thickened folds are identified. When these projections have a very symmetric and uniform appearance, the possibility that they are also caused by a mixture of barium and mucus should be considered. When the edema is more prominent, the mucosal folds become swollen and show a coarsely granular appearance. The edematous and inflamed mucosa forms along the contour symmetric defects that have been referred to as thumb-printing (Fig. 37-14).

Subacute stage

In the subacute stage additional roentgenologic features supervene because of continued ulcerations, beginning fibrosis, and mucosal regeneration. The mucosa assumes a more nodular appearance, and the polypoid pattern becomes more prominent. The inflammatory polyps are usually small and uniform in appearance (Figs. 37-5, 37-15 to 37-17). They may, however, be large, scattered, and irregular. Tiny comma-shaped radiolucent defects between the larger polypoid lesions are probably caused by the pedicles. Areas of more intense ulceration produce a marked irregularity of the contours, which simulates a neoplasm, especially when it is distributed over a short segment. As a rule, the symmetric appearance described previously is maintained. In patients with minimal bowel involvement the haustral pattern may be unaffected. More often the haustra are distorted and irregular and are associated with some degree of rigidity. In the subacute stage these findings become more evident because of the continued inflammatory process and the more distinct narrowing of the lumen caused by rigidity.

Sinus tracts or fistulas are not a feature of ulcerative colitis but are common in granulomatous colitis.

Chronic stage

In the chronic stage fibrosis, epithelial regeneration, and pseudopolyposis are the prominent features (Figs. 37-18 and 37-19). The end result is a shortening of the bowel, depression of the flexures, narrowing of the bowel lumen, and rigidity. Again, symmetry of the involved area is conspicuous. The contours are relatively smooth because of the marked fibrosis and healing of the ulcerations. The haustra are absent, and the bowel has a tubular, rigid appearance. The flexures may be so contracted that a carcinoma is simulated. At this stage of the disease the roentgenologic appearance usually remains fixed and unvarying despite clinical exacerbation or remission. The mucosa reveals a high degree of atrophy with evidence of reepithelial-

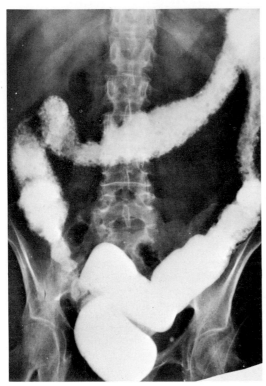

Fig. 37-16. Universal ulcerative colitis. The rectum and sigmoid appear normal. The remainder of the bowel is involved with a moderately severe inflammatory process characterized by narrowing, rigidity, absent haustral markings, slight irregularity of the contour, and numerous inflammatory polyps. By sigmoidoscopy the rectum and lower sigmoid were seen to be minimally involved. Because of the normal roentgenographic appearance of the rectum and sigmoid, there may be difficulty in the differentiation of this type of case from granulomatous colitis. Clinical features were those of ulcerative colitis.

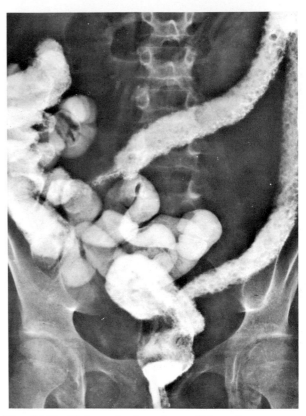

Fig. 37-17. Universal ulcerative colitis, subacute stage. The entire colon is involved with an inflammatory process characterized by moderate narrowing, rigidity, absent haustral markings, and inflammatory polyps. The terminal ileum is normal.

ization. When roentgenograms are made at serial intervals during the course of the disease, one is astonished at the degree of shortening of the colon in the chronic stage of ulcerative colitis. It is remarkable that in a disease that is primarily mucosal, cicatrization and contraction are so pronounced.

In some patients, in the chronic stage, the bowel remains fairly distensible with little shortening and absent haustral markings with no evidence of a mucosal pattern. This appearance has been referred to as chronic, burnt-out ulcerative colitis (Fig. 37-20).

An interesting feature in the diagnosis, especially of early or minimal ulcerative colitis, is the appearance of the descending colon. Normally this portion of the bowel may have no haustral pattern and, because of spasm, may display features that can be confused with inflammatory changes. In the absence of obvious features of ulcerative colitis in other segments of the bowel a definite diagnosis of a lesion in the descending colon may be impossible.

Extension of ulcerative colitis with involvement of the entire colon can occur from a process that is initially limited to one segment. However, in patients with the disease confined to the rectum or left side of the colon, no roentgenologic evidence may be shown to indicate involvement of the remainder of the colon despite repeated observations over a long period of time.

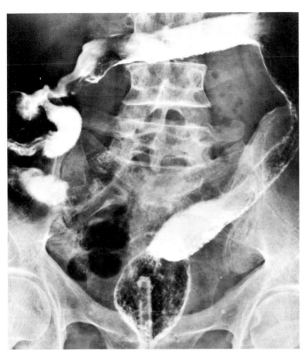

Fig. 37-18. Universal chronic ulcerative colitis. There is a marked degree of narrowing, rigidity, and shortening. The mucosal pattern is absent; there are a few inflammatory polyps. Shortening of the right side of the colon is marked and the anatomic landmarks are difficult to identify. The terminal ileum is elevated.

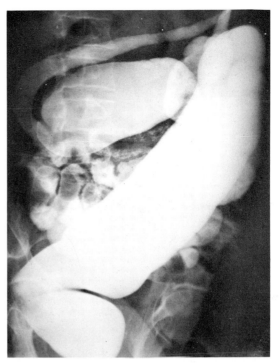

Fig. 37-19. An unusual case of the chronic phase of segmental ulcerative colitis involving the right side of the colon. The right side of the colon has a tubular, pipestem appearance, with enormous dilatation of the terminal ileum. The tubular, rigid, symmetric appearance is in contrast to the asymmetric appearance of granulomatous colitis. Confinement of the inflammatory process to the right side is unusual for ulcerative colitis.

Toxic dilatation of the colon

One of the most dramatic and ominous episodes that may occur in the course of ulcerative colitis is the rapid development of extensive colonic dilatation.[24] This occurs in both acute and chronic phases of the disease and can be associated with extreme toxicity. A portion, or almost all, of the diseased colon becomes tremendously dilated. The distended, tender, silent abdomen is an indication that the bowel is about to perforate. Pathologic examination at this time shows extensive dilatation and thinning of the colonic wall associated with ragged ulceration. Distinct acute inflammatory changes, associated with areas of necrosis, are noted in all the layers of the colon. There is no evidence of organic obstruction in the toxic dilatation of ulcerative colitis. The exact mechanism responsible for the colonic distention is unknown.

In most cases of toxic dilatation, a simple film of the abdomen is sufficient for diagnosis, and a barium enema examination is unnecessary. In the anteroposterior films of the abdomen, taken with the patient lying on his back, the portion of colon most prominently distended is the transverse colon (Figs. 37-21 and 37-22). This is true in part because with the patient supine air in the column rises to the highest segment. The distal descending colon and the sigmoid are less frequently distended. It is uncommon to find distention of the rectum, although the ulcerative process practically always involves this portion of the bowel. An erect or lateral decubitus view may be taken to exclude the presence

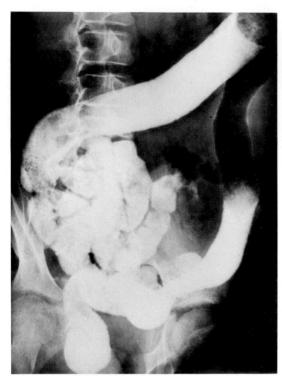

Fig. 37-20. Universal ulcerative colitis, chronic phase. This appearance of narrowing, rigidity, absent mucosal markings, with little shortening, has been referred to as chronic burnt-out ulcerative colitis.

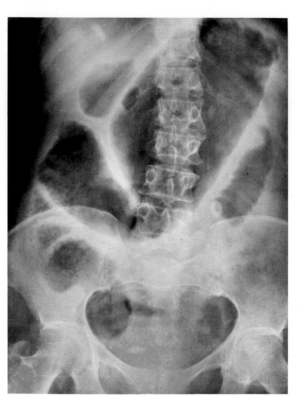

Fig. 37-21. Toxic dilatation of the colon in ulcerative colitis. There is remarkable segmental distention of the transverse colon, with irregular contours. The haustral markings are absent, and there are numerous nodular projections within the lumen.

of free air. Such films will also show fluid levels in the colon and it is fairly characteristic of this condition that the fluid levels are few in number and long. The caliber of the distended segments may be very great. A striking roentgenologic feature is the fact that despite distention the lengths of the visualized segments are relatively normal. The hepatic and splenic flexures are normally situated, and identification of the visualized portion of the colon is not difficult. It is possible that the plastic exudate prevents the bowel from becoming elongated or contracted. The picture of marked distention associated with undistended or relatively narrowed portions of colon in between is in contrast to that seen in mechanical obstruction, in which the colon proximal to the site of obstruction is uniformly distended and often markedly redundant. The roentgenologic appearance of the bowel is sufficient for diagnosis. In the segments involved the normal haustral pattern is absent

(Figs. 37-23 and 37-24). In less involved portions the haustra may appear thickened. Superimposed on the contour there may be innumerable broad-based, nodular, pseudopolypoid projections that extend into the lumen of the bowel (Figs 37-22 and 37-25). Between the soft tissue projections, air-filled crevices, which in some instances have a serrated or toothlike configuration, may be identified. These presumably are the result of deep ulcerations. Peritonitis, at least of a localized nature, with plastic serosal exudate, is usually present in these patients. There is no evidence of fluid in the abdomen. The changes described may develop in a very short period of time. When a free perforation occurs, air is readily identified under the diaphragm. It is not unusual in these patients for a considerable amount of air to accumulate under both leaves of the diaphragm and throughout the abdomen.

On occasion a barium enema examination is

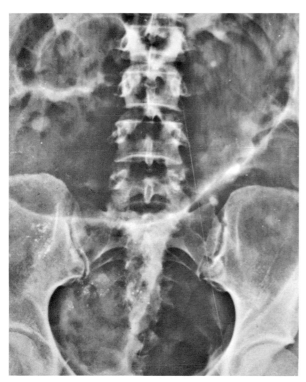

Fig. 37-22. Toxic dilatation in ulcerative colitis. There is marked distention of the transverse colon and midportion of the descending colon. The haustral markings in these regions are absent, with numerous polypoid projections caused by large inflammatory polyps. There is considerable irregularity of the contour of the bowel.

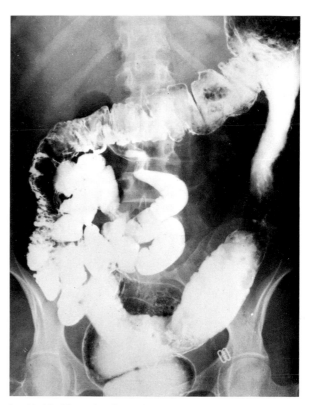

Fig. 37-23. Chronic ulcerative colitis. The barium enema examination shows the moderately severe changes of ulcerative colitis from splenic flexure to rectum. The sigmoid is moderately dilated. The right side of the colon is minimally involved.

performed in patients who have toxic dilatation. Because of the high incidence of spontaneous perforation in toxic dilatation, barium enema examination is contraindicated. Nevertheless, this examination has been attempted in several instances without apparent complications, probably because it is impossible to introduce large quantities of barium without inducing evacuation. The examiner also finds it useless to continue the examination because of the large amount of secretions and air within the colon. However, the barium may outline some of the features (Figs. 37-26 and 37-27), which consist of distention, obliteration of the haustral and mucosal pattern, irregularity of the contour with multiple deep projections indicative of ulceration, and numerous nodular pseudopolypoid intraluminal projections. There may be shortening and lack of redundancy of the colon and an inability of the colon to contract because of loss of tone.

Benign strictures and carcinoma

When rigid criteria of a stricture are utilized, benign strictures in ulcerative colitis are uncommon.[21] The term "stricture" is applied to a localized, rigid, filiform narrowing that has produced some antegrade obstruction. On roentgenologic examination the strictures have a typically benign appearance, with a concentric lumen, smooth contours, and fusiform, pliable, tapering margins (Figs. 37-28 and 37-29). The bowel proximal to the stricture is minimally dilated, and during evacuation the colon empties well. Occasionally, however, the lumen of the stricture is slightly eccentric, with irregularity of the contours and mucosa simulating a carcinoma (Fig. 37-30). Rarely, a small sinus tract is demonstrated, extending laterally from the distal portion of the stricture. Despite the roentgenologic findings of chronic ulcerative colitis, microscopic examination frequently reveals active inflammation at the site of the stric-

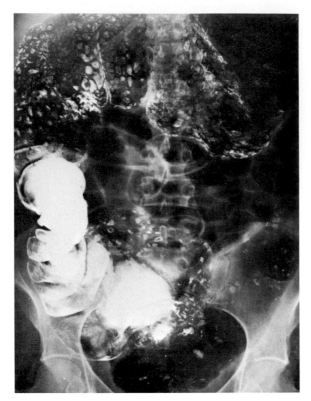

Fig. 37-24. Toxic dilatation of the colon; same patient as in Fig. 37-23, 3 days later. At this time there is huge distention of the transverse colon. The distention of the sigmoid has increased, but the caliber of the descending colon is unchanged. The appearance of the barium in the transverse colon suggests that there is marked ulceration and that there are numerous inflammatory polyps.

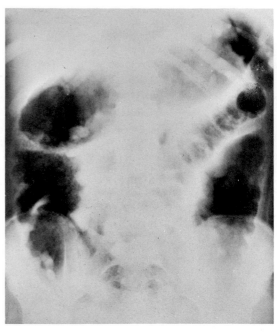

Fig. 37-25. Mild toxic dilatation of the colon. There is slight dilatation of the transverse colon and a segment of descending colon. The inflammatory polyps are large and striking. There is also considerable irregularity of the bowel in both these areas, indicating severe ulceration.

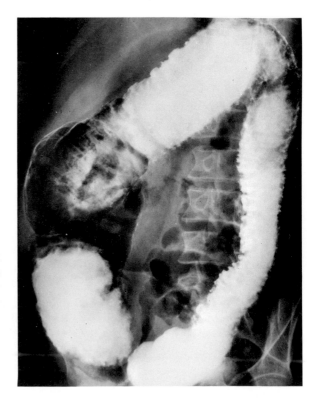

Fig. 37-26. Barium enema examination of a patient with mild toxic dilatation. There is diffuse involvement of the colon, with innumerable ulcerations along the contours producing a serrated appearance. The dilatation in this case is not as extreme as in the usual case of toxic dilatation of the colon.

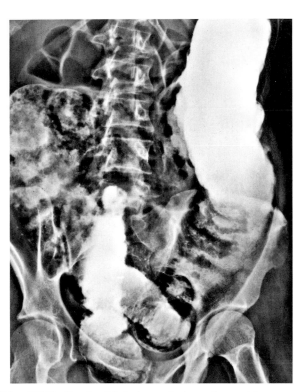

Fig. 37-27. Toxic dilatation of the colon with an attempted barium enema examination. The considerable secretions obscure the details observed in toxic dilatation. A barium enema examination in these cases is frequently futile and is unnecessary for diagnosis.

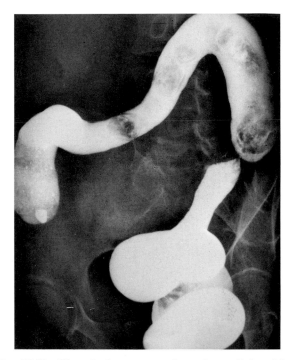

Fig. 37-28. Chronic burnt-out ulcerative colitis with a benign stricture. There is a fusiform, tapering stricture with a concentric lumen and smooth contours, measuring 1.5 cm. in length in the middescending colon. There is a moderate degree of dilatation proximal to the stricture, with retained stool and secretions. The entire colon is involved with chronic burnt-out ulcerative colitis.

ture and immediately proximal and distal to it.

The genesis of stricture in ulcerative colitis is not certain. Traditionally it has been supposed that the stricture represents a localized area of fibrosis. It has been shown, however, that the striking pathologic findings at the site of a stricture are hypertrophy and contraction of the muscularis mucosae.[6] Unlike lesions associated with fibrosis, such strictures might be expected to be reversible, and indeed disappearance of strictures in ulcerative colitis has been described on follow-up roentgenographic examination.[15]

Frequently, areas of spasm are seen in ulcerative colitis and require differentiation from strictures. In these cases we administer 10 mg. propantheline (Pro-Banthine) intravenously. This dose reduces or eliminates spasm, when this is present, or permits better delineation of a stricture. If the lumen is concentric and the margins are smooth, the lesion may be presumed benign. If the lumen is eccentric and the margins are irregular, a carcinoma must be suspected.

An interesting situation occurs when the right side of the colon is shortened, with stricturing of the ileocecal valve and colonization and dilatation of the terminal ileum. The anatomic landmarks become so distorted that the irregular, stenotic ileocecal region suggests a carcinoma in the colon. The dilated terminal ileum could easily be mistaken as a segment of colon and a narrowed ileocecal valve for a carcinoma (Figs. 37-31 and 37-32).

Carcinoma of the colon developed in 6% of our patients who had ulcerative colitis. In two thirds of these the colitis was chronic and burnt out. In one third the colitis was active, with evidence of ulceration and inflammatory polyps. In some patients the carcinoma is present as a filiform stricture with none of the typical roent-

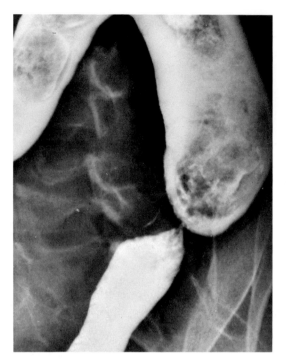

Fig. 37-29. Spot film of the benign stricture shown in Fig. 37-28.

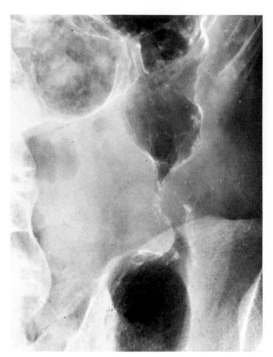

Fig. 37-30. Benign stricture in chronic ulcerative colitis. There is a slightly irregular stricture measuring 3.5 cm. in length in the proximal descending colon. A sinus tract extends laterally from the distal portion of the stricture. There is minimal proximal dilatation. It is impossible in this case to make a definite diagnosis of benign or malignant stricture. Pathologic examination revealed a benign stricture.

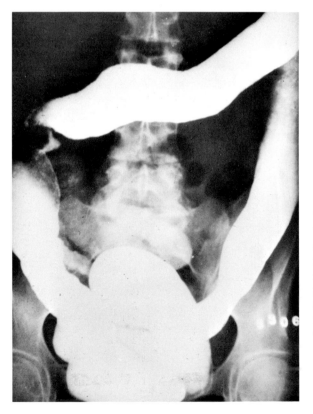

Fig. 37-31. Benign stricture in chronic ulcerative colitis. The right side of the colon is notably shortened, with complete disappearance of a normal cecum and ascending colon. There is stricturing and irregularity of the ileocecal valve, with dilatation of the terminal ileum. Failure to recognize the dilated terminal ileum may result in a mistaken diagnosis of a carcinoma. Operative findings were ulcerative colitis with a benign stricture of the ileocecal valve.

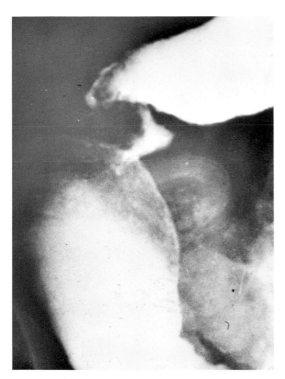

Fig. 37-32. Spot film of the benign stricture shown in Fig. 37-31.

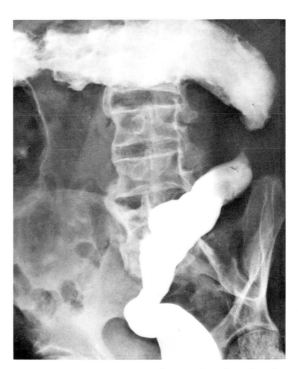

Fig. 37-33. Carcinomatous stricture in chronic ulcerative colitis. The stricture involves the proximal descending colon. The lumen is eccentric, the contours are irregular, and there is moderate dilatation of the proximal bowel. An irregular stricture in ulcerative colitis must be considered a carcinoma until proved otherwise.

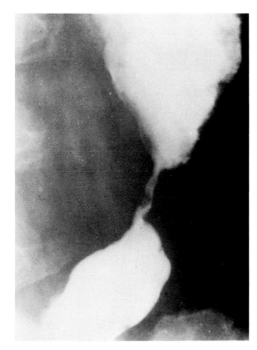

Fig. 37-34. Spot film of the malignant stricture shown in Fig. 37-33.

genologic alterations associated with a carcinoma. The roentgenologic findings in these patients include a narrowed segment, usually measuring from 2 to 6 cm. in length, with an eccentric lumen, irregular contours, and flattened, rigid, tapered margins (Figs. 37-33 to 37-38). There is a moderate degree of dilatation of the proximal bowel, with evidence of increased secretions and retained stool. Clinically, symptoms of colonic obstruction are a prominent feature. The distal transverse colon, descending colon, and the rectum are the most frequent sites of carcinomatous strictures in our series of cases. The atypical roentgenologic features are probably caused by the associated inflammatory disease and the submucosal location of the carcinomas. Pathologic study shows the deep layers of fibrous tissue to be infiltrated by scirrhous carcinoma. An irregular stricture in the presence of chronic ulcerative colitis should be considered as a carcinoma until proved otherwise.

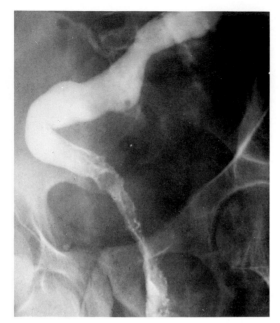

Fig. 37-35. Carcinoma of the rectum with ulcerative colitis. An irregular narrowing of the entire rectum caused by a carcinoma in a patient with chronic burnt-out ulcerative colitis. Numerous nodular defects are also identified in the strictured area.

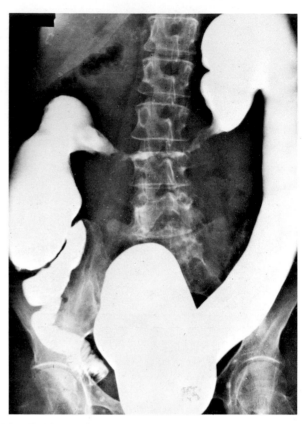

Fig. 37-36. Carcinomatous stricture in chronic burnt-out ulcerative colitis.

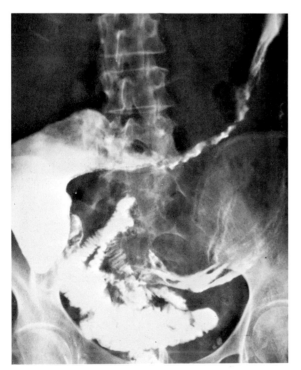

Fig. 37-37. Evacuation film of the stricture shown in Fig. 37-36.

In the remaining patients the carcinoma, in spite of the underlying ulcerative colitis, demonstrated the typical roentgenologic alterations associated with a malignancy and presented no problem in differential diagnosis (Fig. 37-39).

Backwash ileitis

Statistics of the rate of involvement of the ileum in patients with ulcerative colitis vary from 5% to 30%. In our series involvement of the ileum occurred in approximately 10% of the patients. The involvement of the mucosa is minimal and the length of involvement variable (from 4 to 20 cm.). There is no significant narrowing of the bowel lumen. The contours are smooth or slightly serrated. The amount of secretions and motor activity are minimally increased (Fig. 37-40). The findings in the ileum are limited in degree and extent even when the roentgenologic alterations in the colon are marked.

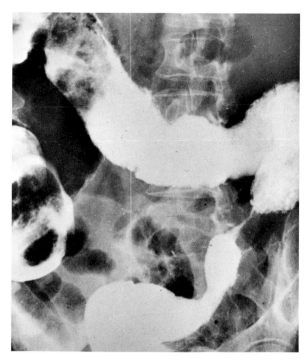

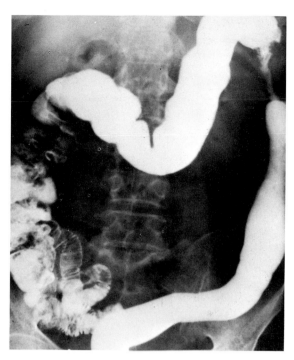

Fig. 37-38. Carcinomatous stricture in chronic ulcerative colitis. There is an irregular stricture involving the proximal descending colon, with an eccentric lumen and marked dilatation of the proximal bowel. The entire colon is involved with burnt-out ulcerative colitis.

Fig. 37-39. Carcinoma in chronic burnt-out ulcerative colitis. The classical appearance of a carcinoma is noted in the proximal descending colon.

In an occasional case of backwash ileitis the distinction from regional enteritis may be difficult. More extensive ulceration of the mucosa may produce spasm with narrowing and rigidity, and in these patients differential diagnosis may be impossible (Fig. 37-41).

Reversibility in ulcerative colitis

Not infrequently, since serial examinations are performed in patients with ulcerative colitis, there appears to be considerable healing of the inflammatory process with a marked reversibility in the appearance of the colon (Figs. 37-42 and 37-43). The narrowing of the lumen has been reported to disappear, the haustral pattern to return to normal, and the inflammatory polyps to vanish. When these cases are analyzed, however, it becomes apparent that not all of them demonstrate true reversion. The narrowing may have been caused by an acute stage, when there was considerable associated spasm and irrita-

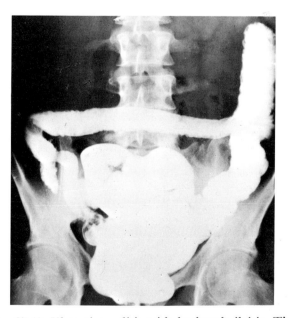

Fig. 37-40. Ulcerative colitis with backwash ileitis. The terminal ileum is distensible, associated with minimal irregularity of the contour and increased secretions. The narrowing and rigidity usually associated with regional enteritis are absent. The inflammatory process involving the colon is evident.

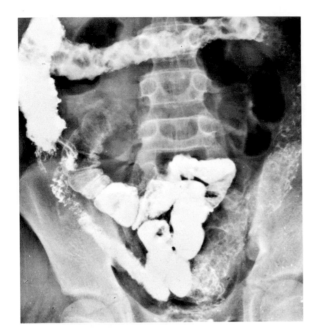

Fig. 37-41. Diffuse ulcerative colitis with backwash ileitis. The backwash ileitis in this case is usually extensive and mimics regional enteritis. There is a moderate degree of narrowing and rigidity, with slight irregularity of the contour and thickening of the mucosal folds. The more extensive involvement of the ileum in this case suggests granulomatous disease. At operation, however, the findings were those of ulcerative colitis and backwash ileitis.

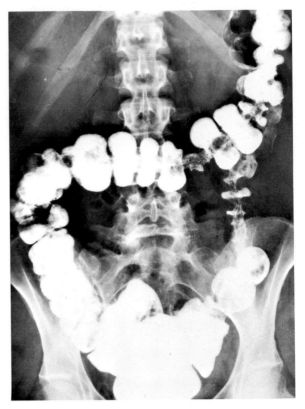

Fig. 37-42. Reversibility in ulcerative colitis. The same patient as in Figs. 37-1 and 37-2, 6 months later. There has been a remarkable reversibility in the appearance of the colon. There is no roentgenographic evidence of an inflammatory process. The haustral markings are within normal limits. A moderate amount of stool is present in the colon because of incomplete preparation.

bility. Actual fibrotic narrowing may never have been present. The reappearance of a normal haustral pattern may also be misleading because the haustra, especially when irregular and thick, can represent pseudohaustrations produced by underlying severe inflammatory disease. Nevertheless, reversibility, to some degree, is an established feature of ulcerative colitis.

On the other hand, it should be noted that at any time in the course of ulcerative colitis an acute flare-up may occur, with a marked change in the roentgenologic appearance of the inflamed bowel. This is most dramatically seen in patients with minimal involvement when subtle roentgenologic alterations become florid, with rapid development of severe ulcerations and pseudopolyps.

Differential diagnosis
Familial polyposis

The colon in a patient with ulcerative colitis may contain a tremendous number of pseudo-polyps. As a result, the appearance may sometimes be confused with familial polyposis.[25] In a majority of cases of ulcerative colitis associated with pseudopolyps there is some roentgenologic evidence of an inflammatory process manifested by the absence or irregularity of the haustral markings, narrowing of the lumen, longitudinal shortening of the colon, and ulceration of the mucosa (Figs. 37-44 and 37-45). On the contrary, in the cases of familial polyposis that we have studied, no evidence is usually found of an inflammatory process in a roentgenologic examination, despite the presence on pathologic examination of minimal inflammatory changes in many of these cases. It should be noted that differentiation between the two entities based upon the appearance of the polyps themselves is unreliable (Figs. 37-46 and 37-47).

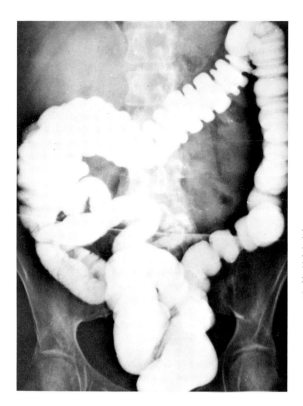

Fig. 37-43. Reversibility in ulcerative colitis. The same patient as in Figs. 37-10 and 37-11, 1 year later. The ileum and colon now appear normal. Reversibility is a feature that is more commonly identified in ulcerative than in granulomatous colitis.

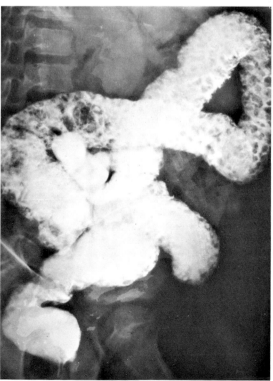

Fig. 37-44. Ulcerative colitis with inflammatory polyps simulating familial polyposis. Numerous inflammatory polyps are distributed throughout the colon. The narrowing, rigidity, and shortening are evidence of an inflammatory process and differentiate the findings from familial polyposis. Differential diagnosis on the basis of the appearance of the polyps alone is impossible.

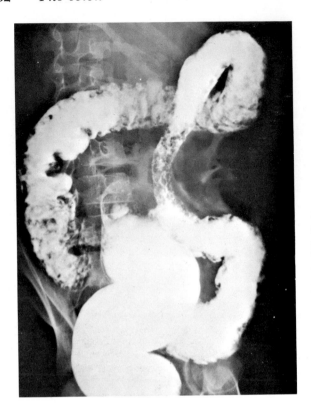

Fig. 37-45. Ulcerative colitis with inflammatory polyps simulating familial polyposis. In this case it is very difficult to differentiate the findings from familial polyposis. There is, however, slight narrowing and lack of distensibility of the transverse and descending colon. Note the lack of involvement of the rectum.

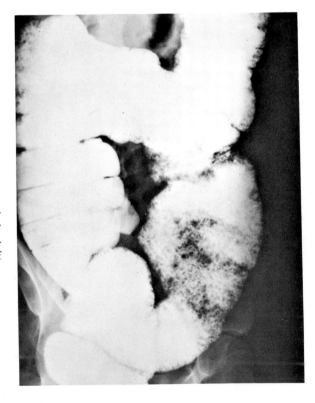

Fig. 37-46. Typical appearance of familial polyposis involving the entire colon. The polyps are more readily distinguishable on the left side. The bowel is more distensible than is usually noted. There is no evidence of an inflammatory process.

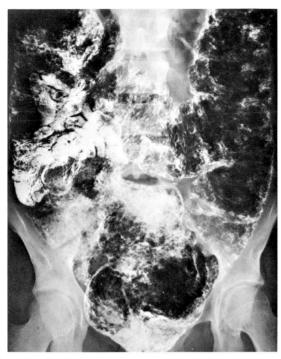

Fig. 37-47. Air study of the same patient as in Fig. 37-46. The tremendous numbers of polyps are again identified. Individual pedicles are difficult to delineate.

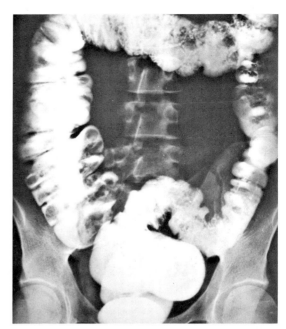

Fig. 37-48. Ulcerative colitis simulating familial polyposis. There is so little evidence of an inflammatory process in this case that differential diagnosis with familial polyposis would be impossible without previous films that demonstrate the characteristic changes of ulcerative colitis. The filling defects were constant and caused by polyps rather than by feces.

A perplexing situation can develop in an occasional case of ulcerative colitis in which the inflammatory process heals and the roentgenologic changes return to normal, except for the large number of inflammatory polyps (Figs. 37-48 to 37-52). In these cases involvement by the ileum with backwash ileitis may aid in differentiation. Familial polyposis rarely involves the small bowel.

Cathartic colon

The roentgenologic findings of cathartic colon[10,22] may be difficult to differentiate from burnt-out ulcerative colitis (Figs. 37-53 and 37-54). In cathartic colon the right side reveals the more extensive alterations. These consist of absent or diminished haustral markings, bizarre contractions, and inconstant areas of narrowing. The bowel is moderately distensible, and after evacuation barium is frequently retained within the colon. The mucosal pattern, when identified, is usually linear, with no evidence of ulceration. In severe cases the left side of the colon may also be involved, but the sigmoid and rectum are usually normally distensible. The terminal ileum can manifest changes similar to those in the right side of the colon for varying lengths. The ileocecal valve is frequently flattened and gaping. Shortening of the colon occurs, especially on the right side, but the flexures are usually normally situated. Fluoroscopically, and on the films, tubular areas of narrowing may be identified. These reveal a concentric lumen with tapering margins and no evidence of rigidity. The areas of narrowing are inconstant and may disappear during a single examination.

GRANULOMATOUS COLITIS

Patients with granulomatous colitis, like those with ulcerative colitis, may have fever, abdominal cramps, and diarrhea or constipation.[11,16] Gross blood in the stools, however, is unusual, and when it does occur it tends to be infrequent

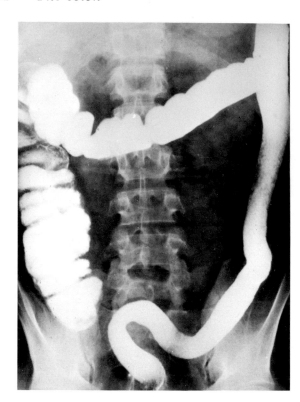

Fig. 37-49. Universal ulcerative colitis involving predominantly the transverse colon, descending colon, and rectum.

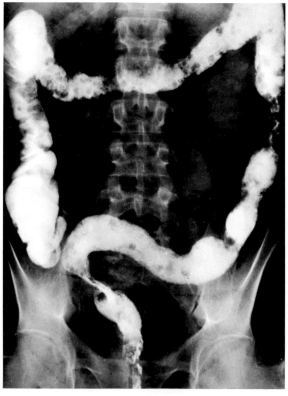

Fig. 37-50. The same patient as in Fig. 37-49, 1 year later. There is more marked involvement of the colon. Numerous large inflammatory polyps can be identified.

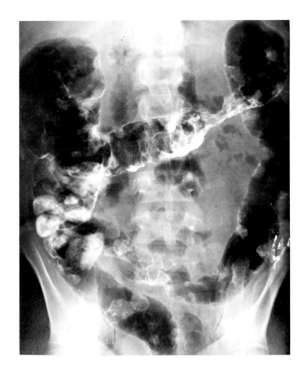

Fig. 37-51. The same patient as in Figs. 37-49 and 37-50, 3 years later. Air study again reveals the large inflammatory polyps. There is narrowing in the distal transverse colon, sigmoid, and rectum. The remainder of the bowel is more distensible than on the previous examination.

Fig. 37-52. Same patient as in Figs. 37-49 to 37-51, 6 years after the initial examination. There is now a carcinomatous stricture of the rectum and a carcinoma of the sigmoid. The remainder of the colon reveals a remarkable reversion in the appearance of the inflammatory process; after colectomy and microscopic study the pathologist had difficulty in determining whether the findings were caused by familial polyposis or ulcerative colitis. The serial roentgenographic films demonstrating the presence of ulcerative colitis were helpful in arriving at the final diagnosis of chronic ulcerative colitis with two superimposed carcinomas.

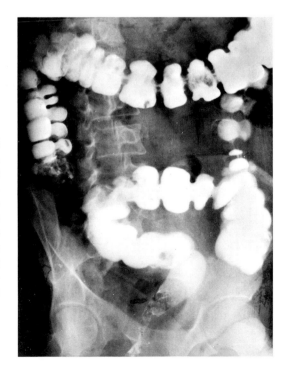

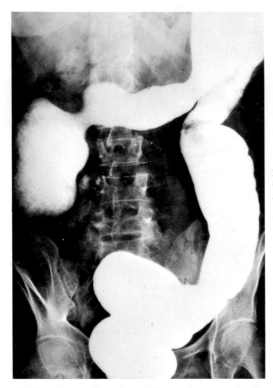

Fig. 37-53. Cathartic colon. There is normal distensibility with complete absence of the haustral markings. The findings are more obvious on the right side of the colon. Areas of narrowing are inconstant.

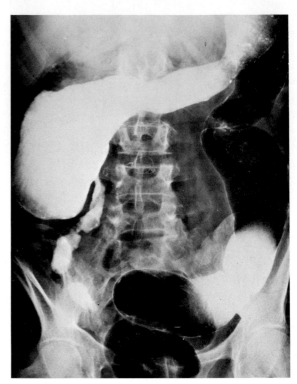

Fig. 37-54. Cathartic colon simulating burnt-out ulcerative colitis. Similar findings may also be seen in the ileum.

and not a prominent feature of the illness. Perianal fistulas and anorectal disease are common in granulomatous colitis and, as has been observed in regional enteritis, they may appear before any of the other clinical features of the disease. Extracolonic manifestations are less common than in ulcerative colitis. Although the rectum may be involved in granulomatous disease,[7] the process tends to be right-sided and segmental and tends to spare the rectum. Therefore, a normal sigmoidoscopy of a patient with colitis is strongly suggestive of granulomatous disease. Clinical distinction between ulcerative and granulomatous disease in the appearance of an involved rectum may be difficult, but an irregularly inflamed, cobblestone surface, if present, suggests the latter.[18] Rectal biopsy reaching the submucosa may yield granulomas. Carcinoma of the colon has only occasionally been reported in association with granulomatous colitis. An increase in the reported incidence of

carcinoma of the small bowel in patients with long-standing regional enteritis suggests that an increased incidence of colonic carcinoma with granulomatous colitis may also be reported with time. Free perforation of the colon into the peritoneal cavity is rare, even though minute, sealed-off perforations are characteristic of the granulomatous disease process.

The medical treatment of granulomatous colitis is similar to that of ulcerative disease and is largely symptomatic and supportive. Corticosteroids are useful in management but are less likely to induce a full remission than in ulcerative colitis. In some patients with granulomatous colitis the disease runs a relatively low-grade and indolent course with moderate disability. When surgery is required in these patients it is usually for obstruction. In other patients the course of the disease is more severe; fistula formation and sinus tracts are common, and infection and chronic toxicity become indications for surgery.

The problem of surgical treatment is more complicated in granulomatous than in ulcerative disease. In ulcerative colitis the disease is curable at the expense of total colectomy and ileostomy. In granulomatous disease of the small intestine (regional enteritis), lengths of bowel that appear normal at operation may become involved in granulomatous disease after resection or bypass procedures. Such recurrence develops in at least half the patients. Similar recurrence has also been noted in patients with granulomatous disease of both ileum and colon (ileocolitis). It appears at present, for reasons not yet clear, that when surgery is performed on patients with granulomatous colitis in whom the small bowel is normal the recurrence rate is considerably less. Nevertheless, since the pathology of small bowel and colonic granulomatous disease is the same, the risk of postoperative spread of disease must be kept in mind. For this reason, patients with granulomatous colitis, like those with regional enteritis, are managed medically as long as possible, and surgery is reserved for complications or for prolonged disability.

The lesions characteristic of regional enteritis may be seen in any segment of the colon with or without associated disease in the small intestine. The colon may be involved in granulomatous disease in one of several ways. First, the colon alone may be the site of primary granulomatous disease, sometimes in its entirety, but more frequently in segmental fashion, with the rectum and sigmoid being spared. Second, in addition to granulomatous disease of the colon there may be involvement, usually simultaneous in onset, of the small bowel. The diseased area in the colon may be continuous with that in the ileum, or it may occur as a skip lesion with normal intervening bowel. Third, the colon may become involved with granulomatous disease only after an operation has been performed for regional ileitis. In this case the diseased segment of colon is usually immediately adjacent to an anastomosis. Finally, the colon may be involved directly by fistula formation from a loop of bowel that is the site of regional ileitis. Such fistulas, in our experience, are usually without significance so far as subsequent development of granulomatous colitis is concerned; the disease does not appear to spread, and the area heals when the diseased small bowel has been removed and the fistula closed.

Therefore, the colon itself can be involved in a primary granulomatous process, or both the colon and the small bowel, usually the ileum, can be the site of granulomatous disease. We have termed such associated involvement "granulomatous ileocolitis." The term "ileocolitis" is used only to describe granulomatous disease and does not refer to ulcerative colitis with backwash ileitis. As has been noted, the ileal involvement in ulcerative colitis does not alter the course of the colonic disease or its management and is therefore of little clinical significance. We believe that regional ileitis and ulcerative colitis are associated only rarely and by chance. Pending full understanding of the etiologic agents involved, it seems reasonable that when regional ileitis is present the associated inflammatory disease in the colon should be granulomatous. This has been the case in recent studies.

Not every segmental colitis, however, is granulomatous. Ulcerative colitis can at times be present in segmental, right-sided, or atypical forms and may be associated with minimal inflammatory changes in the terminal ileum. These lesions must be differentiated from granulomatous colitis and ileitis. Amebiasis, intestinal tuberculosis, ischemic colitis, and scirrhous carcinoma may all manifest roentgenographic features suggestive of granulomatous colitis. These entities are discussed under the heading of "differential diagnosis."

The pathology of granulomatous colitis is similar to that of regional enteritis.[14,17] There is a chronic inflammation extending through the entire wall involving primarily the submucosa. The bowel wall is thick and rigid, with narrowing of the lumen that may lead to stricture formation. Ulcers are deep and tend to be present as long linear ulcerations intersecting with deep transverse ulcers or fissures. The intervening mucosa is swollen, and the luminal surface has a coarsely nodular appearance that has been likened to that of a cobblestone road. "Skip lesions," segments of disease separated by a length of normal bowel, are frequently seen. Involvement of the bowel wall itself may be asymmetric rather than circumferential. Loops of involved gut may adhere to each other or to loops of normal bowel. Fistulas between loops of bowel or to other viscera are common, and intra-abdominal abscesses may be present. When the

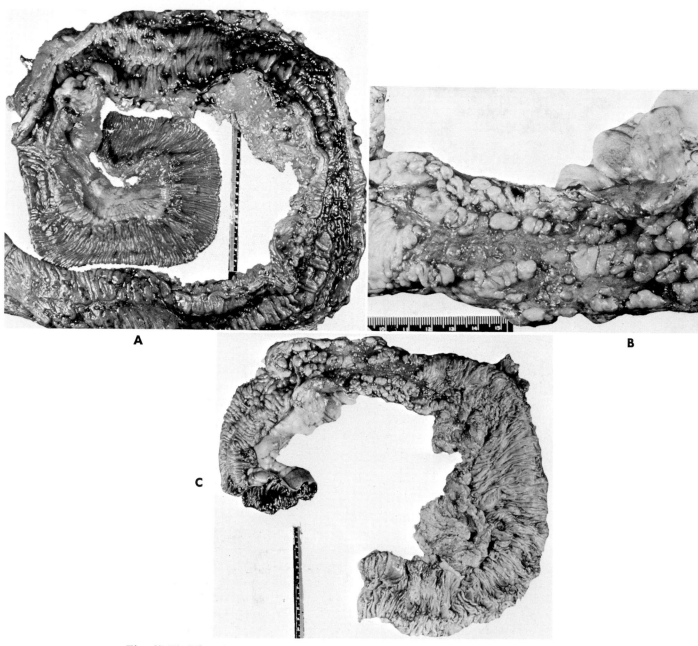

Fig. 37-55. The characteristic pathologic features of granulomatous colitis are demonstrated in this group of surgical specimens. Cobblestoning, longitudinal ulcerations, skip lesions, stricturing, and thickening of the bowel wall are seen. In **D** the pathologic features in the terminal ileum and the right side of the colon are similar.

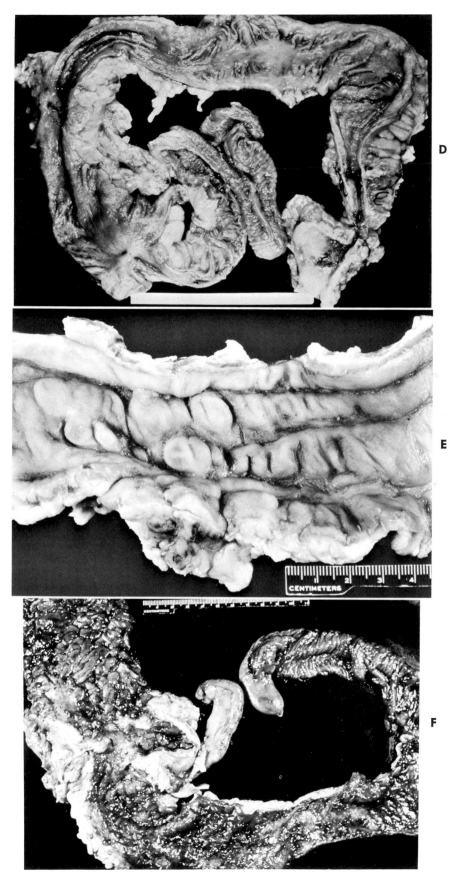

Fig. 37-55, cont'd. For legend see opposite page.

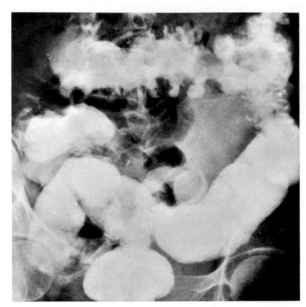

Fig. 37-56. Granulomatous colitis. There is marked irregularity of the contours, caused by numerous large sac-like ulcerations. The left side of the colon is normal.

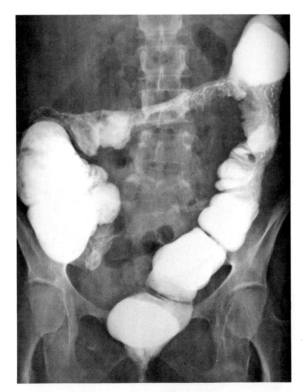

Fig. 37-57. Granulomatous colitis. There is narrowing and irregularity of the transverse and proximal descending colon. Pseudodiverticula and pleating of the folds are seen along the medial aspect of the proximal descending colon. This case represents a later stage of involvement from Fig. 37-56.

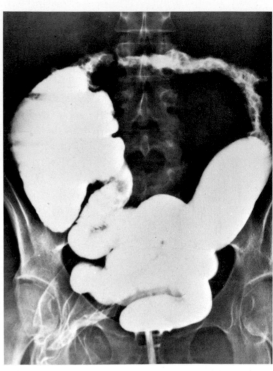

Fig. 37-58. Granulomatous colitis. There is more marked narrowing and irregularity of the transverse colon and proximal descending colon, with considerable dilatation of the right side of the colon. The characteristic segmental distribution is identified.

ileum as well as the colon is involved in this inflammatory process, the condition is called "granulomatous ileocolitis" (Fig. 37-55).

Histologic examination shows a chronic inflammatory reaction most prominent in the submucosa but extending through the bowel wall, with edema and fibrosis. The ulcers are deep and extend through the serosa as sealed-off perforations to which adjacent viscera may adhere. The characteristic histologic feature is the presence of noncaseating granulomas with Langhans' giant cells and epithelioid cells. Especially when ulceration is severe, granulomas may be scanty or absent, but a diagnosis of granulomatous disease is warranted if the other characteristic pathologic features are present. Regional lymph nodes may be enlarged and on section show characteristic granulomas.

Roentgenologic features

Roentgenographic features characteristic of granulomatous colitis are essentially those seen

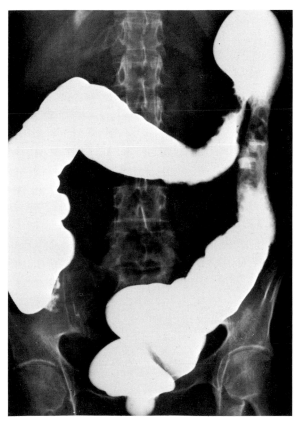

Fig. 37-59. Granulomatous colitis. There are two skip lesions, one in the distal transverse colon and the second in the proximal descending colon, with normal intervening bowel. The contour is irregular and there are large inflammatory polyps.

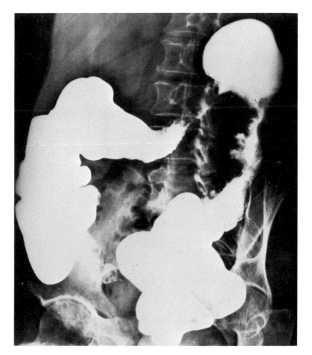

Fig. 37-60. Same patient as in Fig. 37-59. One year later the skip lesions are again identified. At this time pseudodiverticula are seen in the descending colon, reflecting asymmetric involvement.

in regional enteritis of the small bowel.[32] They include skip lesions, longitudinal ulcerations, transverse fissures, deep ragged ulcerations, eccentric involvement and pseudodiverticula, narrowing or stricture formation, pseudopolypoid changes producing a coarse cobblestone pattern, internal fistulas, and sinus tracts (Figs. 37-56 to 37-73).

In early or minimally involved cases many of the typical roentgenographic features of granulomatous disease may not be seen. Instead, there are single or multiple nodular defects or irregularity and rigidity of the contour of a short segment (Fig. 37-74). Sometimes these nodules are associated with tiny ulcerations (Fig. 37-74, *A*). These minimal changes can easily be obscured by filling and distention of the colon or by overlapping adjacent bowel. Study of the mucosal

pattern after evacuation is helpful in these cases; it may reveal thickening or nodularity of the mucosa with an irregular ropelike appearance (Figs. 37-75 to 37-78). Although small areas of ulceration may be difficult to identify, their presence may be suggested by straightening or rigidity of a segment or by the presence of pseudodiverticula on the opposite wall. These conditions occur because ulceration produces spasm and contraction, and the opposite uninvolved wall therefore becomes folded. The small ulcers combine to produce large longitudinal ulcerations or gutters, which are frequently multiple. When this condition is associated with transverse linear ulcerations it produces the characteristic cobblestone pattern (Fig. 37-79).

The transverse ulcers may penetrate beyond the contour of the bowel in such a way that they appear in profile as numerous long, thin spicules perpendicular to the long axis of the bowel or as sinus tracts (Figs. 37-80 to 37-82). They are most frequent between the terminal ileum and the cecum (Fig. 37-83) and may ultimately lead to intramural abscesses (Fig. 37-

Text continued on p. 1003.

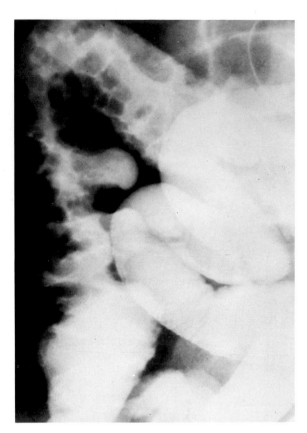

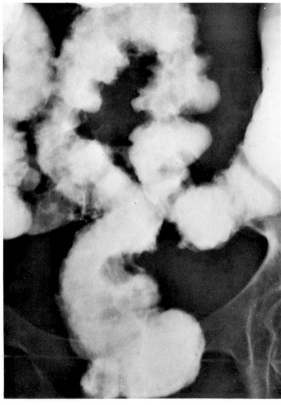

Fig. 37-61. Granulomatous colitis. This spot film of the right side of the colon demonstrates transverse and linear ulceration. Large inflammatory polyps, narrowing, rigidity, and irregular contours are present.

Fig. 37-62. Granulomatous colitis. This spot film of rectum and sigmoid shows submucosal nodules, associated with irregularity of the contour, narrowing, and rigidity. The submucosal nodules probably represent tiny ulcerations with surrounding edema. The thickening of the submucosa also plays a role in the genesis of these nodules.

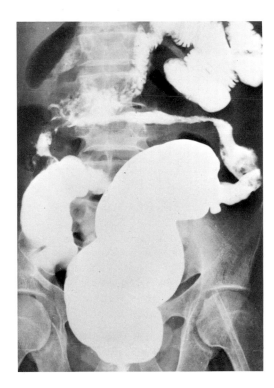

Fig. 37-63. Granulomatous colitis. There is a fistulous communication between a narrowed transverse colon and the duodenum. Fistulas are a feature of granulomatous colitis rather than ulcerative colitis.

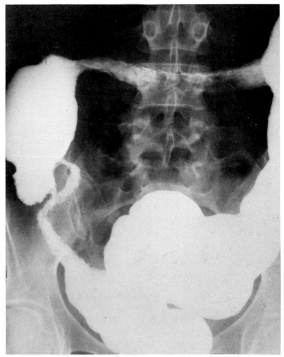

Fig. 37-64. Granulomatous ileocolitis. There is simultaneous and similar involvement of the ileum and the right side of the colon, characterized by narrowing and rigidity of the ileum and transverse colon. The ascending colon is fairly distensible. The left side of the colon is normal.

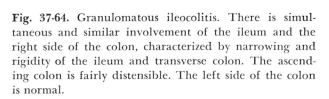

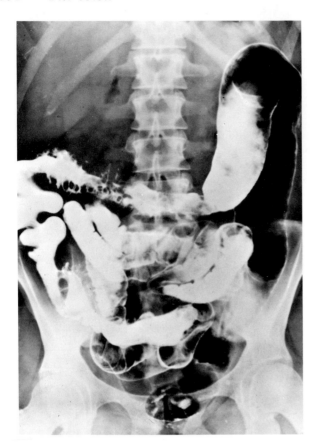

Fig. 37-65. Granulomatous ileocolitis. The ileum and the right side of the colon are involved. Transverse ulcerations and inflammatory polyps are seen in the right side of the transverse colon. A small fistulous communication from the ileum to the cecum is noted. The left side of the colon is normal.

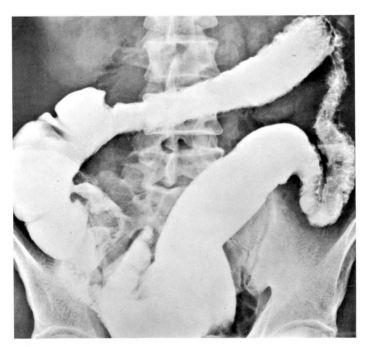

Fig. 37-66. Granulomatous ileocolitis. The findings are severe in the descending colon, where there is narrowing, rigidity, and marked ulceration. The inflammatory process is segmental. The unevenness of involvement is characteristic of granulomatous disease.

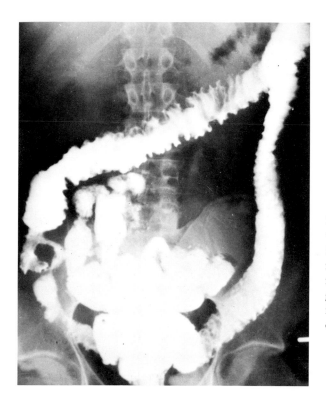

Fig. 37-67. Granulomatous ileocolitis. The ileum is involved with typical regional enteritis. The entire colon is involved with an inflammatory process. The vertical, rigid folds in the transverse colon, associated with irregularity of the contour, are more characteristic of granulomatous disease. The involvement of the terminal ileum with regional enteritis also indicates that the disease in the colon is granulomatous.

Fig. 37-68. Granulomatous ileocolitis. There is narrowing, rigidity, and irregularity of the contour of the terminal ileum and the colon. The findings are more marked on the right side of the colon.

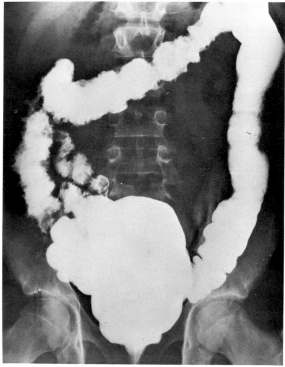

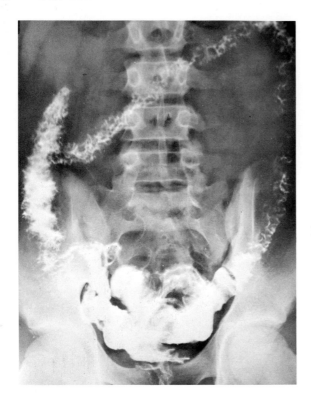

Fig. 37-69. Evacuation film. Same patient as in Fig. 37-68. The mucosa is thickened, hazy, and irregular, with numerous small nodules. The nodular appearance is in contrast to the thickened symmetric mucosal folds seen in ulcerative colitis. The extent of involvement in this case is better determined on the evacuation film.

Fig. 37-70. Regional enteritis with extension into the colon. The terminal ileum is involved with the characteristic findings of regional enteritis. The colon appears normal.

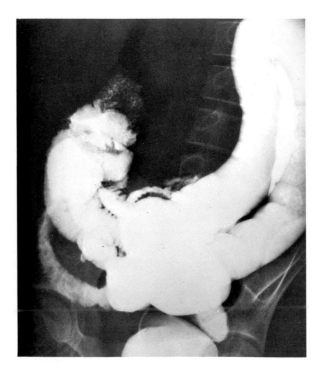

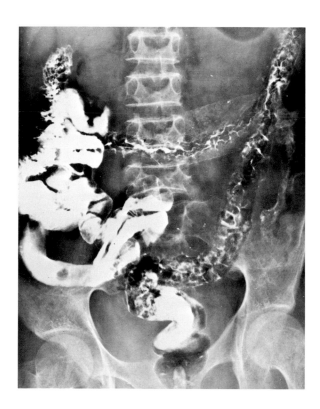

Fig. 37-71. Evacuation film of the patient in Fig. 37-70, taken 1 year later. There is marked involvement of the entire colon, with a sinus tract extending lateral to the descending colon. The mucosa has a cobblestone appearance, with numerous transverse and longitudinal ulcerations. This type of extension is uncommon in granulomatous disease.

Fig. 37-72. Granulomatous ileocolitis. The inflammatory process involves primarily the right side of the colon. There is a skip lesion in the terminal ileum. In the absence of the characteristic findings of regional enteritis, a definite diagnosis of granulomatous disease in the colon would be difficult.

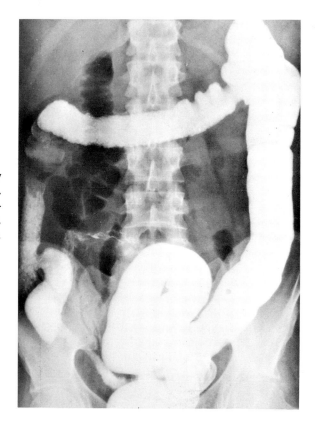

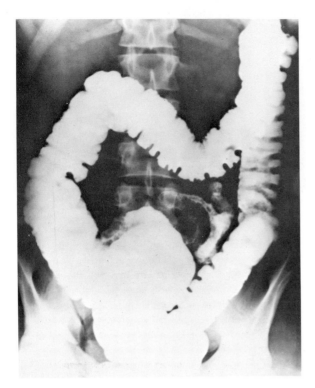

Fig. 37-73. Granulomatous ileocolitis. The roentgenographic findings in the ileum are caused by regional enteritis. In the colon the findings are minimal and characterized by slight flattening of the contours and minimal distortion of the haustral markings. The findings in the terminal ileum indicate that the subtle findings in the colon are caused by granulomatous colitis.

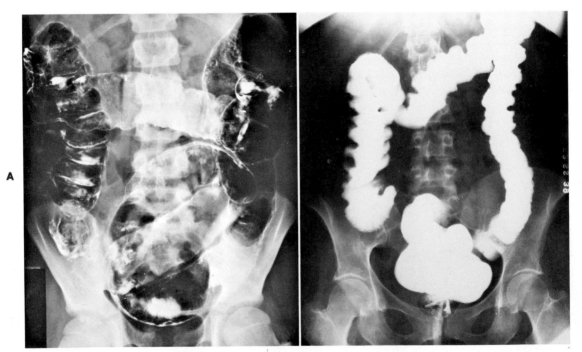

Fig. 37-74. A, Granulomatous colitis. The colon, except for the rectum, is diffusely involved. A moderate degree of spasm was noted during fluoroscopy, and the haustral markings are absent or irregular. Of particular interest are the tiny ulcerations associated with nodular defects that are seen along the contour of the bowel. B, Granulomatous colitis involving the transverse colon. There is minimal involvement of the inferior aspect of the transverse colon, characterized by irregularity and nodular filling defects. The findings are partially obscured by the over-filling of the colon with air. These minimal findings are frequently better identified on a motility film or evacuation film.

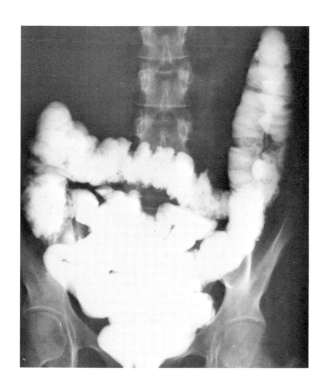

Fig. 37-75. Granulomatous colitis. There is minimal involvement of the right side of the colon, with irregularity of the contours and small nodular defects. The findings are more marked in the distal transverse colon. There is some rigidity and lack of distensibility.

Fig. 37-76. Evacuation film. Same case as in Fig. 37-75. The mucosal pattern has an irregular cobblestone appearance. Several small skip lesions, indicated by the pseudodiverticula, are identified.

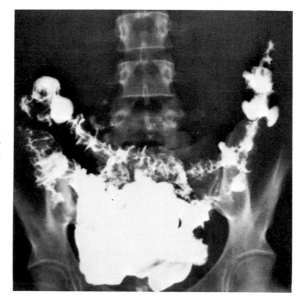

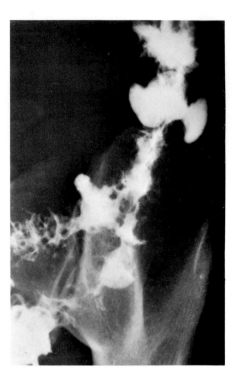

Fig. 37-77. Spot film of the patient in Fig. 37-76. The nodular, cobblestone, ropelike configuration of the mucosal pattern is again seen associated with multiple small pseudodiverticula.

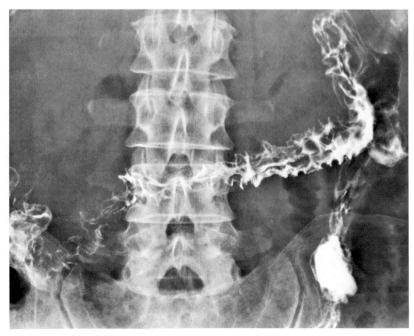

Fig. 37-78. Evacuation film in granulomatous colitis. The nodular cobblestone configuration typical of granulomatous colitis is seen.

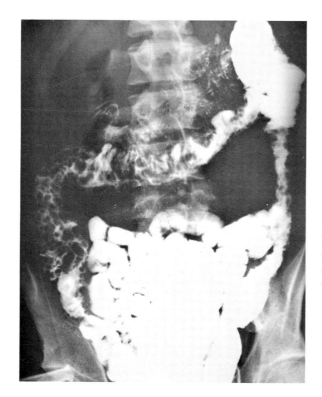

Fig. 37-79. Granulomatous ileocolitis. There is marked cobblestoning, produced by the longitudinal and transverse ulcerations, with narrowing and rigidity of the colon. The rectum is normal. The involvement of the ileum was seen simultaneously to the involvement of the colon. This has been true in most of our cases.

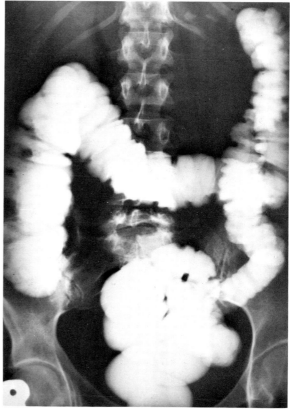

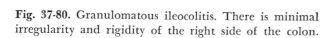

Fig. 37-80. Granulomatous ileocolitis. There is minimal irregularity and rigidity of the right side of the colon.

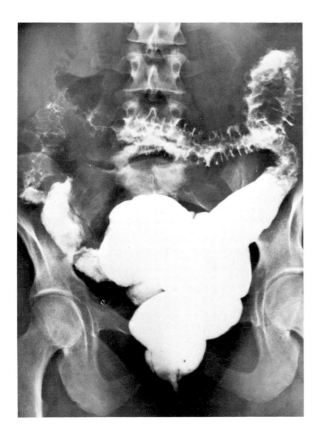

Fig. 37-81. Same case as in Fig. 37-80, 6 months later. There are marked longitudinal and transverse ulcerations involving the right side of the colon and the proximal descending colon. The terminal ileum is also involved. The rectum, sigmoid, and lower descending colon are normal.

Fig. 37-82. Same case as in Figs. 37-80 and 37-81, 1 year after the first film. There is more extensive involvement, with a fistulous communication between the splenic flexure and the colon. The distal transverse colon is markedly ulcerated, with gross irregularity and distortion of the contour. Distinct involvement may occur in a relatively short period of time.

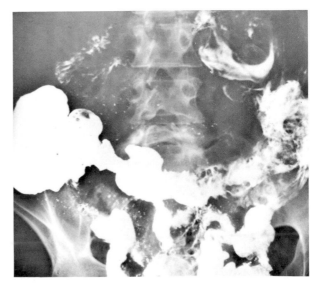

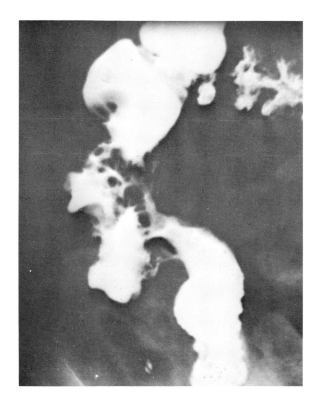

Fig. 37-83. Granulomatous ileocolitis. There are characteristic intramural sinus tracts and fistulas extending from the terminal ileum to the right side of the colon. These tracts are typical of granulomatous disease.

84). These abscesses at times are large, producing a marked irregularity of the contour of the bowel. When they penetrate into the adjacent loops, fistulas are formed (Fig. 37-82). Intestinal fistulas are less frequent in granulomatous disease of the colon, however, than in regional enteritis. In late stages of granulomatous disease, the entire mucosa may be sloughed off because of the diffuse ulceration. In those cases in which the bowel is diffusely and symmetrically involved and there are no typical features of granulomatous disease, differentiation from ulcerative colitis may be impossible, especially in the absence of characteristic features in the small intestine (Figs. 37-85 to 37-87).

Since extensive thickening of the bowel secondary to intramural fibrotic changes is common in granulomatous colitis, irregular stenotic segments and strictures are frequently seen (Figs. 37-88 to 37-93). Occasionally granulomatous colitis is present as a single stricture of the colon (Fig. 37-94). When this stricture is eccentric and associated with overhanging edges, differentiation from a carcinoma may be impossible. In most cases, however, there is additional evidence of involvement of the bowel in the form of skip lesions, further strictures, or other identifying features of granulomatous disease.

Granulomatous colitis can also resemble burnt-out ulcerative colitis, except for its more frequent segmental distribution, usually right sided. There is minimal narrowing or rigidity, associated with absent haustral markings and effacement of the mucosa. These cases probably represent minimal degrees of involvement with little scarring (Fig. 37-95). They present themselves at a time when none of the typical roentgenographic features of granulomatous colitis is present.

Because the chronic inflammation is transmural and tends to thicken the wall, the colon involved with granulomatous colitis would appear to be an unlikely candidate for the development of severe dilatation and threatened perforation. In the more active and early forms of the disease, however, before fibrosis has become a conspicuous feature, moderate degrees of dilatation have been observed.[12] These cases

Text continued on p. 1009.

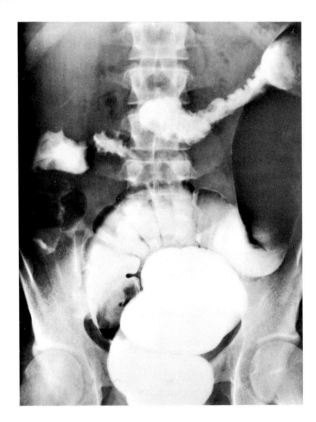

Fig. 37-84. Granulomatous colitis. There is marked segmental involvement of the colon, with a large irregular ulceration in the midtransverse colon.

Fig. 37-85. Granulomatous ileocolitis. The roentgenographic appearance of the colon in this case may be seen in either granulomatous or ulcerative colitis. The superficial longitudinal ulceration without deformity and scarring shown in this case is not a differential feature. This can be identified in both ulcerative and granulomatous colitis. However, the involvement of the terminal ileum with typical regional enteritis enables the radiologist to make a diagnosis of granulomatous ileocolitis.

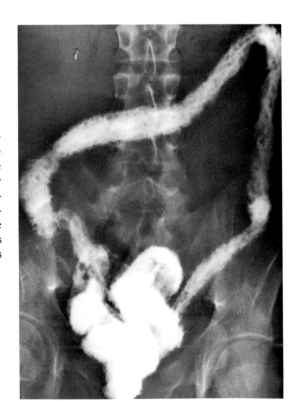

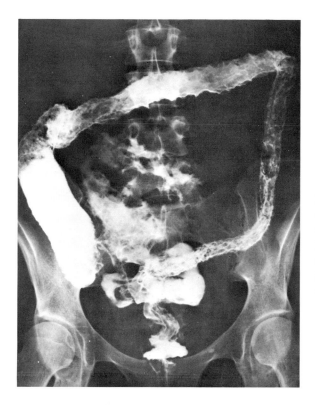

Fig. 37-86. Granulomatous ileocolitis. There is diffuse ulceration of the entire colon. This type of diffuse involvement can be seen in both ulcerative and granulomatous colitis. In this case there is a perforation from the terminal ileum with a large fistulous communication. This finding is associated with granulomatous disease rather than ulcerative colitis.

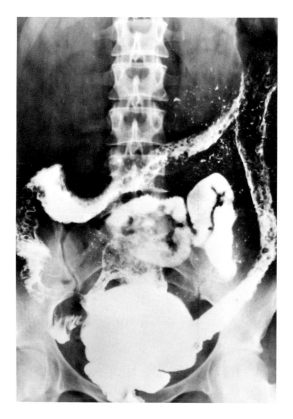

Fig. 37-87. Granulomatous ileocolitis. The findings in the colon could be those of ulcerative or granulomatous colitis. The findings in the ileum, with fistula formation, marked narrowing, and rigidity are those of regional enteritis, and therefore the process is granulomatous ileocolitis.

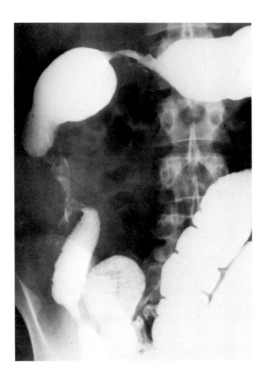

Fig. 37-88. Granulomatous ileocolitis. Multiple smooth strictures in granulomatous ileocolitis. To the present time these strictures have not been associated with a carcinoma.

Fig. 37-89. Granulomatous colitis. There are multiple strictures characteristic of granulomatous colitis.

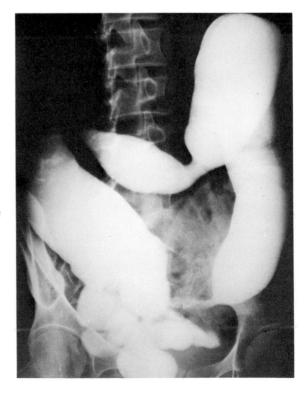

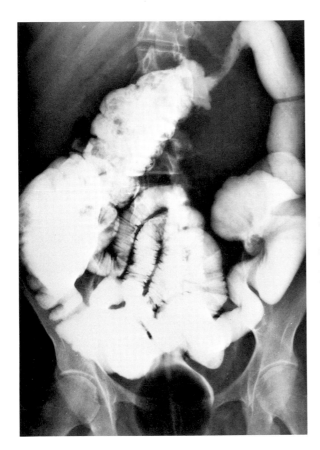

Fig. 37-90. Granulomatous colitis. The distal half of the transverse colon is considerably narrowed. A skip lesion is seen in the middescending colon, characterized by pseudodiverticula formation, pleating of the bowel, and distinct irregularity. In the absence of multiple strictures, differentiation of a single stricture from a carcinoma may be difficult.

Fig. 37-91. Granulomatous colitis. There are two areas of narrowing in the colon, secondary to granulomatous disease. In the absence of multiple areas of involvement, a single lesion can easily mimic a carcinoma.

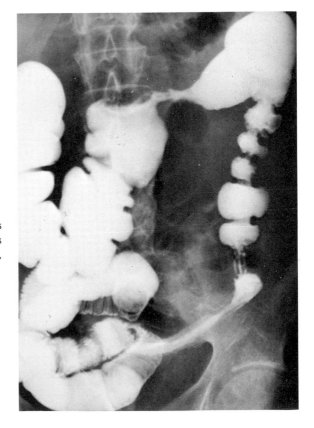

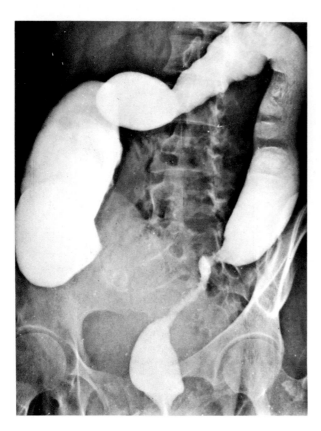

Fig. 37-92. Granulomatous colitis. There is involvement of the entire colon with an inflammatory process and a stricture in the sigmoid. Differentiation of this case from a carcinoma in ulcerative colitis in difficult. (See also Fig. 37-93.)

Fig. 37-93. Postevacuation roentgenograph of the same case as in Fig. 37-92 reveals involvement of the terminal ileum with granulomatous disease, indicating that the stricture is probably benign.

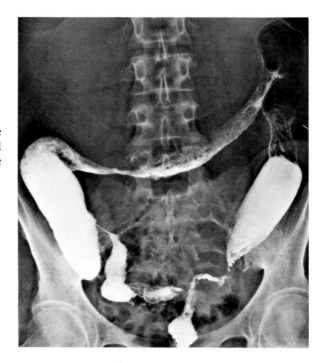

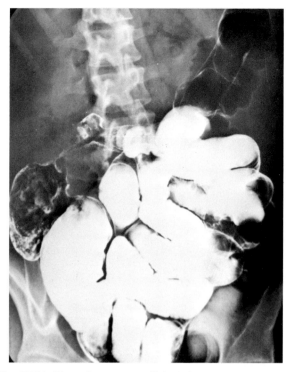

Fig. 37-94. Granulomatous colitis. There is a single stricture involving the right side of the colon. Differentiation of this lesion from a carcinoma is impossible.

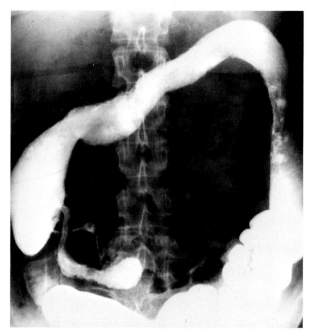

Fig. 37-95. Granulomatous ileocolitis. The findings in the colon mimic burnt-out ulcerative colitis. The presence of a fistula in the terminal ileum is characteristic of regional enteritis. The findings in the colon therefore are caused by granulomatous colitis.

are frequently associated with deep abscesses and sinus tracts, and the findings have usually been confined to the transverse colon. The markedly distended colon observed in toxic dilatation of ulcerative colitis has not been seen in our patients, although it has been reported by others.[9,20]

It is well known that recurrence of granulomatous disease in colon or small bowel may develop after surgery. Linear extension of disease in the absence of surgery, however, is uncommon in our experience, although it does occur. Normal areas between skip lesions may become diseased, and a minimally involved colon with multiple skin lesions may become severely and diffusely ulcerated in a short time.

Marked reversibility may be observed in serial examinations of patients with granulomatous disease.[13] Usually this change has followed a course of therapy with steroids in a patient with active and acute disease. The profound submucosal edema may disappear, producing an ap-

pearance indistinguishable from that of a normal colon. Unlike ulcerative colitis, in which occasionally even the chronic changes of a shortened colon may return to normal, resolution in the more chronic cases of granulomatous colitis has not been observed.

INFLAMMATORY DISEASE OF THE STOMA

Since ileostomy and colectomy are performed for both ulcerative and granulomatous colitis, the appearance of postoperative inflammatory disease in the ileum proximal to the stoma is of importance. Such "prestomal ileitis" is of two varieties. One is related to obstruction of the stoma, a mechanical problem associated with narrowing or retraction of the ileostomy. This abnormality is termed "ileostomy dysfunction." The other type of prestomal ileitis is extension of granulomatous disease. Ileostomy dysfunction may be seen after surgery for both ulcerative and granulomatous colitis. Development of the

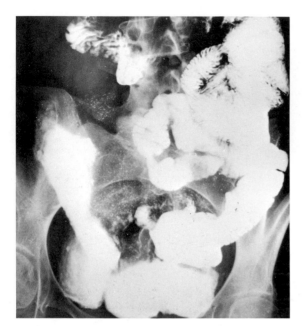

Fig. 37-96. Ileostomy dysfunction. The ileum proximal to the stoma is slightly dilated, with increased secretions and slight irregularity of the contour. There is no evidence of narrowing or rigidity. The findings here are caused by obstruction at the stoma.

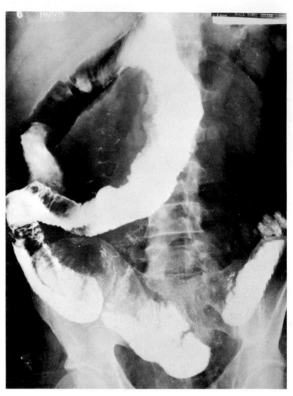

Fig. 37-97. Ileostomy dysfunction. The slight dilatation of the ileum is associated with increased secretions and irregularity of the contour. The findings are secondary to ileostomy dysfunction.

granulomatous process in the region of the stoma is seen only if surgery was performed for granulomatous disease. In our own series of cases, prestomal granulomatous ileitis has been seen with increasing frequency in patients with preoperative disease in both ileum and colon. We have seen this complication much less commonly in those patients in whom the preoperative disease was confined to the colon.

In ileostomy dysfunction the ileum is dilated and there are abundant secretions. The folds are slightly thickened and ulcerations are minimal. (Figs. 37-96 and 37-97). When prestomal granulomatous ileitis develops, however, the roentgenographic findings are identical to those of regional enteritis (Fig. 37-98).

GRANULOMATOUS COLITIS AND DIVERTICULITIS

Diverticulitis may be confused with granulomatous colitis, especially when granulomatous disease is confined to the sigmoid. Granulomatous colitis is not uncommon in middle-aged and elderly patients, an age group in which diverti-

culosis and diverticulitis are also often found. On occasion the two diseases may coexist.

In granulomatous colitis the involved segment tends to be long—usually 10 cm. or longer—whereas in diverticulitis the segment is usually short, perhaps 3 to 6 cm. in length. The abscesses of granulomatous colitis often have a triangular shape, but at times they may be difficult to distinguish from coexistent diverticula. In the ulcerating mucosa of granulomatous colitis the folds are straightened, perpendicular, and associated with a thick wall and intraluminal secretions; in a perforated diverticulum the abscess usually creates an extramural defect or an arcuate configuration of the folds that stretch over the abscess. The transverse fissures and marked mucosal edema of granulomatous colitis produce a stepladder configuration; in diverticulitis there are no transverse fissures and the folds tend to be arcuate rather than straightened.

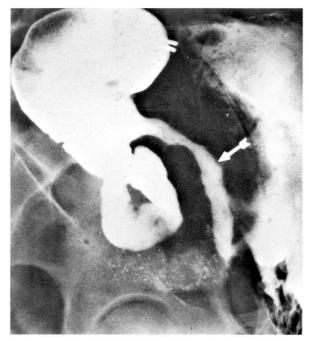

Fig. 37-98. Granulomatous ileitis after ileostomy for granulomatous ileocolitis. The ileum adjacent to the ileostomy is narrowed and rigid. The findings here are in contrast to the findings seen in ileostomy dysfunction and are caused by extension of the granulomatous process after surgery.

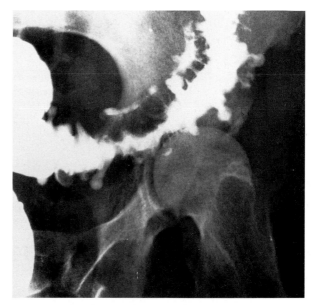

Fig. 37-99. Granulomatous colitis. The sigmoid is involved, with an inflammatory process characterized by narrowing of the lumen, rigidity, and thickening of the folds. There is a long intramural fistulous tract on the medial aspect of the sigmoid associated with multiple transverse fissures and abscesses. An occasional diverticulum is seen at the distal margin of the sigmoid.

A characteristic sign of granulomatous colitis is the presence of a long fistulous tract in the submucosa or the muscular layers, parallel to the lumen of the bowel (Figs. 37-99 and 37-100). This tract, which has been noted for many years in patients with inflammatory disease of the colon, has previously been attributed to diverticulitis with multiple perforations of diverticula and development of tracking in the bowel wall. Such multiple simultaneous perforations of diverticula seem unlikely occurrences, however, and pathologic examination of resected specimens containing the long fistulous tract have revealed the typical lesions of granulomatous colitis.[23]

Differential diagnosis
Amebiasis

Especially when it produces skip lesions, amebiasis may resemble the roentgenographic findings of granulomatous colitis. When the lesion is diffuse, however, it more frequently suggests the changes of ulcerative colitis. The alterations are uniform and symmetrical, and involvement of the rectum is common. Usually, however, amebiasis is a low-grade, chronic process with the changes confined to the cecum. Any inflammatory process of the cecum may produce narrowing, so the cone-shaped configuration so commonly associated with amebiasis is merely an indication of inflammation. The differential diagnosis includes other localized lesions such as appendiceal abscess.

Ischemic colitis

Ischemic colitis is easily differentiated from granulomatous colitis by the characteristic acute episode of abdominal pain and bleeding and by the rapid progression of roentgenographic findings from a stage of inflammatory edema, which may mimic both ulcerative and granulomatous colitis, to resolution or to stenosis. The

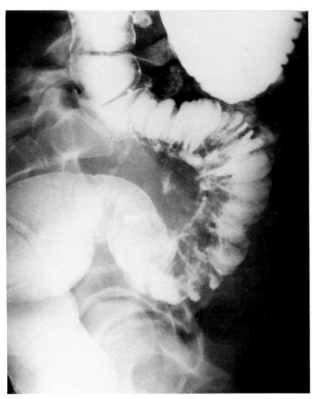

Fig. 37-100. Granulomatous colitis. A long intramural fistulous tract with multiple transverse fissures is seen.

sequence of events rarely requires more than 1 to 6 weeks. If the patient is examined roentgenologically at any particular phase of this process, the roentgenographic appearance may suggest inflammatory disease. Pseudosacculations are not uncommon residuals of ischemia. Histologic findings at biopsy or necropsy may suggest either ulcerative or granulomatous colitis.[19]

Scirrhous carcinoma of the colon

Long segments of colon, usually sigmoid, may be involved with carcinoma in a linitis plastica or scirrhous presentation. The differential diagnosis from a single segment of granulomatous colitis may be difficult. In carcinoma, however, nodularity is prominent and the inflammatory mucosal alterations of granulomatous colitis are usually not seen.

Tuberculosis

It is impossible to differentiate tuberculosis from granulomatous ileocolitis. In those in-stances in which the inflammatory process is confined to the distal ileum and proximal colon, tuberculosis must be considered. Cases of intestinal tuberculosis are sometimes associated with a normal roentgenogram of the chest.

REFERENCES

1. Colp, R.: A case of nonspecific granuloma of the terminal ileum and cecum, Surg. Clin. N. Amer. 14:443, 1934.
2. Crohn, B. B., Ginzburg, L., and Oppenheimer, G. D.: Regional ileitis; a pathological and clinical entity, J.A.M.A. 99:1323, 1932.
3. Crohn, B. B., and Yarnis, H.: Regional ileitis, ed. 2, New York, 1958, Grune & Stratton, Inc.
4. Dalziel, T. K.: Chronic interstitial enteritis, Brit. Med. J. 2:1068, 1913.
5. Ginzberg, L., Marshak, R. H., and Eliasoph, J.: Regional jejunitis, Surg. Gynec. Obstet. 111:1, 1960.
6. Goulston, S. J. M., and McGovern, V. J.: The nature of benign strictures in ulcerative colitis, New Eng. J. Med. 281:290, 1969.
7. Gray, B. K., Lockhart-Mummery, H. E., and Morson, B. C.: Crohn's disease of the anal region, Gut 6:515, 1965.
8. Harris, F. I., Bell, G. H., and Brunn, G.: Chronic cicatrizing enteritis; regional ileitis (Crohn), Surg. Gynec. Obstet. 57:637, 1933.
9. Hawk, W. A., and Turnbull, R. B., Jr.: Primary ulcerative disease of the colon, Gastroenterology 51:802, 1966.
10. Heilbrun, N.: Roentgen evidence suggesting enterocolitis associated with prolonged cathartic abuse, Radiology 41:486, 1943.
11. Janowitz, H. D., Lindner, A. E., and Marshak, R. H.: Granulomatous colitis, J.A.M.A. 191:825, 1965.
12. Javett, S. L., and Brooke, B. N.: Acute dilatation of the colon in Crohn's disease, Lancet 2:126, 1970.
13. Jones, J. H., Lennard-Jones, J. E., and Young, A. C.: Reversibility of radiological appearance during clinical improvement in colonic Crohn's disease, Gut 10:738, 1969.
14. Jones-Williams, W.: Histology of Crohn's syndrome, Gut 5:510, 1964.
15. Kolodny, M.: Reversible right colonic strictures in chronic ulcerative colitis, Radiology 97:83, 1970.
16. Lindner, A. E., Marshak, R. H., Wolf, B. S., and Janowitz, H. D.: Granulomatous colitis; a clinical study, New Eng. J. Med. 269:379, 1963.
17. Lockhart-Mummery, H. E., and Morson, B. C.: Crohn's disease (regional enteritis) of the large intestine and its distinction from ulcerative colitis, Gut 1:87, 1960.
18. Lockhart-Mummery, H. E., and Morson, B. C.: Crohn's disease of the large intestine, Gut 5:493, 1964.
19. Margulis, A. R.: Radiology of ulcerative colitis, Radiology 105:251, 1972.
20. Margulis, A. R., Goldberg, H. I., Lawson, T. L., Montgomery, C. K., Rambo, O. N., Noonan, C. D., and Amberg, J. R.: The overlapping spectrum of

ulcerative and granulomatous colitis; a roentgeno-graphic-pathologic study, Amer. J. Roentgen. 113: 325, 1971.

21. Marshak, R. H., Bloch, C., and Wolf, B. S.: The roentgen findings in strictures of the colon associated with ulcerative and granulomatous colitis, Amer. J. Roentgen. **90**:709, 1963.

22. Marshak, R. H., and Gerson, A.: Cathartic colon, Amer. J. Dig. Dis. **5**:724, 1960.

23. Marshak, R. H., Janowitz, H. D., and Present, D. H.: Granulomatous colitis in association with diverticula, New Eng. J. Med. **283**:1080, 1970.

24. Marshak, R. H., Korelitz, B. I., Klein, S. H., Wolf, B. S., and Janowitz, H. D.: Toxic dilatation of the colon in the course of ulcerative colitis, Gastro-enterology **38**:165, 1960.

25. Marshak, R. H., Moseley, J. E., and Wolf, B. S.: The roentgen findings in familial polyposis with special emphasis on differential diagnosis, Radiology **80**:374, 1963.

26. Marshak, R. H., and Wolf, B. S.: Chronic ulcera-tive granulomatous jejunitis and ileojejunitis, Amer. J. Roentgen. **70**:93, 1953.

27. Marshak, R. H., and Wolf, B. S.: Roentgen findings in regional enteritis, Amer. J. Roentgen. **74**: 1000, 1955.

28. Moseley, J. E., Marshak, R. H., and Wolf, B. S.: Regional enteritis in children, Amer. J. Roentgen. **84**:532, 1960.

29. Present, D. H., Lindner, A. E., and Janowitz, H. D.: Granulomatous disease of the gastrointestinal tract, Ann. Rev. Med. **17**:243, 1966.

30. Slaney, G.: Hypersensitivity granulomata and the alimentary tract, Ann. Roy. Coll. Surg. Eng. **31**: 249, 1962.

31. Van Patter, W. N., Bargen, J. A., Dockerty, M. B., Feldman, W. H., Mayo, C. W., and Waugh, J. M.: Regional enteritis, Gastroenterology **26**:347, 1954.

32. Wolf, B. S., and Marshak, R. H.: Granulomatous colitis (Crohn's disease of the colon); roentgen features, Amer. J. Roentgen. **88**:662, 1962.

38 | Diverticular disease of the colon

Ifor Williams
†**Felix G. Fleischner**

The late Felix Fleischner was one of several workers in a variety of disciplines who, during the early 1960s, took a new look at diverticular disease of the colon. As he had done on previous occasions, he approached the roentgenologic problem from a personal study of pathologic specimens to produce a new synthesis that invited his colleagues to think again.

Despite the 1970 publication of a textbook on smooth muscle[6] as well as a description of electrical activity of both the colon[11] and Auerbach's plexus,[60] fundamental knowledge of the organization of contraction in the colon is rudimentary and we are still forced to use such terms as "spasm" and "contracture." In 1910

Keith, a curator of a pathology museum, gave a demonstration, using a handful of specimens of diverticular disease, which was so comprehensive that little of real importance has been added to the present day.[25]

Although diverticula of the colon had been known to pathologists for a long time before 1898, Graser observed that diverticula were found at the center of inflammatory masses adjacent to the sigmoid; diverticula of the colon had previously been mistaken for neoplasms.[22] Brewer, Mayo, and Moynihan confirmed his findings.[5,34,39] The introduction of the barium enema and the observation of symptomless diverticula of the left colon by DeQuervain,[12] Case,[9] Carman,[7] and Spriggs and Marxer[47a] led to the concept of diverticulosis. Since then the distinction between diverticulosis and diverticulitis has been emphasized. A few investigators had observed the thick wall of the involved segment and had postulated spasm or hypertrophy of muscle as an important feature. In 1963 and 1964 radiologists,[17,56] pathologists,[37] and surgeons,[1,42] measuring intraluminal pressures, together produced new evidence of a muscular dysfunction that is now believed to be a feature of the disease of more fundamental importance than either diverticula or inflammation. It is the explanation of the roentgenographic deformities in terms of the muscular dysfunction that is of interest to the radiologist.

ETIOLOGY

The incidence of this disease, as measured by the presence of diverticula discovered in persons who are given barium enema, is high. Carroll,[8] Welch,[52] and McCune and associates[33] have conservatively estimated that of sixty million persons in the United States who are over 40 years of age, about six million will develop diverticulosis. Of those with diverticulosis about 20% will suffer from diverticulitis, requiring proper diagnosis and treatment. The figures from the Mayo Clinic for diverticulosis are

---

†Deceased.

8.5% of 47,000 enemas.[44] More recent series give a higher figure—one third of all enemas at the Massachusetts General Hospital,[53] for example. Hughes, in a prospective study of hospital autopsies in Australia, states that 48% of patients over the age of 50 have some diverticula.[24] There are no reliable accounts of a congenital form; indeed, below the age of 35 the disease is uncommon and below 30 it is rare. This is the standard teaching, but Evans and Dawson have documented nine cases of operatively proved diverticulitis in persons under the age of 40.[15] It is conceivable that the disease is becoming more frequent and appearing at an earlier age. Roughly equal numbers of males and females appear in the series, and there is no striking difference in incidence between the sexes.

These figures are compiled from industrially advanced nations and are in complete and striking contrast to those from rural countries and the Far East. Reports from Korea,[26] Japan,[26] Iran[50] and the Near East,[28] parts of Africa,[3] and South America[26] emphasize the rarity, even total absence, of diverticula in these populations. Other considerations of incidence are racial factors and food and eating habits. Painter has summarized the worldwide distribution and historical appearance, linking it to lack of roughage in the diet. In England, he argues, the great increase in diverticula followed the introduction of white bread made from refined flour to replace the previous coarse brown flour.

According to Hughes,[24] there is no correlation with obesity, hypertension, or gallstones, although no one has yet established statistically satisfactory criteria for the existence of Saint's triad. Gallstones, hiatus hernia, and diverticular disease are all common diseases of maturity and old age; and for two at least, diagnostic criteria for their presence are open to wide observer variation.

A curious and interesting association is the occurrence of diverticulitis in young people under the age of 20 who suffer from Marfan's disease, in which connective tissue is known to be at fault.[35]

METHOD OF EXAMINATION

It is valuable to inspect the plain abdominal film carefully, not so much for diverticulosis as for diverticulitis. A poorly contoured mass sur-

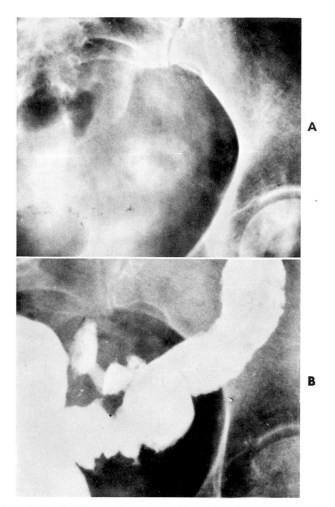

Fig. 38-1. A, Plain abdominal film. An irregular gas shadow is visible in the pelvis, on the left, surrounded by an ill-defined soft tissue mass. **B,** By barium enema a communicating pelvic abscess from a perforated diverticulum is found to have caused the gas shadow.

rounded by gas-filled bowel loops or obscuring of the standard fat lines suggests a localized inflammatory process. An irregularly shaped gas deposit in an unaccustomed place, although it does not permit a definite diagnosis of a paracolic abscess secondary to a ruptured diverticulum, would support a clinical suspicion, encourage further investigation, and determine the line of such an investigation (Fig. 38-1).

Solitary diverticula and diverticulosis are usually incidental findings not particularly looked for. They are best found in the routine examination by barium enema in which proper positioning, compression films, and postevacuation roentgenograms have been used in order to display every colonic part free from superimposition. Standard preparation will help to remove retained fecal matter from most diverticula.

Suspected or established diverticulitis deserves a special note. Diverticulitis as presently understood is not an inflammation in a diverticulum but rather a rupture of a diverticulum with intramural or localized pericolic abscesses, rarely with direct peritoneal communication. Because every added straining may contribute to spread of the inflammation, the examination should be performed with proper care. The preparation should be limited to a carefully applied water enema, and the barium enema itself should be performed without undue pressure, forceful distention of the colon, or undue compression of the tender area in the patient's left lower quadrant. If extravasation of barium is observed the examination should be discontinued. It is not advisable to force more barium through the perforation in order to see how far the extravasate will go. This information might be provided on later films after spontaneous spreading of the barium. Although it is undesirable, extravasation is not usually considered to be a catastrophe. Extravasation occurs usually through a preexisting rupture into a preformed paracolic abscess or fistulous tract identified as such by this same examination. In the rare case of a frank extravasation into the peritoneal cavity one should keep in mind that, in addition to the fecal peritonitis, barium sulfate in the peritoneal cavity is apt to cause extensive adhesions. For this reason barium should not be used whenever a frank perforation originating from the colon is known to exist or is seriously suspected. In this case any one of the tri-iodinated water-soluble contrast media should be used instead of barium sulfate.

Spasm is a major factor in diverticulitis. Films of the sigmoid colon taken during the early filling stages may show gross narrowing and irregularity, only to disappear at further filling or after the administration of smooth-muscle relaxants.

THE DIVERTICULA

Colonic diverticula of the common type are acquired herniations of mucosa and muscularis mucosae through the muscularis propria. Some at least are reducible hernias, and most radiologists have seen sacs in the early filling stage that completely vanish at full distention. Sacs seen easily during one enema may never appear during a subsequent one, a feature that makes assessment of the natural history of the disease very uncertain. In size they vary from tiny V-shaped protrusions to the rare giant ones several centimeters across; commonly they are from 3 to 10 mm. in diameter in the distended state.

The circular muscle of the colon is fasciculated[40] and is arranged in small packets very roughly comparable to washers around a bolt. It is between the fasciculi that the mucosa extrudes with no apparent damage to the muscle, which is pushed aside and thrown up into small hillocks on each edge of the opening (Fig. 38-2). Between the taeniae is a thin but quite definite layer of longitudinal muscle, and fibers from this are sometimes carried over the top of the smaller sacs. The details of this and the radiologic counterpart are shown in Fig. 38-2. The neck of the sac where it crosses the wall is quite short, but the distortion of the lumen in the saw-tooth sign may give the false appearance of a long neck.

Diverticula are found in all regions of the large bowel with the exception of the rectum, although rarely a single one may be visible just distal to the rectosigmoid junction. By far the most common site is the left side of the colon and especialy the sigmoid, but patients may have only scattered ones in the transverse or ascending portions. It is common practice to describe a group with sacs limited to the cecal area, but this is clinical convenience and there is little evidence of a real difference.[24] The cecum is the site of saccular outpouching, which may retain barium, of the whole muscle wall, but this type bears no relationship to diverticula.[24]

In the sigmoid, which has been better studied, the sacs arise from the side walls of the intestine in four rows,[47] one on each side of the mesenteric taenia and one on the mesenteric side of each antimesenteric taenia. They never penetrate the taeniae themselves, but in the short antimesenteric zone emerge very much smaller sacs or pinpoint protrusions (Fig. 38-3, *B*). The classical account has always stated that the sites of protrusion are determined by the points of weakness in the walls at the entry of blood ves-

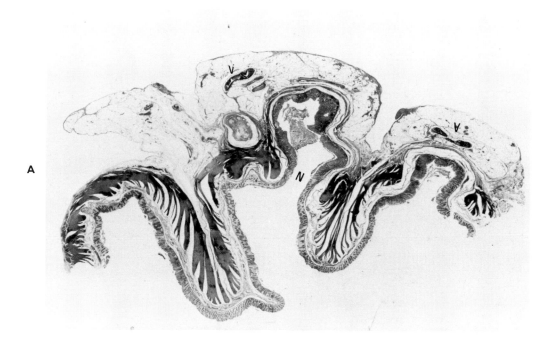

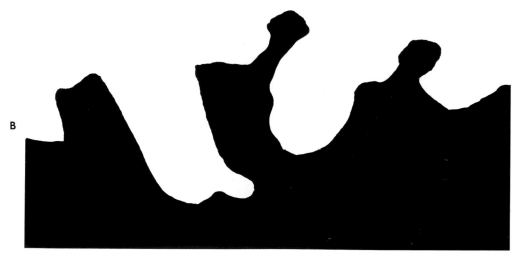

Fig. 38-2. A, A longitudinal section of the colon wall through two folds of diverticular disease. Note that the folds are composed of an infolding of the whole wall, the circular muscle is fasciculated, two diverticula open in this section, and the circular muscle at the neck, **N,** is pushed aside and heaped up. The vessels, **V,** are in close relationship to the apex of the sacs. The fine layer over the apex of the sacs is in this case a mixture of fibrous tissue and longitudinal muscle. **B,** The roentgenologic counterpart, one side of a saw-tooth sign. (From Williams, I.: Brit. J. Radiol. **38:**440, 1965.)

sels. Many workers have injected the blood vessels of the colon and have shown a close relationship of the arteries to the sacs, but none of the techniques were good enough to prove that the artery went through the wall at exactly the same point as the mucosal herniation emerged. The literature has many diagrams but no histologic section of such an exact relationship. Against this view has been the experience of several workers who at dissection of the colon could not find an artery of any size in the right place. This argument, which has been going on for many years, has been largely solved by the work of Tagliacozzo and Virno, who reviewed the literature and with their own studies indicated that both sets of observations are correct.[48,49] The arteries (Fig. 38-6) arise from the mesenteric arcade as (1) short vessels that penetrate the mesenteric taenia or nearby lateral wall, or (2) the long straight arteries that course around the lateral walls, dividing into two or three branches, and then immediately penetrate the muscle wall just on the mesenteric side of the antimesenteric taenia. As they reach the submucosa they divide and rapidly form a submucosal plexus.

Tagliacozzo and Virno's view is summarized diagrammatically in Fig. 38-4. Increase in pressure in the lumen also raises the pressure in the submucosal layer and forces out the artery with its related loose connective tissue. At this stage the mucosa is still within the lumen and quite smooth. As the extrusion increases, the connective tissue attachments drag the mucosa into the gap and the stage is set for direct pressure from the lumen onto the narow opening in the muscle. As more and more mucosa herniates outward the artery is pushed away from the wall and comes to lie over the apex of the sac. At the neck of the sac only small, and thus hard to see, branches remain. I (I.W.) have observed the stage of vascular herniation only, with a smooth intact lumen below, on four occasions to occur on distention of the lumen; this has been illustrated histologically by Arfwidssen as well.[1] Fig. 38-5 shows the histology of this stage. Inflammation spreading to a sizable artery at the apex of the sac is responsible for the massive hemorrhage that sometimes occurs in diverticulitis.

Unfortunately, this simple story cannot explain everything. Some sacs appear in the mid-

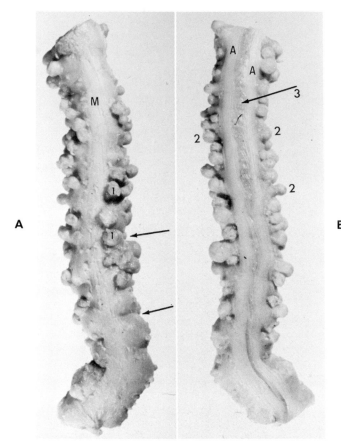

Fig. 38-3. A fixed, distended specimen of diverticulosis of the sigmoid with the fat dissected away. **A,** View from the mesenteric aspect with a single taenia, **M,** visible. **B,** The antimesenteric view, with two taeniae, **A,** close together. **C** and **D,** The views of each side. Note that the infoldings are on the longer lateral walls (arrows). The antimesenteric zone is short and has the tiny antimesenteric sacs, **B3,** and seen in profile in **C3.** The lateral diverticula are in two rows, near the mesenteric taenia, **1,** and near the antimesenteric taenia, **2.** Additional ones seen in **C** and **D** lie outside these rows on the convexity of the haustra.

dle of the haustrum where, as in the antimesenteric zone, there are no penetrating vessels. A second mechanism has been postulated, for which there is isolated histologic evidence.[14,15,58] The muscular dysfunction in its shortening of the colon crumples the circular layer in the same way that a coat sleeve wrinkles when it is raised up the arm. This cracks the circular layer in a circumferential fashion and leads to a weak zone through which the mucosa herniates.

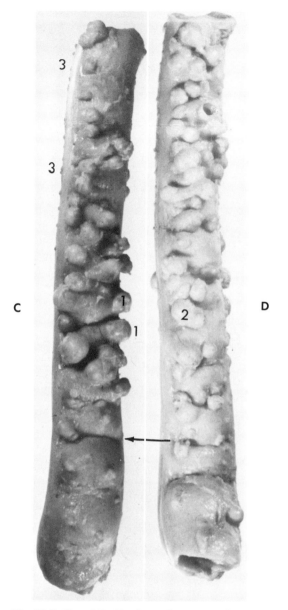

Fig. 38-3, C and D. For legend see opposite page.

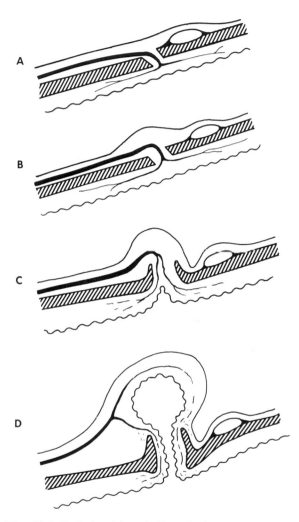

Fig. 38-4. Relationship of diverticula to blood vessels. **A,** Penetrating branch of a long artery, piercing the circular muscle close to the antimesenteric taenia. It divides on entering the submucosa. **B,** Pressure in the lumen raises the pressure in the submucosal space and forces out the artery and nearby submucosa, while the mucosa stays normally within the lumen. **C,** With further expulsion of the vessels the submucosal attachments drag the mucosa into the gap. **D,** The final state with the main artery over the apex of the sac. At the neck in the muscular gap, only small inconspicuous branches remain. (Modified from Tagliocozza, S., and Virno, F.: Vascular relationships of diverticula of the colon; morphological study, Ann. Ital. Chir. **38**:420, 1961.)

Diverticula are visible roentgenologically as anything from a tiny point to the common round appendage on a short neck. Distended, the sac itself is spherical or ovoid, rarely bilobed. Greater irregularities raise the possibility of inflammation. If there is much fecal material in the sac, only a coating of barium on the wall is visible, resulting in the flask shadow (Fig. 38-27). Plugging of the neck of the sac by feces allows filling of a short blunt protrusion from

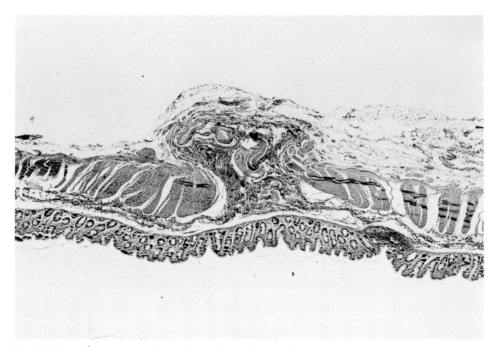

Fig. 38-5. Early stage of diverticula formation. The surgical specimen was distended, and small protrusions appeared. Some contained tiny peaks of mucosa but in some, including this one, only vessels herniated outward. The section shows a smooth mucosa but a small hump where the artery and related submucosa has been pushed outward. Note that on the right hand of the opening the circular muscle has already turned outward. Fig. 38-17 shows the specimen from which this section was obtained.

the lumen. The ease of filling depends on the degree of distention and the amount of contraction of the muscle wall. The larger ones seem to fill more readily on the postevacuation film, and older textbooks speak of the follow-up examination as the most certain method of demonstration.

It seems paradoxical that the distinction of diverticula from polyps should cause difficulties. However, it occasionally does so with double-contrast visualization of the colon. There is no difficulty if the diverticulum and polyp are seen in profile. However, in the face-on view either, the diverticulum or the polyp may cast a perfect circular linear shadow. There is, however, a minute difference according to Welin's observation. The circular line in diverticulum has a sharp outer edge and a fuzzy, blurred inner edge. In a small sessile polyp with a flattened top the inner edge of the line is rather sharp and the outer edge is fading. This difference is sometimes distinct enough to lead to a definite diagnosis, but in many instances it cannot

be relied upon. It is best to identfy a polyp as a soft tissue mass protruding into the gas-filled intestine by better positioning (projection), steroscopic views, a modified degree of distention of the bowel, or repeated barium enema examination. These procedures may involve great technical difficulties, more so since polyps occur in the presence of diverticula, but their recognition is important, particularly in the presence of rectal bleeding.

Beranbaum and Beranbaum have published a useful paper on the diagnosis of polyps in the distorted sigmoid colon of diverticular disease, stressing the need for great technical competence.[2] They insist that one film showing a polyp convincingly should outweigh the failure to show it on other films of the same area.

ROENTGENOLOGY AND SIGNIFICANCE OF MUSCULAR DISORDER

One of the striking features of operative specimens of diverticular disease is the thickness of the muscle in the affected area. The taeniae

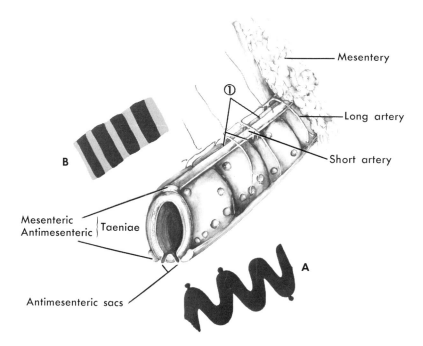

Fig. 38-6. Diagram of the anatomy of the sigmoid colon, as described in the text. **A,** The roentgenograph in the line of the mesentery showing the saw-tooth sign and sacs on the horizon. **B,** The roentgenograph at right angles to the mesentery, showing no diverticula and half-shadow bars.

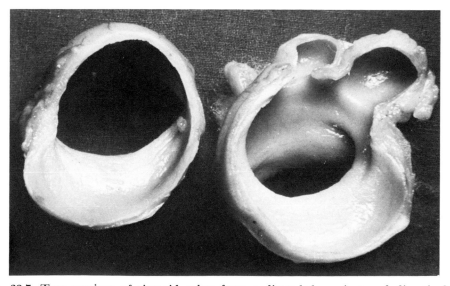

Fig. 38-7. Two portions of sigmoid colon from a distended specimen of diverticulosis above a carcinoma of the rectum. When viewed from the lumen it is possible to appreciate the crescentic shape of the interhaustral folds. In the example on the right the second fold in the background points in the opposite direction. The diverticula arise from the haustral convexity approximately opposite to the fold. A 3 mm. polyp is visible on the specimen on the left.

are prominent and tough, the circular muscle is thick and very convoluted, and the nearby mesentery is bunched up and firmer than normal.[37] This finding can be appreciated in the sigmoid but is apparently not recognizable in the rest of the colon. It can be present in the absence of inflammation (Fig. 38-26) and contributes a great part of the palpable mass that is felt at operation, even if an abscess is additionally present.

The key to the understanding of the nature of this mass and of the roentgenograms is the anatomy of the sigmoid colon, which is an asymmetrical structure and cannot be regarded as a simple cylinder (Fig. 38-6). The three taeniae are arranged in the form of an isosceles triangle, one under the mesentery and two close together, enclosing the short antimesenteric zone to form the base. The lateral walls, each between the mesenteric taenia and one antimesenteric taenia, are long and flexible, and it is these walls that bend inwards to form the interhaustral folds. The folds are deep on one lateral wall but fade away as they pass around the circumference, so that the haustra opposite are quite smooth and well distended. Folds alternate from side to side down the length of the intestine (Figs. 38-3 and 38-10), and when viewed from the lumen are crescent shaped (Fig. 38-7). Diverticula emerge from the lateral walls as already discussed (Figs. 38-3 and 38-6). It is seen at once that X-rays in the line of the mesentery will travel down the interhaustral folds and show the diverticula on the horizon, while in those films taken at right angles to the mesentery the sacs will be hidden behind the barium-filled lumen and the interhaustral folds will show as half shadow bars. This visually striking difference is illustrated in Fig. 38-8, in which a Chassard-Lapine view in the line of the mesentery is compared with an oblique supine view. In routine work the rays are coming at largely unpredictable angles to a mobile S-shaped loop of intestines and interpretation will not always be so easy.

It was the radiologists Goulard and Hampton[21] and Wolf, Khilnani, and Marshak[59] who unraveled the meaning of this picture. They argued that in diverticulosis the interhaustral folds were deeper and closer together than they should be and that the essential feature was that the colon failed to elongate fully. The sigmoid

A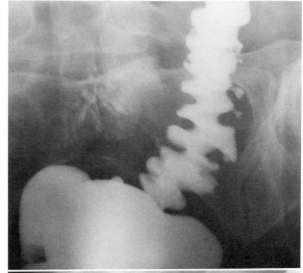

B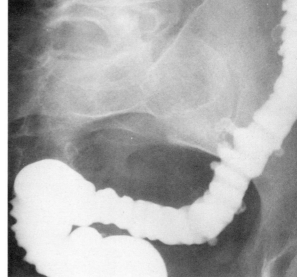

Fig. 38-8. A, Chassard-Lapin view showing a saw-tooth sign and diverticula on the horizon. **B,** Oblique supine view at the same state of filling, with the transverse portion of the sigmoid corresponding to the segment shown in **A.** Note that the sacs are not visible and that the interhaustral folds are shown as half-shadow bar-shaped bands across the lumen. These are also visible in the portion of the sigmoid ascending out of the pelvis.

and its mesentery can be compared to a fan (Fig. 38-9) in which the diseased portion is not fully opened. It thus contains more muscle, nerve cells, mucosa, and blood vessels per unit length than does the normal, while the mesenteric fat is bunched up to form a palpable thickening. Thus at operation the affected segment is

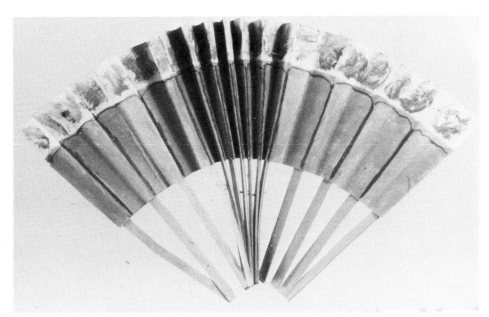

Fig. 38-9. The sigmoid colon and its mesentery can be compared to a fan in which the diseased portion is not fully opened. Thus the mesentery will be thicker and the bowel will contain more muscle, fat, nerves, mucosa, and blood vessels per unit length in the affected segment.

shorter than normal. Roentgenologically, the muscle can still be seen to contract and relax,[56] but it will not elongate fully, although the histologists offer no explanation of these features.

The best descriptive term is a contracture as defined for voluntary muscle by Gasser, "a term without definition, convenient in its vagueness for the various states of muscle shortening, themselves not well understood, but in which there is a real or fancied difference from tetanic contraction."[18] Fleischner, who was aware of the extreme variability of the roentgenologic signs in life during a single enema but realized that they could also be found at autopsy, expressed much the same idea in the phrase "spasm which persists becomes permanent,"[36] The most important change from the radiologist's point of view is the shortening of the colon, since it gives rise to the recognizable roentgenologic signs; but the pathologists speak of hypertrophy of circular muscle as an important constituent of some specimens.[1,37]

On occasion the haustra crumple in addition to the interhaustral folds and give an irregular spiked outline to the lumen (Fig. 38-10). This has been argued to also be a manifestation of shortening.[58] Crescents from both sides pass across the antimesenteric wall. Although low in height at this point they are twice as numerous and can give a spiky outline to one side of the bowel (Fig. 38-11). The disruption of the antimesenteric wall can also take the form of ridges and troughs (Fig. 38-12), and this can give a unilateral crenated edge.[31,58] These patterns, which are often seen in the lower descending colon above a sigmoid obviously the site of diverticular disease, are called in the English literature prediverticular patterns and are a problem in interpretation only when they appear in the absence of diverticula elsewhere.[20] They are perhaps best regarded as examples of the muscular disorder of diverticular disease without diverticula, a disease state that is hard to diagnose and rarely sufficiently important to warrant operation.[1,16,37]

DIVERTICULITIS

In its strict meaning "diverticulitis" implies the presence of inflammation, although the word is also used to indicate diverticular disease with symptoms. Histologically, the inflammation starts in the mucosa of the diverticulum and is predominantly lymphocytic in nature.[37] Spreading of the disease to involve the mucosa

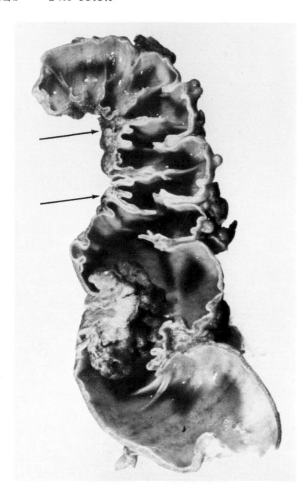

Fig. 38-10. Resection for carcinoma of the rectum seen in the lower half. The roentgenologic diagnosis was easy, in spite of the presence of diverticula below the growth. Above the carcinoma is the typical alternating pattern of interhaustral folds. On the wall between the arrows the fold pattern is more frequent and less regular.

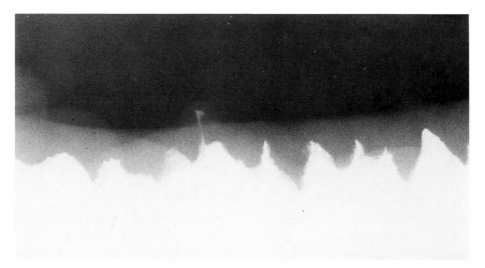

Fig. 38-11. Roentgenograph of a distended operative specimen, with the antimesenteric border on the horizon. Closely packed spikes and rounded convexities cause this palisade sign. A tiny diverticulum has broken through at one point. The length of this intestine is 23 mm.

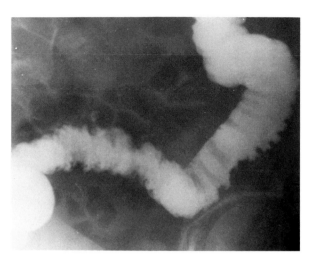

Fig. 38-12. The transverse portion of the sigmoid is the site of diverticular disease. In the ascending portion of the sigmoid there are no sacs, but one border is castellated. This unilateral crenated border is a manifestation of the muscular shortening, even though no sacs are visible in the area.

of the neck or the lumen does occur, but very rarely.[29] Fleischner and Ming make the important point that the result is the development of tiny perforations that rapidly heal to produce a scar of small dimensions, often involving only part of the circumference of a sac (Fig. 38-13).[34] One can see from Fig. 38-13 that the roentgenologic demonstration of this tiny deformity is very difficult; however, it is of sufficient size to cause the pathologist to label the specimen as an example of diverticulitis. If the microperforation enlarges and fails to heal, bowel contents escape, leading to abscess formation that may then track across the peritoneal cavity to other structures or enter the retroperitoneal space. In the fully developed clinical picture of a patient with elevated temperature and a high leukocyte count, together with a left iliac fossa mass, the diagnosis of inflammation is easy. But most cases do not come into this category. Morson's series of 155 surgical specimens makes this point very clearly.[37] All patients with a diagnosis of diverticulitis, were operated on, yet of the specimans one third showed no sign of inflammation

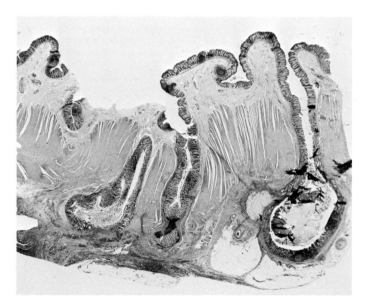

Fig. 38-13. Photomicrograph of a specimen of sigmoid, showing two perforated diverticula. The mucosa is intact except for the sites of perforations. The muscularis is markedly thickened. In the diverticulum on the right a small paradiverticular abscess is surrounded by a fibrous wall. In the left diverticulum an epithelialized scar at the bottom of the diverticulum and extensive subserous fibrosis indicate an old healed perforation and peridiverticulitis. (Original magnification ×5.5.)

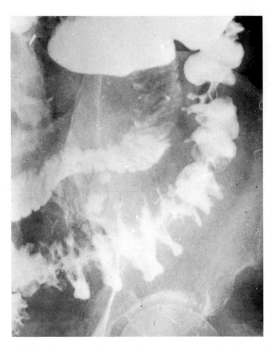

Fig. 38-14. In a patient with repeated episodes of diverticular ruptures an abscess above the sigmoid had formed and broken through into an adjacent ileal loop. This loop filled with barium through the sigmoidoileal fistulous system.

past or present, and four had no diverticula. The obverse is also true. In Hughes' series of ninety-nine cases found at autopsy, four had histologically active inflammation, yet the patients complained of no symptoms and the diagnosis was not considered before death.[24] It is likely from the pathology that there will be a group of cases, possibly a distressingly high proportion, in which the inflammation is difficult or impossible to show by radiologic means. As yet, published papers have made little attempt to assess roentgenologic accuracy.

If inflammation develops around a solitary diverticulum situated in the ascending or transverse colon, the patient is usually operated on as an emergency with the diagnosis of appendicitis or cholecystitis. The diagnosis of diverticulitis is considered more often in the sigmoid colon. In the absence of indications of severe peritonitis medical management is undertaken, including a diagnostic enema some days later. Two groups of signs lead to the diagnosis of inflammation, one concerned with demonstrating the presence of a hole in the intestine wall and the other with the presence of an extrinsic abscess.

Air under the diaphragm and a fistula from the diseased sigmoid to the small bowel (Fig. 38-14) or bladder (Fig. 38-15) are reliable indi-

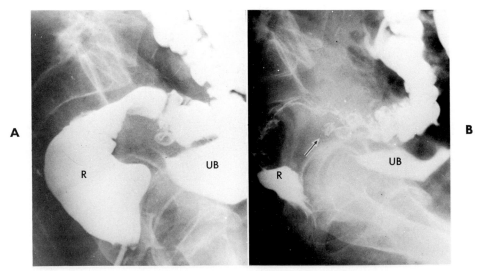

Fig. 38-15. A, Prerectal diverticular abscess, clinically first believed to be a prostatic lesion. The urinary bladder is also filled with opaque medium. **B,** The blown-out collapsed diverticulum next to an intact one. **R** indicates rectum; **UB** is the urinary bladder.

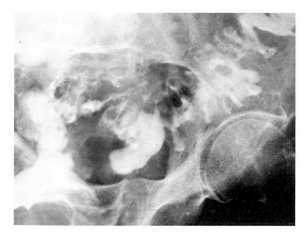

Fig. 38-16. A larger perforation abscess originating from the midsigmoid extends down into the left pelvic space.

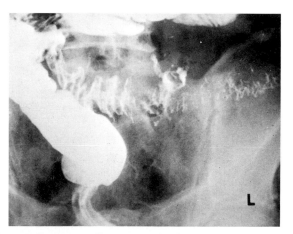

Fig. 38-17. A small communicating paracolic abscess after diverticular rupture at the upper aspect of the sigmoid.

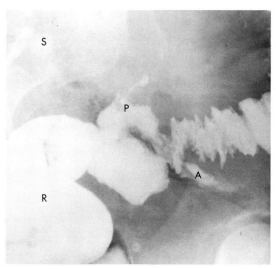

Fig. 38-18. Postevacuation roentgenogram, lateral view. Diverticular perforation abscesses extend in anterior, **A**, and posterior, **P**, direction. **R** is rectum; **S** is sacrum.

cators of diverticulitis if carcinoma can be excluded. Most nontraumatic sigmoidovesical fistulas in the elderly result from diverticulitis, as do about one third of sigmoidovaginal fistulas.[60]

The leak of barium may be quite easy to see; an irregular sinus track (Figs. 38-16 and 38-17), a fuzzy cloud of barium (Fig. 38-18), or a thin streak (Fig. 38-19) mark the spot. Easy to miss (Figs. 38-20 and 38-21) are the small leaks leaving a tiny dot of barium some distance from the lumen, which very much like a calcified lymph node or a bit of contrast medium on the patient's skin. These may first be recognized on the postevacuation film, and quick refilling with multiple spot films may be necessary to show the exact relationship of the lumen.

The presence of an extrinsic pressure deformity is presumptive evidence of an abscess or fibrosis. The inflammation may completely occlude the mouth of the sac so that it does not fill. A gross deformity of one or more of the normally spherical sacs (Figs. 38-21 and 38-22) is very suggestive of present or past inflammation, and the diagnosis is made more certain if there is a previous examination for comparison. Large abscesses displace the colon or indent it in the fashion characteristic of extrinsic masses (Figs. 38-23 and 38-24). More difficult is the detection of additional deformity in the presence of major muscular dysfunction. Films must be exposed in the stage of full filling or after administration of smooth-muscle relaxants, since the spasm of the early filling stage usually relaxes and the initial impression of extrinsic pressure vanishes. Even gross deformities may be the result of muscular contracture either alone or with tiny areas of inflammation (Figs. 38-25 to 38-27). Fleischner's case (Fig. 38-28) is fairly typical of what many people would accept as indicating extrinsic abscesses, but it is hard to give any real guide to this problem.

RELATIONSHIP TO IRRITABLE COLON SYNDROME

The irritable colon syndrome is an old clinical concept known under a variety of names

Text continued on p. 1032.

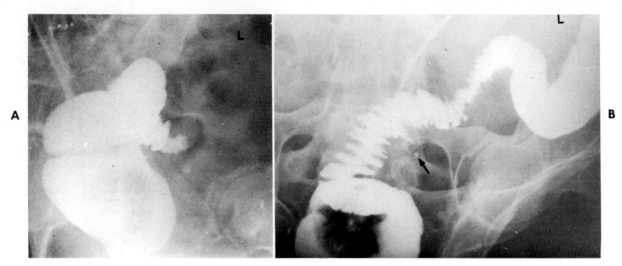

Fig. 38-19. A, Acute condition within the abdomen in a man 50 years of age. Complete obstruction at the rectosigmoid junction was encountered at barium enema study. At the immediate laparotomy a left pelvic abscess was found and drained and a transverse colostomy established. **B,** Nine days later, with the patient greatly improved, the sigmoid had opened. An extravasated barium speck (arrow) indicated the site of rupture. The sigmoid was resected 3 months later.

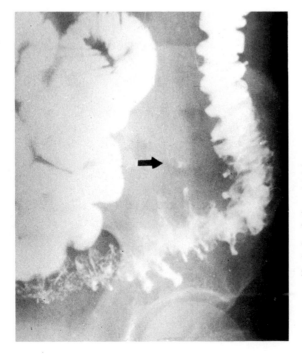

Fig. 38-20. In this patient, who had experienced slight lower abdominal tenderness, free gas was found beneath the diaphragm. Two days later a colon examination was undertaken in the search for the site of perforation. This postevacuation film showed an elongated haustrum-diverticulum in the proximal sigmoid. The arrow points to an isolated barium fleck, evidence of a small, confined extravasation.

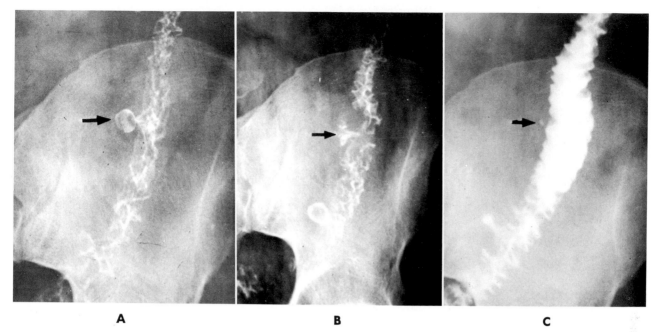

A   **B**   **C**

Fig. 38-21. A, Two diverticula in the descending colon. **B,** Eight months later, during an attack of acute diverticulitis, the upper diverticulum has ruptured and collapsed, and some barium has spilled. Local swelling of the colonic wall forms a cushion-like mass. **C,** Two months later, after full recovery of the patient, there is no visible trace of irregularity in the colonic wall at the site of the self-amputated divericulum. A persistent barium fleck signals the residual minute scar surrounding the extravasated matter.

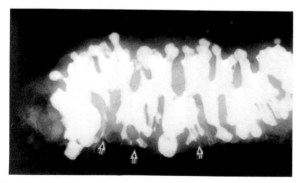

Fig. 38-22. Surgical specimen of the sigmoid of a patient with well-documented episodes of diverticulitis, the last with free gas beneath the diaphragm only 5 months before surgery. Several diverticula (arrows) are irregular and pointed. The pathologic description was: "Diverticulosis and chronic diverticulitis with focal ruptures. The tissue around those diverticula is thickened and shows chronic inflammation with widespread foreign body giant cell reaction." This inconspicuousness of the residues is the rule rather than the exception.

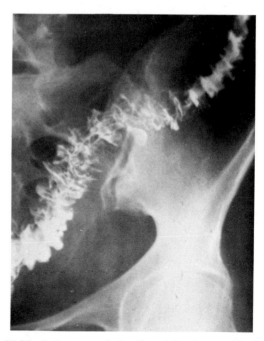

Fig. 38-23. A large, sealed off pelvic abscess displacing the sigmoid upward as any adnexal mass may do. The proximal sigmoid is slightly compressed, its lower contour irregular, and one diverticulum is visible in this area. This abscess originated from a ruptured sigmoid diverticulum; it was successfully drained and the sigmoid resected.

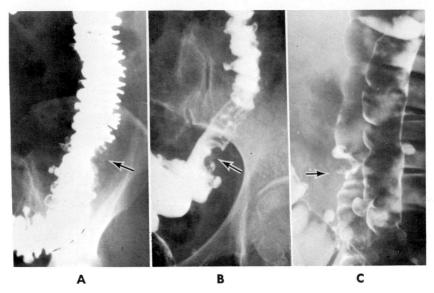

A **B** **C**

Fig. 38-24. A and **B,** Localized mural swelling in the lower descending colon at the site of a ruptured diverticulum. The laterally bulging paracolic fat line, suggesting an extra-colonic mass, was better observed on the original films. **C,** A similar lesion in the upper descending colon, visualized by double-contrast technique.

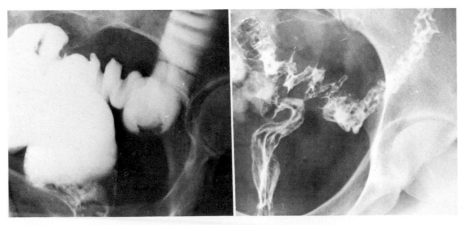

Fig. 38-25. Colon examination of a 42-year-old woman with a history of alternating diarrhea and constipation. Crowded, thick haustral folds and few diverticula were found in the sigmoid, either full or after the patient had defecated. The diagnosis was spastic colon and diverticula.

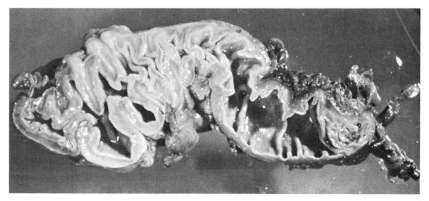

Fig. 38-26. Surgical specimen of the sigmoid taken from the patient in Fig. 38-25, resected for obstruction in the course of spastic colon syndrome. Thick muscular folds in accordion arrangement cause marked shortening and narrowing of the lumen and chamber formation. A few diverticula without inflammation were also found.

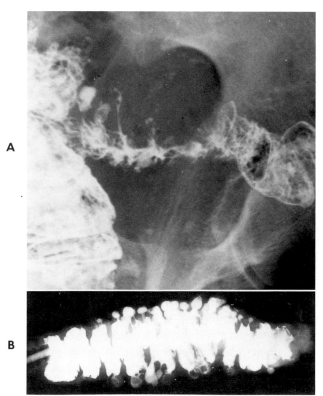

Fig. 38-27. A, Roentgenograph showing a narrowed area with an intact mucosal pattern. There are obvious sacs distally and a partially filled sac in the middle zone. The long thin line of barium is the remnant of a haustrum leading to a sac. No smooth muscle relaxant was used here. B, The surgical specimen. Only histologic inflammation is visible. Note that the haustral pattern is very crowded, and in life only a small central channel is visible.

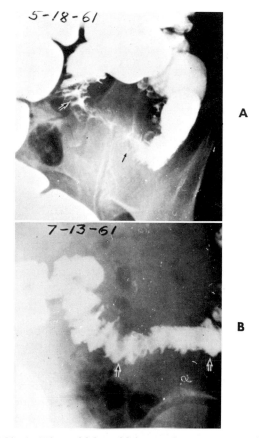

Fig. 38-28. A, The midsigmoid is grossly narrowed, with funneling at both ends, and has a distorted mucosal pattern. This narrow loop was seen and felt to lie in the center of the tender mass in the left lower quadrant. B, Two months later, after laparotomy with draining of a left pelvic abscess and establishment of a transverse colostomy, the narrow portion has opened up, with irregularities still persisting. Arrows indicate the identical portions in A and B.

such as spastic colon, mucous colitis, colonic neurosis, and many more. Despite the support given to it by some great authorities, this syndrome has had a twilight existence in academic medicine, largely because of the difficulties of definition and the absence of diagnostic laboratory tests.

Truelove and Reynell hold that three categories of patients can be identified.[51] In the first type the dominant symptom is diarrhea that lasts from a few hours to several weeks. Between attacks the bowel movements may be normal or loose. In the second type, often called spastic colon, the dominant symptom is pain, usually in the left iliac fossa and of a continuous nature with colicky exacerbations. The pain may be associated with an urge to defecate, which brings relief. But evacuation is incomplete and patients complain of constipation although passing more than the usual number of stools, small in size, and classically ribbon shaped. An excess of mucus is a feature in some. In the third type pain with alternating diarrhea and constipation are present. A similar syndrome may persist for years after an attack of dysentery. It has been common practice to attribute this disease to psychologic disturbances, a view somewhat upset by Weser and his colleagues.[54] They found a group of patients fitting the clinical criteria for the irritable colon syndrome, who had a deficiency of lactase in the small bowel and whose diarrhea resulted from their failure to metabolize lactose. Even so, large numbers of patients still do not have a demonstrable abnormality and the irritable colon syndrome remains a necessary clinical grouping.

The roentgenologic changes in this disease were described by Golden.[19] The left side of the bowel is narrower than usual; stripping waves during the filling stage are vigorous and repeated and may even prevent filling. The haustral folds are crowded together and persistent. Lumsden and his colleagues' radiologic criteria are very similar, although they categorized them from a series of barium enemas on patients who underwent no preparation.[30] Intraluminal recordings in patients with this disease who have pain show increase in frequency and size of the pressure waves, and according to Arfwidsson, similar results are obtained in diverticular disease.[1] In diverticular disease Painter and Truelove have found that pressure does not increase in the resting state, but rather after eating or after the injection of neostigmine (Prostigmin) bromide. The technical problems of recording intraluminal pressures are presently the subject of much discussion, and exactly what conclusions can be drawn from such experiments is a matter of argument. Many would agree that they indicate increased activity of muscle and at the very least support for the idea that diverticula are of the pulsion type.

The irritable colon syndrome and diverticular disease have similar symptoms, roentgenologic findings and intraluminal pressure measurements. At the present time it is impossible to make a distinction between them in every patient. The problem is highlighted by Boles and Jordan, who in a paper on the natural history of diverticulosis asserted that pure diverticulosis was not responsible for symptoms.[4] They take roentgenograms of all patients with symptoms of the irritable colon syndrome. For the proposition that patients who have the irritable colon syndrome later develop diverticular disease in greater numbers or a more severe form than the normal population, the evidence remains minimal. On the basis of clinical impression Edwards[14] thought that they did not, although Fleischner in the first edition of this book argued strongly that they did. The physician who needs to project his own confidence to the patient having symptoms may have to take a stand on this point, but the radiologist can justifiably take an uncommitted view.

NATURAL HISTORY

Recent discoveries indicate that uncertainties of clinical diagnosis and the difficulties of comparing barium enemas make past attempts to determine the natural history of colonic diverticular disease of little value. Most of what has been written is confined to recording the clinical sequelae of a single attack of diverticulitis. On the radiologic side, Boles and Jordan[4] believed that in 70% of patients the disease progressed, whereas Horner,[23] following up 183 patients for an average period of 5 years, found that in 129 (70%) there was no progression.

COMPLICATIONS
Peritonitis

Usually the peritonitis that follows perforation is very localized, but free spread can occur. In aged patients this is a complication with a high mortality. Collections of pus may subsequently form in the peritoneum in any of the common sites, or it may be retroperitoneal around the kidneys or the rectum. The reparative powers of the abdominal cavity are well known, and at the time of elective surgery weeks or months after the acute incident only the smallest residues may be visible. Certainly the roentgenologic detection of these minor changes is an uncommon event.

Bleeding

Bleeding is minor and intermittent although not rare in diverticular disease, and with this symptom the need to exclude carcinoma and polyps becomes more important than ever. In the aged and often in those with colons that have many diverticula and little muscular abnormality, a special type of bleeding occurs. It is unheralded and profuse, leading to exsanguination if treatment is not vigorous. In the past, blind resections of large parts of the colon have been undertaken for this complication, and arteriography to detect the bleeding point, which may be in a single diverticulum, is an obvious future approach.

Obstruction

Complete large-bowel obstruction, even in diverticulitis, is rare, which is a surprising observation if the radiologic appearances at barium enema are taken at their face value. It may be impossible to force barium retrograde past the sigmoid of a patient with diverticulitis who the same day is having normal bowel movements.[55] Angulation of a small-bowel loop adherent to the inflamed sigmoid may result in small-bowel obstruction.

Fistulas

The fistulas to bladder, vagina, and small bowel have already been illustrated. In view of the recent accounts of granulomatous colitis superimposed on diverticular disease, it is perhaps worth considering this combination in the presence of fistulas.[46]

Ulcerative colitis

When this mucosal disease is superimposed on diverticulosis the prognosis becomes grave.[12] Multiple pericolic abscesses occur. Ulceration of mucosa beyond the sigmoid is a clue to the diagnosis.

CLASSIFICATION

The concepts of diverticulosis and diverticulitis are firmly established in the minds of most physicians and are entrenched in the literature, so that the abandonment of these two names would be virtually impossible, although the present idea of three elements—a muscular dysfunction, sacs, and inflammation—makes them hard to defend. Morson's large series has simply crystallized the feeling of many physicians and surgeons that the clinical diagnosis of the state of inflammation is much less certain than older textbooks would have one believe.[37] Many use diverticular disease as an all-embracing term, implying the muscular abnormality and most often the presence of sacs but leaving the possibility of inflammation deliberately vague. The radiologist can be a little more descriptive, quantifying the sacs in degrees from few to very numerous and making an attempt to assess the degree of shortening. In the absence of clear indications of inflammation at barium enema, the radiologist can leave the decision of what emphasis to give to the symptoms in the hands of the clinician.

At the other end of the scale is the question of the degree and persistence of roentgenographic deformity necessary to establish the presence of diverticular disease. A saw-tooth sign with no sacs, persistently present in a local area of the sigmoid in an otherwise normal colon, is a rare finding. Usually it is found with prediverticular patterns in the descending portion, and a distinction from spastic colon may be impossible. All radiologists are aware that a saw-tooth deformity can be a transient finding in a normal enema. Fortunately, the problem has little importance in routine clinical work, and most hospital staffs quickly reach accord on minimum criteria for radiologic diverticular disease. Without such understanding confusion can occur.

DIFFERENTIAL DIAGNOSIS
Carcinoma

There is little to add to Schatzki's list in consideration of the problem of the narrowed segment.[45] Carcinoma tends to create a short narrowing, with shoulders at each end and obviously destroyed mucosa. In diverticular disease the narrowing is usually longer, the ends are funneled, and the mucosa is preserved. Tiny sharp spikes where the barium enters the rem-

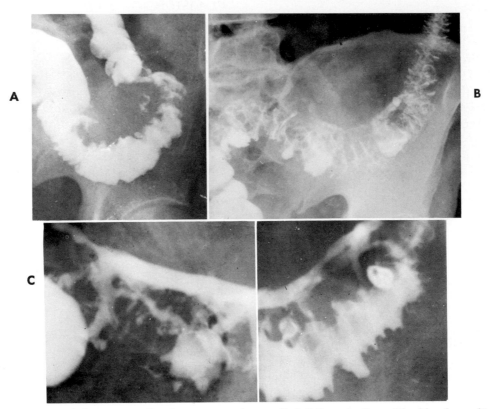

Fig. 38-29. A long paracolic abscess, sometimes called "dissecting" or "double channel" abscess. **A,** The sigmoid loop as it fills at the beginning of the barium enema examination. **B,** Barium, having leaked through several diverticular ruptures, fills a chain of communicating abscesses and forms a long channel parallel to the colonic lumen. **C,** Composite of two spot films to show the numerous fistulas and the long paracolic abscess. There is now evidence that this form of abscess is indicative of the development of granulomatous colitis.

nants of the compressed haustra on the edges of the narrowed zone suggest diverticular disease, as does the presence of a solitary sac in the narrowed area (Fig. 38-27). Funneled ends in carcinoma can result from spread of the growth outside or the development of an abscess. The best possible technique and the least spasm are necessary for the difficult case and for the demonstration of small growths within an area already distorted by the muscular dysfunction. Morton and Goldman give statistics of accuracy of differentiation of diverticulitis from carcinoma, based on pre-1962 techniques.[38] They support the concept that the distinction is usually easy, sometimes difficult, and occasionally impossible.

Granulomatous colitis

Two recent papers have explored the diagnosis of granulomatous colitis grafted on diverticular disease and suggest that some examples of this combination have been missed in the past. According to Marshak and his colleagues, the fissures of granulomatous colitis may look like the deformed haustra of diverticular disease.[32] They believe that the long subserous abscess track (Fig. 38-29), long called diverticulitis, is pathognomonic of granulomatous colitis. Schmidt and associates advise that fistulas, extension of ulceration out of the sigmoid, and irregular spikes should alert one to the possibility of granulomatous disease.[46]

Ischemic colitis

When the colon becomes acutely ischemic the patient may have pain, fever, and rectal bleeding, and diverticulitis is a possible clinical diagnosis. Roentgenologically, a limited length of large bowel is involved and the sigmoid is not immune. From the published pictures, both diverticulitis and ischemic colitis have isolated roentgenologic features in common. Half shadow bars and deformities of the wall resembling thumbprints are two such, but so far little difficulty has been recorded when the total pattern is considered.

REFERENCES

1. Arfwidsson, F.: Pathogenesis of multiple diverticula of the sigmoid colon in diverticular disease, Acta Chir. Scand. (Suppl.) **342**:1, 1964.
2. Deranbaum, J. L., and Deranbaum, E. R.: Small polypoid lesions associated with spastic diverticulosis, Dis. Colon Rectum **8**:78, 1965.
3. Bohrer, S. P.: Hiatus hernia and diverticulosis in Nigeria, New Eng. J. Med. **272**:695, 1965.
4. Boles, R. S., Jr., and Jorden, S. M.: The clinical significance of diverticulosis, Gastroenterology **35**:579, 1958.
5. Brewer, G. E.: The etiology of certain cases of left-sided intra-abdominal suppuration-acute diverticulitis, Amer. J. Med. Sci. **134**:482, 1907.
6. Bülbering, E., Brading, A., Jones, A., and Tomita, T., editors: Smooth muscle, London, 1970, Edward Arnold.
7. Carman, R. D.: Roentgenologic findings in 3 cases of diverticulitis of the large bowel, Ann. Surg. **61**:343, 1915.
8. Carroll, P. T.: Diverticula, diverticulosis and diverticulitis of the colon; indications for operation and refinement of surgical technic, Dis. Colon Rectum **4**:88, 1958.
9. Case J. T.: Roentgen study of colonic diverticula, Amer. J. Roentgen. **21**:207, 1929.
10. Chaudhary, N. A., and Truelove, S. C.: The irritable colon syndrome; a study of the clinical features, predisposing causes and prognosis in 130 cases. Quart. J. Med. **31**:307, 1962.
11. Christensen, J., Caprilli, R., and Lund, G.: Electric slow waves in circular muscle of cat colon, Amer. J. Physiol. **217**:771, 1969.
12. Collins, D. C.: The grave prognosis of ulcerative colitis engrafted on diverticulitis coli, Amer. J. Gastroent. **35**:222, 1961.
13. DeQuervain, F.: Zur Diagnose der erworbenen Dickdarmdivertikel und der Sigmoiditis diverticularis, Deutsche Ztschr. Chir. **128**:67, 1914.
14. Edwards, H. C.: Diverticula of the colon and vermiform appendix; Hunterian lecture, Lancet **1**:221, 1934.
15. Evans, W. E., and Dawson, R. G.: Diverticulitis in the young adult, Amer. Surg. **36**:518, 1970.
16. Fleischner, F. G., and Ming, S. C.: Revised concepts on diverticular disease of the colon, II. So-called Diverticulitis; diverticular sigmoiditis and peridiverticulitis; diverticular abscess, fistula, and frank peritonitis, Radiology **84**:599, 1965.
17. Fleischner, F. G., Ming, S. C., and Henken, E. M.: Revised concepts on diverticular disease of the colon, I. Diverticulosis; emphasis on tissue derangement and its relation to the irritable colon syndrome, Radiology **83**:859, 1964.
18. Gasser, H. S.: Contractures of skeletal muscle, Physiol. Rev. **10**:35, 1930.
19. Golden, R.: Diagnostic roentgenology, vol. 2, New York, 1936, Thomas Nelson & Sons.
20. Goligher, J. C.: Surgery of the anus, rectum and colon, ed. 2, London, 1967, Baillière, Tindall & Cassel.
21. Goulard, A., Jr., and Hampton, A. O.: Correlation of the clinical, pathological and roentgenological findings in diverticulitis, Amer. J. Roentgen. **72**:213, 1954.
22. Graser, E.: Entzündliche Stenose des Dickdarmes, bedingt durch Perforation multipler falscher Divertikel, Centralbl. Chir. **25**:140, 1898.
23. Horner, J. L.: Natural history of diverticulosis, Amer. J. Dig. Dis. **3**:343, 1958.
24. Hughes, L. E.: Postmorten survey of diverticula disease of the colon, Gut **10**:336, 1969.
25. Kieth, A.: Diverticula of the alimentary tract of congenital or obscure origin, Brit. Med. J. **1**:376, 1910.
26. Kim, E. H.: Hiatus hernia and diverticulum of the colon—their low incidence in Korea, New Eng. J. Med. **271**:764, 1964.
27. Leader, A. G., and Stell, R. D.: Urologic diagnosis and the urologic examination. In Campbell, M. F., editor: Urology, ed. 2, vol. 1, Philadelphia, 1963, W. B. Saunders Co.
28. LeMay, M.: Personal communication.
29. Lumb, G. D., and Protheroe, R. H. B.: Mucosal inflammatory spread in diverticulitis and ulcerative colitis, Arch. Pathol. **62**:185, 1956.
30. Lumsden, K., Chaudhary, N. A., and Truelove, S. C.: The irritable colon syndrome, Clin. Radiol. **14**:54, 1963.
31. Marcus, R., and Watt, J.: The radiological appearances of diverticula in the antimesenteric intertaenial area of the pelvic colon, Clin. Radiol. **16**:87, 1965.
32. Marshak, R. H., Janowitz, H. D., and Present, D. H.: Granulomatous colitis in association with diverticula, New Eng. J. Med. **283**:1080, 1970.
33. McCune, W. S., Lovine, V. M., and Miller, D.: Resection and primary anastomosis in diverticulitis of the colon, Ann. Surg. **145**:683, 1957.
34. Mayo, W. J., and Wilson, L. B.: Acquired diverticulitis of the large intestine, Surg. Gynec. Obstet. **5**:8, 1907.
35. Mielke, J. E., Becker, K. L., and Gross, J. B.: Diverticulitis of the colon in a young man with Marfan's syndrome, Gastroenterology **48**:379, 1965.
36. Ming, S. C., and Fleischner, F. G.: Diverticulitis of the sigmoid colon; Reappraisal of the pathology and pathogenesis, Surgery **58**:627, 1965.
37. Morson, B. C.: The muscle abnormality in diverticular disease of the sigmoid colon, Brit. J. Radiol. **36**:385, 1963.
38. Morton, D. L., and Goldman, L.: Differential diagnosis of diverticulitis and carcinoma of the sigmoid colon, Amer. J. Surg. **103**:55, 1962.
39. Moynihan, B. G. A.: Mimicry of malignant disease of large intestine, Brit. Med. J. **2**:1817, 1906.
40. Pace, L., and Williams, I.: The organisation of the muscular wall of the human colon, Gut **10**:325, 1969.

41. Painter, N. S.: Diverticular disease of the colon—a disease of Western civilization, D. M. **3:**57, 1970.

42. Painter, N. S.: The etiology of diverticulosis of the colon with special reference to the action of certain drugs on the behaviour of the colon, Ann. Roy. Coll. Surg. Eng. **34:**98, 1964.

43. Painter, N. S., Truelove, S. C., Adran, G. M., and Tuckey, M.: Segmentation and localization of intraluminal pressures in the human colon, with special reference to the pathogenesis of colonic diverticula, Gastroenterology **49:**169, 1965.

44. Pemberton, J. de J., Black, B. M., and Maino, C. R.: Progress in the surgical management of diverticulitis of the sigmoid colon, Surg. Gynec. Obstet. **85:**523, 1947.

45. Schatzki, R.: The roentgenologic differential diagnosis between cancer and diverticulitis of the colon, Radiology **34:**657, 1940.

46. Schmidt, G. T., Lennard-Jones, J. E., Morson, B. C., and Young, A. C.: Crohn's disease of the colon and its distinction from diverticulitis, Gut **9:**7, 1968.

47. Slack, W. W.: The anatomy, pathology, and some clinical features of diverticulitis of the colon, Brit. J. Surg. **50:**185, 1962.

47a. Spriggs, E. I., and Marxer, O. A.: Multiple diverticula of the colon, Lancet **1:**1067, 1927.

48. Tagliacozzo, S., and Virno, F.: The vascularisation of the colon wall; morphological study, Ann. Ital. Chir. **38:**301, 1961.

49. Tagliacozzo, S., and Virno, F.: Vascular relationships of diverticula of the colon; morphological study, Ann. Ital. Chir. **38:**420, 1961.

50. Thomas, S. F.: Radiologic manifestations of gastrointestinal disease in South Central Iran. Paper presented at the Annual Meeting of the Radiologic Society of North America, Chicago, November, 1964.

51. Truelove, S. C. E., and Reynell, R. C.: Diseases of the digestive system, Philadelphia, 1963, F. A. Davis Co.

52. Welch, C. E.: Diverticulitis of the colon, Amer. J. Gastroent. **29:**374, 1958.

53. Welch, C. E., Allen, A. W., and Donaldson, G. A.: An appraisal of resection of the colon for diverticulitis of the sigmoid, Ann. Surg. **138:**332, 1953.

54. Weser, E., Rubin, W., Ross, L., and Sleisinger, M. H.: Lactase deficiency in patients with the "irritable colon syndrome," New Eng. J. Med. **273:**1070, 1965.

55. Wigh, R., and Swenson, P. C.: Roentgenologic aspects of diverticulitis and its complications, Amer. J. Surg. **82:**587, 1951.

56. Williams, I.: The resemblance of diverticular disease of the colon to a myostatic contracture, Brit. J. Radiol. **38:**437, 1965.

57. Williams, I.: Mass movements (mass peristalsis) and diverticular disease of the colon, Brit. J. Radiol. **40:**2, 1967.

58. Williams, I.: Diverticular disease of the colon without diverticula, Radiology **89:**401, 1967.

59. Wolf, B. S., Khilnani, M., and Marshak, R. H.: Diverticulosis and diverticulitis; roentgen findings and their interpretation, Amer. J. Roentgen. **77:**726, 1957.

60. Wood, J. D.: Electrical activity from single neurons in Auerbach's plexus, Amer. J. Physiol. **219:**159, 1970.

61. Wychulis, A. R., and Pratt, J. H.: Sigmoidovaginal fistulas; a study of 37 cases, Arch. Surg. **92:**520, 1966.

Colonic polyps 39

James E. Youker
Wylie J. Dodds
Sölve Welin

The detection of polyps of the colon remains a challenge to the radiologist despite changing concepts on the possible role of this lesion in the development of colon cancer. Approximately 20 years ago in the campaign against cancer of the colon the slogan was, "Polyp detection is cancer prevention." This statement was based on the assumption that in most instances carcinoma of the colon developed from adenomatous polyps. Hence, it was thought that the radical removal of these polyps would constitute a real prophylaxis against cancer of the colon. More recently, serious questions have been raised concerning the validity of this theory.

Adenomatous polyps of the colon are a common lesion, the incidence of which varies tremendously depending on the method of detection. For instance, at the Cancer Prevention Center in Chicago 50,000 proctoscopic examinations revealed the presence of polyps in 7.9% of the patients examined.[44] Polyps were revealed in 15% of 1,000 consecutive proctoscopies by Walske and his colleagues.[58] On 1,552 combined proctoscopic and roentgenologic examinations Gianturco and Miller found polyps in 2.7%.[20] Enquist noted polyps in 19.2% of 1,462 patients examined by both proctoscopy and double-contrast enema at the Cancer Detection Center of the University of Minnesota.[17] Using the same diagnostic methods. Rosensweig and Horwitz found polyps in 24.2% of 777 patients studied.[45]

Early in the 1920s roentgenologists realized that for the diagnosis of small colonic tumors the standard barium enema examination was unsatisfactory. Even with roentgenographic examination alone the results vary considerably depending largely on the technique used. With the ordinary barium enema examination polypoid neoplasms with a diameter of 1 cm. and less escape detection.[60] In an effort to improve these results the barium enema examination has undergone refinements and modifications.

With the so-called mucous membrane relief technique (tannic acid and barium enema), tumors as small as 10 mm. in diameter have been demonstrated. Christie and his co-workers reported polyps in 40 of 4,226 patients examined by this technique.[10]

With the Gianturco high kilovoltage technique and diluted barium, Wietersen found polypoid growths in 31 patients on 1,000 consecutive examinations; 24% of these were malignant based on the histologic criteria of that time.[66] By using pressure spot films as well as a high kilovoltage technique Jarre and Figiel reported an 8% incidence of colonic polyps proximal to the rectosigmoid junction.[28]

The double-contrast method was adopted in Malmö, Sweden, in 1953 because of the great theoretical advantages it offered in the diagnosis of small colonic lesions. For its routine use, however, four conditions had first to be satisfied: (1) adequate cleansing of the intestine; (2) preparation of the intestinal mucosa to permit a thin, uniform coating by the contrast material; (3) rapid evacuation of the colon to avoid delay between the various steps of the examination; and (4) not more than 20 minutes in the examining room for the entire procedure. The Malmö modification of the double-contrast technique meets these requirements. It differs from other methods by directly preparing the intestine for the examination and represents a considerable refinement in the roentgenographic examination of lesions in the large bowel.

With the Malmö technique, 12.5% of the patients examined have been found to have polypoid tumors.[62] Most of the examinations were done because of bowel symptoms, but others were part of a more extensive investigation for suspected cancer. This combination represented the usual hospital type of patient material.

Because of the astonishingly high rate of polyps discovered by the Malmö technique of barium enema, an effort was made to compare this method with the incidence of polypoid lesions of the colon in necropsy material. In this manner a rough estimate could be made of the number of polyps present in the colon, which are actually demonstrated by barium enema. Polypoid tumors were found in 11.3% of 671 necropsies done in Malmö in 1956.[67] A second study from 1958 to 1961 revealed colonic tumors in 12.5% of 3,398 necropsies.[16] Necropsies were performed on virtually 100% of the patients who died in the hospital. The number of colonic polyps detected with the double-contrast enema method suggests that in Malmö it is as high as that noted at necropsy.

Other autopsy series from the United States in which the colonic mucosa was closely scrutinized for very small polyps report a considerably higher incidence of polyps. Arminski found that 41.3% of the adults over 20 years of age undergoing autopsy at the Grace Hospital in Detroit, Michigan, had adenomatous polyps of the colon or rectum.[2] Blatt found adenomatous polyps in 38.8% of colons removed at autopsy from persons over 30 years of age.[6] In both of these series,

at least 50% of polyps found were less than 4 mm. in diameter and would have been difficult to detect on barium enema examination.

PREPARATION FOR ROENTGENOGRAPHY

Residual feces and mucus interfere greatly with the correct roentgenologic diagnosis of colonic lesions. The most important prerequisite for improved diagnostic results is a colon that is free of all solids and fluids.

The widespread belief that complete cleansing of the intestine is impossible was dispelled by the advent of contact laxatives. These insoluble compounds are not absorbed in the intestine and hence do not produce systemic toxicity. The exact mode of action of these drugs is not yet understood. Probably they act directly upon the mucosa of the large bowel through a local reflex. Their action on the small intestine is minimal.

Despite these contact laxatives, the results of the double-contrast examination of the large bowel were still not satisfactory. The bowel never became entirely clean. Furthermore, the barium did not coat the mucous membrane satisfactorily.

To improve mucosal coating, tannic acid was blended with a contact laxative (bisacodyl) to form bisacodyl tannex (Clysodrast).

The addition of tannic acid has several advantages. Because tannic acid is irritating, it stimulates contraction of the entire colon and acts as a powerful laxative. It acts as an astringent, precipitates protein, and inhibits the secretion of mucus and the transudation of fluid into the lumen of the colon. This helps the barium to adhere to the bowel wall, resulting in a uniform coating without artifacts, bubbles, or flaking.

The concentration of tannic acid recommended for use in enemas has varied between 0.25% and 3%. Too low a concentration has no effect. Excessive abdominal cramps and syncope result if the concentration is too high. Moreover, tannic acid is a potent hepatotoxin. In Malmö, the concentration of tannic acid used for the cleansing enema is 0.25% and for the barium enema, 0.75%.

A lively controversy regarding the safety of tannic acid has been stimulated in North America by the reports of deaths after its use in barium enemas.[33,38] As a result, the Food and Drug Administration of the United States prohibited the use of tannic acid in enemas. Recently, tannic acid in the form of bisacodyl tannex has again been released for use in enemas provided certain restrictions are rigidly adhered to. A complete discussion of the current state of tannic acid usage appears elsewhere in this text.

The combining of tannic acid with the contact laxative in bisacodyl tannex represented an advance, but in some instances mucus production was still excessive. Therefore, oral atropine was given; this not only decreased the intestinal secretions, but also diminished the painful contractions induced by the laxative.

An additional advantage of pretreatment with atropine is that it protects against hypotension, which may rarely occur. Special caution is necessary in hypertensive patients receiving drugs that partially block the normal bioregulatory systems.

The preparations for roentgenographic examination of the large bowel vary considerably in different radiology departments. In Malmö the following method is used: The day before the examination the patient eats lightly of easily digestible food. Two tablespoonfuls of castor oil are given before noon, and an enema of water is administered that evening. On the morning of the examination toast and a cup of coffee or tea are permitted. On arrival at the radiology department the patient is given atropine orally, from 0.25 to 1 mg., depending on his age (Table 39-1). A half hour after administration of the atropine an enema is given containing both water and bisacodyl tannex. This preparatory enema with the added bisacodyl tannex is given by specially trained persons well acquainted with the importance of the procedure. The enema is given slowly, and during it the patient lies first on his left side, then on his stomach, then on his right side, and finally on his back. When retention of the enema is difficult the patient is placed in a supine position on a bed pan, with his coccyx slightly elevated. This position plus frequent reassurance may result in complete instillation and retention of the enema.

The routine use of this double-contrast method requires certain modifications in the physical plan of the radiology department. A special room for the cleansing enema, easy access to toilets, and rooms with cots are necessary in departments doing many colon examinations.

In children the dose of atropine (Table 39-1) and the amount of contact laxative-tannic acid preparation is reduced according to the age and weight (Table 39-2). Common salt is added to the enema in infants to obtain an isotonic solution and thereby decrease the risk of water resorption.

Table 39-1. Premedication of oral atropine

Age in years	Quantity
3 to 6	0.25 mg.
6 to 9	0.50 mg.
9 to 12	0.75 mg.
over 12	1.00 mg.

Table 39-2. Cleansing enema

Age in years	Bisacodyl tannex	Salt +	Water
3 to 6	¼ pkg.	2 teaspoons	1.0 liter
6 to 9	½ pkg.	3 teaspoons	1.5 liters
9 to 12	¾ pkg.	3 teaspoons	1.5 liters
12 to 18	1 pkg.	3 teaspoons	1.5 liters
Adults	1 pkg.	4 teaspoons	2.0 liters

DIFFERENTIATION OF TRUE POLYPOID LESIONS FROM EXTRANEOUS MATERIAL

By far the most common material confused with polypoid tumors on barium enema examination is fecal material (Fig. 39-1, *A*). Usually fecal material is freely movable, but occasionally it adheres so firmly to the bowel mucosa that it resembles a broad-based polyp. The irregular shape of the feces and the uneven barium coating usually excludes this diagnosis. However, differentiation of feces and polyps may be impossible even after modern methods of cleansing the bowel have been used. In these cases repetition of the examination may be necessary.

Air bubbles also cause confusion in interpretation (Fig. 39-1, *B*). They are characterized by a thin, gradually fading barium margin surrounding the radiolucent air bubble. Frequently several extremely small air bubbles are clustered about a larger one. According to Stevenson and his co-workers slow insufflation of air is more likely to result in multiple air bubbles.[52] When water of increased hardness is used in

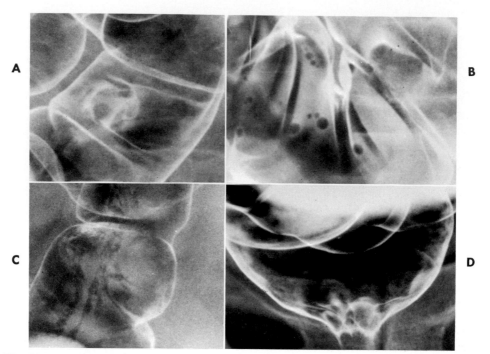

Fig. 39-1. A, Extraneous material mimicking colonic polyps. Fecal material characterized by irregular shape and changing position. Note the absence of an identifiable base. **B,** Air bubbles identified by the gently fading margin of barium and the presence of many small satellite bubbles. **C,** Mucous strands demonstrating long irregular branching defects and seen in association with fecal material. **D,** Hemorrhoids showing filling defects associated with linear shadows of veins.

preparing the barium mixture, fewer air bubbles are formed. Kendig has added 4 tablespoons of calcium lactate to each liter of barium mixture to harden the water.[31]

Oil bubbles from excessive castor oil or from mineral oil may give an appearance similar to that of air bubbles. To avoid this, excessive lubricating agents should not be used on the enema tube tip.

Occasionally, long, slender strands are seen within the barium; these represent mucus (Fig. 39-1, C). Their length may suggest the presence of Ascarides. When the changing widths of these mucous strands and the associated fecal material are recognized, their identification becomes simple.

The lumbar spinous processes, focal skeletal changes, calcified blood vessels or lymph nodes, and genitalia all may be misinterpreted as polyps when their shadows are superimposed on the colon. However, these calcific and boney densities can be rotated away from the colon in different projections.

The examiner must be aware of the appearance in the rectal area of the round open tip of the enema tube. Internal hemorrhoids, which also produce filling defects in the rectum, are usually associated with the linear shadows of the veins from which they arise (Fig. 39-1, D).

When barium-coated diverticula are seen to protrude beyond the bowel wall, they do not create a diagnostic problem. A barium-coated, air-filled diverticulum superimposed on the lumen of the bowel, however, may be confusing. Exclusion of a polyp is simple when an air-fluid level is seen within the diverticulum (Fig. 39-2). There is another sign of great value in differentiating diverticula from polypoid tumors of the colon (Fig. 39-2). The ring of barium coating a diverticulum has a smooth, well-defined outer border and an irregular inner surface. Conversely, the barium coating a polyp is smooth on its inner border and poorly defined on the outer. This difference occurs because the barium is inside the diverticulum; hence, the outer surface

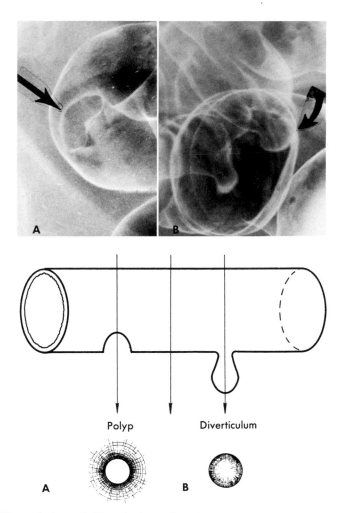

Fig. 39-2. Differentiation of diverticula and polypoid tumors. **A,** The arrow points to the sharp inner border of barium encircling a sessile polyp. **B,** The sharp outer border of barium (arrow) is confined by the wall of a diverticulum. A second diverticulum shows an air-fluid level. (From Welin, S.: Radiologe **2**:87, 1962; and from Youker, J. E., and Welin, S.: Radiology **84**:610, 1965.)

of the barium ring is smooth where it is confined by the mucosal surface of the diverticulum. The fecal stream is in contact with the inner surface of the barium ring and so it appears irregular and blurred. The situation is the opposite in a polypoid tumor, where the barium is outside the polyp. At its points of contact with the mucosal surfaces of the polyp the inner border of the barium ring is smooth.

However, in a few rare but confusing instances a pedunculated polyp may have the appearance of a diverticulum with a distinct outer border and a fuzzy indistinct inner margin. Friedland and Poole have pointed out that manual pressure over a diverticulum during an air

contrast study may result in a decrease in its size and an increase in the amount of barium within the diverticulum.[19] These changes aid in the identification of the lesion as a diverticulum.

DIFFERENTIATION OF BENIGN AND MALIGNANT LESIONS

The double-contrast method has become a valuable adjunct in the roentgenologic diagnosis of polyps, even those that measure only a few millimeters in diameter.

Morphologic types of polyps

Polypoid tumors can be classified as three morphologic types (Fig. 39-3): the sessile, the in-

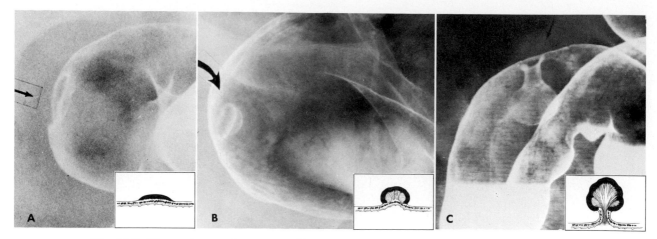

Fig. 39-3. Illustrations and corresponding roentgenograms demonstrate the three forms of polyps produced during pedicle formation. **A,** The flat plaque of adenomatous tissue forms a sessile polyp. **B,** Heaping of the tissue causes a protuberant mass with a broad base, which represents the intermediate form. **C,** Classic pedunculated polyp. (From Youker, J. E., and Welin, S.: Radiology 84:610, 1965.)

termediate or protuberant, and the pedunculated. The roentgenologic criteria for each of these types are individually characteristic and can be differentiated by the appearance of the base of the polyp.[71]

Often the *sessile* polyp is extremely flat and, therefore, difficult to differentiate from the mucosa of the colonic wall (Fig. 39-3, *A*). When viewed face-on, these polyps appear more or less rounded; in profile they may protrude only slightly into the lumen of the colon. The histology of these neoplasms certainly cannot be determined in the early stages. It may represent a slowly growing, benign, noninfiltrating adenomatous polyp or a rapidly infiltrating malignant tumor invading the deeper layers of the bowel.

In the *intermediate* type of polyp (Fig. 39-3, *B*) the adenomatous tissue is heaped into a protuberant mass, its broad base resting on the bowel wall. Its appearance imparts the impression that the process of traction has not progressed long enough to produce a stalk. On microscopic section, however, a central fibrous core, representing the potential stalk, is usually seen in the protuberant polypoid tumor. In the intermediate or protuberant type of polyp there is a small recess between the base of the polyp and the bowel wall. This recess is filled with barium during the air contrast barium enema examination. Barium also coats the body of the polyp, and hence, two white rings are created

on the roentgenogram. The relationship of these rings to each other is determined by the angle at which the roentgen ray beam strikes the barium-coated, broad-based polyp. When the polyp is viewed face-on, the ring of barium over the polyp and the ring about the base are superimposed, giving a single circle (Fig. 39-4, *A*). When seen in profile, the broad attachment of the polyp to the wall is demonstrable (Fig. 39-4, *D*). Viewed tangentialy, the thinner barium covering the polypoid body is overlapped by the denser white ring of barium in the recess about the base. The relationship between these two barium rings may be changed considerably by small variations of the angle of the roentgen ray (Fig. 39-4, *B* and *C*). An analogy can be made to a bowler hat in which the barium-coated body of the polyp represents the crown and the barium around the base, the brim.

Adenomatous polyps of the third type are *pedunculated,* particularly those situated in the descending and sigmoid colon. Welch[61] and Scarborough[46] considered the formation of a stalk to be the result of peristaltic waves associated with the effect of the fecal stream. Traction is thereby exerted on the polyp so that the normal mucosa is drawn out into a stalk. According to Castleman and Krickstein, the development of this pedicle is favored by the fact that adenomas are usually small and not infiltrative.[9] The plaque of adenomatous tissue may, therefore,

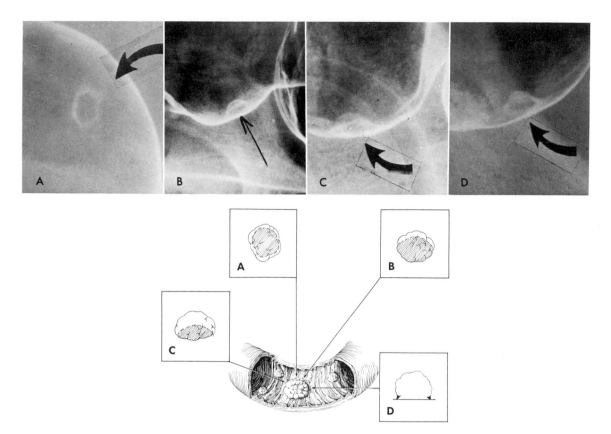

Fig. 39-4. Broad-based polypoid tumor. The roentgenographic image of the intermediate polyp varies according to the angle at which the beam traverses the polyp. **A,** View from directly above, in which a single circle is produced. **B,** Tangential roentgen-ray beam produces the "hat sign," with the barium encircling the base superimposed on the rim of barium coating the body of the polyp. **C,** A slightly different angle of beam produces a different image. **D,** Polyp in profile. (From Youker, J. E., and Welin, S.: Radiology **84:** 610, 1965.)

be lifted up by the traction of the fecal stream until the base becomes drawn out into a stalk (Fig. 39-3, *C*). Although not all agree with this concept of the passive production of a pedicle, it does explain the formation of three different roentgenographic images.

The pedicle of the polyp may be identified in profile either by its thin coating of barium surrounded by air (Fig. 39-3, *C*), or as a negative shadow in an area of residual barium.

When the roentgen ray beam passes parallel to the long axis of the pedicle, the barium-coated pedicle appears as a small white circle within the larger circle of barium covering the body of the polyp. This appearance is analogous to a bull's eye or a target (Fig. 39-5, *A, B, C,* and Fig. 39-14).

The pedunculated polyps usually present no diagnostic difficulty. Occasionally interpretation may be in error and a polyp with a stalk be falsely diagnosed as the broad-based intermediate type. Such an error occurs when the body of the pedunculated polyp lies against the colonic wall, creating a barium ring at the point of contact. In these cases, the pedicle lies parallel to the bowel wall, and its presence may not be appreciated.

Demonstration of the pedicle or the broad base establishes definitely that a polypoid tumor is present and rules out foreign material as a cause of the filling defect.

Colonic polyps and malignancy

The controversy over the role of polyps in colonic malignancy has been very succinctly expressed by Margulis in a recent editorial in

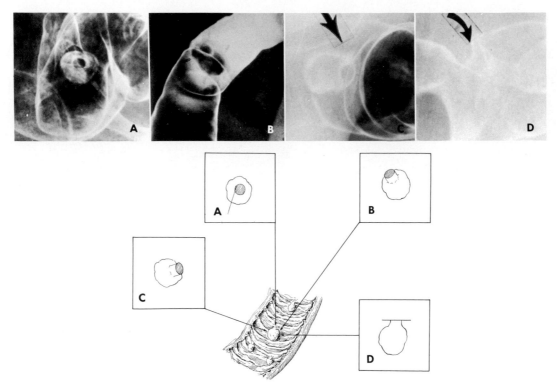

Fig. 39-5. Varying angles of the roentgen-ray beam in relation to the pedicle of a polypoid tumor produce different roentgenographic images. **A,** The target sign, which is produced when the roentgen-ray beam is directed parallel (arrow) to the long axis of the pedicle. **B,** An eccentric target sign is produced by the roentgen-ray beam crossing the pedicle and polyp at a tangent. **C,** A slightly different projection. **D,** The pedicle is shown in profile when the roentgen-ray beam passes at right angles to the long axis of the pedicle. Note the tugging on the bowel wall by the pedicle. (From Youker, J. E., and Welin, S.: Radiology **84:**610, 1965.)

which he states, "The significance of colonic polyposis, its relation to cancer, its treatment, and even the importance of its detection has been in a state of flux for more than twenty years."[35]

Many authors have expressed the view that adenomatous polyps are potentially malignant.[15,56,59] They have stated further that there are histologic or cytologic criteria for determining whether an adenoma has undergone malignant degeneration. They, therefore, regard the neoplasm as a stage in the development of a malignant lesion and consider the formation as definitely precancerous. Death from colonic cancer of almost all untreated patients with familial polyposis is considered as evidence of an intimate connection between adenoma and carcinoma.

Other investigators consider malignant degeneration to be very rare and point out that colonic cancer in children occurs infrequently, whereas polyps are relatively common. Ackerman and del Regato have expressed the opinion that adenomas have no essential part in the development of cancer.[1] Still another group considers malignancy to be present from the beginning in every tumor.[4]

Recently, there has been a shift in emphasis from the theory that adenocarcinoma of the colon may develop from adenomatous polyps to the concept of an abnormal mucosa that gives rise to both polyps and cancer in the presence of appropriate carcinogens. An example of such an abnormal mucosa is multiple familial polyposis of the colon in which adenomatous polyps and cancer frequently coexist.

Electron microscopic and autoradiographic studies of human hyperplastic and adenomatous polyps of the colon by Kaye and associates have demonstrated immaturity of the pericryptal fibroblast sheath of the adenomatous polyp.[29] This parallels the immaturity of the overlying adenomatous epithelium and indicates that both epithelial and mesenchymal components of the adenomatous mucosa are involved.

Several carcinogens have been shown to produce colon carcinoma in rats.[8] In many of these rats the carcinogen has resulted in the simultaneous formation of carcinomas, colonic polyps, and villous adenomas.[8] The action of the bacterial flora of the intestine is necessary to activate at least one type of carcinogen.

Dietary habits and the restricted consumption of cellulose in advanced countries may explain some geographic and cultural differences in the incidence of colonic cancer. Conceivably, the slower transit time of bowel contents in the person with a low cellulose diet permits a longer exposure of the bowel mucosa to possible carcinogens.[35]

A very exciting possibility for the detection of cancer of the colon is the development by Gold of an assay for tumor-specific antigens in human digestive tract cancer.[22] Although there have been false-positive results, this assay may permit the identification of cancer of the gastrointestinal tract. The detection of the exact site of the cancer in the patient with a positive assay represents a challenge to the radiologist of potentially staggering proportions. This entire subject was well reviewed in the July, 1971, issue of *Cancer* in a report on The First National Conference on Cancer of the Colon and Rectum held in January, 1971, under the sponsorship of The American Cancer Society.

Whatever opinion is favored regarding malignancy or potential malignancy of polyps, it is well known that about 95% of the polypoid tumors of the colon are of the adenomatous type. In view of the frequency of adenomatous polyps one may seriously wonder whether "polyp detection is cancer prevention." The important question, therefore, is whether a small polypoid tumor is benign or malignant. Unfortunately, this question cannot always be answered, but certain characteristics of the polyp are suggestive and serve as a useful and practical guide in determining malignancy.

Criteria of malignancy

Size. One of these criteria is the size of the polyp. An analysis of the diameter of polyps in reexamined patients has shown the critical roentgenographic diameter to be 10 mm.[64] The probability of malignancy in a polypoid tumor increases progressively when the diameter exceeds 10 mm. Spratt found only one cancer in 91 tumors under 1.24 cm. in diameter.[50] However, 12% of tumors with a diameter between 1.24 and 1.97 cm. were cancerous, as were all lesions over 3 cm. in diameter. Grinnell in a review of resected adenomatous polyps and papillary adenomas of the colon and rectum also found a sharply increased incidence of cancer as the polypoid tumors increased in size.[24] There was a 1.9% incidence of cancer in 693 tumors less than 0.9 mm. in diameter; 5% in 364 tumors 1 to 1.4 cm. in diameter, and 22.7% in 185 tumors 1.5 to 1.9 cm. in diameter.

Tumors smaller than 10 mm. in diameter and which in roentgenograms appear benign may be observed safely by serial studies. However, even among very small tumors, carcinomas may be expected. Therefore, all patients with lesions of this size should be reexamined every 6 months for 2 years, and then at longer intervals. In view of the slow growth of such tumors, double-contrast enema studies at shorter intervals are not necessary.

Rate of growth. Another useful observation in evaluating malignancy is the rate of tumor growth. This rate of growth is a biologically important feature of all neoplasms. It recently has received increased attention, and there has been great improvement in our knowledge of the growth rates of various tumors.

In 1959 Blum used ultraviolet rays on rats to induce skin cancer.[7] He recorded the time required from the first exposure to the development of the skin cancer. Measurements of tumor growth were correlated with time, which indicated that tumor progression was geometric. Mottram performed similar experiments, using tar instead of ultraviolet rays, which demonstrated the same geometric progression.[40]

The increase in size of pulmonary metastasis from carcinoma of the colon and rectum was studied in twenty-two patients by Collins and his co-workers.[12] Serial roentgenograms of the chest were obtained at various intervals. These metastatic neoplasms also progressed geomet-

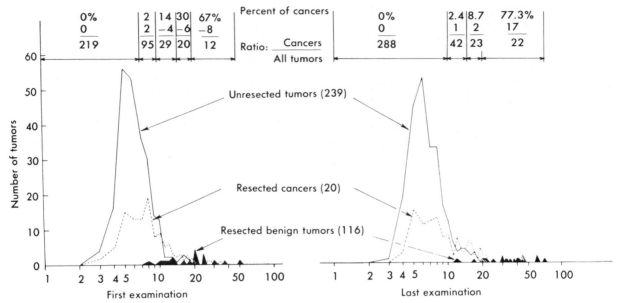

	Percent of cancers			
0%		2	14	30	67%
0		2	−4	−6	−8
219		95	29	20	12

	0%		2.4	8.7	77.3%
	0		1	2	17
	288		42	23	22

Ratio: Cancers / All tumors

Unresected tumors (239)

Resected cancers (20)

Resected benign tumors (116)

Number of tumors

First examination   Last examination

Diameter of (mm.) tumors of the large intestine and rectum measured on serial double contrast barium enemas

Fig. 39-6. The frequency distribution of the diameters of 375 colonic tumors measured on the first and last of a series of double-contrast enema studies. The upper scale gives the frequency of known cancers observed in the bracketed size ranges. Resected benign tumors and cancers were observed for an average of 834 days and the unresected tumors for an average of 939 days. (From Welin, S., Youker, J., and Spratt, J. S.: Amer. J. Roentgen. **90:**673, 1963.)

rically, and the time necessary for a doubling of their volume was constant. This "doubling time" varied in different patients and was much slower than had been anticipated. The "mean doubling time" was 116 days for the human pulmonary metastasis. Collins also postulated that the doubling time should be the same for primary and secondary tumors in each case.

In 1961 Spratt and Ackerman reported a single case of carcinoma of the colon.[51] The rate of growth of the tumor was studied by nine double-contrast enema examinations over a 7½-year period. In this instance the doubling time was 636 days.

In Malmö, 263 patients with 375 polypoid tumors of the large intestine were followed with serial double-contrast enema studies. The tumors were measured, and the time between examinations was recorded. Of the 375 tumors, 136 were excised from 109 patients. Histologic sections of these excised tumors were reviewed and classified independently by four pathologists. Their classifications were matched to the rates of growth observed for various tumors.

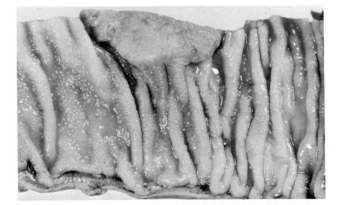

Fig. 39-7. Semicircle of a spreading plaque of cancer having a uniform thickness. The cancer approximated the geometric shape of a cylinder, maintaining uniform height, whereas the diameter of its circular base enlarged in all directions. (From Welin, S., Youker, J., and Spratt, J. S.: Amer. J. Roentgen. **90:**673, 1963.)

Most early cancers of the colon and rectum proliferate over the mucosal surface of the bowel as circumferentially spreading plaques (Fig. 39-7) of a rather constant height. It is possible, therefore, to relate the measurements of the diameters to changes in tumor volume. Tumor growth measurements made from roentgenograms in effect measure the net results of new cell formation, cell death, surface desquamation, and cell dissemination by way of the bloodstream. This recording of the dynamic growth changes in colonic polyps is not possible with any other method.

The results in the Malmö study were expressed both as absolute linear growth and as doubling time. By roentgenographically measuring the diameters of polypoid tumors at repeated roentgenologic examinations, the time necessary for doubling of tumor volume could be calculated. Doubling time, therefore, is a meaningful expression of geometric growth rate. From the data accumulated in the Malmö studies, it was not possible to determine whether polypoid tumors grow at a linear or a geometric rate (Fig. 39-8).

The carcinomas are distinctly predominant in the more rapid growth rate range, with a doubling time of between 138 and 1,155 days (Fig. 39-9). This corresponds to a linear diametrical rate of growth of between 0.0003 and 0.025 mm. a day, which represents an extremely slow rate of growth (Fig. 39-10). Even the most rapidly growing cancer would require 100 days to increase in diameter by 2.5 mm. At this growth rate a tumor the size of a Lieberkühn's gland would take 6 to 8 years to attain a diameter of 60 mm.

Adenomatous polyps tended to grow more slowly than the carcinomas, at a rate that did not vary with the presence of atypical cellular changes. However, the growth rate of some adenomatous polyps was as rapid as cancer. Hence, it cannot be concluded with certainty from the growth rate alone whether a neoplasm of the large bowel or rectum is malignant. By statistical analysis, however, the probability of malignancy can be estimated from the growth rate even when the polyp is very small.

Such analysis showed in the Malmö study that when the doubling time is more than 1,155 days the probability of cancer is only 1% to 2%. With a doubling time of 300 to 1,155 days the probability increases to 19% to 29%, and with a doubling time of fewer than 300 days it is 35%. Therefore, any increase in the size of a polypoid tumor must be considered as an absolute indication for operation (Fig. 39-11). Similar findings have been reported by Figiel and co-workers.[18]

Morphologic changes. The roentgenographic demonstration of a stalk or pedicle 2 cm. or more in length almost always indicates a benign polyp.[25,37] Very rare exceptions have been reported with metastases to regional lymph nodes from a focus of invasive cancer confined to the head of a pedunculated adenomatous polyp. Polypoid cancer may be pedunculate, but in these cases the pedicle is usually thick, short, and irregular.

A morphologic change to which much importance must be attached is a constant indentation at the base of the tumor. Such a dimpling or indentation of the colonic wall in the tangential view at the site of origin of the polyp almost

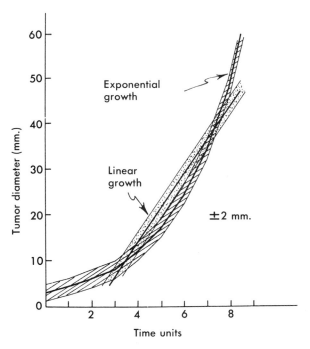

Fig. 39-8. Overlap of straight line and exponential diametric growth curves, with an error in diametric measurement of 2 mm. during five-eighths of the time required for a tumor to grow from a diameter of 3 mm. to a diameter of 60 mm. (From Welin, S., Youker, J., and Spratt, J. S.: Amer. J. Roentgen. **90:**673, 1963.)

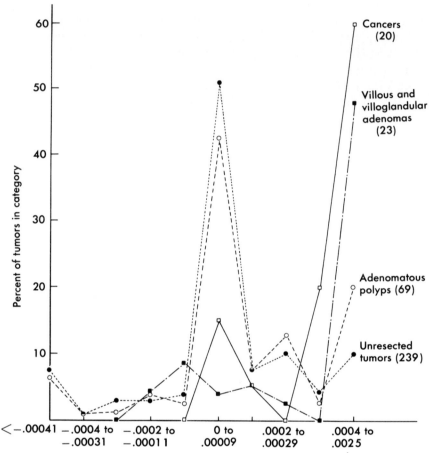

Fig. 39-9. Patterns of exponential diametric tumor growth. (From Welin, S., Youker, J., and Spratt, J. S.: Amer. J. Roentgen. 90:673, 1963.)

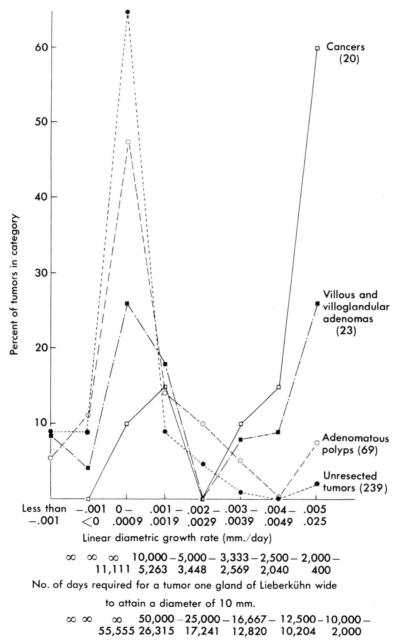

Fig. 39-10. Patterns of linear diametric tumor growth. (From Welin, S., Youker, J., and Spratt, J. S.: Amer. J. Roentgen. **90**:673, 1963.)

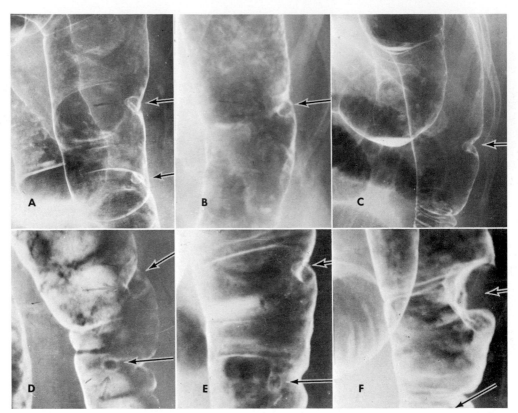

Fig. 39-11. Over 3½ years of observation by double-contrast enema studies, a polypoid tumor of 8 mm. grew into a 32 mm. symptomatic carcinoma in a 65-year-old man (upper arrow). This tumor had, from the first observation, marginal infiltration and indentation of the tumor base, the roentgenologic diagnostic signs of cancer, when viewed tangentially Simultaneously, a second polypoid tumor (lower arrow) showed neither growth nor infiltration during the period of observation. **A,** November 18, 1953; **B,** April 29, 1954; **C,** December 13, 1954; **D,** January 7, 1956; **E,** March 7, 1956; **F,** May 13, 1957. (From Welin, S., Youker, J. ,and Spratt, J. S.: Amer. J. Roentgen. **90**:673, 1963.)

always indicates that the polyp is malignant (Fig. 39-12).[64,72] This change is not pathognomonic since a local inflammatory process can, theoretically, produce a similar picture. The indentation is, however, so common in cancer that it is now regarded as an absolute indication for surgical removal. In many patients we have been able to follow the development of such an indentation (Fig. 39-11). Although this change is important as a positive sign, its absence does not exclude the possibility of malignant degeneration. Its value as a diagnostic sign applies only to broad-based polyps. Pedunculated polyps may exhibit a similar indentation at the base as the result of traction.

Another change, demonstrable only by the double-contrast method and useful in the evaluation of malignancy, is an irregular surface of the polypoid tumor. A rough, cauliflower-like surface instead of a smooth surface is found more often in carcinomas than in benign polyps (Fig. 39-13).[72]

The likelihood of malignancy is greater when the width of the base of a polyp is greater than the height on the profile view and when the face on outline of the neoplasm is oval (Fig. 39-14).

Sentinel polyps

Even in patients with large stenotic cancers of the colon, the double-contrast technique is extremely important. Not only are size, position, and shape of the tumor better evaluated, but this method also permits the discovery of any adjacent or so-called sentinel polyps (Fig. 39-14).

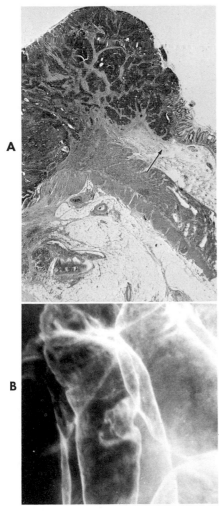

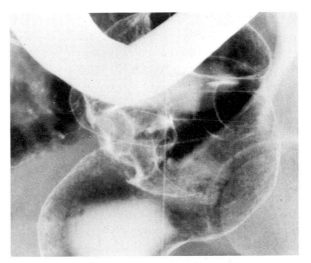

Fig. 39-13. Small carcinoma, demonstrating the rough surface of the tumor frequently found in carcinoma.

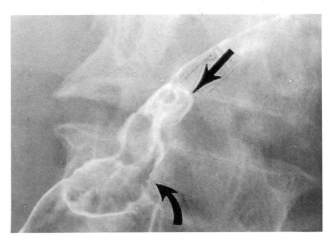

Fig. 39-14. The lower arrow shows a small sessile cancer with the length of the tumor exceeding the height. The upper arrow shows an adjacent benign pedunculated polyp demonstrating the target sign. (From Youker, J. E., and Welin, S.: Radiology 84:610, 1965.)

Fig. 39-12. A, Histologic picture of a small cancer that grew from a diameter of 8 mm. to a diameter of 32 mm. over 1,474 days of observation by double-contrast enema studies. The roentgenologic diagnosis of cancer was made when this tumor was 9 mm. in diameter because of the roentgenographic evidence of marginal infiltration. The tendency of a cancer to undermine normal mucosa adjacent to the neoplasm (arrow) is discernible by roentgenographic examination if the base of the cancer is viewed in a tangential projection during a double-contrast enema study. **B,** Another small malignant polyp demonstrating indentation of the base. This indentation is highly suggestive of malignancy. Benign polyps with a pedicle may also indent the base because of traction. (From Welin, S., Youker, J., and Spratt, J. S.: Amer. J. Roentgen. **90:**673, 1963.)

In studies of colonic carcinoma, sentinel polyps were present in 30% of the patients. Many of these polyps showed the same histologic malignant changes as the primary tumor. The histologic examination of excised sentinel polyps of seventy patients showed frank cancer in ten. Of the remaining sixty nonmalignant polyps, fifty-three demonstrated atypical cellular changes on histologic examination. A considerable distance may separate the site of the sentinel polyp from the more advanced carcinoma.

Roentgenography and proctoscopy in rectal diagnosis

Formerly, lesions of the rectum and the distal part of the sigmoid were considered to belong in the special domain of the proctologist. The role of the roentgenologist in evaluating this area was a subordinate one. This situation no longer holds true. With the Malmö technique the rectum and distal sigmoid are the parts of the colon that are most adequately and accurately diagnosed (Figs. 39-4 and 39-19). The roentgenologic examination should precede the proctoscopy so that it may act as a guide to the proctologist. Otherwise, polyps on the anterior wall and above Houston's valves may sometimes be overlooked at proctoscopy.

All polyps within reach of the protoscope should be removed whether or not they produce symptoms. The possibility of their being malignant is too great to allow them to remain, and visual inspection will not with certainty exclude malignancy.

We consider surgical removal indicated in all cases of polyps when: (1) their diameters measure more than 10 mm.; (2) invasive growth is seen at their base; (3) breadth of polyps is greater than height; (4) size of the polyps has increased during follow-up examination; (5) the surface of the polyps is irregular; (6) the polyps are multiple; (7) the polyps are within reach of the proctoscope.

All other polypoid neoplasms, in which the roentgenograms do not indicate immediate operation, are reexamined at 6, 12, and 24 months. All patients who have been operated on for a colonic cancer are requested to return for reexamination within 3 months. The patients are then reexamined once a year or, if considered necessary, more often.

EXTRINSIC LESIONS

Certain extrinsic lesions may press upon the colon and mimic intrinsic polypoid tumors.[43] One such extrinsic lesion, included here because of its roentgenographic similarity to polyps, is endometriosis. Although most common during the fifth decade of life,[53] it has been reported in patients as old as 67 and 69 years.[11] The lesions of endometriosis are usually found in the rectum and sigmoid, but implants may rarely occur in the cecal area. The characteristic roentgenographic appearance is that of a sharply margined

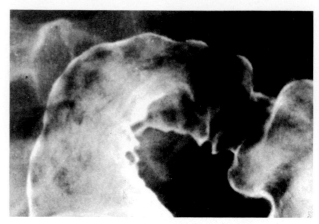

Fig. 39-15. A typical case of endometriosis, showing an extraluminal pressure defect with intact mucosa.

defect that may compress the lumen but rarely encompasses it (Fig. 39-15).[49] The colonic mucosa over the lesion remains intact. The diagnosis of endometriosis may be strongly suspected when these roentgenographic changes are associated with the typical clinical complaints of tenderness and rectal bleeding at the time of menstruation. It should be added that endometriosis of the pelvic serosa may also produce a characteristic deformity of the bowel at the rectosigmoid junction.[54]

Particularly frequent as extrinsic causes of filling defects in the cecum are lesions of the appendix, such as abscess, granuloma, carcinoma, carcinoid, or mucocele.[5] Appendiceal abscess or granuloma can often be suspected by the nature of the clinical picture. The diagnosis of mucocele of the appendix may be suggested when a sharply defined, polypoid, intraluminal mass is demonstrated in the cecum in the absence of appendiceal filling. Calcification is frequently seen in the mucocele and may aid in making the diagnosis. A similar lesion that must be considered in the differential diagnosis of polypoid defects of the cecum is an invaginated stump of the appendix after an appendectomy. It creates a polypoid lesion at the tip of the cecum that is indistinguishable from a true intraluminal tumor.

A large, round, and smooth filling defect with intact mucosa at the ileocecal valve area may occur because of a submucosal fatty infiltration of the valve leaflets. This lipomatosis of the ileocecal valve is often asymptomatic, representing a coincidental finding at barium enema examination. In other cases there may be vague abdominal distress, cramping pain, or even nausea and vomiting. The entity predominates in women and is uncommon under 40 years of age.[27] Lipoma of the ileocecal valve, which is much less frequent, can be differentiated histologically from this lesion because of the demarcating capsule of the lipoma. The radiologic diagnosis can be made with some assurance if barium can be refluxed back into the terminal ileum. Roentgenograms obtained after evacuation of the barium enema may demonstrate radial folds in the shape of a star. These folds probably represent prolapsed ileal mucosa. Lasser and Rigler stated that roentgenograms obtained before the introduction of the barium enema showed an increased radiolucency at the valve site because of the high fat content of this lesion.[32]

POLYPOID LESIONS OF THE COLON
Adenomas

The benign adenomatous lesions of the colon can be divided into two main groups—the adenomatous polyps, and papillary or villous adenomas.[25] There exists a variant of these two types, containing histologic elements of each, which Spjut has called a "villoglandular polyp."[64]

Adenomatous polyps are the most common benign tumors of the colon encountered by the radiologist. The very small growths, less than 4 mm. in diameter, often are hyperplastic or mucosal polyps rather than adenomatous polyps and should be considered as degenerative changes in the colonic mucosa and not neoplastic.[2,47]

The benign villous adenoma or papillary adenoma accounts for about 2.5% of all tumors of the colon and rectum.[26] Turell and Brodman, however, state that as many as 15% of the polyps within reach of the sigmoidoscope are villous.[57] This lesion has attracted attention because of its high incidence of malignant degeneration.[65] According to Grinnell and Lane, the incidence of cancer in adenomatous polyps less than 1 cm. in diameter is 0.6% compared to 12.5% in the villous adenomas of the same size.[25,47] Classically, the lesion is a large, broad-based mass that spreads over the bowel wall in a carpet-like fashion. It is most common in the rectum. About 10% of the tumors are pedunculated, and therefore the lesion must be differentiated from other

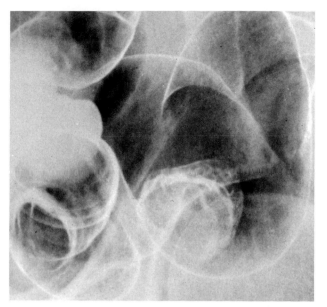

Fig. 39-16. A villous adenoma, polypoid in shape, showing a lacelike pattern because of contrast material caught between villous fronds.

polypoid tumors of the colon. Barium caught between the villous strands of the tumor appears on the roentgenogram either fine and lacelike or coarse, irregular, and warty (Fig. 39-16).[63,68] This appearance when present helps differentiate the villous tumors from other adenomatous polyps. Unfortunately, only one third of these lesions exhibit findings typical or suggestive of villous tumors.[30] The more proximal the lesion the less likely it is to have a typical villous appearance.[30] Prediction of malignancy based on the roentgenographic appearance of the tumor is not possible.[55]

There is a group of less common benign tumors of the bowel that must also be considered in any discussion of polypoid lesions of the colon.

Lipomas

Lipomas are the next most common benign tumors of the colon after adenomas. They predominate in women and in the later years of life. The roentgenographic appearance is characteristic enough to enable identification in a significant number of cases.[21,36,69] Most lipomas are submucosal.[21] They are more frequent in the ascending colon and cecum but may occur on the left side of the colon.[42] A stalk may form from prolonged fecal traction as the lipoma in-

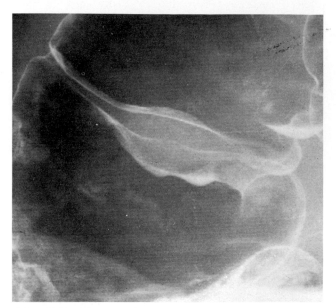

Fig. 39-17. Lipoma of the ascending colon. This lesion is characterized by a smooth surface and relative radiolucency.

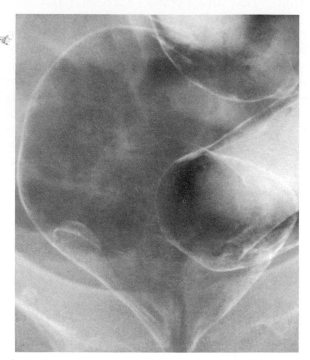

Fig. 39-18. A small carcinoid tumor of the rectum demonstrating the hat sign.

creases in size. Intussusception has been reported, with the pedunculated lipoma representing the nidus.[21] Rectal bleeding, the result of ulceration of the surface of the lipoma, may be the presenting symptom.

The roentgenographic appearance is that of a smooth, sharply outlined, relatively radiolucent polypoid lesion with intact mucosa (Fig. 39-17). The relative radiolucency has stimulated considerable controversy. Ginzburg and his colleagues expressed the opinion that it is the result of low radiodensity of the fat.[21] According to Margulis and Jovanovich only a very thin layer of barium adheres to the smooth surface of the lipoma, resulting in the appearance of a relatively radiolucent lesion on air-contrast barium enema examination.[36] These authors advocate plain water enemas and roentgen ray exposure at low kilovoltage to accentuate the increased radiolucency of the lipoma. Wolf, Melamed, and Khilnani have suggested the diagnosis of lipoma by comparing the change in shape of these soft fatty tumors between the filled film of the barium enema and the postevacuation film.[69] They also state that a pedicle develops only when the lipomas are large, and that these pedicles tend to be wider than those of adenomatous polyps.

Carcinoid tumors

The third most frequent lesion of the colon is the carcinoid. This tumor has stimulated great interest because of its variable malignancy and the specific clinical syndrome associated with metastatic carcinoid in the liver. Carcinoid tumors develop most frequently in young and middle-aged adults. This type of tumor originates in the deep layers of the mucosa or submucosa and appears initially as a small sessile growth.[53] The tumors may become pedunculated. They are more common in the appendix (90%)[14] and, as stated previously, are among the causes of extrinsic pressure on the cecum.

The rectum is the next most common site of carcinoid, followed by the areas of the cecum and ileocecal valve, respectively. The rectal lesions are usually small and rarely metastasize (2 of 37).[53] They cannot be differentiated from adenomatous polyps on air-contrast studies (Fig. 39-18). Carcinoid lesions elsewhere in the colon metastasize more frequently (9 of 12).[53] Those that metastasize have a roentgenographic appearance reminiscent of adenocarcinoma or lymphoma with a large, bulky, frequently ulcerated tumor often with a prominent extraluminal mass.[48]

Leiomyomas

Less common are the leiomyomas of the colon. They occur much more often in the stomach and small intestine than in the colon. According to Golden and Stout the incidence in the colon is greatest in the rectum, followed by that in the cecum.[23] Four gross pathologic types are described by MacKenzie, McDonald, and Waugh.[34] These are: (1) intracolic, appearing as polypoid defects on barium enema examination and occasionally even pedunculated; (2) extracolic; (3) circumferential; and (4) dumbbell tumors, polypoid defects in the lumen with extraluminal soft tissue density adjacent to the bowel wall. The characteristic picture of a deeply ulcerated lesion with massive bleeding, which is encountered in the stomach and small intestine, is rarely seen in the colon.[53] Certainty of differentiation between a leiomyoma and a leiomyosarcoma is not possible on the barium enema examination. Meszaros has stressed that the larger size, the higher incidence of deep ulceration, and the presence of an extraluminal mass suggest a leiomyosarcoma.[39]

Lymphangiomas

Among the very rare lesions of the colon is lymphangioma. The lesion consists of fluid-filled cystic masses with endothelium-lined walls. It is usually intramural, and the mucosa over the lesion is intact. However, lymphangiomatous tumors may have a stalk.[41] Arnett and Friedman demonstrated a lymphangioma in the ascending colon that disappeared completely on distention of the bowel.[3] Apparently, this disappearance was the result of the soft, easily compressible consistency of the lesion. A similar compressibility has been noted in cavernous hemangiomas and lipomas. Hemangiomas are usually multiple, often contain radiopaque phleboliths, and may cause exsanguinating rectal bleeding.

Extremely rare benign tumors

A number of other extremely rare benign tumors[53] deserve only to be listed. These include fibroma, enterogenous cysts, endothelioma, and granular cell myoblastoma. Most of these tumors are located submucosally or intramurally, their mucosa is intact, and their roentgenographic appearance is that of a benign lesion.

The so-called "benign lymphoma" is a lesion restricted to the rectum.[53] This tumor consists of well-differentiated lymphoid tissue, usually in the form of a sessile polyp, but occasionally pedunculated. Roentgenographic differentiation from adenomatous polyps is impossible. Development of lymphosarcoma from these lesions has not been proved.

POLYPOSIS SYNDROMES

Although the prevalence of gastrointestinal polyposis syndromes is low, during their careers most radiologists will see one or more patients with intestinal polyposis. More than 300 cases of multiple familial polyposis and Peutz-Jeghers syndrome, respectively, and about 200 cases of Gardner's syndrome have been documented in the medical literature. Undoubtedly, many patients with these syndromes are not reported. The results of two independent studies suggest that the incidence of multiple familial polyposis in the United States is about 1 in 7000 to 8000 live births.[100,101] Peutz-Jeghers syndrome has been estimated to occur at about the same frequency as familial multiple polyposis.[95] In the pediatric age group, juvenile polyps are the most common polypoid lesion found in the colon. Turcot's syndrome and Cronkhite-Canada syndrome, although rare, are well defined clinical entities.

The radiologist plays an important role in the diagnosis and evaluation of the gastrointestinal polyposis syndromes. Many patients with unsuspected alimentary tract polyposis are referred for roentgenographic examination because of gastrointestinal symptoms. The polyposis syndromes should be considered when (1) a gastrointestinal polyp is identified in a young patient, (2) two or more polyps are demonstrated in any patient, or (3) a colon carcinoma is present in a patient less than 40 years old. A high index of suspicion is imperative because failure to recognize polyposis coli syndromes associated with the development of malignancy not only inevitably results in tragedy for the patient but also delays detection of other afflicted family members. Elective colon resection results in clinical cure for these patients. Other polyposis syndromes such as Peutz-Jeghers syndrome and Cronkhite-Canada syndrome are equally important to diagnose accurately so that appropriate management may be rendered.

Gastrointestinal polyposis syndromes that affect the colon may be classified into hereditary or nonhereditary types as in the following outline.

A. Hereditary
1. Familial multiple polyposis
2. Gardner's syndrome
3. Peutz-Jeghers syndrome
4. Turcot's syndrome
B. Nonhereditary
1. Cronkhite-Canada syndrome
2. Juvenile polyposis
   (sometimes hereditary)

The three major hereditary syndromes—familial multiple polyposis, Gardner's, and Peutz-Jeghers—are all characterized by autosomal dominant inheritance. Consequently, approximately half the offspring of individuals with these syndromes will be afflicted and no sex predilection occurs. Turcot's syndrome appears to be transmitted by an autosomal homozygous recessive gene, a fact that helps account for the great rarity of the syndrome. Cronkhite-Canada syndrome is nonfamilial, and the majority of patients with juvenile polyposis have a normal family history.

Familial multiple polyposis

Familial multiple polyposis is characterized by hereditary transmission, polyposis coli, and the eventual development of colon carcinoma. This disease, recognized since Cripp's description in 1882,[79] is the best-known hereditary gastrointestinal polyposis syndrome and serves as a prototype with which other polyposis syndromes can be compared. Large numbers of patients with multiple polyposis studied by Dukes and Veal reveal an autosomal dominant mechanism of inheritance.[84,109] The abnormal gene has high penetrance, estimated to be about 80%. Approximately two thirds of afflicted individuals have a family history of colonic polyps or carcinoma, and about one third represent sporadic cases.[109]

The onset of clinical symptoms usually occurs during the third or fourth decades of life, with an average age of about 30 years. Clinical symptoms include vague abdominal pain, diarrhea, bloody stools, weight loss, or prolapse of a polyp through the rectum. Occasionally, the disorder is associated with electrolyte depletion significant enough to cause weakness or protein-losing enteropathy, which results in hypoalbuminemia and edema. A high percentage of individuals with clinical symptoms have an existing colon carcinoma or develop a large-bowel malignancy within 2 years.[109]

The gastrointestinal polyps are numerous, range from pinhead lesions to 1 cm. or more in size, and may be sessile or pedunculated. The rectum and left colon are more frequently involved than is the right colon, but often the entire colonic mucosa is carpeted with myriads of polyps so that normal mucosa is not seen. Involvement of the small bowel or stomach or both occurs in less than 5% of the patients. This generalized form of polyposis has been termed "diffuse familial polyposis."[112] The polyps in patients with familial multiple polyposis generally arise during the first or second decade of life but are not usually evident until after puberty. Occasionally, the polyps develop for the first time in afflicted individuals over 40 years of age. On histologic examination the polyps are indistinguishable from the common solitary adenomatous polyps found in the general adult population. Occasionally, villous adenomas or inflammatory polyps may also be present.

Colon cancers arise about 15 years after the onset of polyposis, a time interval similar to that recorded for the development of colon cancer after the onset of chronic ulcerative colitis. As a rule, colon cancers develop in patients with familial multiple polyposis between the ages of 20 to 40 years and are practically unknown below the age of 20 years.[92] Colon carcinoma develops in nearly 100% of untreated patients. The natural history of the disease in untreated patients is death from metastatic disease by the age of 45 years, the average age being 40 years.[109]

Although sigmoidoscopic findings are nearly always positive when the roentgenographic examination of the large bowel demonstrates polyps,[92] a colon examination should be performed in all suspected patients in order to document the size, number, and distribution of polyps, and to search for carcinoma (Fig. 39-19). The polyps can be identified on barium enema examination as multiple punctate eminences that impart a serrated or saw-tooth contour to the intraluminal column of barium, or as larger filling defects 1 to 2 cm. in diameter.[94] Some of the lesions may have pedicles. In many instances the polyps are most numerous in the left colon. Involvement of the terminal ileum is

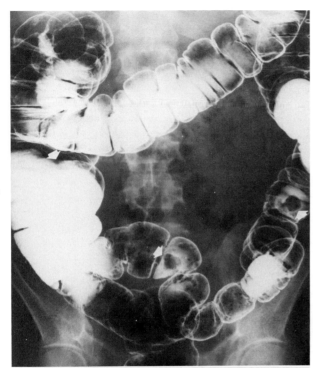

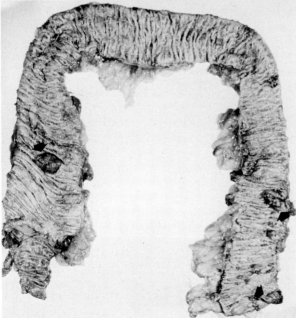

Fig. 39-19. Familial multiple polyposis. **A,** A pneumocolon examination demonstrates numerous 2 to 5 mm. polyps and three 1.5 to 2.0 cm. polypoid carcinomas (arrows). **B,** Gross specimen of resected colon. Myriads of small polyps are seen along with the three polypoid carcinomas (arrows).

unusual. Small, elusive polyps, 1 to 2 mm. in diameter, may be hidden by barium but are often elegantly shown on pneumocolon examination. Carcinomas may appear as polypoid filling defects, areas of symmetrical, segmental narrowing, or typical annular lesions with overhanging margins. Multiple carcinomas are common.

Because colon carcinoma will invariably develop in virtually all patients with familial multiple polyposis, the need for early and accurate diagnosis in affected individuals and subsequent family screening cannot be overstressed. Familial multiple polyposis should be regarded as a curable disease. The colon is a dispensable organ, not necessary for useful life, and colon carcinoma is entirely preventable if patients with familial multiple polyposis are identified when they are young and prophylactic colectomy is performed.[91] Generally, surgery can be deferred until the patients are in their late teens or early twenties. Total colectomy with an ileorectal anastomosis is a suitable operation for reliable patients who will return for follow-up proctoscopic examination. In some patients the rectal polyps regress following colectomy.[77] Recurrent rectal polyps may be eradicated by cautery.

Gardner's syndrome

In a series of articles written between 1950 and 1953, Gardner and co-workers[85] described a syndrome featuring autosomal dominant inheritance, multiple soft tissue tumors, osteomatosis, polyposis coli, and a potential for colon malignancy. Patients with Gardner's syndrome seek medical treatment for cosmetic deformities caused by the soft tissue or bony lesions, dental abnormalities, or abdominal symptoms. Symptoms referable to the colon are similar to those described for patients with familial multiple polyposis. In some instances the patients have complaints of excessive scar formation (keloids) or symptoms of bowel obstruction caused by peritoneal adhesions.

The cutaneous lesions consist of sebaceous or inclusion cysts, which are most numerous on the scalp and back but which may be present on the face or extremities. Benign mesenchymal tumors include fibromas, lipomas, lipofibromas, leiomyomas, and neurofibromas.[78] Malignant sarcomas, such as fibrosarcomas or leiomyosarcomas are unusual but do occur. The fibrous tissue in

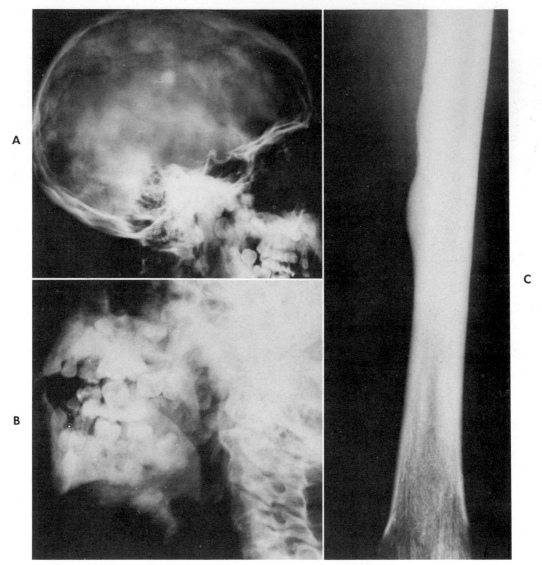

Fig. 39-20. Boney abnormalities associated with Gardner's syndrome. **A,** Multiple osteomas of skull. **B,** Osteomatosis of the mandible. **C,** Localized cortical thickening of the femur.

patients with Gardner's syndrome often has a pronounced tendency toward proliferation, thereby resulting in desmoid tumors, keloids, hypertrophied scars, mammary fibromatosis, peritoneal adhesions, mesenteric fibrosis, and retroperitoneal fibrosis. Fibrous tissue proliferation may arise either spontaneously or in response to injury or surgery.

Localized areas of dense bone (osteomas), appearing as exostoses or enostoses, are commonly present in the maxilla, mandible, or skull (Fig. 39-20, *A* and *B*).[113] Localized bony overgrowth may cause cosmetic deformity. The long bones,

particularly the femur and tibia, are frequently abnormal and demonstrate localized cortical thickening, wavy cortical thickening (Fig. 39-20, *C*), or exostoses.[76] The long bones may also be slightly shortened and bowed.[113] Dental abnormalities, commonly present, include odontomas, unerupted supernumerary teeth, hypercementosis, and a tendency toward numerous caries. The patients often require dental prosthesis at an early age. Both the bone and soft tissue lesions often appear before or during puberty, and may precede the development of polyps.

The intestinal polyps are usually limited to

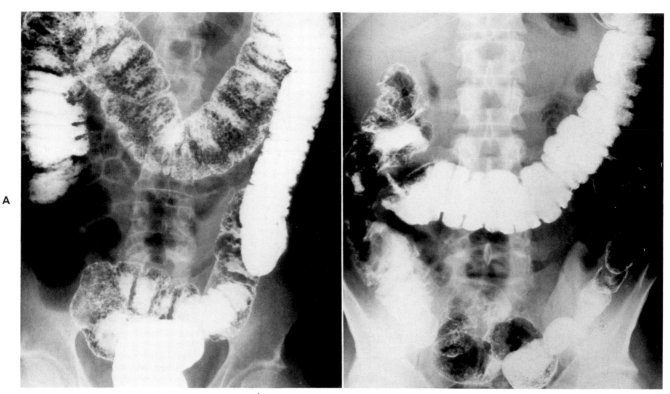

Fig. 39-21. Gardner's syndrome. Colon examinations in two afflicted individuals from the same family. **A,** Myriads of small polyps carpet the colon. **B,** An annular hepatic flexure carcinoma is present. Numerous small polyps are seen in the sigmoid. (Courtesy Dr. Alvin A. Watne.)

the colon. Extracolonic polyps in the small bowel or stomach occur in less than 5% of the patients; however, lymphoid hyperplasia of the terminal ileum, commonly present in Gardner's syndrome, may cause a cobblestone appearance that simulates multiple adenomas. The polyps generally appear during the teens and increase in number during the third and fourth decades of life, often resulting in carpeting of the entire colon (Fig. 39-21, *A*). On gross and histologic examination the polyps do not differ from the adenomatous polyps present in patients with familial multiple polyposis. Furthermore, virtually all patients with Gardner's syndrome eventually develop colon carcinoma if the colon is not removed (Fig. 39-21, *B*). In untreated patients with colon carcinoma, the average age at death is 41 years, which is essentially identical to that of patients with familial multiple polyposis from large-bowel cancer.[111]

McKusick has suggested that the respective genes causing Gardner's syndrome and familial polyposis may be alleles occurring at the same chromosomal locus.[96] Smith hypothesizes that Gardner's syndrome and familial multiple polyposis represent opposite poles of a disease spectrum produced by a single pleotrophic gene with varying expressivity.[105] Contrary to earlier opinions,[96] the colonic polyps associated with the two syndromes do not appear to differ in growth pattern, distribution and number, histologic features, or malignant potential. Incomplete manifestations of Gardner's syndrome occur in individual patients or some families. Polyposis coli may be accompanied by only the soft tissue or bony lesions. Conversely, patients with familial multiple polyposis have a tendency to develop desmoid tumors[105] and small-bowel adhesions.[93] Whatever the relationship between Gardner's syndrome and familial polyposis may be, the threat of colon malignancy is identical, and prophylactic colectomy should be performed when

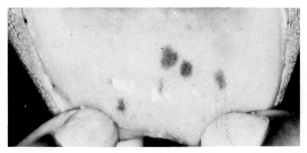

Fig. 39-22. Peutz-Jeghers syndrome. Pigmented macules, characteristic of the syndrome, are present on the mucosal surface of the lower lip.

patients afflicted with either syndrome are about 20 years of age.

Peutz-Jeghers syndrome

In 1921 Peutz described the association of mucocutaneous pigmentation and gastrointestinal polyposis in members of a Dutch family.[99] The syndrome remained generally unrecognized, however, until 1949 when Jeghers and co-workers reported 10 patients with the syndrome and documented a mendelian dominant mode of inheritance.[88] Peutz-Jeghers syndrome is worldwide in distribution and has no racial predilection. About 50% of the reported cases have a family history of the syndrome, whereas the remaining 50% are sporadic.[73]

The characteristic mucocutaneous pigmented lesions usually develop during infancy or early childhood[75] and are present in nearly all Peutz-Jeghers patients. Unless the lesions are specifically looked for, however, they often are not noticed by either the patient or the physician. The mucocutaneous lesions appear as brown or black, oval or slightly irregular, macules that are 1 to 5 mm. in diameter. The lesions are most common on the lips, particularly the mucosal surface of the lower lip (Fig. 39-22) and on the buccal mucosa. Pigmentation occurs less frequently on the face or volar aspect of the hands and feet. Dissociation between the skin lesions and gastrointestinal polyposis is unusual.[81,82]

The clinical symptoms are usually related to gastrointestinal polyposis. The most common clinical symptom is cramping, abdominal pain caused by intussusception.[83] Most of the intussusceptions are transient but some persist and cause significant small-bowel obstruction. Rectal bleeding, or melena, occurs in about 30% of the

patients, but massive gastrointestinal bleeding is rare. Chronic hypochromic anemia secondary to low-grade intestinal blood loss is commonly present. In some instances prolapse of a rectal polyp brings the patient to clinical attention.

The polyps in patients with Peutz-Jeghers syndrome occur predominantly in the alimentary tract but are occasionally located in the urinary[106] or respiratory tract. The small bowel is involved in more than 95% of the patients, the colon and rectum in about 30%, and the stomach in about 25%. The polyps are multiple and range in size from 0.1 to 3 cm. Myriad 1 to 2 mm. nodules may be present in the small bowel, but carpeting has not been observed in the stomach or colon. The small bowel and gastric polyps, once considered precancerous adenomas, are currently regarded as benign hamartomatous malformations without malignant potential.[73,82] Most colonic polyps in patients with Peutz-Jeghers syndrome, however, are proliferative mucosal lesions that are indistinguishable from adenomatous polyps.[97] Gastrointestinal carcinomas in patients with Peutz-Jeghers syndrome have been reported to occur in the stomach and colon (the usual sites of gastrointestinal tract carcinoma) and the duodenum.[83] Carcinoma is rare in the small bowel. The incidence of gastrointestinal carcinoma in patients with Peutz-Jeghers syndrome is probably greater than that in the general population.[83]

On roentgenographic examination, jejunal or ileal polyps, often associated with intussusception, are usually demonstrated during a carefully performed small-bowel examination, utilizing compression and appropriate spot films.[86] Colonic polyps, when present, number from two to a dozen or more (Fig. 39-23, *A*). Diffuse carpeting of the colon has not been observed. The colonic lesions are often pedunculated. Sessile lesions greater than 1.0 to 1.5 cm. in diameter, lesions demonstrating rapid growth, or annular lesions (Fig. 39-23, *B*) should be regarded as suspicious for carcinoma.

Patients with Peutz-Jeghers syndrome benefit from supportive, conservative treatment. Indiscriminant prophylactic resection of intestine may cause death from malabsorption. Surgery should be reserved for patients with persistent obstruction, severe bleeding, or suspected malignancy. During operation the surgeon should sacrifice as little bowel as possible.[82]

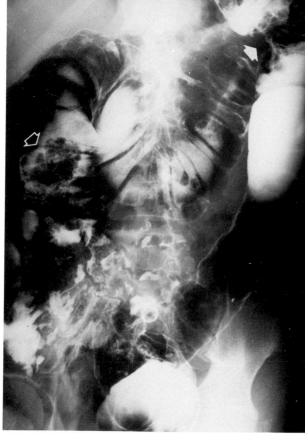

Fig. 39-23. Colon lesions in Peutz-Jeghers syndrome. **A,** The arrows identify three benign sigmoid polyps. No other colon lesions were present. **B,** A constricting carcinoma (arrow) is seen in the splenic flexure. The resected specimen also demonstrated about a dozen small polyps and a sessile hamartoma, 6 cm. in diameter, located in the cecum (open arrow).

Turcot syndrome

An association between polyposis coli and central nervous system tumors was suggested by Turcot and co-workers in 1959.[108] To date, seven patients (six from two families) with the syndrome have been documented.[74] The fact that neither brain tumors nor colonic polyps appeared in the parents of affected individuals suggests an autosomal recessive mode of inheritance.

In each patient clinical symptoms developed during the second decade and consisted predominantly of either diarrhea caused by colonic polyps or seizures secondary to a brain tumor. Most of the patients died as a result of their central nervous system malignancy.

The polyps are multiple, range in diameter from 0.1 to 3 cm., and are limited to the rectum and colon. The polyps appear to be benign adenomas, but histologic description has been incomplete. Colon carcinoma developed in two patients. The majority of central nervous system tumors have been supratentorial glioblastomas.

Cronkhite-Canada syndrome

In 1955, Cronkhite and Canada[80] described two patients with generalized gastrointestinal polyposis associated with ectodermal abnormalities. Twelve more isolated case reports have appeared in the literature, and we have recently seen one additional patient.[89,98] The disorder develops during middle or old age (average age 62 years, range 42 to 75), and shows no sexual, familial, racial, or geographic predilection.

The most common presenting symptom is diarrhea of several month's or more duration. The stools are watery, often containing blood or mucus or both. The diarrhea is usually accompanied by anorexia, vomiting, abdominal pain, and severe weight loss. Marked weakness results from electrolyte loss and hypocalemia often causes tetany. Protein is also lost in the stool, and most patients develop peripheral edema secondary to hypoalbuminemia. The ectodermal abnormalities, which are invariably present, include alopecia, brownish hyperpigmentation, and atrophy of the fingernails and toenails.

Roentgenographic examination demonstrates multiple gastric and colonic polyps (Fig. 39-24). More than half the patients have evidence of small-bowel polyps that may be accompanied by thickened mucosal folds and increased intralu-

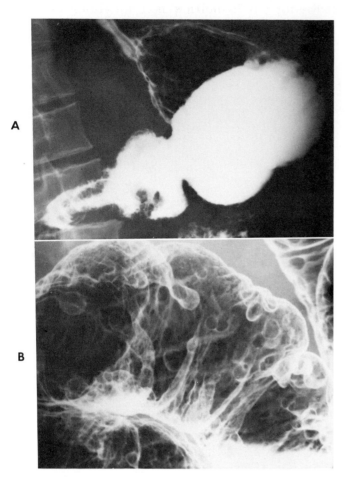

Fig. 39-24. Cronkhite-Canada syndrome. **A,** Hundreds of polypoid lesions, pinhead in size, mammillate the distal half of the stomach. Several larger polypoid lesions are also present in the antrum. **B,** Spot film of splenic flexure. Numerous polypoid lesions are well shown.

minal fluid. Esophageal polyps have been described in two patients.

On histologic examination the polyps once regarded as adenomas reveal inflammatory changes of the juvenile type.[89,90] Villous atrophy or cystlike dilatation of glands, as seen in Menetrier's disease, may be present. The lesions do not appear to be associated with any potential for gastrointestinal malignancy.

In females the disease generally has an inexorable, downhill course resulting in death from inanition and cachexia within 6 to 18 months after onset of the diarrhea. In males a tendency exists for remission.

Juvenile polyposis

Juvenile polyps, although occasionally present in adults, are so called because they generally develop during childhood. These polyps, also called retention or inflammatory polyps, have characteristic gross and histologic features that distinguish them from adenomatous polyps and cellular hamartomas. The juvenile polyp usually has a smooth, round contour, whereas adenomatous polyps often have a fissured, lobulated appearance. The polyps are soft in consistency, and, on cut surface, reveal many cystic spaces filled with mucin. The predominant histologic feature is abundant connective tissue stoma that contains cystic structures lined with epithelium. Numerous inflammatory cells may be present. These lesions are nonneoplastic and are not associated with malignancy.

Juvenile polyps are seen in several different clinical conditions; they may occur as: (1) isolated colonic polyps in children; (2) multiple lesions that may involve the stomach and small bowel in addition to the colon; (3) numerous lesions carpeting the colon in babies; (4) inflammatory polyps coexisting with colonic polyps in patients with familial multiple polyposis; and (5) the underlying intestinal lesions in Cronkhite-Canada syndrome.

Most juvenile polyps develop as isolated colonic lesions in children less than 10 years of age. The lesions are solitary in about 75% of the cases and, when multiple, seldom number more than several.[104] The family history is generally normal. Rectal bleeding is the most common presenting symptom; other symptoms include rectal prolapse, abdominal pain, and diarrhea.[87] On barium enema the polyps are identified as roundish filling defects, often pedunculated, which are located most commonly in the rectum or sigmoid. Because the lesions are benign and have a tendency toward autoamputation or regression (Fig. 39-25), surgical treatment is not warranted in the absence of severe bleeding or intussusception.

Occasionally, numerous juvenile polyps develop in the colon[110] and in some instances, also in the small bowel or stomach.[103] This form of juvenile polyposis is often familial and may be encountered in teenagers and adults as well as in children. Mild rectal bleeding is the most common clinical symptom. A rare, nonfamilial juvenile polyposis syndrome associated with

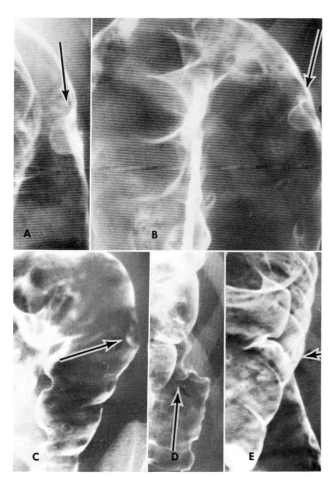

Fig. 39-25. Regression in diameter of a polyp in a 5-year-old child from 9 mm. to 4 mm. during 4½ years of observation. Similar though less striking regression has been observed in adults. **A,** December 21, 1953; **B,** August 8, 1955; **C,** January 31, 1956; **D,** August 16, 1957; **E,** February 10, 1958. (From Welin, S., Youker, J., and Spratt, J. S.: Amer. J. Roentgen. **90:**673, 1963.)

bloody diarrhea, anemia, hypoproteinemia and edema has been described in infants less than 1 year of age.[102,107] The six isolated cases reported have all occurred in males.[107] Symptoms developed during the first few months of life and the children died prior to 18 months of age.

Differential diagnosis

The gastrointestinal polyposis syndromes are usually easily separated from one another (Table 39-3). Once the radiologist suspects the diagnosis of a polyposis syndrome, the specific syndrome can often be established by obtaining a family history and performing an abbreviated

Table 39-3. Summary of features characterizing gastrointestinal polyposis syndromes

Syndrome	Symptom onset usual age (yrs.)	Hereditary transmission	Distribution Stomach	Distribution Small bowel	Distribution Colon	Histology	Additional features	Prognosis
Multiple polyposis	15 to 30	Dominant	Less than 5%	Less than 5%	100%	Adenomas		Colon carcinoma
Gardner's	15 to 30	Dominant	~ 5%	~ 5%	100%	Adenomas	Soft tissue tumors, osteomatosis	Colon carcinoma
Peutz-Jeghers	10 to 30	Dominant	25%	95%	30%	Cellular hamartomas	Pigmented skin lesions	With or without G.I. tract carcinoma
Turcot's	Teens	Recessive	—	—	100%	Adenomas	C.N.S. tumors	C.N.S. tumors
Cronkhite-Canada	40 to 70	None	100%	Less than 50%	100%	Inflammatory glandular dilatation	Alopecia, onychia, hyperpigmentation. Diarrhea with protein and electrolyte losses	Death often of cachexia
Juvenile polyps (common type)	Less than 10	Usually none	—	—	100%	Inflammatory	Diarrhea with protein loss possible	Regression, autoamputation

physical examination to search for soft tissue tumors, mucocutaneous pigmentation, or other ectodermal abnormalities. Roentgenographic examination of the entire gastrointestinal tract is necessary to determine the number, size, and distribution of polyps, and to identify, when present, associated gastrointestinal malignancy. This information is helpful in differential diagnosis and in planning therapy.

In some instances, overlaps between the established polyposis syndromes may occur, such as those described between familial multiple polyposis and Gardner's syndrome. Additionally, some pedigrees demonstrate a familial modification of the general features of a given syndrome. For example, families with Peutz-Jeghers syndrome may show a polyp distribution differing from the average values listed in Table 39-4. In one family, polyps were located predominantly in the small bowel and stomach[75]; whereas, in another family the polyps were located primarily in the small bowel and colon.[81]

In addition to being separated from one another, polyposis syndromes affecting the colon also need to be distinguished from other conditions that cause multiple filling defects in the large bowel: retained fecal material, pseudopolyposis secondary to inflammatory colitis, nodular lymphoid hyperplasia, benign lymphoid hyperplasia, ganglioneuromatosis, lipomatous polyposis, pneumatosis intestinalis, and lymphosarcoma. Full knowledge of the clinical, laboratory, and roentgenographic findings for a given patient usually permits accurate diagnosis of the underlying condition. In some instances differentiation between the above conditions is dependent on histologic examination of tissue material.

REFERENCES

1. Ackerman, L. V., and del Regato, J. A.: Cancer: diagnosis, treatment, and prognosis, ed. 4, St. Louis, 1970, The C. V. Mosby Co.
2. Arminski, T. C., and McLean, D. W.: Incidence and distribution of adenomatous polyps of the colon and rectum based on 1,000 autopsy examinations, Diseases of the colon and rectum, vol. 7, 1964, J. B. Lippincott Co.
3. Arnett, N. L., and Friedman, P. S.: Lymphangioma of the colon; roentgen aspects, Radiology 67:882, 1956.
4. Bacon, H. E., Laurens, J., and Peale, A. R.: Histopathology of adenomatous polyps of the colon and rectum, Surgery 29:663, 1951.
5. Bartone, N. F., Grieco, R. V., and Vasilas, A.: Roentgen signs in lesions affecting the caecum, Amer. J. Roentgen. 84:285, 1960.
6. Blatt, L. J.: Polyps of the colon and rectum; incidence and distribution, Dis. Colon Rectum 4:277-282, 1961.
7. Blum, H. F.: On the mechanism of cancer induction by ultraviolet radiation. III, The growth curve, J. Nat. Cancer Inst. 23:337, 1959.
8. Burdette, W. J.: Carcinoma of the colon and antecedent epithelium, Springfield, Ill., 1970, Charles C Thomas, Publisher.
9. Castleman, B., and Krickstein, H. Z.: Do adenomatous polyps of the colon become malignant? New Eng. J. Med. 267:469, 1962.
10. Christie, A. C., Coe, F. O., Hampton, A. O., and Wyatt, G. M.: Value of tannic acid enema and post-evacuation roentgenograms in examination of the colon, Amer. J. Roentgen. 63:657, 1950.
11. Colcock, B. P., and Lamphier, T. A.: Endometriosis of the large and small intestine, Surgery 28:997, 1950.
12. Collins, V. P., Loeffler, K., and Tivey, H.: Observations on growth rates of human tumours, Amer. J. Roentgen. 76:988, 1956.
13. Cremin, B. J., and Louw, J. H.: Polyps in the large bowel in children, Clin. Radiol. 21:195-200, 1970.
14. Dockerty, M. B.: Carcinoids of the gastrointestinal tract, Amer. J. Clin. Path. 25:794, 1955.
15. Dockerty, M. B.: Pathologic aspects in the control of spread of colonic carcinoma, Proc. Mayo Clin. 33:157, 1958.
16. Ekelund, G.: On cancer and polyps of colon and rectum, Acta Path. Microbiol. Scand. 59:165, 1963.
17. Enquist, I. F.: The incidence and significance of polyps of the colon and rectum, Surgery 42:681, 1957.
18. Figiel, L. S., Figiel, S. J., and Wietersen, F. K.: Roentgenologic observations of growth rates of colonic polyps and carcinoma, Acta Radiol. [Diagn.] (Stockholm) 3:417, 1965.
19. Friedland, G. W., and Poole, G. J.: False-positive "Eccentric target sign" on barium-air contrast enema examination, Radiology 99:67, 1971.
20. Gianturco, C., and Miller, G. A.: Routine search for colonic polyps by high-voltage radiography, Radiology 60:496, 1953.
21. Ginzburg, L., Weingarten, M., and Fischer, M. G.: Submucous lipoma of the colon, Ann. Surg. 148:767, 1958.
22. Gold, P., and Freedman, S. O.: Demonstration of tumor-specific antigens in human colonic carcinomata by immunological tolerance and absorption techniques, J. Exp. Med. 121:439, 1965.
23. Golden, T., and Stout, A. P.: Smooth muscle tumors of the gastrointestinal tract and retroperitoneal tissues, Surg. Gynec. Obstet. 73:784, 1941.
24. Grinnell, R. S.: The chance of cancer and lymphatic metastasis in small colon tumors discovered on x-ray examination, Ann. Surg. 159:132-138, 1964.
25. Grinnell, R. S., and Lane, N.: Benign and malignant adenomatous polyps and papillary adenomas of the colon and rectum, an analysis of 1,856

tumors in 1,335 patients, Inter. Abstr. Surg. **106:** 519-538, 1958.

26. Hines, M. O., Hanley, P. H., Ray, J. E., and Bralliar, M.: Villous tumors of the colon and rectum, Dis. Colon Rectum **1:**128, 1958.
27. Hultén, J.: Lipomatosis of the ileocaecal valve, Acta Chir. Scand. **129:**104, 1965.
28. Jarre, H. A., and Figiel, S. J.: Refinements in radiologic diagnosis of colonic disease. In Rajewsky, B., editor, Proceedings of Ninth International Congress of Radiology, Munich, 1959, vol. 1, Stuttgart, 1961, Georg Thieme Verlag.
29. Kaye, G. I., Pascal, R. R., and Lane, N.: The colonic pericryptal fibroblast sheath: Replication, migration, and cytodifferentiation of mesenchymal cell system in adult tissue, Gastroenterology **60:**515, 1971.
30. Kaye, J. J., and Bragg, D.: Unusual roentgenologic and clinicopathologic features of villous adenomas of the colon, Radiology **91:**799-806, 1968.
31. Kendig, T.: Personal communications.
32. Lasser, E. C., and Rigler, L. G.: Ileocecal valve syndrome, Gastroenterology **28:**1, 1955.
33. Lucke, H. H., Hodge, K. E., and Patt, N. L.: Fatal liver damage after barium enemas containing tannic acid, Canad. Med. Ass. J. **89:**1111, 1963.
34. MacKenzie, D. A., McDonald, J. R., and Waugh, J. M.: Leiomyoma and leiomyosarcoma of the colon, Ann. Surg. **139:**67, 1954.
35. Margulis, A. R.: The changing concepts of colonic polyposis, Amer. J. Roentgen. **113:**386, 1971.
36. Margulis, A. R., and Jovanovich, A.: The roentgen diagnosis of submucous lipomas of the colon, Amer. J. Roentgen. **84:**1114, 1960.
37. Marshak, R. H.: The pedunculated adenomatous polyp, Amer. J. Dig. Dis. **10:**958-967, 1965.
38. McAlister, W. H., Anderson, M. S., Bloomberg, G. R., and Margulis, A. R.: Lethal effects of tannic acid in the barium enema, Radiology **80:**765, 1963.
39. Meszaros, W. T.: Leiomyosarcoma of the colon, Amer. J. Roentgen. **89:**766, 1963.
40. Mottram, J. C.: On the origin of tar tumours in mice, either from single cells or many cells, J. Path. Bact. **40:**407, 1935.
41. Ochsner, S. F., Ray, J. E., and Clark, W. H.: Lymphangioma of the colon, Radiology **72:**423, 1959.
42. Pemberton, J. de J., and McCormack, C. J.: Submucous lipomas of colon and rectum, Amer. J. Surg. **37:**205, 1937.
43. Phillips, W. M., Remine, W. H., Beahrs, O. H., and Scudamore, H. H.: Benign lesions of the cecum simulating carcinoma, J.A.M.A. **172:**1465, 1960.
44. Portes, C., and Majarakis, Y.: Proctosigmoidoscopy-incidence of polyps in 50,000 examinations, J.A.M.A. **163:**411, 1957.
45. Rosensweig, J., and Horwitz, A.: Adenomatous tumours of the colon and rectum; the importance of early detection and treatment, Amer. Surg. **24:**515, 1958.
46. Scarborough, R. A.: The relationship between polyps and carcinoma of the colon and rectum, Dis. Colon Rectum **3:**336, 1960.
47. Seaman, W. B.: Disease of the colon: new concepts, old problems, Radiology **100:**251-269, 1971.
48. Shulman, H., and Giustra, P.: Invasive carcinoids of the colon, Radiology **98:**139-144, 1971.
49. Spjut, H. J., and Perkins, D. E.: Endometriosis of the sigmoid colon and rectum, Amer. J. Roentgen. **82:**1070, 1959.
50. Spratt, J. S., and Ackerman, L. V.: Relationship of the size of colonic tumors to their cellular composition and biological behavior, Surg. Forum **10:**56, 1960.
51. Spratt, J. S., and Ackerman, L. V.: The growth of a colonic adenocarcinoma, Amer. Surg. **27:**23, 1961.
52. Stevenson, C. A., Moreton, R. D., and Cooper, E. M.: The nature of fictitious polyps of the colon, Amer. J. Roentgen. **63:**89, 1950.
53. Stout, A. P.: Tumors of the colon and rectum (excluding carcinoma and adenoma). In Turell, R., editor: Diseases of the colon and anorectum, vol. 1, Philadelphia, 1959, W. B. Saunders Co.
54. Theander, G., and Wehlin, L.: Deformation of the rectosigmoid junction in the pelvis endometriosis, Acta Radiol. (Stockholm) **55:**241, 1961.
55. Turek, R., Davis, W. C., Welson, W. J., and Olson, R. O.: The roentgenographic diagnosis of villous tumors of the colon, Amer. J. Roentgen. **113:**349-351, 1971.
56. Turell, R.: Colonic adenomas, Amer. J. Surg. **76:**783, 1948.
57. Turell, R., and Brodman, H. R.: Adenomas of colon and rectum. In Turell, R., editor: Diseases of the colon and anorectum, vol. 1, Philadelphia, 1959, W. B. Saunders Co.
58. Walske, B., Hamilton, J., and Kisner, P.: From benign polyp to carcinoma, Arch. of Surg. (Chicago) **70:**318, 1955.
59. Wagensteen, O. H.: Cancer of the colon and rectum; with special reference to (1) earlier recognition of alimentary tract malignancy; (2) secondary delayed re-entry of the abdomen in patients exhibiting lymph node involvement: (3) subtotal primary excision of the colon; (4) operation in obstruction, Wisconsin Med. J. **48:**591, 1949.
60. Weber, H. M.: The roentgenologic demonstration of polypoid lesions and polyposis of the large intestine, Amer. J. Roentgen. **25:**577, 1931.
61. Welch, C. E.: The treatment of polyps of the colon, Surg. Gynec. Obstet. **93:**368, 1951.
62. Welin, W.: Results of the Malmö technique of colon examination, J.A.M.A. **199:**369-371, 1967.
63. Welin, S., and Lórinc, P.: Das Röntgenbild des villösen (zottenförmigen) Tumors im Bereich des Colons, Radiologe **2:**107, 1962.
64. Welin, S., Youker, J., and Spratt, J. S.: The rates and patterns of growth of 375 tumours of the large intestine and rectum observed serially by double contrast enema study (Malmö technique), Amer. J. Roentgen. **90:**673, 1963.
65. Wheat, M. W., and Ackerman, L. V.: Villous adenomas of the large intestine, Ann. Surg. **147:**476, 1958.
66. Wietersen, F. K.: High kilovoltage method of investigation of the colon as a routine roentgenologi-

cal procedure, Amer. J. Roentgen. **77**:690, 1957.

67. Winblad, S., and Frieberg, S.: Observations on the pathology of polyps of the colon, Acta Path. Microbiol. Scand. **III** (Supp.):89, 1956.

68. Wolf, B. S.: Roentgen diagnosis of villous tumors of the colon, Amer. J. Roentgen. **84**:1093, 1960.

69. Wolf, B. S., Melamed, M., and Khilnani, M. T.: Lipoma of the colon, J. Mount Sinai Hosp. N.Y. **21**:80, 1954.

70. Yates, C. W.: Double contrast studies of the colon; polyps in children, Southern Med. J. **46**:315, 1953.

71. Youker, J. E., and Welin, S.: Differentiation of true polypoid tumors of the colon from extraneous material; a new roentgen sign, Radiology **84**:610-615, 1965.

72. Youker, J. E., Welin, S., and Main, G.: Computer analysis in the differentiation of benign and malignant polypoid lesions of the colon, Radiology **90**:794-797, 1967.

73. Bartholomew, L. G., Moore, C. E., Dahlin, D. C., and Waugh, J. M.: Intestinal polyposis associated with mucocutaneous pigmentation, Surg. Gynec. Obstet. **115**:1, 1962.

74. Baughman, F. A., Jr., List, C. F., Williams, J. R., Muldoon, J. P., Segarra, J. M., and Volkel, J. S.: The glioma-polyposis syndrome, New Eng. J. Med. **281**:1345, 1969.

75. Burdick, D., Prior, J., and Scanlon, G. T.: Peutz-Jeghers syndrome: clinical-pathologic study of a large family with a 10 year follow-up, Cancer **16**:854, 1963.

76. Chang, C. H., Platt, E. D., Thomas, K. E., and Watne, A. L.: Bone abnormalities in Gardner's syndrome, Amer. J. Roentgen. **103**:645, 1968.

77. Cole, J. W., McKalen, A., and Powel, J.: The role of ileal contents in the spontaneous regression of rectal adenomas, Dis. Colon Rectum **4**:413, 1961.

78. Coli, R. D., Moore, J. P., La Marche, P. H., De Luca, F. G., and Thayer, W. R.: Gardner's syndrome: a revisit to the previously described family, J. Dig. Dis. **15**:551, 1970.

79. Cripps, H.: Two cases of disseminated polyps of the colon, Trans. Path. Soc. London **33**:165, 1882.

80. Cronkhite, L. W., Jr., and Canada, W. J.: Generalized gastrointestinal polyposis: an unusual syndrome of pigmentation, alopecia, and onychotrophia, New Eng. J. Med. **252**:1011, 1955.

81. Dodds, W. J., Schulte, W. J., Godard, J. E., Hogan, W. J., and Hensley, G.: Investigation of a large negro family with Peutz-Jeghers syndrome, Gastroenterology **60**:651, 1971.

82. Dormandy, T. L.: Gastrointestinal polyposis with mucocutaneous pigmentation (Peutz-Jeghers syndrome), New Eng. J. Med. **256**:1093, 1957.

83. Dozois, R. R., Judd, S., Dahlin, D. C., and Bartholomew, L. G.: The Peutz-Jeghers syndrome: is there a predisposition to the development of intestinal malignancy, Arch. Surg. **98**:509, 1969.

84. Dukes, C. E.: Familial intestinal polyposis, Ann. Roy. Coll. Surg. Eng. **10**:293, 1952.

85. Gardner, E. J., and Richard, R. C.: Multiple cutaneous and subcutaneous lesions occurring simultaneously with hereditary polyposis and osteomatosis, Amer. J. Hum. Genet. **5**:139, 1953.

86. Godard, J. E., Dodds, W. J., Phillips, J. C., and Scanlon, G. T.: Peutz-Jeghers syndrome: clinical and roentgenographic features, Amer. J. Roentgen. **113**:316, 1971.

87. Holgersen, L. O., Miller, P. E., and Zintel, H. A.: Juvenile polyps of the colon, Surgery **69**:288, 1971.

88. Jeghers, H., McKusick, V. A., and Katz, K. H.: Generalized intestinal polyposis and melanin spots of the oral mucosa, lips and digits: a syndrome of diagnostic significance, New Eng. J. Med. **241**:933, 1949.

89. Johnson, K., Soergel, K. H., Hensley, G. T., Dodds, W. J., and Hogan, W. J.: Evaluation of gastrointestinal function in a patient with Cronkhite-Canada syndrome, Gastroenterology. In Press.

90. Johnston, M. M., Vosburgh, J. W., Wiens, A. T., and Walsh, G. C.: Gastrointestinal polyposis associated with alopecia, pigmentation, and atrophy of the fingernails and toenails, Ann. Intern. Med. **56**:935, 1962.

91. Kennedy, B., Dodds, W. J., Schulte, W., and Hensley, G.: Familial multiple polyposis: a "curable" disease, Wisconsin J. Med. **70**:230, 1971.

92. Lockhart-Mummery, H. E.: Intestinal polyposis, Practitioner **203**:620, 1969.

93. Lockhart-Mummery, H. E.: Intestinal polyposis: the present position, Proc. Roy. Soc. Med. **60**:381, 1967.

94. Marshak, R. H., Mosely, J. E., and Wolf, B. S.: The roentgen findings in familial polyposis with special emphasis on differential diagnosis, Radiology **80**:374, 1963.

95. McConnell, R. B.: The genetics of gastrointestinal disorders, London, 1966, Oxford University Press.

96. McKusick, V. A.: Genetic factors in intestinal polyposis, J.A.M.A. **182**:271, 1962.

97. Morson, B. C.: Some peculiarities in the histology of intestinal polyps, Dis. Colon Rectum **5**:337, 1962.

98. Orimo, H., Fujita, T., Yoshikawa, M., Takemoto, T., Matsuo, Y., and Nakao, K.: Gastrointestinal polyposis with protein-losing enteropathy, abnormal skin pigmentation and loss of hair and nails (Cronkhite-Canada Syndrome), Amer. J. Med. **47**:445, 1969.

99. Peutz, J. L. A.: Ober een zeer merkwaardige, geo-combineerde familaire Polyposis van de Slymvliezen van den Tractus intestinalis met die van de Neuskeelholte en Gepaard met eigen aardige Pigmentaties van Huiden Slijmvliezen, Nederl. Maandschr. Geneesk. **10**:134, 1921.

100. Pierce, E. R.: Some genetic aspects of familial multiple polyposis of the colon in a kindred of 1,422 members, Dis. Colon Rectum **11**:321, 1968.

101. Reed, T. E., and Neel, J. V.: A genetic study of multiple polyposis of the colon (with an appendix deriving a method of estimating relative fitness), Amer. J. Hum. Genet. **7**:236, 1955.

102. Ruymann, F. B.: Juvenile polyps with cachexia: report of an infant and comparison with Cronkhite-Canada syndrome in adults, Gastroenterology **57**:431, 1969.

103. Sachatello, C. R., Pickren, J. W., and Grace, J. T.: Generalized juvenile gastrointestinal polyposis: a hereditary syndrome, Gastroenterology **58:**699, 1970.

104. Silverberg, S. G.: "Juvenile" retention polyps of the colon and rectum, J. Dig. Dis. **15:**617, 1970.

105. Smith, W. G.: Multiple polyposis, Gardner's syndrome and desmoid tumors, Dis. Colon Rectum **1:**323, 1958.

106. Sommerhaug, R. G., and Mason, T.: Peutz-Jeghers syndrome and ureteral polyposis, J.A.M.A. **211:**120, 1970.

107. Soper, R. T., and Kent, T. H.: Fatal juvenile polyposis in infancy, Surgery **69:**692, 1971.

108. Turcot, J., Després, J., and St. Pierre, F.: Malignant tumors of the central nervous system associated with familial polyposis of the colon: report of two cases, Dis. Colon Rectum **2:**465, 1959.

109. Veale, A. M. O.: Intestinal Polyposis, Cambridge, 1965, Cambridge University Press.

110. Veale, A. M. O., McColl, I., Bussey, H. J., and Morson, B. C.: Juvenile polyposis coli, J. Med. Genet. **3:**5, 1966.

111. Watne, A. L., Johnson, J. G., and Chang, C. H.: The challenge of Gardner's syndrome, Cancer **19:**266, 1969.

112. Yonemoto, R. H., Slayback, J. B., Byron, R. L., and Rosen, R. B.: Familial polyposis of the entire gastrointestinal tract, Arch. Surg. **99:**427, 1969.

113. Ziter, M. H.: Roentgenographic findings in Gardner's syndrome, J.A.M.A. **192:**158, 1965.

40 | Colonic malignancy

Frederic E. Templeton

ETIOLOGY

Why the colon is a frequent site of cancer has not been established. Apart from ulcerative colitis and a few hereditary diseases, no relationship between colonic carcinoma and other diseases has been established. Some authors postulate that certain drugs or foods modified by the liver become carcinogenic and are secreted into the bile. After entering the colon these substances stimulate neoplasia by direct contact with mucosal cells through the medium of feces. This assumption is supported by experimental data. Mice injected intramuscularly with carcinogens develop both benign and malignant colonic neoplasms. More work is necessary before the assumption is accepted or rejected.[62] Urine may also contain a colonic carcinogen. Tumor of the colon is reported in ureterocolic anastomosis performed to relieve ureteral obstruction.[27]

The role heredity plays is difficult to establish in isolated instances but is easily established in familial polyposis and Gardner's, Turcot's, and Peutz-Jeghers syndromes.[1,26,34]* Not established in either hereditary polyposis or in simple colonic polyposis is the relationship between benign polyps and malignancy.[17,37]

TYPES OF EXAMINATION

Carcinoma of the gastrointestinal tract not explored at surgery can be detected by endoscopy, radiography, cytology, and angiography. For colonic carcinoma cytology is unreliable and angiography is limited. Endoscopy (proctoscopy and sigmoidoscopy) and radiography complement each other. One examination should not be done without the other.

Endoscopy

Over 50% of the colonic carcinomas lie in the distal colon within the range of the rigid sigmoidoscope (Fig. 40-1). With the use of the flexible fiberscope the percentage of carcinomas discovered should be higher. More of the lower colon can be visualized as this instrument, which can be tied into a knot without losing the image, is manipulated around the flexures, especially the rectosigmoid. On rare occasions the instrument is threaded to the cecum. Usually the instrument cannot be manipulated above the pelvic colon because the sigmoid is too redundant (Fig. 40-2).

Radiology

The radiologist looks for a carcinoma in those portions of the colon above the reach of the

---

*Familial polyposis is probably of autosomal, nonsexlinked, dominant transmission. The incidence of heterozygotes for polyposis at birth is one in 66,850 in the St. Louis area.[7] Gardner's syndrome is associated with neoplasms of the skin, subcutaneous tissues, and bone. Turcot's syndrome is a combination of colonic polyps and brain tumor. It is an autosomal recessive mechanism of inheritance.[6] Peutz-Jeghers syndrome is associated with cutaneous lesions. The intestinal lesions are hamartomas. Carcinomatous change is rare.

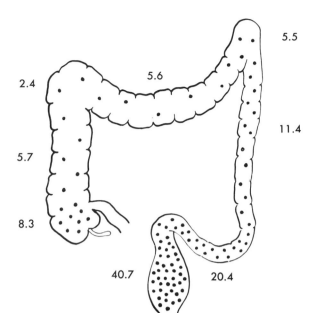

Fig. 40-1. Relative distribution, in percent, of adenocarcinoma occurring in the several segments of the colon. (From Berk, J. E., and Haubrich, W. S.: Malignant tumors of the colon and rectum. In Bockus, H. L., editor: Gastroenterology, ed. 2, Philadelphia, 1964, W. B. Saunders Co.)

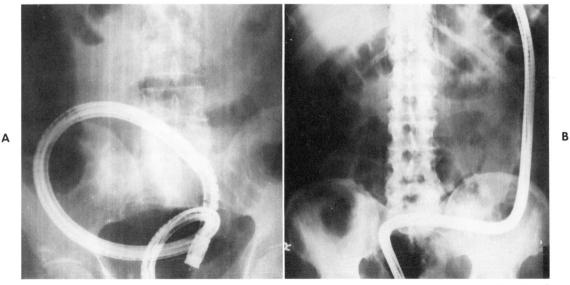

Continued.

Fig. 40-2. A, A flexible fibroscope has been manipulated past tight curves of a redundant sigmoid. The end lies at about the junction of the descending sigmoid. **B,** In a different patient the fibroscope has been passed to the splenic flexure. The patient, who had had the cecum and part of the sigmoid removed for primary carcinomas, was being reevaluated because of chronic diarrhea. **C,** The same colon examined in **B** is depicted with barium. The only abnormality encountered is a stricture 60 cm. from the anus, the site of an end-to-end anastomosis after removal of a sigmoidal neoplasm. Because the colonoscope often stretches the bowel more than the enema, distances of a lesion from the rectum cannot be related to distances estimated from the barium enema. (Courtesy Dr. Alvin Thompson.)

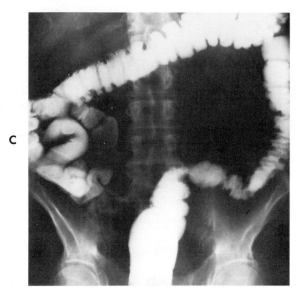

Fig. 40-2, cont'd. For legend see p. 1069.

proctoscope. This is usually above the rectosigmoid bend at the level of the third sacrovertebral body, which marks the reflection of the peritoneum. Rarely does a radiologist find a tumor of the rectum not observed by an experienced proctologist or not felt by digital examination by the clinician. Weber summed up the relationship between the referring physician and the roentgenologist: "I believe . . . it is a mistake for the roentgenologist to assume responsibility of diagnosis for that portion of the intestinal tract within the range of the proctoscope and wrong for his counterparts to ask him to do so."[58]

An important adjunct to roentgenologic examination of the colon is the survey film. The film gives much information. Calcified concretions in viscera and calcifications in arteries, lymph nodes, and tumors are recorded. Gas may outline a tumor, indicate obstruction or perforation of the bowel, or lie in the wall of the intestine (pneumatosis cystoides) (Fig. 40-3). The advantage of the survey film is reemphasized in order that the examiner not overlook an important part of the examination.

ROENTGENOLOGIC PATHOLOGY
Types of carcinoma

The types of carcinomas in the gastrointestinal tract are polypoid, ulcerative, or infiltrative. Appearances vary; they may be small, large, ragged, smooth, localized, infiltrating, or multiple. Others are annular and stenosing.

The cell from which a neoplasm arises rarely influences the architecture of the lesion. Therefore, differentiation of cancer from other lesions can on occasions be difficult or impossible by roentgenography. However, the usual moderately differentiated adenocarcinoma is characterized by an abrupt transition from tumor to normal adjacent mucosa.[42] Other tumors infiltrate and appear as inflammations.

Special types of adenocarcinoma are mucoid, colloid, squamous, and villous adenocarcinomas. In the highly malignant mucoid and colloid carcinomas the cells do not lose their function. Although mucus in the stools may be increased, the tumor cannot be differentiated from the usual adenocarcinomas at roentgenologic examination. Scirrhous carcinoma and villous adenocarcinomas have different roentgenologic characteristics and are described separately.

Neoplasms arising from mesothelial tissue are sarcomas. The most common of these rare tumors are the lymphosarcomas and the leiomyosarcomas. As in adenocarcinoma, these tumors produce a variety of patterns.

Growth and diagnosis of carcinoma

Not known is the manner by which tumors grow. No large series of patients in whom life

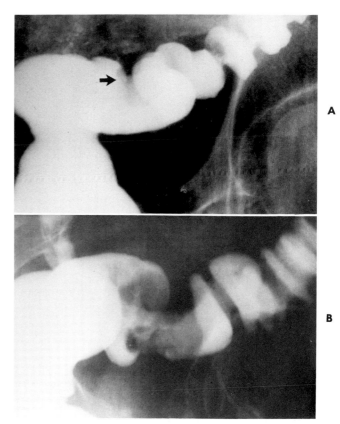

Fig. 40-4. A, At the first examination a tiny globose tumor lies clamped, crab-fashion about a pseudohaustrum. The lesion seems to bridge and broaden the apex of the haustral crease (arrow). Often pseudohaustra are not opposed with indentations on the opposite wall and do not extend in a circumferential manner. **B,** A typical annular ulcerating carcinoma was found at the same site 3 years later. (Courtesy Dr. John Walker.)

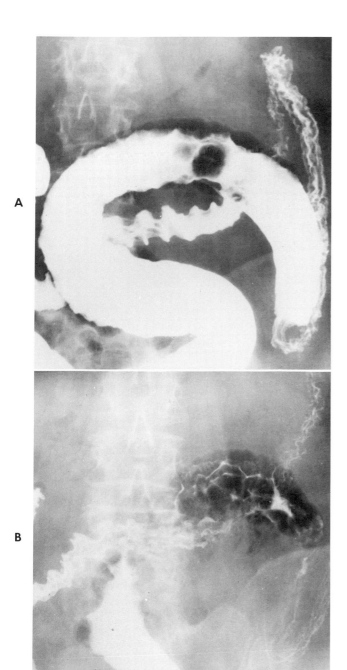

Fig. 40-3. Pneumatosis cystoides. **A,** The barium-filled colon. **B,** After partial evacuation. Gas in the wall forms a translucent cuff about the barium in the sigmoid colon. Usually pneumatosis occurs in inflammatory disease. Only rarely is the condition observed in neoplasm. In this case transmural (Crohn's) disease was the diagnosis.

cycles of tumors have been followed has been published. By comparing observations on tumors that are missed and observed later or by watching tumors grow in patients either by endoscopy, radiography, or biopsy the life cycles of adenocarcinomas are postulated.

Radiologists describe instances of adenocarcinomas in the early stages of growth. In thirty-one patients having two or more examinations performed 6 or more months apart, Walker found that early tumors produce tiny, spherical, smoothly contoured intraluminal defects.[56] As the lesions grow they bridge the apices of small haustral creases. The creases seem to be pseudohaustration produced by an infolding of the submucosa and possibly the muscularis. Invasion of the tunica propria or the muscularis is not

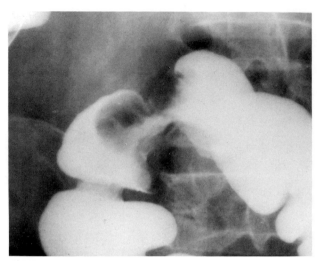

Fig. 40-5. Encircling carcinoma of the hepatic flexure involves a short segment. Sharp shelflike margins are present. The narrow central segment is irregular, and no mucosal folds are visible.

likely in the early stages, since several of the tumors take as long as 10 years to develop into full-blown neoplasms (Fig. 40-4). In an early carcinoma, Schinz, Baensch, and Friedl found that one side of a broadened haustrum was irregular.[53] The pattern was similar to that of Walker's examples.[56]

The pathologic description of the early stages correlates with the radiologic observations. Perrett and Truelove state that many cancers arise in thickenings of the mucosa—the carcinoma in situ.[47] Robbins agrees and records that the early lesions are small, elevated, button-like, polypoid masses.[51] For a long time the lesions remain superficial and are small areas of asymptomatic cancerous transformation.

As the tumor grows it spreads in all directions, forming either a flattened, sessile, raised plaque or a rounded, polypoid, fungating mass. The flat sessile tumor invades the deeper structures, thickens and stiffens the walls, and destroys the muscle. Peristalsis and local contractions are obliterated. Encroaching on the blood supply, the center of the tumor becomes necrotic and ulcerates. Often by this time the tumor surrounds and narrows the lumen. The common annular ulcerating variety with overhanging edges results (Fig. 40-5).[42]

Infrequently the growth breaks through the bowel wall into pericolic fat or spreads into

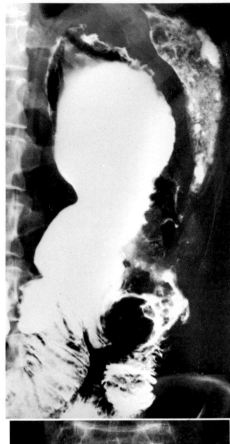

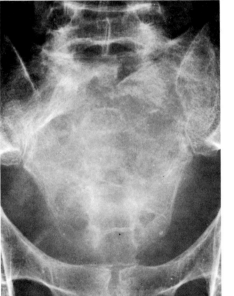

Fig. 40-6. A, A fistula between a neoplasm of the descending colon and jejunum appeared during an examination of the small bowel. **B,** Destruction of the anterior part of the sacrum from adenocarcinoma of the rectum. In some areas, particularly on the left side, the posterior portion has also been destroyed.

regional lymph nodes or neighboring organs (Fig. 40-6). Soiling the peritoneal cavity will cause peritonitis.[51]

Most carcinomas are moderately differentiated adenocarcinomas. These tumors develop from a small sessile or polypoid lesion to a full-grown polypoid or annular ulcerating lesion in 1 to 2 or more years. Roentgenologically, the transitions from the tumors to normal adjacent mucosa is often abrupt and is indicated by overhanging edges. Slightly elevated masses with smooth surfaces that stiffen and indent the walls are characteristic of infiltrating growths. In the early stages cancers associated with inflammation and the scirrhous carcinomas escape detection, because the transition from normal to abnormal bowel is indistinct.

Fungating polypoid carcinoma

The polypoid fungating carcinomas probably begin as flat sessile or polypoid masses that grow

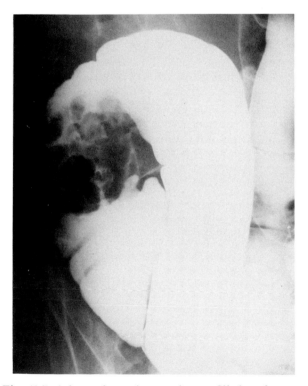

Fig. 40-7. A large, fungating carcinoma fills but does not obstruct the lumen of the ascending colon. These tumors may produce no symptoms other than iron deficiency anemia. Sometimes blood cannot be detected in the stool. Therefore if the colon is not examined in patients having unexplained iron deficiency anemia, the tumor may go undetected for months or even years.

into the lumen. These tumors, which are usually located in the cecum, ascending colon, and rectum, become bulky, fissured, friable, and ulcerative. They weep blood slowly and cause anemia (Fig. 40-7).[2]

In the barium-filled colon the masses show clearly when excess barium is pushed away with pressure or when air is added after the colon is partially evacuated or drained. The size, shape, and position of the tumor is not changed by compressing or distending the lumen (Fig. 40-8).

Tumors of the cecum and ascending colon not invading the ileocecal sphincter obstruct late, even though some reach diameters of 8 or 10 cm.[6] Both the large caliber of the bowel and the liquid aliment, delivered from the small intestine, allow the fecal stream to pass through the small channels created by the large masses. When the ileocecal sphincter is obliterated early, obstruction is the first sign of trouble (Fig. 40-9).

Polypoid lesions occasionally fill the rectum. Accessible by proctoscopic and digital examination, they rarely are as large as some cecal tumors. Unfortunately the rectal masses are more invasive than the cecal. Discovering them when they are smaller than the cecal masses gains little as far as curative results are concerned (Fig. 40-10).

Annular ulcerating cancers

The small-calibered transverse, descending, and sigmoidal segments of the bowel are favorite locations for the annular ulcerating cancer. The tumor infiltrates around as well as along the colonic wall and does not form a bulky mass. When first seen at roentgenographic examination, the tumor is rarely more than 4 or 5 cm. long. Overhanging edges, sharply defined against the adjacent mucosa, are characteristic. The central lumen is narrow, ragged, and devoid of folds (Fig. 40-11).[4,53] Occasionally the lesion is longer than 4 or 5 cm. (Fig. 40-15).

Occasionally a carcinoma will encircle either the ascending colon or the rectum. Before it encircles the lumen, the tumor is often obscured in the anteroposterior view of the filled colon but shows as an indentation in the oblique and lateral projections. A sharp border divides the healthy mucosa from the tumor (Fig. 40-12).[4]

If the tumor is accompanied by an inflamed mucosa, the sharp distinction between unin-

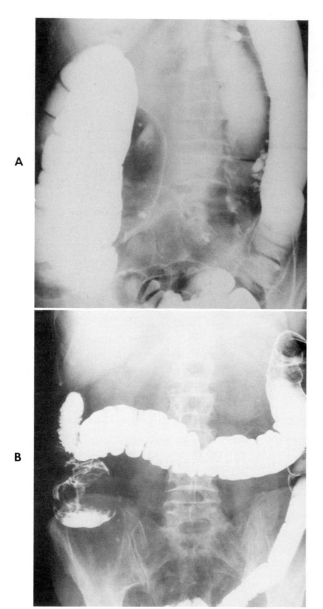

Fig. 40-8. Carcinoma of the cecum. A 76-year-old wo-man noticed blood in the stools and felt a mass in the right side of her abdomen. Her hematocrit reading was 29%. **A,** In a filled colon a mass in the cecum is obscured by barium, which overdistends the cecum. **B,** After par-tial evacuation the colon shortened and a large tumor involving all but a small portion of the lateral wall of the cecum is evident. The upper and lower margins are sharply defined against the adjacent normal mucosa. At fluoroscopy the tumor could be moved about. The size and contours of the tumor did not change with pressure and appeared similar to the above pattern on spot films. This illustrates the value of palpation, spot roentgenography, and the postevacuation film.

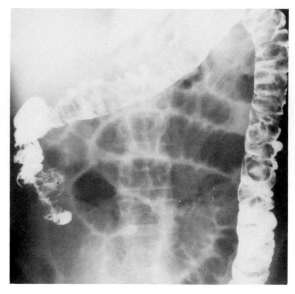

Fig. 40-9. A carcinoma of the cecum obstructs the ileo-cecal sphincter. The ileum is distended with gas. The colon contains much fecal material. Oral cathartic was contraindicated and enemas were of no value. This il-lustrates that in obstruction valuable information can be obtained even if the colon contains fecal material.

volved tissue and tumor is not evident. Problems in differential diagnosis from inflammation arise.

Certain physiologic phenomena occur and vary the appearance of lesions. At evacuation the colon shortens and fine folds appear. As the colon shortens, loops of bowel hidden by other loops appear. Valuable information is added to that obtained from the barium-filled colon. Ab-normal patterns sometimes stand out sharply against the normal (Fig. 40-13).

Parallel thick folds often extend transversely across the colon immediately distal to the tumor. The length of the segment involved with these folds is rarely more than 7 or 8 cm. This condi-tion, called fibrillation, is an early sign of intus-susception, which does not progress. Fibrillation is caused by the contraction of the longitudinal muscle and the tenia.[4] The pattern must not be confused with the fine transverse folds that pre-cede most mass evacuation contractions. The fibrillated region is not invaded by tumor and is easily distended. With distention, the fibrillation disappears and the lumen becomes smooth. Fib-rillation also occurs in both the annular ulcer-ating and the polypoid tumors (Fig. 40-14).

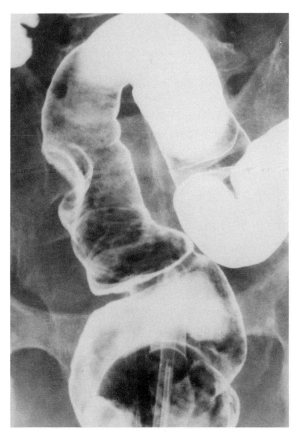

Fig. 40-10. Small symptomless adenocarcinoma discovered at proctoscopic examination. The patient had no symptoms but had noted red blood in the stool. The concave broad base of the tumor suggests malignancy. Biopsy confirmed the diagnosis of adenocarcinoma.

Squamous carcinomas

Squamous carcinoma arising from squamous cells is a disease of the anus and not the colon. However, few instances of squamous carcinoma apparently arising from cellular rests are reported in the rectum. These cells produce raised sessile masses. Differentiation from other tumors is made at biopsy.

Scirrhous carcinoma

Although often seen in the stomach, scirrhous carcinoma or linitis plastica rarely occurs in the colon. As in the stomach, the walls, by diffuse infiltration, become thick and rigid. Early lesions are easily overlooked. The infiltrate produces no narrowing or obvious stiffening of the walls and is confined to one side of the colonic lumen, usually the mesenteric. The involved

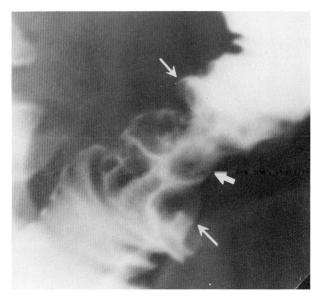

Fig. 40-11. Annular adenocarcinoma of the lower descending colon. The mucosa is replaced by a polypoid mass lying within an ulcer (large arrow). The tissue immediately surrounding the central mass is rendered polypoid by submucosal invasion by the tumor. The extremities of the lesion are sharply defined against the normal intestine, the walls of which "overhang" (small arrows). Accordion-like folds below the tumor indicate a small element of intussusception, a condition rarely encountered in inflammation.

segment is wavelike and does not have the regular indentations produced by normal haustra. The contour cannot be changed by distention or palpation.

As the lesion progresses the infiltrate spreads circumferentially as well as longitudinally. The lumen narrows. Eventually a segment of bowel 10 to 30 cm. long with a lumen of 1 to 3 cm. in diameter develops. As in the early stages, the configuration is constant, does not respond to peristalsis or local contractions, and cannot be changed by increasing intraluminal pressure, by using relaxing drugs, by having the patient evacuate, or by palpation.

The fixed mucosal pattern is distorted and irregular. Masses and deep ulcers are uncommon. At the center of the lesion most folds are erased by the infiltrate. Toward the extremities of the lesion the mucosa thickens and produces a coarse cobblestone appearance with star-shaped linear collections of barium.[61] The pattern sometimes resembles the "fingerprint" patterns of infarcted bowel.

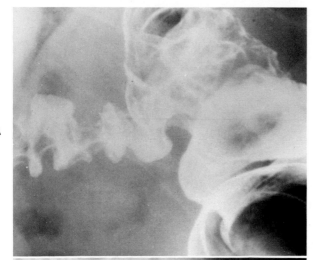

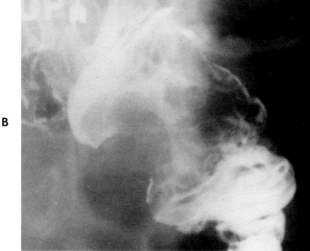

Fig. 40-12. Annular ulcerating carcinoma. **A,** The lesion involves the descending colon immediately distal to the splenic flexure. In an anteroposterior projection the tumor is not clearly defined when the lumen is distended with barium and air. **B,** Using pressure, spot roentgenography, and a slightly different angle the characteristics of the tumor appear. Normal mucosa overhangs both ends of the medial aspect of the tumor giving an "applecore" effect. The ragged lumen is devoid of folds. The lateral wall of the colon is not yet involved, and distended when the lumen filled with barium and air. This distention was one reason that the tumor failed to show up well in **A.**

In the far-advanced stages the interior of the irregular lumen is smooth. In all cases the ends of the lesion fade gradually into the normal bowel. Thick walls, which are thicker than those of contracted normal and inflamed colons, are characteristic of the lesion. Unfortunately, the thickness of colonic walls cannot always be determined at roentgenologic examination.

Scirrhous carcinoma of the stomach may spread to the colon. For this reason the stomach should be examined when a diffuse infiltrate is encountered in the sigmoid or the transverse colon. Scirrhous carcinoma of the stomach, spreading to the colon either by drop metastasis to the sigmoid or by direct invasion through the gastrocolic ligament to the transverse colon, can imitate a primary lesion.

Scirrhous carcinomas constitute about one third of the tumors occurring in ulcerative colitis.[41] In ulcerative colitis this carcinomatous defect is difficult or impossible to differentiate from long benign stricture and is not recognized before it metastasizes or invades other organs (Fig. 40-15).

Cloacogenic carcinoma is a rare but highly malignant lesion arising from the cloacogenic zone of the anorectal junction (Fig. 40-16).

Calcifications in adenocarcinoma

Occasionally calcifications in adenocarcinoma of the colon occur. The calcifications are rare, usually occur in large tumors, and are found on plain films along the course of the colon. The calcifications are curvilinear, mottled, or both. Calcifications also appear in the metastatic lesions to lymph nodes and to the liver (Fig. 40-17). All the recorded cases are from mucoid carcinomas, perhaps because the mucus-producing glands cause stones. The pancreas and the salivary and prostatic glands are examples. Calcifications probably are more common than roentgenologically indicated. The resolution of films used at routine roentgenologic examinations is insufficient to depict the small punctate densities.[23]

COMPLICATIONS

Cancer of the colon causes important complications, such as obstruction, perforation, invasion of the adjacent tissue, and intussusception. Of these possibilities, obstruction is common and on occasions may be the first indication of a diseased bowel.

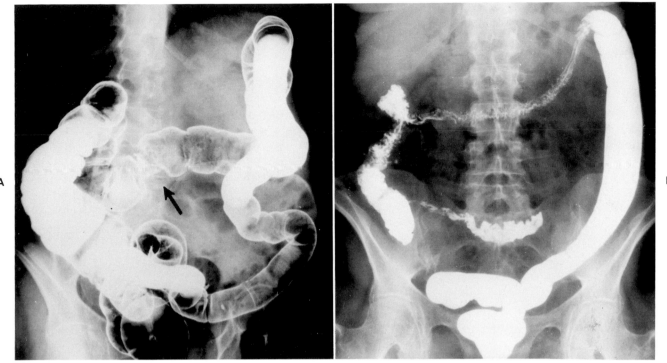

Fig. 40-13. A, A half-moon–shaped pattern presents on the inferior aspect of the transverse colon (arrow). **B,** After evacuation fine normal mucosal pattern is obliterated in the region of the abnormality observed in **A** (arrow). The inferior margin straightens, probably because adjacent normal intestinal wall does not balloon out over the edges of the mass. This illustrates one of the fine points in evaluating the postevacuation film. A nonulcerating sessile adenocarcinoma was found at surgery.

Obstruction

Obstruction produced by a carcinoma that surrounds and narrows the lumen occurs frequently in the descending and sigmoidal segments of the bowel. Narrowing and eventual obstruction is often assisted by inflammation, fibrosis, and impacted fecal material.

Signs of obstruction are slow to develop. The colon proximal to obstruction fills with aliment arriving from the small bowel. The cecum and the ascending portion balloon out and are evident as large collections of gas or mixtures of gas and fecal material. If the ileocecal sphincter does not resist the pressures built in the colon, gas distends the terminal ileum as well.

The site and cause of obstruction can sometimes be observed on a survey film, especially if the offending lesion is in the proximal portion of the colon. The closer the obstruction is to the ileocecal sphincter, the earlier are the signs of obstruction (Figs. 40-9 and 40-18).

Obstruction in the region of the splenic flexure is difficult to assess. Often the normal colon distal to the splenic flexure contracts and the portion proximal remains distended. The same is true in some tumors of the sigmoid. The colon distal to the splenic flexure distends and then contracts, forcing fecal material past the sigmoidal tumor. The transverse and ascending portions remain distended. On a survey film taken when the descending colon is contracted, the examiner postulates obstruction at the splenic flexure. He misses the carcinoma of the sigmoid when giving a barium enema if that carcinoma is not obvious or is hidden in redundant loops of bowel (Fig. 40-19). The interplay of blocking and passing of fecal material through the narrowed lumen produces alternating constipation and diarrhea.

Ogilvie described a syndrome in which the transverse colon was dilated and the descending colon and sigmoid collapsed. In each instance

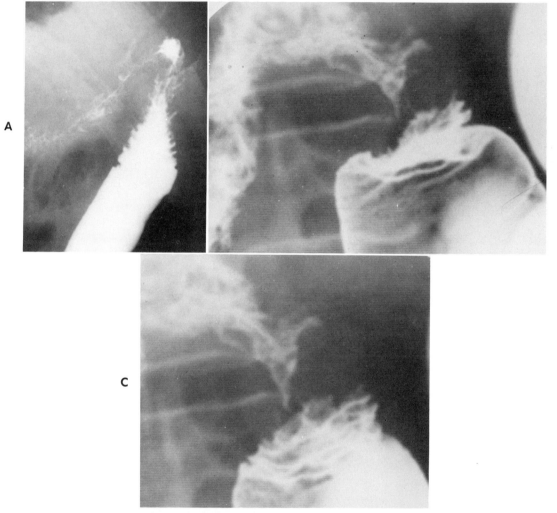

Fig. 40-14. Fibrillation of the colon. **A,** The fine transverse folds that precede a mass evacuation contraction and cause serrated borders are termed "fibrillation." These folds are produced by contraction of the longitudinal muscle, which, in peristalsis, reacts shortly before the circular muscle. **B** and **C,** Two phases of fibrillation forming in front of an annular ulcerating carcinoma. In these cases the fibrillation is produced not only by contraction of longitudinal muscle attempting to peel the mucosa back over the tumor but also by buckling of the mucosa as the tumor is forced into the lumen by contracting circular muscle behind the tumor. Whatever the cause of these patterns, the patterns are similar to, if not identical to, those observed in the early phases of intussusception. Fibrillation indicates that the mucosa is not invaded by neoplasm.

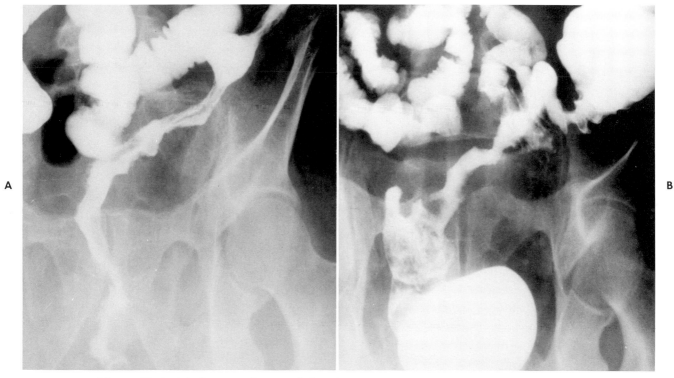

Fig. 40-15. A, Scirrhous carcinoma of the distal portion of the colon. **B,** An unusually long, differentiated, ulcerating adenocarcinoma, not associated with ulcerative colitis, involves the sigmoid. Pronounced ulceration causes the ragged appearance. Unlike scirrhous carcinoma the extremities of the lesion are sharp against adjacent normal mucosa.

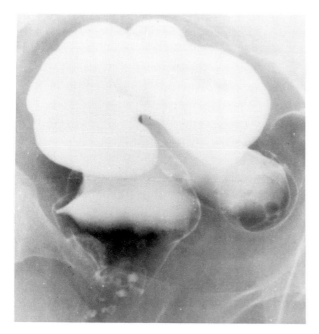

Fig. 40-16. Cloacogenic carcinoma, oblique view, A finely ulcerated 2 cm. mass located at the anorectal junction is well seen on the air contrast study. This type of plaque lesion is typical. Lesions arising from the remnants of the anal ducts may be higher in location and indistinguishable from carcinoma of the rectum. (From Glickman, M. G., and Margulis, A. R.: Cloacogenic carcinoma, Amer. J. Roentgen. **107:**175, 1969.)

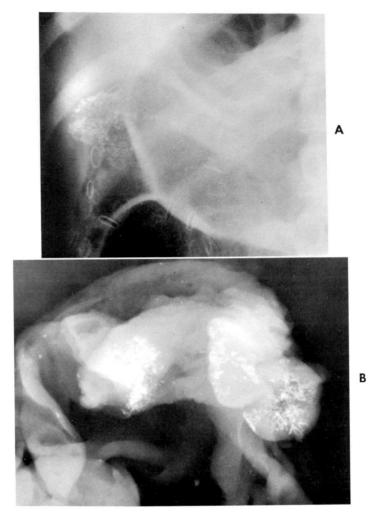

Fig. 40-17. A, Coarse calcification in a mucinous adenocarcinoma of the hepatic flexure. The oval shadows are produced by watermelon seeds. **B,** Specimen shows the calcification more clearly. (Courtesy Dr. F. F. Zboralske.)

the symptoms strongly suggested obstruction of the splenic flexure. Carcinoma was suspected. At laparotomy the colon was normal, but the celiac plexus was invaded by carcinoma from another source, probably the pancreas. Ogilvie reasoned that the abrupt change from a dilated colon proximal to the collapsed bowel at the splenic flexure was the result of different innervations.[15,44] At the splenic flexure the vagus nerve ceased and the sacral nerve took over. The arterial supply that carried the sympathetic nerves also changed. The superior mesenteric artery supplied the transverse colon and the inferior mesenteric artery the descending colon. Because of the differences in innervations, the motor function of the proximal segment of the

bowel was not smoothly transferred to the distal segment.

Perhaps there is something to this reasoning. On two occasions I have encountered large, obstructing scybala, lodged proximal to an end-to-end anastomosis, which had to be removed surgically after removal of the carcinoma from the splenic flexure. The slight narrowing caused by the anastomosis was not considered in itself sufficient to explain the scybala.

In similar obstructions the barium enema is necessary to locate the site and to determine the cause. Only with the barium enema can the site of obstruction be determined and the proper treatment be outlined (Fig. 40-20).

Most obstructing tumors are sharply defined

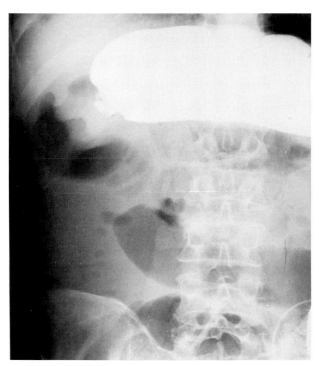

Fig. 40-18. Obstructing adenocarcinoma. The carcinoma obstructing the colon at the hepatic flexure is evident between gas proximal and barium distal to the lesion. On the proximal side a dimple indenting the lumen entering the tumor is filled with gas.

against the normal adjacent mucosa. The distal shoulders of the lesion stand out against barium injected from below. Often some barium mixture enters the narrowed lumen. Impacted fecal material is forced upwards out of the lumen. The "ball valve" action of the impaction explains why the barium mixture is forced retrograde past the lesion and why fecal material is held above the lesions for varying periods of time (Fig. 40-21).

Bezoars have been confused with carcinoma in the stomach but rarely elsewhere. Fronstien and Hutchinson described an obstructing trichobezoar lodged above a narrowed sigmoid from which diverticula protruded.[24] Carcinoma was considered prior to surgery. At autopsy after a colostomy, a bezoar consisting of fine hairs was embedded in feces and impacted against a sclerosing diverticulitis.

Perforation

Adenocarcinoma can erode through the colonic wall, perforate and release colonic content

into the peritoneal cavity or into the adjacent organs, or burrow into the adjacent abdominal wall. Perforation into the peritoneal cavity causes an acute episode recognized clinically. Because of the acute process the patient is not examined with a barium enema. Perforation into the adjacent organs does not produce an acute episode (Fig. 40-6).

After acute symptoms subside a barium enema may safely be given. Barium sometimes escapes from the bowel into a walled-off abscess or into an invaded organ. Water-soluble mixtures are not used unless free peritoneal perforation is suspected. They are hypertonic, stimulate peristalsis, and do not produce the contrasting shadows of barium. So far I have experienced no problem with barium. However, I do not examine the patient in acute distress, and I do not force barium with excessive pressure (2 feet of water pressure is enough). Excessive pressure is difficult to produce unless a self-retaining catheter is used; normally, the rectum is a built in safety valve.

The roentgenologist should not force the barium mixture through a narrow stricture that is causing obstruction into the lumen above the lesion, which is usually distended with fecal material and fluid. He chances perforating the bowel. In some long-standing obstructions the mucosa above the obstructed site is inflamed, ulcerated, easily perforated, and resembles ulcerative colitis.[49] Furthermore, surgeons find it difficult to operate upon a bowel that is filled with barium. Many surgeons prefer to explore the rest of the bowel at operation rather than have the radiologist look for a second tumor.

Intussusception

Adenocarcinoma and other masses may produce intussusception, in which one part of the bowel invaginates into that immediately adjoining. The outer or sheathing segment is the intussuscipiens and the inner invaginated segment is the intussusceptum.

In the adult the nidus for intussusception is usually a tumor. A long mesentery and a not entirely understood combination of contracting circular and longitudinal muscles of the bowel cause the tumor to enter the lumen of the adjacent portion of bowel. The bowel and attached mesentery and glands are pulled along as the intussusception progresses. The mesentery and

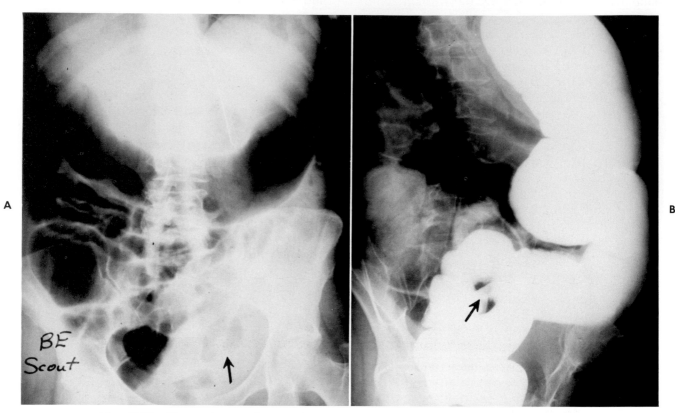

Fig. 40-19. Obstructing carcinoma of the sigmoid. **A,** On a survey film of a patient clinically suspected of having an obstructing carcinoma, the ascending small intestine and the transverse colon are distended with gas. The descending colon and sigmoid are collapsed. The significance of the inverted U shaped pattern was not appreciated (arrow). **B,** With barium enema the sigmoid and descending colon fill easily. When barium entered the gas-distended transverse segment, the examination was aborted. The splenic flexure was normal. Oglivie's syndrome was suggested. At operation an annular adenocarcinoma of the sigmoid was found. On hindsight the inverted U indicated on the scout film was gas in the lumen of the tumor, which, after barium was administered, was seen through the filled redundant loops of sigmoid (arrow).

glands lie between the intussuscipiens and the intussusceptum.[21]

The direction of the intussusception may be either toward the rectum (isocolic) or toward the cecum (rectocolic).[20,30] The first form is frequent, starts anywhere in the bowel, and travels for varying distances depending upon the anatomic arrangement of the bowel and mesentery. A tumor arising in the small intestine can prolapse into the colon, progress for a long distance, and simulate colonic carcinoma (Fig. 40-22). Tumors of the cecum have progressed the length of the bowel and have prolapsed through the rectum. The rectocolic form of intussusception is rare (Fig. 40-23).

Although intussusception usually is secondary to tumor, intussusception of normal structures may occur. The sigmoid can enter the rectum under certain conditions. These predisposing conditions are: (1) a long mobile mesentery, (2) a rectosigmoid junction held immobile by the sacral and pelvic fascia, and (3) an unusually narrow sigmoid lumen compared to the rectum.[25] Intussusception without tumor has also been observed at roentgenographic examination in the region of the hepatic flexure. Intussusception is commonly seen at postmortem examination, and transient intussusception without tumor is observed at surgery. Tumor, if present, is evident after the intussusception is reduced.

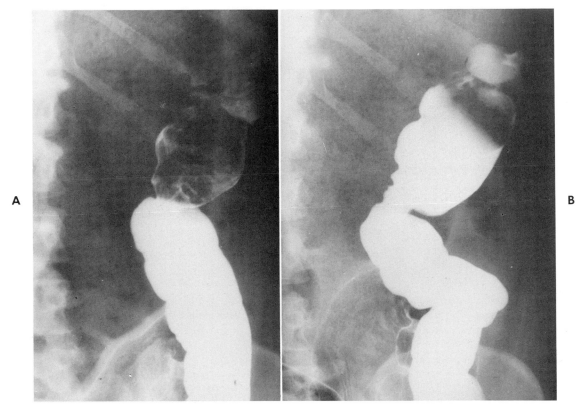

Fig. 40-20. Scyballa causing obstruction. **A,** A large mass appears as a tumor, partially obstructing the upper descending colon. **B,** With enema, the fecal nature of the mass was proved when barium forced the mass upward. Stool softener and enema relieved the patient of the mass.

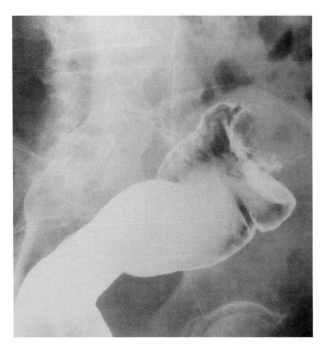

Fig. 40-21. Carcinoma obstructing the sigmoid. The patient had experienced intermittent abdominal cramps, constipation, and diarrhea. The survey film did not suggest obstruction. The barium enema could not be forced above a mass involving the sigmoid. The pattern of the mass, bulging into the sigmoid and barium entering but not passing through the lumen are characteristics of an annular ulcerating carcinoma. Compare with Fig. 40-18.

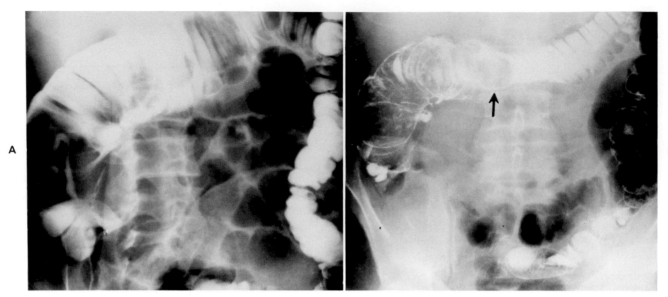

Fig. 40-22. Intussusception of small-bowel tumor into the colon. **A,** A long mass extends from the cecum into the midtransverse colon. The cecum marked by the appendix was not involved. Later, using only barium the mass proceeded retrogradely ahead of the enema but could not be forced through the ileocecal sphincter. **B,** After partial evacuation the mass returned to the midtransverse colon (arrow). The backward and forward movement of the lesion indicated intussusception. At surgery the tumor causing the intussusception arose from the small intestine 9 cm. from the sphincter and had traveled through the ileocecal sphincter dragging the small intestine after it. For this reason the cecum and the appendix were not involved by the lesion.

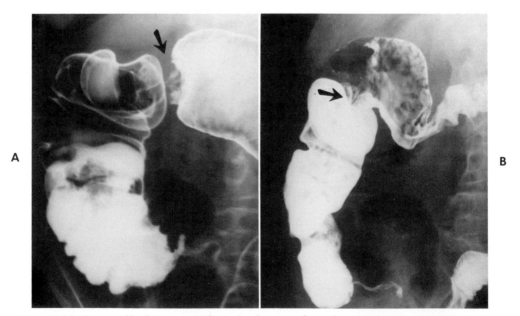

Fig. 40-23. Rectocolic intussusception. **A,** An annular adenocarcinoma presents in the proximal transverse colon (arrow). **B,** On the postevacuation film the tumor invaginates retrogradely into the ascending colon. Folds in the distal segment gather together and point toward the ascending colon (arrow). At surgery an adenocarcinoma arising in the transverse colon had intussuscepted into the ascending colon.

Intussusception of the appendix into the cecum, which is uncommon, may suggest cecal carcinoma. Howard and associates reported two such cases, reviewed the literature, and described the conditions favoring appendiceal intussusception.[28] In both patients, a woman and a man, roentgenographs of the barium-filled cecum indicated a slightly lobulated polypoid mass in the appendiceal region. The appendix did not show on roentgenographs and was not seen at surgery. At pathologic examination of the resected specimens, invagination of the appendix was found.

Pneumatosis cystoides intestinalis

Pneumatosis cystoides intestinalis, gas in the intestinal wall, is reported in association with colonic carcinoma. Apparently gas passes through fissures produced by the carcinoma and dissects between layers of uninvaded wall. At roentgenologic examination longitudinal cyst-like gaseous collections parallel the long axis of the bowel. Occasionally a cyst ruptures and allows gas to escape into the peritoneal cavity (Fig. 40-3).[8]

DIFFERENTIAL DIAGNOSIS

Carcinoma of the colon must be differentiated from many conditions that simulate its appearance. These are variations of normal and abnormal bowel.

Normal variations

An ileocecal sphincter having thickened lips and a submucosa infiltrated with fat appears large and resembles a polypoid mass that can be mistaken for cancer. The situation is sometimes amplified by ileal mucosa prolapsing through the sphincter.[16] Hawley and Mithoefer[29] reported two patients operated upon for "filling defects" in the ileocecal region. At surgery the ileum protruded into the cecum. In one patient, a 70-year-old woman, the mass was soft, sessile, lobulated, and measured 3 cm. in diameter. There was no edema of the prolapsed mucosa or ileocecal sphincter. The surgeon reduced the lesion digitally. It reoccurred when pressure was released. The patient recovered uneventfully.

Ten years later Felson and Wiot stated that another physician, believing that carcinoma of the cecum was present, operated on the same patient.[17] The original diagnosis of prolapsing ileal mucosa was confirmed.

Mistaking a large ileocecal valve for carcinoma is avoided by recognizing the different patterns of the normal valve. When the cecum is compressed by palpation, the valve appears in profile or face-on. In profile the normal valve produces an elongated tapering lucent pattern in the medial wall of the cecum about 4 or 5 cm. from the cecal tip. Indentation or haustrum in the opposite wall of the cecal lumen is rare. Often a thread of barium extends through the center of the structure. This thread represents barium in the lumen and if watched enlarges as barium flows retrograde into the ileum. If the cecum is incompletely rotated the ileocecal valve appears in profile on the lateral aspect of the cecum.

In the face-on view the valve presents a round translucency in the barium mixture. The size is changed by applying and releasing pressure. Often barium in the lumen causes a target-like pattern. A few folds radiate from the center. By turning the patient either to the left or right the valve can be brought into profile.

The ileocecal valve invaded by a carcinoma is irregular and cannot be changed by palpation because of rigidity. Sometimes a mass is palpated through the abdominal wall. The tumor may narrow the lumen and cause partial or complete obstruction.

Spasm, the failure of a small segment to relax, often occurs in many segments of the colon, particularly in the transverse and descending portions early in the examination. Usually the patterns disappear, and the bowel assumes a normal appearance by the time the rest of the colon is examined. Occasionally the spasm persists and resembles an annular carcinoma. In spasm fine parallel folds are traced through the narrowed lumen. In tumors the folds are destroyed and the lumen is irregular. The ends of the tumor are undercut by invading carcinoma. The ends of spasms taper. If the pattern persists and the examiner is unsure of his diagnosis, propantheline (Pro-Banthine) bromide to relax the spasm is suggested by some authors. The usual dose is 30 mg. intramuscularly. I use the drug infrequently. It is not always effective, and patients, especially those past middle age, may suffer adverse effects. A second barium enema or an examination a day or two later, although inconvenient for the patient, usually solves the problem and avoids the possibility of an unpleasant reaction.

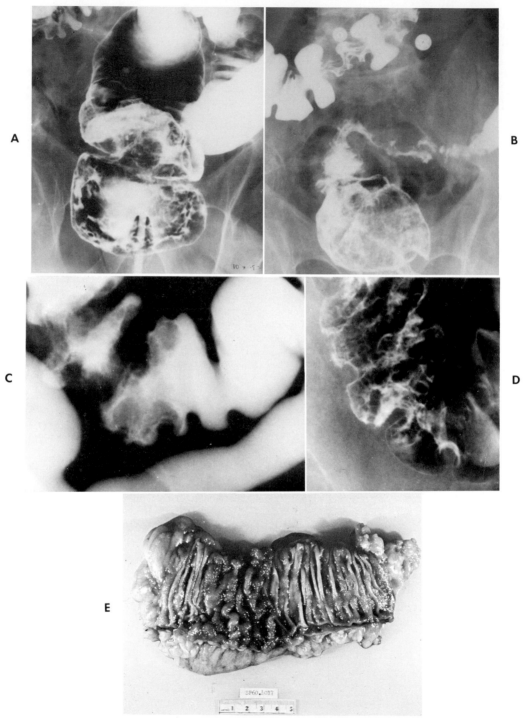

Fig. 40-24. A and **B,** Villous adenoma. **A,** A large mass, which looks like a barium-soaked sponge, fills the rectum. **B,** At evacuation the tumor is smaller, having been squeezed by the contraction of the bowel. **C** to **E,** Villous tumor. **C,** Large lobulated mass involves a long segment of the transverse colon. Although almost filling the lumen, the colon was not obstructed. **D,** Air contrast study reveals the lobulated surface with intervening clefts. The wall has distended. **E,** Specimen reveals the thickened folds of mucosa.

Sometimes small piling up of mucosa over an indentation of a haustrum causes a small, irregular, flat polypoid defect. The pattern, usually seen in the double-contrast examination at fluoroscopy, can be pressed out by palpation. The location of the shadow and the absence of infiltration of the walls indicate the normal state of the bowel.

Studying haustral patterns sometimes gives clues to the presence of a small carcinoma. Haustra are usually symmetrical. An indentation on one wall is accompanied by a similar indentation in the opposite wall. If a haustrum appears on one wall and not on the other, or is irregular, special care should be given in order to be sure that a neoplasm does not exist.

Abnormal conditions
Villous adenomas

Villous adenomas are papillary tumors consisting of long slender projections of mucosa called fronds. The tumors arise from epithelial cells and not glands and are not pedunculated. They occur anywhere in the colon but are usually found in the rectum. The lesions are sessile and bulky and may surround the lumen of the bowel. They are soft and easily molded by contractions of the bowel and can be missed by palpation. The mass of the tumor rarely obstructs the bowel and can produce intussusception.[36]

At roentgenologic examination the tumors are recognized by linear streaks produced by barium lodged between the fronds and are particularly evident on films recorded after evacuation. The patterns produced are likened to a barium-soaked sponge (Fig. 40-24).

Some villous adenomas cause dehydration, hypocalcemia, azotemia, and circulatory distress. Often mucus precedes the normal stool in the morning. The amount of mucus relates directly to the surface area of the growth and not to a peculiarity of the neoplasm. The patient compensates for the loss of electrolytes for many years. Eventually the tumor becomes so large that compensation is ineffectual.[9,36] Bleeding is frequent. The lesions are usually single, and malignant degeneration is common. The frequency with which malignancy is reported depends upon the diligence of the pathologist examining the specimen. Histologic and gross examination of the lesion must be correlated in order to make the correct evaluation.[45]

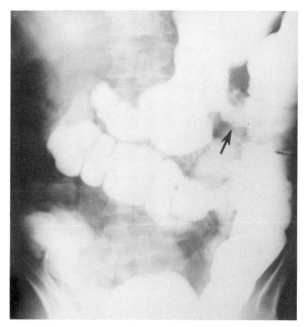

Fig. 40-25. A carcinoma of the stomach invaded the descending colon, producing a gastrocolic fistula (arrow). The lesion was demonstrated by barium enema. The patient was not aware of trouble until her breath became obnoxious and she began having large foul-smelling stools that contained fat. Bacteria entering the small bowel from the colon produced a malabsorption syndrome.

Some villous adenomas, especially those arising in the right side of the colon, do not have a spongelike appearance. Without electrolyte imbalance they are indistinguishable from other masses.[54]

Colon invaded by tumors arising in adjacent structures

Tumors spreading from adjacent organs may invade the colon and appear as primary colonic tumors. These carcinomas arise from the stomach, gallbladder, duodenum, kidney, and even the pancreas. Gastric carcinoma invading the colon through the gastrocolic ligament may cause gastrocolic fistula. In these instances primary tumors of the colon are sometimes reported when the original lesion is in the stomach (Fig. 40-25).

Carcinoma arising in the cervix, vagina, ovaries, and urinary bladder can invade the rectum and sigmoid. Radiation therapists routinely ask for examinations of the colon in "staging"

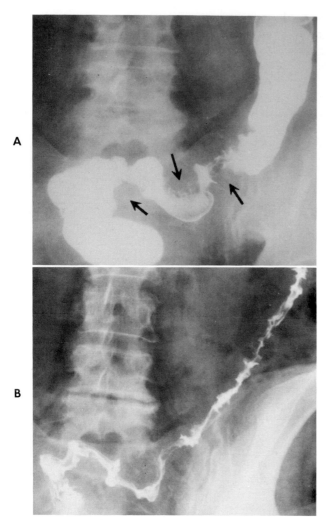

Fig. 40-26. Carcinoma of the breast metastasizing to colon. **A,** Three polypoid indentations deformed the lower descending colon (arrows). **B,** After partial evacuation intact folds in the region of the tumors became apparent. At surgery three masses were felt in the wall of the lower portion of the descending colon. Many nodules were scattered over the peritoneum. Histologically, the pattern of the peritoneal masses resembled that of the original tumor. Subserosal and probably intramural metastatic tumors to the colon was the surgical diagnosis.

lesions of the urogenital tract. The patterns presented may appear as a primary carcinoma of the lower colon. The differentiation is made by knowing that a lesion exists in the originating organ.

In carcinoma of the cervix a rectovaginal fistula is a serious complication. Although colonic carcinoma does involve neighboring structures, the symptoms of colonic carcinoma usually bring the patient to the physician before other structures are involved. Rectovaginal fistulas as presenting lesions usually originate from carcinoma of the vagina or uterus rather than from carcinoma of the colon. On barium enema with the patient in lateral position, the fistula appears as a channel emerging from the anterior wall of the rectum or inferior aspect of the sigmoid. If the fistula is large, barium will flood the vagina.

Invasion of the colon by adjacent tumors is not as common as it was in the past. Patients seek help sooner. Better urography and cholangiography, the intravenous injection of contrast material into arteries and veins, and improved roentgenographic equipment have all played a role in the early detection of important lesions.

Metastasis to the colon from carcinoma occurring outside the abdominal cavity is uncommon. The abnormalities produced by metastatic carcinoma are usually multiple and eccentrically located. They may obstruct the lumen. If the examiner does not know of a primary carcinoma elsewhere he may diagnose either primary neoplasm or inflammatory disease if diverticula are present. Sharply defined "shelving" margins observed in the primary annular ulcerating carcinoma are absent in the few metastatic lesions reported. The intramural nature of the lesion and intact mucosa is appreciated when the colon is partially distended (Fig. 40-26).

Endometriosis

Endometrial tissue (adenomyosis) sometimes invades and deforms the colon in women who have not borne children or who have had only one child. The implants respond to hormonal influence. The symptoms are exaggerated during menstruation and regress when ovarian stimulation is removed. With each exacerbation fibrosis is produced. Eventually fibrosis becomes pronounced, fixes the deformity, and permanently narrows the bowel. The relationship between symptoms and the menstrual cycle eventually disappears.

The sigmoid colon and the rectosigmoid junction above the reflection of the peritoneum at the level of the third sacral segment is the usual site of the tumor. The tumor, seen in lateral projection, causes a curved, sharply defined indentation fixed on the anterior wall of the rectosigmoid junction. The latter pattern is expected

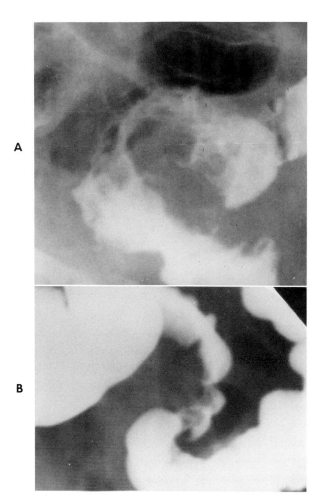

Fig. 40-27. Endometriosis invading the colon. **A,** A mass on the anterior wall of the rectosigmoid narrows the lumen. The lesion was found 1 week after the patient was operated on for endometriosis. The surgeon had explored the region and stated that no tumor was present. At a second operation the mass proved to be an abscess involving the anterior aspect of the rectosigmoid. Although the mass in the patient was not a neoplasm, the pattern is common in people having endometriosis and other polypoid tumors. Tumors at the rectosigmoid bend are easily missed at roentgenologic examination if good lateral views of the rectosigmoid are not obtained. **B,** The midsigmoid is narrowed by invasion of the inferior wall by endometrial tissue. The superior wall is not invaded and the extremities of the lesions are not as distinct as they usually are in annular ulcerating carcinoma. These variations indicate that the pattern is caused by tissue invading from without; in this case endometrial tissue.

since the tumor invades from the cul-de-sac. Because of the sharp bend that occurs at rectosigmoid the lumen narrows and the lesion may easily be overlooked (Fig. 40-27, *A*).

Lesions located more proximally in the sigmoid colon cause an irregularly narrowed channel within which folds are identified. The ends of the lesion are not sharp against the normal portion of bowel. If colonic diverticula are present the differentiation from scarring produced by diverticulitis is not possible by roentgenography.

Endometriosis can invade the mucosa and cause bleeding, but rarely produces multilobulated masses resembling adenocarcinomas. The prominent, undermined, or overhanging edges seen in carcinoma do not usually occur in endometriosis (Fig. 40-27, *B*).

The cecum is rarely the site of endometrial implants. The cecal tip is indented by an intramural extramucosal smooth nodular mass. Constriction and kinking of the cecum seldom occurs. The lesion is differentiated from other conditions by recognizing that symptoms are aggravated during the menstrual cycle.

Intussusception of the sigmoid into the rectum and of the cecum into the ascending colon as a result of endometriosis has been reported.[19]

Carcinoid

Carcinoid is an incidental finding unless the tumor causes obstruction (Fig. 40-26). It is often low-grade malignant. Although the appendix and the small bowel are preferred sites, carcinoid tumors occur elsewhere in the colon, especially in the cecum. As in other tumors, carcinoid rarely causes obstruction of the cecum but can obstruct the narrower transverse and descending segments of the colon and may act as a nidus for intussusception. Flushing, the distinctive characteristic of the carcinoid syndrome, occurs rarely. Often the tumor cannot be differentiated roentgenographically from a polypoid adenocarcinoma. When small, carcinoid tumors and adenocarcinoma may be smooth and sessile. When large, only carcinoma becomes ulcerated and fissured (Fig. 40-27).

Sarcomas

Sarcomas of the colon are infrequently encountered. The lesions are either localized to an organ such as the colon or are diffuse and

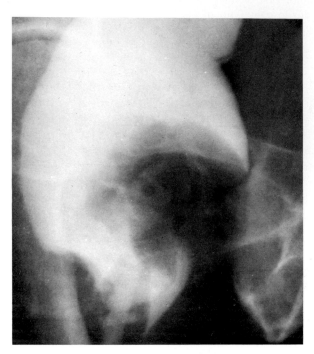

Fig. 40-28. Large, sessile, lobulated mass with a broad base protrudes into the rectum. The upper border forms a sharp acute angle with the rectal wall. This was an undifferentiated sarcoma.

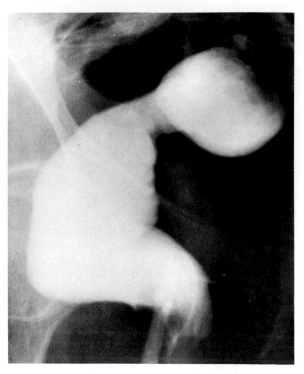

Fig. 40-29. A lymphoma contricts the rectosigmoid. Transition to the normal mucosa is not discrete and the walls are less rigid than in adenocarcinoma. Roentgenologic differentiation from adenocarcinoma may not be possible.

part of systemic disease. The usual types are lymphosarcoma, reticulum cell sarcoma, and leiomyosarcoma. The lesions can occur anywhere in the colon but commonly involve the cecum and the rectosigmoid. Often the solitary lesions are beyond the range of the proctoscope and are recognized at exploratory laparotomy, biopsy, or necropsy. The usual diagnosis before histologic diagnosis is carcinoma or inflammatory disease.

A few signs may suggest solitary sarcoma. Constitutional symptoms are fewer than in carcinoma. The mass palpated through the abdomen or seen at roentgenographic examination can be large without causing symptoms. On occasion the patient sees his physician because he has felt a mass in his abdomen. Signs of bowel distress and blood in the stool are often absent.

As in carcinoma the localized sarcomas are polypoid, ulcerating, annular, and infiltrating. The polypoid form produces an irregular or smooth mass that protrudes into the lumen (Fig. 40-28). At palpation the mass often feels

larger than it appears at fluoroscopy because, unlike most polypoid carcinomas, the tumor grows outward from the lumen as well as into the lumen. Some tumors ulcerate. The result is a large, irregular ulcer, surrounded by a thick rolled margin.[33] Like carcinoma, the sarcomatous ulcer can perforate and spill colonic contents into the peritoneal cavity.[50]

In the annular lymphomas the transition to the normal mucosa is gradual and the wall less rigid than in carcinoma (Fig. 40-29). Invasion of the ileocecal sphincter causes obstruction. Like carcinomas, the sarcomas, especially those occurring in the cecum and ascending colon, can give rise to intussusception.

The diffuse type of sarcoma is difficult to differentiate from inflammatory disease. Long segments or the entire bowel are involved. With enema the bowel distends. Haustra may be normal, widened, or obliterated. In the incompletely distended colon or after partial evacuation an irregular cobblestone pattern is superimposed on coarse mucosal folds. Sometimes the prominent folds appear matted and "cerebriform." The colon is not rigid. The folds can be deformed but not obliterated by pressure. With extensive disease, small polypoid lesions appear and resemble the pseudopolyps of ulcerative colitis. Lymphomas, however, do not produce small ulcerations and shortening of the colon, changes that indicate advanced inflammatory disease.

In my limited experience with infiltrating colonic lymphoma, the lesions resemble inflammation. This is particularly true in Hodgkin's disease. As in Crohn's disease, "skip" lesions occur and are associated with lesions in the small intestine. The diagnosis is made by finding evidence of the lymphoma in the chest or peripheral nodes.

Confusing infiltrating lymphosarcoma with inflammatory disease is a common error. Winkelstein and Levy state that to the inexperienced eye lymphosarcoma resembles ulcerative colitis or carcinoma at sigmoidoscopy.[59] However, the mucosa has a characteristic convoluted, cerebriform appearance. The mucosa is not involved until late in the disease.

Federman and associates reported a patient having a reticulum cell sarcoma of the entire colon that was treated for 15 years as ulcerative colitis.[16] Proctoscopic findings were not described, and no tissue for biopsy was removed. Had biopsy been performed the correct diagnosis probably would have been established early in the disease.

Other types of sarcomas have been described. Fibrosarcomas are sessile and usually circumscribed. Angiosarcomas can be of various sizes and shapes and may constrict the lumen. They should be observed by angiography. Malignant melanosarcomas, usually located in the rectum, are often large and undergo ulceration and necrosis.

Leiomyoma and leiomyosarcoma are indistinguishable from one another at roentgenologic examination unless metastases are present. Most myomatous tumors protrude into the colonic lumen, whereas a few grow outwards into the peritoneal cavity; others grow in both directions. Less commonly, the tumor grows circumferentially, producing a constriction. The roentgenographic appearance is that of a mass with intact overlying mucosa. Occasionally, at the crown of the mass a large penetrating ulcer occurs. The margins of the mass are sharply demarcated, and the angle formed by the mass and the adjacent mucosa is sharp. These features also occur in other intraluminal tumors and are not diagnostic of myomatous neoplasms. Intussusception, which is common, may prevent roentgenologic identification of the mass. Less commonly the tumors produce mechanical obstruction. The constricting lesions sometimes resemble carcinoma but involve a longer segment of bowel than most common adenocarcinomas.

When first detected, myomatous tumors of the colon are frequently large, and a mass is usually palpable. They may, by their size, displace adjacent organs.[55]

Radiation injury

Radiation to the pelvis, especially the cervix, uterus, and prostate, can damage the rectum and sigmoid. In the early stages acute inflammation, resulting in thickened folds, ulceration, and stricture, does not present a problem to the diagnostic radiologist. The problem arises when the patient returns several months or years later with complaints relating to the bowel. At roentgenologic examination a segment of rectum or sigmoid is narrowed, smooth, and rigid. The distance between the rectum and sacrum is increased and measures 2 or more cm.

A narrowed segment 5 to 15 cm. long and having the ends merge gradually with normal bowel is almost assuredly the result of radiation injury. Vasculitis produced by radiation is probably the initiating cause. Malignant change of the intestinal tract injured by radiation is so rare that it must be considered a curiosity.[46] Long segments of abnormal bowel are surely the result of radiation injury (Fig. 40-30, *A*). Unless follow-up studies are available, it is often difficult from single examinations to exclude recurrence of tumor.

A short, sharply defined, narrowed segment in a patient having no history of bowel damage during radiation is probably a carcinoma.

Ischemia of the bowel

Arterial or venous obstruction causes a long lesion starting with marked edema of the bowel and resolving into a narrowed, foldless segment. Without history or knowledge of the acute phase, the differentiation from scirrhous carcinoma is difficult. The lumen of the resolved

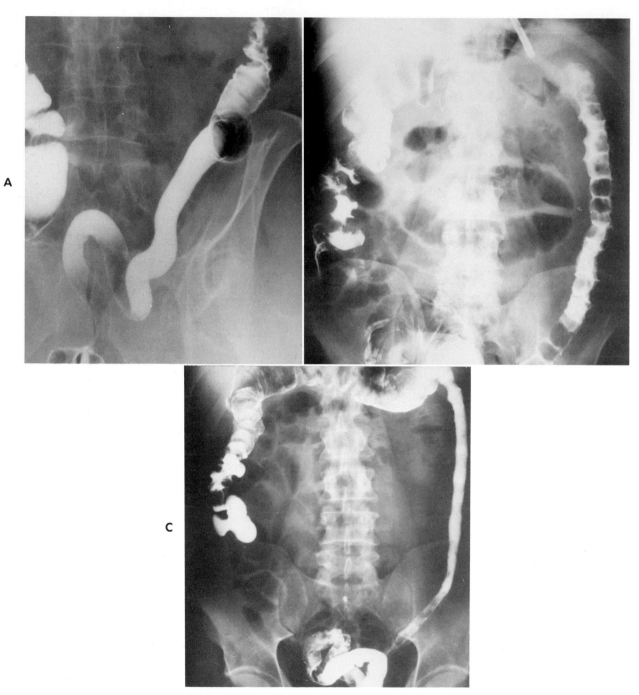

Fig. 40-30. A, Radiation injury to the rectosigmoid. Three months after irradiation to the pelvis for carcinoma of the cervix, the rectosigmoid became smooth and narrow. **B,** After a vascular insult to the inferior mesenteric artery the mucosa of the descending colon is edematous and produces "large polypoid" masses. **C,** The same patient 10 days later. The lumen is narrowed and smooth. The resemblance is similar to the radiation injury indicated in **A** and to scirrhous carcinoma (Fig. 40-15).

ischemic segment is narrow and pliable at palpation and does not enlarge when the enema pressure is increased. When the pressure is released the lumen of the bowel decreases slightly. The caliber of the lumen in advanced stages of scirrhous carcinomas does not change with changes in enema pressure. The outline of the lumen is ragged and stiff. In rare instances lesions confined to segments of the colon supplied by a given artery should suggest infarction (Fig. 40-30, *B* and *C*).

Rare lesions

Tumors of the appendix. Tumors of the appendix on occasions indent and invade the tip of the cecum. The tumors appear at the origin of the appendix, located 3 or 4 cm. below the ileocecal sphincter on the medial aspect of the cecum. The tumors are carcinoid, carcinoma, mucocele, myxoglobulosis, tumors of mesenchymal origin, and endometrial transplants. Masses of the cecal tip after the appendix is removed are usually granulomas. Appendiceal tumors often produce a circular arrangement of folds caused by a puckering of the mucosa, scar, or intussusception.[28]

Myxoglobulosis is an uncommon variant of mucocele and may obstruct the appendix. The appendix becomes cystlike. At roentgenologic examination a sharply defined mass indents the medial cecal wall. The margins are abrupt and angular, a characteristic of intramural extramucosal lesion. The cecum is displaced by the mass, and the mucosa is not invaded. Calcified, faceted, or annular bodies move about within the cyst and layer in the upright position. The calcifications differ from the punctate variety found in colloid carcinoma of the colon.[19]

Duplication. Duplications of a segment of colonic lumen occur anywhere and cause tumorlike structures that indent, displace, or even obstruct the colon. The condition usually involves the cecum and rectum and consists of isolated lesions arising from embryologic rests in the wall of the bowel. The duplication arises from the main lumen and produces a diverticulum-like structure. If the lumen is closed off it causes a cyst (Fig. 40-31). Cysts rarely cause intussusception. When the cysts are adjacent to the rectum, the rectum is displaced forwards and upwards from the sacrum. A similar situation occurs in presacral teratomas and lipomas. All

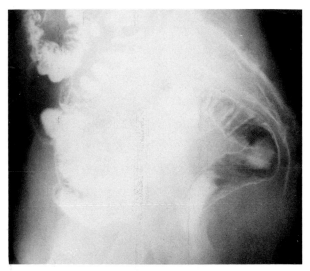

Fig. 40-31. A retrorectal mass was removed from this patient, and the pathologist reported a cloacal cyst. However, in view of the posterior location of the lesion, the pathologist stated that duplication was also a possibility.

tumors are best seen in a lateral projection of the rectosacral region and appear similar, except that in some instances the lipoma casts the characteristic radiolucent shadow of fat.

Colitis cystica profunda. Colitis cystica profunda is rarely recognized and must be separated from colitis cystica superficialis, a condition that is pathognomonic of pellagra.[10] The latter produces no roentgenologic signs. The former invades the submucosa. Submucosal cysts lie in edematous mucosa and produce nodular, polypoid, or cauliflower-like patterns. Ulcers are rare. The multiple polyps, similar to polyposis localized to the rectum, occur from 5 to 12 cm. from the anus and cover either a small area or spread around the rectum causing strictures.[57]

An example of colitis cystica profunda was reported by the Armed Forces Institute of Pathology. A polyp overlying submucosal glands and cysts was mistakenly called colloid carcinoma.[13] Differentiation by studying only the cells and not the distribution of glandular tissue in the walls of the colon indicated the correct diagnosis.

No roentgenologic pattern is distinct for the condition. In studying biopsies of polyps or cysts the condition should be kept in mind so as not to call a benign lesion malignant and subject the patient to unnecessary surgery.

Solitary ulcer. Solitary ulcer, which resembles adenocarcinoma, is so rare that it must be treated as a pathologic curiosity. One ulcer was discovered in the cecum by a barium enema.[5]

According to pathologic descriptions, the patient consults his physician because of acute abdominal distress.[7,31,40] The symptoms often resemble perforated appendix. With that diagnosis surgery is performed. Barium enema is not given because of the acute symptoms and signs of perforation.

At surgery the appendix is normal. Opposite the ileocecal sphincter lies an indurated mass thought to be perforated adenocarcinoma. The right colon is resected. Only at pathologic examination is the true nature of the lesion recognized.

If a roentgenologist examines a patient having a simple ulcer before perforation he will probably encounter the following patterns. In the early stages the ulcer, which looks like that seen in the stomach or duodenum, appears usually on the anterior wall of the cecum within a few centimeters of the ileocecal sphincter. The tissue around the ulcer is indurated and firm. In the advanced state the induration forms a mass that protrudes into the bowel. The mass measures 5 or more cm. in diameter. On the mucosal surface in the center of the mass protrudes a deep funnel-shaped ulcer measuring 1 or 2 cm. The margins of the ulcer are firm and raised, without undercutting. The mass resembles neoplasm that stenoses and eventually obstructs the intestine. Some bleed.

Most solitary ulcers occur in the cecum. A few are reported in other sections of the colon and rectum. Naiken and Rochman reported an ulcer in a patient with rectal bleeding.[43] A lesion interpreted as carcinoma was found in the transverse colon. At pathologic examination four discrete, benign, annular ulcers were found, separated by normal mucosa. All had indurated serpiginous edges.

The cause is unknown. Inflamed diverticulum has been suggested but has not been proved. "Stasis" is considered, probably because shallow ulcers commonly form in the bowel behind long-standing obstruction. However, ulcers behind the obstruction are not surrounded with firm indurated tissue.

Pseudotumors. Pseudotumors caused by pressure of external masses or by adhesions may mimic carcinoma. These extraneous masses are abnormal, such as a large ovary, or are normal, such as a barium-filled, redundant, distended sigmoid. The patterns are differentiated from colonic lesions by distending the colon, especially the cecum, which is the most common site of pseudotumors, with air after barium has been administered. As the cecum distends, the walls balloon out and become smooth and the "tumor" disappears.[39]

Two conditions that can be mistaken for tumor are a loop of bowel that, seen on end, may look like a polyp, or spasm of the bowel, particularly in the transverse and descending colon, which may mimic annular neoplasm.

INFLAMMATIONS AND CANCER
Ulcerative colitis and carcinoma

Carcinoma is a serious complication of ulcerative colitis. The incidence of neoplasm increases with severity and the length of time the patient has the disease. In most instances the neoplasm does not appear in the first 10 years but becomes increasingly frequent in people who have the disease for 10 years or longer.[38] When discovered by a radiologist the carcinoma is advanced, and the usual signs of carcinoma with sharp overhanging edges are obscured by the surrounding diseased tissue. Since long-standing ulcerative colitis gives rise to strictures, all strictures should be suspected of carcinoma. Carcinomas that involve long lengths of bowel are often scirrhous and comprise about 30% of the carcinomas arising in ulcerative colitis. Because these carcinomas involve long segments of bowel they are recognized after the bowel becomes rigid, narrow, and irregular. Mucosal patterns within the lumen do not help differentiate ulcerative colitis from carcinoma because the patterns appear similar (Fig. 40-15).

Carcinoma and diverticulitis

In diverticulitis healing produces fibrotic tissue, which contracts, forms a narrow lumen, and looks like carcinoma. Obstruction may result. In cancer the involved segment is short and narrow. Diverticula and folds within the involved segment are absent, victims of the neoplastic infiltration. The overhanging shoulder of ulcerating adenocarcinoma may show (Fig. 40-32). In diverticulitis the invaded segment is often longer and narrow. The change is usually caused

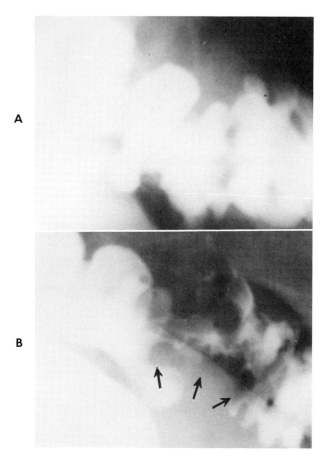

Fig. 40-32. Carcinoma and diverticulitis. **A,** Many diverticula protrude from the sigmoid with no evidence of carcinoma. **B,** Three years later a carcinoma obliterated many of the diverticula. Arrows mark the involved segment. (**A** and **B** are identical projections of the same segment of bowel.)

by surrounding inflammation, produced by a diverticulum that has perforated. The folds within the involved segment are irregular and diverticula can be identified. The extremities of the lesion gradually merge with the irregular folds produced by diverticulosis. Sometimes a fistula or abscess fills with barium.

A neoplasm accompanied by marked inflammation cannot be differentiated from diverticulitis. The inflamatory tissue adjacent to the mucosa obliterates the sharp margins of the tumor.

Solitary cecal diverticulitis may simulate carcinoma if the inflammation is not acute. The surgeon not sure of his clinical diagnosis requests a barium enema. The radiologist finds a lesion on the anterior wall. The lesion may contain the fecalith sometimes observed on the

survey film. The pattern is similar to that caused by solitary ulcer, but usually the surrounding inflammation is not pronounced and deep ulcer does not exist. The lesion is considered by some surgeons to be a congenital reduplication connecting with the bowel and not the acquired diverticulum seen elsewhere in the bowel.

Not all authors agree that congenital diverticula are the sole cause of cecal diverticulitis.[3] Not uncommonly, one or more symptomless diverticula are encountered in the cecum associated with diverticula elsewhere in the colon. In every way the cecal diverticula appear similar to the acquired diverticula so frequently found in the sigmoid. After inflammation begins, differentiation between congenital and acquired diverticula is not possible even at pathologic examination.

Other inflammatory lesions

Other inflammatory lesions simulate carcinoma and are so rare that detailed description is unnecessary. They are lymphogranuloma venereum, syphilis, actinomycosis, and amebic colitis.

More common are tuberculosis and transmural colitis or Crohn's disease. Tuberculosis may be misinterpreted as carcinoma of the cecum. The terminal ileum is involved in only the advanced cases of tuberculosis, and therefore "cecal tuberculosis" is a better term than "ileocecal tuberculosis." The roentgenologic differentiation of tuberculosis confined to the cecum and terminal ileum is the same as that used for Crohn's disease. The two diseases appear similar. Elongated ulcers and ridges cause an irregular lumen. The lumen may narrow and stenose. The final diagnosis is made by finding tuberculosis elsewhere, usually the lungs. Bacilli are found in the stools.[35] Crohn's disease is indicated by skip lesions and is rarely associated with carcinoma.[47] Fig. 40-33 depicts an unusual granuloma diagnosed as carcinoma at roentgenologic examination.

Pelvic lipomatosis

Pelvic lipomatosis is a benign disease manifested by increased deposition of fat in the pelvis. It can produce colon and bladder deformities, mimicking those caused by widespread pelvic neoplasms.

The soft tissue of the pelvis appears radio-

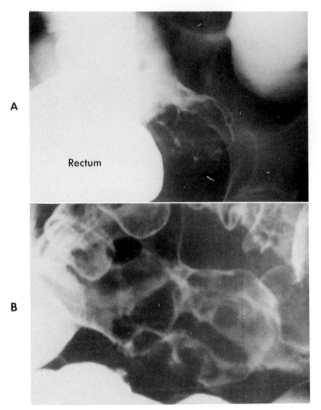

Fig. 40-33. Localized granuloma of the sigmoid. **A,** The lesion overlying the pelvic brim is partially obstructed by the rectum. **B,** On spot films the polypoid lobular nature of the lesion is evident. At roentgenologic examination polypoid adenocarcinoma of the sigmoid was diagnosed. At pathologic examination no evidence of carcinoma was found. The tissue consisted of inflammation and fibrosis interspersed with granulomas. No evidence of granulomatous disease was found elsewhere in the gastrointestinal tract at roentgenologic examination or at surgical exploration.

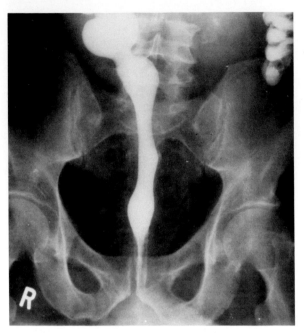

Fig. 40-34. Elongated, narrow, and extrinsically impressed rectosigmoid in a patient with pelvic lipomatosis. There is an ill-defined radiolucency of the soft tissues of the pelvis. (From Moss, A. A., Clark, R. E., Goldberg, H. I., and Pepper, H. W.: Pelvic lipomatosis: a roentgenographic diagnosis, Amer. J. Roentgen. **115:** 411-419, 1972.)

lucent. The bladder is usually vertically elongated. The disease usually occurs in males (29 of 30 reported cases). The disease has been reported occurring at any age, including childhood. Hypertension is a frequent complication.

Histologically, there is no evidence of neoplasm. The findings are of normal mature adipose tissue.

RECURRENT CARCINOMA

The patient who has had a carcinoma removed is subject to recurrent carcinoma elsewhere in the bowel as well as at the operative site.

In some persons with colonic carcinoma the distal colon is removed and colostomy established. In others local resection is performed and continuity is reestablished by end-to-end anastomosis. In each person the colon left after surgery should be examined.

How often should the colon be reexamined? Probably once a year is sufficient.[48] Most cancers do not grow rapidly and do not metastasize in the first year. The frequency (1 year) of examination holds true for familial polyposis and Peutz-Jeghers, Gardner's, and Turcot's syndromes. In these syndromes colonic polyps become malignant. Those people who have a genetic strain for familial polyposis and who have not developed polyps by the age of 40 will probably not develop polyps or malignancy.[37]

Carcinomas may recur at the site of an end-to-end anastomosis. The recurrence probably results from implantation of cells left in the lumen or from incompletely removed tumors. In two instances Fleischner and Berenberg noted a

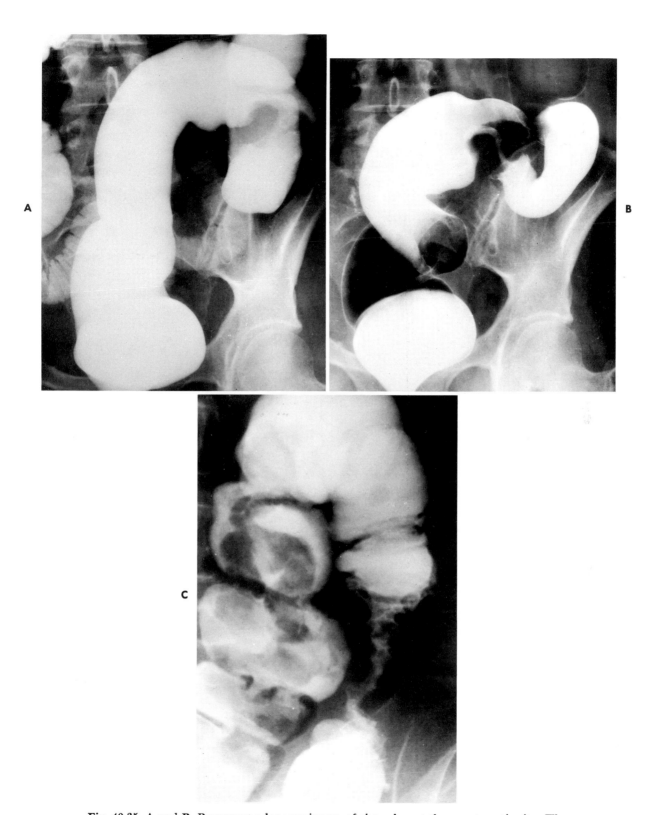

Fig. 40-35. A and **B,** Recurrent adenocarcinoma of the colon at the anastomotic site. The neoplasm has completely encircled the colon at this site. The displacement of the tumor with change in position of the patient indicates that it is not adherent to the adjacent abdominal wall. **C,** Recurrent adenocarcinoma at the anastomotic site. A long segment of colon is constricted with intact but thickened mucosa proximally, indicating submucosal extension.

tumor on the ileal side of an ileocolic anastomosis.[22] In another instance a suture thread was found in the center of a recurrent tumor. These findings suggest that carcinoma becomes implanted during the anastomosis.

Annular constriction with sharp ends and appearing similar to a primary tumor indicates recurrence. A small bandlike stricture with pliable margins of the adjacent lumen is probably caused by scar tissue. Sometimes the recurrent carcinoma involves only one side of the bowel. The examiner cannot be certain if the appearance is caused by recurrent carcinoma or scar tissue. In case of doubt exploratory laparotomy is indicated even if liver scans are normal. It is unwise to wait a month to see if a change occurs. I have found that a base line study done shortly after the examination is of no value. Scar and regeneration of soft tissue often produces pronounced changes (Fig. 40-35).

REFERENCES

1. Achord, J. L., and Proctor, H. D.: Malignant degeneration, and metastasis in Peutz-Jegher's syndrome, Arch. Intern. Med. 3:498, 1963.
2. Aylett, S.: Surgery of the cecum and colon, Edinburgh 1954, E. & S. Livingston.
3. Bennett-Jones, M. J.: Primary solitary diverticulitis of the cecum, a report of 3 cases, with review of 17 recorded cases, Brit. J. Surg. 25:66, 1937.
4. Berg, H. H.: Röntgenuntersuchung am Innenrelief des Verdauugskanals, Leipzig, 1930, Georg Thieme Verlag.
5. Bombi, G.: Policlinico (sez-Prot) 36:1550, 1929.
6. Cantor, M. O., and Reynolds, R. P.: Gastrointestinal obstruction, Baltimore, 1957, The William & Wilkins Co.
7. Cromer, C. D. L.: Benign ulcer of the cecum, Amer. J. Dig. Dis. 13:230, 1946.
8. Cutler, D., and others: Pneumotosis cystoides intestinalis, report of 22 cases, Amer. J. Proctol. 20:261, 1969.
9. Davis, E. J. and others: Villous adenomas of the rectum and sigmoid colon with severe fluid and electrolytic depletion, Ann. Surg. 155:806, 1962.
10. Denton, J.: Colitis cystica profunda, Amer. J. Trop. Med. 5:173, 1925.
11. Dryfuss, J. R., and Janower, M. J.: Radiologic examination of the colon, Baltimore, 1969, The William & Wilkins Co.
12. Edwards, C. L., and Hayes, R. L.: Scanning malignant neoplasm with gallium 67, J.A.M.A. 212:1182, 1970.
13. Edwards, C. L., and Hayes, R. L.: Tumor scanning with ^{67}Ga citrate, J. Nucl. Med. 10:103, 1969.
14. Epstein, S. E., and others: Colitis cystica profunda, Amer. J. Clin. Path. 45:186, 1966.
15. Falk, W. S., and Rogers, J. C. T.: Familial polyposis, 25 year follow-up, Arch. Surg. 96:962, 1968.
16. Federman, J., and others: Malignant lymphoma of over 15 years duration masquerading as ulcerative colitis, Amer. J. Roentgen. 89:771, 1963.
17. Felson, B., and Wiot, J. F.: Some interesting right lower quadrant entities, Radiologic Clinics of North America, Philadelphia, 1969, W. B. Saunders Co.
18. Flemming, C.: Retrograde intussusception, Lancet 2:1136, 1937.
19. Fitzwilliams, D. C. L.: Pathology and etiology of intussusception, Lancet 1:628, 1908.
20. Fleischner, F. E., and Berenberg, A. L.: Recurrent carcinoma of the colon at the site of anastomosis: roentgen observations, Radiology 66:540, 1956.
21. Fletcher, B. D., and others: Calcified adenocarcinoma of the colon, Amer. J. Roentgen. 101:301, 1967.
22. Fronstein, M. H., and Hutcheson, J. B.: Trichobezoar as a cause of obstruction of the colon, Amer. Surg. 33:475, 1966.
23. Gardner, E. G., and Richards, R. C.: Multiple cutaneous and subcutaneous lesions occurring simultaneously with hereditary polyposis and osteomatosis, Amer. J. Hum. Genet. 5:139, 1953.
24. Grant, E.: Sigmoidal rectal intussusception and the unstable colon, Amer. J. Dig. Dis. 19:19, 1952.
25. Haney, M. J., and McGarity, W. E.: Ureterosigmoidostomy and neoplasms of the colon, J.A.M.A. 103:69, 1971.
26. Hawley, C., and Mithoefler, J.: Ileal prolapse, Radiology 54:380, 1950.
27. Howard, R. J., and others: Intussusception of the appendix simulating carcinoma of the cecum, Arch. Surg. 101:520, 1970.
28. Janower, M. J., and others: Cancer of the gastrointestinal tract in young people, Radiologic Clinics of North America, Philadelphia, 1969, W. B. Saunders Co.
29. Jones, F.: Colonic pseudo-obstruction, Ogilvie's syndrome, clinical gastroenterology, ed. 2, Philadelphia, 1963, F. A. Davis Co.
30. Lewis, E. E.: A case of retrograde intussusception occurring during life, Brit. J. Surg. 23:683, 1936.
31. Lipton, S., and Reisman, E. D.: Simple ulcer of the cecum, Amer. J. Surg. 134:279, 1951.
32. Lower, J. D., and others: Accuracy of roentgen examination in detecting carcinoma of the colon, Dis. Colon Rectum 8:170, 1960.
33. Lumsden, K., and Truelove, S. C.: Radiology of the digestive system, Philadelphia, 1965, F. A. Davis Co.
34. Lynch, H. T., and Kruch, A. J.: Heredity and adenocarcinoma of the colon, Gastroenterology 53:517, 1967.
35. Marionotti, G., and others: Radiologic aspects of intestinal tuberculosis in the ileocecal tract and colon, Rev. Clin. Tuber. 40:22, 1967.
36. Mc Kittrick, L. S., and Wheelock, F. C.: Carcinoma of colon, Springfield, Ill., 1954, Charles C Thomas, Publisher.
37. McKusick, V. A.: Genetic factors in intestinal polyps, J.A.M.A. 182:271, 1962.

38. McMillan, W. O., and others: Problem of cancer in ulcerative colitis, Southern Med. J. **61**:526, 1968.

39. Matter, B., and Rotke, K. H.: Pseudotumors—radiographic findings in the colon, Radiol. Diagn. **10**:573, 1969.

40. Maynard, J.: Solitary ulcer of the cecum, Guy. Hosp. Rep. **116**:39, 1967.

41. McQueeney, A. J., and others: Primary scirrhous carcinoma of the colon, Amer. J. Roentgen. **101**:306, 1967.

42. Mulligan, R. M.: Syllabus of human neoplasms, Philadelphia, 1951, Lea & Febiger.

43. Naiken, V. S., and Rackman, R.: Giant ulcer of the transverse colon, J.A.M.A. **217**:344, 1971.

44. Ogilvie, H.: Large intestinal colic due to sympathetic deprivation, Brit. Med. J. **672**:671, 1948.

45. Olson, R. O., Davis, W. C.: Villous adenomas of the colon, benign or malignant, Arch. Surg. **38**:487, 1969.

46. Parker, R. G.: Personal communication.

47. Perrett, A. D., and Truelove, S. C.: Chronic disease and carcinoma of the colon, Brit. Med. J. **2**:466, 1968.

48. Prevot, R.: Grundriss der Röntgenologie des Magen-Darmeanals, Hamburg, 1948, H. H. Nolke Verlag.

49. Rankin, F. W., and Stephens, A.: Cancer of the colon and rectum, ed. 2, Springfield, Ill., 1950, Charles C Thomas, Publishers.

50. Ritvo, M., and Shauffar, I. A.: Gastrointestinal diagnosis, Philadelphia, 1952, Lea & Febiger.

51. Robbins, S. L.: Pathology, Philadelphia, 1967, W. B. Saunders Co.

52. Rosato, F. E., and others: Nonmetastatic cutaneous manifestations of cancer of the colon, Amer. J. Surg. **117**:227, 1969.

53. Schinz, H. R., Baensch, W. E., and Friedl, E.: Roentgen diagnostics, Translated by Case, J. T., New York, 1952, Grune & Stratton, Inc.

54. Tung, C. H. K., and Goldman, H.: The incidence and significance of villous changes in adenomatous polyps, Amer. J. Clin. Path. **53**:21, 1970.

55. Valdes-Depena, A. M., and Stein, G. N.: Morphologic pathology of the alimentery tract, Philadelphia, 1970, W. B. Saunders Co.

56. Walker, J. H.: Growth patterns of colon carcinoma, Bull. Mason. Clin. **25**:11, 1971.

57. Wayte, D. M., and Helwig, E. B.: Colitis cystica profunda, Amer. J. Clin. Path. **48**:159, 1967.

58. Weber, H. M.: Diagnosis of early intestinal cancer, Amer. J. Roentgen. **64**:929, 1950.

59. Winkelstein, A., and Levy, M.: Lymphosarcoma of the intestines, Gastroenterology **1**:1093, 1943.

60. Wolf, B. S., and Marshak, R. H.: Roentgen features of diffuse lymphosarcoma of the colon, Radiology **75**:733, 1960.

61. Wolf, S. W., and Marshak, R. H.: Linitis plastica or diffusely infiltrating type of carcinoma of the colon, Radiology **81**:502, 1963.

62. Wynder, E. L., and Shigematsue, T.: Environmental factors of the colon and rectum, Cancer **20**:1520, 1967.

Part VII

The pancreas and the lesser sac

Pathology of the pancreas | 41

Harlan J. Spjut
Antonio Navarrete

Lesions of the pancreas and biliary tract are important not only in themselves but because of involvement of adjacent organs. A lesion that commonly impinges upon nearby structures is the pancreatic pseudocyst. Pseudocyst usually follows an episode of pancreatitis or trauma. Pseudocysts in adults usually follow acute or chronic pancreatitis, and pseudocysts in children are usually related to trauma. The lesion is found in the head or body, or both, and only rarely confined to the tail of the pancreas. Because of the location, pseudocysts may displace the stomach anteriorly, displace the transverse colon, or extend into the pelvis and even into the mediastinum. Ordinarily, pseudocysts are unicameral and their wall is fibrous and devoid of an epithelial lining.[2]

Pseudocysts comprise approximately three fourths of the cysts of the pancreas, with the remainder being true cysts. True cysts have an epithelial lining. They are generally classified as congenital or acquired cysts; under the latter there are retention cysts, parasitic cysts, and cysts that may accompany neoplasms.[9]

PANCREATITIS

Acute pancreatitis is commonly associated with alcoholism but other factors such as pancreatic duct obstruction, reflux of bile, trauma, autoimmunization, and infection are individually or in combination important in the cause of pancreatitis. Grossly, the pancreas is usually enlarged, firm, and edematous, with chalky white areas of fat necrosis. If vessel necrosis occurs there will be focal or extensive extravasation of blood (hemorrhagic pancreatitis). Roentgenographically, the majority of patients have no abnormalities, about one third will have evidence of ileus, and a few will have calcific densities in the pancreatic area.[4]

Suppurative pancreatitis may result from infection in a neighboring organ, such as appendicitis or perforated peptic ulcer. According to Steedman and associates the most common cause

PANCREATITIS

MALFORMATIONS

CARCINOMA

ISLET CELL TUMORS

of suppuration (abscess) in the pancreas is preceding pancreatitis.[13] Most of the abscesses were located in the left subphrenic or retroperitoneal spaces, having originated in the body or tail of the pancreas. Usually, the roentgenograms demonstrate displacement of parapancreatic organs.

In chronic pancreatitis there is progressive destruction of parenchyma with fibrous replacement of parenchyma, duct obliteration, or duct dilatation. More than half of the patients have roentgenographically detectable calcification in the pancreatic area. The small or large ducts contain calculi; interstitial calcification is infrequent (Fig. 41-1).[8]

MALFORMATIONS

Annular pancreas is a rare anomaly that is apparently caused by a failure of fusion between the ventral and dorsal buds of the developing pancreas. The ventral bud develops independently and surrounds the second portion of the duodenum. There may be sufficient constriction to produce symptoms, or the lesion may be found coincidentally. At times the constriction may be severe enough that the lesion is diagnosed during infancy.

Aberrant pancreas is found in approximately 2% of autopsies. Favorite locations of aberrant pancreas are the stomach, duodenum, jejunum, Meckel's diverticulum, and ileum. Aberrant pancreas in other viscera is a rare finding. Usually the nodule, which is yellowish, is located

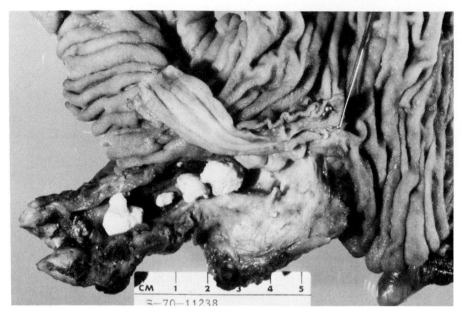

Fig. 41-1. Chronic pancreatitis. Calculi are seen in the dilated pancreatic duct. The surrounding pancreas is fibrous. Methodist Hospital S-70-11238.

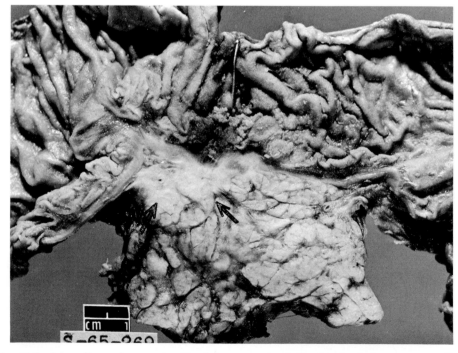

Fig. 41-2. A small carcinoma (outlined by arrows) of the head of the pancreas. Even though the carcinoma is small, the duodenal wall is invaded. Lymph nodes contained metastatic carcinoma. The probe is in the ampulla of Vater. BTGH #65028.

in the mucosa or submucosa of the bowel and occasionally may be found in the serosa or the muscularis.[5]

CARCINOMA

Carcinoma of the pancreas causes approximately 8 deaths per 100,000 population in the United States each year. During the past two decades there has been an increase in the number of deaths caused by carcinoma of the pancreas.[1] With rare exceptions carcinoma of the pancreas is a disease of adulthood, there being only some 22 cases reported in childhood.[6]

Approximately two thirds of the carcinomas of the pancreas occur in the head of the pancreas; the remainder occur in the body and tail or involve the pancreas diffusely. Grossly, the lesion usually presents as a hard ill-defined enlargement, commonly causing obstruction of the duct of Wirsung and the common bile duct. (Fig. 41-2). Much of the firmness of the cancer is caused by a frequently occurring fibrosis and chronic inflammation. Histologically, the majority of carcinomas of the pancreas are adenocarcinomas with varied degrees of differentiation and are probably ductal in origin. Occasional tumors have been reported that were thought to have been of acinar cell origin. A few carcinomas of the pancreas have been described that were squamous cell carcinomas or mixed squamous cell and adenocarcinomas. Metastases from carcinoma of the pancreas are frequent to regional lymph nodes, liver, lung, peritoneum, and the adrenal glands. The duodenum is frequently invaded in specimens that have been studied after surgical resection. The lesions may be associated with ulceration of the duodenal mucosa.[3,7,11,12]

A variant of carcinoma is the cystadenocarcinoma of the pancreas. Benign lesions designated as cystadenomas of the pancreas have also been described. There are fewer than 100 cases of cystadenomas and cystadenocarcinomas reported in the literature. These lesions are usually well encapsulated, lobulated, multicystic, and involve the body or tail. An interesting feature is the occurrence of the majority of these in women. In a few instances the capsule is calcified and may be so identified roentgenographically. Approximately 80% of these lesions present as a palpable upper abdominal mass and may reach 30 cm. in size. Histologically, these are often well-differentiated adenocarcinomas, some of which produce large quantities of mucin. In contrast to the ordinary carcinoma of the pancreas the cystadenocarcinoma is usually slow to metastasize and has a relatively good prognosis.[5,14]

ISLET CELL TUMORS

Islet cell tumors are most common in the body and tail of the pancreas, and approximately 10% are multiple. Unless functional, they are usually discovered by chance either at surgical exploration or at autopsy. Functional and nonfunctional tumors are histologically indistinguishable. Those associated with the Zollinger-Ellison syndrome have been designated as nonbeta cell tumors. The others, which are insulin-producing tumors, may demonstrate beta granules with proper staining techniques. Malignant islet cell tumors are difficult to differentiate from those that are benign unless metastases have occurred or there is infiltration into the surrounding organs or tissues. Capsular invasion or blood vessel invasion have not in themselves been considered evidence of overt malignancy. These carcinomas are compatible with a long life even in the presence of metastases.[10]

REFERENCES

1. American Cancer Society, 1971 Cancer facts and figures, New York, 1970, The Society.
2. Becker, W. F., Pratt, H. S., and Ganji, H.: Pseudocysts of the pancreas, Surg. Gynec. Obstet. **127**:744, 1968.
3. Bell, E. T.: Carcinoma of the pancreas, Amer. J. Path. **33**:499, 1957.
4. Cogbill, C. L., and Song, K. T.: Acute pancreatitis, Arch. Surg. **100**:673, 1970.
5. Frantz, V. K.: Tumors of the pancreas, Washington, D. C., 1959, Armed Forces Institute of Pathology.
6. Grosfeld, J. L., Clatworthy, H. W., Jr., and Hamoudi, A. B.: Pancreatic malignancy in children, Arch. Surg. **101**:370, 1970.
7. Halpert, B., Makk, L., and Jordan, G. L., Jr.: A retrospective study of 120 patients with carcinoma of the pancreas, Surg. Gynec. Obstet. **121**:91, 1965.
8. Hermann, R. E.: Clinical aspects of pancreatitis, Postgrad. Med. **36**:135, 1964.
9. Howard, J. M., and Jordan, G. L.: Surgical diseases of the pancreas, Philadelphia, 1960, J. B. Lippincott Co.
10. Kernen, J. A., Scofield, G., Koucky, C., Benitez, R. E., and Ackerman, L. V.: Long survival with islet cell carcinoma of the pancreas, Amer. J. Clin. Path. **39**:137, 1963.
11. MacMahon, H. E., Brown, P. A., and Shen, E. M.:

Acinar cell carcinoma of the pancreas with subcutaneous fat necrosis, Gastroenterology 49:555, 1965.

12. Perez, C. A., Sturim, H. S., Kouchoukos, N. T., and Kamberg, S.: Some clinical and radiographic features of gastrointestinal histoplasmosis, Radiology **86**:482, 1966.

13. Steedman, R. A., Doering, R., and Carter, R.: Surgical aspects of pancreatic abscess, Surg. Gynec. Obstet. **125**:757, 1967.

14. Warren, K. W., and Hardy, K. I.: Cystadenocarcinoma of the pancreas, Surg. Gynec. Obstet. **127**:734, 1968.

Examination of the pancreas | 42

Arthur R. Clemett

Evidence of pancreatic disease may be found in a variety of conventional or routine roentgenographic examinations, including chest, abdomen, extremities, gastrointestinal series, barium enema, intravenous pyelogram, and indirect (oral or intravenous) cholangiograms. In addition, several special procedures have been employed in the roentgenographic evaluation of the pancreas. These are "special" in that they may entail significant risk or patient discomfort, may require special skills or equipment, or can be done only in conjunction with a surgical procedure. These techniques include direct cholangiography, hypotonic duodenography, selective arteriography, splenoportography, retropneumoperitoneum with tomography, and direct pancreatography. The number and diverse character of these techniques indicate that there is as yet no reasonably simple, safe, specific method of roentgenographic examination of the pancreas.

It is impossible to assess, in any scientific fashion, the comparative merits and faults of the conventional examinations and special procedures. This would require study of a large number of patients with suspected pancreatic disease, each to be examined by all techniques—obviously an impossibility, even if the required time, money, and spartan group of patients could be found. Appraisal of the various methods of examination, then, is necessarily subjective and must be based to some extent on critical evaluation of the medical literature.

Most reports emphasize a single special technique. Careful study all too often suggests that extensive commitment to a single technique either produces consummate skill in interpretation of the findings or, alternatively, a pronounced unconscious bias for the procedure. It is not rare for illustrations, even with the aid of line drawings and arrows, to strain the credulity of the reader. The special procedures considered here have been constantly refined, but despite occasional extravagant claims of their value, no one technique is clearly the method of choice in roentgenographic examination of the pancreas.

In actual practice roentgenographic evaluation of the pancreas is based on a synthesis of clinical data and the findings of several roentgenographic procedures. Radioisotope scanning[64] and ultrasonic scanning[52] are sometimes useful adjuncts. These various procedures should be regarded as complementary rather than competitive. Each one must be evaluated and used in terms of its ease of application, hazards, patient discomfort, expected result, and diagnostic accuracy.

Since diagnosis is often by indirect means it should be realized that the pancreas in vivo may have considerable mobility. It must also be appreciated that the adult human pancreas may vary considerably in size, shape, proportion, position, and disposition in the body. Some measure of this variability is illustrated in Fig. 42-1, which shows three pancreatograms from a series of postmortem in situ injection studies.

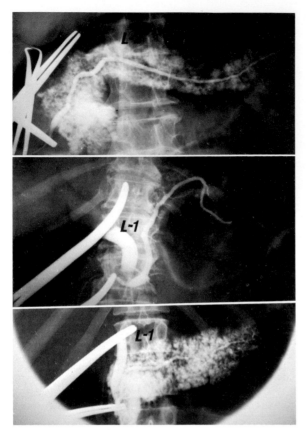

Fig. 42-1. Postmortem diatrizoate (Hypaque) sodium injections of the undisturbed pancreas through a catheter in the main pancreatic duct. Common bile duct and duodenal papilla are clamped. Note the variations in these three examples selected from thirty-five such studies.[126]

PLAIN FILM STUDIES

Significant chest abnormalities in acute pancreatitis have been noted in from 14% to almost 50% of cases.[38,114] Although nonspecific, these findings contribute to the diagnosis as well as to the prognosis of the disease. The mediastinum may be an unusual site of presentation of a pancreatic pseudocyst.[75]

Intramedullary fat necrosis in bones resulting from pancreatitis is well known pathologically[106] and roentgenologically.[43,54,68] Identification of typical bone infarcts or aseptic necrosis of the femoral or humeral head sometimes provides the first clue to the diagnosis of chronic pancreatitis.

Abdominal films make limited contributions to the diagnosis of acute pancreatitis.[123] Ab-

normalities are noted in one third to two thirds of cases, depending on the series cited. A variety of signs have been described that, on analysis, have the common feature of a lack of specificity. Gas abscess, pancreatic calculi, and the rarely recognized mottled shadows of disseminated fat necrosis[9] are virtually the only certain plain film signs of pancreatic disease. The former is rare and the latter infrequently found in acute pancreatitis, although Stein and co-workers noted pancreatic calculi in 17% of sixty-six patients with acute pancreatitis.[114] Diffuse pancreatic calculi are considered the hallmark of chronic or relapsing pancreatitis, although occasional patients will have neither signs nor symptoms of pancreatic disease.[59] Calcification in the wall of pancreatic cysts has been noted.[26,91] The slow-growing, usually bulky cystadenomas and cystadenocarcinomas are the only pancreatic neoplasms to calcify with significant frequency (about 10%).[7] On rare occasions, however, calcification has been observed in both adenocarcinomas and islet cell tumors.[18,60,91] Phlebolith-like calcifications have been reported in cavernous lymphangioma of the pancreas.[28]

GASTROINTESTINAL SERIES

Despite its many deficiencies, the conventional upper gastrointestinal study is a basic roentgenographic examination for detection of pancreatic disease. Somewhat limited, recumbent examination done early in the course of acute pancreatitis yields positive findings in 70% to 90% of cases.[10,108] Frequency of detection of pancreatic tumors has varied from 24%[35] (increased to 57% on retrospective study) to 77%[105] in different reports. An overall diagnostic accuracy of 40% to 50% is a likely average to be expected, considering many series,* and allowing for the retrospective nature of some of these.

The fundamental purpose of the examination is to seek evidence of pancreatic enlargement or tumefaction. To accomplish this certain modifications or additions to the usual procedure are useful. These include study in the true lateral projection for evidence of enlargement of the body and tail of the pancreas. Several techniques have been devised for this, particularly cross-table lateral films with air contrast studies with

---

*See references 8, 17, 23, 44, 47, 51, and 88.

the patient in the prone position or barium studies with the patient in the supine position. For convenience and simplicity, however, upright films are recommended since complementary frontal and lateral projections are readily obtained. Lateral films, made with the patient in the decubitus position, without corresponding complementary frontal projections, should be interpreted with great care, for significant shifts in position of the viscera can occur with this posture.

Many attempts have been made to recognize pancreatic and other retroperitoneal masses by determination of retrogastric space measurements. Results have been controversial. Even those claiming the value of measurements admit that the standards vary with body habitus and that measurements are unreliable in the presence of obesity, previous surgery, hernias involving the omentum, hepatomegaly, ascites, and emphysema.[107] One statistical study supports the widespread belief that measurements per se have little validity, and only extrinsic pressure effects on the posterior stomach wall have diagnostic significance.[49]

The "pad effect" is a valuable sign of enlargement of the body of the pancreas and refers to the effacement of the gastric antrum and, at times, the adjacent duodenal bulb with or without extrinsic deformity of the contours of these structures.[19] Often it can only be elicited with care, and it must be differentiated from other extrinsic pressure effects, such as those made by the spine or an enlarged liver. Frequently the pad sign is best demonstrated by carefully graded compression with the patient in the semierect position (Fig. 42-2, *A*). It may disappear with the patient in this position because of the caudad position of the antrum. Conversely, it may be lost if the patient is fully recumbent because of the cephalad stomach position and poor filling of the antrum.

Gross enlargement of the duodenal loop is actually rather infrequent with pancreatic disease and is usually found with pancreatic cysts (Fig. 42-3), pseudocysts (Fig. 43-17), and large slow-growing tumors such as the cystadenoma. The loop is a rather variable structure and slight degrees of enlargement are difficult to recognize with confidence. A high transverse stomach in a heavyset patient readily creates the illusion of a large loop where, in fact, it is normal. Recog-

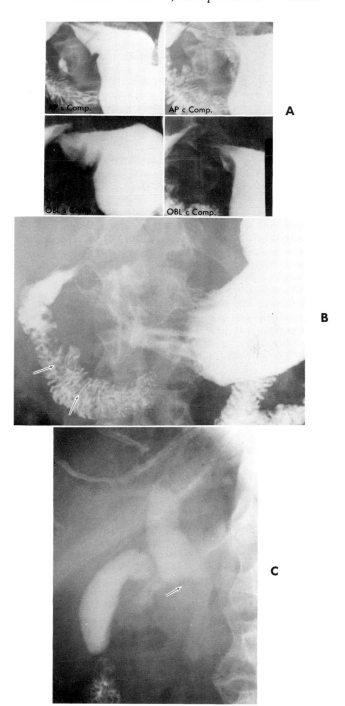

Fig. 42-2. Carcinoma of the head of the pancreas. Patient not jaundiced despite large tumor measuring 8 by 8 by 6 cm. **A,** Pad effect demonstrated by graded compression with patient in semierect position. **B,** Duodenal changes on P-A film, with patient in prone position, consisting of double contour (arrows) and slight deformity of the medial mucosal folds and the small diverticulum. **C,** Oral cholecystogram showing partial common duct obstruction at the level of the upper margin of the pancreatic mass (arrow).

nition that the widened loop is a poor sign of carcinoma of the pancreas[21] has led to repeated emphasis of the minor and at times rather subtle changes in the duodenum produced by enlargement of the head of the pancreas.[51,105] These include flattening and indentation of the medial wall, formation of double margins, deformity and displacement of diverticula, and alteration of the height, width, and direction of the mucosal folds on the medial aspect of the duodenum (Figs. 42-2, *B,* 42-11, *A,* and 42-12, *A*). Recognition of these changes is considerably enhanced by the use of serialographic exposures of the duodenal loop to supplement the fluoroscopic spot films and radiographs of the usual examination. Irregular contraction of the duodenum is another subtle finding that has been observed,[105] and this is best demonstrated by cineroentgenography of the duodenal loop.

The dilated retroduodenal segment of the common duct may deform the duodenal bulb or postbulbar area, and this has been stressed as an important sign of tumor of the head of the pancreas.[51] Dilatation of the intrapancreatic and intramural segments of the common duct, however, may produce all of the signs just described and create the false impression of a substantial mass in the head of the pancreas. Small tumors of the distal common duct (Fig. 42-4) or papilla of Vater (Fig. 42-5), as well as distal impaction of a gallstone (Fig. 42-10), may be responsible for this infrequent diagnostic pitfall. The importance of an adequate cholangiogram in differential diagnosis here is obvious.

In the usual clinical setting pancreatic enlargement when once identified presents few problems in differential diagnosis. Based on the gastrointestinal roentgenographic features

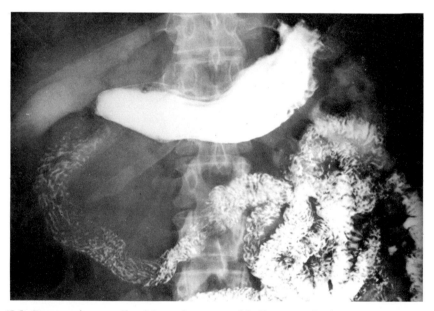

Fig. 42-3. Pancreatic cyst, lined by columnar epithelium, producing enlargement of duodenal loop.

Fig. 42-4. Small carcinoma of the distal common bile duct mistaken for a large tumor of the head of the pancreas. **A,** Early spot film showing extrinsic pressure on duodenum and distortion of the mucosal folds. **B,** Later a distorted and deformed diverticulum fills (arrow). **C,** Diagrammatic representation of autopsy findings. Tumor, **a,** measured 0.6 cm. in diameter and common bile duct, **b,** 2.7 cm. Pancreatic duct, **c,** not involved.

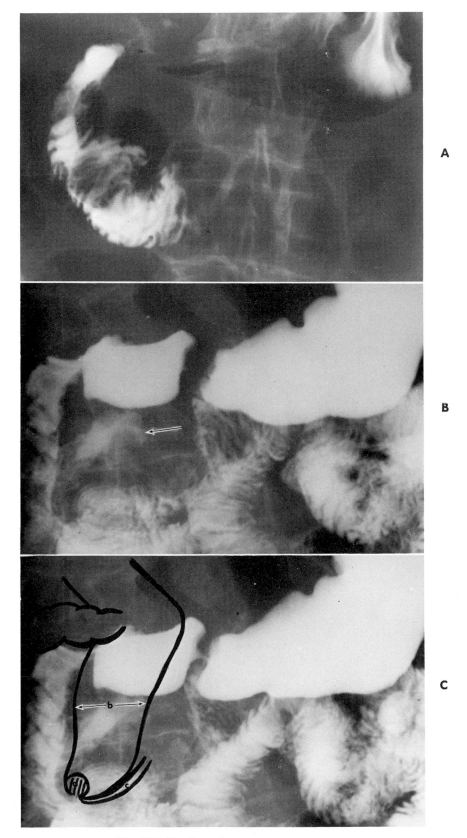

Fig. 42-4. For legend see opposite page.

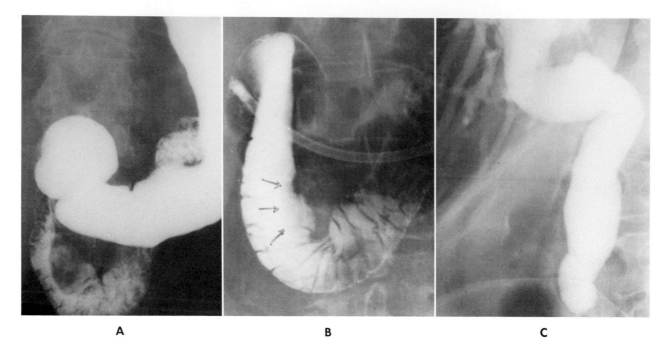

A   B   C

Fig. 42-5. Carcinoma of the papilla of Vater with obstructive jaundice. **A,** Prominent extrinsic defect on second portion of duodenum. **B,** Defect (arrows) is less conspicious on hypotonic duodenogram suggesting a compressible stricture. **C,** Percutaneous cholangiogram confirms the defect to be a greatly dilated common bile duct secondary to a very small tumor of the papilla.

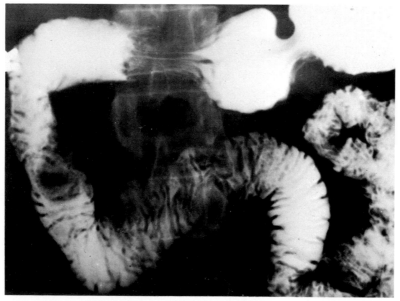

Fig. 42-6. Extrinsic defect, second portion of duodenum, resulting from gallstone impacted in distal common bile duct.

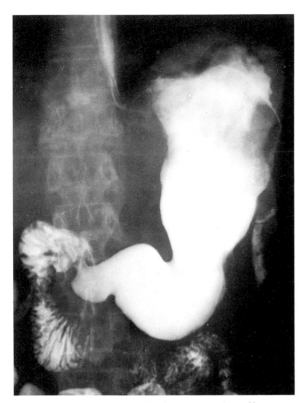

Fig. 42-7. Carcinoma of tail of pancreas invading upper half of the body of the stomach.

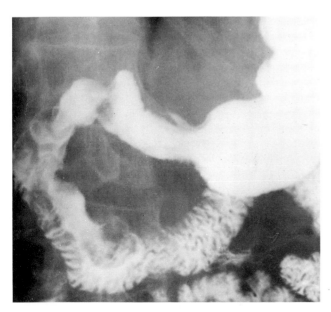

Fig. 42-8. Carcinoma of head of pancreas invading duodenum with ulceration.

alone, however, it is usually impossible to differentiate pancreatitis and pseudocyst from tumor. In fact, much of the evident pancreatic enlargement in carcinoma cases may be a result of secondary pancreatitis. Grossly evident pancreatitis has been noted in one fourth[78] to one third[88] of carcinoma cases, although the inflammatory process tends to be confined to the gland. Pancreatic carcinoma and pancreatic calculi may coexist, and pseudocyst occurs as a rare complication of pancreatic carcinoma.[78] Extension of a pancreatic inflammatory process to any segment of the alimentary canal tends to produce mucosal edema (see Figs. 42-9, *A*, 42-10, 42-19, and 42-20), and this feature favors the diagnosis of pancreatitis. Extension of carcinoma is by mural or mucosal infiltration, occasionally with ulceration (Figs. 42-7 to 42-9). This type of extension may make differential diagnosis of the site of tumor origin impossible, and this problem has been noted in 7% of a large series of pancreatic cancers.[23]

HYPOTONIC DUODENOGRAPHY

Basically, hypotonic duodenography is a refinement of the barium examination of the duodenum. The technique consists of intubation of the duodenum and examination with direct injection of barium and air after induction of hypotonia with anticholinergic drugs.[55] Duodenal intubation is quickly and easily done in virtually all patients with the styletted tubes that are now available.[13,37] Several anticholinergic drugs have been used. The intramuscular injection of 30 to 60 mg. of propantheline (Pro-Banthine) bromide regularly produces a marked hypotonia of the duodenum, which usually lasts for several minutes, during which time the examination is completed. The principal side effects are dryness of mucous membranes and tachycardia. Fluid restriction and voiding prior to the procedure largely prevents the acute urinary retention that may occur in patients with prostatism.[32] Glaucoma and significant cardiovascular disease are the major contraindications.

The use of topical anesthetic agents in the duodenum is often advocated, but adequate hypotonia is readily achieved with the anticholinergic drugs alone. The Indianapolis group has recently reported on the use of glucagon (2 mg. administered intravenously) for hypotonic duodenography. The method is effective and vir-

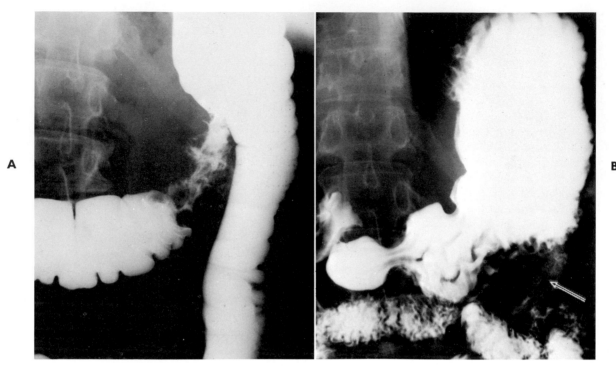

Fig. 42-9. **A,** Carcinoma of body of pancreas invading distal transverse colon with extensive ulceration. **B,** Mural invasion of greater curvature of the stomach by the same lesion. Residual barium in colon ulceration (arrow).

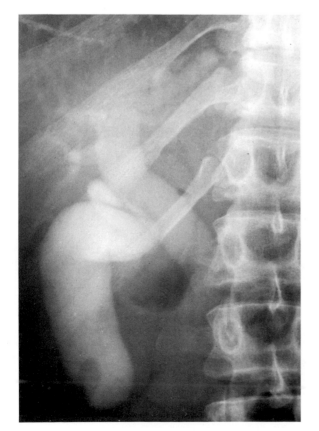

Fig. 42-10. Carcinoma of the head of the pancreas. Partial common bile duct obstruction demonstrated by intravenous cholangiogram.

tually free of complications.[74] A "tubeless" technique may be employed, but the inability to control the amounts of air and barium results in a less than optimal examination.

Hypotonic duodenography is an adjunct to the conventional gastrointestinal examination. It may permit recognition of subtle changes that are equivocal on routine examination, but the procedure often serves the most important function of dispelling findings of the routine examination that are considered suspicious. At times the nature of a deforming mass can be suggested by its changed appearance on hypotonic duodenography (Fig. 42-5). Detailed knowledge of normal duodenal anatomy is essential to proper interpretation of the hypotonic duodenogram.[37] There is nothing inherent in the technique that improves differential diagnosis of the abnormalities recognized.[14,103] The combined use of hypotonic duodenography and percutaneous cholangiography further refines diagnostic accuracy of lesions in and about the head of the pancreas.

BARIUM ENEMA AND INTRAVENOUS PYELOGRAM

The posterior peritoneal reflection of the transverse mesocolon lies along the anterior inferior surface of the body of the pancreas, and the tail of the pancreas as a rule extends to the splenic hilum lying anterior to the left kidney and posterior to the splenic flexure of the colon. As a result of these anatomic relationships, pancreatic inflammatory processes and tumors may extend to involve the colon (Figs. 42-9 and 42-10) or the left kidney. In the colon, pancreatitis infrequently may cause segmental areas of spasm, mucosal edema, pericolonic fibrosis, and adhesions.[109] Pancreatic tumor or pseudocyst may compress, distort, or displace the left kidney and ureter, thus simulating primary renal disease, particularly when hematuria occurs.[22,73]

INDIRECT CHOLANGIOGRAPHY

Common bile duct visualization by the oral or the more usual intravenous technique has very limited usefulness in the diagnosis of pancreatic disease. The cases with diagnostic anatomic changes in the duct are the ones in which the excretion and visualization of the contrast agent are likely to be poor or absent. At times evidence of partial duct obstruction is seen in the absence of clinical jaundice (Figs. 42-2, *C*

and 42-10).[127] The nature of the lesion producing the obstruction can seldom be determined, however, either because of poor roentgenographic definition of the distal duct or the nonspecific character of the findings in the rare cases where visualization occurs. On at least one occasion, though, intravenous cholangiography demonstrated abrupt angulation of the common duct and pronounced right lateral convexity of its intrapancreatic segment and permitted the diagnosis of pancreatic carcinoma.[66] Moderate changes of this nature, however, have also been described in pancreatitis (see Fig. 42-12, *B*).[104]

DIRECT CHOLANGIOGRAPHY

By the time diagnosis is made, carcinoma of the head of the pancreas usually completely obstructs the common bile duct at its site of entry into the pancreas. The proximal duct and intrahepatic branches are severely dilated. The distal duct has either a characteristic caudal convexity (Fig. 42-11, *B*)[39] or a jagged, notched apperance (Fig. 42-12, *B*),[34] which is probably the roentgenographic counterpart of the puckering of the dilated duct at the site of obstruction described by surgeons.[78] One report of a small tumor causing a hooklike deformity of the intrapancreatic segment of the duct has been published.[41] The common bile duct lies in a groove on the dorsal aspect of the head of the pancreas and a tongue of pancreatic tissue usually completely covers its posterior surface.[63] In about one of eight cases, however, the posterior surface of the duct is free of pancreatic tissue, and this variation probably explains the absence of jaundice and complete duct obstruction with some large tumors of the head of the pancreas (Fig. 42-2, *C*).

Demonstration of a well-defined tumor edge, intraluminal extension of a mass, or a short segmental stenosis will usually differentiate bile duct tumor from a primary pancreatic lesion.[24] Similarly, when an obstructing lesion can be shown to be relatively small and located in the distal duct, tumor of the duodenal papilla or so-called ampulla of Vater can be distinguished (Fig. 42-5).[36] Stones in the distal common duct are readily recognized. Chronic pancreatitis tends to produce a characteristic cholangiographic appearance consisting of a long, tapered narrowing of the distal duct, moderate dilatation of the duct proximal to the pancreas, and

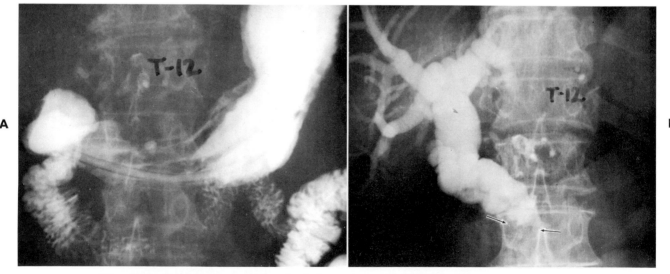

Fig. 42-11. Carcinoma of the head of the pancreas. **A,** Elongation and widening of mucosal folds on medial aspect of the second portion of the duodenum. **B,** Characteristic blunt obstruction of the common bile duct at the upper margin of the pancreas (arrows) on a percutaneous transhepatic cholangiogram. Partial filling of a distended gallbladder, **a** on this upright film.

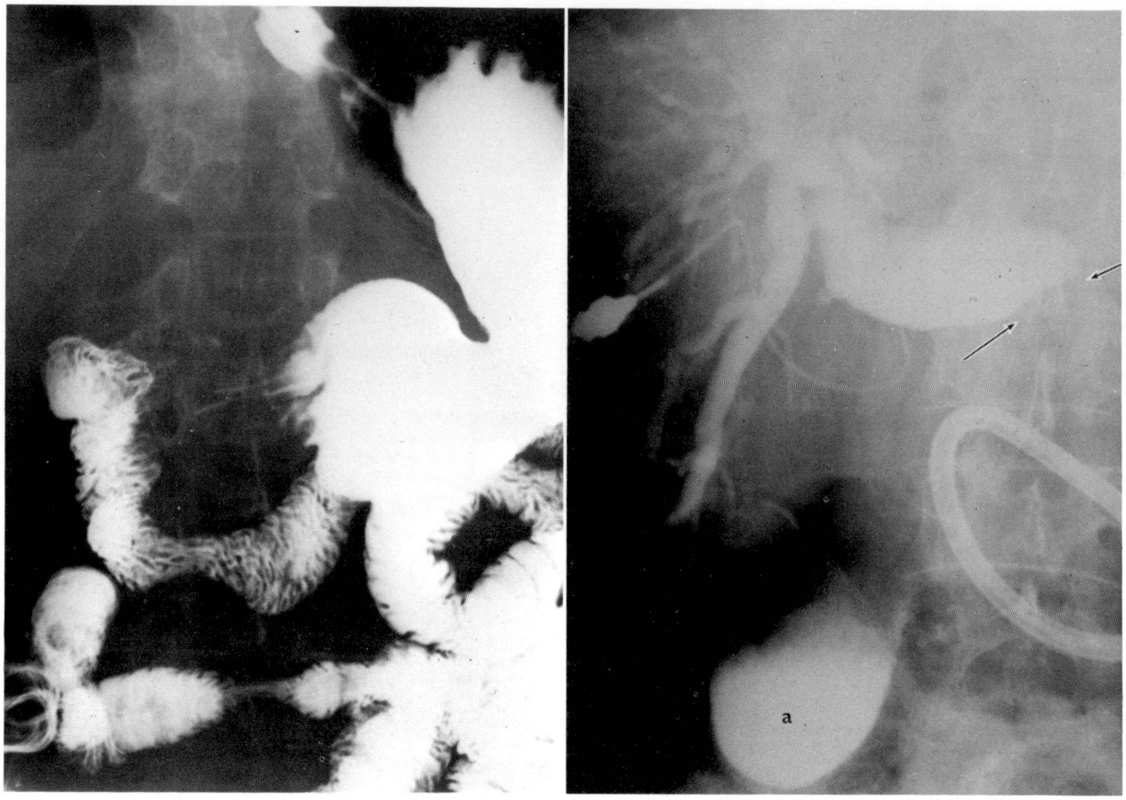

Fig. 42-12. Carcinoma of the head of the pancreas. **A,** Double contour, medial aspect of the second portion of the duodenum, with slight elongation and widening of the mucosal folds here. **B,** Complete obstruction of the common bile duct on operative cholangiogram. The jagged or notched contour at the site of obstruction (arrows) resulted from the folds produced by the puckering of the duct where it entered the tumor.

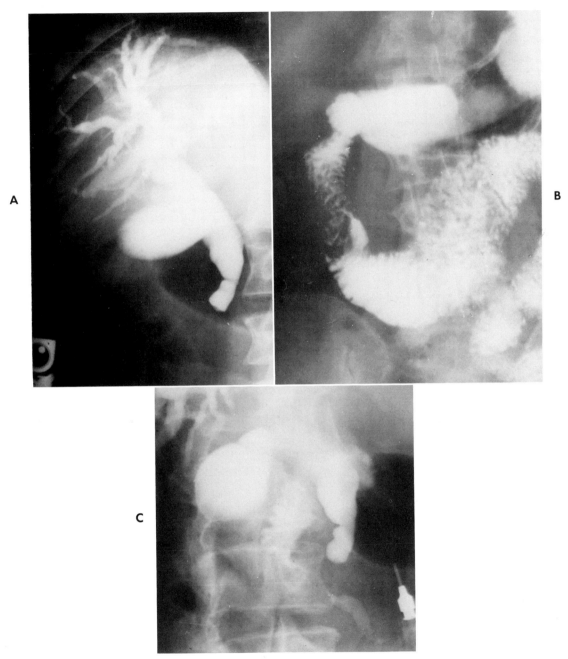

Fig. 42-13. Carcinoma of pancreas. **A,** Percutaneous cholangiogram demonstrating non-specific obstruction of the distal common bile duct caused by carcinoma of the common duct, pancreas, or papilla. **B,** Ulceration of the medial aspect of the second portion of the duodenum virtually excludes a common duct primarily. **C,** Spot film shows the duct obstruction to be some distance from the ulceration, indicating a large tumor that is likely to be a primary pancreatic lesion.

little or no dilatation of the intrahepatic ducts (Figs. 43-9, *D* and 43-22, *B*).

Direct cholangiography provides considerable precision in the diagnosis of disease in and about the head of the pancreas, particularly when complemented by gastrointestinal examination.[36] In the jaundiced patient percutaneous transhepatic cholangiography is usually the most valuable diagnostic procedure. It should be performed on any patient in whom surgery is contemplated for possible obstructive jaundice. Contraindications are few. In fact, absolute refusal of surgical intervention can be regarded as the only contraindication to percutaneous cholangiography.

SELECTIVE ARTERIOGRAPHY

Despite the complex blood supply of the pancreas and numerous anatomic variations, selective arteriography has become a standard technique for evaluation of pancreatic disease. Selective celiac and superior mesenteric arteriography comprises the basic examination. Inflation of the stomach with air is a helpful adjunct. Simultaneous celiac and superior mesenteric artery injections have been advocated,[6,70,71] but "superselective" studies of gastroduodenal and splenic arteries or even smaller branches result in superior examinations.[93] Modification of blood flow with balloon catheters[94] or pharmacologic agents[12] may furthur improve visualization.

Selective arteriography has been applied to the pancreas primarily for the diagnosis of adenocarcinoma, since the conventional roentgenographic features so often fail in this disease. The spectrum of opinion regarding its usefulness is very wide, varying from expressions of poor diagnostic accuracy on the one hand[40,81] to the method of choice for the diagnosis of carcinoma on the other.[70] Angiography may yield the correct diagnosis of pancreatic carcinoma in many cases where other means have failed. Unfortunately, with rare exceptions this has not permitted diagnosis of resectable lesions because the angiographic abnormalities are late manifestations of carcinoma.[82]

Angiographic signs of pancreatic carcinoma include arterial encasement, pathologic vessels, arterial obstructions, tumor opacification, vascular displacement, splenic or portal vein obstruction, hepatic metastases, and gallbladder enlargement.[15] Encasement is the most frequent ab-

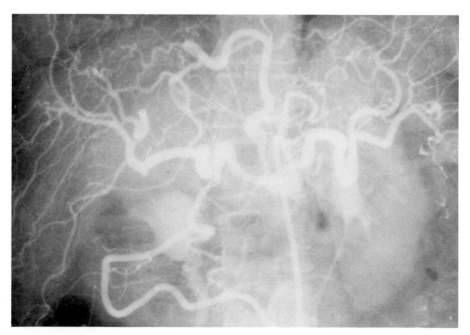

Fig. 42-14. Inoperable carcinoma of pancreas with encasement of gastroduodenal, common hepatic, accessory left hepatic, and proximal splenic arteries.

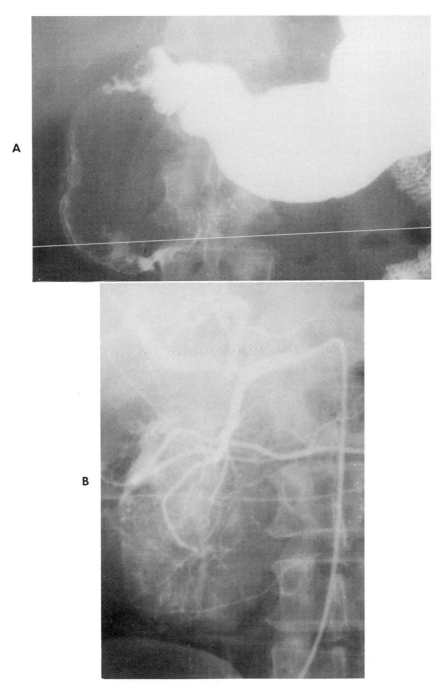

Fig. 42-15. Primary carcinoma of pancreas. **A,** Large mass with ulceration. **B,** Vascular tumor on selective angiography.

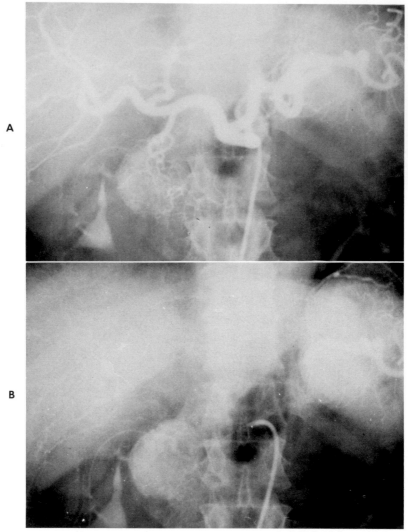

Fig. 42-16. Zollinger-Ellison syndrome with large, vascular, islet cell carcinoma of head of pancreas.

normality recognized. It may be smooth or serrated and serpiginous. The latter type is considered typical of carcinoma,[81,95] whereas smooth encasement must be accompanied by other signs to make a confident diagnosis. Adenocarcinoma of the pancreas is usually avascular, and clear demonstration of tumor staining of tumor vessels is unusual[100] but does occur in some cases (Fig. 42-15). Vascular displacement is often difficult to recognize[15] and is usually minimal because of the infiltrating character of most pancreatic cancers.[81]

Pancreatitis and atherosclerosis are the greatest problems in the differential diagnosis of pancreatic angiographic abnormalities. Several other conditions may produce changes similar to those of pancreatic carcinoma. These include carcinoma of the papilla of Vater, carcinoma of the common bile duct, carcinoma of the stomach, metastases to peripancreatic lymph nodes, penetrating peptic ulcers, postoperative changes, and arteritis.[95] Even gallstones impacted in the common bile duct have been confused with small pancreatic tumors on angiographic study.

Islet cell tumors are often vascular, and angiography is usually the method of choice for demonstrating these lesions. About 75% can be expected to be revealed by tumor staining.[72]

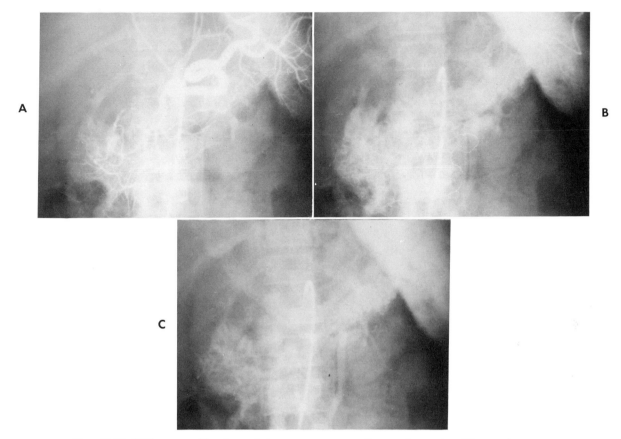

Fig. 42-17. Diffuse opacification of the pancreas on celiac angiography. The patient was a chronic alcoholic with no clinical or laboratory evidence of pancreatic disease.

Lesions as small as 1 cm. have been recognized.[62] Some islet cell tumors have no significant endocrine function but most are insulinomas. Other endocrine functions occur, and angiographic study for islet cell tumor is indicated in the Zollinger-Ellison syndrome,[45] WDHA (watery diarrhea hypokalemia achlorhydria) syndrome,[67] carcinoid syndrome,[29] and in the search for ACTH-secreting tumors.[121] The homogeneous staining of accessory spleens must not be confused with islet cell tumor. Other differential diagnostic problems that have been noted include hyperplastic lymph node, a few cases of recurrent pancreatitis, and bleeding into a pancreatic pseudocyst.[62]

Tumor staining is a regular feature of cystadenoma and cystadenocarcinoma,[92,115] and in these bulky tumors aortography may be adequate for diagnosis.[11] Large abnormal arteries and veins are found as well, and the tumor staining may be irregular when the cystic component is prominent.[119] Smooth encasement can occur in benign cystadenoma, but truncation of arteries is a feature of cystadenocarcinoma.[2] The rare pancreatic sarcomas also show tumor stains.[77,97]

Increased vascularity is sometimes present in the wall of pancreatic pseudocysts. Displacement of vessels, however, is the usual finding, and erosion of the splenic artery can result in deposition of contrast media into the cysts.[57] Nonspecific arterial abnormalities similar to atherosclerosis occur in pancreatitis. "Beading" of intrapancreatic arteries is said to be a more specific change, but this, like the statement that angiographic diagnosis is possible in 50% of cases, seems a rather extravagant claim.[96] Diffuse alterations of intrapancreatic vessels in chronic pancreatitis versus the focal character of the abnormalities caused by carcinoma may be important in differential diagnosis.[100] Splenic vein stenosis or occlusion complicates some cases of chronic pancreatitis.

Increased vascularity and pancreatic enlargement have been described in some cases of acute pancreatitis.[1,100] Normal variation is so great, however, that objective changes can only be documented by serial studies of individual patients.[1] Striking vascularity of the pancreas is not infrequent in chronic alcoholics with no evidence of pancreatic disease (Fig. 42-17).

SPLENOPORTOGRAPHY

The splenic vein lies adjacent to the posterior-superior margin of the body and tail of the pancreas and unites with the superior mesenteric vein behind the neck of the pancreas to form the portal vein. This anatomic relationship readily explains the distortion and partial or complete splenic vein occlusion that may occur with pancreatic tumors[16,27,98] or pseudocysts.[120] Pancreatitis may cause splenic vein thrombosis without pseudocyst formation. In a series of ninety-five patients with pancreatitis studied by splenoportography, Rösch and Herfort found two partial and two complete splenic vein occlusions.[99] In most of their other cases, they noted abnormalities consisting of slight deformities or dilatation of the splenic vein and delayed blood flow. In patients with suspected pancreatic disease, nevertheless, splenoportography is generally performed for the usual indications of suspected portal hypertension, gastric or esophageal varices, or explained splenomegaly. The procedure is indicated to evaluate the operability of pancreatic carcinoma, since demonstration of significant displacement or invasion of the portal or splenic vein is an almost certain sign of inoperability.[27]

RETROPNEUMOPERITONEUM WITH TOMOGRAPHY

Retropneumoperitoneum with tomography for visualization of the pancreas has been used in several European centers,[41,55,61,71] but has been tried only sporadically in the United States.[69,79] There are many technical variations, but the basic method consists of retroperitoneal injection of gas, gas inflation of the stomach, and body section radiography in the sagittal and coronal planes. Axial transverse laminograms with the patient in the upright position have

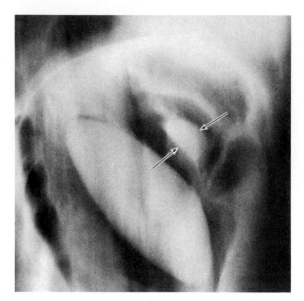

Fig. 42-18. Normal body of the pancreas (arrows) demonstrated by retropneumoperitoneum and tomography. (Courtesy Dr. J. Frimann-Dahl.)

also been done to outline the pancreas in the horizontal plane. European radiologists have generally used oxygen for retroperitoneal injection, whereas carbon dioxide has been favored in the United States because of its greater safety. Gas volumes have varied from 600 to 2,400 ml. Measures ancillary to the basic procedure have included (1) simultaneous pneumoperitoneum,[69] (2) concurrent introduction of iodinated contrast media into the stomach, urinary tract, and biliary system,[79] and (3) intravenous injection of iodinated contrast agents and secretin which, it is claimed, opacifies the pancreas.[61]

The outlines of the normal pancreas can be well shown by this method (Fig. 42-18). Cysts and tumors have been demonstrated, but there has been no determination of the minimum size necessary for confident recognition. Mosely demonstrated a pancreatic mass in seventeen patients by retropneumoperitoneum and tomography, but the gastrointestinal examination also revealed abnormalities in all of these patients.[79] The procedure causes significant patient discomfort,[55] provides no basis for accurate determination of the nature of a pancreatic mass, and fails when an inflammatory process or tumor infiltration has obliterated the potential spaces about the pancreas.

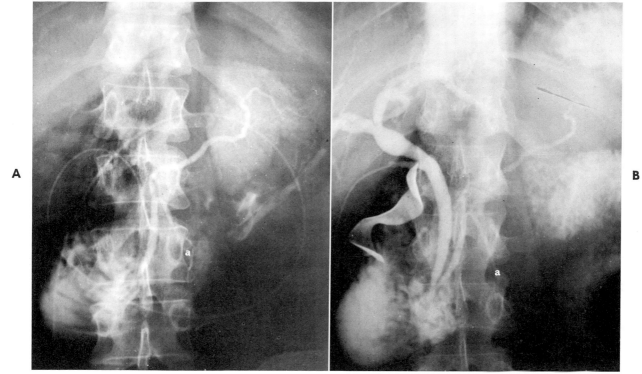

Fig. 42-19. Normal operative pancreatogram by common duct injection and reflux. **A,** Catheter malposition opposite the pancreatic duct orifice on the first injection resulted in filling of the secondary branches and acini in the tail of the pancreas. No evidence of pancreatitis. **B,** Repeat examination with the common duct catheter in proper position. The large, oblique branch from the uncinate process, **a,** is a frequent normal finding in pancreatography.

PANCREATOGRAPHY

Direct injection of contrast media into the duct system gives the best roentgenographic demonstration of the pancreas. This was formerly done only at operation or postoperatively. With the development of the fiberoptic duodenoscope direct catheterization of the duct can now be accomplished in most patients.[85]

Operative pancreatography is usually done by duodenotomy with transpapillary catheterization of the pancreatic duct, resection of the tail of the pancreas with injection into the duct transected here, or direct needling of a dilated duct palpated at surgery.[53] The latter procedure is used infrequently. Transpapillary catheterization of the main pancreatic duct is readily accomplished as a rule, and sphincterotomy is seldom necessary.[50,53,65] Some surgeons, however, perform sphincterotomy routinely.[30,58] Postoperative examination is possible when a catheter has been left in the main pancreatic duct for drainage. Such catheters may be looped in the duodenum and brought out alongside a common duct T tube[30] or exteriorized directly through the wall of the duodenum, which is sutured to the anterior parietal peritoneum.[65]

Pancreatography may also be accomplished by injection into the common duct with reflux into the pancreatic duct. Reflux of some degree occurs in about 40% of direct cholangiographies.[50] Administration of morphine intravenously[48] or intraduodenal instillation of 0.1N hydrochloric acid[117] increases the frequency and extent of this reflux. Satisfactory pancreatograms may be obtained by reflux in over two thirds of the cases attempted.[48]

Transduodenal pancreatography has been criticized as dangerous because of the risk of causing acute pancreatitis.[90] This occurs infrequently, and causality is difficult to establish, since most

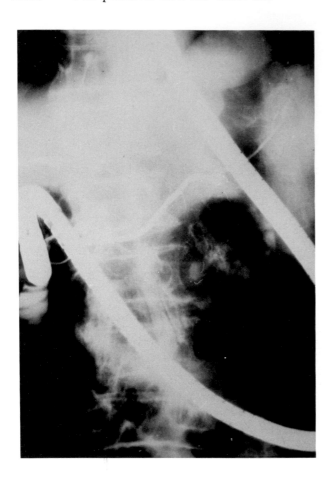

Fig. 42-20. Peroral pancreatogram. Catheter entering the papilla is obscured on this film by the duodenoscope. (Courtesy Dr. Itaru Oi.)

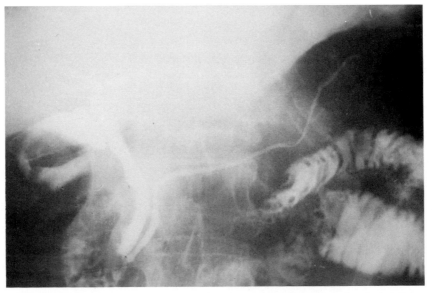

Fig. 42-21. Normal peroral pancreatocholangiogram after removal of duodenoscope. (Courtesy Dr. Itaru Oi.)

of these patients have had a sphincterotomy as well. Transient elevations of serum amylase without symptoms are common, being noted in 20% to 50% of patients.[50] Those most experienced with operative pancreatography consider it quite safe if proper technique is used.[31,58]

The key to safe technique is avoidance of duct distention. Overinjection causes opacification of secondary ducts, parenchymal staining, and extravasation of contrast media.[118] Pancreatography by common duct injection and reflux is generally safe, since sphincter resistance is overcome before dangerous pancreatic duct pressures occur,[48] but the technique is still subject to occasional technical errors (Fig. 42-19). Amounts of contrast media recommended for transpapillary operative pancreatography vary from 0.5 to 5.0 ml.[30,50,58,65,118] A loose fit of the catheter is important to allow excess contrast material to flow into the duodenum. Acetrizoate (Urokon) sodium and iodopyracet (Diodrast) were the contrast agents originally used for pancreatography,[30,65] but these have been supplanted by 50% diatrizoate (Hypaque) sodium. The latter is recommended since it has been shown both in vitro and in vivo not to activate trypsinogen.[33]

Peroral pancreatography via the duodenoscope has many advantages over operative pancreatography. The patient is awake and able to cooperate. Examination is done with fluoroscopic control. The amount of contrast media needed, a volume that will obviously vary from patient to patient, can be accurately determined. This visual control and the patient's reaction to the injection should obviate the risk of significant pancreatitis from the procedure, although a transient rise in serum amylase is common.

Some groups perform the procedure under general anesthesia and thus lose some advantages of the peroral method.[56,116] Most patients, however, tolerate duodenoscopy amazingly well with only mild sedation even for periods in excess of 1 hour. Identification of the papilla of Vater is generally quite easy, but training and practice are necessary to develop the skill required for cannulation of the duct. In experienced hands successful cannulation can be expected in about 75% of cases or even more.[25,84]

Pancreatography has been utilized primarily for evaluation of recurrent or chronic pancreatitis. Strictures and dilatation of the main pancreatic duct, stones,[3] and periductal fibrosis af-

fecting secondary ducts are readily demonstrated. The origin, spread, and persistence of pseudocysts can be evaluated, and these lesions may be demonstrated after being missed by surgical exploration. The diagnosis of chronic pancreatitis can be confirmed by the roentgenographic findings, and pancreatography is invaluable in determining the proper surgical procedure in chronic pancreatitis.

A few pancreatic carcinomas have been demonstrated by the technique of pancreatography.[3,48,50,65,86] Complete duct obstruction is present in some cases, but diagnostic changes are evident in others. These consist of partial obstruction of the main pancreatic duct, localized deformity of the duct, absence of secondary ducts at the level of the tumor, and marked dilatation of the main pancreatic duct proximal to the tumor.[86] With increased utilization of peroral pancreatography the differential features of carcinoma and pancreatitis will probably be greatly refined.

EXPERIMENTAL METHODS OF PANCREATIC VISUALIZATION

This subject was reviewed in 1965[89] and in 1968,[112] and Table 42-1 contains a partial compilation of the more notable efforts to produce roentgenographic visualization of the pancreas. All of these efforts have basically failed. Their very variety again indicates the unsatisfactory nature of existing methods for roentgenographic examination of the pancreas.

Table 42-1. Experimental techniques for roentgenographic visualization of the pancreas

I. Augmentation of existing clinical methods
    A. Intra-arterial trypsin injection with arteriography and retropneumoperitoneum[51,71]
    B. Intravenous secretin with selective arteriography[68]

II. Pancreatic duct opacification by physical and/or pharmacologic methods
    A. Contrast reflux from duodenum[27,30]
    B. Reflux pancreatography in dogs[122] and cats[101]
    C. Contrast reflux from common duct by use of iodipamide sodium, morphine, and cholecystokinin[80]

III. Pancreatic parenchyma opacification by intravenous methods
    A. Iodinated aniline dyes[87]
    B. Halogenated zinc compounds[79]

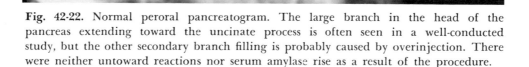

Fig. 42-22. Normal peroral pancreatogram. The large branch in the head of the pancreas extending toward the uncinate process is often seen in a well-conducted study, but the other secondary branch filling is probably caused by overinjection. There were neither untoward reactions nor serum amylase rise as a result of the procedure.

REFERENCES

1. Aakhus, T., Hofsli, M., and Vestad, E.: Angiography in acute pancreatitis, Acta Radiol. **3**:119, 1969.
2. Abrams, R. M., Beranbaum, E. R., Beranbaum, S. L., and Ngo, N. L.: Angiographic studies of benign and malignant cystadenoma of the pancreas, Radiology **89**:1028, 1967.
3. Andersson, A., Edstrom, C., Saltzman, G. F., and Schampi, B.: Concretions in the pancreatic duct diagnosed by cholangiography, Acta Radiol. **8**:183, 1969.
4. Arner, O., Hagberg, S., and Seldinger, S. I.: Percutaneous transhepatic cholangiography: puncture of dilated and nondilated bile ducts under roentgen television control, Surgery **52**:561, 1962.
5. Baum, M., and Howe, C. T.: Hypotonic duodenography in the diagnosis of carcinoma of the pancreas and its further use when combined with percutaneous cholangiography and pancreatic scintiscanning, Amer. J. Surg. **115**:519, 1968.
6. Baum, S., Roy, R., Finkelstein, A. K., and Blakemore, W. S.: Clinical application of selective celiac and superior mesenteric arteriography, Radiology **84**:279, 1965.

7. Becker, W. F., Welsh, R. A., and Pratt, H. S.: Cystadenoma and cystadenocarcinoma of the pancreas, Ann. Surg. **161**:845, 1965.
8. Beeler, J. W., and Kirklin, B. R.: Roentgenologic findings accompaning carcinoma of the pancreas, Amer. J. Roentgen. **67**:576, 1952.
9. Berenson, J. E., Spitz, H. B., and Felson, B.: The abdominal fat necrosis sign, Radiology **100**:567, 1971.
10. Bergkvist, A., and Seldinger, S. I.: Contrast roentgenography in differential diagnosis between perforated ulcer and acute pancreatitis, Acta Chir. Scand. **118**:137, 1959.
11. Bieber, W. P., and Albo, R. J.: Cystadenoma of the pancreas: its arteriographic diagnosis, Radiology **80**:776, 1963.
12. Bierman, H. R., Zion, D. E., Stulberg, H. J., and Silberman, E. L.: Arterial patterns of pancreatic lesions, Angiology **20**:13, 1969.
13. Bilbao, M. K., Frische, L. H., Dotter, C. T., and Rosch, J.: Hypotonic duodenography, Radiology **89**:438, 1967.
14. Bilbao, M. K., Rösch, J., Frische, L. H., and Dotter, C. T.: Hypotonic duodenography in the

diagnosis of pancreatic disease, Seminars Roentgen. 3:280, 1968.

15. Bookstein, J. J., Reuter, S. R., and Martel, W.: Angiographic evaluation of pancreatic carcinoma, Radiology 93:757, 1969.

16. Bookstein, J. J., and Whitehouse, W. M.: Splenoportography, Radiol. Clin. N. Amer. 2:447, 1964.

17. Broadbent, T. R., and Kerman, H. D.: One hundred cases of carcinoma of the pancreas: a clinical and roentgenological analysis, Gastroenterology 17:163, 1951.

18. Brunschwig, A.: Large islet-cell tumor of the pancreas, Surgery 9:554, 1941.

19. Cnui, J. T.: Roentgenology of pancreatic disease, Amer. J. Roentgen. 44:485, 1940.

20. Castiglioni, G. C., and Petronio, R.: Percutaneous intrahepatic cholangiography as a diagnostic aid in posthepatic jaundice, Surgery 56:635, 1964.

21. Cattell, R. B., Warren, K. W., and Au, F. T. C.: Periampullary carcinomas: diagnosis and surgical management, Surg. Clin. N. Amer. 39:781, 1959.

22. Chamberlin, G. W., and Imber, I.: Pyelography for the diagnosis of lesions of the body and tail of the pancreas, Radiology 63:722, 1954.

23. Chiat, H., and Faegenburg, D. H.: Illusory neoplasms of the stomach and duodenum as a manifestation of carcinoma of the pancreas, Radiology 74:771, 1960.

24. Clemett, A. R.: Carcinoma of the major bile ducts, Radiology 84:894, 1965.

25. Cotton, P. B., Blumgart, L. H., Davies, G. T., Pierce, J. W., Almon, P. R., Burwood, R. J., Lawrie, B. W., and Read, A. E.: Cannulation of Papilla of Vater via fiber-duodenoscope, Lancet 1:53, 1972.

26. Desmond, A. M., and Robinson, M. R. G.: Solitary cyst in the head of the pancreas, Brit. J. Surg. 57:209, 1970.

27. DeWeese, M. S., Figley, M. M., Fry, W. J., Rapp, R., and Smith, H. L.: Clinical appraisal of percutaneous splenoportography, Arch. Surg. (Chicago) 75:423, 1957.

28. Dodds, W. J., Margolin, F. R., and Goldberg, H. I.: Cavernous lymphangioma of the pancreas, Radiol. Clin. Biol. 38:267, 1969.

29. Dollinger, M. R., Ratner, L. H., Shamoian, C. A., and Blackbourne, B. D.: Carcinoid syndrome associated with pancreatic tumors, Arch. Intern. Med. 120:575, 1967.

30. Doubilet, H., Poppel, M. H., and Mulholland, J. H.: Pancreatography: techniques, principles, and observations, Radiology 64:325, 1955.

31. Doubilet, H., Poppel, M. H., and Mulholland, J. H.: Pancreatography, Ann. N. Y. Acad. Sci. 78:829, 1959.

32. Eaton, S. B., Benedict, K. T., Ferrucci, J. T., and Fleischli, D. J.: Hypotonic duodenography, Radiol. Clin. N. Amer. 8:125, 1970.

33. Elmslie, R. G., White, T. T., and Magee, D. R.: Pancreatography with particular reference to the activation of pancreatic enzymes, Surg. Gynec. Obstet. 117:405, 1963.

34. Evans, J. A.: Specialized roentgen diagnostic techniques in the investigation of abdominal disease, Radiology 82:579, 1964.

35. Eyler, W. R., Clark, M. D., and Rian, R. L.: An evaluation of roentgen signs of pancreatic enlargement, J.A.M.A. 181:967, 1962.

36. Ferris, E. J., Joison, J., Shapiro, J. H., and Byrne, J. J.: Percutaneous transhepatic cholangiography, Amer. J. Roentgen. 92:1131, 1964.

37. Ferrucci, J. T., Benedict, K. T., Page, D. L., Fleischli, D. J., and Eaton, S. B.: Radiographic features of the normal hypotonic duodenogram, Radiology 96:401, 1970.

38. Fishbein, R., Murphy, G. P., and Wilder, R. J.: The pleuropulmonary manifestations of pancreatitis, Dis. Chest 41:392, 1962.

39. Flemma, R. J., Schauble, J. F., Gardner, C. E., Anlyan, W. G., and Capp, M. P.: Percutaneous transhepatic cholangiography in the differential diagnosis of jaundice, Surg. Gynec. Obstet. 116:559, 1963.

40. Fredens, M., Egebald, M., and Nielsen, F. H.: The value of selective angiography in the diagnosis of tumors in pancreas and liver, Radiology 93:765, 1969.

41. Frimann-Dahl, J.: Radiology in tumours of the pancreas, Clin. Radiol. 12:73, 1961.

42. Gayliss, H., and Gunn, K.: Transduodenal cholangiography, Surg. Gynec. Obstet. 100:249, 1955.

43. Gerle, R. D., Walker, L. A., Achord, J. L., and Weens, H. S.: Osseous changes in chronic pancreatitis, Radiology 85:330, 1965.

44. Goswitz, J. T.: Carcinoma of the pancreas: a comprehensive review of 173 cases emphasizing inadequacy of our diagnostic techniques, Ohio Med. J. 57:1255, 1961.

45. Gray, R. K., Rösch, J., and Grollman, J. H.: Arteriography in the diagnosis of islet-cell tumors, Radiology 97:39, 1970.

46. Greenfield, H., Segal, L. H., and DeFrancis, N.: Attempted visualization of the pancreatic ducts by ampullary reflux, Gastroenterology 29:280, 1955.

47. Halpert, B., Makk, L., and Jordan, G. L., Jr.: A retrospective study of 120 patients with carcinoma of the pancreas, Surg. Gynec. Obstet. 121:91, 1965.

48. Hayes, M. A.: Operative pancreatography, Surg. Gynec. Obstet. 110:404, 1960.

49. Herbert, W. R., and Margulis, A. R.: Diagnosis of retroperitoneal masses by gastrointestinal roentgenographic measurements: a computer study, Radiology 84:52, 1965.

50. Hess, W.: Surgery of the biliary passages and the pancreas, Princeton, 1965, D. Van Nostrand Co., Inc.

51. Hodes, P. J., Pendergrass, E. P., and Winston, N. J.: Pancreatic, ductal, and Vaterian neoplasms: their roentgen manifestations, Radiology 62:1, 1954.

52. Holm, H. H.: Ultrasonic scanning in the diagnosis of space-occupying lesions of the upper abdome, Brit. J. Radiol. 44:24, 1971.

53. Howard, J. M., and Short, W. F.: An evaluation of pancreatography in suspected pancreatic disease, Surg. Gynec. Obstet. 129:319, 1969.

54. Immelman, E. J., Bank, S., Krige, H., and Marks,

I. N.: Roentgenologic and clinical features of intramedullary fat necrosis in bones in acute and chronic pancreatitis, Amer. J. Med. **36**:96, 1964.

55. Jacquemet, P., Liotta, D., Mallet-Guy, P.: The early radiological diagnosis of diseases of the pancreas and ampulla of Vater: Elective exploration of the ampulla of Vater and the head of the pancreas by hypotonic duodenography, Springfield, Ill., 1965, Charles C Thomas, Publisher.

56. Jeanpierre, R., Laurent, J., Bas, M., Fays, J., Dornier, R., Bigard, M., Vicari, F., Gaucher, P., and Heully, F.: Catheterisme de l'ampoule de Vater au cours des examens duodenoscopiques, Arch. Franc. Mal. Appar. Dig. **60**:525, 1971.

57. Kadell, B. M., and Riley, J. M.: Major arterial involvement by pancreatic pseudocysts, Amer. J. Roentgen. **99**:632, 1967.

58. Keddie, N., and Nardi, G. L.: Pancreatography; a safe and effective technic, Amer. J. Surg. **110**:863, 1965.

59. Kelley, M. L., Jr., Squine, L. F., Boynton, L. C., and Logan, V. W.: Significance of pancreatic calcification, New York J. Med. **57**:721, 1957.

60. Kendig, T. A., Johnson, R. M., and Shackford, B. C.: Calcification in pancreatic carcinoma, Ann. Intern. Med. **65**:122, 1966.

61. Kisseler, B., Leistner, G. H., and Barth, E.: A new method for the roentgenologic opacification of the pancreas, Radiology **83**:6. 1964.

62. Korobkin, M. T., Palubinskas, A. J., and Glickman, M. G.: Pitfalls in arteriography of islet-cell tumors of the pancreas, Radiology **100**:319, 1971.

63. Kune, G. A.: Surgical anatomy of common bile duct, Arch. Surg. (Chicago) **89**:995, 1964.

64. Landman, S., Polcyn, R. E., and Gottschalk, A.: Pancreas imaging—Is it worth it? Radiology **100**:631, 1971.

65. Leger, L.: Surgical contrast visualization of the pancreatic ducts with a study of pancreatic external secretion, Amer. J. Dig. Dis. **20**:8, 1953.

66. Levene, G., and Scheff, S.: Intravenous cholangiography as an aid in diagnosis of carcinoma of the head of the pancreas, Radiology **68**:714, 1957.

67. Lopes, V. M., Reis, D. D., and Cunha, A. B.: Islet-cell adenoma of the pancreas with reversible watery diarrhea and hypokalemia, Amer. J. Gastroent. **53**:17, 1970.

68. Lucas, P. F., and Owen, T. K.: Subcutaneous fat necrosis, polyarthritis and pancreatic disease, Gut **3**:146, 1962.

69. Ludin, H., and Asch, T.: The normal lateral pneumotomographic appearance of the pancreas, Radiology **72**:197, 1959.

70. Lunderquist, A.: Angiography in carcinoma of the pancreas, Acta Radiol. [Diagn.] (Stockholm) **235** (Supp.):1, 1965.

71. Macarini, N., and Oliva, L.: Neue Wege zur Pankreasdarstellung, Fortschr. Röntgenstr. **86**:55, 1957.

72. Madsen, B., and Hansen, E. S.: Correlation between angiographic diagnosis and histology of pancreatic insulomas, Brit. J. Radiol. **43**:185, 1970.

73. Marshall, S., Lapp, M., and Schulte, J. W.: Lesions of the pancreas mimicking renal disease, J. Urol. **93**:41, 1965.

74. Miller, R. E., Chernish, S. M., Scholz, N. E., and Rosenak, B. D.: Hypotonic duodenography with glucagon. To be published in Radiology, July 1973.

75. McClintock, J. T., McFee, J. L., and Quimby, R. L.: Pancreatic pseudocyst presenting as a mediastinal tumor, J.A.M.A. **192**:573, 1965.

76. McCune, W. S., and Stambro, W. W.: Visualization of the pancreas by aortography, Ann. Surg. **150**:561, 1959.

77. Meaney, T. F., and Buonocore, E.: Arteriographic manifestations of pancreatic neoplasm, Amer. J. Roentgen. **95**:720, 1965.

78. Mikal, S.: Operative criteria for diagnosis of cancer in a mass of the head of the pancreas, Ann. Surg. **161**:395, 1965.

79. Mosely, R. D., Jr.: Diagnosis of tumors of the pancreas with the aid of pneumoretroperitoneal pancreatography and splenoportography, Amer. J. Roentgen. **80**:967, 1958.

80. Mosely, R. D., Jr.: Roentgen diagnosis of pancreatic disease, Arch. Intern. Med. (Chicago) **107**:31, 1961.

81. Nebesar, R. A., and Pollard, J. J.: A critical evaluation of selective celias and superior mesenteric angiography in the diagnosis of pancreatic diseases, particularly malignant tumor: facts and "Artefacts", Radiology **89**:1017, 1967.

82. Nusbaum, M., Baum, S., Kuroda, K., and Blakemore, W. S.: Selective mesenteric arteriography in the diagnosis of pancreatic lesions, Amer. J. Gastroent. **48**:421, 1967.

83. Ödman, P.: Percutaneous selective angiography of the celiac artery, Acta Radiol. **159** (Supp.):1, 1958.

84. Oi, I.: Personal communication.

85. Oi, I., Takemoto, T., and Nakayama, K.: "Fiberduodenoscopy" early diagnosis of cancer of the Papilla of Vater, Surgery **67**:561, 1970.

86. Patel, J., and Lataste, J.: Ducto-pancreatography in discrimination between pancreatitis and pancreatic cancer, Presse Med. **62**:652, 1954.

87. Paul, R. E., Miller, H. H., Kahn, P. C., Callow, A. D., Edwards, T. L., and Patterson, J. F.: Pancreatic angiography, with application of subselective angiography of the celiac or superior mesenteric artery to the diagnosis of carcinoma of the pancreas, New Eng. J. Med. **272**:2285, 1965.

88. Perez, C., Powers, W. E., Holtz, S., and Spjut, H. J.: Roentgenologic-pathologic correlation of resectable carcinoma of the pancreatico-duodenal region, Amer. J. Roentgen. **94**:438, 1965.

89. Peskin, G. W., and Johnson, C.: Pancreatic visualization, Amer. J. Med. Sci. **249**:223, 1965.

90. Pollock, A. V.: Pancreatography in the diagnosis of chronic relapsing pancreatitis, Surg. Gynec. Obstet. **107**:765, 1958.

91. Poppel, M. H.: Roentgen manifestations of pancreatic disease, Springfield, Ill., 1951, Charles C Thomas, Publisher.

92. Ranninger, K., and Saldino, R. M.: Arteriographic

diagnosis of pancreatic lesions, Radiology **86**:470, 1966.

93. Reuter, S. R.: Superselective pancreatic angiography, Radiology **92**:74, 1969.

94. Reuter, S. R.: Modification of pancreatic blood flow with balloon catheters: a new approach to pancreatic angiography, Radiology **95**:57, 1970.

95. Reuter, S. R., Redman, H. C., and Bookstein, J. J.: Differential problems in the angiographic diagnosis of carcinoma of the pancreas, Radiology **96**:93, 1970.

96. Reuter, S. R., Redman, H. C., and Joseph, R. R.: Angiographic findings in pancreatitis, Amer. J. Roentgen. **107**:56, 1969.

97. Rösch, J., and Bret, J.: Arteriography of the pancreas, Amer. J. Roentgen. **94**:182, 1965.

98. Rösch, J., and Herfort, K.: Contribution of splenoportography to the diagnosis of diseases of the pancreas. I, Tumorous diseases, Acta Med. Scand. **171**:251, 1962.

99. Rösch, J., and Herfort, K.: Contribution of splenoportography to the diagnosis of diseases of the pancreas. II, Inflammatory diseases, Acta Med. Scand. **171**:263, 1962.

100. Rösch, J., and Judkins, M. P.: Angiography in the diagnosis of pancreatic disease, Seminars Roentgen. **3**:296, 1968.

101. Rosenbaum, H. D., Barker, E. G., Gibson, D. E., and Griffen, W. O.: Reflux pancreatography. Experimental observations in the cat, Invest. Radiol. **6**:321, 1971.

102. Rubaum, N. J., and Shohl, T.: X-ray visualization of the pancreas, Ann. Surg. **153**:246, 1961.

103. Rubinstein, Z. J., Bank, S., Marks, I. N., and Psillos, C.: Hypotonic duodenography in chronic pancreatitis, Brit. J. Radiol. **44**:142, 1971.

104. Sachs, M. D., and Partington, P. F.: Cholangiographic diagnosis of pancreatitis, Amer. J. Roentgen. **76**:32, 1956.

105. Salik, J.: Pancreatic carcinoma and its early roentgenologic recognition, Amer. J. Roentgen. **86**:1, 1961.

106. Scarpelli, D. G.: Fat necrosis of bone marrow in acute pancreatitis, Amer. J. Path. **32**:1077, 1956.

107. Schultz, E. H., Jr.: Measurements of the retrogastric space, Radiology **84**:58, 1965.

108. Schultz, E. H., Jr.: Aids to diagnosis of acute pancreatitis by roentgenologic study, Amer. J. Roentgen. **78**:607, 1957.

109. Schwartz, S., and Nadelhaft, J.: Simulation of colonic obstruction at the splenic flexure by pancreatitis; roentgen features, Amer. J. Roentgen. **78**:607, 1957.

110. Shaldon, S., Barber, K. M., and Young, W. B.: Percutaneous transhepatic cholangiography, a modified technique, Gastroenterology **42**:371, 1962.

111. Shapiro, R.: Experimental opacification of the pancreas: a preliminary report, Radiology **69**:690, 1957.

112. Shapiro, R.: Radiopacification of the pancreas: a review of experimental efforts, Seminars Roentgen. **3**:318, 1968.

113. Silverman, J., and Hill, B. J.: Intravenous pancreatography—a negative result, Radiology **81**:596, 1963.

114. Stein, G. N., Kalser, M. H., Sarian, N. N., and Finkelstein, A.: An evaluation of the roentgen changes in acute pancreatitis: correlation with clinical findings, Gastroenterology **36**:354, 1959.

115. Swanson, G. E.: A case of cystadenoma of the pancreas studied by selective angiography, Radiology **81**:592, 1963.

116. Takagi, K., Ikeda, S., Nakagawa, Y., Kumakura, K., Maruyama, M., Someya, N., Takada, T., Takekoshi, T., and Kin, T.: Endoscopic cannulation of the Ampulla of Vater, Endoscopy **2**:107, 1970.

117. Thal, A. P., Goott, B., and Margulis, A. R.: Sites of pancreatic duct obstruction in chronic pancreatitis, Ann. Surg. **150**:49, 1959.

118. Trapnell, J. E., and Howard, J. M.: Transduodenal pancreatography: an improved technique, Surgery **60**:1112, 1966.

119. Van Cangh, P. J., and Thorlakson, R. H.: Cystadenoma of the pancreas, Canad. J. Surg. **11**:63, 1968.

120. Varriale, P., Bonanno, C. A., and Grace, W. J.: Portal hypertension secondary to pancreatic pseudocysts, Arch. Intern. Med. (Chicago) **112**:89, 1963.

121. Vieweg, W. V. R., Graber, A. L., and Cerchio, G. M.: Pancreatic islet cell carcinoma with hyperinsulinism and probable, ectopic ACTH-MSH secretion, Arch. Intern. Med. **124**:731, 1969.

122. Waldron, R. L., Bragg, D. G., Daly, W. J., and Seaman, W. B.: Experimental reflux pancreatography and cholangiography, Radiology **88**:357, 1967.

123. Weens, H. S., and Walker, L. A.: The radiologic diagnosis of acute cholecystitis and pancreatitis, Radiol. Clin. N. Amer. **2**:89, 1964.

124. Wiechel, K. L.: Percutaneous transhepatic cholangiography, Acta Chir. Scand. **330** (Supp.):1, 1964.

125. White, T., and McGee, D. F.: Attempted opacification of the pancreas with the use of iodinated dyes, Radiology **72**:238, 1959.

126. Wilson, C. S.: In situ pancreatography in postmortem material, Yale School of Medicine, 1963.

127. Wise, R. E.: Intravenous cholangiography, Springfield, Ill., 1962, Charles C Thomas, Publisher.

43 | Nonneoplastic disease of the pancreas

Arthur R. Clemett

CONGENITAL ANOMALIES

Congenital anomalies of the pancreas are rare, but the duct system is subject to several anatomic variations. There is no complete agreement on the frequency of these variations. The apparent discrepancies may reflect variations in the techniques used for the anatomic studies. A collective result of several studies* indicates that the duct of Wirsung and the common bile duct form a single channel in 60% to 70% of cases, that the duct of Santorini is present and communicates with the duct of Wirsung about half of the time, and that the duct of Santorini is the main pancreatic duct in 2% to 10% of individuals. A dilatation or ampulla of the common channel seldom occurs, but it is common in the duct of Santorini just before its junction with the duodenum.[77]

---

*See references 17, 24, 56, 77, 83, 117, and 134.

1130

Annular pancreas

Annular pancreas is the only congenital anomaly of the gland proper that occurs with significant frequency. There are incomplete varieties, but in the usual case the duodenum is completely surrounded by a band of pancreatic tissue. Pancreatic tissue may sometimes infiltrate the muscularis propria of the duodenum.[23] The degree of mechanical obstruction produced is variable, ranging from none in the asymptomatic patient to high-grade stenosis or complete obstruction. Indeed, annular pancreas first seen in the neonatal period is commonly associated with duodenal atresia,[3,48] and the roentgenographic findings here are typical of the latter lesion. Most other childhood cases are recognized because the anomaly produces significant partial obstruction. Although the obstruction is sometimes nonspecific in character, roentgenographic diagnosis is usually possible by identification of the typical bandlike deformity of the second duodenum, which is often somewhat eccentric. The short constrictions caused by extrinsic peritoneal bands or mucosal diaphragms permit differential diagnosis from these lesions.[48] Extrinsic compression of the second duodenum by hyperplastic lymph nodes has been reported to simulate annular pancreas in childhood.[39]

Over half of the cases of annular pancreas are first detected in adult life.[23] Some are asymptomatic (Fig. 43-1). Chronic low-grade obstruction may cause presenotic dilatation of the duodenum.[80,126] There is high incidence of duodenal ulcer (approximately 30%) associated with annular pancreas in adults (Fig. 43-2).[23] Low-grade obstruction and the typical location of the papilla of Vater distal to the ring of pancreatic tissue are significant etiologic factors. Pancreatitis occurs in about 15% of patients with annular pancreas and may be complicated by pseudocyst formation.[23] The reason for the high incidence in pancreatitis is unknown, but minor trauma[132] and inadequate drainage[23] of the ring of pancreatic tissue have been suggested as possible causes.

Pancreatography will reveal the ductal anatomy of annular pancreas. Bypass procedures are the favored treatment, since division of the annular pancreas frequently results in pancreatic fistulas.[47]

Aberrant pancreas

Aberrant pancreatic tissue has been found in many sites—esophagus,[97] stomach, duodenum, small intestine, Meckel's diverticulum, transverse colon, mesentery, spleen, gallbladder, bile ducts, liver, and mediastinum.[101] Most of these, however, occur in the stomach and duodenum, and the great majority of lesions detectable by roentgenographic studies are located in the gastric antrum or duodenal bulb. These intramural lesions are most frequently submucosal, but any or all layers of the stomach wall may be involved.[70] They are usually smaller than 2.5 cm. in diameter,[28,101] and multiple lesions are not uncommon. The usual roentgenographic appearance is that of a small, well-defined intramural mass with a central dimple or umbilication representing the orifice of a ductlike structure. Sometimes actual filling of a short duct may occur.[28] When the central umbilication or duct can be identified and differentiated from

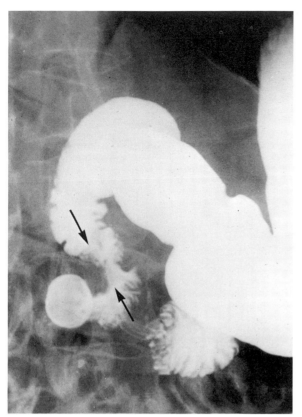

Fig. 43-1. Asymptomatic annular pancreas associated with a lateral duodenal diverticulum in an adult.

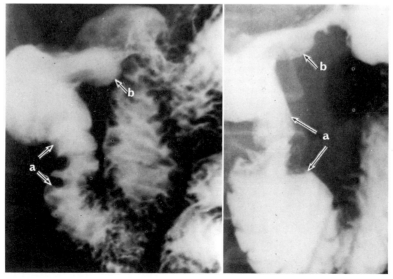

Fig. 43-2. Annular pancreas, **a,** in an adult with low-grade duodenal obstruction and large duodenal ulcer, **b.**

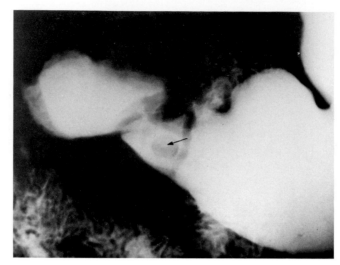

Fig. 43-3. Aberrant pancreas in gastric antrum. Central umbilication (arrow) resulting from a ductlike structure permitted correct preoperative diagnosis.

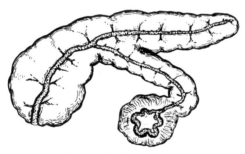

Foregut duplication

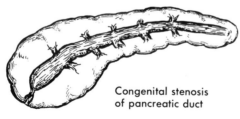

Congenital stenosis
of pancreatic duct

Fig. 43-4. Diagrammatic representation of rare congenital anomalies of the pancreas. The muscular sac in the foregut duplication is lined by gastric mucosa. Severe congenital stenosis of the main pancreatic duct is associated with neonatal meconium ileus.

an ulcer, a conclusive diagnosis is possible (Fig. 43-3). Eklof found characteristic roentgenographic changes in twenty-one of twenty-five proved cases.[28] These lesions are occasionally associated with gastric ulcers,[70] and they are potentially subject to all of the pathologic processes of the pancreas proper.[87]

Other anomalies

There are two additional congenital pancreatic anomalies of real or potential roentgenologic importance even though they are very rare. These are foregut duplication of the pancreas and congenital stenosis of the main pancreatic duct (Fig. 43-4).

Foregut duplications

The reported foregut duplications have occurred in children and have caused significant symptoms.[12,45] Pathologically, the lesions are thick-walled, muscular sacs lined by gastric epithelium. They are connected to the pancreas and have a well-defined duct system. In one case the entire anomaly was demonstrated by operative pancreatography,[45] and in another the communicating duct was shown by this technique after excision of the duplication.[12]

Congenital stenosis

The congenital stenoses are found in newborn infants dying after operation for meconium ileus.[49,58] Gross examination reveals that the distal pancreatic duct is completely occluded and histologic examination shows that it was replaced in one case by multiple slitlike structures.[49] Pronounced cystic dilatation of the pancreatic ducts is present proximal to the obstruction. The parenchyma shows acinar atrophy and fibrosis. Despite some similarities, this condition is distinct from cystic fibrosis in which the typical pathologic findings occur after the second month of life.[84] Diagnosis of congenital stenosis of the pancreatic duct is theoretically possible by direct pancreatography done by needle puncture of a dilated duct at surgery. This lesion may be related to the less severe stenoses of the sphincter of Oddi or pancreatic duct, which have been described as rare causes of pancreatitis in children.[45]

Cystic fibrosis (mucoviscidosis)

Cystic fibrosis is, of course, now recognized as a hereditary systemic disease, a generalized disorder of the exocrine glands. The name derives from the fact that the pathologic changes in the pancreas were the first to be noted, and pancreatic achylia is a prominent feature of the disease. It is noteworthy, however, that the loss of pancreatic exocrine function may occur gradually over several months or years and is not necessarily complete.[84]

Extra-alimentary manifestations of the disease —the well-known pulmonary lesions, sinus disease, hypertrophic pulmonary osteoarthropathy, and retarded growth and maturation[121]—will not be considered here. In about 15% of patients with cystic fibrosis meconium ileus develops in the neonatal period.[133] The roentgenographic features of this disorder are described in Chapter 58. An identical obstructive disorder, so-called meconium ileus equivalent, occasionally occurs in older children with cystic fibrosis and is often related to the cessation of pancreatic enzyme substitution therapy.[19]

Calcified concretions have been found histologically in cystic fibrosis and on rare occasion they have been demonstrated roentgenologically.[16,82,133] The small-bowel pattern is often abnormal. Thickened, clubbed, or effaced mucosal folds in the duodenum and jejunum are the most constant findings. Moderate dilatation of the small bowel is present in some cases (Fig. 43-5). Other noteworthy gastrointestinal manifestations of cystic fibrosis include the rare occurrence of duodenal ulcer,[4] rectal prolapse in about 15% of patients, an increased incidence of intussusception in older children,[133] the occurrence of pneumatosis cystoides intestinalis that is probably related to the pulmonary disease,[133] a hypoplastic-appearing gallbladder,[30] nonvisualization of the gallbladder on oral cholecystog-

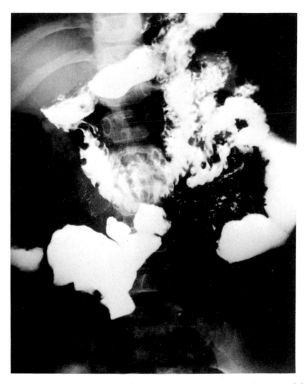

Fig. 43-5. Abnormal small-bowel pattern in a 7-year-old child with cystic fibrosis. The duodenal and jejunal mucosal folds are thickened, clubbed, or effaced. Some dilatation of the bowel is present as well.

raphy in about 20% of patients,[86] and development of biliary cirrhosis complicated by portal hypertension with esophageal varices. Tucker and co-workers found the latter complication in two of 175 patients studied.[121]

In older patients with cystic fibrosis the colon may present a striking appearance. On plain films it is usually abundantly filled or even slightly distended by a mottled or foamy appearing fecal mass. Adequate cleansing is seldom obtained for barium enema examination and evacuation of the enema is usually poor. Multiple poorly defined filling defects are present, many of which are adherent to the mucosa (Fig. 43-6, *A*). These are collections of abnormal mucus. Even when the enema is completely evacuated the mucosal pattern is abnormal. The folds are thickened and increased in number, giving the impression of a hyperplastic mucosa (Fig. 43-6, *B*). This appearance is best explained by rectal biopsy specimens that have shown increased numbers of goblet cells and crypts that are

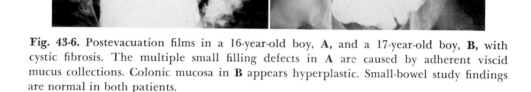

Fig. 43-6. Postevacuation films in a 16-year-old boy, **A,** and a 17-year-old boy, **B,** with cystic fibrosis. The multiple small filling defects in **A** are caused by adherent viscid mucus collections. Colonic mucosa in **B** appears hyperplastic. Small-bowel study findings are normal in both patients.

widely dilated and packed with mucus.[88] The latter changes may be evident grossly in biopsy specimens and certainly produce an increase in the mucosal surface area.

ACUTE PANCREATITIS

Pathologic appearances of acute pancreatitis are exceedingly variable, ranging from interstitial edema to extensive necrosis with hemorrhage and widespread peritoneal fat necrosis. Clinical diagnosis is often difficult, and suspicion of pancreatitis is usually confirmed by elevated serum amylase determinations. Unfortunately, normal enzyme values may be present late in the course of severe pancreatitis and elevated values occur at times in several other acute abdominal disorders. Roentgenographic examination of the abdomen and chest contributes to the recognition of less than half of the cases of acute pancreatitis, this by virtue of the demonstration of several nonspecific findings that may accompany the disease.[108,130] Positive diagnosis of acute pancreatitis on plain abdominal films is possible only in a very small percentage of cases.

Primary manifestations

In severe pancreatitis the gland may be enlarged to three or four times normal size. In the infrequent instance when this enlargement can be confidently recognized on plain films a positive diagnosis of pancreatitis is possible. This is particularly true if there is supporting evidence such as duodenal ileus and pancreatic calculi, as shown in Fig. 43-7.

A mottled pattern of the soft tissues about the pancreas and the rest of the abdomen is a rare phenomenon caused by extensive peritoneal fat necrosis.[9,130] The faint densities measure 1 to 3 cm. in diameter. They have been related to the formation of insoluble calcium soaps in the areas of fat necrosis.[75] Calcification is not seen roentgenologically, however, and it was not present histologically in one case studied.[8] The mottled pattern may be a result of the roentgenographic contrast between the necrotic foci and the surrounding normal adipose tissue.

Suppuration may complicate the course of acute pancreatitis and pancreatic abscesses may be expected in 1.0% to 1.5% of cases of acute pancreatitis.[31,113] With gas-forming organisms a so-called gas abscess of the pancreas is produced (Figs. 43-8 and 43-9). In some series gas has been present in the majority of pancreatic abscesses.[29] There may be either a single cavity containing gas and fluid or a collection of mottled gas shadows in the region of the pancreas.[2] The

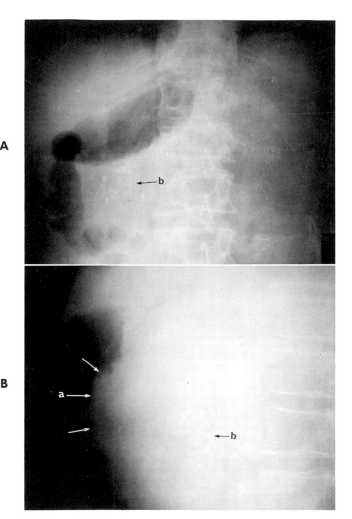

A

B

Fig. 43-7. Acute hemorrhagic pancreatitis. **A,** Left lateral decubitus film; **B,** cross-table lateral film. There is evidence of a retrogastric mass, **a,** duodenal ileus, and edema of the duodenal mucosa. Despite the obvious pancreatic calcification, **b,** there was no previous history of pancreatitis.

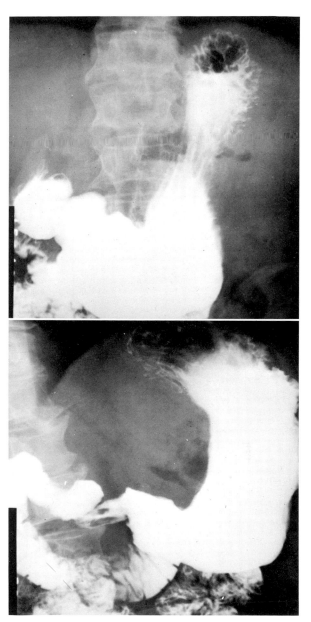

Fig. 43-8. Gas abscess of pancreas. The suppurative process was resolved by antibiotic therapy. Active pancreatitis persisted, however, and was subsequently found to be secondary to a pancreatic carcinoma.

process commonly extends to involve the lesser peritoneal sac[130] but may also spread to the retroperitoneal space and flank.[34] In some instances the gas abscess will become apparent only on serial examinations, and it may be clearly recognized only after contrast studies are done.[32]

The foregoing findings provide the basis for a positive plain film diagnosis of acute pancreatitis. Pancreatic calcification is certain evidence of a diseased pancreas, and its identification in an appropriate clinical setting certainly suggests the diagnosis of acute pancreatitis. Acute cholecystitis, perforated peptic ulcer, and similar

disorders obviously can and do occur in patients with pancreatic calcification, however, and the identification of calcification alone does not therefore permit a prior diagnosis of acute pancreatitis. In most series of acute pancreatitis cases calcification is an infrequent finding, but its incidence has been noted to be as high as 17%.[115]

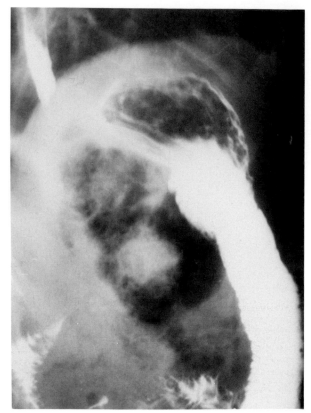

Fig. 43-9. Gas abscess of the pancreas. Previous gastric resection of Billroth II type.

Secondary manifestations

Acute pancreatitis may be attended by several secondary manifestations, some functional and some anatomic, the frequency and intensity of which tend to parallel the severity of the primary inflammatory process. Those form the basis for several roentgenographic "signs" and findings that have been described in and may contribute to the diagnosis of acute pancreatitis.[92,94,115] These include irritability, spasm, paresis, and mucosal edema of the stomach, duodenum, and segments of the colon; swelling of the duodenal papilla; paralytic ileus, particularly when confined to the jejunum; obliteration of kidney and psoas margins by retroperitoneal extension of the inflammatory process; ascites; elevation and restricted motion of the diaphragm, especially on the left; pleural effusions; discoid atelectasis; and lower lobe bronchopneumonia. These changes are all quite nonspecific, the actual diagnostic value of many is questionable, and some are readily recognized only with contrast studies.

Sentinel loop

An isolated distended loop of small bowel reflecting an early paralytic ileus, designated the "sentinel loop," has been popularized in the medical literature as a significant clue to the diagnosis of acute pancreatitis. Stein and coauthors reported this in 55% of their patients with acute pancreatitis,[115] while Weens and Walker noted a well-defined sentinel loop in less than 10%.[130] It occurred with equal frequency in their patients with acute cholecystitis. The term sentinel loop, in fact, was originally applied in cases of acute appendicitis and cholecystitis.[65] This finding may occur in a great variety of acute abdominal disorders.

Colon cut-off sign

"Colon cut-off sign" is another phrase that has captured medical fancy and is frequently cited as useful plain film evidence of acute pancreatitis. As originally described in a small number of patients by Price[96] and by Stuart,[118] the term referred to the absence of gas in the transverse colon, which was thus "cut-off" from the gasfilled hepatic and splenic flexures. This was attributed to spasm of the transverse colon induced by the inflammatory process extending between the leaves of the transverse mesocolon.

Brascho and co-workers later used the same term to describe gaseous distention of the transverse colon with collapse of the descending colon.[13] They reported this in twenty-eight of fifty-four cases of acute pancreatitis and ascribed the transverse colon gas to atony of this segment. Weens and Walker found this appearance in but one of fifty unselected cases of acute pancreatitis.[130] Distal transverse colon obstruction may be simulated in pancreatitis by segmental colon spasm in the acute phase or fibrosis and adhesions in the later stages.[109] This, however, is a rare event. Considering the normal occurrence of transverse colon gas and the unspectacular appearance of the published cases, it seems likely that this colon cut-off sign has little diagnostic validity or usefulness.

Chest abnormalities

Chest abnormalities were found by Fishbein and coauthors in 14% of 155 patients with a clinical diagnosis of acute pancreatitis.[33] Pleural effusion was present in 6%. Fluid accumulation in the left pleural space is most frequent in acute pancreatis, but effusions can occur on either or both sides. The amylase content of the aspirated pleural fluid is almost invariably elevated, with the level exceeding that of the serum.

Contrast examination of the gastrointestinal tract

Several studies have shown that contrast examination of the gastrointestinal tract greatly improves the roentgenographic diagnosis of acute pancreatits. Significant anatomic or functional abnormalities may be found in 70% to 90% of cases, and positive findings are more frequent when the examination is done early in the course of the disease. Bergkvist and Seldinger studied twenty-six patients with acute pancreatitis by upper gastrointestinal examination within 48 hours of the onset of symptoms.[10] Pancreatic enlargement was recognized in ten patients. The abnormality most frequently noted was duodenal paresis, which was readily recognized in twenty-four of the twenty-six patients. This observation is corroborated by the experience of others.[108,130] Spasm or irritability of the duodenum occurs infrequently, although this was the most prominent of several nonspecific changes described by Poppel in cases of mumps complicated by pancreatitis.[94]

Swollen duodenal papilla

A swollen duodenal papilla is an important sign of pancreatitis (Fig. 43-16), but it may occur in other conditions.[92] The normal papilla averages 1.5 cm. in length and 0.5 cm. in width.[95] The range of normal variation is such, however, that recognition of minor degrees of enlargement may be difficult. Submucosal edema of the duodenum is a common and prominent feature in acute pancreatitis (Fig. 43-10).[108,130] The same propensity for edema formation occurs in other segments of the alimentary tract secondarily involved by extension of the pancreatic inflammatory process (Fig. 43-12). When acute pancreatitis is complicated by formation of pseudocysts that adhere to and displace the stomach, edema of the adjacent gastric mucosa is a characteristic finding (Figs. 43-22 and 43-23). Obstruction of the second[14,110] and third[111] portions of the duodenum are rare complications of acute pancre-

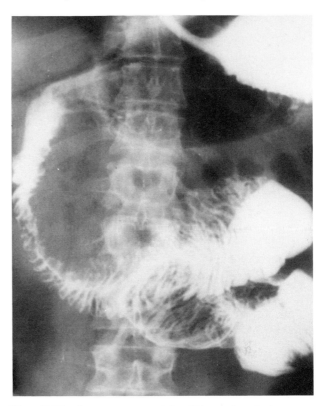

Fig. 43-10. Acute pancreatitis. There is obvious enlargement of the head of the pancreas and submucosal edema of the adjacent duodenum.

atitis that have been demonstrated by gastrointestinal examination.

Oral cholecystograms

Oral cholecystograms are frequently obtained to differentiate suspected acute cholecystitis and acute pancreatitis. A normal study excludes the diagnosis of cholecystitis. The diagnostic significance of nonvisualization of the gallbladder is uncertain in this situation, since in about half of those patients with acute pancreatitis and normal gallbladders, visualization is not accomplished.[123] After subsequent convalescence this group can be shown to have normally functioning gallbladders. In about one third of patients with acute pancreatis, intravenous cholangiograms fail to visualize either the bile ducts or the gallbladder.[130] The intravenous study is helpful only when it provides positive evidence of cholecystitis or demonstrates a normal gallbladder.

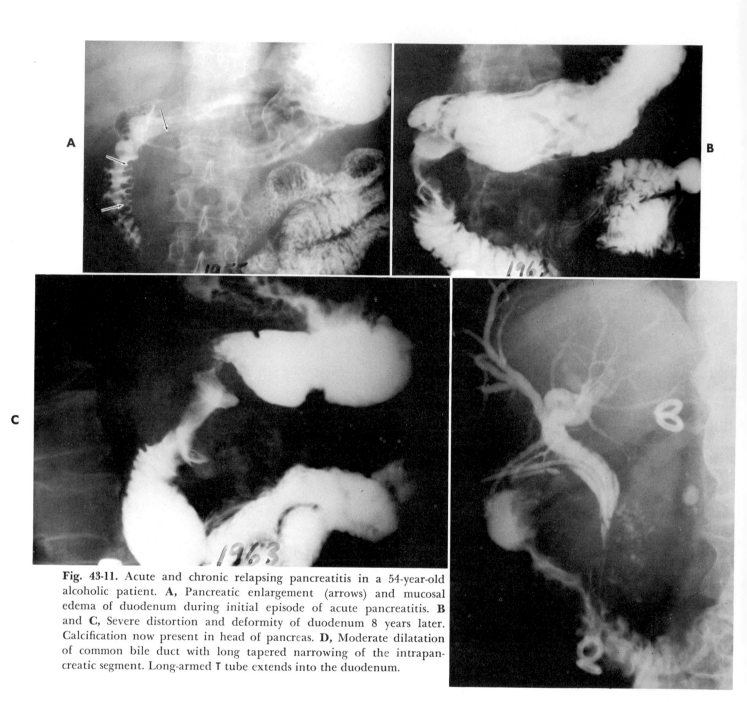

Fig. 43-11. Acute and chronic relapsing pancreatitis in a 54-year-old alcoholic patient. **A,** Pancreatic enlargement (arrows) and mucosal edema of duodenum during initial episode of acute pancreatitis. **B** and **C,** Severe distortion and deformity of duodenum 8 years later. Calcification now present in head of pancreas. **D,** Moderate dilatation of common bile duct with long tapered narrowing of the intrapancreatic segment. Long-armed T tube extends into the duodenum.

Factors influencing diagnosis

Patients with acute pancreatitis are rarely subjected to pancreatography while the disease is active. Total obstruction of the main pancreatic duct may be demonstrated (Fig. 43-13). The characteristic roentgenographic finding of acute pancreatitis is diffuse parenchymal opacification.[21] This can occur in focal areas of inflammation or the entire gland may be involved.

Parenchymal opacification is believed to result from changes in permeability of the duct epithelium. Injection of 70% iodopyracet (Diodrast) has been shown to induce this change in the normal pancreas, and a repeat injection within a few minutes then results in parenchymal opacification.[22] With single injections some care must be exercised in equating parenchymal opacification with acute pancreatitis. Errors in

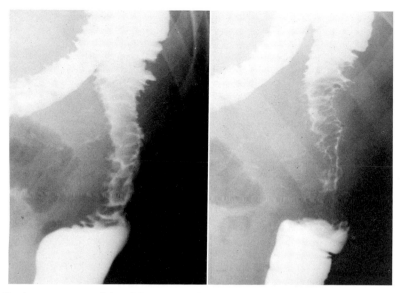

Fig. 43-12. Acute pancreatitis with extension of inflammatory process to splenic flexure causing spasm and pronounced submucosal edema.

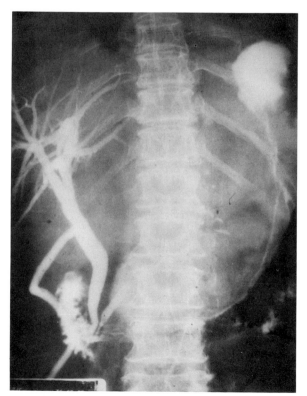

Fig. 43-13. Acute pancreatitis. There is diffuse homogeneous staining of the head of the pancreas with contrast medium. The pancreatic duct is completely obstructed to retrograde flow.

technique may result in excessive injection pressures that can cause opacification of the normal pancreas (see Fig. 43-19).

A great many factors have been implicated in the cause of acute pancreatitis.[26] In adults biliary tract disease and alcoholism are the two most commonly associated conditions. Roentgenographic evaluation of the biliary tract should be considered routine in the study of the patient with acute pancreatitis.

Concomitant pancreatitis is frequent with pancreatic carcinoma. In one half of the carcinoma cases studied by Mikal there was some evidence of associated pancreatitis, and gross fat necrosis was found in one fifth of these patients.[76] At times the pancreatitis may dominate the clinical picture. Sarles and co-workers in a study of 205 cases of acute and chronic pancreatitis found carcinoma obstructing the main duct to be the etiologic factor in three patients.[105] In obscure or puzzling cases of pancreatitis this possibility should be considered, and it is a cogent argument for operative pancreatography in these patients (Fig. 43-14).

Acute pancreatitis is uncommon in children, and in most cases the cause is unknown.[11] In contrast to adults, in children associated biliary tract disease is rare. Nonpenetrating trauma to the abdomen is clearly the cause in a few cases.[64]

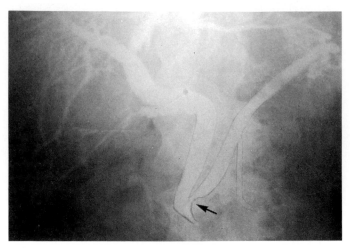

Fig. 43-14. Investigation of acute pancreatitis. Operative cholangiopancreatogram (retouched) obtained after two episodes of acute pancreatitis in a 50-year-old woman. Partial obstruction and dilatation of the main pancreatic duct caused by extrinsic pressure (arrow) from a primary pancreatic carcinoma measuring less than 1 cm. in diameter.

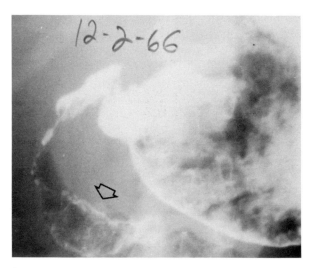

Fig. 43-15. Acute pancreatitis caused by calcified stone in distal common bile duct (arrow) of a child. The gallbladder was normal. Symptoms and swelling of the pancreas resolved with spontaneous passage of the calculus.

More frequently the disease is caused by infestation with *Ascaris lumbricoides*.[11] One or several worms may be demonstrated in the duodenum by gastrointestinal examination in these cases.[38] In instances of fatal necrotizing pancreatitis the parasites may be found in the pancreas itself.[27,79] Ascariasis is also a rare cause of pancreatitis in adults, and the disease results from

the mechanical effects of adult worms in the common bile duct or the pancreatic duct.[90]

The Chinese liver fluke, *Clonorchis sinensis*, has also been noted to reside in the pancreatic ducts and cause pancreatitis.[72] Parasitic infestation, furthermore, may promote primary stone formation in the bile ducts, which in turn can cause pancreatitis (Fig. 43-15). The mechanical derangements of primary duodenal diseases, such as Crohn's disease[63] or intraluminal duodenal diverticulum,[81] have also been implicated as causes of pancreatitis, presumably caused by the reflux of duodenal contents into the duct.

CHRONIC PANCREATITIS
Pancreatic calcification

Pancreatic calcification is the most important roentgenographic manifestation of chronic pancreatis. Its true incidence is uncertain. Warren and Veidenheimer found pancreatic calcification in 31% of 291 patients with a clinical diagnosis of chronic relapsing pancreatitis.[128] Sarles and coauthors noted calcification roentgenologically in 76% of sixty-two patients in whom the diagnosis of chronic pancreatitis was confirmed by histologic examination.[105] They found no instances of primary lithiasis of the duct of Wirsung, although this has been described as a common initial event in the genesis of extensive calcification.[128] The calcification has two forms, the

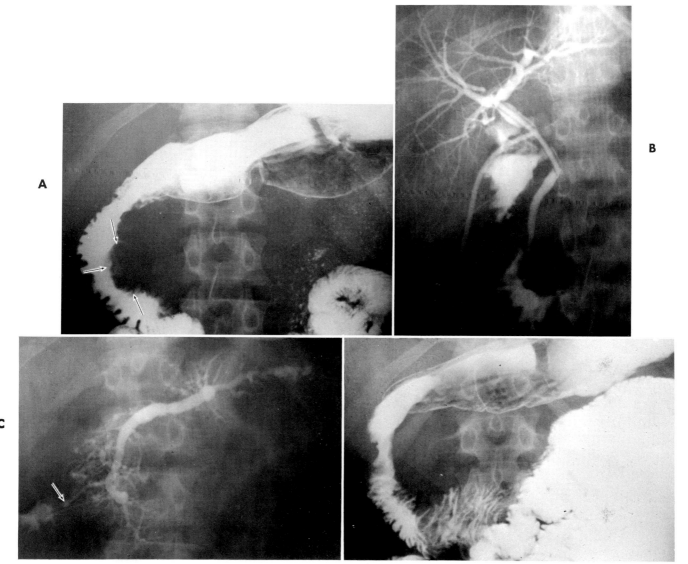

Fig. 43-16. Acute and chronic relapsing pancreatitis. **A,** Swelling of duodenal papilla during acute episode (arrows). **B,** Lateral bowing of intrapancreatic segment of common duct on operative cholangiogram 2 weeks later. **C,** Operative pancreatogram with changes of chronic pancreatitis. Note ampulla-like dilatation at end of duct of Santorini (arrow). **D,** Residual duodenal deformity 2 years later. Faint calcifications now present in head of pancreas.

most frequent of which is calcium carbonate concretions in ducts of varying size.[60] Otherwise, calcification occurs in the form of hydroxyapatite in areas of fat necrosis in the pancreatic parenchyma.

The time required for calcification to occur and become evident on roentgenographic examination is unknown. In the patient illustrated in Fig. 43-11 calcification was noted 8 years after the initial clinical episode of pancreatitis,

whereas in the case shown in Fig. 43-16 calcification occurred 2 years after the first clinical attack. The pancreatogram (Fig. 43-16, *C*) at the time of this initial episode, however, already showed changes of chronic pancreatitis. In a small number of patients (probably 10% to 15%) pancreatic calcification will be noted in the absence of past or present symptoms of pancreatitis.[55,73]

In adults pancreatic calcification is associated

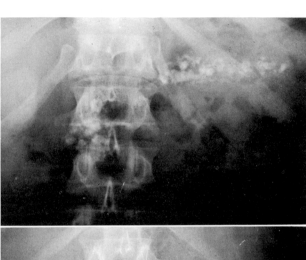

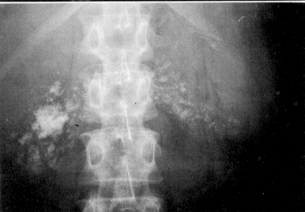

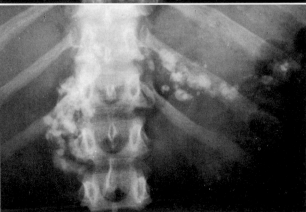

Fig. 43-17. Extensive pancreatic calcification in three different patients.

with a high incidence of alcoholism.[85] In children calcification is a rare finding although it has been recorded in cystic fibrosis,[16,82,133] chronic recurrent pancreatitis,[91] in association with alcoholism and malnutrition,[107] and with protein malnutrition in the absence of symptoms of pancreatitis.[52]

Pancreatic calcifications may be focal or diffuse and they vary in character from tiny punctate deposits to large dense aggregates (Fig. 43-17). When tiny and few in number they are often overlooked, especially when obscured by the spine on frontal projections. Differential diagnosis of biliary calculi, renal stones, hepatic and splenic calcifications, costal cartilage calcification, and calcified lymph nodes usually presents few problems. On occasion it may be difficult or impossible to differentiate calcific plaques in the aorta or its upper abdominal branches.

Roentgenograms demonstrating calcification provide a useful profile of the patient with chronic pancreatitis. An increase in the extent of calcification signifies progressive disease. The complication of pseudocyst formation may be evident by changes in position of the calcifications (Fig. 43-18). Pancreatic calculi have been implicated as a rare cause of gastrointestinal hemorrhage, either by erosion into the duodenum or by causing bleeding into the main pancreatic duct.[127] An increased incidence of pancreatic carcinoma has been shown in patients with chronic pancreatitis and calcification of the gland.[7,89] In one remarkable case the development of a pancreatic carcinoma was attended by the partial disappearance of the pancreatic calcification demonstrated 3 years earlier.[122] Although this was suggested as a useful sign of carcinoma, other instances of the spontaneous disappearance of pancreatic calcification have been noted in the absence of carcinoma.[5,114]

Examination

Gastrointestinal examination is normal in most cases of chronic pancreatitis. Minor alterations of the duodenal contour will be evident sometimes and these changes are reputed to be recognized frequently when hypotonic duodenography is employed.[51] In a few instances chronic pancreatitis produces extensive distortion and deformity of the duodenum (Fig. 43-11), and symptomatic duodenal obstruction may occur (Fig. 43-26).

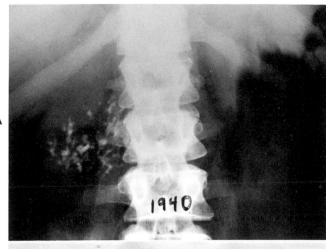

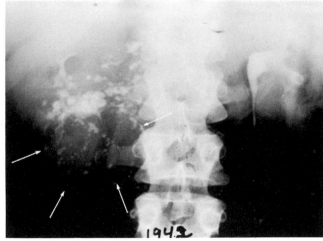

Fig. 43-18. A, Chronic pancreatitis with extensive calcification. **B,** Development of a pseudocyst (arrows) in the head of the pancreas is clearly evident by the change in position of the calcifications 2 years later.

Intravenous cholangiography reveals evidence of partial common bile duct obstruction in some cases of chronic pancreatitis.[135] Features more characteristic of the disease, however, are usually shown only by direct cholangiography. In some instances there is abrupt angulation of the common duct and a right lateral convexity of its intrapancreatic segment (Fig. 43-16, *C*). A more typical pattern, however, consists of a long, tapered narrowing of the distal duct within the pancreas, moderate dilatation proximal to this, and normal intrahepatic ducts (Figs. 43-11, *B* and 43-26, *B*).[103] Sarles and co-workers found this pattern to some degree in sixty-three of eighty

cholangiographies in patients with chronic pancreatitis.[105]

A normal main pancreatic duct will be shown by pancreatography in some patients with chronic pancreatitis (19% and 24% in some studies).[54,105] In most cases, though, dilatation, tortuosity, irregular contours, and single or multiple stenoses will be demonstrated.[46] On rare occasions nonopaque calculi may be demonstrated as the cause of recurrent pancreatitis (Fig. 43-19). Duct stenosis and irregular contours are reliable evidence of chronic pancreatitis. A not infrequent pattern consists of a long tapered stenosis of the main duct in the head of the pancreas, with moderate proximal ductal dilatation (Fig. 43-20). This must be differentiated from carcinoma where the stenosis is more abrupt and there is very marked dilatation proximal to the obstruction.

The diameter of the normal pancreatic duct may vary from 1 to 9 mm.[134] The caliber of the duct tends to increase with advancing age. Millbourn found the mean maximum diameter to be 3.5 mm. in the third decade and this value was increased to 5.5 mm. after age 70.[77] There is some correlation of common duct and pancreatic duct size (a ratio of 2:1 being a crude rule of thumb), which may help in the recognition of pathologic dilatation. In the considerable experience of Sarles and co-workers pancreatic duct dilatation in chronic pancreatitis was always caused by obstruction, with duct stenoses being twice as frequent a cause as stones.[105]

Other evidence of chronic pancreatitis by pancreatography includes filling of many secondary and tertiary branches and acinar opacification.[46,54,120] The alterations in the secondary branches are often striking and frequently provide the most convincing evidence of chronic pancreatitis (see Figs. 43-16, *C*, and 43-26, *C*). The dilated, irregular, tortuous ducts are quite unlike the thin, smooth, straight secondary branches of the normal pancreas. Stenoses regularly occur at the junction of the branches with the main pancreatic duct. The pathologic basis for this change may be either irregular periductal fibrosis[105] or metaplasia of the duct epithelium or both.[100]

PANCREATIC PSEUDOCYST

Pancreatic pseudocysts are encapsulated collections of exudate, blood, and secretions that

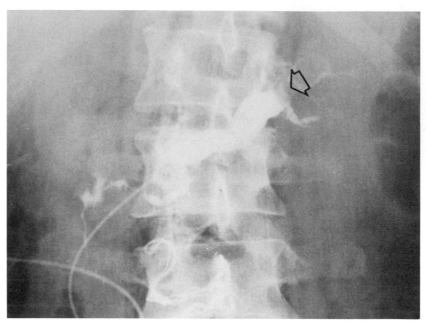

Fig. 43-19. Nonopaque stone (arrow) in a dilated main pancreatic duct caused recurrent pancreatitis until removed surgically.

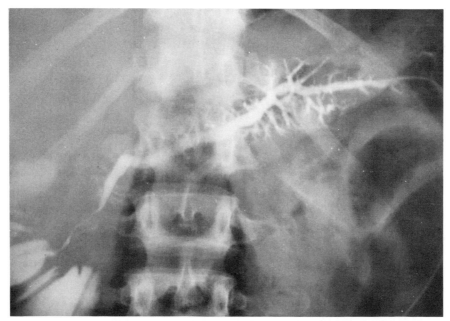

Fig. 43-20. Chronic relapsing pancreatitis. There is a long, tapered stricture of the main pancreatic duct in the head of the pancreas with moderate ductal dilatation proximal to this. The secondary ducts have some mild stenosis and irregularities.

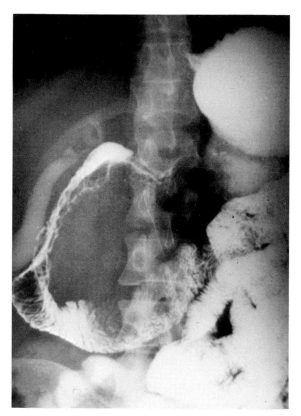

Fig. 43-21. Chronic pancreatitis with pseudocyst in the head of the pancreas.

result from pancreatic necrosis or rupture of ducts and acini. The walls are composed of granulation and fibrous tissue and the inner lining is often necrotic. Initially the contents consist largely of blood and exudate, but later as blood is destroyed and active inflammation subsides, the pseudocyst may contain almost pure pancreatic juice. Pseudocysts may be small and entirely intrapancreatic in location, but with extension beyond the confines of the gland they may attain large size. In either location the pseudocyst nearly always communicates with the pancreatic duct system.[46]

Most pseudocysts in adults are secondary to pancreatitis. These may occur in the course of a single episode of acute pancreatitis, but more frequently they develop insidiously in chronic relapsing pancreatitis.[53] Some pseudocysts in adults result from trauma, and nonpenetrating abdominal trauma is the most important etiologic factor in children.[20,57] At times there may be an interval of several months between the

injury and the onset of symptoms resulting from the pseudocyst. Most pancreatic carcinomas cause at least partial duct obstruction, and it is not surprising, therefore, that pseudocyst formation complicates a few tumors (5% in one series).[76]

The roentgenographic manifestations of pseudocysts are variable and obviously depend on the size of the lesion, its site of origin, and the extent of migration of the inflammatory process. Lesions of sufficient size occurring in and about the pancreas are readily recognized by their compression and displacement of the adjacent stomach and duodenum (Figs. 43-21 to 13-23), as well as displacement of the transverse colon by larger lesions. Sometimes accurate differentiation of pseudocysts from lesions of adjacent organs may be difficult or impossible as in those cases, for instance, of pancreatic pseudocysts simulating intrarenal masses.[41,116] Calcification of the wall of a chronic pseudocyst does occur on rare occasions.[129]

Sometimes the migration of inflammatory products and pancreatic secretions is such that the main bulk of the pseudocyst may be quite remote from the pancreas proper (Fig. 43-24).[93] Mediastinal pseudocysts result from the migration of inflammatory products and pancreatic secretions through either the esophageal or aortic hiatus of the diaphragm.[36,71] Rarely the mediastinal mass may cause mechanical impairment of cardiac function.[131] Major displacements of the esophagus above and the stomach below the diaphragm are the usual findings,[35,99] but in some cases conventional examinations will only reveal the mediastinal mass.[61] The remote lesions may defy accurate roentgenographic diagnosis unless pancreatography demonstrates communication between the mass and the pancreatic duct system (Figs. 43-25 and 43-26). Further extension of mediastinal pseudocyst into the soft tissues of the neck has been observed.[119]

COMPLICATIONS OF PANCREATITIS AND PSEUDOCYSTS

Extra-abdominal fat necrosis has long been known to occur in acute and chronic pancreatitis. In an autopsy study Scarpelli found histologic evidence of intramedullary fat necrosis of bone in 10% of patients with acute or subacute pancreatitis.[106] These cases had widespread intra-

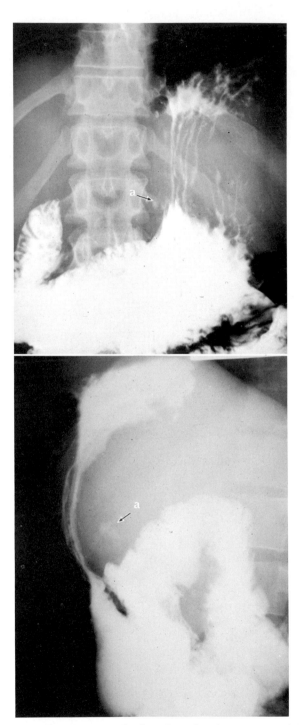

Fig. 43-22. Acute and chronic relapsing pancreatitis with acute pseudocyst of the tail of the pancreas. Pseudocyst is adherent to stomach with edema of adjacent gastric mucosa. Calcifications of body of pancreas, **a.**

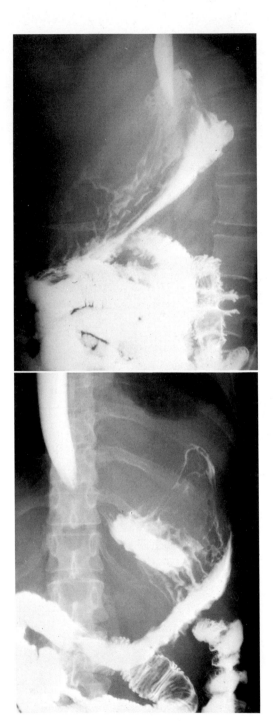

Fig. 43-23. Acute pancreatitis with pseudocyst in lesser peritoneal sac and left pleural effusion.

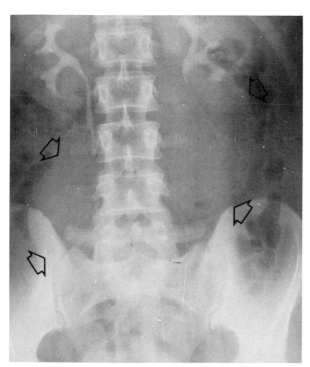

Fig. 43-24. Pancreatic pseudocyst (arrows) following trauma. This inframesocolic collection probably resulted from injury to the uncinate process of the pancreas.

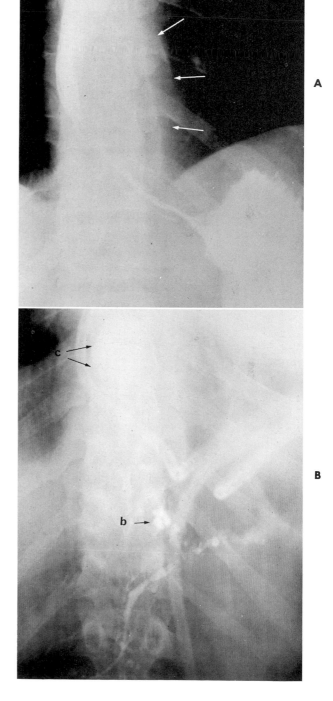

Fig. 43-25. Chronic pancreatitis with mediastinal pseudocyst. **A,** lower mediastinal mass deviating esophagus to the right and causing dysphagia developed after 3 months of recurrent bilateral pleural effusions. **B,** Operative pancreatogram with evidence of chronic pancreatitis, a small peripancreatic pseudocyst, **b,** and leakage of some contrast medium into the mediastinal pseudocyst, **c.**

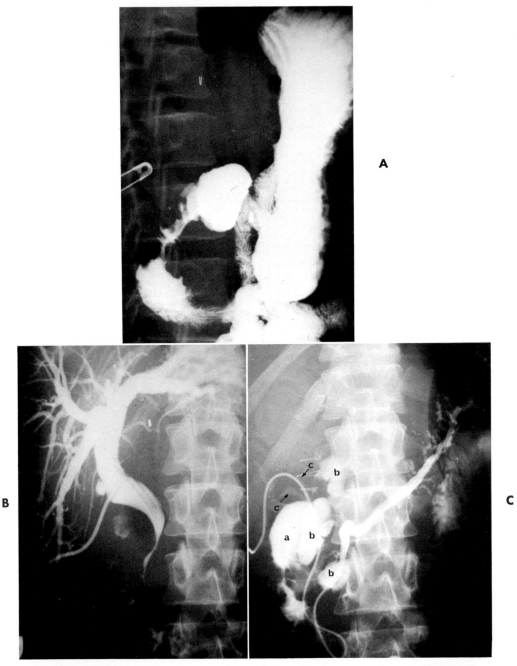

Fig. 43-26. Chronic pancreatitis. **A,** Distortion, deformity, and high-grade duodenal obstruction requiring gastroenterostomy. **B,** T tube cholangiogram. **C,** Postoperative pancreatogram. Pancreatic duct catheter looped in duodenum, inserted in common bile duct, and exteriorized with the T tube. Duodenum, a, pseudocysts, b, in and about head of pancreas, faint opacification of common duct, c. Maximum diameter of main pancreatic duct 7 mm. Pronounced irregularities and stenoses of secondary branches.

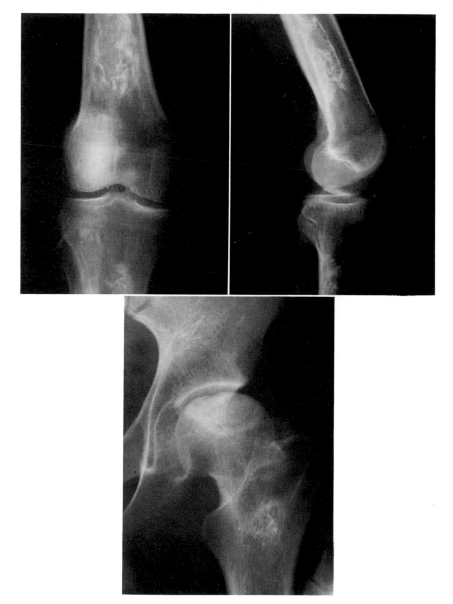

Fig. 43-27. Medullary bone infarcts and aseptic necrosis of femoral head in patients with chronic relapsing pancreatitis.

abdominal fat necroses or other extra-abdominal lesions as well. Only in recent years has the roentgenographic evidence of these bone lesions been recognized.[37,50,68]

Sclerotic intramedullary bone lesions, roentgenologically identical to bone infarcts, have been the most common finding in chronic pancreatitis. These are most frequent in the distal femur and proximal tibia, but they may occur elsewhere (Fig. 43-27). Aseptic necrosis of the humeral and femoral heads has also been noted.

In a few cases focal destructive lesions have been found in the long bones. These medullary lesions erode the adjacent cortex and may cause periosteal reaction. Serial examinations have shown slow resolution of this process without subsequent sclerosis.[50,112] These lesions may be caused by medullary fat necrosis,[6] medullary ischemia,[1] or both.

Splenic vein occlusion is a rare but well-recognized complication of pancreatic disease. Thrombosis may occur as a result of pancreatitis,[102] and pancreatic pseudocysts at times occlude the vein by direct compression.[124] Splenomegaly, gastric varices, and esophageal varices may result, although the latter may be absent when collateral pathways adequately circumvent the obstruction between the spleen and the portal vein. The combination of splenomegaly and gastric varices in the absence of evidence of liver dysfunction and esophageal varices should suggest a possible pancreatic lesion.

In addition to pleural effusions acute pancreatitis may be associated with pericardial effusion.[66] Intractable massive ascites is a rare complication of acute pancreatitis. There is a high incidence of subacute pancreatitis and pseudocyst in these patients, and lymphatic obstruction is probably a major factor in the pathogenesis of the ascites.[25] Stenosing colon lesions in and about the splenic flexure are rare complications of pancreatitis. These may spontaneously resolve but sometimes cause chronic obstruction.[78,109] Arterial and venous thromboses adjacent to areas of fat necrosis may result in intestinal infarction,[18,42] and renal failure caused by bilateral renal artery thrombosis in acute pancreatitis has been reported.[125] Erosion of splenic artery aneurysms with hemorrhage through the pancreatic duct has been reported, and most of these patients have had chronic pancreatitis.[104]

Pancreatic pseudocysts are subject to several complications of interest to the radiologist. These include common bile duct obstruction,[40] gastrointestinal hemorrhage,[98] massive hemorrhage into the cyst,[15] ascites,[69] rupture into the portal vein with generalized fat necrosis,[136] intraperitoneal rupture with clinical signs of peritonitis, rupture into the thoracic cavity,[74] spontaneous rupture into the stomach[44] and duodenum,[67] and simultaneous rupture into the stomach and colon with formation of a gastrocolic fistula.[46]

REFERENCES

1. Achord, J. L., and Gerle, R. D.: Bone lesions in pancreatitis, Amer. J. Dig. Dis. **11**:453, 1966.
2. Agnos, J. W., and Holmes, R. B.: Gas in the pancreas as a sign of abscess, Amer. J. Roentgen. **80**:60, 1958.
3. Atallah, N. K., and Melhem, R. E.: Annular pancreas in infancy, Amer. J. Roentgen. **90**:740, 1963.
4. Aterman, K.: Duodenal ulceration and fibrocystic pancreas disease, Amer. J. Dis. Child. **101**:210, 1961.
5. Baltaxe, H. A., and Leslie, E. V.: Vanishing pancreatic calcifications, Amer. J. Roentgen. **99**:642, 1967.
6. Bank, S., Marks, I. N., Farman, J., and Immelman, E. J.: Further observations on calcified medullary bone lesions in chronic pancreatitis, Gastroenterology **51**:224, 1966.
7. Barthalomew, L. G., Gross, J. B., and Comfort, M. W.: Carcinoma of pancreas associated with chronic relapsing pancreatitis, Gastroenterology **35**:473, 1958.
8. Baylin, G. J., and Weeks, K. D.: Some roentgen aspects of pancreatic necrosis, Radiology **42**:466, 1944.
9. Berenson, J. E., Spitz, H. B., and Felson, B.: The abdominal fat necrosis sign, Radiology **100**:567, 1971.
10. Bergkvist, A., and Seldinger, S. I.: Contrast roentgenography in differential diagnosis between perforated ulcer and acute pancreatitis, Acta Chir. Scand. **118**:137, 1959.
11. Blumenstock, D. A., Mithoefer, J., and Santulli, T. V.: Acute pancreatitis in children, Pediatrics **19**:1002, 1957.
12. Bradbeer, J. E.: Unusual foregut anomaly: Extragastric pouch communicating with pancreatic duct, Brit. J. Surg. **46**:603, 1958.
13. Brascho, D. J., Reynolds, T. N., and Zanca, P.: Radiographic "colon cut-off sign" in acute pancreatitis, Radiology **79**:763, 1962.
14. Brust, R., and Chen, K-C.: Acute hemorrhagic pancreatitis complicated by duodenal obstruction: report of a case, Amer. J. Roentgen. **87**:732, 1962.
15. Buckham, C. A.: Arterial hemorrhage in pseudocyst of pancreas, Arch. Surg. (Chicago) **92**:405, 1966.
16. Caffey, J.: Pediatric x-ray diagnosis, ed. 4, Chicago, 1961, Year Book Medical Publishers, Inc.
17. Carroll, S. E.: Anatomical studies of ampulla of Vater, Canad. J. Surg. **6**:149, 1963.
18. Collins, J. J., Peterson, L. M., and Wilson, R. E.: Small intestinal infarction as a complication of pancreatitis, Ann. Surg. **167**:433, 1968.
19. Cordonnier, J. K., and Izant, R. J.: Meconium ileus equivalent, Surgery **54**:667, 1963.
20. DiCenso, S., Ginsburg, S. B., and Snyder, W. H., Jr.: Pancreatic pseudocysts in childhood, Surg. Gynec. Obstet. **119**:1049, 1964.
21. Doubilet, H., Poppel, M. H., and Mulholland, J. H.: Pancreatography: techniques, principles, and observations, Radiology **64**:325, 1955.
22. Doubilet, H., Poppel, M. H., and Mulholland, J. H.: Pancreatography, Ann. N. Y. Acad. Sci. **78**:829, 1959.
23. Doubilet, H., and Worth, M. H., Jr.: Pseudocyst of annular pancreas demonstrated by operative pancreatography, Surgery **58**:824, 1965.
24. Dowdy, G. S., Jr., Waldron, G. W., and Brown, W. G.: Surgical anatomy of the pancreatobiliary ductal system, Arch. Surg. (Chicago) **84**:1, 1962.
25. Dreiling, D. A.: The lymphatics, pancreatic ascites, and pancreatic inflammatory disease, Amer. J. Gastroent. **53**:119, 1970.
26. Dreiling, D. A., Janowitz, H. D., and Perrier, C. V.:

Pancreatic inflammatory disease: a physiologic approach, New York, 1964, Hoeber Medical Division, Harper & Row, Publishers.

27. Duncan, N. A.: Pancreatitis due to Ascariasis, Brit. Med. J. 1:905, 1948.
28. Eklof, O.: Accessory pancreas in the stomach and duodenum: clinical features, diagnosis and therapy, Acta Chir. Scand. 121:19, 1961.
29. Evans, F. C.: Pancreatic abscess, Amer. J. Surg. 117:537, 1969.
30. Esterly, J. R., and Oppenheimer, E. H.: Observations in cystic fibrosis of the pancreas. I, The gallbladder, Bull. Johns Hopkins Hosp. 110:247, 1962.
31. Fallinger, J. L., Robbins, T. B. and Pickens, D. R.: Abscesses of the pancreas, Surgery 60:964, 1966.
32. Felson, B.: Gas abscess of pancreas, J.A.M.A. 163:637, 1957.
33. Fishbein, R., Murphy, G. P., and Wilder, R. J.: The pleuropulmonary manifestations of pancreatitis, Dis. Chest 41:392, 1962.
34. Fisher, M. S.: Three unusual cases of pancreatitis, Brit. J. Radiol. 34:788, 1961.
35. Galligan, J. J., and Williams, H. J.: Pancreatic pseudocysts in childhood, Amer. J. Dis. Child. 112:479, 1966.
36. Gee, W., Foster, E. D., and Doohen, D. J.: Mediastinal pancreatic pseudocyst, Ann. Surg. 169:420, 1969.
37. Gerle, R. D., Walter, L. A., Achord, J. L., and Weens, H. S.: Osseous changes in chronic pancreatitis, Radiology 85:330, 1965.
38. Gilbert, M. G., and Carbonnell, M. L.: Pancreatitis in childhood associated with Ascariasis, Pediatrics 33:589, 1964.
39. Gilroy, J. A., and Adams, A. B.: Annular pancreas, Radiology 75:568, 1960.
40. Gonzalez, L. L., Jaffe, M. S., Wiot, J. F., and Altemeier, W. A.: Pancreatic pseudocyst: a cause of obstructive jaundice, Ann. Surg. 161:569, 1965.
41. Gorder, J. L., and Stargardter, F. L.: Pancreatic pseudocysts simulating intrarenal masses, Amer. J. Roentgen. 107:65, 1969.
42. Griffiths, R. W., and Brown, P. W.: Jejunal infarction as a complication of pancreatitis, Gastroenterology 58:709, 1970.
43. Grollman, A. I., Goodman, S., and Fine, A.: Localized paralytic ileus, an early roentgen sign in acute pancreatitis, Surg. Gynec. Obstet. 91:65, 1950.
44. Guyer, P. B., and Amin, P. H.: Radiological demonstration of spontaneous rupture of pancreatic pseudocysts, Brit. J. Radiol. 43:342, 1970.
45. Hendren, W. H., Greep, J. M., and Patton, A. S.: Pancreatitis in childhood: experience with 15 cases, Arch. Dis. Child. 40:132, 1965.
46. Hess, W.: Surgery of the biliary passages and the pancreas, Princeton, 1965, D. Van Nostrand Co., Inc.
47. Heymann, R. L., and Whelan, T. J.: Annular pancreas: demonstration of the annular duct on cholangiography, Ann. Surg. 165:470, 1967.
48. Hope, J. W., and Gibbons, J. F.: Duodenal obstruction due to annular pancreas, Radiology 63:473, 1954.
49. Hurwitt, E. S. and Arnheim, E. E.: Meconium ileus associated with stenosis of the pancreatic duct, Amer. J. Dis. Child. 64:443, 1942.
50. Immelman, E. J., Bank, S., Krige, H. and Marks, I. N.: Roentgenologic and clinical features of intramedullary fat necrosis in bones in acute and chronic pancreatitis, Amer. J. Med. 36:96, 1964.
51. Jacquemet, P., Liotta, D., and Mallet-Guy, P.: The early radiological diagnosis of diseases of the pancreas and ampulla of Vater: elective exploration of the ampulla of Vater and the head of the pancreas by hypotonic duodenography, Springfield, Ill., 1965, Charles C Thomas, Publisher.
52. Joffe, N.: Pancreatic calcification in childhood associated with protein malnutrition, Brit. J. Radiol. 36:758, 1963.
53. Kaiser, G. C., King, R. D., Kilman, J. W., Lempke, R. E., and Schumaker, H. B.: Pancreatic pseudocysts: an evaluation of surgical management, Arch. Surg. (Chicago) 89:275, 1964.
54. Keddie, N., and Nardi, G. L.: Pancreatography: a safe and effective technic, Amer. J. Surg. 110:863, 1965.
55. Kelley, M. L., Jr., Squine, L. F., Boynton, L. C., Logan, V. W.: Significance of pancreatic calcification, New York J. Med. 57:721, 1957.
56. Kelly, T. R., and Troyer, M. L.: Pancreatic ducts and postoperative pancreatitis, Arch. Surg. (Chicago) 87:614, 1963.
57. Kilman, J. W., Kaiser, G. C., King, R. D., and Schumaker, H. B., Jr.: Pancreatic pseudocysts in infancy and childhood, Surgery 55:455, 1964.
58. Kornblith, B. A., and Otani, S.: Meconium ileus with congenital stenosis of the main pancreatic duct, Amer. J. Path. 5:249, 1929.
59. Kune, G. A.: Surgical anatomy of common bile duct, Arch Surg. (Chicago) 89:995, 1964.
60. Lagergren, C.: Calcium carbonate precipitation in the pancreas, gallstones, and urinary calculi, Acta Chir. Scand. 124:320, 1962.
61. Laird, C. A., and Clagett, O. T.: Mediastinal pseudocyst of the pancreas in a child: report of a case, Surgery 60:465, 1966.
62. Leger, L.: Surgical contrast visualization of the pancreatic ducts with a study of pancreatic external secretion, Amer. J. Dig. Dis. 20:8, 1953.
63. Legge, D. A., Hoffman, H. N., and Carlson, H. C.: Pancreatitis as a complication of regional enteritis of the duodenum, Gastroenterology 61:834, 1971.
64. Leistyna, J. A., Macaulay, J. C.: Traumatic pancreatitis in childhood: report of a case and a review of the literature, Amer. J. Dis. Child. 107:644, 1964.
65. Levitin, J.: Scout film of the abdomen, Radiology 47:10, 1946.
66. Lipson, J. D., and Stephenson, H. E.: Pancreatitis complicated by pericardial effusion and cardiac tamponade, Arch. Surg. 103:414, 1971.
67. Littmann, R., Pchaczevsky, R., and Richter, R. M.: Spontaneous rupture of a pancreatic pseudocyst into the duodenum, Arch. Surg. 100:76, 1970.

68. Lucas, P. F., and Owen, T. K.: Subcutaneous fat necrosis, polyarthritis and pancreatic disease, Gut **3**:146, 1962.

69. MacLaren, I. F., Howard, J. M., and Jordan, G. L.: Ascites associated with a pseudocyst of the pancreas, Arch. Surg. **93**:301, 1966.

70. Martinez, N. S., Morlock, C. G., Dockerty, M. B., Waugh, J. M., and Weber, H. M.: Heterotopic pancreatic tissue involving the stomach, Ann. Surg. **147**:1, 1958.

71. McClintock, J. T., McFee, J. L., and Quimby, R. L.: Pancreatic pseudocyst presenting as a mediastinal tumor, J.A.M.A. **192**:573, 1965.

72. McFadzean, A. J. S., and Yeung, R. T. T.: Acute pancreatitis due to clonorchis sinensis, Trans. Roy. Soc. Trop. Med. Hyg. **60**:468, 1966.

73. McGeorge, C. K., Widmann, B. P., Ostrum, H., and Miller, R. F.: Diffuse calcification of the pancreas, Amer. J. Roentgen. **78**:599, 1957.

74. Merikas, G., Stathopoulos, G., and Katsas, A.: Painless pancreatic pseudocyst ruptured into the thoracic cavity, Gastroenterology **54**:101, 1968.

75. Merner, T. B.: Acute pancreatis with peritoneal fat necrosis—roentgen diagnosis, Amer. J. Roentgen. **80**:67, 1958.

76. Mikal, S.: Operative criteria for diagnosis of cancer in a mass of the head of the pancreas, Ann. Surg. **161**:395, 1965.

77. Millbourn, E.: Calibre and appearance of the pancreatic ducts and relevant clinical problems: a roentgenologic and anatomical study, Acta Chir. Scand. **118**:286, 1960.

78. Mohiuddin, S., Sakiyalak, P., Gullick, H. D., and Webb, W. R.: Stenosing lesions of the colon secondary to pancreatitis, Arch. Surg. **102**:229, 1971.

79. Moore, M. P.: The pathologic aspects of Ascariasis, Southern Med. J. **47**:825, 1954.

80. Moresi, H. J., and Ochsner, S. F.: Megabulbus of the duodenum in the adult: report of a case associated with annular pancreas and ulceration, Amer. J. Dig. Dis. **9**:170, 1964.

81. Nance, F. C., Cocchiara, J., and Kinder, J. L.: Acute pancreatitis associated with an intraluminal duodenal diverticulum, Gastroenterology **52**:544, 1967.

82. Neuhauser, E. B. D.: Cited by Tucker, A. S., Mathews, L. W., and Doershuk, C. F.: Roentgen diagnosis of complications of cystic fibrosis, Amer. J. Roentgen. **89**:1048, 1963.

83. Newman, H. F., Weinberg, S. B., Newman, E. B., and Northrup, J. D.: The papilla of Vater and distal portions of the common bile duct and duct of Wirsung, Surg. Gynec. Obstet. **106**:687, 1958.

84. O'Flynn, M. E., and Rowley, W. F.: Development of pancreatic function and cystic fibrosis, Pediat. Clin. N. Amer. **12**:655, 1965.

85. Owens, J. L., Jr., and Howard, J. M.: Pancreatic calcification: Late sequel in natural history of chronic alcoholism and alcoholic pancreatitis, Ann. Surg. **147**:326, 1958.

86. Ozonoff, M. B., and Tappan, V.: Gallbladder structure and function in cystic fibrosis. To be published.

87. Palmer, E. D.: Benign intramural tumors of the stomach, Medicine **30**:81, 1951.

88. Parkins, R. A., Eidelman, S., Rubin, C. E., Dobbins, W. O., III, and Phelps, P. C.: The diagnosis of cystic fibrosis by rectal suction biopsy, Lancet **7313**:851, 1963.

89. Pauline-Netto, A., Dreiling, D. A., and Barnofsky, I. D.: Relationship between pancreatic calcification and cancer of pancreas, Ann. Surg. **151**:530, 1960.

90. Pham, B. T.: Acute pancreatitis due to Ascaris lumbricoides in common bile duct, West. J. Surg. **67**:270, 1959.

91. Plechas, N. P.: Chronic recurrent pancreatitis in childhood: case report, Arch. Surg. (Chicago) **81**:883, 1960.

92. Poppel, M. H.: The roentgen manifestations of relapsing pancreatitis, Radiology **62**:514, 1954.

93. Poppel, M. H.: Some migratory aspects of inflammatory collections of pancreatic origin, Radiology **72**:323, 1959.

94. Poppel, M. H., and Berow, C.: Roentgen manifestations of pancreatitis complicating mumps, Amer. J. Roentgen. **61**:219, 1949.

95. Poppel, M. H., and Jacobson, H. G.: Roentgen aspects of the papilla of Vater, Amer. J. Dig. Dis. **1**:49, 1956.

96. Price, C. W. R.: The colon cut-off sign in acute pancreatitis, Med. J. Aust. **1**:313, 1956.

97. Razi, M. D.: Ectopic pancreatic tissue of esophagus with massive upper gastrointestinal bleeding, Arch. Surg. (Chicago) **92**:101, 1966.

98. Reinhoff, W. F.: III: An evaluation of pancreatic cysts treated at the Johns Hopkins Hospital, Surgery **47**:188, 1960.

99. Reynes, C. J., and Love, L.: Mediastinal pseudocyst, Radiology **92**:115, 1969.

100. Rich, A. R., and Duff, G. L.: Experimental and pathological studies on the pathogenesis of acute hemorrhagic pancreatitis, Bull. Johns Hopkins Hosp. **58**:212, 1936.

101. Rooney, D. R.: Aberrant pancreatic tissue in the stomach, Radiology **73**:241, 1959.

102. Rösch, J., Herfort, K.: Contribution of splenoportography to the diagnosis of diseases of the pancreas. II, Inflammatory diseases, Acta Med. Scand. **171**:263, 1962.

103. Sachs, M. D., and Partington, P. F.: Cholangiographic diagnosis of pancreatitis, Amer. J. Roentgen. **76**:32, 1956.

104. Sandblom, P.: Gastrointestinal hemorrhage through the pancreatic duct, Ann. Surg. **171**:61, 1970.

105. Sarles, H., Sarles, J-C., Camatte, R., Muratore, R., Gaini, M., Guien, C., Pastor, J., and LeRoy, F.: Observations in 205 confirmed cases of acute pancreatitis, recurring pancreatitis, and chronic pancreatitis, Gut **6**:545, 1965.

106. Scarpelli, D. G.: Fat necrosis of bone marrow in acute pancreatitis, Amer. J. Path. **32**:1077, 1956.

107. Schmidt, B. J., Barreto, H. P. B., Barbante, P. J., Ramos, O. L., Concone, M. C. M., Queiroz, A. S., and Carvalho, A. A.: Pancreatic lithiasis due to malnutrition and alcoholism in a child, J. Pediat. **65**:613, 1964.

108. Schultz, E. H., Jr.: Aids to diagnosis of acute pancreatitis by roentgenologic study, Amer. J. Roentgen. **89**:825, 1963.

109. Schwartz, S., and Nadelhaft, J.: Simulation of colonic obstruction at the splenic flexure by pancreatitis: roentgen features, Amer. J. Roentgen. **78**:607, 1957.

110. Sheikh, H.: Duodenal ischaemia complicating acute pancreatitis, Brit. Med. J. **1**:1539, 1965.

111. Simon, M., and Lerner, M. A.: Duodenal compression by the mesenteric root in acute pancreatitis and inflammatory conditions of the bowel, Radiology **79**:75, 1962.

112. Sperling, M. A.: Bone lesions in pancreatitis, Ann. Med. **17**:334, 1968.

113. Stoodman, P. A., Doering, R., and Carter, R.: Surgical aspects of pancreatic abscess, Surg. Gynec. Obstet. **125**:757, 1967.

114. Stein, G. N.: X-ray investigation of the pancreas. In Bockus, H. L., editor: Gastroenterology, vol III, ed. 2, Philadelphia, 1965, W. B. Saunders Co.

115. Stein, G. N., Kalser, M. H., Sarian, N. N., and Finkelstein, A.: An evaluation of the roentgen changes in acute pancreatitis: correlation with clinical findings, Gastroenterology **36**:354, 1959.

116. Stept, L. A., Johnson, S. H., Marshall, M., and Price, S. E.: Intrarenal pancreatic disease, J. Urol. **106**:15, 1971.

117. Sterling, J. A.: The common channel for bile and pancreatic ducts, Surg. Gynec. Obstet. **98**:420, 1954.

118. Stuart, C.: Acute pancreatitis: preliminary investigation of a new radiodiagnostic sign, J. Fac. Radiol. **8**:50, 1956.

119. Sybers, H. D., Shelp, W. D., and Morrissey, J. F.: Pseudocyst of the pancreas with fistulous extension into the neck, New Eng. J. Med. **278**:1058, 1968.

120. Thal, A. P., Goott, B., and Margulis, A. R.: Sites of pancreatic duct obstruction in chronic pancreatitis, Ann. Surg. **150**:49, 1959.

121. Tucker, A. S., Mathews, L. W., and Doershuk, C. F.: Roentgen diagnosis of complications of cystic fibrosis, Amer. J. Roentgen. **89**:1048, 1963.

122. Tucker, D. H., and Moore, I. B.: Vanishing pancreatic calcification in chronic pancreatitis: a sign of pancreatic carcinoma, New Eng. J. Med. **268**:31, 1963.

123. Kaden, V. G., Howard, J. M., and Doubleday, L. C.: Cholecystographic studies during and immediately following acute pancreatitis, Surgery **38**:1082, 1955.

124. Varriale, P., Bonanno, C. A., and Grace, W. J.: Portal hypertension secondary to pancreatic pseudocysts, Arch. Intern. Med. **112**:89, 1963.

125. Vogel, R. M., and Keohane, M.: Renal vascular abnormalities in acute pancreatitis, Arch. Intern. Med. **119**:610, 1967.

126. Walko, R.: Contribution to the roentgen diagnosis of annular pancreas with reports of two cases, one with an unusually large duodenal dilatation, Fortschr. Geb. Rontgenstr. **92**:401, 1960.

127. Ward, W. W., Collier, H. S., and Griswold, R. A.: Massive gastrointestinal hemorrhage due to pancreatic lithiasis, Amer. J. Surg. **109**:476, 1965.

128. Warren, K. W., and Veidenheimer, M.: Pathologic considerations in the choice of operation for chronic relapsing pancreatitis, New Eng. J. Med. **266**:323, 1962.

129. Weber, J. M., Blumen, L. J., Wilson, W. L.: Uncommon cases of pancreatic disease, Amer. J. Gastroent. **53**:132, 1970.

130. Weens, H. S., and Walter, L. A.: The radiologic diagnosis of acute cholecystitis and pancreatitis, Radiol. Clin. N. Amer. **2**:89, 1964.

131. Weidmann, P., Rutishauser, W., Siegenthaler, W., and Senning, A.: Mediastinal pseudocyst of the pancreas, Amer. J. Med. **46**:454, 1969.

132. Whelan, T. J., Jr., and Hamilton, G. B.: Annular pancreas, Ann. Surg. **146**:252, 1957.

133. White, H., and Rowley, W. F.: Cystic fibrosis of the pancreas: Clinical and roentgenographic manifestations, Radiol. Clin. N. Amer. **1**:539, 1963.

134. Wilson, C. S.: In situ pancreatography in postmortem material, thesis. Yale School of Medicine, New Haven, 1963.

135. Wise, R. E.: Intravenous cholangiography, Springfield, Ill., 1962, Charles C Thomas, Publisher.

136. Zeller, M., and Hetz, H. H.: Rupture of a pancreatic cyst into the portal vein. Report of a case of subcutaneous nodular and generalized fat necrosis, J.A.M.A. **195**:869, 1966.

44 | Neoplasms of the pancreas

Alexander R. Margulis

CARCINOMA

Carcinoma is by far the most common neoplasm of the pancreas. It is a relatively common tumor; of all carcinomas, 0.85% are estimated to be in the pancreas.[42,87] According to a statistical report published in 1971, pancreatic cancer is the second most common malignant disease of the gastrointestinal tract.[80] In the United States it trails by a far margin the incidence of carcinoma of the large bowel, but it exceeds that of the esophagus, liver and biliary tract, and stomach. In a study of 13,500 necropsies, carcinoma in the pancreas was found in 0.51%.[10,39] Pancreatic carcinoma is a disease of middle and older age, with approximately 60% of the victims being between the ages of 50 and 69 years. It is not uncommon, however, in patients even in their twenties.[17,39] The disease predominates in males, with a ratio reported as from 2:1 to as high as 7 : 1.[20,42,83]

The prognosis of carcinoma of the pancreas is extremely grave. The first 5-year survival after surgical treatment of a carcinoma of the head of the pancreas was reported in 1951.[54] Cattell, Warren, and Au reported a 9% 5-year survival of patients who had undergone radical operation for carcinoma of the head of the pancreas.[18] Although this 9% statistic is often quoted, it actually represents only four patients of a group of forty-five. This group of forty-five was part of a total of eighty-one patients. Only sixteen patients surviving 5 years after surgical treatment were reported in 1959.[86] As late as 1963, a single case report of a 5-year survival for carcinoma of the head of the pancreas appeared.[91]

Carcinoma of the body and tail of the pancreas comprises approximately 25% of all carcinomas of the pancreas.[84] The prognosis for this condition is even worse than that for carcinoma of the head of the pancreas. To my knowledge, no series of 5-year survivals has been reported for carcinoma of the body and tail of the pancreas.

The reason for this poor prognosis is that the tumor is located in an organ that lies retroperitoneally. It is distant from the digestive tube and organs that can be visualized roentgenologically. The tumor grows insidiously, causing rather vague minimal symptoms. Because these tumors are often missed on roentgenologic examination, a study was done in the University of California San Francisco with inflatable balloons on models resembling pancreas. These balloons were also inserted into necropsy specimens of the pancreas in which the duodenum was intact. The results showed that in order to produce changes in the duodenal loop the "tumor" had to assume large dimensions. As was expected, the farther the "tumor" grew from the duodenal loop, the larger it had to be before it caused changes (Fig. 44-1).[73]

In addition to being located in a relatively silent organ, the pancreatic tumor metastasizes extensively before producing symptoms, because the pancreas has no limiting capsule. An abundance of large arteriovenous and lymphatic vessels is located in the area of the pancreas. Only the thin parietal peritoneum protects the peritoneal cavity from widespread local dissemination.

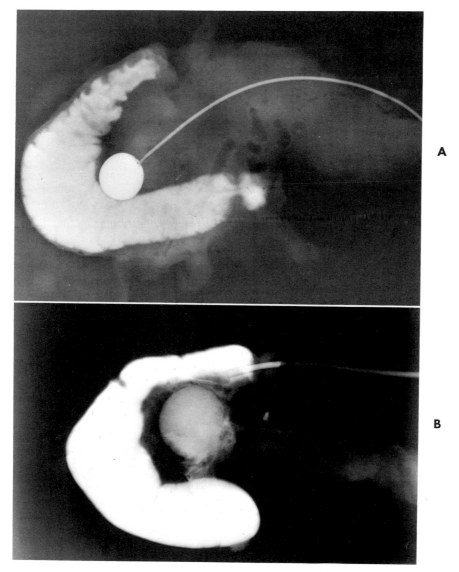

Fig. 44-1. A, Balloon placed in pancreas of a fresh specimen that includes the duodenum and pancreas. The balloon is placed close to the duodenum, and distention with 5 ml. of 10% diatrizoate sodium produces a definite impression. **B,** A balloon filled with water is introduced into the pancreas of another fresh, human specimen of pancreas and duodenum. The balloon is placed in the center of the pancreas, and distention with 30 ml. of water produces no deformity. (From Russell, W. M., and Margulis, A. R.: Amer. J. Roentgen. 94:449, 1965.)

The common symptoms of carcinoma of the pancreas are related to its location. The prognosis of carcinoma of the head of the pancreas is somewhat less grave than that of carcinoma of the body and tail. Because carcinomas of the head of the pancreas are nearer the common bile duct, jaundice or mucosal invasion of the gastrointestinal tract result earlier.

Roentgenography in diagnosis

Except for those seen by vascular techniques, few signs have been added to the original diagnostic roentgenographic signs described by Rigler[68] and Frostberg[34] in spite of continued interest in the subject.* A large number of pub-

*See references 5, 8, 9, 17, 22, 23, 31, 43, 47, 63, 66, 67, 88, 93, and 94.

lished studies intimate that an early diagnosis of this condition is possible by roentgenologic methods.[9,63,75] They give the impression that carcinoma of the pancreatic head can be discovered early enough to improve both the individual patient and the salvage rate. According to these reports it is the close attention that the radiologist gives to refined, minute signs that results in this diagnosis. In reality fine and unobtrusive roentgenologic signs may be diagnosed very early, but these actually represent a late stage of the disease. Frequently the radiologist sees minute signs on the roentgenographs and on fluoroscopy, only to have the surgeon encounter inoperable widespread cancer.

Perez and co-workers reported a study of twenty-nine patients with carcinoma of the pancreaticoduodenal region.[63] In retrospect, Perez concluded that in about 70% of these cases detailed barium studies of the duodenal loop would have provided the diagnosis. All but three lesions in this group measured less than 4 cm. in greatest diameter. In addition the group included carcinomas of the papilla of Vater and of the distal common duct. Despite these facts, twenty-one of the twenty-nine patients were dead within 2 years after operation. Only one patient was alive 2 years after operation, without clinical evidence of local recurrence or metastasis. At surgery, carcinoma of the head of the pancreas had been found in twelve of these patients. All of the lesions in this series could be resected with a one-stage Whipple procedure. Preoperative gastrointestinal roentgenograms and a complete histologic examination of the resected specimen had been included in all.

Early roentgenologic signs of a pancreatic malignant neoplasm are signs of a mass. They vary somewhat, depending on whether the neoplasm is in the head, body, or tail.

Carcinoma of the head of the pancreas

Masses in the head of the pancreas are rarely seen on plain roentgenograms of the abdomen, although a soft tissue mass may be sufficiently large to cause impressions on the air-filled lumen of the gut. Lymphoma, cysts, or pseudocysts will frequently present this appearance in the region of the pancreas as will also widespread carcinoma (Fig. 44-2). When a large gallbladder is present with jaundice, an obstructive process

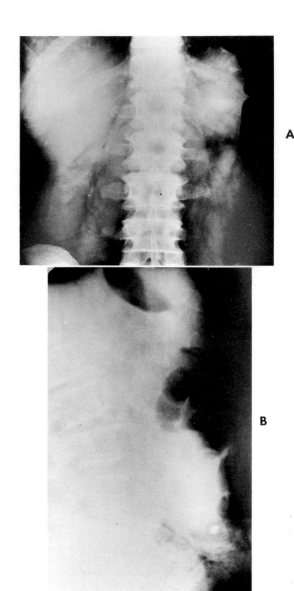

Fig. 44-2. A, Frontal projection of an abdomen, with a large soft tissue mass, of a patient with cystadenoma of the pancreas. The large rounded mass is seen impressing the air-filled duodenum and is seen to be located above the kidneys. B, Lateral projection shows the large soft tissue mass impressing the stomach and duodenum.

should be suspected in either the ampulla or the common duct.

Gastrointestinal studies with barium sulfate are the present conventional method of roentgenologic investigation of the pancreatic area. The ability to detect a mass and its impingement on the barium-filled gut depends on the size of the mass as well as on its proximity to the gut.[73]

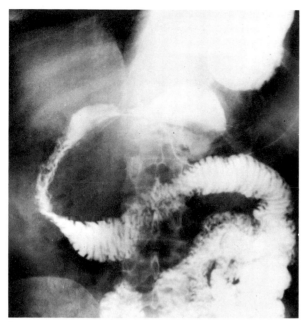

Fig. 44-3. Supine view, taken during a gastrointestinal series, of a patient with carcinoma of the head of the pancreas. The large mass is impressing and partially invading the second portion of the duodenum. The stomach is also impressed. The duodenal loop is considerably larger than normally seen. Such enlarged loops are not commonly seen in carcinoma of the head of the pancreas.

Roentgenologic signs common in larger masses in the head of the pancreas are: (1) enlargement of the duodenal loop, (2) forward displacement of the antrum of the stomach and the second retroperitoneal segment of the duodenum, (3) impression of a mass in the second part of the duodenum, (4) invasion of the duodenum at the area of the pancreatic head, (5) compression of the duodenum by the obstructed and distended common duct, (6) impression by an enlarged gallbladder, and (7) invasion of the stomach. Each of these is discussed in the following paragraphs.

Enlargement of the duodenal loop is a sign reliable only in the presence of large masses, which, as discussed previously, only occasionally represent carcinoma. In the presence of carcinoma these masses usually indicate a huge neoplasm that is widespread (Fig. 44-3). Measurements to establish a normal range of size of the duodenal loop are most difficult, especially in obese subjects with horizontal stomachs. Perez

and colleagues pointed out that appreciable widening of the duodenal sweep may often be the result of pancreatitis surrounding the lesion.[63] The size of the mass that is seen, they stated, does not necessarily reflect the actual size of the tumor. Extremely large duodenal loops, however, indicate a process other than a carcinoma of the head of the pancreas unless the patient is jaundiced and cachectic.

Forward displacement of the second retroperitoneal portion of the duodenum in the lateral view, and of the antrum of the stomach, likewise indicates a large mass in the region of the head of the pancreas (Fig. 44-4). The sign is reliable only if the mass causes a definite convex impression on the duodenum or stomach or both. Recently, interest has revived in measuring the retrogastric space from roentgenographs for the diagnosis of retrogastric tumors.[41,78] Measurements alone, without the impression, are not reliable even when corrected for height and weight of the patient. Lateral and anteroposterior roentgenograms of 200 normal subjects and of 72 patients with proved retrogastric and retroduodenal masses were subjected to nine measurements.[41] The measurements were correlated with the height and weight of the patients. A considerable overlap was shown between values obtained from normal persons and those from patients with proved masses. Impression, as recognized by an experienced radiologist familiar with the appearance of normal organs in various projections, was the most important single factor in determining presence of mass. This appearance was more important than any measurements. Fig. 44-5 shows the distribution of 135 normal persons and thirty-five patients. The minimum distance of stomach to spine was plotted against a ratio of height to weight. The overlap was great except when measurements were such as to indicate that no question existed about the presence of a mass as determined by other criteria.

A new method for accurate measurement of the midline retrogastric and retroduodenal spaces was described by Poole.[65] The patient swallows a half ounce of barium, which is manipulated so that it enters the bulb and the second portion of the duodenum. The antrum is then compressed backward in anteroposterior position with a padded device that contains a coin in the center of the compressing surface.

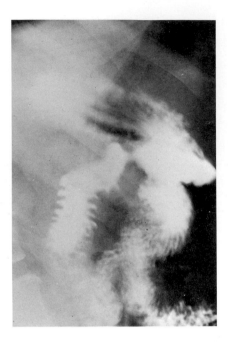

Fig. 44-4. Carcinoma of the head of the pancreas in an asymptomatic male patient. The lesion was unresectable. This right lateral view taken during a gastrointestinal examination shows the stomach, the second portion of the duodenum, and the duodenojejunal juncture to be displaced forward. The second portion of the duodenum is impressed from behind.

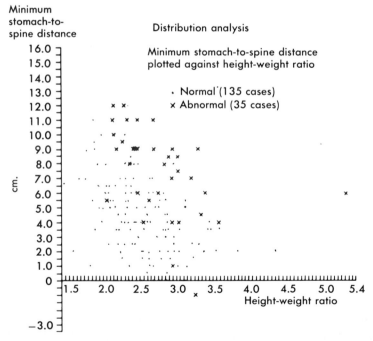

Fig. 44-5. A distribution analysis of 170 cases from a computer study of roentgenographic measurements of retroperitoneal masses. There is a tendency toward separate groupings of normal and abnormal when stomach-to-spine measurements were plotted against the height-weight ratios. The figure is a facsimile of the original IBM plot. (From Herbert. W. W., and Margulis, A. R.: Radiology **84**:52, 1965.)

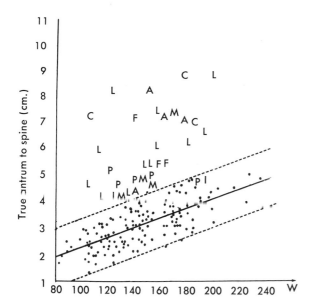

Fig. 44-6. Plot of body weight of 141 normal patients vs. corrected antrum-to-spine distance. Regression line is represented by central double line and the 95% confidence limits by the dotted lines. (From Poole, G. J.: A new roentgenographic method of measuring the retrogastric and retroduodenal spaces: statistical evaluation of reliability and diagnostic utility, Radiology **97**:71, 1970.)

Pressure is applied until the posterior antral surface presses against the retroperitoneal structures. Roentgenograms are obtained in the lateral projection and the coin diameter allows correction for magnification. The measurement of the antrum to anterior surface of the lumbar spine must be correlated with the weight of the patient. Measurements from the posterior surface of the horizontal duodenum to the anterior surface of the lumbar spine were obtained similarly, without applying pressure.

The results on twenty volunteers, 141 normal patients, and thirty-three patients with proved retrogastric masses showed the great value and reproducibility of this method (Fig. 44-6).

Impression of a mass on the second portion of the duodenum, if definite, is a most valuable sign (Fig. 44-3). Occasionally, however, a great deal of experience is required before a mass without invasion or ulceration can be diagnosed definitively (Fig. 44-7). The "inverted 3" sign[34] is a manifestation of this type of impression, but it may also accompany pancreatitis or other masses in this region.

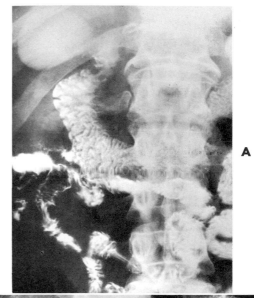

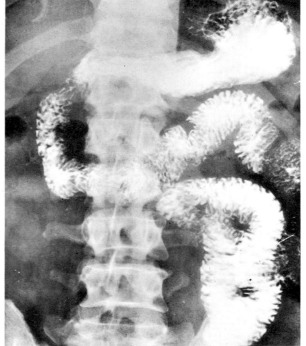

Fig. 44-7. Impression on the second portion of the duodenum by masses in the region of the head of the pancreas. **A,** Definite impression on the second portion of the duodenum is produced by carcinoma of the head of the pancreas. There is stiffening and drawing out of the folds of the duodenum along its medial aspect. The gallbladder is still functioning. **B,** Impression on the second portion of the duodenum by carcinoma of the head of the pancreas, producing a positive Frostberg sign.

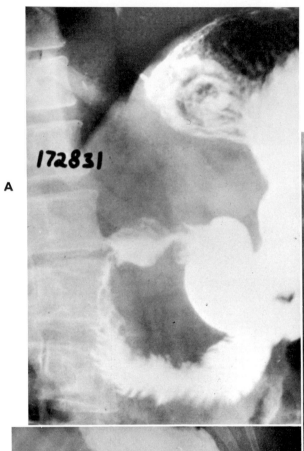

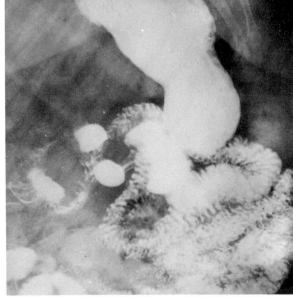

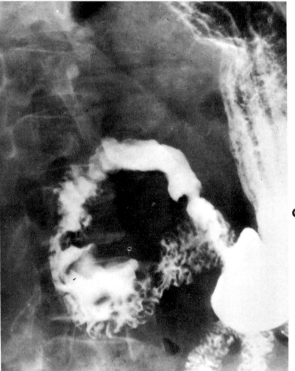

Fig. 44-8. A, Carcinoma of the head of the pancreas invading and destroying the mucosa of the second portion of the duodenum. The stomach is also invaded in the region of the pylorus. **B,** Invasion of the pancreas and duodenum by metastasis from a carcinoma of the kidney. Grossly and roentgenologically the appearance is indistinguishable from a primary carcinoma of the pancreas. The accurate diagnosis could be made only by histologic means. **C,** Large mass involving duodenum and pancreas with irregular, large ulceration in the mass and connecting with the duodenum. The histologic diagnosis of primary carcinoma of the duodenum might be challenged.

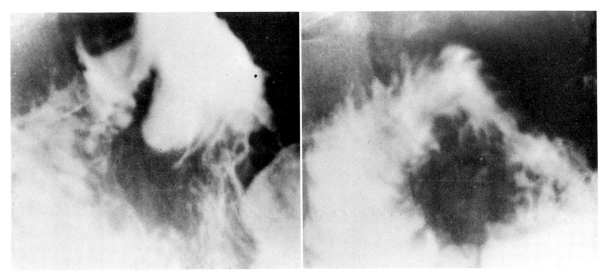

Fig. 44-9. Unresectable carcinoma of the head of the pancreas in a severely jaundiced patient. The characteristic impression on the immediate postbulbar portion of the duodenum by a distended common duct is seen. There is an impression on the duodenum along the medial aspect of the second portion, with stiffening of the folds and formation of a pseudodiverticulum.

Invasion of the duodenum in the area of the pancreatic head is the most reliable sign of a malignant tumor in this region. Frequently, histologic interpretation of these large ulcerating masses may be difficult. The pathologist may have difficulty in deciding whether these lesions represent carcinoma of the head of the pancreas, of the biliary ducts, or of the duodenum itself (Fig. 44-8). Ulceration and irregularity of the mucosa can be overemphasized as diagnostic signs, as in two of the cases reviewed by Perez and his colleagues.[63] Both were carcinomas, one of the pancreas, the other of the ampulla of Vater. Destruction of the mucosa, interpreted roentgenologically, was not confirmed by pathologic examination, which showed only infiltration of the submucosa.

Compression of the duodenum by the obstructed, distended, common duct is an indirect sign suggesting the diagnosis of carcinoma of the head of the pancreas only when it is associated with other roentgenologic and clinical signs (Figs. 44-9 and 44-10). The usefulness of this sign alone is limited because of the variations in length and course of the postbulbar, mesenteric portion of the duodenum.

Impression by an enlarged gallbladder also is only a contributing sign and not a definite primary one. It strengthens the validity of other signs of a mass in the head of the pancreas.

Dilatation of the gallbladder that produces a smooth rounded indentation on the outer aspect of the upper descending duodenum is a reliable roentgenographic finding. Eyler and associates found no false-positive reactions in 100 patients with pancreatic carcinoma.[31] In twenty-seven of thirty-eight enlarged gallbladders found at laparotomy or necropsy, this sign was demonstrated.[90] Eaton and co-workers found only one patient in their series of 300 consecutive patients without demonstrable duodenal, biliary, or pancreatic disease in whom this sign was produced by impression of the colon.[25]

Invasion of the stomach by carcinoma of the head of the pancreas (Fig. 44-11) is not nearly as common as by carcinoma of the body and tail. It does occur, however, and frequently the differential diagnosis may lie between carcinoma of the stomach and carcinoma of the pancreas. If the carcinoma is far advanced and widespread and invasion of the stomach is extensive, determination of the origin of the primary tumor may be difficult for the histologist. If the neoplasm is present only on the posterior wall of the stomach (Fig. 44-12) and is associated with other signs of a mass in the pancreatic head, it

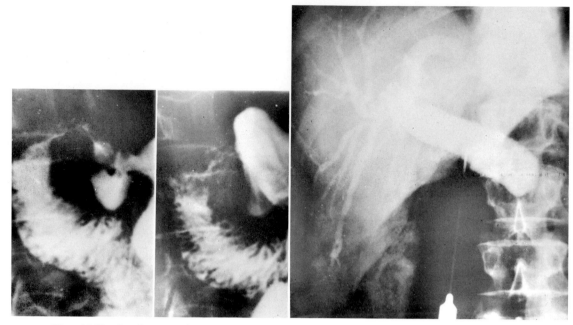

Fig. 44-10. Carcinoma of the head of the pancreas, producing an impression on the second portion of the duodenum with fixation of folds, irregularity of contour, and impression by the dilated common duct on the immediate postbulbar portion. A direct injection of the common duct shows the massive dilatation of this structure.

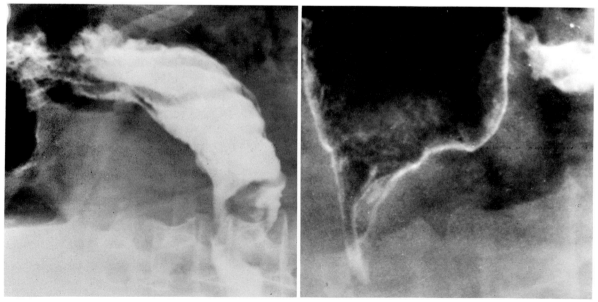

Fig. 44-11. Massive invasion of the antrum of the stomach by carcinoma of the head of the pancreas in two patients.

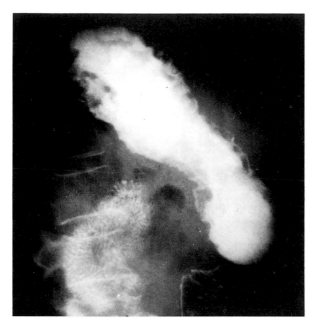

Fig. 44-12. Invasion of the posterior wall of the stomach by carcinoma of the head of the pancreas. It is invasion from the posterior wall by a mass located in the region of the pancreas that makes the distinction from carcinoma of the stomach possible. Large masses involving all the organs in this area present difficulties in making the diagnosis of the primary site of origin.

strongly suggests the roentgenologic diagnosis of carcinoma of the pancreas.

Attention has recently been directed to some early roentgenologic signs.[9,75] In general these signs, especially when several are present, raise the suspicion of a mass in the region of the head of the pancreas. Some of these signs are:

1. Irregular contractions and frequent spasticity of segments of the second or third duodenum
2. Distortion of the mucosal folds in the duodenum, with frequent spikelike fixation (Figs. 44-7, *A*, and 44-10)
3. Fixation of duodenal folds, producing elongation and pseudodiverticula resembling fistulas (This fixation may also be caused by necrosis and resultant ulceration.)
4. Gross irregularity and evidence of invasion of a duodenal diverticulum by a mass[25] (Fixation, rotation, and displacement alone are not reliable signs.)
5. Fixation of the medial wall of the second part of the duodenum so that the concavity appears equal in supine, prone, and oblique projections

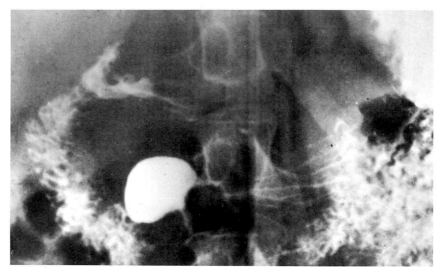

Fig. 44-13. Invasion of a diverticulum of the third portion of the duodenum by carcinoma of the head of the pancreas. If seen in several views, this invasion is a localizing roentgenographic sign of a malignant process in the head of the pancreas. Notice the impression and fixation of folds in the second portion of the duodenum.

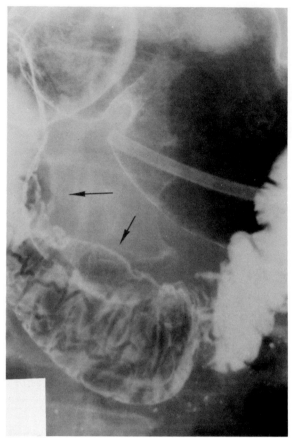

Fig. 44-14. A hypotonic duodenogram in a patient with carcinoma of the pancreas. The large irregular impression on the second portion of the duodenum by the mass (arrows) is shown to excellent advantage.

6. Indentations on the medial border of segments of the second or third portions of the duodenum, produced by nodularities of the pancreas (These indentations may appear as intraluminal masses.)

Hypotonic duodenography

The findings of carcinoma of the pancreaticoduodenal area demonstrated by hypotonic duodenography are essentially the same as with the conventional barium gastrointestinal examination.[24] Signs of invasion of the duodenum by the tumor resulting in spiculation, nodularity, obstruction, and ulceration are more specific and reliable than the signs produced by impression of a mass. As Eaton and co-workers stressed, the value of hypotonic duodenography resides in the technically superior nature of the

examination, and the consistent and accurate demonstration of the pathologic anatomy (Figs. 44-14 and 44-15).

The accuracy of hypotonic duodenography in the diagnosis of pancreaticoduodenal malignancy is significantly better than with conventional barium studies because of the technical excellence of the roentgenograms obtained with the roentgenopharmacologic approach.[13,26] The accuracy of hypotonic duodenography in the diagnosis of these tumors is in the range of 80%, whereas with conventional barium studies it was 57%.

Carcinoma of the body and tail of the pancreas

Carcinomas of the body and tail constitute approximately 25% of the carcinomas of the pancreas. The roentgenologic diagnosis, like the clinical diagnosis, is usually made late and does not affect the outcome. Nevertheless, establishment of a clinical diagnosis is important, because it facilitates the care of the patient during the terminal period of his illness. The roentgenograms of forty-six patients with carcinoma of the body and tail of the pancreas were studied by Mani and his co-workers.[51] These showed that the changes caused by the disease are reflected mainly by deformities in the gastrointestinal tract.

The esophagus may be affected by neoplasm of the body and tail of the pancreas and may be invaded.[82,84] Mani and colleagues noted involvement of the stomach in 41% of their patients. Invasion with fixation of the wall was as common as destruction of the mucosa (Fig. 44-16) either without (Fig. 44-17) or with ulceration. Impression defects (Fig. 44-18) with or without splaying of mucosal folds (Fig. 44-19) also were common but were more difficult to appreciate. These findings, although retrospective in most of the patients, were established and evaluated against 200 consecutive upper gastrointestinal examinations as controls (Tables 44-1 and 44-2).

Carcinomas of the body and tail of the pancreas frequently involved the duodenum, especially the third and fourth portions. Mani and his coauthors observed displacement of the duodenum (Figs. 44-20 and 44-21) in more than one direction in 43% of the patients and invasion in 61%.[51] Partial or complete obstruction

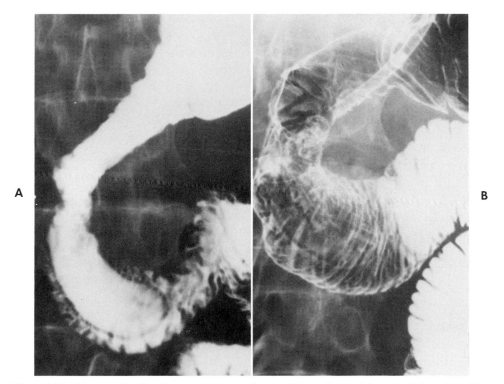

Fig. 44-15. Hypotonic duodenogram in a 57-year-old patient with a painless jaundice. **A,** Spot film from a barium study shows an intraluminal diverticulum of the duodenum to excellent advantage, and a small mass on the medial aspect of the proximal second portion of the duodenum represents a small carcinoma of the head of the pancreas. **B,** Double-contrast spot film of hypotonic duodenogram shows the small carcinoma of the head of the pancreas to excellent advantage. (Courtesy Dr. Charles Rennell.)

of the duodenum, most commonly in the third portion, was often associated with destruction of the mucosa (Fig. 44-22). Ulceration was less common than either obstruction of the lumen or fixation of the wall. Changes produced by an extrinsic mass on the duodenum were found in 60% of the patients.

Frequently, the duodenojejunal juncture and the proximal portion of the jejunum are displaced or invaded by carcinomas of the body and tail of the pancreas. Any fixed irregularity in this area, especially when associated with extrinsic impression, should be carefully evaluated. Malignant lymphoma, metastatic neoplasms, or abscesses can sometimes produce roentgenographic appearances that are indistinguishable from primary carcinoma (Fig. 44-23).

Examinations of the upper gastrointestinal tract with barium sulfate are most helpful in establishing the diagnosis of carcinomas of the body and tail of the pancreas. Occasionally, however, roentgenologic examination also shows significant involvement of the colon.[93] In one study of twenty-four patients who had roentgenologic colon examinations there were changes in the transverse colon or splenic flexure resulting from the neoplasm.[51] Five of the tumors that produced changes in the colon were in the tail and four in the body of the pancreas. In two instances extensive obstruction and invasion simulated a primary colonic carcinoma (Fig. 44-24). Splaying of the mucosal folds of the colon was also seen, as were impressions caused by an extrinsic mass. Occasionally, carcinoma of the body and tail of the pancreas will appear on plain roentgenograms of the abdomen as a soft tissue mass. This appearance usually means that the tumor has spread widely. The mass seen on the

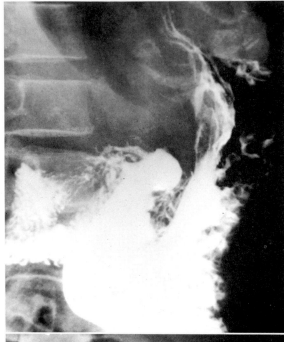

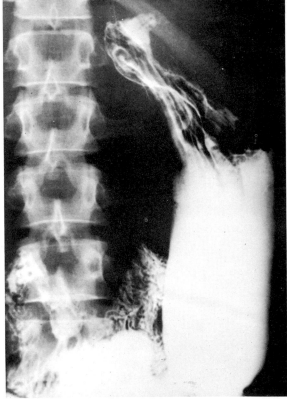

Fig. 44-16. Invasion of the stomach by two carcinomas of the body and tail of the pancreas. No massive ulceration is seen. (From Mani, J. R., Zboralske, F. F., and Margulis, A. R.: Amer. J. Roentgen. **96:**429, 1966.)

roentgenograms is an additive picture of extension of the primary tumor. Frequently the extension involves the head of the pancreas.

The spleen may be enlarged because of partial obstruction of the splenic vein.[52] In 10% of the normal population the left kidney is lower than the right.[77] Mani and associates found the left kidney to be lower in 50% of their patients.[51] In five of twelve of their patients in whom cholecystography was performed the gallbladder could be visualized.

Gastrointestinal cineradiography

Cineradiographic barium examination of the gastroduodenal region is a promising additional technique in the search for elusive pancreatic tumors. Adler and Meyers published results of a prospective study in 61 patients with apparent obstructive jaundice, and concluded that the same findings as in the conventional barium examination were most helpful in their diagnosis.[2] Alterations in motility, such as delayed passage of barium into the duodenum, disordered motility, and retrograde peristalsis were nonspecific findings. The authors' prospective accuracy was 82% for periduodenal malignancy. Their diagnosis was often based on the transient demonstration of a static abnormal finding rather than of abnormal motility.

Arteriography in diagnosis

Ödman first demonstrated the feasibility of selective catheterization of the celiac axis and the superior mesenteric arteries.[58] Since then arteriography of the vessels that supply the pancreas has become possible. Paul and his colleagues have shown the value of the procedure,[62] and this has been further demonstrated by Lunderquist[49] and Rösch,[69] Boijsen,[14] Olsson,[59] Glenn and co-workers,[35] and many others have emphasized ultraselective pancreatic angiography through injection of the gastroduodenal or dorsal artery of the pancreas. The value and accuracy of angiography in the diagnosis of pancreatic carcinoma has been the subject of numerous articles.[16,26,33,56,89] Bookstein and his co-workers expressed the belief that pancreatic angiography, particularly when superselective injections are practiced, is a highly reliable method in the diagnosis of malignant pancreatic neoplasm.[16]

The diagnosis of a carcinoma anywhere in the

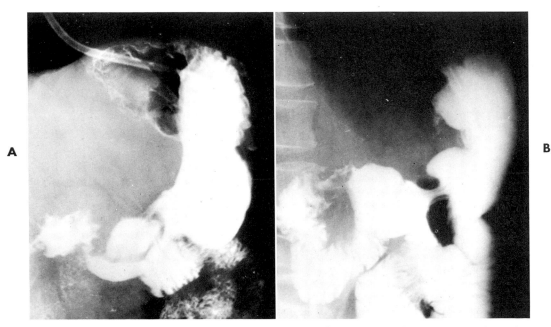

Fig. 44-17. Carcinoma of the body and tail of the pancreas invading the stomach and producing large ulcers in two patients. **A,** There is a large ulcer in the antrum of the stomach. **B,** There is large posterior gastric wall ulceration in the upper portion of the stomach, which is perforating into the lesser sac. (From Mani, J. R., Zboralske, F. F., and Margulis, A. R.: Amer. J. Roentgen. **96:**429, 1966.)

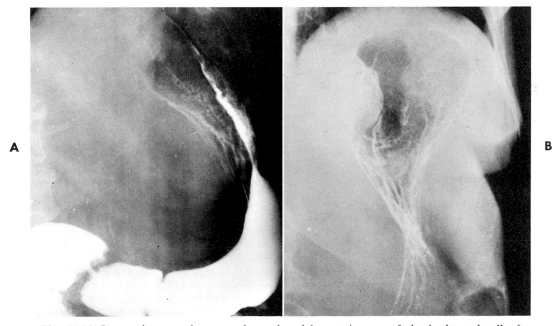

Fig. 44-18. Impressions on the stomach produced by carcinomas of the body and tail of the pancreas. **A,** A huge mass caused by far-advanced carcinoma. **B,** An impression on the fundus of the stomach produced by a lobulated, irregular mass, somewhat resembling a carcinoma of the stomach. (From Mani, J. R., Zboralske, F. F., and Margulis, A. R.: Amer. J. Roentgen. **96:**429, 1966.)

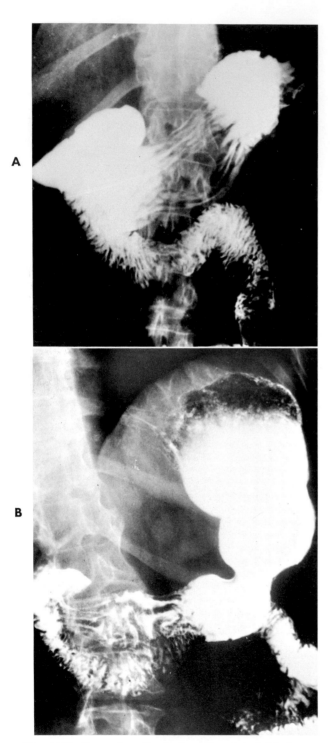

Fig. 44-19. Examples of splaying of gastric folds by posterior impression from carcinomas of the body of the pancreas. (From Mani, J. R., Zboralske, F. F., and Margulis, A. R.: Amer. J. Roentgen. **96**:429, 1966.)

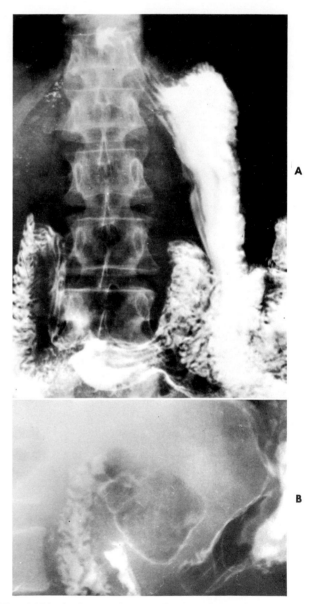

Fig. 44-20. A, Impression on the fourth portion of the duodenum by a carcinoma of the body of the pancreas. The impression is from the medial aspect. **B,** Medial impression and displacement of the fourth portion of the duodenum from the lateral aspect by carcinoma of the body of the pancreas. (From Mani, J. R., Zboralske, F. F., and Margulis, A. R.: Amer. J. Roentgen. **96**:429, 1966.)

Table 44-1. Gastric roentgenographic findings in 46 cases of carcinoma of the body and tail of the pancreas*

Findings	Number of times occurred	Description	
Displacement	31† (67%)	Right	2
		Left	7
		Superior	5
		Inferior	2
		Anterior	25
Invasion	19‡ (41%)	Fixation of wall with intact mucosa and/or edema	11
		Destruction of mucosa and/or ulceration	12
		Obstruction, partial or complete	0
Extrinsic mass	31§ (67%)	Impression defect	30
		Splaying of mucosal folds	6

*Reprinted from Mani, J. R., Zboralske, F. F., and Margulis, A. R.: Amer. J. Roentgen. **96**:429, 1966.
†In several instances displacement occurred in more than one direction.
‡Three cases revealed fixation and destruction of mucosa.
§All six patients with splayed mucosal folds also had impression defects.

Table 44-2. Duodenal roentgenographic findings in 46 cases of carcinoma of the body and tail of the pancreas*

Findings	Number of times occurred	Description	
Displacement	20† (43%)	Right	5
		Left	2
		Superior	2
		Inferior	10
		Anterior	6
Invasion	28‡ (61%)	Fixation of wall with intact mucosa and/or edema	16
		Destruction of mucosa and/or ulceration	6
		Obstruction, partial or complete	19
Extrinsic mass	23§ (50%)	Impression defect	19
		Splaying of mucosal folds	12

*Reprinted from Mani, J. R., Zboralske, F. F., and Margulis, A. R.: Amer. J. Roentgen. **96**:429, 1966.
†In several instances displacement occurred in more than one direction.
‡Several patients had two or more types of invasion.
§In eight patients combined impression and splaying occurred.

pancreas is established by the following criteria:

1. Demonstration of displacement of arteries surrounding and supplying the pancreas (Fig. 44-25). Displacement, however, is difficult to establish and may be more easily evaluated in conjunction with other signs pointing to the same conclusion. Normally the course of the vessels varies.

2. Demonstration of irregular arterial stenosis (Fig. 44-26). This finding is of much more value than demonstration of displacement of arteries and is more specific, although instances of narrowing from inflammatory disease have been observed.[48,57] Nebesar and Pollard,[50] as well as Bookstein and co-workers,[16] stressed the need for differentiation between smooth and irregular arterial narrowing. An irregularly serrated stenosis of a major artery in the pancreatic region is an almost certain sign of encasement by malignancy. Smooth narrowing has little diagnostic

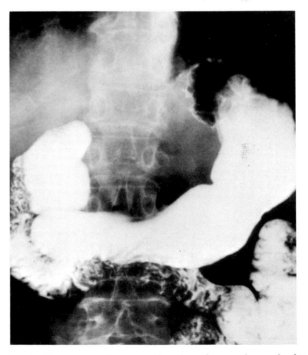

Fig. 44-21. Impression on the fourth portion of the duodenum from below and impression also on the jejunum close to the duodenojejunal juncture by carcinoma of the body and tail of the pancreas, which causes splaying as well as invasion without obstruction. (From Mani, J. R., Zboralske, F. F., and Margulis, A. R.: Amer. J. Roentgen. **96**:429, 1966.)

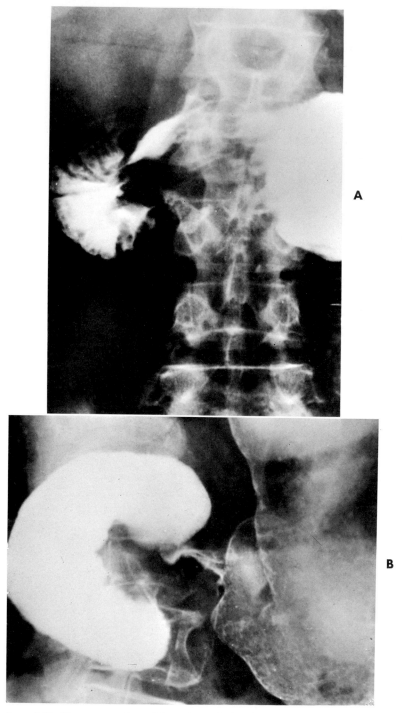

Fig. 44-22. A and **B,** Two examples of invasion of the duodenum by carcinoma of the body and tail of the pancreas with pronounced obstruction of the second and third portions of the duodenum. In **B** it is also seen that the mass invades the antrum of the stomach. (From Mani, J. R., Zboralske, F. F., and Margulis, A. R.: Amer. J. Roentgen. **96:**429, 1966.)

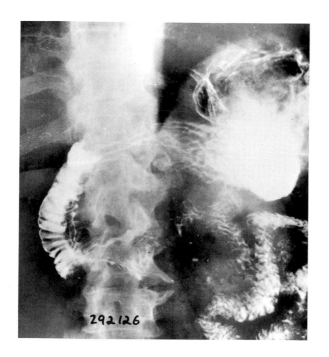

Fig. 44-23. Nonneoplastic abscess in the pancreas connecting with the duodenum by a sinus filled with barium. The mass and the duodenal changes are not distinguishable from a primary carcinoma of the pancreas.

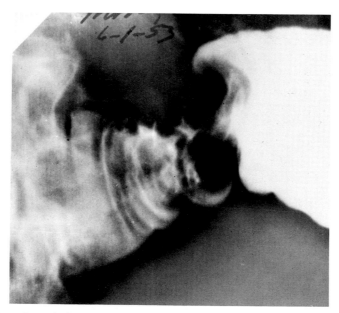

Fig. 44-24. Invasion of the distal transverse colon by carcinoma of the body and tail of the pancreas, simulating a primary carcinoma of the colon. Invasion of the colon is not rare in this condition. (From Mani, J. R., Zboralske, F. F., and Margulis, A. R.: Amer. J. Roentgen. **96:**429, 1966.)

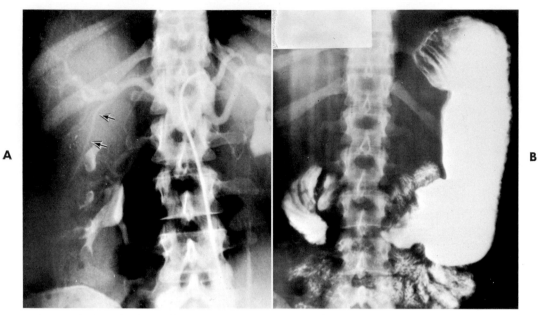

Fig. 44-25. **A,** Selective celiac arteriogram. There is displacement of the gastroduodenal artery by a large mass in the region of the pancreas (arrows). **B,** The findings produced by this carcinoma of the pancreas in the gastrointestinal series with barium were far more dramatic.

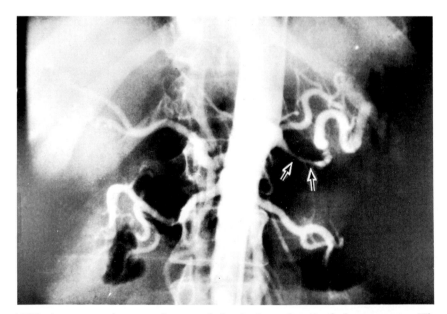

Fig. 44-26. Aortogram in a carcinoma of the body and tail of the pancreas. There is narrowing and irregularity of the splenic artery (arrows). There is dilatation distal to the stenosing lesion.

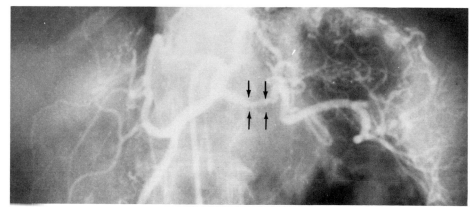

Fig. 44-27. Celiac arteriogram in a patient with carcinoma of the body of the pancreas. The upper gastrointestinal study, of excellent quality, was not diagnostic. The celiac arteriogram shows irregular encasement of the splenic artery (arrows).

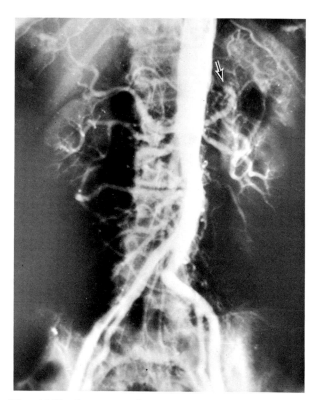

Fig. 44-28. Aortogram in a patient with carcinoma of the body of the pancreas. There is complete occlusion of the distal splenic artery (arrow), with contrast material reaching the spleen by means of multiple, tortuous, collateral vessels.

significance since it may be a sign of atherosclerosis or fibromuscular hyperplasia (Figs. 44-26 and 44-27).

3. Demonstration of complete occlusion of one of the major vessels (Fig. 44-28). Such an occlusion is also seen in inflammatory disease and may also be present after laparotomy and surgical occlusion of the vessels.

4. Demonstration of diseased vessels. Sometimes the vessels that are seen are difficult to identify as tumor vessels. They may, at times, represent anastomoses (Fig. 44-28). In inflammatory disease an increased amount of vascularity is frequently observed. Tumor stain is usually not seen in carcinoma of the pancreas, predominantly a tumor of scirrhous type. Frequently, however, such a stain is seen in tumors of the islets of Langerhans such as insulinoma and nonbeta cell adenoma of the pancreas.[48-50]

5. Demonstration of venous occlusion or irregular compression, or both, during the venous phase of the selective arteriogram. The venous phase often contributes importantly toward the diagnosis of a pancreatic neoplasm.

After the initial enthusiasm for arteriography in the diagnosis of pancreatic neoplasms,[53,69] a period of predictable disenchantment and skepticism followed.[33,56,62,89] A relatively high incidence of false-positive results was noted, particularly when pancreatitis was present, and many authors also reported that they obtained false-negative studies. The incidence of false-negative results was particularly high in the study by Nebesar and Pollard[56]; in seventeen instances of pancreatic carcinoma, the false-negative incidence was 71%. Bookstein and co-authors stressed the value of superselective studies to obtain an accurate diagnosis.[16] They described three patients in whom the diagnostic findings were demonstrated only after the superselective injections. Eaton and associates calculated the prospective accuracy of angiographic diagnosis of cancer of the pancreas from three articles that they reviewed, which included seventy-two patients with that neoplasm.[24] The over-all incidence of true positive results was 62%, of false-positive 25%, and of false-negative 38%.

The results of Bookstein and his co-workers were considerably better.[16] In their series of forty-one patients with carcinoma of the pancreas, the incidence of true positive results was an impressive 76%. Pancreatic angiography thus remains an important roentgenographic technique in the diagnosis of cancer of this organ. It should be performed whenever this diagnosis is strongly suspected clinically in the absence of a positive conventional or hypotonic barium study. Superselective injections can help greatly in patients in whom the usual selective studies are inconclusive.

Selective arteriography of the pancreas will never be capable of screening the large number of patients in whom, theoretically, cure might be achieved. These are the patients with obscure symptoms and signs whose small lesions in silent locations do not permit conclusive results by other methods of examination.

Splenoportography in diagnosis

Splenoportography is of value in the diagnosis of carcinoma of the body and tail of the pancreas. Often it facilitates estimation of extent of tumor. The tumor may displace and deform the adjacent veins, or it may obstruct the splenic vein or its tributaries. It may narrow the splenic or portal vein, producing dilatation proximally. Even relatively small tumors of the body or tail of the pancreas may cause these changes. Carcinomas of the head of the pancreas, however, rarely effect significant changes in the portal vein unless they arise in its immediate proximity. Splenoportography is not recommended for evaluating the extent of change or for establishing the diagnosis of carcinoma of the pancreatic head.[70,71]

The value of splenoportography is sharply limited because it offers no definite diagnostic criteria for differentiation between carcinoma and pancreatitis or pseudocysts (Fig. 44-29).

The splenic venogram is recommended for the venous study of tumors in the pancreas. It is obtained after selective injection of the celiac axis and the superior mesenteric artery. This method permits visualization of the arterial, capillary, and venous beds with performance of only one procedure.

Percutaneous transhepatic cholangiography in diagnosis

Percutaneous transhepatic cholangiography is probably one of the most accurate procedures for positive identification of carcinoma of the head of the pancreas in the jaundiced patient.[29,30,79] This procedure does not, however, provide an early diagnosis. By the time this examination is performed the tumor is usually well advanced. Percutaneous cholangiography does not permit conclusions regarding extent of the tumor. It does reveal the site and appearance of the obstruction, and it permits preliminary planning of the operative procedure. It may be used in conjunction with other methods, such as barium sulfate studies of the upper gastrointestinal tract and selective arteriography. It is valuable in distinguishing between obstructive and unobstructive jaundice and also between the various types of extrahepatic obstruction. The technique of this examination and its results are covered in Chapter 52.

Differential diagnosis

The differentiation of carcinoma of the head of the pancreas from *carcinoma of the ampulla of Vater* is important.[18,90] The prognosis for the latter malignancy is considerably better than for carcinoma of the head of the pancreas.[21] The findings on barium sulfate studies of the upper gastrointestinal tract are usually more localized to the ampullary region. Frequently, an intraluminal mass projects from the papilla into the second portion of the duodenum. The papilla

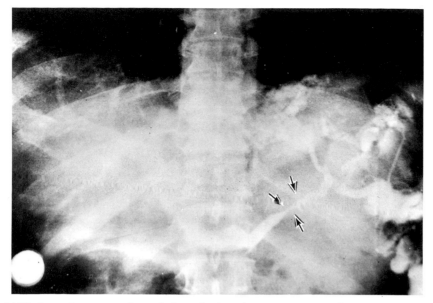

Fig. 44-29. Irregular narrowing of the splenic vein (arrows) seen in a splenoportogram taken of a patient who had pseudocysts of the pancreas and chronic pancreatitis. The narrowing is of the type described for carcinoma of the pancreas. The findings show the nonspecificity of these signs of splenoportography.

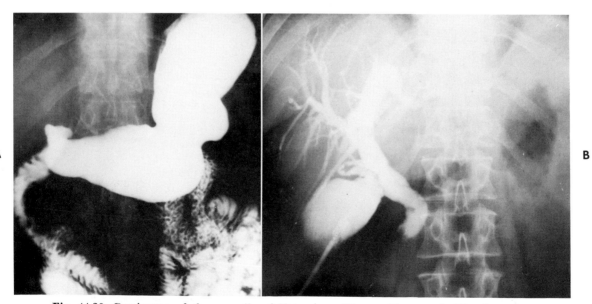

Fig. 44-30. Carcinoma of the ampulla of Vater in a 56-year-old man. **A,** The large impression on the second portion of the duodenum and the mass and ulceration in the region of the papilla are typical of this neoplasm but may also be a manifestation of carcinoma of the head of the pancreas. **B,** Operative cholangiogram through a needle shows dilatation of the ducts and irregular invasion of the common duct not far from the ampulla. This type of invasion cannot be differentiated from carcinoma of the pancreas.

of Vater may be increased in size. Some irregularity in this region or fixation of the mucosal folds surrounding this defect may be present.[43,63,75] Hypotonic duodenography is of particular value in the diagnosis of this neoplasm.

Carcinoma of the papilla of Vater may also appear as an irregular ulceration of the duodenum. This finding is even more common than in carcinoma of the head of the pancreas (Fig. 44-30).[63]

Primary carcinomas of the extrahepatic bile ducts are extremely difficult to differentiate by roentgenologic means from carcinomas of the head of the pancreas. Percutaneous transhepatic cholangiography, occasionally cholecystography, rarely intravenous cholangiography, arteriography, and barium sulfate studies of the upper gastrointestinal tract may localize the lesion in the extrahepatic bile duct.[19] At best, however, this is only indirect evidence for differentiation. Particularly is this true if, on arteriography, the tumor is very small, no change involves the surrounding barium-filled intestine, and transhepatic cholangiography shows complete occlusion of the extrahepatic bile duct.

Carcinoma of the gallbladder may present a difficult differential diagnosis. This neoplasm spreads massively and also involves surrounding structures,[46] in doing so it invades the large bile ducts. Transhepatic cholangiography can frequently permit differentiation from other neoplasms of this region by the type of invasion of the hepatic ducts that it shows.[30]

CYSTADENOCARCINOMA

Cystadenocarcinomas are quite rare. Rutledge and Lischer have found fewer than twenty cases of cystadenocarcinomas reported before 1958.[74] Of the one hundred cases of pancreatic carcinoma reported by Mikal and Campbell only two can be classified as cystadenocarcinomas.[53] Warren and his associates found that in four of five patients with cystadenocarcinomas operated upon the tumors were completely resectable.[90] Of these, four patients were alive and well 4 years after operation. Glenner and Mallory reported on carcinomas of the pancreas originating in cystadenomas associated with papillary proliferations.[36] They expressed the belief that papillary cystadenomas of the pancreas tend toward malignant propensity much as do papillary cystadenomas of the ovary.

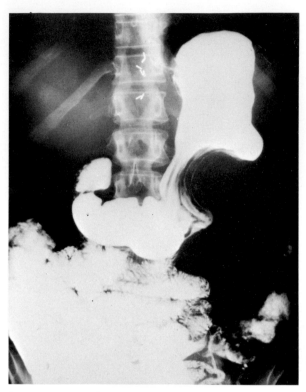

Fig. 44-31. Very large impression on greater curvature of body of the stomach by a large but noninvasive cystadenocarcinoma of the pancreas.

Unless the surrounding structures, particularly the intestine, are invaded, cystadenocarcinomas of the pancreas cannot be differentiated roentgenographically from benign cystadenomas (Fig. 44-31). Primary carcinoma of the pancreas with pseudocyst is much more likely to be diagnosed roentgenologically than is cystadenocarcinoma. The increased vascularity of this tumor in conjunction with other signs of malignancy permits an accurate diagnosis from selective arteriograms. Although most reports in the literature indicate the presence of large displaced arteries with many tortuous branches that enter the tumor and form a rich network of vessels,[1,72] selective arteriography is not always diagnostic.[89]

NONEPITHELIAL MALIGNANT TUMORS

Sarcomas of the pancreas are rare lesions and roentgenographically are indistinguishable from other masses in the head of the pancreas, such as carcinomas. Isolated reports have appeared on leiomyosarcoma[32] and rhabdomyosarcomas of the pancreas. Practically any type of sarcoma may occur in the pancreas.[4,11]

Lymphoma may also involve the pancreas,[44] and only rarely is there a generalized lymphoma of the abdomen that does not involve the pancreas. The roentgenologic diagnosis is not difficult, since the lesions are usually widespread; the differential diagnosis then lies only between widespread metastatic disease and lymphoma.

METASTATIC MALIGNANCY

Metastasis to the pancreas is possible from practically every type of carcinoma (Fig. 44-8, *B*). Carcinomas of the lung, breast, and kidney and malignant melanomas are the most common sources.[92] The establishment of a diagnosis of metastasis is usually impossible without knowledge of the primary tumor. Tumors of adjacent organs, notably carcinoma or leiomyosarcoma of the stomach and carcinoma of the gallbladder or of the colon, also frequently involve the pancreas.[92]

BENIGN EXOCRINE TUMORS

Solid duct adenomas are rare benign tumors that may become as large as 9 cm. in diameter. I have had no experience with roentgenologic procedures for diagnosis of this type of tumor. It should be roentgenographically indistinguishable from a benign cystadenoma of the pancreas.

Cystadenoma of the pancreas is a relatively more common tumor of the pancreas and occurs anywhere within this organ.[64] The tumor can reach considerable size and may be indistinguishable from the much more common pseudocyst. Its distinguishing characteristics are impingement on and displacement of surrounding organs, notably the duodenum (Fig. 44-32), lack of history of pancreatitis or injury, a palpable mass, and the demonstration by aortography and selective arteriography of a rich vascular pattern (Fig. 44-33).[6,7,12,85] Occasionally, cystadenomas of the pancreas show calcification.[40]

NONEPITHELIAL BENIGN TUMORS

Benign pancreatic tumors that originate from supporting tissues are exceedingly rare.[61,81] They include leiomyoma, fibroma, fibromyoma, lymphangioma, hemangioma, neurofibroma, and lipoma among others. The symptoms as well as

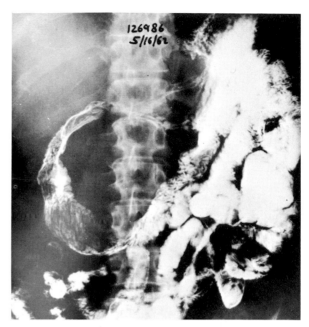

Fig. 44-32. Cystadenoma of the pancreas producing enlargement of the duodenal loop and a great deal of impression on the second and third portions of the duodenum.

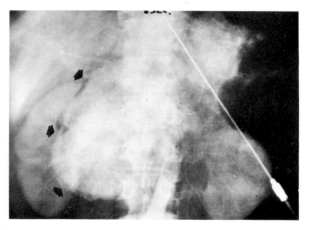

Fig. 44-33. Aortogram showing the extreme vascularity of a cystadenoma involving the head and body of the pancreas (arrows).

the roentgenographic findings point to a growing mass that displaces but does not invade.

ENDOCRINE TUMORS

Insulinomas are usually small, measuring less than 2 cm. in diameter. They present great difficulty of diagnosis by any method other than selective arteriography. By selective arteriogra-

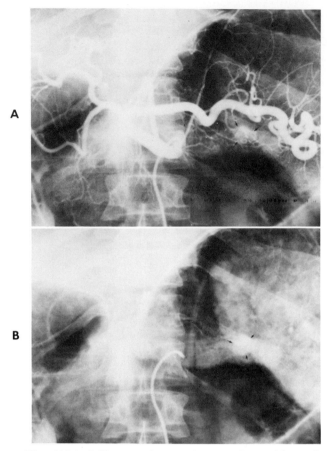

Fig. 44-34. Celiac arteriogram in a patient with an insulinoma. **A,** During the early arterial phase the tumor with its irregular vessels is well outlined in the body of the pancreas (arrows). **B,** During the venous phase the tumor shows a vascular blush (arrows).

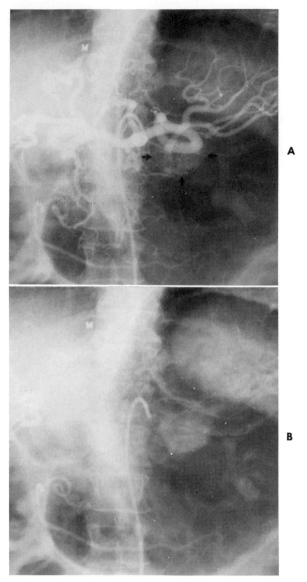

Fig. 44-35. Celiac arteriogram in a patient with Zollinger-Ellison syndrome. **A,** Irregular vessels are seen in the tumor, which is in the body of the pancreas (arrows). **B,** In a later phase of this study, the tumor shows a vascular blush.

phy the tumor appears as an intensely vascular, definitely outlined, rounded mass (Fig. 44-34).[7,49,60] Hyperinsulinism produced by this tumor is correctable by surgical extirpation; therefore it is of great clinical importance to define this tumor accurately in a region where exploration may be difficult. Insulinomas may, however, present difficulties in angiographic diagnosis when their vascularity is not strikingly increased. An arteriogram obtained on only one projection, showing the tumor superimposed on the spine or hidden by other highly vascularized structures, adds further to difficulty.[60] This difficulty, however, can be solved rather easily by photographic subtraction.

Bookstein and Oberman reported that only three of their eight patients with insulinoma had positive arteriograms.[15] Gray and associates reviewed a series of published articles on arteriography in patients with insulinoma.[37] They included, in addition to their own, only those that reported both positive and negative results. They arrived at an overall incidence of 63% in instances of a diagnostic increase in vascularity.

Nonbeta cell tumors of the islets of Langerhans, producing the Zollinger-Ellison syndrome, secrete a gastrin-like substance[38] that produces a syndrome of gastric hypersecretion and hyperacidity, frequently with peptic ulceration and diarrhea.

The tumors themselves are usually small and not detectable by roentgenographic examination. More than 50% of these tumors are malignant[27,28] and metastasize to the liver and spread through the peripancreatic region. The malignancy is low grade, however, and the peptic ulcerations almost always result from gastric hypersecretion and hyperacidity and not from tumor invasion. Visualization by arteriography and retrospection of diagnosis was reported by Ludin and his co-workers.[48] In their patient, vascularity was increased in the liver, to which the tumor had metastasized as well as in the primary tumor of the tail of the pancreas.

Selective superior mesenteric and celiac arteriography certainly appears to be a worthwhile procedure whenever the diagnosis of the Zollinger-Ellison syndrome is established by other means (Fig. 44-35). Indirect roentgenologic findings have been dealt with elsewhere in this text. These findings are hypersecretion, large gastric folds, abnormal pattern of small bowel, duodenal dilatation, and peptic ulceration of the stomach, duodenum, postbulbar area, or even jejunum.[3,55,76]

Islet cell tumors have been described that do not secrete either insulin or the substance resulting in the Zollinger-Ellison syndrome. These tumors can be detected roentgenologically if they are large enough to involve surrounding structures.[45] Most other tumors of the islets of Langerhans not producing symptoms remain undetected until necropsy and are of no roentgenologic significance. Islet cell tumors producing diarrhea but not gastric hypersecretion or hyperchlorhydria can occur. The severe diarrhea associated with these tumors may lead to severe hypokalemia. The syndrome has been described as pancreatic cholera. The hormone secreted by the tumor has not yet been identified.

REFERENCES

1. Abrams, R. M., Beranbaum, E. R., Beranbaum, S. L., and Ngo, N. L.: Angiographic studies of benign and malignant cystadenoma of the pancreas, Radiology 89:1028, 1967.
2. Adler, D. C., and Meyers, H. E.: Cineradiographic examination of the upper gastrointestinal tract in obstructive jaundice, J.A.M.A. 199:709, 1967.
3. Amberg, J. R., Ellison, E. H., Wilson, S. D., and Zboralske, F. F.: Roentgenographic observations in the Zollinger-Ellison syndrome, J.A.M.A. 190:185, 1964.
4. Amunni, G. F.: Il profilo anatomo-isto-patologico dei tumori mesenchimali primitivi maligni del pancreas; contributo casistico; sarcoma fuso-cellulare e linfosarcoma, Arch. Ital. Mal. Appar. Dig. 18:79, 1952.
5. Anacker, H.: Kritische Bewertung der röntgenologischen Untersuchungsmethoden zur Pankreasdiagnostik, Radiologe 5:312, 1965.
6. Bång, I.: Ein angiographisch diagnostizierter Fall von Cystadenoma Pancreatis, Radiologe 5:287, 1965.
7. Baum, S., Roy, R., Finkelstein, A. K., and Blakemore, W. S.: Clinical application of selective celiac and superior mesenteric arteriography, Radiology 84:279, 1965.
8. Beeler, J. W., and Kirklin, B. R.: Roentgenologic findings accompanying carcinoma of pancreas, Amer. J. Roentgen. 67:576, 1952.
9. Beranbaum, S. L.: Carcinoma of the pancreas; a bidirectional roentgen approach, Amer. J. Roentgen. 96:447, 1966.
10. Berk, J. E.: Diagnosis of carcinoma of the pancreas, Arch. Intern. Med. (Chicago) 68:525, 1941.
11. Berman, J. K., and Levene, N.: Sarcoma of the pancreas, Arch. Surg. (Chicago) 73:894, 1956.
12. Bieber, W. P., and Albo, R. J.: Cystadenoma of the pancreas; its arteriographic diagnosis, Radiology 80:776, 1963.
13. Bilboa, M. K., Rösch, J., Frische, L. H., and Dotter, C. T.: Hypotonic duodenography in the diagnosis of pancreatic disease, Seminars Roentgen. 3:280, 1968.
14. Boijsen, E.: Selective pancreatic angiography, Brit. J. Radiol. 39:481, 1966.
15. Bookstein, J. J., and Oberman, H. A.: Appraisal of selective angiography in localizing islet-cell tumors of the pancreas, Radiology 86:682, 1966.
16. Bookstein, J. J., Reuter, S. R., and Martel, W.: Angiographic evaluation of pancreatic carcinoma, Radiology 93:757, 1969.
17. Broadbent, T. R., and Kerman, H. D.: One hundred cases of carcinoma of the pancreas; clinical and roentgenologic analysis, Gastroenterology 17:163, 1951.
18. Cattell, R. B., Warren, K. W., and Au, F. T. C.: Periampullary carcinomas; diagnosis and surgical management, Surg. Clin. N. Amer. 39:781, 1959.
19. Clemett, A. R.: Carcinoma of the major bile ducts, Radiology 84:894, 1965.
20. D'Aunoy, R., Ogden, M. A., and Halpert, B.: Carcinoma of pancreas; analysis of 40 autopsies, Amer. J. Path. 15:217, 1939.
21. Dennis, C., and Varco, R. L.: Survival for more than 5 years after pancreato-duodenectomy for cancer of the ampulla and pancreatic head, Surgery 39:92, 1956.
22. Dodds, W. J., and Zboralske, F. F.: Roentgenographic diagnosis of pancreatic neoplasms, Seminars Roentgen. 3:242, 1968.
23. Eaton, S. B., Benedict, K. T., Jr., Ferrucci, J. T., Jr., and Fleischli, D. J.: Hypotonic duodenography, Radiol. Clin. N. Amer. 8:125, 1970.

24. Eaton, S. B., Ferrucci, J. T., Jr., and Benedict, K. T., Jr.: A comprehensive evaluation of radiologic exploration of the pancreas, CRC Critical Rev. Radiol. Sci. 1:166, 1970.
25. Eaton, S. B., Ferrucci, J. T., Jr., Margulis, A. R., and Weens, H. S.: Unfamiliar roentgen findings in pancreatic disease, Amer. J. Roentgen. In press.
26. Eaton, S. B., Fleischli, D. J., Pollard, J. J., Nebesar, R. A., and Potsaid, M. S.: Comparison of current radiologic approaches to the diagnosis of pancreatic disease, New Eng. J. Med. 279:389, 1968.
27. Ellison, E. H., and Carey, L.: Diagnosis and management of Zollinger-Ellison syndrome, Amer. J. Surg. 105:383, 1963.
28. Ellison, E. H., and Wilson, S. D.: The Zollinger-Ellison syndrome; re-appraisal and evaluation of 260 registered cases, Amer. Surg. 160:512, 1964.
29. Evans, J. A.: Specialized roentgen diagnostic technics in the investigation of abdominal disease, Radiology 82:579, 1964.
30. Evans, J. A., Glenn, F., Thorbjarnarson, B., and Mujahed, Z.: Percutaneous transhepatic cholangiography; discussion of the method and report of 25 cases, Radiology 78:362, 1962.
31. Eyler, W. R., Clark, M. D., and Rian, R. L.: An evaluation of roentgen signs of pancreatic enlargement, J.A.M.A. 181:967, 1962.
32. Feinberg, S. B., Margulis, A. R., and Lober, P.: Roentgen findings in leiomyosarcoma of the pancreas, Minnesota Med. 40:505, 1957.
33. Fredens, M., Egeblad, M., Holst-Nielsen, F.: The value of selective angiography in the diagnosis of tumors in pancreas and liver, Radiology 93:765, 1969.
34. Frostberg, N.: Characteristic duodenal deformity in cases of different kinds of peri-vaterial enlargement of pancreas, Acta Radiol. (Stockholm) 19:164, 1938.
35. Glenn, F., Evans, J. A., Halpern, M., and Thorbjarnarson, B.: Selective celiac and superior mesenteric arteriography, Surg. Gynec. Obstet. 118:93, 1964.
36. Glenner, G. G., and Mallory, G. K.: The cystadenoma and related malfunctional tumors of the pancreas; pathogenesis, classification, and significance, Cancer 9:980, 1956.
37. Gray, R. K., Rösch, J., and Grollman, J. H., Jr.: Arteriography in the diagnosis of islet-cell tumors, Radiology 97:39, 1970.
38. Gregory, R. A., Tracy, H. J., French, J. M., and Sircus, W.: Extraction of a gastrin-like substance from a pancreatic tumor in a case of Zollinger-Ellison syndrome, Lancet 1:1045, 1960.
39. Gullick, H. D.: Carcinoma of pancreas; a review and critical study of 100 cases, Medicine 38:47, 1959.
40. Haukohl, R. S., and Melamed, A.: Cystadenoma of pancreas; report of 2 cases showing calcification, Amer. J. Roentgen. 63:234, 1950.
41. Herbert, W. W., and Margulis, A. R.: Diagnosis of retroperitoneal masses by gastrointestinal roentgenographic measurements; a computer study, Radiology 84:52, 1965.
42. Hick, F. K., and Mortimer, H. M.: Carcinoma of pancreas, J. Lab. Clin. Med. 19:1058, 1934.
43. Hodes, P. J., Pendergrass, E. P., and Winston, N. J.: Pancreatic, ductal and vaterian neoplasms; their roentgen manifestations, Radiology 61:1, 1954.
44. Jackson, H., Jr., and Parker, F., Jr.: Hodgkin's disease and allied disorders, New York, 1947, Oxford University Press, Inc.
45. Kalish, P. E., and Shapiro, B.: Islet cell carcinoma of the pancreas producing obstructive jaundice, Ann. Surg. 158:222, 1963.
46. Khilnani, M. T., Wolf, B. S., and Finkel, M.: Roentgen features of carcinoma of gallbladder on barium-meal examination, Radiology 79:264, 1962.
47. Larsen, K. A., and Pedersen, A.: Roentgenologic findings in stomach and duodenum in cancer of pancreas, Acta Radiol. (Stockholm) 45:459, 1956.
48. Ludin, H., Enderlin, F., Fahrländer, H. J., and Scheidegger, S.: Failure to diagnose Zollinger-Ellison syndrome by pancreatic arteriography; report of a case, Brit. J. Radiol. 39:494, 1966.
49. Lunderquist, A.: Angiography in carcinoma of the pancreas, Acta Radiol. [Diagn.] (Stockholm) 235 (Suppl.):1, 1956.
50. Madsen, B.: Demonstration of pancreatic insulomas by angiography, Brit. J. Radiol. 39:488, 1966.
51. Mani, J. R., Zboralske, F. F., and Margulis, A. R.: Carcinoma of the body and tail of the pancreas, Amer. J. Roentgen. 96:429, 1966.
52. Marks, L. J., Weingarten, B., and Gerst, G. R.: Carcinoma of tail of pancreas associated with bleeding gastric varices and hypersplenism, Ann. Intern. Med. 37:1077, 1952.
53. Mikal, S., and Campbell, A. J. A.: Carcinoma of pancreas; diagnostic and operative criteria based on 100 consecutive autopsies, Surgery 28:963, 1950.
54. Miller, E. M., and Clagett, O. T.: Survival 5 years after radical pancreatoduodenectomy for carcinoma of head of pancreas, Ann. Surg. 134:1013, 1951.
55. Missakian, M. M., Carlson, H. C., Huizenga, K. A.: Roentgenographic findings in Zollinger-Ellison syndrome, Amer. J. Roentgen. 94:429, 1965.
56. Nebesar, R. A., and Pollard, J. J.: A critical evaluation of selective celiac and superior mesenteric angiography in the diagnosis of pancreatic diseases, particularly malignant tumor: facts and artefacts, Radiology 89:1017, 1967.
57. Ödman, P.: Pancreatic angiography. In Abrams, H. L., editor: Angiography, vol, 2, Boston, 1961, Little, Brown and Company.
58. Ödman, P.: Percutaneous selective angiography of main branches of aorta (preliminary report), Acta Radiol. (Stockholm) 45:1, 1956.
59. Olsson, O.: Angiographie bei Pankreastumoren, Radiologe 5:281, 1965.
60. Olsson, O.: Angiographie in drei Fällen von Insuloma Pancreatis, Radiologe 5:286, 1965.
61. Pack, G. T., Trinidad, S. S., and Lisa, J. R.: Rare primary somatic tumors of the pancreas, A.M.A. Arch. Surg. 77:1000, 1958.
62. Paul, R. E., Jr., Miller, H. H., Kahn, P. C., Callow, A. D., Edwards, T. L., Jr., and Patterson, J. F.: Pancreatic angiography, with application of subselective angiography of the celiac or superior mesenteric

artery to the diagnosis of carcinoma of the pancreas, New Eng. J. Med. **272**:283, 1965.

63. Perez, C. A., Powers, W. E., Holtz, S., and Spjut, H. J.: Roentgenologic-pathologic correlation of resectable carcinoma of the pancreatico-duodenal region, Amer. J. Roentgen. **94**:438, 1965.

64. Piper, C. E., Jr., ReMine, W. H., and Priestley, J. T.: Pancreatic cystadenomata; report of 20 cases, J.A.M.A. **180**:648, 1962.

65. Poole, G. J.: A new roentgenographic method of measuring the retrogastric and retroduodenal spaces: statistical evaluation of reliability and diagnostic utility, Radiology **97**:71, 1970.

66. Poppel, M. H.: Roentgen manifestations of pancreatic disease, Springfield, Ill., 1951, Charles C Thomas, Publisher.

67. Poppel, M. H., Jacobson, H. G., and Smith, R. W.: The roentgen aspects of the papilla and ampulla of Vater, Springfield, Ill., 1953, Charles C Thomas, Publisher.

68. Rigler, L. G.: Diagnosis of extra-gastro-intestinal abdominal masses, Radiology **21**:229, 1933.

69. Rösch, J.: Röntgenuntersuchung und Einsatz der Methoden bei Pancreaserkrankungen, Radiologe **5**: 257, 1965.

70. Rösch, J.: Die Splenoportographie in der Diagnostik der Pankreaserkrankungen, Radiologe **5**:274, 1965.

71. Rösch, J., and Herfort, K.: Contribution of splenoportography to the diagnosis of diseases of the pancreas, I. Tumorous diseases, Acta Med. Scand. **171**: 251, 1962.

72. Rösch, J., and Judkins, M. P.: Angiography in the diagnosis of pancreatic disease, Seminars Roentgen. **3**:296, 1968.

73. Russell, W. M., and Margulis, A. R.: Impression on the duodenal loop resulting from tumor of the pancreas; a roentgenographic evaluation, Amer. J. Roentgen. **94**:449, 1965.

74. Rutledge, R., and Lischer, C. E.: Papillary cystadenocarcinoma of the pancreas, Texas J. Med. **54**:89, 1958.

75. Salik, J. O.: Pancreatic carcinoma and its early roentgenologic recognition, Amer. J. Roentgen. **86**: 1, 1961.

76. Schlaeger, R., LeMay, M., and Wermer, P.: Upper gastrointestinal tract alterations in adenomatosis of endocrine glands, Radiology **75**:517, 1960.

77. Schorr, S., Aviad, I., Birnbaum, D., and Loewenthal, M.: Pyelography as an aid for diagnosis of liver cirrhosis with a study of normal position of kidneys, Amer. J. Roentgen. **88**:1142, 1962.

78. Schultz, E. H., Jr.: Measurements of the retrogastric space, Radiology **84**:58, 1965.

79. Seldinger, S. I.: Percutaneous transhepatic cholangiography, Acta Radiol. (Stockholm) **253** (Suppl.): 1966.

80. Silverberg, E., and Holleb, A. I.: Cancer statistics, 1971, CA **21**:13, 1971.

81. Skapinker, S.: Fibromyoma of the pancreas, Ann. Surg. **156**:976, 1962.

82. Sloan, L. E., and Wharton, G. K.: Cancer of pancreas, Amer. J. Gastroent. **21**:441, 1954.

83. Smith, B. K., and Albright, E. C.: Carcinoma of body and tail of pancreas: report of 37 cases studied at State of Wisconsin General Hospital from 1925-1950, Ann. Intern. Med. **36**:90, 1952.

84. Strang, C., and Walton, J. N.: Carcinoma of body and tail of pancreas, Ann. Intern. Med. **39**:15, 1953.

85. Swanson, G. E.: A case of cystadenoma of the pancreas studied by selective angiography, Radiology **81**:592, 1963.

86. Tendler, M. J., and Livermore, G. R., Jr.: Role of biopsy and radical operation in the management of carcinoma of the head of the pancreas; report of a case surviving for seven years, Ann. Surg. **150**:290, 1959.

87. Thamsen, L., Hjorth, N., Christensen, A. R., and Bjørneboe, M.: Cancer of pancreas; clinical and pathological study, Acta Med. Scand. **139**:28, 1950.

88. Tucker, D. H., and Moore, I. B.: Vanishing pancreatic calcification in chronic pancreatitis; a sign of pancreatic carcinoma, New Eng. J. Med. **268**:31, 1963.

89. Voorthuisen, A. E. van: Disappointments in angiographic examination of the pancreas, Radiol. Clin. **41**:47, 1971.

90. Warren, K. W., Cattell, R. B., Blackburn, J. P., and Nora, P. F.: A long-term appraisal of pancreaticoduodenal resection for peri-ampullary carcinoma, Ann. Surg. **155**:652, 1962.

91. Weber, A. O.: Carcinoma of head of pancreas with spread to local lymph nodes; five-year survival after radical pancreaticoduodenectomy, J.A.M.A. **186**:150, 1963.

92. Willis, R. A.: The spread of tumours in the human body, ed. 2, London, 1952, Butterworth & Co., Ltd.

93. Willy, R. G., and Drymalski, G. W.: Carcinoma of tail of pancreas; roentgenographic aspects—2 case reports. Quart. Bull. Northwestern Univ. Med. School **25**:276, 1951.

94. Wise, R. E., and Johnston, D. O.: Roentgenologic diagnosis of malignancy of pancreas, Surg. Clin. N. Amer. **36**:699, 1956.

45 | The lesser peritoneal sac

Harry Z. Mellins

ANATOMY

PATHOLOGY

ROENTGENOLOGIC FINDINGS
  Signs of free air
  Signs of fluid
  Signs of abscess formation
  Displacement of the stomach
  Use of contrast medium
  Signs of internal herniation

Because of the deep and protected position of the lesser peritoneal sac, there are few localized symptoms of disease in this area, and physical examination of the area is difficult. Roentgenologic contributions to the diagnosis of lesser sac disease are therefore important. Because the lesser sac has a recognizable shape and some surfaces formed by opacifiable organs, it can be outlined roentgenologically, and pathologic changes within it can be recognized.

ANATOMY

The peritoneum of the anterior abdominal wall may be traced upward, starting arbitrarily at the umbilicus. The round ligament (ligamentum teres) is the vestige of the umbilical vein and runs posteriorly and upward from the umbilicus to end at the left branch of the portal vein. As it draws away from the anterior abdominal wall it pulls a fold of peritoneum with it to create the falciform ligament. The peritoneum of the anterior abdominal wall covers the undersurface of the diaphragm. From the posterior aspect of the diaphragm the peritoneum runs downward and forward on the right as the anterior layer of the coronary ligament of the liver and on the left as the anterior layer of the triangular ligament of the liver (Fig. 45-1). It continues along the superior surface of the liver, around the sharp anterior margin and on to the undersurface.

On the right the peritoneum along the under-surface of the right lobe of the liver becomes, posteriorly, the posterior layer of the right coronary ligament. It continues downward over the right suprarenal gland and kidney to the duodenum and right colic flexure. Continuing medially in front of the inferior vena cava, it is continuous with the posterior wall of the lesser peritoneal sac.

On the left, the peritoneum covers the lower surface of the quadrate lobe, the undersurface and lateral surfaces of the gallbladder, and the inferior and posterior borders of the left lobe. It is then reflected from the undersurface of the left lobe as the inferior layer of the left triangular ligament and from the porta hepatis and the fossa for the ductus venosus to the lesser curvature of the stomach and the first 2.5 cm. of the duodenum as the anterior layer of the hepatogastric and hepatoduodenal ligaments. Together these ligaments constitute the lesser omentum. Traced to the right, the peritoneum of the anterior surface of the lesser omentum turns around the hepatic artery, bile duct, and portal vein and becomes continuous with the anterior wall of the lesser peritoneal sac. Traced downward it covers the anterosuperior surface of the stomach and the beginning of the duodenum and is carried down to a large free fold, the gastrocolic ligament or greater omentum, which invests the colon. Above the colon it continues as the transverse mesocolon and thus reaches the posterior abdominal wall at the level of the pancreas.

The peritoneum forming the anterior wall of the lesser sac runs downward and laterally to the lesser curvature of the stomach and the duodenum. Continuing laterally it covers the posterior surface of the stomach and is reflected onto the spleen as the posterior layer of the anterior sheet of the greater omentum, or the posterior surface of the gastrosplenic ligament.

The peritoneum that forms the posterior wall of the lesser sac covers the anterior surface of the inferior vena cava, the celiac artery, the pancreas, the left suprarenal gland, and the left kidney. From the kidney it is reflected onto the

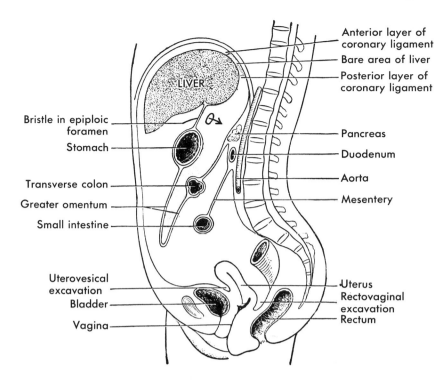

Fig. 45-1. Diagrammatic representation of the sagittal section of the abdominal cavity, showing the relationships of the lesser peritoneal sac. (From Goss, C. M., editor: Gray's anatomy of the human body, ed. 27, Philadelphia, 1959, Lea & Febiger.)

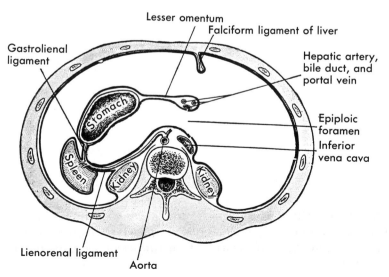

Fig. 45-2. Diagrammatic representation of the transverse section of the abdominal cavity at the epiploic foramen. (From Goss, C. M., editor: Gray's anatomy of the human body, ed. 27, Philadelphia, 1959, Lea & Febiger.)

spleen as the deep layer of the splenorenal ligament. The left lateral boundary of the lesser peritoneal sac is therefore the pedicle of the spleen, where the gastrosplenic and the splenorenal ligaments come together (Fig. 45-2).

The body and fundus of the stomach are in contact with the diaphragm and the spleen. To the right of the fundus the upper portion of the posterior surface is in contact with the left kidney, the left suprarenal gland, and the diaphragm. The inferior portion of the posterior surface of the stomach is in contact with the pancreas; the splenic artery, as it runs along the upper border of the pancreas; the transverse mesocolon; and the transverse colon. These structures together form the stomach bed. They lie immediately behind the posterior wall of the lesser peritoneal sac, which separates them from the stomach.

Gas or fluid may collect in any of four intraperitoneal subphrenic spaces: on the right, in the suprahepatic space and in the hepatorenal space; on the left, in the combined suprahepatic–anterior subhepatic space and in the lesser sac.

PATHOLOGY

A variety of disease processes in the organs that form the boundaries of the lesser sac may be responsible for invasion of this space by air, exudate, gastrointestinal contents, blood, and tumors. Occasionally, infection in the lesser sac may lead to pulmonary and pleural infection.

Stomach. Perforation of ulcers of the anterior wall of the stomach may be sealed or covered by adjacent organs such as the liver or greater omentum. If the perforation is free, diffuse peritonitis may occur as gastric air and fluid enter the greater peritoneal cavity. Penetrating ulcers of the posterior wall of the stomach may set up sufficient reaction to cause fibrous adhesions between the peritoneum of the anterior surface and that of the posterior surface of the lesser peritoneal sac. When perforation occurs the ulcer penetrates into the substance of the pancreas. If, however, the lesser peritoneal sac is not obliterated by the reaction to the penetrating ulcer, perforation of an ulcer of the posterior wall will lead to the evacuation of air and fluid into the lesser sac (Figs. 45-3 and

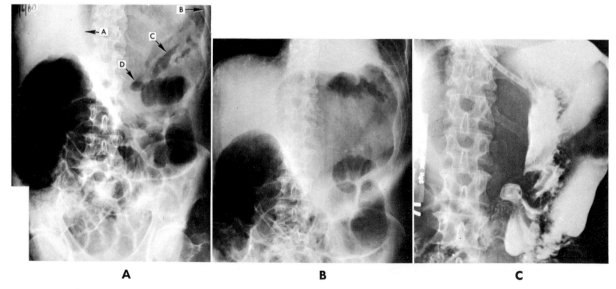

A	**B**	**C**

Fig. 45-3. A, Perforated posterior wall gastric ulcer in a middle-aged man. Note the right border of the lesser sac, *A*, the left border, *B*, gastric rugae outlined by air in the stomach, *C*, and the ulcer crater, *D*. **B,** Erect film showing the right, superior, and left borders of the lesser sac. **C,** Film showing the stomach, ulcer crater, and left side of the lesser sac demonstrated by aqueous contrast medium. (Courtesy Dr. H. Friedman.)

45-5). It may produce an air-containing abscess, which older authors called pyopneumothorax subphrenicus.[21] A case of a loculated abscess of the lesser peritoneal sac after perforation of a benign ulcer in the antrum of the stomach was documented by Taveras and Golden.[26]

Laceration of the stomach by blunt abdominal trauma is rare, probably because the stomach has a thick wall and is a freely movable organ. On occasion, however, particularly when the stomach is decidedly distended after the intake of a large amount of food or fluid, blunt abdominal trauma may lead to rupture of the stomach, with emptying of the gastric contents into the lesser sac if the laceration is posterior (Fig. 45-4).

Herniation of the gastric fundus into a localized eventration of the left dome of the diaphragm has resulted in a gastric perforation 2 cm. long with extravasation of gastric contents into the lesser sac.[19]

Congenital weakness of the stomach in newborn infants may lead to idiopathic rupture of the stomach.[5,27] If the laceration is posterior, the lesser sac will be exposed to the gastric contents. Because of the large amounts of swallowed air at this age, pneumoperitoneum of the lesser sac results (Fig. 45-10).

Duodenum. Perforation of ulcers of the posterior wall can lead to involvement of the lesser sac.[22] Theoretically, any lesion leading to gas or fluid in the greater peritoneal sac might be expected to involve the lesser sac by way of the foramen of Winslow. Actually, this must be very rare.

Gallbladder. Complications after gallbladder surgery may lead to involvement of the lesser sac or the lesser omentum. Morrison reported a case in which bile, leaking around a drainage tube placed in the cystic duct after a cholecystectomy, found its way into the foramen of Winslow and caused bile peritonitis in the lesser sac with effusion of over 1,000 ml. of fluid, while the greater peritoneal cavity remained dry.[19] Extravasation of fluid between the leaves of the lesser omentum after gallbladder surgery can result in a large cystic expansion of the lesser omentum.

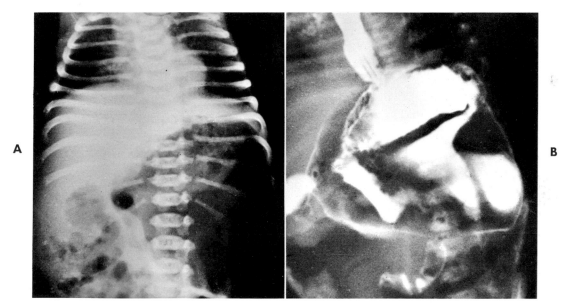

Fig. 45-4. A, Spontaneous rupture or perforation of the posterior wall of the stomach in a newborn infant. **B,** Aqueous contrast medium from the stomach entered the lesser sac through the perforation and empties through the foramen of Winslow. (Courtesy Dr. C. Berman.)

Seven proved cases of gallbladder herniation through the foramen of Winslow into the lesser sac have been reported.[8,28] The largest series is that of Vint[28] who documented four cases diagnosed roentgenologically and confirmed at operation, as well as twenty-seven additional roentgenologically characteristic cases that are unconfirmed. Herniation is more likely to occur when the patient is upright or prone, whereas reduction frequently occurs when the supine or right lateral recumbent positions are assumed. If the gallbladder is incarcerated the symptoms are likely to be those of acute cholecystitis. In the presence of free herniation and spontaneous reduction, transient vague abdominal discomfort may be the only symptom.

Liver. Trauma to the liver may lead to bleeding into either the greater or lesser peritoneal sac. Dietz reported a case of injury to the left lobe of the liver with the formation of a lesser sac hematoma. Differentiation from a huge subcapsular liver hematoma is difficult.[9]

Pancreas. The complications of acute hemorrhagic or chronic recurrent pancreatitis often lead to involvement of the lesser peritoneal sac. The roentgenologic findings in two cases of lesser peritoneal sac abscess resulting from pancreatic necrosis were described by Bittdorf in 1913.[3] A long air-fluid level was seen under the elevated left dome of the diaphragm in both cases, and in one of them the gastric air bubble was absent. A similar case with an air fluid level 7 cm. long and anterior displacement of the stomach was reported by Samuel in 1950.[24] Lesser sac abscesses following acute pancreatic necrosis are also manifested as multiple small gas bubbles.[9]

Newman and Frische describe an abscess in the lesser peritoneal sac that indented the posterior wall of the fundus and body of the barium-filled stomach, simulating a gastric neoplasm.[20] Similarly, pseudocysts of the pancreas may also indent the lumen of the stomach and simulate an intrinsic lesion.

Kopf describes the case of a 10-year-old boy who sustained a blow to his epigastric region that produced a tumor mass in the left upper quadrant.[15] No roentgenograms are described by Kopf, but at operation a large effusion was found in the lesser peritoneal sac and a fibrin plug occluded the foramen of Winslow.

Pancreatic hemorrhage may lead to retro-peritoneal bleeding. In some instances the peritoneal covering is broken and the blood fills the lesser peritoneal sac. The hemorrhage may be related to acute pancreatitis, but at times the cause is not clear (Fig. 45-8).

Kidney. Left perinephric abscess may lead to involvement of the lesser peritoneal sac. The kidney is often surrounded by pus, and usually the abscess cavity is extensive. It may extend in various directions. It has been described as bursting into the pleura or extending down the psoas muscle. Bluth has observed a middle-aged woman with diabetes and urinary tract infection who developed a perinephric abscess that burrowed into the lesser peritoneal sac (Fig. 45-6). Dietz documented a lesser sac gas abscess as a complication of left perinephric abscess in a 58-year-old man with diabetes, alcoholism, and cirrhosis.[9]

Small and large intestines. A leaking retrocolic gastrojejunostomy, perforation of a marginal ulcer in a retrocolic gastrojejunostomy, and perforation of the anterior surface of the transverse colon can cause involvement of the lesser peritoneal sac.[29]

The most common intestinal lesion involving the lesser sac is herniation through the epiploic foramen. Over ninety cases have been reported. In two thirds, the predominant viscus involved was the small intestines, and in the other third, the colon.[23] An anomaly of mesenteric length, intestinal rotation, or fixation of the right half of the colon must be present for herniation to occur. Roberts emphasizes that obstruction is of the closed loop type and that there may be two closed loops if the terminal ileum that is herniated acts as a taut strap occluding the transverse colon or if only the transverse colon is involved while the ileocecal valve is competent.[23]

Chest. Two cases of colon bacillus pneumonia occurring as complications of lesser peritoneal sac abscesses have been reported by Faegenburg and co-workers.[11]

ROENTGENOLOGIC FINDINGS
Signs of free air

Filling of the lesser sac with gas, such as occurs after perforation of a posterior gastric ulcer (Figs. 45-3 and 45-5), laceration of the stomach (Figs. 45-4 and 45-10), or extension of a perinephric gas abscess, demonstrates the characteristic shape of the lesser sac (Fig. 45-6). The

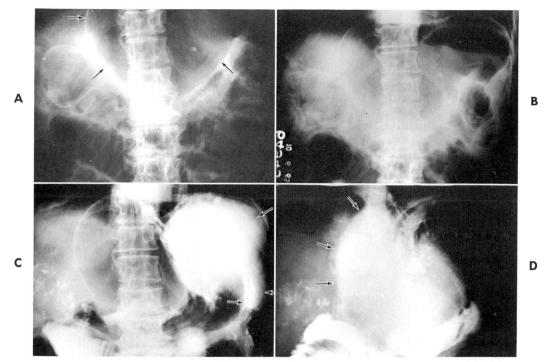

Fig. 45-5. Huge lesser curvature ulcer in a male patient. **A,** The posterior portion of the ulcer perforated into the lesser sac, and simultaneously the anterior portion perforated into the greater sac. The upper arrow indicates the falciform ligament, and the lower arrows outline the lesser sac collection. **B,** An erect film shows the margins of the lesser sac. Note that the superior pole of the spleen is not outlined, as it would be if the air on the left were in the greater sac. **C,** Aqueous contrast medium extravasated through the perforated posterior wall ulcer accumulates in the dependent left side of the lesser sac (arrows). **D,** Contrast medium displaced to the right by gravity demonstrates the right border of the lesser sac (arrows).

right border of the gas collection is a curved line slightly to the right of the lumbar spine. It is in the expected location of the common bile duct or the portal vein, which demarcates the right border of the lesser omentum and hence the lesser sac. The superior margin of the gas shadow is projected slightly below the highest portion of the diaphragm, because the lesser sac abuts against the diaphragm in its posterior and therefore more caudal level. The left border of the lesser sac is somewhat inside the inner border of the ribs, at the hilus of the spleen, where the gastrosplenic and splenorenal ligaments meet. The inferior border of the lesser sac varies in its level and depends upon the extent of fusion of the anterior and posterior leaves of the greater omentum. The inferior border tends to run inferiorly and to the left.

It may be as high as the lower border of the stomach and as low as the level of the true pelvis (Figs. 45-4, *B,* and 45-10).

Smaller collections of air, insufficient to fill the entire lesser sac are more difficult to localize than collections that assume the normal size and shape of the lesser sac. If these smaller collections are within the lesser sac, a lateral view in which the stomach contains either air or opaque contrast medium will show them to lie posterior to the stomach. If the gas collection is anterior to the stomach and under the diaphragm, it is in the anterior subphrenic space and hence in the greater peritoneal sac (Fig. 45-7). Free gas collections in the midline, just under the diaphragm, regularly turn out to represent these greater peritoneal sac collections rather than gas in the superior recess of the lesser sac.

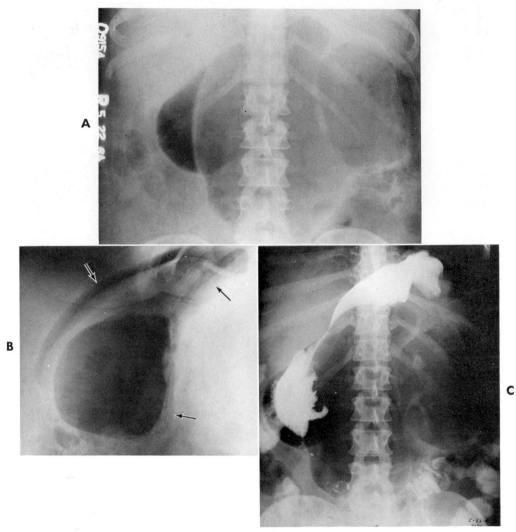

Fig. 45-6. A, Diabetes mellitus and urinary tract infection in a middle-aged woman. Note three large gas collections. **B,** Dorsal decubitus film of the same patient showing anterior displacement of the gas-filled stomach (white arrow) by a gas collection in the lesser sac (black arrows). This is the large central gas collection in **A. C,** Typical displacement of the stomach by lesser sac gas collection. Note the left perinephric gas collection. Operation revealed a left perinephric gas-forming abscess perforating into the lesser sac. (Courtesy Dr. I. Bluth.)

If there is gas in both the lesser and greater peritoneal sacs, it may be difficult to recognize the lesser sac involvement. Visualization of the falciform ligament on the supine film or demonstration of gas under the right dome or both domes of the diaphragm will establish the presence of free air in the greater sac. Concomitant lesser sac involvement may be established by recognizing the typical shape of the gas-filled lesser sac or by giving the patient an aqueous contrast medium orally and filling the lesser sac by way of a gastric perforation or laceration (Fig. 45-5).

Signs of fluid

Anterior displacement of the stomach by a mass of the density of water should suggest the possibility of fluid in the lesser sac or a retroperitoneal mass (Fig. 45-8). It may be impossible to distinguish between the two. If barium sul-

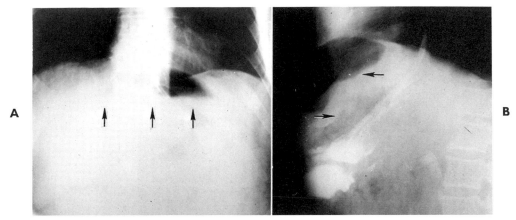

Fig. 45-7. A, Erect film showing a large midline gas collection under the diaphragm in a patient with a perforated anterior wall gastric ulcer. **B,** Lateral view taken after opacification of the stomach showing the large midline gas collection to be within the greater peritoneal sac, in the anterior subphrenic space (upper arrow). The gas collection directly in front of the stomach is in the left anterior subhepatic space (lower arrow).

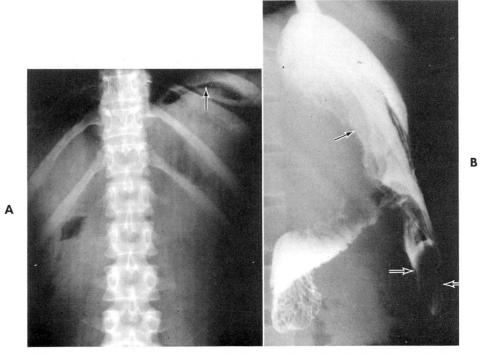

Fig. 45-8. A, Concavoconvex gas shadow in the gastric fundus, indicating a retrogastric mass (arrow). The patient, a young woman, was being treated with corticosteroids for polyarteritis nodosa when she developed cramping epigastric pains with intermittent hematemesis and melena. A tender mass was palpated in the left uppr quadrant of the abdomen. **B,** Lateral film of the stomach revealing a lobulated retrogastric mass of lesser sac collection. At operation multiple hematomas and free blood were found in the lesser sac, but the bleeding site could not be found. (Courtesy Dr. F. Henley.)

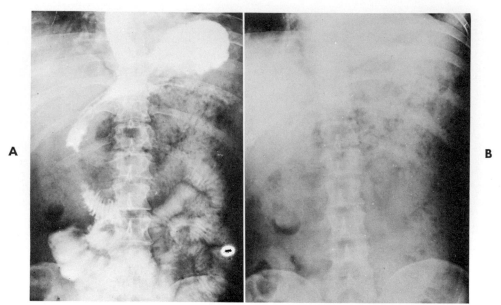

Fig. 45-9. A, An extensive gas abscess of the pancreas, with involvement of the lesser sac. The stomach is axially rotated anteriorly and upward. **B,** Abscess bubbles, which tend to be confined to the lesser sac.

fate or other opaque media are given by mouth, visualization of downward displacement of the duodenojejunal junction tends to favor a retroperitoneal mass rather than a lesser sac collection.

Signs of abscess formation

Lesser sac abscesses may manifest themselves roentgenologically as innumerable small gas bubbles (Fig. 45-9) or as larger gas collections with fluid levels. Walled-off abscess collections secondary to perforation of a posterior wall gastric ulcer usually demonstrate a long fluid level in a large gas collection. The abscess that follows pancreatic necrosis can be either of the long air-fluid level type or of the multiple disseminated gas bubble variety.

Displacement of the stomach

The two fixed points of the gastrointestinal tract in the vicinity of the stomach are the esophageal hiatus in the diaphragm and the junction of the first and second portions of the duodenum, where the duodenum becomes retroperitoneal. The stomach can therefore be likened to a bucket handle. Filling of the lesser sac, or any retrogastric lesion, will displace the body of the stomach anteriorly, superiorly, and

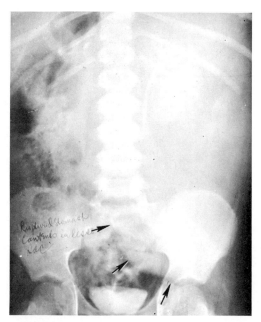

Fig. 45-10. Traumatic rupture of the stomach in a child after a full meal. At operation the lesser sac was full of fluid gastric contents. Note the oblique lower margin of the lesser sac projected over the left side of the pelvis.

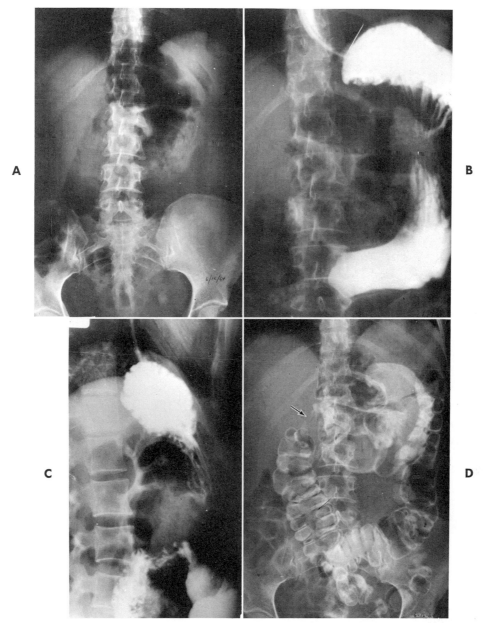

Fig. 45-11. A, Symptoms of intermittent intestinal obstruction in a female patient. Note the midline gas collection suggesting a cecal volvulus. **B** and **C,** Views showing that the cecum is medial and posterior to the stomach. **D,** Delayed film showing the contrast-filled cecum in the lesser sac with the gas-filled ileum above it. The arrow indicates the portion of colon traversing the foramen of Winslow. (Courtesy Dr. R. W. Perrin.)

usually to the right (Figs. 45-6, *C*, 45-9, *A*, 45-10, and 45-12, *B*). Theoretically, a large lesser sac collection might bulge the lesser omentum anteriorly, and a large collection in the inferior portion of the lesser sac might bulge the anterior leaf of the greater omentum anteriorly. Perforation of either omentum, with a collection anterior to it, might therefore displace the stomach posteriorly. In the great majority of cases lesser sac collections displace the stomach anteriorly.

Use of contrast medium

Opacification of the stomach with contrast material, followed by films in the frontal and lateral position, is the best way to demonstrate whether a gas or fluid collection lies medial to and behind the stomach and hence is in the lesser peritoneal sac (Figs. 45-6, *B*, 45-8, *B*, and 45-11, *B* and *C*). If the possibility of perforation of the stomach exists, iodinated contrast media should be given by mouth. If the stomach has indeed perforated posteriorly the contrast material will enter the lesser sac and demonstrate its typical configuration and borders (Figs. 45-3, *C*, 45-4, *B*, 45-5, *C* and *D*).

Signs of internal herniation

Gas- or fluid-filled loops of small intestine or ascending colon may be suspected of being in the lesser sac if they are projected medial to the lesser curvature of the stomach (Figs. 45-11, *A*, and 45-12, *A*). If a lateral view of the abdomen, with opacification of the stomach, demonstrates the gas- or fluid-filled intestinal loops to lie posterior to the stomach, the diagnosis is confirmed (Figs. 45-11, *B* and *C*). Evidence concerning the segment of intestine involved and the nature of the obstructing mechanism may be provided by barium enema examination. There may be a narrowing of the transverse colon at the junction of its middle and proximal thirds (Fig. 45-11, *D*), possibly with an axial twist in the mucosal pattern (Fig. 45-12, *C*) where the colon goes through the epiploic foramen. On the other hand, there may be an extrinsic oblique band of compression at the junction of the middle and proximal thirds of the transverse colon where a taut strap of small intestine passes over the colon anteriorly on its way to the epiploic foramen (Fig. 45-13).

Herniation of the gallbladder through the foramen of Winslow may be demonstrated on frontal roentgenographs of combined gallbladder and upper gastrointestinal studies. The gallbladder lies medial to the duodenal bulb and can be seen to be draped over the apex of the bulb. If the herniation is reduced by manual pressure under fluoroscopic control, the gall-

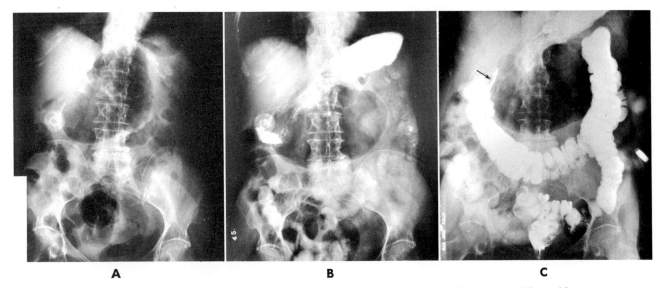

| A | B | C |

Fig. 45-12. A, Symptoms in a male patient, suggesting intestinal obstruction. The midline gas collection in the upper abdomen suggests a cecal volvulus. **B,** Displacement of the barium-filled stomach. **C,** An axial twist of the colon where it enters the lesser sac through the foramen of Winslow. (Courtesy Dr. J. J. McCort.)

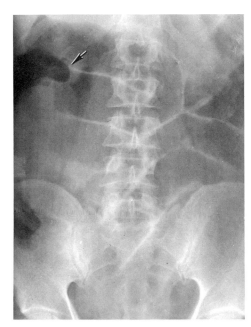

Fig. 45-13. Extrinsic compression of the colon (arrow) by a taut strap of small bowel passing to the epiploic foramen in a case of internal hernia.

bladder will be seen to travel up and over the apex of the duodenal bulb, rather than simply swinging in an arc anterior to the bulb like a "mobile" or left-sided gallbladder.

REFERENCES

1. Agnos, J. W., and Holmes, R. B.: Gas in the pancreas as a sign of abscess, Amer. J. Roentgen. **80**:60, 1958.
2. Bannen, J. E.: Investigation of free gas in the peritoneal cavity, Brit. J. Radiol. **18**:390, 1945.
3. Bittdorf, A.: Uber Abszesse im Saccus Omentalis nach Pankreasnekrose, Mitt. Grenzgeb. Med. Chir. **26**:109, 1913.
4. Blevis, L. S., and Van Patten, H. T.: Hernia through the foramen of Winslow, Canad. Med. Ass. J. **88**:89, 1963.
5. Braunstein, H.: Congenital defect of gastric musculature with spontaneous perforation; report of five cases, J. Pediat. **44**:55, 1954.
6. Cimmino, C. V.: Lesser sac hernia via the foramen of Winslow, Radiology **60**:57, 1958.
7. Cimmino, C. V., and Sholes, D. M., Jr.: Gas in the lesser sac in perforated peptic ulcer, Amer. J. Roentgen. **68**:19, 1952.
8. Dardik, H., and Cowen, R.: Herniation of the gallbladder through the epiploic foramen into the lesser sac, Ann. Surg. **165**:644, 1967.
9. Dietz, M. W.: Lesser peritoneal sac abnormalities, Missouri Med. **66**:106, 1969.
10. Erskine, J. M.: Hernia through the foramen of Winslow, Surg. Gynec. Obstet. **125**:1093, 1967.
11. Faegenburg, D., Saperstein, R., Christ, H., and Mishrick, A.: Colon bacillus pneumonia: a complication of lesser sac abscess, Amer. J. Roentgen. **107**:300, 1969.
12. Felson, B.: Gas abscess of the pancreas, J.A.M.A. **163**:637, 1957.
13. Hollenberg, M. S.: Radiographic diagnosis of hernia into lesser peritoneal sac through the foramen of Winslow, Surgery **18**:498, 1945.
14. Khilnani, M. T., Lautkin, A., and Wolf, B. S.: Internal hernia through the foramen of Winslow, J. Mount Sinai Hosp. N. Y. **26**:188, 1959.
15. Kopf, H.: Traumatische Bursa-omentalis "Zyste," Zbl. Chir. **79**:1997, 1953.
16. Lavarde, J., and Chevret, R.: Contribution a l'etude radiologique des occlusions; hernie etranglée de l'hiatus de Winslow, Presse Med. **57**:562, 1949.
17. McLaughlin, J. S.: Giant omental syst; case report with emphasis on radiological diagnosis, Amer. Surg. **30**:125, 1964.
18. Mitchell, G. A. G.: The spread of acute intraperitoneal effusions, Brit. J. Surg. **28**:291, 1940.
19. Morrison, M. C.: Radiological findings in lesser sac effusion, Canad. Med. Ass. J. **52**:474, 1945.
20. Newman, H., and Frische, L. H.: Lesser omental abscess simulating gastric neoplasm; report of a case, Radiology **69**:567, 1957.
21. Osler, W.: The principles and practice of medicine, ed. 8, New York, 1916, D. Appleton and Company.
22. Parker, J. J., and Mikity, V. G.: Radiographic diagnosis of intestinal perforation in early infancy, Calif. Med. **104**:35, 1966.
23. Roberts, P. A. L.: Hernia through the foramen of Winslow, Guy Hosp. Rep. **102**:253, 1953.
24. Samuel, E.: Pancreatic abscess; its radiological features, S. Afr. Med. J. **24**:420, 1950.
25. Smoot, J. L.: Hernia through the foramen of Winslow, Ann. Surg. **136**:1040, 1952.
26. Taveras, J. M., and Golden, R.: Roentgenology of the abdomen. In Golden, R., editor: Diagnostic roentgenology, Baltimore, 1961, The Williams & Wilkins Co.
27. Vargas, L. L., Levin, S. M., and Santulli, T. V.: Rupture of stomach in newborn infant, Surg. Gynec. Obstet. **101**:417, 1955.
28. Vint, W. A.: Herniation of the gallbladder through the epiploic foramen into the lesser sac: radiologic diagnosis, Radiology **86**:1035, 1966.
29. Walker, L. A., and Weens, H. S.: Radiological observations on the lesser peritoneal sac, Radiology **80**:727, 1963.

Part VIII

The liver and the biliary tract

Pathology of the gallbladder and bile ducts | 46

Harlan J. Spjut
Antonio Navarrete

ANOMALIES

Anomalies of the gallbladder may vary from complete absence to septate duplication to complete duplication. Duplications are important usually only in the face of acquired disease. Rarely heterotopic gastric mucosa is found in the gallbladder or bile ducts.[17]

ROKITANSKY-ASCHOFF SINUSES

A common abnormality of the gallbladder is Rokitansky-Aschoff sinuses. These sinuses represent outpouchings of the mucosa into or through the muscularis. When present there is associated generalized adenomyomatosis, cholecystitis and frequently lithiasis. Occasionally, the sinuses are visible roentgenographically.[8]

CHOLELITHIASIS

Ten percent to 20% of gallstones contain enough calcium to be radiopaque. Stones may be classified as (1) pure—cholesterol, calcium, or bile pigments; (2) mixed—a mixture of cholesterol, calcium bilirubinate, and, rarely, calcium carbonate; and (3) combined—a shell of mixed stone with a center of cholesterol. Mixed stones comprise about 80% of all gallstones.[14]

Several factors have been related to the formation of stones: bile stasis, infection, metabolic defect, and hemolytic disorders. Recently an alteration of the plasma membrane of the bile canaliculus has been proposed as important in stone formation. It is suggested that there is an increase in the amount of cholesterol passing through the membrane. Another possibility is an alteration of the cholesterol-phospholipid ratio, again at the plasma membrane level.[2]

CHOLECYSTITIS

With either acute or chronic cholecystitis approximately 90% of the resected gallbladders contain stones. Acute cholecystitis is often engrafted upon chronic cholecystitis. In the acute disease suppuration and edema may greatly thicken the wall. This may progress to extensive necrosis of the gallbladder wall or gangrenous cholecystitis. Perforation of the acutely inflamed gallbladder is still an important cause of mortality.

Much of the alteration of the gallbladder in the chronic disease is caused by fibrosis that thickens the wall. The mucosa is flattened and Rokitansky-Aschoff sinuses are usually present.

It should be remembered that acute and chronic cholecystitis as well as lithiasis may occur in childhood.[6]

NEOPLASTIC DISEASES

Benign neoplasms of the gallbladder are uncommon. Among those that may be detected roentgenographically are the papillomas, the sessile adenomas, and the adenomyoma.

Seldom is carcinoma of the gallbladder diagnosed preoperatively. First, it is an uncommon lesion (0.4% to 4.6% of biliary tract operations), and second, there are no specific symptoms. However, in patients in their 70s who have biliary tract disease about 10% have a neoplasm in the biliary tract. Thus, such patients should be given careful examinations.

Most carcinomas of the gallbladder are adenocarcinomas, with a few epidermoid carcinomas and mixed adenocarcinoma-epidermoid carcinomas. The tumors may be papillary, nodular, or diffusely infiltrative. The carcinomas directly invade the liver and contiguous structures. Metastasis to regional lymph nodes is common. The disease is advanced by the time a diagnosis is made. For all practical purposes, the survivors of gallbladder carcinoma are those in whom the lesion is discovered incidentally in a cholecystectomy specimen.[5]

SCLEROSING CHOLANGITIS

The cause of sclerosing cholangitis is unknown; however, infection is considered as the major etiologic possibility. The disease occurs more frequently in males than females, and the ages range from 21 to 67 years. It is not necessarily associated with gallbladder or liver disease although either or both may be present. Grossly, the entire duct system or just the common duct may be involved. The lesion has been described as being cordlike, stenotic, thick-walled, or even nodular. Calculi are usually not present in the ducts. Microscopically, there is chronic inflammation and fibrosis of the submucosa, and the other layers of the ducts with the mucosa usually remaining intact. Recently a relationship between sclerosing cholangitis and Reidel's struma and fibrous retroperitonitis has been described.[1,16]

CHOLEDOCHAL CYST

Cystic dilatation of the common duct (choledochal cyst) has been seen in all ages although the lesion seems to dominate in children and young adults; it is more frequent in females than in males. The lesion is considered to be a congenital malformation and occurs most often in the lower biliary tree. The size is variable, but it may become large enough to displace the stomach. Four types have been described: (1) cystic dilatation of the common duct, (2) diverticulum of the common duct, (3) dilatation of the intraduodenal portion of the common duct, and (4) multiple cystic alterations of the intrahepatic and extrahepatic ducts. The first of the four types comprises 88% of choledochal cysts. Histologically, the cyst wall consists of fibrous tissue with a few smooth muscle fibers. The inner surface is bile stained, and only rarely is epithelium identified. The wall may be calcified.[11]

Patients with choledochal cysts often have an abdominal mass and jaundice and are operated upon for these findings. Rarely an adenocarcinoma will arise in a choledochal cyst. Two were reported by Macfarlane and Glenn[12]; they occurred in women ages 65 and 28.

BENIGN AND MALIGNANT TUMORS

Papillomas of the papilla or of the common duct in addition to causing obstruction of the biliary tree may protrude into the duodenum and present a defect when viewed roentgenographically. The lesions may be rounded, soft, and papillary; histologically, they are benign, epithelial papillary lesions that may be cystic.[3] The ampulla may be obstructed by inflammation of the papilla (papillitis) as described by Nardi and Acosta.[13] In addition, obstruction has been associated with polypoid hyperplasia and inflammation of the duodenum in the vicinity of the papilla.[7]

Carcinoma of the biliary duct system may involve the cystic, hepatic, or common duct with the lesions being most frequent in the common hepatic and common bile ducts. Grossly, the carcinomas often infiltrate the duct wall and invade the surrounding tissues and viscera. The surfaces, when viewed, may have a granular or lobate appearance. Some of the lesions may be soft and papillary. Histologically, the carcinomas are fairly well-differentiated adenocarcinomas with an occasional one having a squamous component. The lesions may be dominantly papillary in their histologic configuration. More than one half of the carcinomas in the lower duct system will have spread beyond the ducts at time of operation.[9,15] The prognosis of carcinomas of the extrahepatic ducts is poor (1.6% 5-year survival) in contrast to carcinoma of the papilla of Vater. In the latter the 5-year survival is 39%.

Carcinomas located at the bifurcation of the main hepatic ducts have a slightly different life history than would be expected for a lesion in an area that makes its resection difficult, if not impossible. Even in those cases that are not resected, patients may live with the disease for many months. Grossly, the tumors are usually firm, well localized, and apparently slow growing. They may be present in the duct system as intramural tumors that are annular or occasionally bulky and friable. Microscopically, they are well-differentiated adenocarcinomas often with a major fibrous component.[10]

Rarely, a mesenchymal tumor arises in the bile ducts. Sarcoma botryoides (embryonal rhabdomyosarcoma) may arise in the common duct and greatly distend and obstruct the duct. The few patients who have had this tumor have fared poorly.[4]

REFERENCES

1. Bartholomew, L. G., Cain, J. C., Woolner, L. B., Utz, D. C., and Ferris, D. O.: Sclerosing cholangitis, New Eng. J. Med. **269**:8, 1963.
2. Bouchier, I. A. D.: Gallstone formation, Lancet **1**:711, 1971.
3. Cattell, R. B., Braasch, J. W., and Kahn, F.: Polypoid epithelial tumors of the bile ducts, New Eng. J. Med. **266**:57, 1962.
4. Davis, G. L., Kissane, J. M., and Ishak, K. G.: Embryonal rhabdomyosarcoma (sarcoma botryoides) of the biliary tree, Cancer **24**:333, 1969.
5. Frank, S. A., and Spjut, H. J.: Inapparent carcinoma of the gallbladder, Amer. Surg. **33**:367, 1967.
6. Glenn, F., and Hill, M. R., Jr.: Primary gallbladder disease in children, Ann. Surg. **139**:302, 1954.
7. Griffen, W. O., Jr., Schaefer, J. W., Schindler, S., Hyde, G., and Bryant, L. R.: Ampullary obstruction by benign duodenal polyps, Arch. Surg. **97**:444, 1968.
8. Halpert, B.: Significance of the Rokitansky-Aschoff sinuses, Amer. J. Gastroent. **35**:534, 1961.
9. Jordon, G. L., Jr., and Simons, B. E.: Carcinoma of the ampulla of Vater, Texas Med. **66**:70, 1970.
10. Klatskin, G.: Adenocarcinoma of the hepatic duct at its bifurcation within the porta hepatis, Amer. J. Med. **38**:241, 1965.
11. Lee, S. S., Min, P. C., Kim, G. S., and Hong, P. W.: Choledochal cyst; a report of nine cases and review of the literature, Arch. Surg. **99**:19, 1969.
12. Macfarlane, J. R., and Glenn, F.: Carcinoma in choledochal cyst, J.A.M.A. **202**:1003, 1967.
13. Nardi, G. L., and Acosta, J. M.: Papillitis as a cause of pancreatitis and abdominal pain, Ann. Surg. **164**:611, 1966.
14. Rains, A. J. H.: Gallstones, Ann. Roy. Coll. Surg. Eng. **29**:85, 1961.
15. Van Heerden, J. A., Judd, E. S., and Dockerty, M. B.: Carcinoma of the extrahepatic bile ducts, Amer. J. Surg. **113**:49, 1967.
16. Warren, K. W., Athanassiades, S., and Monge, J. I.: Primary sclerosing cholangitis, Amer. J. Surg. **111**:23, 1966.
17. Welling, R. E., Krause, R. J., and Alamin, K.: Heterotopic gastric mucosa in the common bile duct, Arch. Surg. **101**:626, 1970.

47 | Roentgenology of the liver and bile ducts

Arthur R. Clemett

The liver, in a sense, is a sponge with an intricate skeleton composed of blood vessels, bile ducts, and lymphatics. Precise diagnosis of many liver diseases is possible because roentgenologic techniques permit opacification of hepatic arteries, portal veins, hepatic veins, bile ducts, and even hepatic lymphatics under certain circumstances. Gross alterations of liver size and shape are evident on plain films and conventional gastrointestinal studies. Radioisotope scanning provides more precise definition of contour and readily demonstrates defects of structure even though this technique lacks the resolution of special roentgenographic methods.

The various roentgenologic procedures should be regarded as complementary rather than competitive, for not only should the proper combination of examinations yield the diagnosis but also the result of one examination may aid in interpretation of another study (Fig. 47-1).[28,70,190]

The internal architecture of the liver is segmental,[158] quite analogous to that of the lung, and basic knowledge of this anatomy is sometimes essential for accurate diagnosis of diseases of the liver and bile ducts. Hepatic arteries, portal vein branches, and bile ducts follow the segmental pattern (Fig. 47-2), but the hepatic veins have an arrangement unrelated to the segmental distribution. The major hepatic veins are the right, middle, and left, but numerous variations and supplemental veins may be encountered.[54]

CONGENITAL LESIONS

Anomalies of the liver and biliary atresia are described in Chapter 57. Most diseases considered here are clearly congenital, but classification of some is arbitrary, since the cause is uncertain.

Biliary hypoplasia

Biliary hypoplasia, a poorly understood condition, is probably related to so-called intrahepatic biliary atresia.[19] The cause is unknown. Destruc-

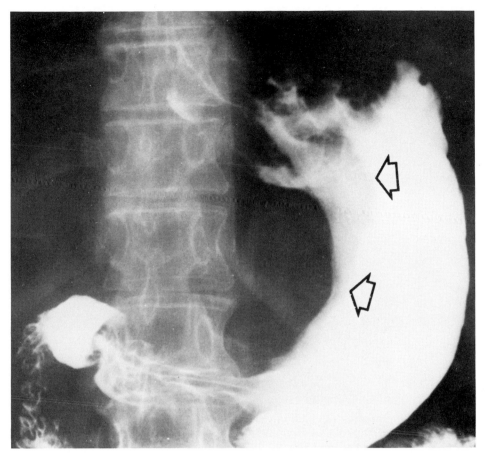

Fig. 47-1. Liver abscess of the left lobe that causes the extrinsic pressure defect on the stomach characteristic of left lobe enlargement.

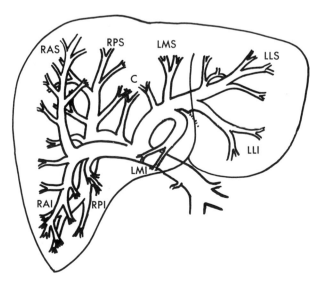

Fig. 47-2. Diagram of segmental anatomy of intrahepatic portal veins. The right and left lobes are divided by a plane extending from the gallbladder fossa to the inferior vena cava. **RAS,** Right anterior superior; **RAI,** right anterior inferior; **RPS,** right posterior superior; **RPI,** right posterior inferior; **LMS,** left medial superior; **LMI,** left medial inferior (the quadrate lobe in classical anatomy); **LLS,** left lateral superior; **LLI,** left lateral inferior; **C,** Caudate lobe.

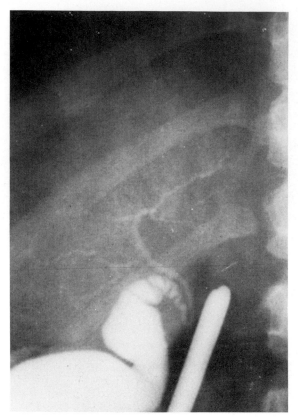

Fig. 47-3. Biliary hypoplasia in a 7-year-old child. Operative cholangiogram with clamp on common bile duct shows reflux into the diminutive intrahepatic ducts.

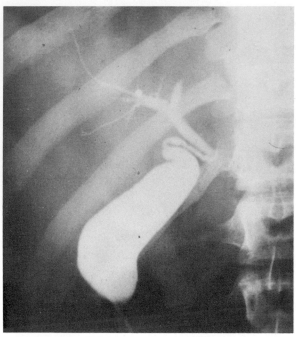

Fig. 47-4. Benign recurrent cholestasis in a 16-year-old patient. Operative cholangiogram with pressure on common duct shows normal common hepatic duct with narrowing and attenuation of intrahepatic tributaries.

tion of the duct system by inflammation and bile stasis has been suggested as the cause, along with primary dysplasia.[86] This entity raises the question of a real difference between what is termed "neonatal hepatitis" and "intrahepatic biliary atresia."

In its severe form the extrahepatic duct system may be hypoplastic, but the characteristic anatomic finding is a hypoplastic intrahepatic duct system. The ducts are diminutive and sometimes fibrotic.[137] The pathologic anatomy is evident on the operative cholangiogram (Fig. 47-3). Intralobular bile ducts are diminished in number on liver biopsy[203] or even absent in some samples obtained.[179] Cholestasis is frequent, and inflammation and fibrosis may vary from none[179] to severe.[73] The clinical course is quite variable. Jaundice is often intermittent but may be absent in some patients and severe in others. The prognosis is generally more favorable than in biliary atresia. Long survival with good health is pos-

sible if the complications of secondary biliary cirrhosis and portal hypertension do not occur.

Benign recurrent cholestasis

The cause of benign recurrent cholestasis is unknown, but it is included here because of the many similarities to the biliary hypoplasia of children. Most of the reported cases have been in adults, but by history the onset of recurrent episodes of jaundice is often in childhood and a congenital basis has been suggested.[197] All known causes of cholestasis have been excluded in the cases reported. Cholangiograms have been reported as normal,[218] but review of several of the original films has shown attenuation of the intrahepatic bile ducts to be a consistent feature of the disease (Fig. 47-4). In addition to cholestasis, liver biopsy specimens show diminished numbers of small bile ducts.[123] As the name implies, the clinical course of the disease is quite mild.

Bile duct variations

The segmental anatomy of the bile ducts is schematically illustrated in Fig. 47-5. A number of variations may occur in the junctional arrangement of the segmental or divisional ducts (Fig. 47-6). Knowledge of the segmental anatomy of the bile ducts and these variations is vital to both surgeon and radiologist[207] in order to avoid the biliary fistula that occurs with accidental transection of aberrant ducts.[221]

Congenital diaphragm of the common hepatic duct

Very few cases of congenital diaphragm of the common hepatic duct have been reported. Histologically, these thin webs or diaphragms may have a structure similar in all respects to the common hepatic duct wall[154] or may be fibrous with isolated areas of cartilage, large nerves, and vascular channels.[65] There is no doubt of the congenital nature of this lesion; but, curiously, clinical manifestations appear late, from the second to the fifth decade of life in reported cases. Partial obstruction and a weblike defect in the common hepatic duct are the characteristic roentgenologic features (Fig. 47-7). Bile stasis, stone formation, and secondary biliary cirrhosis are the complications that eventually cause clinical symptoms.

Congenital bronchobiliary fistula

Congenital bronchobiliary fistula is probably the result of union of an anomalous bronchial bud with an anomalous bile duct bud in the 5- to 6-week-old embryo or a foregut duplication extending from the laryngotracheal outgrowth to the hepatic diverticulum of the 6- to 7-week-old embryo. The condition is very rare. The fistulas originate at or near the carina and usually terminate at the level of left hepatic duct. In addition to respiratory and bile duct epithelium, the fistula may contain esophageal mucosa.[215]

Clinically, cough productive of yellow or green sputum is present from the first days of life, and signs of atelectasis or pneumonia appear. Diagnosis is made by endoscopy, bronchography, or cholecystocholangiography.[61] Successful surgical excision of the fistula is curative.

Choledochal cyst

Choledochal cyst is the most common congenital lesion of the bile ducts, with over 600 cases having been reported.[89] About one case per year may be encountered in large medical

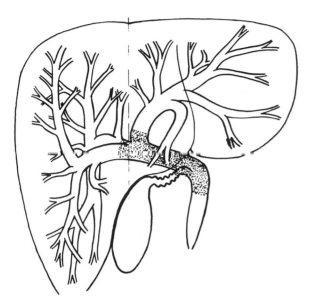

Fig. 47-5. Segmental anatomy of bile ducts. Shaded portion indicates area in which numerous variations in junctional arrangement occur.

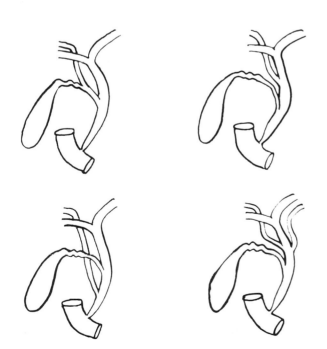

Fig. 47-6. Some bile duct variations as determined in 400 consecutive biliary operations.[88]

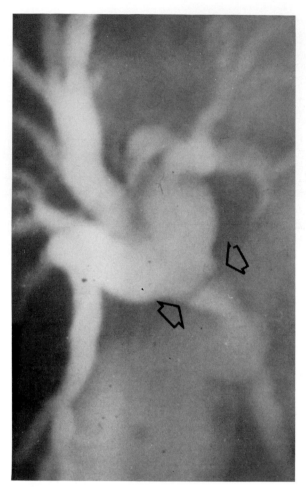

Fig. 47-7. Congenital diaphragm of common hepatic duct in a 41-year-old patient (arrows). (Courtesy Dr. Jack Wittenberg.)

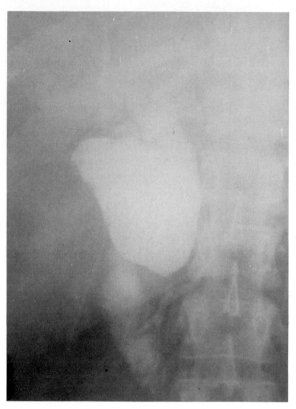

Fig. 47-8. Choledochal cyst in a 26-year-old patient. Operative cholangiogram after cholecystectomy. Note that the distal common duct enters the main pancreatic duct some distance proximal to the duodenal papilla.

centers.[88,131] Females are affected four times as often as males.[131] About half the patients are less than 10 years old.[8,131] It is unusual, however, to find the lesion in infants,[67] and it is rare in newborns, although it has been reported.[235] Many cases occur in young adults and even a few in the aged.

The usual lesion consists of segmental dilatation of the common bile duct and adjacent portions of the common hepatic duct and cystic duct (Fig. 47-8). Separate areas of segmental dilatation of intrahepatic and extrahepatic ducts are rare variants of choledochal cysts.[60,98,103] Diverticulum-like structures, both extrahepatic and intrahepatic, are also included under the classification of choledochal cysts. These comprise about 1% of the reported cases.[8] The so-

called choledochocele involves only the intramural portion of the duct and is lined on both sides with duodenal mucosa.[107,176] It is best regarded as a duplication cyst of the duodenum.[52,176]

Clinically, the triad of abdominal pain, jaundice, and a right upper quadrant mass is considered classical for choledochal cysts. The manifestations are exceedingly variable, however, and patients may have chronic pain alone or mild jaundice and a mass evident only on careful roentgenologic examination.

A right upper quadrant mass may be present on plain films. The usual finding on gastrointestinal examination is anterior displacement of the second portion of the duodenum by an extrinsic mass. If the right kidney is normal this

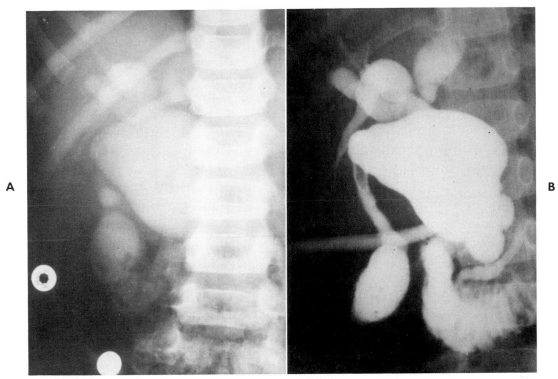

Fig. 47-9. Choledochal cyst in a 7-year-old child. **A,** Intravenous cholangiogram. **B,** Operative cholangiogram. Note that the distal common duct enters the lateral aspect of the main pancreatic duct about 2 cm. proximal to the duodenal papilla.

is almost diagnostic of choledochal cyst. A choledochocele is an intramural mass in the region of the duodenal papilla.[52,107,176] Oral cholecystocholangiography and intravenous cholangiography may opacify choledochal cysts,[35,97,98,103,189] usually in patients with relatively normal liver function tests. Direct cholangiography best demonstrates the extent of the cyst and relationships of the remaining duct system (Fig. 47-9).

Histologically, the cyst wall is usually fibrous without an epithelial lining,[89,114] even in the newborn with choledochal cyst.[235] That the lesion is congenital is a standard statement totally lacking in proof. Theories of pathogenesis include localized spontaneous perforation of the common bile duct,[35] mechanical kinking of the duct with secondary obstruction, valvelike folds, primary weakness of the wall, and primary congenital malformation.[114] The few roentgenologic studies demonstrating the complete anatomy of the duct system have consistently demonstrated an anomaly of the junction of the common duct and the main pancreatic duct (Figs. 47-8 and

47-9).* The common bile duct enters into the lateral aspect of the pancreatic duct some distance proximal to the duodenal papilla. This anomaly, which may be found in the absence of choledochal cyst,[113] precludes a sphincteric mechanism at the common duct–pancreatic duct junction and favors reflux of pancreatic juice into the common duct because pancreatic duct pressure exceeds common duct pressure.[18] This explains the high amylase content of choledochal cysts[8,18] and suggests that the choledochal cyst is acquired as the result of recurrent localized cholangitis.[18] Other cases tentatively classified as choledochal cyst may be secondary to unrecognized trauma with localized perforation of the duct system or may have been misclassified (Fig. 47-10).

The accepted surgical therapy of choledochal cyst is free anastomosis of the cyst to the intestine, either cyst-duodenostomy or cyst-jejunostomy. The usual complications of the disease include stone formation and recurrent cholangitis,

---

*See references 18, 75, 97, 98, 114, and 189.

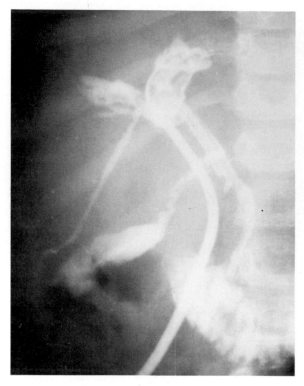

Fig. 47-10. Intrahepatic choledochal cyst (?) in a 4-year-old child. The catheter is in a cystic dilatation of intrahepatic bile ducts. The filling defect is inspissated bile. No obstructing lesion was found. A fibrous wall without epithelium was present on biopsy. Perhaps this lesion should be classified as Caroli's disease.

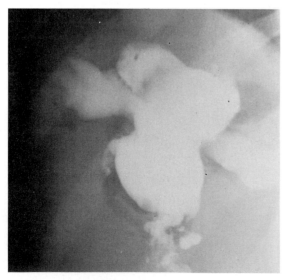

Fig. 47-11. Caroli's disease. Segmental saccular dilatation of intrahepatic bile ducts demonstrated on T tube cholangiogram. (Courtesy Dr. John A. Evans.)

which may in some instances progress to biliary cirrhosis and even to portal hypertension.[67] Perforation causing bile peritonitis may occur.[75,103] There is a significant incidence of bile duct carcinoma in choledochal cyst.[138] Some tumors are present at the time the cyst is first recognized,[15] although others develop months or years after surgical treatment.[226] In contrast to the usual bile duct carcinoma, these tumors tend to be quite aggressive and metastasize early and widely.

Caroli's disease

The cardinal features of "Caroli's disease," or "communicating cavernous ectasia," are segmental saccular dilatation of intrahepatic bile ducts, a predisposition to biliary calculus formation and cholangitis, and absence of cirrhosis or portal hypertension.[164] The disease is familial and may be evident at birth, but most cases of this rare entity are recognized in young adults. The symptoms of abdominal pain and fever are caused by stone formation and cholangitis. The course remains relatively benign until recurrent cholangitis results in liver abscesses, the most common cause of death in these patients.[164] Secondary biliary cirrhosis may also occur.[87]

There may be roentgenologic evidence of liver enlargement and defects in the liver scan can result from the dilated intrahepatic bile ducts. Oral and intravenous cholangiography may reveal stones, but the definitive diagnosis is usually made only by direct cholangiography (Figs. 47-11 and 47-12).[164]

Intrahepatic cystic dilatation of bile ducts has been associated with (extrahepatic) choledochal cyst,[76] and some authors regard it is a variant of choledochal cyst.[138] Caroli's disease, however, is probably a distinctly separate entity. Some reported cases have shown features of congenital hepatic fibrosis[101]; these diseases may be related. In most instances, however, Caroli's disease is readily distinguished on clinical and pathologic grounds. In congenital hepatic fibrosis the communicating cystic malformations involve smaller intrahepatic bile ducts and fibrosis predominates, causing portal hypertension, which is the essential clinical feature of the disease.[78,93,106]

DIFFUSE LIVER DISEASES
Hepatomegaly

Gross hepatomegaly is readily recognized on plain films, supplemented by gastrointestinal

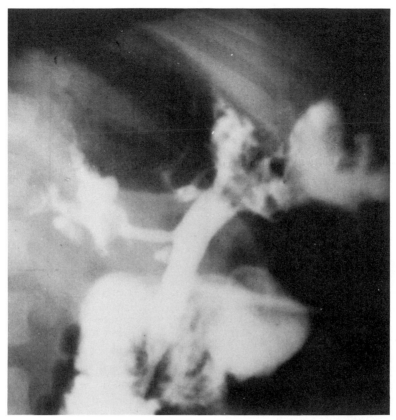

Fig. 47-12. Caroli's disease with stone formation in a 3-year-old child. (Courtesy Dr. Donald Babbitt.)

studies, and may be caused by a large number of diffuse diseases or by one or multiple focal lesions such as abscesses, cysts, or tumors. The diffuse lesions seldom have characteristic appearances on special studies. Scans reveal hepatomegaly with either homogeneous distribution of the radioactivity or irregular, "patchy" uptake. Exceptionally, diffuse infiltrative lesions such as Gaucher's disease may simulate metastatic tumor on liver scan (Fig. 47-13).

With liver enlargement caused by diffuse disease, arteries are stretched and elongated and irregular distribution of contrast may occur in the sinusoidal phase in such diverse conditions as cirrhosis and fatty liver, collagen disease,[6] sarcoidosis,[117] and chronic active hepatitis (Fig. 47-14). These appearances may be quite indistinguishable from multiple small metastases or multiple abscesses.[6] Diffuse infiltrative lesions often cause elongation and narrowing of intrahepatic bile ducts (Fig. 47-15). In some instances associated abnormalities in other organs such as

bone (Fig. 47-16), spleen, lungs, heart, or gastrointestinal tract may provide clues to the nature of the liver disease.

Cirrhosis

Roentgenologic findings in cirrhosis vary with the stage of the disease. The liver may be large, with the features of diffuse hepatomegaly described above. When collapse, contraction, and scarring become prominent, the hepatic artery branches of the affected area become tortuous or "corkscrew" in appearance. Regenerating nodules cause stretching of hepatic artery branches. Contraction of the right lobe with extensive regeneration of the left is a common pattern in cirrhosis (Fig. 47-17), but a dominant regenerating nodule may be found in other locations (Fig. 47-18).

Hepatic veins are relatively delicate structures with meager supporting elements. Cirrhosis causes severe alterations in hepatic vein structure before significantly affecting portal vein

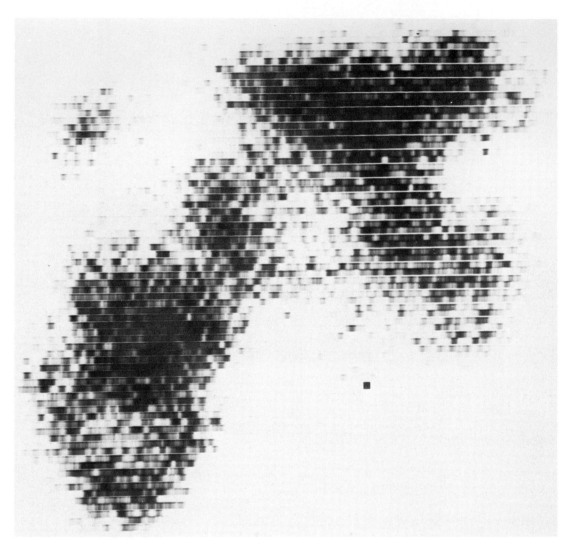

Fig. 47-13. Gaucher's disease in a 36-year-old patient. The defects on liver scan simulate metastatic carcinoma.

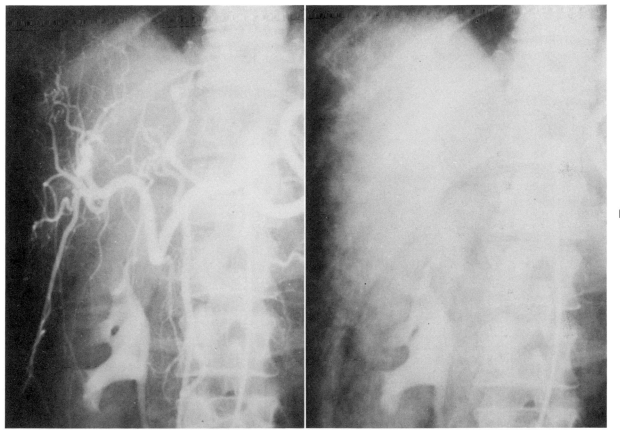

Fig. 47-14. Chronic active hepatitis. **A,** Arterial phase reveals stretching of arteries in the lower portion of the right lobe and tortuous vessels in the upper portion because of some contraction of the liver. **B,** Irregular distribution of contrast in sinusoidal phase.

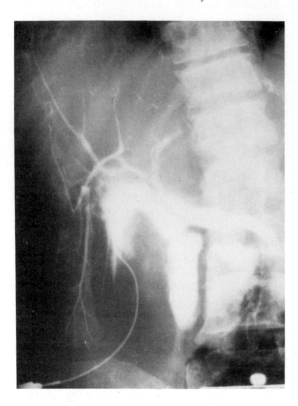

Fig. 47-15. Myelofibrosis with marked hepatomegaly. Percutaneous transhepatic cholangiogram reveals elongated and attenuated intrahepatic ducts and a normal extrahepatic duct system. Hepatomegaly was caused by myeloid metaplasia and passive congestion.

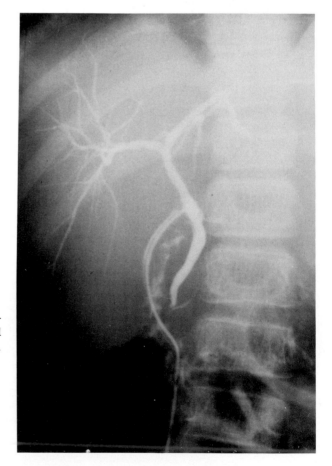

Fig. 47-16. Thalassemia with extramedullary hematopoiesis in the liver. Intrahepatic ducts are elongated and narrowed. Note the changes in the lumbar spine.

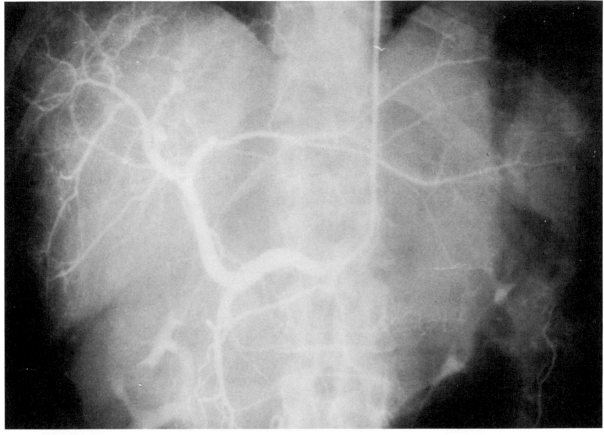

Fig. 47-17. Cirrhosis. The arteries in the right lobe are tortuous and distorted because of contraction, whereas those on the left are elongated and narrowed because of regenerating nodules.

branches. These changes, which may be demonstrated by free and wedged hepatic venography, consist of loss of branching, loss of tapering, and deformity of the veins (Fig. 47-19). These findings have a positive correlation with the severity of progressive cirrhosis.[210] Hepatic venous bed distortion by regenerating nodules is the source of the outflow obstruction in cirrhosis, but the venographic deformities do not necessarily correlate with portal hypertension.[210]

In biliary cirrhosis, diffuse narrowing and diminished branching of intrahepatic bile ducts is frequent.[132] Similar changes occur in Laennec's cirrhosis (Fig. 47-20). The extrahepatic ducts are normal.

Radioisotope scans reveal the size and shape of the cirrhotic liver. Uptake may be homogeneous but is usually irregular or patchy in character. This is caused by scarring, variations in uptake by regenerating nodules, and the con-trast between hepatic parenchyma and vascular spaces (see Fig. 47-21). ^{99m}Tc sulfur colloid scans show increased uptake in spleen and bone marrow compared to the liver,[190] and the relative difference reflects the severity of liver disease.

Hepatic outflow obstruction in cirrhosis causes a rise in hepatic interstitial pressure, which in turn induces an increase in bile flow[134] and hepatic lymph formation. A twofold to one hundredfold increase in thoracic duct flow may be found in cirrhosis. Lymphangiography reveals the thoracic duct diameter, normally 1 to 5 mm., to be increased, and the duct is tortuous.[53,206] Intrahepatic injection of contrast media results in a high incidence of lymphatic visualization in cirrhosis.[38] Lymphatic visualization also occurs frequently in a variety of other primary liver diseases (Fig. 47-22) and in extrahepatic bile duct obstruction. In fact, with

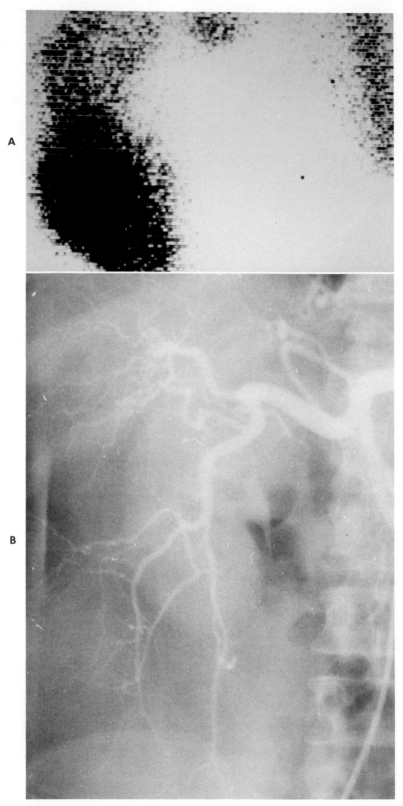

Fig. 47-18. Cirrhosis of the liver with palpable right flank mass. **A,** Liver scan shows increased uptake in the mass and patchy uptake in the remainder of the liver. **B,** Arteriogram identifies the mass as a regenerating nodule in a Reidel's lobe.

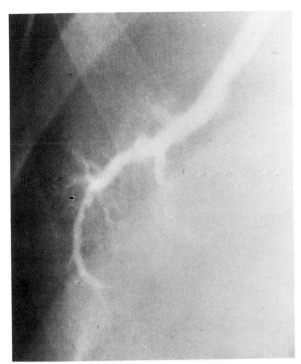

Fig. 47-19. Hepatic venogram in severe cirrhosis, showing marked distortion and deformity of hepatic vein.

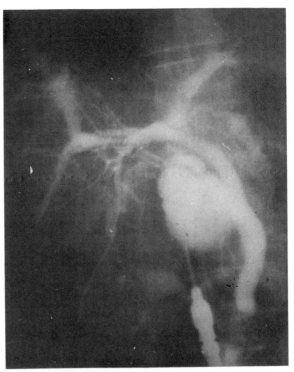

Fig. 47-20. Cirrhosis with jaundice. The extrahepatic duct system is normal, whereas the intrahepatic ducts are elongated and narrowed.

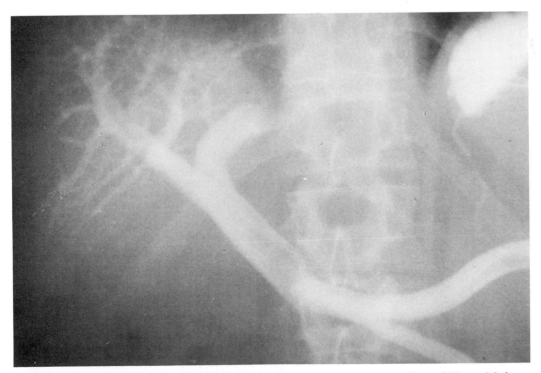

Fig. 47-21. Cirrhosis. Splenoportogram shows contracted right lobe and nonfilling of left lobe because of the effect of gravity.

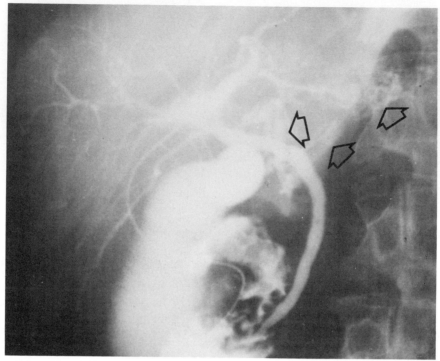

Fig. 47-22. Chronic active hepatitis. Percutaneous cholangiogram excludes bile duct obstruction. There is extensive filling of dilated hepatic lymphatics (arrows).

an injection-withdrawal technique for percutaneous cholangiography, there is lymphatic visualization in over 10% of cases.[41]

VASCULAR DISEASES
Portal hypertension

The hemodynamics of portal hypertension are described in Chapter 53. Cirrhosis, of course, is the major cause of portal hypertension in the United States. Several other entities must be considered in any given case, especially when liver function is relatively normal. These include schistosomiasis,[22,44] portal vein thrombosis, splenic vein thrombosis, hepatic vein obstruction, sarcoidosis,[160] hepatoportal sclerosis, congenital hepatic fibrosis, partial nodular transformation of the liver,[204] hepatic artery–portal vein shunts,[80] cystic fibrosis,[77] and portal vein aneurysm.[94,227]

Budd-Chiari syndrome

The majority of hepatic vein occlusions or obstructions go unnoticed because of the rapid development of collateral circulation. This is often so effective that significant hepatic con-

gestion or hemodynamic alterations do not occur. The clinical features of the less frequent *symptomatic* hepatic vein obstruction, the Budd-Chiari syndrome, depend on the rapidity and extent of the venous obstruction. Hepatomegaly and ascites are the major manifestations. Jaundice is relatively infrequent and often mild when it occurs. In some cases portal hypertension and its consequences are prominent clinical features.

Budd-Chiari syndrome may be caused by thrombosis of hepatic veins or the intrahepatic vena cava, webs or membranes in this part of the cava, venous obstruction by tumors, cysts, or abscesses, and even mechanical derangement secondary to torsion of the liver by diaphragmatic hernia.[39] The cause of hepatic vein thrombosis is unknown in a majority of cases. Specific causes include polycythemia vera,[170] chronic leukemia,[174] hepatic vein invasion by *Aspergillus* in leukemia patients,[249] poisoning by *Senecio* alkaloids,[139] oral contraceptives,[57,214] and trauma. Hepatocarcinoma and metastastic carcinoma are the usual tumors causing the syndrome, but any mass obstructing hepatic

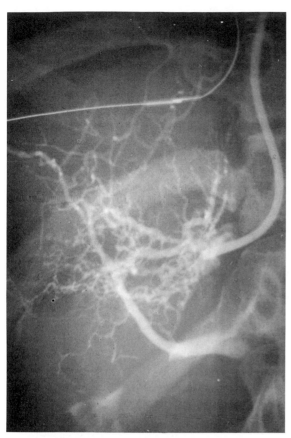

Fig. 47-23. Budd-Chiari syndrome. Injection into a portal vein reveals the "spider's web" pattern and filling of another hepatic vein through collaterals.

venous return can produce this, such as renal carcinoma invading the cava, leiomyosarcoma of the inferior vena cava,[112,213] or right atrial myxoma.[63]

Webs or diaphragms of the intrahepatic vena cava as causes of the Budd-Chiari syndrome are important because they are amenable to surgical cure. They are relatively infrequent in the western world but have been reported to cause one third of the cases of Budd-Chiari syndrome in Japan. The pathogenesis of these lesions is sometimes obscure. Many seem to be congenital, with gradual fibrosis and constriction of the lumen finally leading to symptoms,[196,96] whereas others are clearly secondary to venous thrombosis.[236]

Arterial portography and splenoportography are usually inconclusive in establishing the diag-

nosis of Budd-Chiari syndrome. Inferior vena cavography followed by catheter exploration of the hepatic vein orifices should be done in all cases. Hepatic vein injections may reveal distortion of the veins, strictures, webs, or thrombi. Collateral hepatic venous pathways may be demonstrated. In the "spider's web" network pattern (Fig. 47-23), the vessels do not correspond to any normal hepatic venous pattern, a fact that is considered pathognomonic of the Budd-Chiari syndrome.[126] Intraparenchymal angiography can demonstrate thrombotic, neoplastic, and membranous obstructions of hepatic veins and vena cava.[184]

Hepatoportal sclerosis

Intrahepatic portal vein obstruction in the absence of cirrhosis or other specific causes of portal vein obstruction has been designated by many terms including "hepatoportal sclerosis,"[159] "idiopathic portal hypertension,"[29] "primary portal hypertension,"[223] "noncirrhotic intrahepatic portal hypertension,"[250] "noncirrhotic portal fibrosis,"[29] "intrahepatic portal vein occlusion,"[223] and "obliterative portal venopathy."[167] The disease is not rare. It accounts for up to 16% of cases in some series of patients with portal hypertention,[250] and it seems to be particularly prevalent in India.[29,167]

The liver in hepatoportal sclerosis is typically firm but not nodular. Minor portal tract fibrosis is the rule (Fig. 47-24), fairly extensive fibrosis may be present sometimes, but in other cases architectural changes are subtle and recognized only by irregularity of hepatic vein distribution.[250] There are no regenerating nodules, bile duct proliferation, or necrosis. The fundamental lesion is in the intrahepatic portal veins, and it may have an irregular, patchy distribution. There is subendothelial thickening.[167,250] This suggests organized thrombi in some cases,[29] and recanalized thrombi are clearly evident in other cases (Fig. 47-25).[167,223] Evidence of extrahepatic portal vein abnormalities such as fibrous thickening, calcification, or partial thrombosis is present in about one fifth of cases.[29,250] Speculation as to the cause has included primary phlebosclerosis[159] and intrahepatic pylephlebitis secondary to intra-abdominal sepsis.[29,223]

Clinically, some patients present with splenomegaly only, but all eventually show evidence of portal hypertension. Liver function tests are

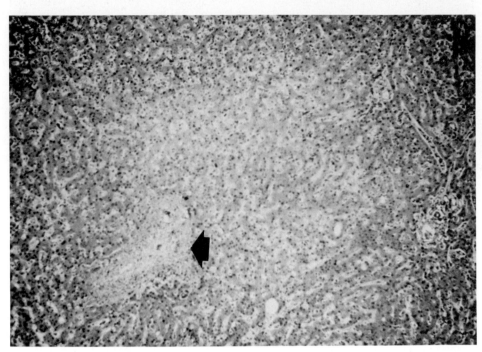

Fig. 47-24. Hepatoportal sclerosis. The liver is relatively normal but there is minimal fibrosis in the portal area (arrow). The vein is occluded by organized thrombus.

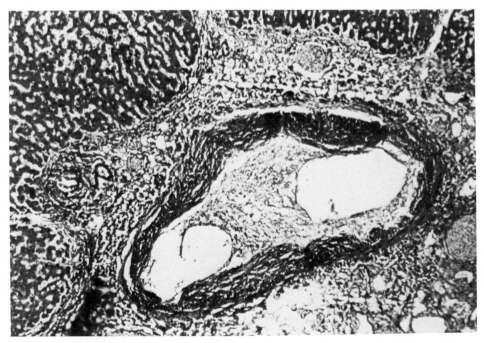

Fig. 47-25. Hepatoportal sclerosis; recanalized thrombus in larger intrahepatic portal vein.

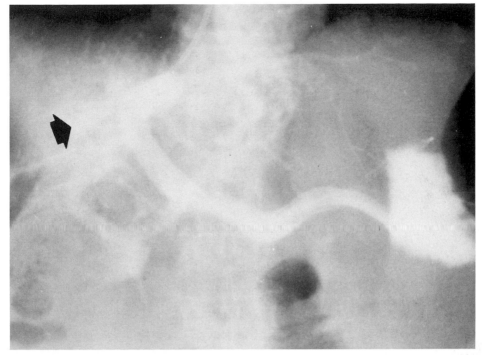

Fig. 47-26. Hepatoportal sclerosis. Splenoportogram reveals evidence of portal hypertension and relatively normal intrahepatic portal vein branches on the left. There is a complete loss of segmental architecture in the right lobe and some large vessels show abrupt truncation (arrow).

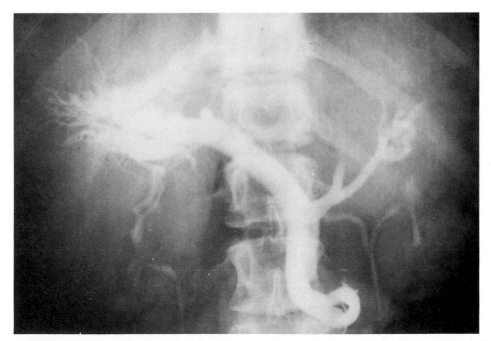

Fig. 47-27. Hepatoportal sclerosis. Operative portogram shows patent extrahepatic portal vein. Splenectomy several years previously accounts for the small splenic vein. The normal segmental anatomy of the intrahepatic portal veins is replaced by a cluster of collateral vessels.

usually normal or only slightly deranged. Hemodynamic studies indicate a presinusoidal obstruction. The differential diagnosis includes other causes of intrahepatic portal vein obstruction—congenital hepatic fibrosis,[93] partial nodular transformation of the liver,[204] sarcoidosis,[160] and schistosomiasis.[44] These patients tolerate portosystemic shunt surgery well and have a much better prognosis than the cirrhotic patient with portal hypertension.[250]

Careful evaluation of the intrahepatic portal vein branches on a technically good splenoportogram should differentiate hepatoportal sclerosis from cirrhosis in most cases, except those in which very small peripheral veins are occluded by thrombi.[223] There is gross irregularity of the intrahepatic portal venous pattern, and large segmental branches may show abrupt truncation by thrombi (Fig. 47-26). In some cases portal vein to portal vein collaterals are prominent (Fig. 47-27). Similar or identical roentgenologic findings have been noted in schistosomiasis[44] and partial nodular transformation of the liver,[204] and theoretically they might also be present in congenital hepatic fibrosis and sarcoidosis.

Hepatic artery aneurysm

Hepatic artery aneurysms are classified as true or false aneurysms. Etiologic factors, listed here in order of frequency,[81] are infection,[6] atherosclerosis,[149] external[42,82] or operative[28] trauma, and specific vascular diseases such as periarteritis nodosa[31,116] or necrotizing angiitis associated with drug abuse.[84] The lesions may also be congenital.

Clinical consequences depend upon the size or rupture of the aneurysm. These lesions may compress the common hepatic or common bile duct and cause jaundice.[149] The vascular lesions in periarteritis can cause hematomas and infarcts of the liver.[31,116] Intraparenchymal rupture with subsequent entry into bile ducts produces hemobilia,[82] sometimes with jaundice. Extrahepatic rupture can result in massive hemobilia or hemoperitoneum,[225] retroperitoneal hemorrhage, or rupture into the duodenum or stomach.[81] Rupture into a portal vein with subsequent hepatic artery–portal vein fistula may be compatible with long survival.[191] Congenital aneurysms with hepatic artery–portal vein fistulas may result in portal hypertension[141] and ascites.[216] One such case caused chronic mesenteric vascular insufficiency and infarction by a combination of portal hypertension and superior mesenteric artery "steal" caused by the shunting.[80]

As in any other aneurysm, calcification does occur but is quite rare.[108] Large aneurysms may reveal themselves by extrinsic pressure on adjacent structures.[33] Accurate diagnosis, of course, depends on angiography.

INCREASED DENSITY OF LIVER

Deposit of sufficient concentrations of elements of high atomic number results in visualization of the liver because of its increased roentgenographic density. Iron, atomic number 26, is probably the most frequent cause of this phenomenon. Excess body burden of iron comes from three sources: (1) increased absorption in hemochromatosis,[64] (2) multiple transfusions in patients with refractory anemias, and (3) increased dietary iron.[110]

In the first form, hemochromatosis, the liver is said to be increased in density while the spleen is not.[64] In transfusional hemosiderosis, the density of the spleen tends to be greater,[202] but there are exceptions (Fig. 47-28). Visualization of the shrunken spleen of sickle cell anemia, of course, is caused by another mechanism.[105] The third form is known as "Bantu siderosis" because it is so prevalent among the South African Bantu.[110] Over 50% of adults are affected. Excessive dietary iron stems from food preparation in iron containers, especially acid-fermented cereals and the native "Kaffir beer." Greater iron losses in women because of menstruation and significantly higher beer consumption by men account for the greater incidence of siderosis in males. Increased density of both liver and spleen is usual in this form of hemosiderosis.[110]

Thallium intoxication has also been reported to cause increased roentgenographic density of the liver.[79] Most cases of thallium poisoning are caused by accidental or suicidal ingestion of rodenticides. The lethal dose is 0.2 to 1.0 gm. Although the concentration of the element per gram of liver is relatively small, the high atomic number of 81 probably accounts for the liver opacification.

Thorium, atomic number 90, is the other principal element causing diffuse liver opacifi-

Fig. 47-28. Transfusional hemosiderosis in a patient with thalassemia. The increased density caused by iron deposition permits visualization of the left lobe of the liver and recognition of ascites by separation of the right lobe from the lateral abdominal wall. The arrows indicate the margins of the right and left lobes.

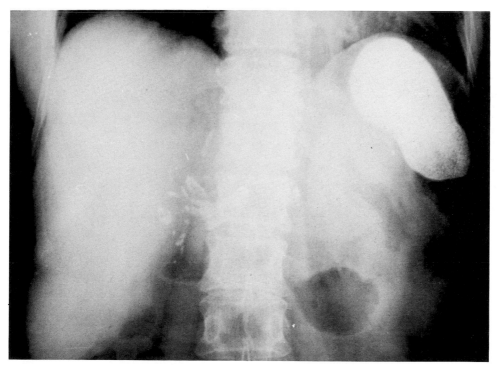

Fig. 47-29. Old thorium dioxide (Thorotrast) injection. There is a reticular pattern in the liver and a stippled pattern in the spleen and regional lymph nodes. The small dense spleen and opacified lymph nodes indicate that injection occurred several years earlier.

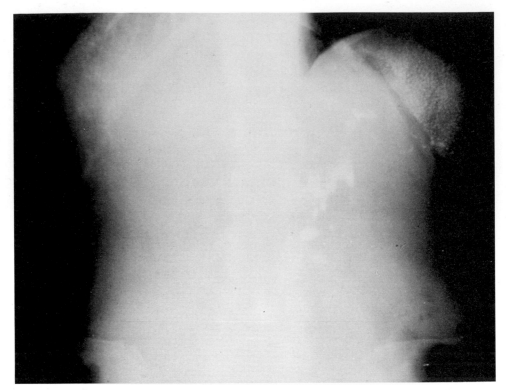

Fig. 47-30. Hemangioendothelial sarcoma 22 years after thorium dioxide injection. Very little residual thorium dioxide is present in the markedly enlarged liver. The opacified lymph nodes are displaced to the left by the large liver tumor.

cation. Following intravascular injection of colloidal thorium dioxide (Thorotrast) about 70% is found in the liver, 30% in the spleen, and the remainder in other tissues, principally bone marrow and abdominal lymph nodes. Thorium dioxide has a reticular pattern in the liver and a stippled appearance in the spleen (Fig. 47-29). The pattern slowly changes with time. Liver density diminishes and spleen density increases, in part because of shrinkage of the liver. Lymph nodes draining these organs become opacified. In patients given thorium dioxide to evaluate therapy of metastatic liver carcinoma, the earliest opacification of lymph nodes was noted 7 months after injection.[222] Thorium dioxide is notorius for causing liver tumors. These develop after a mean latent period of 15 years but some take as long as 30 years.[115] About 50% of these tumors are hemangioendothelial sarcomas (Fig. 47-30), and the remainder are hepatocarcinomas and cholangiocarcinomas.[106]

Table 47-1. Hepatic calcifications

Tuberculosis,[13] histoplasmosis, gumma,[5,45]* brucellosis*
Granulomatosis of childhood
Echinococcal cyst, 33%
Old pyogenic or amebic abscess[45]
Portal venous thromboemboli[24,205]
Hepatic artery aneurysm[108]*
Intrahepatic calculi
Posteclampsia,* capsule of regenerating nodules in cirrhosis*
Congenital cyst[45,144]*
Cavernous hemangioma, 10% of "giant" hemangiomas[3]
Infantile hemangioendothelioma[162,201]
Hepatoblastoma (children), 10% to 20%
Cholangiocellular carcinoma[7,157]
Metastatic tumor
    Mucinous carcinoma of colon, stomach,* breast
    Ovarian carcinoma (psammoma bodies)
    Melanoma,[119]* pleural mesothelioma,[177]* osteosarcoma,[172]*
      adrenal rest tumor,* carcinoid,* leiomyosarcoma.*

*Very rare or single case report.

LIVER CALCIFICATIONS

The causes of liver calcifications are summarized in Table 47-1. Many patterns are typical, for example, the ringlike configuration of cysts and the stippled calcification of mucinous carcinoma metastases. There are exceptions, however, and the pattern of calcification alone seldom permits a confident diagnosis.

INFLAMMATORY LESIONS
Hepatitis

In viral hepatitis roentgenologic findings vary with the stage and severity of the disease. In early hepatitis the liver is enlarged, and patchy uptake on liver scans is caused by scattered areas of necrosis. If the disease progresses to chronic active hepatitis or postnecrotic cirrhosis, some portions of the liver become contracted, with local arterial tortuosity reflecting this event (Fig. 47-14, *A*).

Tuberculosis

The liver is regularly involved in miliary tuberculosis, but localized tuberculosis of the liver is quite rare in the western world, although sporadic cases are reported.[66] It seems relatively frequent in the Philippines, where six to seven cases per year of localized hepatobiliary tuberculosis have been encountered in a single hospital.[13] The disease was twice as frequent in males as females with the peak incidence in the second decade of life. Some patients were jaundiced but fever, weight loss, and hepatomegaly were the principal clinical findings. The liver was often hard and nodular, simulating carcinoma. Hepatic calcifications were present in 48% of these patients and 66% of the patients had concomitant pulmonary tuberculosis.

Chronic granulomatous disease of childhood

Chronic granulomatous disease of childhood is one of the familial polymorphonuclear leukocyte dysfunction syndromes characterized by a defect in microbicidal activity causing prolonged intracellular survival of phagocytized bacteria. Clinically, there is the onset in childhood of recurrent chronic infections, most notably suppurative lymphadenitis, pyoderma, pneumonias, hepatic abscesses, osteomyelitis, and other suppurative infections. Boys are affected most frequently and most severely. Indeed, "fatal granulomatosis of childhood"[30] was originally believed to affect boys exclusively,[36] but it is now known to affect girls as well. The disease in girls is milder. Relative defects in neutrophil function have been demonstrated in some, but not all,[147] asymptomatic mothers of affected boys, and this is consistent with a recessive, sex-linked mode of transmission. The genetic mechanism in girls is less certain.[17]

The pathologic findings are those of chronic infection in which granuloma formation is common and caseation and suppuration do occur. Pulmonary infection is almost invariable, and autopsy studies reveal a high incidence of liver involvement.[36] An additional pathologic feature is infiltration of the reticuloendothelial system with pigmented lipid histiocytes. The infiltration is quite variable in extent and is unrelated to the site of infectious lesions.[36]

Reviews of the roentgenologic features of chronic granulomatous disease have stressed chronic pulmonary infections, hilar lymphadenopathy, pleural effusion, osteomyelitis, and hepatosplenomegaly as the principal findings.[219,248] Liver calcifications (Fig. 47-31) have been present in four of five cases that I have seen,[91] and this feature was the key to the original roentgenologic diagnosis of chronic granulomatous disease in several of these patients. The calcifications may be florid (Fig. 47-32) or rather subtle (Fig. 47-33), particularly early in this chronic disease. Sporadic case reports mention liver calcifications in chronic granulomatous disease,[129,145,169] but these have been curiously absent in the larger series.[219,248] Calcification has also been mentioned in abdominal and cervical lymph nodes, spleen, and pulmonary granulomas.[74] Liver scans reveal decreased uptake in regions of abscesses or granulomatous lesions,[17,169] and angiography has shown the abscesses to be avascular centrally with hypervascularity about the margins.[169]

Liver abscess—pyogenic, amebic, fungal

The mortality of unrecognized and untreated liver abscess is 100%.[12,181] In almost all cases diagnosis is possible with present roentgenologic techniques. Analysis of several large series[12,25,173] reveal that abscesses are multiple in about half of the cases. Most are pyogenic, about 10% amebic, and 1% to 2% fungal. General sepsis causes about 30% of cases and over 40% are secondary to infection in the portal vein drain-

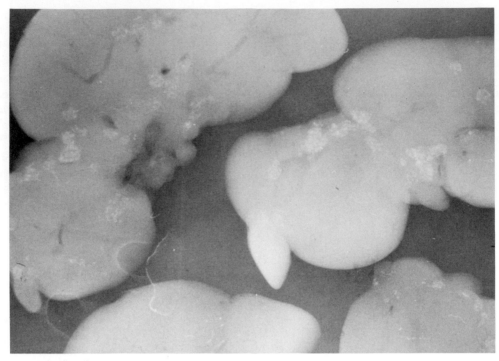

Fig. 47-31. Chronic granulomatous disease of childhood, autopsy specimen. Multiple areas of calcification are present throughout the liver, which is grossly deformed as a result of scarring from the multiple hepatic abscesses.

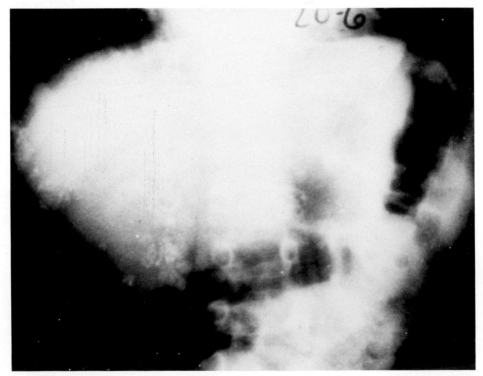

Fig. 47-32. Chronic granulomatous disease of childhood. Dense calcifications can be seen throughout the liver in this 11-year-old boy.

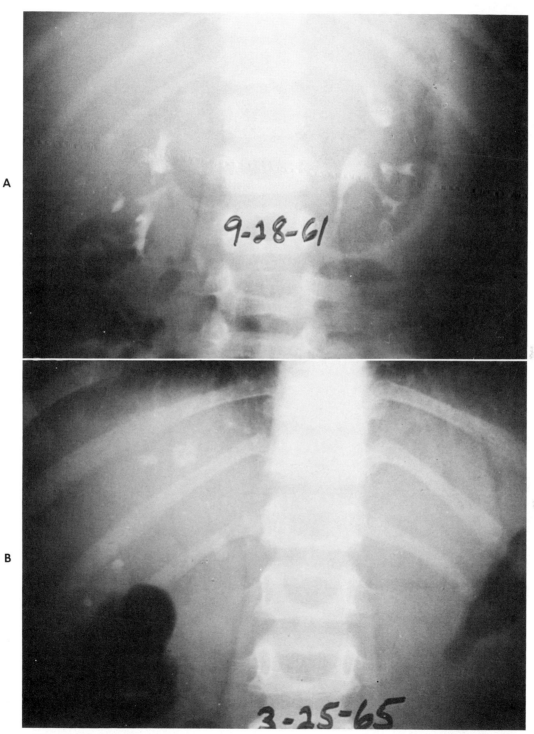

Fig. 47-33. Chronic granulomatous disease of childhood. Faint liver calcifications were originally overlooked in this little girl being evaluated for fever of unknown origin. **A,** Calcifications were clearly evident in September 1961 and had increased in density 4 years later, **B.**

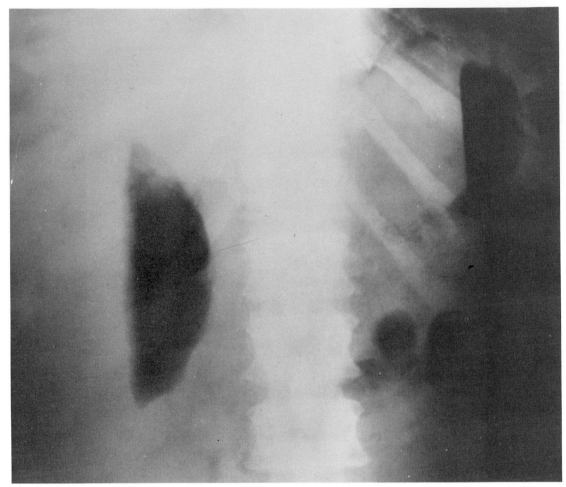

Fig. 47-34. Gas-containing abscess of liver. Taken in right lateral decubitus position. (Courtesy Dr. W. Seaman.)

age area. About 20% are caused by bile duct disease with some element of obstruction. Gallstones are the most common cause here,[59] but some cases are caused by tumor and a few by benign stricture. The remaining cases of liver abscess are caused by direct extension of adjacent inflammatory lesions, infected tumor, or trauma.

Plain film findings include hepatomegaly, loss of the hepatic angle, gallbladder distention, elevation of the right diaphragm, pleural effusion, and right lower lobe atelectasis or infiltration.[198] Identification of gas in the abscess (Fig. 47-34) is a rare event usually asociated with *Klebsiella* infections.[68] Abscesses cause negative defects on liver scans, and arteriography reveals displace-

ment of arteries and avascular defects (Fig. 47-35). There may be a rim of increased vascularity about the margins of the abscess depending on the intensity of the inflammatory reaction here. Arteriography is more sensitive than scanning in detection of small abscesses (Fig. 47-36). Amebic abscesses have the same characteristics as pyogenic lesions.[234] Most patients with amebic liver abscess do *not* have a history of intestinal amebiasis or show clinical and radiologic evidence of this.[193]

Complications of liver abscess include septicemia, rupture into the right subphrenic space, rupture with generalized peritonitis, empyema, and common hepatic duct obstruction.[12] The less frequent lesions of the left lobe can rupture

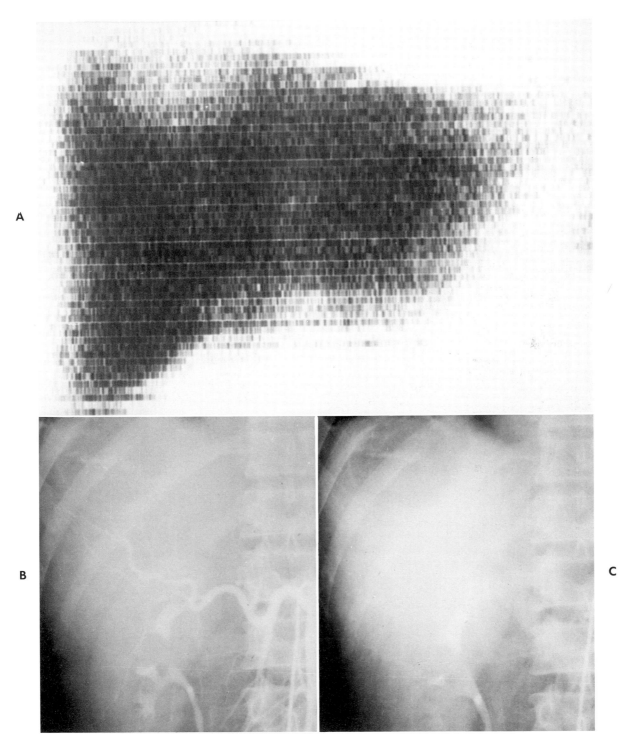

Fig. 47-35. Liver abscess. **A,** Defect high in right lobe of liver. **B,** Arteries are stretched about the lesion. **C,** Negative defect is evident in sinusoidal phase, and there is a rim of increased density at the margins of the lesion.

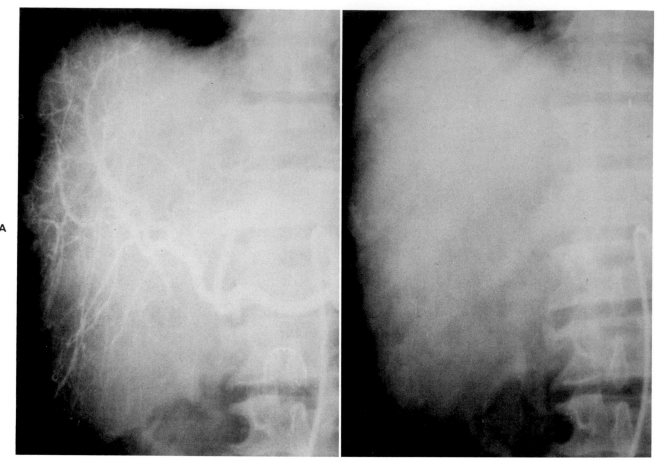

Fig. 47-36. Multiple small liver abscesses. **A,** There is deviation of some smaller arteries. **B,** Small lucent defects are present in the sinusoidal phase. [99m]Tc sulfur colloid scan was negative in this case.

into either pleural space or the pericardium, causing acute cardiac tamponade.[34] Hemobilia secondary to abscess has been recorded, and on the angiogram in this instance there was diffusion of contrast media into the abscess cavity.[232]

Sclerosing cholangitis—primary and secondary

In some cases of long-standing common bile duct stones, the intrahepatic bile ducts proximal to the lesion become narrowed, straightened, and attenuated (Fig. 47-37). This is caused by a secondary sclerosing cholangitis. Primary sclerosing cholangitis is a rare lesion,[156] which, nevertheless, is an important cause of right upper quadrant pain and jaundice. Criteria for diagnosis include generalized thickening and stenosis of extrahepatic and intrahepatic ducts,

absence of calculi and exclusion of previous biliary surgery, primary biliary cirrhosis, and malignancy.[47,99] It has been argued that the presence of calculi should not exclude this diagnosis when the stones are clearly a coincidental finding.[237]

Pathologically, the extrahepatic ducts, and to some extent the intrahepatic ducts, are involved in a diffuse fibrosing process that may be patchy in some cases. The walls of extrahepatic ducts are greatly thickened by the fibrosis and nonspecific inflammatory reaction. The mucosa is usually intact. At operation, there are often adhesions about the foramen of Winslow, edema of tissues in the porta hepatis, hyperplastic lymph nodes, and the common bile duct is thickened and cordlike. Pouting of the mucosa after incision of the duct is sometimes noted.[99]

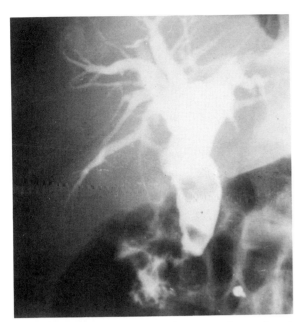

Fig. 47-37. Choledocholithiasis and secondary sclerosing cholangitis. Percutaneous cholangiogram reveals dilated common duct containing many stones and narrowing, straightening, and attenuation of the smaller intrahepatic bile ducts.

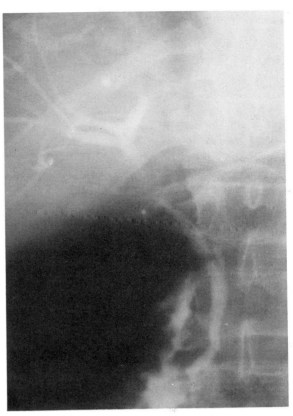

Fig. 47-38. Primary sclerosing cholangitis. There is diffuse narrowing of the intrahepatic and extrahepatic ducts.

Many cases of primary sclerosing cholangitis, perhaps one half, occur in patients with chronic ulcerative colitis.[229,237] Pancreatitis has also been associated.[199] The cause of primary sclerosing cholangitis is unknown; speculation as to causation includes bacterial infection in the portal system and an auto-immune reaction.[47] The latter is further suggested by other associated diseases including regional enteritis,[4,16] retroperitoneal fibrosis,[21] Reidel's struma,[21] follicular lymph node hyperplasia, and orbital pseudotumor.[240] Treatment consists of biliary decompression, where feasible, and corticosteroid therapy. Complete regression of the lesions may occur.[157] The mortality, however, is significant, and some patients develop a secondary biliary cirrhosis. The prognosis, though, is probably better than that of primary biliary cirrhosis.[229]

In primary sclerosing cholangitis, intravenous cholangiography is usually unsuccessful[237] or detail of duct anatomy is inadequate to recognize the lesion.[124] Direct cholangiography reveals either diffuse narrowing of the extrahepatic and intrahepatic ducts or multiple strictures of varying lengths, most often without much proximal dilatation.[127] Percutaneous transhepatic cholangiography usually fails when there is diffuse ductal narrowing (Fig. 47-38) but may succeed when the disease is patchy and focal areas of relative dilatation are present. When there is a single, short, segmental stricture, usually with considerable proximal dilatation, the clinical and pathologic diagnosis of primary sclerosing cholangitis is always suspect, since these cases, with very rare exceptions,[62] are eventually proved to be bile duct carcinomas.[40] Such examples are present in most series of primary sclerosing cholangitis cases.[199,229,237]

PARASITES

Other than amebic abscess, the most important parasitic diseases affecting the liver and bile ducts are schistosomiasis, echinococcal cyst, ascariasis, and infestation by the liver flukes, *Fasciola hepatica* and *Clonorchis sinensis.* Schistosomiasis is an important cause of presinusoidal portal hypertension and has been known to cause bile duct strictures in some instances.[118] The Chinese liver fluke, *Clonorchis sinensis*, resides in the bile ducts. Clonorchiasis is usually a benign disease,[211] but it can cause secondary biliary cirrhosis, cholangitis, and primary choledocholithiasis. The parasite may be visualized at times on direct cholangiography as a linear, curved, or comma-shaped lucency measuring about 2 cm. in length.

Echinococcal cyst

Man is an accidental intermediate host of the dog tapeworm, *Taenia echinococcus*. The embryos reach the body through the gastrointestinal tract and are filtered through the liver and lungs, thus accounting for the more frequent involvement of these organs. Growth of the cyst is slow, often taking years to develop. The more common *Echinococcus granulosus* tends to produce one or a few large cysts, whereas *Echinococcus multilocularis* is more invasive and produces multiple small cysts.[244] The patient's geographic and ethnic origins are importane clues for diagnosis. Eosinophilia is present in some cases. A positive result of Casoni's test usually establishes the diagnosis of echinococcal infection although false-positive and false-negative results do occur.

Radiologic procedures are essential for the preoperative diagnosis of echinococcal disease. The frequency of calcification of the cyst is difficult to determine but seems to be about 33%.[152,244] The cysts produce negative defects on liver scans. Arteriography reveals displacement of arteries (Fig. 47-39) and sharply circumscribed negative defects. A well-defined rim of increased density about the margins of the cyst is a common but not invariable angiographic feature.[20,152,188] This is undoubtly caused by the inflammatory reaction of the host, compression of liver parencyhma, or some combination of these two. Calcification is said to denote an inactive cyst, but this is not strictly true. It is likely, however, that dense calcification and absence of the rim of increased vascularity favor an inactive cyst. Occasionally, cholangiography will demonstrate the cyst communicating with the bile ducts.[231] Such patients may have pain and intermittent jaundice from discharge of scolices and hooklets into the ducts.

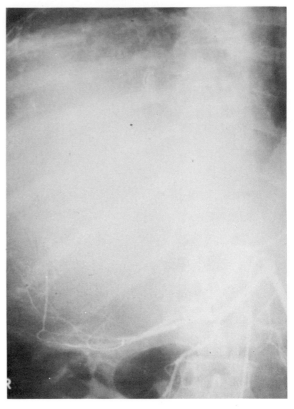

Fig. 47-39. Large cchinococcal cyst in right lobe of liver, with marginal calcification and arterial displacement.

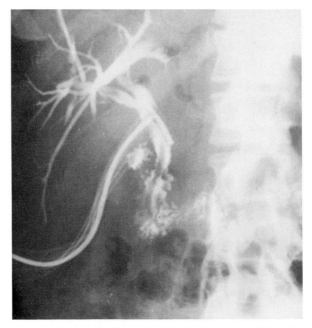

Fig. 47-40. *Ascaris lumbricoides* in common bile duct and second portion of the duodenum.

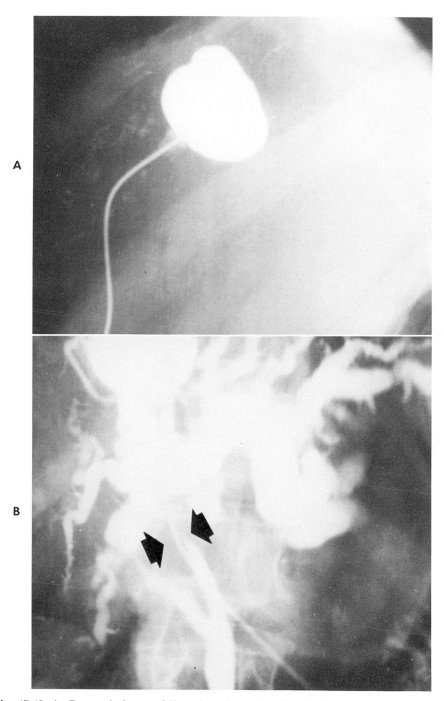

Fig. 47-41. A, Congenital cyst of liver found incidentally during percutaneous cholangiogram. The cyst had no communication with the dilated intrahepatic bile ducts proximal to the scirrhous carcinoma of the common hepatic duct. **B,** Previous cholecystectomy (arrows).

Ascariasis

Invasion of the biliary tract by *Ascaris lumbricoides* does occur, especially with heavy infestation. Adult ascarids may be demonstrated on intravenous cholangiograms[48] and are readily recognized on direct cholangiography (Fig. 47-40). Biliary tract infestation, furthermore, is related to primary intrahepatic calculi. This disease entity is fairly prevalent in the orient[142,241] and in South America.[43] The patients tend to be younger than the usual cholelithiasis population and many have the onset of symptoms in childhood.[43] Heavy *Ascaris* infestation is common, and with careful studies *Ascaris* eggs or immature worms can often be demonstrated as the nidus of the stone.[43] Such cases have been reported in the United States.[185] Investigation for parasitic infestation seems warranted in any case of primary intrahepatic calculi, particularly in youngsters.

LIVER CYSTS
Solitary liver cyst

Solitary liver cysts may be incidental findings (Fig. 47-41) or may be present as a right upper quadrant mass with pressure symptoms. They are said to be four times as frequent in females as males and the right lobe of the liver is involved twice as often as the left.[180] Most are lined by cuboidal epithelium,[144] ciliated epithelium has been noted in some,[49] and other cysts have a fibrous wall without identifiable epithelium.[180] Calcification has been noted in the wall of the cyst histologically[49] and is sometimes evident on abdominal films.[45] Diagnosis has been made by demonstration of a rounded lucent defect on tomograms of the liver following intravenous injection of a large dose of contrast media.

Polycystic disease of liver

Polycystic disease of the liver is rare and generally conceded to be congenital in origin. The cysts originate from bile duct structures and contain clear fluid. The polycystic liver usually develops progressively and is rarely detected in childhood. Exceptions to this generalization are those rare cases in which the disease causes portal hypertension.[200] Polycystic liver disease usually becomes clinically evident in the fourth or fifth decade. This diagnosis should be suspected in the patient with hepatomegaly and multiple defects on liver scan who is clinically well and has normal liver function tests. Angiography will establish the diagnosis by demonstrating displaced arteries and sharply marginated lucent defects in the capillary phase (Fig. 47-42).

About half of the patients also have polycystic kidney disease,[155] and this association should help establish the diagnosis. The reverse is less frequent and only one fourth of the patients with polycystic kidney disease have polycystic liver disease.

Cavernous hemangioma

Cavernous hemangioma is the most common benign liver tumor.[3] Small hemangiomas are often incidental findings on angiography done for other reasons (Fig. 47-43), at surgery, or autopsy. Some are associated with the Rendu-Osler-Weber disease. They may be single or multiple. Some lesions present as large hepatic masses, and calcification occurs in about 10% of these.[3] It has been stated that the calcification is characteristic in type, consisting of trabeculations or spicules of calcium radiating from a central point. This appearance (the description of which bears a striking resemblance to hemangioma of bone) is seldom found in reality. Most reproductions do not reveal any characteristic pattern to the calcifications in liver hemangiomas.[56]

Large hemangiomas produce negative defects on liver scans. Blood pool scanning has been advocated to identify hemangiomas,[69] but it is likely that this will fail in many cases because of the extensive sclerotic component of this lesion. Angiography readily demonstrates the characteristic features of cavernous hemangioma. The feeding vessels tend to be large, arteries are displaced by the tumor mass, and irregular lakes of contrast media are present and persist throughout the examination (Fig. 47-44).[1] The large number of bizarre vascular spaces at times causes confusion with hepatocarcinoma, but the displacement of arteries in hemangioma in contrast to the vessels entering the lesion in hepatoma and the persistence of contrast in the vascular lakes should readily distinguish these lesions in most instances.[151]

The dramatic complication of this lesion is spontaneous rupture with hemoperitoneum, which may be fatal.[163]

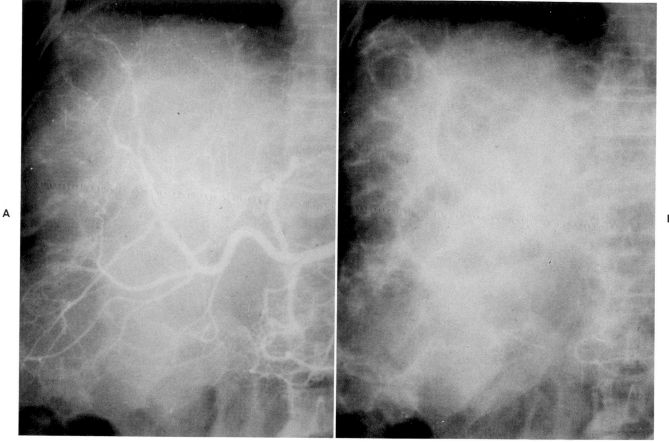

Fig. 47-42. Polycystic disease of liver. **A,** Smaller arteries are displaced by the cyst. **B,** Rounded, smooth defects of varying size are present throughout the liver in the sinusoidal phase.

Infantile hemangioendothelioma

These cellular tumors are also known as capillary hemangiomas of the liver.[230] They are quite rare but may cause hepatomegaly and congestive heart failure in infancy. The high output failure is caused by shunting of blood from hepatic artery to hepatic veins. Calcification may occur in the lesion.[201] Diagnosis is established by angiography. There are large feeding vessels that are stretched and distorted and fail to taper. Fairly dense hepatic vein opacification is a characteristic diagnostic feature (Fig. 47-45).[162]

If shunting is not severe or can be controlled by surgical excision or hepatic artery ligation, spontaneous involution of the tumor is the rule.[51] Some tumors have features of both the cavernous and capillary hemangioma.[23]

Hamartomas

Hamartomas are rather rare benign tumors, which may be composed primarily of bile duct elements, liver cells, lymphatics, vascular elements or a mixture of these.[128] Most hamartomas found in adults contain mixed elements. The patients are usually in good health and have no symptoms caused by the tumor. On arteriography, these lesions may have enlarged, irregular and tortuous feeding vessels.[6,162] A diffuse homogeneous tumor blush is usual, although irregular staining may occur because of the variable tissue components in the tumor. Cystic elements are prominent in some cases (Fig. 47-46), and a defect may be present on liver scan.

The mesenchymal cystic hamartoma of infants and children is usually present as an asymp-

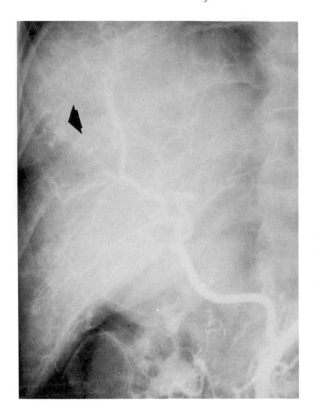

Fig. 47-43. Small hemangioma of liver found incidentally during investigation for colonic bleeding. Patient had a vascular malformation of the right colon. Vascular lakes (arrow) filled during arterial phase and persisted late in the examination.

tomatic abdominal mass.[111] Most of these are avascular on angiography,[169] but some of these lesions may show areas of tumor staining reflecting their cellular and vascular components.[10]

Liver cell adenoma

Lesions in liver cell adenoma are very rare and may be encountered accidentally or cause symptoms by virtue of their size. They may be multiple. The scarce reports of liver scans indicate variable results. Uptake of ^{131}I rose bengal and ^{99m}Tc sulfur colloid were about the same as normal liver in one case,[192] whereas a negative defect was present on an [198]Au scan in another.[175] Angiographic findings include stretching and tortuosity of small arteries, some neovascularity, and diffuse homogeneous staining of the tumor (Fig. 47-47). A reticular pattern of small veins was a prominent feature in one case.[175]

Focal nodular hyperplasia

The many synonyms for this focal nodular hyperplasia indicate its obscure nature. It has been called adenoma, mixed adenoma, benign hepatoma, solitary hyperplastic nodule, focal nodular cirrhosis, solitary cirrhotic liver nodule, cholangiohepatoma, isolated nodule of regenerative hyperplasia, pseudoneoplasm, and focal nodular hyperplasia.[247] This rare lesion of unknown cause occurs mostly in females. It is usually found incidentally at operation or autopsy but occasionally may appear clinically as a relatively asymptomatic upper abdominal mass.[95,143]

Grossly, the typical lesion is a circumscribed, gray-white, subcapsular nodule, with many fibrous trabecular strands tending to divide the lesion into smaller nodules. At operation it is often mistaken for metastatic tumor. Histologically, there is a pseudocapsule and the bulk of the lesion is composed of regenerating liver nodules, with fibrosis in central and portal areas. The latter contain proliferating bile ducts and some lymphocytic infiltration. These features distinguish focal nodular hyperplasia from adenoma of the liver. The histology is similar to that of partial nodular transformation of the liver.[204] This entity, however, is distinctly dif-

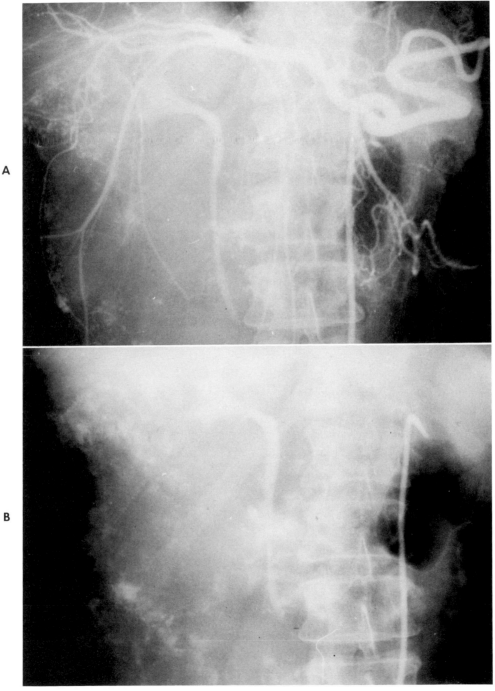

Fig. 47-44. Hemangioma of the liver. **A,** Arteriogram reveals stretching of arteries about the masses and filling of vascular lakes. **B,** These signs persist in the late phase of the examination. (Courtesy Dr. Ray Abrams.)

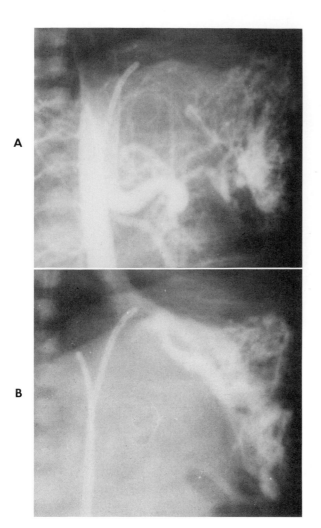

Fig. 47-45. Infantile hemangioendothelioma. A, Aortogram, lateral view. The celiac axis is huge and supplies a vascular liver tumor. B, Hepatic veins draining the tumor are densely opacified on later film. (Courtesy Dr. Ralph Littwin.)

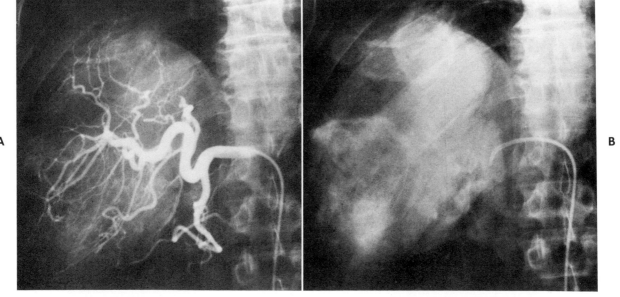

Fig. 47-46. Hamartoma of liver in a 59-year-old man. A, Smaller hepatic arteries are displaced and distorted by tumor mass. B, Later film shows diffuse staining and multiple cystic lesions.

Fig. 47-47. Adenoma of liver. **A,** The feeding vessels are rather tortuous but otherwise unremarkable. **B,** Diffuse homogeneous tumor stain is present later in examination. (Courtesy Dr. R. F. Colapinto.)

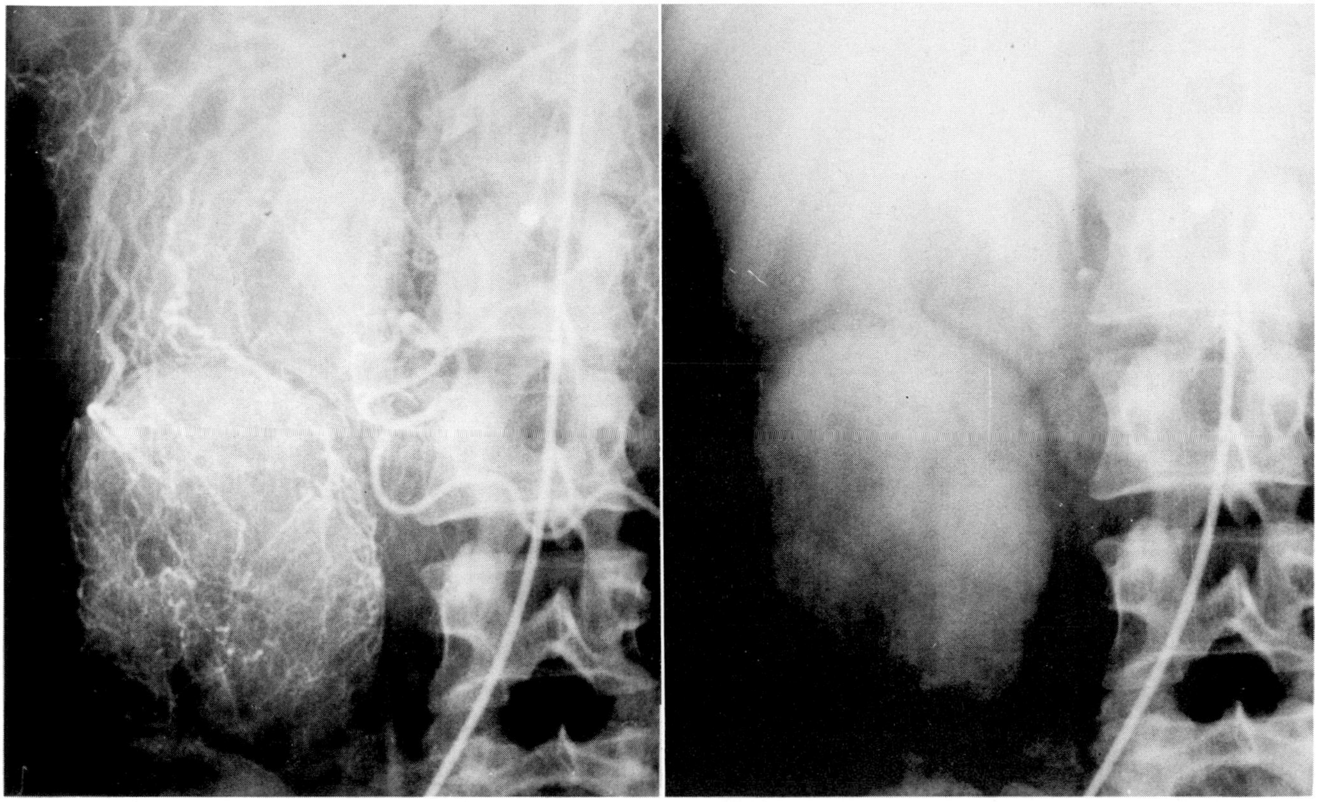

ferent in that the nodules are multiple, centrally located, and encroach upon major portal vein branches causing presinusoidal portal hypertension.

The activity of the nodule on liver scan is probably rather variable. Decreased activity over the lesion has been noted once with ^{131}I rose bengal,[247] but the scan may be rather unremarkable even with a large lesion (Fig. 47-48). On angiography, the feeding vessels are widened and tortuous and there is a diffuse homogeneous tumor stain (Fig. 47-49).[14] The angiographic appearance is identical to that of adenoma and of some hamartomas. The absence of vascular lakes differentiates the lesion from hemangioma. Distinction from hepatocarcinoma may be difficult in some instances.

MALIGNANT LIVER TUMORS

A practical classification of malignant liver tumors is given in Table 47-2.

Hepatocarcinoma

Hepatocarcinoma is much more frequent in Africa and Asia than it is in Europe and North America.[135] About 70% of cases in the United States occur in patients with cirrhosis,[109] but this association is much less frequent in oriental countries.[135] Most patients are adults, but the tumor does occur in children, sometimes in association with biliary atresia and secondary biliary cirrhosis.[171] The major symptoms are right upper quadrant pain and weight loss, but a few patients have bone pain caused by osseous metastases,[109] shock from massive intraperitoneal hemorrhage from the tumor,[100] or obstructive jaundice caused by sloughing of necrotic tumor into the bile ducts.[72]

A large liver, sometimes with obvious irregularity, may be found on plain films. Defects caused by the tumor can be demonstrated on thorium dioxide hepatography,[27] but arteriography and scanning are the two most important

A

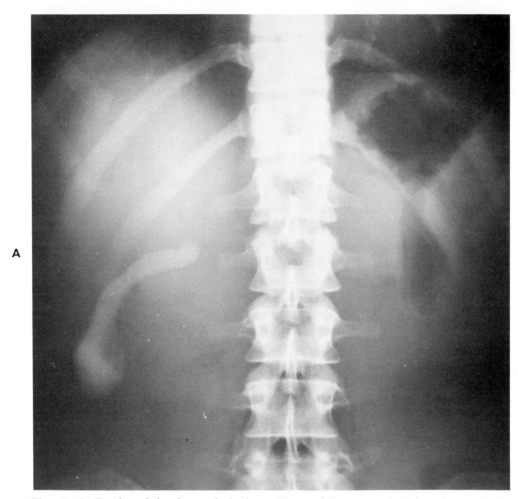

Fig. 47-48. Focal nodular hyperplasia in a 24-year-old woman. **A,** Distortion and deformity of gallbladder by mass in right lobe of liver. **B,** Displacement of feeding vessels and some irregularity of small vessels. **C,** Diffuse homogeneous stain persists late in examination. (Courtesy Dr. Al Crossett.)

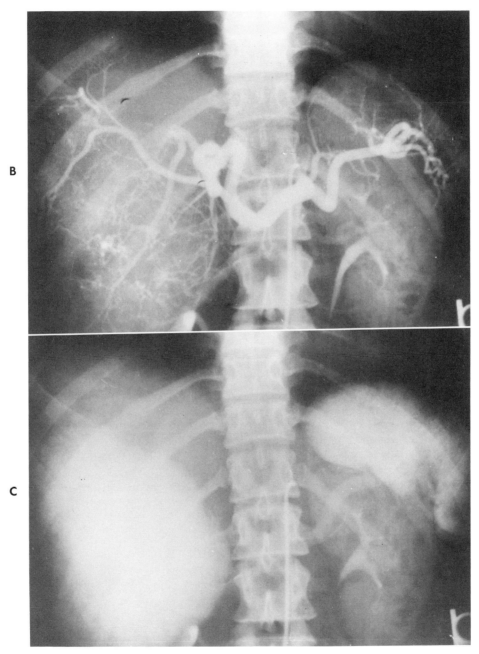

Fig. 47-48, cont'd. For legend see opposite page.

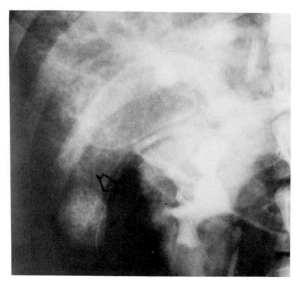

Fig. 47-49. Focal nodular hyperplasia, an incidental finding on arteriography done for other purposes. This late film also shows the wall of the gallbladder.

Table 47-2. Classification of malignant liver tumors

Malignant hepatoma	Approximate relative incidence[46]
Hepato (cellular) carcinoma	75%
Hepatoblastoma	7%
Cholangio (cellular) carcinoma	6%
Mixed hepatocholangiocarcinoma	12%
Primary sarcomas	
Metastatic carcinoma and sarcoma	

diagnostic procedures.[109] On [99mTc] sulfur colloid scans the tumor causes an area of decreased or absent uptake. [67Ga] citrate uptake is increased in most vascular hepatomas and shows equilibrated uptake in the other hepatomas.[220] Uptake of [75Se]-selenomethionine is also increased in hepatocarcinoma.[58] Combinations of radioisotope scans improve diagnostic accuracy but are not specific for hepatocarcinoma because [67Ga] citrate uptake and [75Se]-selenomethionine uptake may also be increased in some metastases, lymphosarcoma, and abscesses.[58,130,220] Exceptional hepatomas may be so well differentiated functionally that there is equilibrated uptake of [131I] rose bengal.[208]

Hepatocarcinomas are very vascular tumors and with angiography show vascular proliferation, tumor staining, and arteriovenous shunting. The hypervascularity is usually massive, involving the entire tumor (Fig. 47-50), but it may be arborescent or basket-like in some cases in which there is displacement of arteries and proliferation of fine vessels at the tumor margins.[121] Angiography also differentiates the three gross forms of hepatocarcinoma—uninodular or diffuse types.[71] Obstruction, deviation, or compression of the portal vein is common in hepatoma (Figs. 47-51 and 47-52, A) and is more likely to occur with hepatocarcinoma than with metastatic tumor.[238] Hepatic vein invasion is also frequent and hepatocarcinoma frequently causes the Budd-Chiari syndrome (Fig. 47-52). Some hepatomas are said to be avascular on angiography,[187] but most of these are either necrotic tumors or examples of mixed hepatocellular-cholangiocellular carcinoma.

Vascular metastases can usually be distinguished from the diffuse form of hepatocarcinoma in the clinical setting. Well-differentiated hepatomas with a more normal vascularity may be difficult to distinguish from some hamartomas, adenomas, and focal nodular hyperplasia. The good health of the latter patients may aid in the distinction. The presence in serum of alpha-fetoglobulin aids in the diagnosis of hepatocarcinoma. This serologic test is positive in 60% to 90% of cases of hepatocarcinoma and is negative in cholangiocarcinoma.[135] It is fairly specific for hepatocarcinoma, but high titers also occur in embryonal tumors and have been noted with metastatic gastric and prostatic carcinoma,[9,125,153] as well as in Indian children with cirrhosis.[168]

Hepatoblastoma

This embryonal tumor may be epithelial in type or contain mixed epithelial and mesodermal elements. It should be distinguished from hepatocarcinoma, which also occurs in children but is less frequent than hepatoblastoma in this age group.[102] The hepatoblastoma, furthermore, occurs in younger children, the usual age range being from birth to 3 years. Calcification of the tumor (Fig. 47-53) is moderately frequent (about 12%) in contrast to hepatocarcinoma in which this does not occur. Angiography reveals tumor neovascularity and tumor staining identical to hepatocarcinoma.[162]

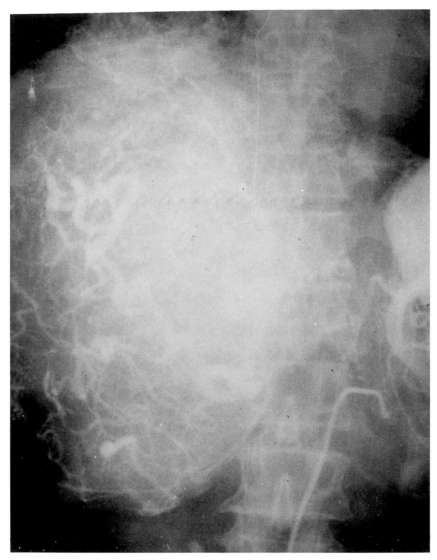

Fig. 47-50. Hepatocarcinoma, multinodular type.

The prognosis is better than with hepatocarcinoma, and about 20% of the hepatoblastomas are curable by surgical resection.[102]

Cholangiocellular carcinoma

"Cholangiocellular carcinoma" is the preferable term for this hepatoma of bile duct origin, since its synonyms, "cholangioma" and "cholangiocarcinoma," have also been used to designate bile duct carcinoma, which is a quite different tumor originating from the larger bile ducts. The cholangiocellular carcinoma usually has a prominent fibrotic component and on angiography is a relatively avascular tumor showing stretched or encased arteries (Fig. 47-54, *A*). If vascular proliferation is present, it is minimal. The intrahepatic bile ducts are also encased or obstructed by the tumor (Fig. 47-54, *B*). Calcification does occur in this tumor and may be recognized on plain films.[7,157]

Sarcomas

Primary sarcomas of the liver are very rare tumors arising from mesodermal elements. The hemangiosarcoma, the malignant counterpart of hemangioendothelioma, has similar angiographic features. These vascular masses have large sinusoidal pools similar to the benign

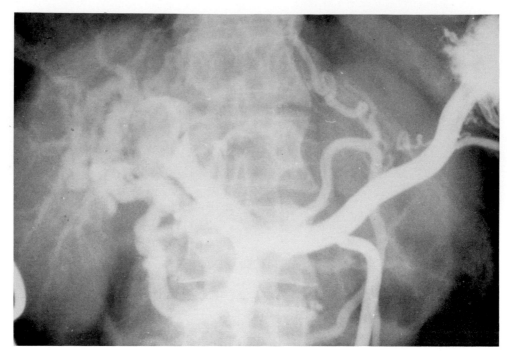

Fig. 47-51. Splenoportogram showing hepatocarcinoma invading and obstructing the portal vein.

tumor but differ in that encasement of arteries may also be present.[162] Primary leiomyosarcoma is a rare lesion that presents with hepatomegaly, shows a defect on liver scan, and rather surprisingly is a relatively avascular lesion on angiography.[246] The hemangioendotheliosarcoma, which may actually arise from Kupffer cells, is usually associated with administration of thorium dioxide and may be recognized as a defect in the reticular pattern of thorium dioxide in the liver.[182] Other primary sarcomas include fibrosarcoma, rhabdomyosarcoma, and malignant mesenchymoma.[182] A case of primary osteosarcoma in a patient with hemochromatosis has been reported in which tumor bone was evident histologically but not seen on x-ray.[148]

Metastatic tumor

This is the most common liver tumor, and metastatic disease may or may not cause hepatomegaly. Displacement and deformity of the gallbladder sometimes identifies the liver masses. Calcification, particularly in mucinous carcinoma, may aid in specific diagnosis. The usual mucinous carcinoma calcification consists of myriads of tiny, punctate densities (Fig. 47-55),

which sometimes defy certain recognition. Exceptionally, the calcification may be dense or cystic in character. Calcification also occurs in other metastatic tumors (Fig. 47-56 and Table 47-1).

If the metastases are large enough they are readily recognized on liver scans. Angiographic findings are variable and generally reflect the arteriographic features of the primary tumor, although tumor necrosis may modify this. The usual vascular metastases are carcinoid (Fig. 47-57), islet cell carcinoma, choriocarcinoma, leiomyosarcoma, and hypernephroma,[178,187] whereas moderate vascularity may be found in seminoma, adrenal carcinoma, endometrial carcinoma, some colon and breast tumors, and rare pancreatic carcinomas.[178] Metastatic carcinoma causes displacement and distortion of bile ducts, obstruction of larger ducts, and nonfilling of smaller peripheral ducts (Fig. 47-58).[133]

BILE DUCT CARCINOMA

Bile duct carcinomas are fairly common; several cases per year may be encountered in large medical centers.[85] There are geographic variations in frequency varying from one bile

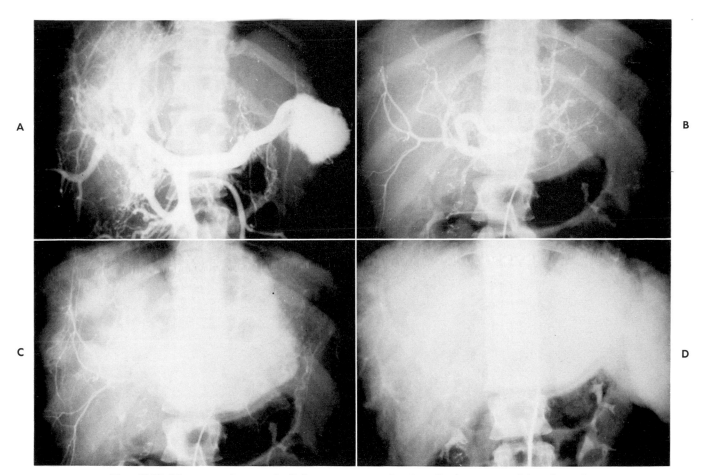

Fig. 47-52. Hepatocarcinoma. **A,** Splenoportogram showing displacement of intrahepatic portal veins and portal hypertension. **B** and **C,** The bulk of the tumor is in the left lobe with multiple nodules in the right lobe of the liver. **D,** Opacification of intrahepatic portal vein branches in the right lobe on late phase caused by development of Budd-Chiari syndrome.

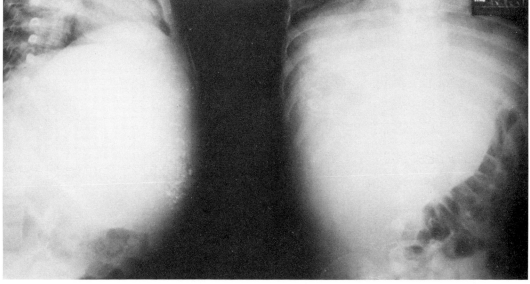

Fig. 47-53. Hepatoblastoma in a 1-year-old infant.

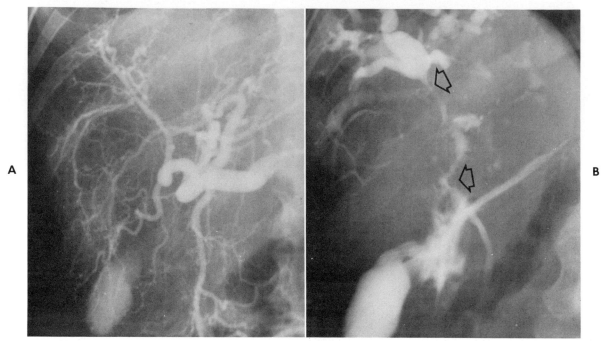

Fig. 47-54. Cholangiocellular carcinoma. **A,** Encasement and distortion of intrahepatic arteries without tumor neovascularity. **B,** Encasement and high-grade obstruction of intrahepatic bile ducts by the large tumor between the arrows. (Courtesy Dr. Barry Held.)

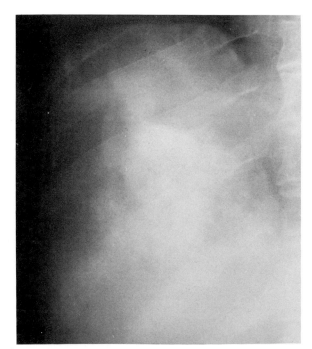

Fig. 47-55. Calcified mucinous carcinoma from the colon.

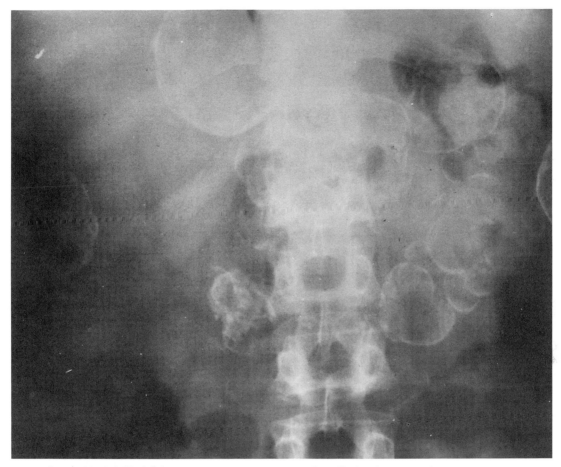

Fig. 47-56. Calcified leiomyosarcoma metastases, primarily in the stomach. (Courtesy Dr. David Inkeles.)

duct carcinoma for every eight pancreatic carcinomas in New Haven, Connecticut,[40] to one bile duct carcinoma for each pancreatic carcinoma in Glasgow, Scotland.[32] These tumors are most frequent in the fifth to eighth decades of life but do occur in younger individuals. There is an association with chronic ulcerative colitis. In one large series of ulcerative colitis patients, 0.7% developed bile duct carcinoma,[186] and the youngest patients (17 years and 22 years) with primary bile duct carcinoma also had chronic ulcerative colitis.[85]

The tumors arise in the larger bile ducts; the site of tumor origin determined from the combined data of two large series[217,233] is as follows:

1. Left or right hepatic duct, 13%
2. Common hepatic duct, 37%
3. Junction of cystic and common hepatic duct, 15%
4. Cystic duct, 6%
5. Common bile duct, 33%

A few tumors are polypoid intraluminal lesions (Fig. 47-59) and some are bulky tumor masses (Fig. 47-60). These types are mainly cellular adenocarcinomas. The most common lesion, however, is the small scirrhous carcinoma (Fig. 47-61).[40,242] These are often well differentiated adenocarcinomas in which the pathologic diagnosis may be difficult because of the normal occurrence of glandular structures in the bile duct wall.

Rarely, oral cholecystocholangiography may demonstrate a bile duct tumor, but oral or intravenous methods are likely to fail because of nonvisualization or poor detail when visualiza-

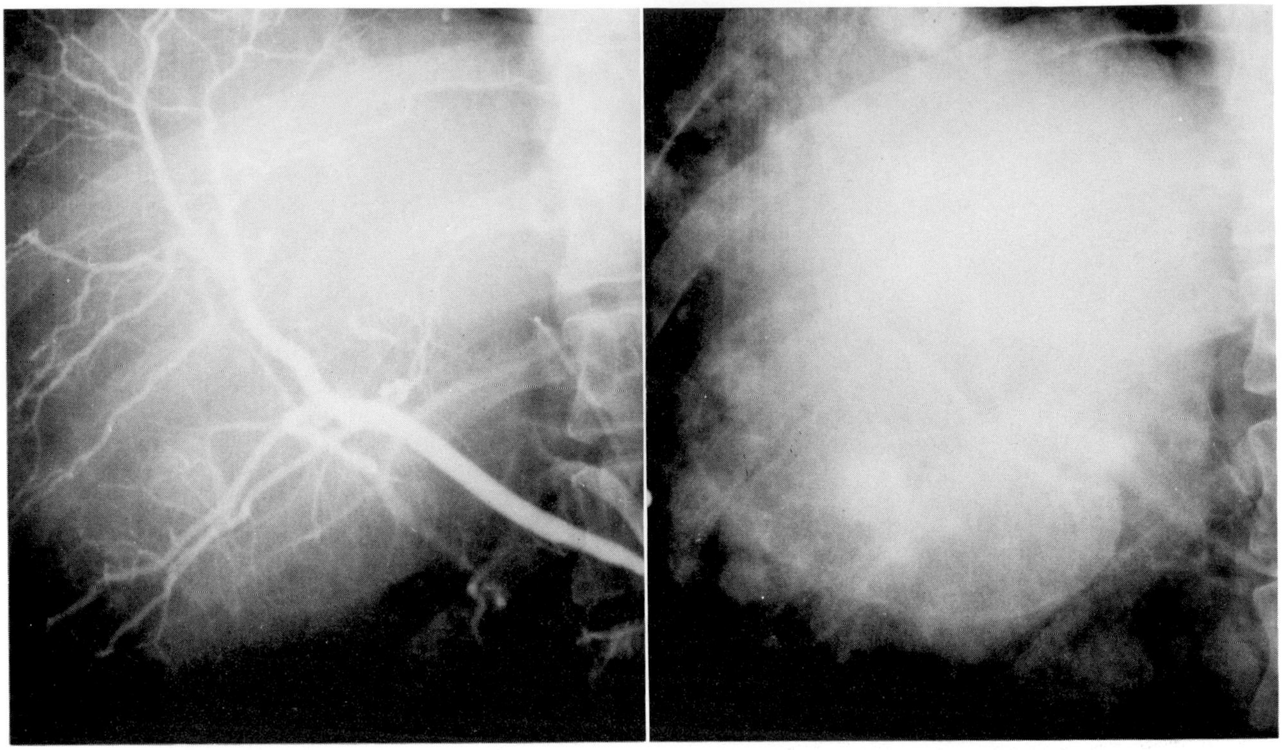

Fig. 47-57. Vascular metastases caused by metastatic carcinoid. (Courtesy Dr. Gus Seliger.)

tion does occur.[40] The diagnosis is usually easy with direct cholangiography. It is axiomatic that a short stricture of the bile ducts, in the absence of a known cause such as surgical trauma, is a scirrhous carcinoma unless proved otherwise (Figs. 47-62 and 47-63). The tumor is usually slow growing and tends to extend along the axis of the ducts, resulting in some larger lesions (Fig. 47-64). Problems in differential diagnosis arise when the tumor causes total obstruction of the duct. Liver scans in bile duct carcinoma cases may reveal patchy or mottled uptake, which is usually caused by dilated intrahepatic bile ducts rather than by metastases.[242] Selective arteriography reveals tiny, thin tumor vessels with irregular encasement or obstruction of arteries.[120] These changes, however, can be quite subtle and may be mimicked by inflammatory lesions.

Some special features of bile duct carcinoma are of importance and deserve mention. Successful surgical resection is only rarely possible,[161] but many of these patients have long periods of good health if surgical measures can control biliary obstruction.[122] This is particularly true in the very slow growing lesions, some of which have been originally and erroneously diagnosed as primary sclerosing cholangitis.[11] The other important aspect of bile duct carcinoma is the high incidence of diagnostic failure, both surgical and radiologic, in common hepatic duct tumors (Fig. 47-65).[40,242] Most of these lesions high in the porta hepatis are evident only after extensive dissection (Fig. 47-63), but some of them in more accessible locations are also missed (Figs. 47-64 and 47-65). These overlooked common hepatic duct tumors present a fairly typical clinical syndrome[122] characterized by one or more unrevealing operations for obstructive jaundice where the liver is found to be tense or turgid and the gallbladder and common duct are empty or collapsed. The use of preoperative percutaneous transhepatic cholangiography should prevent this error.

Differential diagnosis of bile duct carcinoma

Stricture or accidental surgical ligation of bile ducts can give a cholangiographic picture identical to the small scirrhous carcinoma (Fig. 47-66).

Text continued on p. 1251.

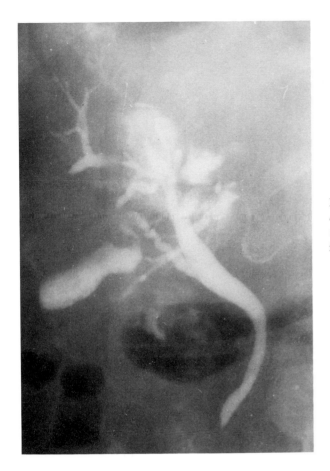

Fig. 47-58. Metastatic carcinoma shown by percutaneous cholangiogram. The tumor is obstructing numerous intrahepatic ducts and the smaller biliary radicals failed to fill. (Courtesy Dr. Barry Held.)

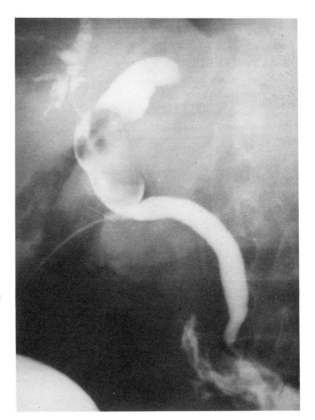

Fig. 47-59. Polypoid carcinoma of the common hepatic duct.

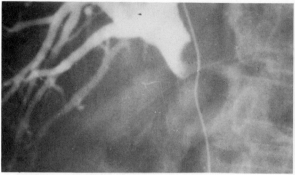

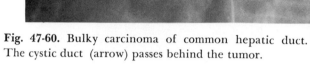

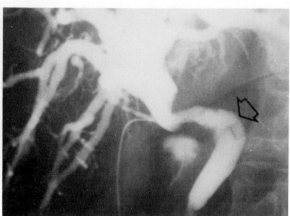

Fig. 47-60. Bulky carcinoma of common hepatic duct. The cystic duct (arrow) passes behind the tumor.

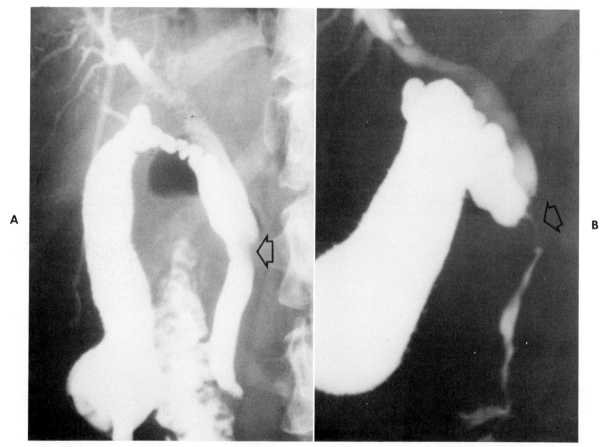

Fig. 47-61. Scirrhous carcinoma at junction of cystic and common hepatic ducts. **A,** A small defect (arrow) is present at the junction of the ducts and there is some dilatation of the common hepatic duct proximal to this. The lesion was overlooked on this injection through a cholecystostomy tube. **B,** Several months later a well-defined scirrhous carcinoma with overhanging edges is present at this site (arrows).

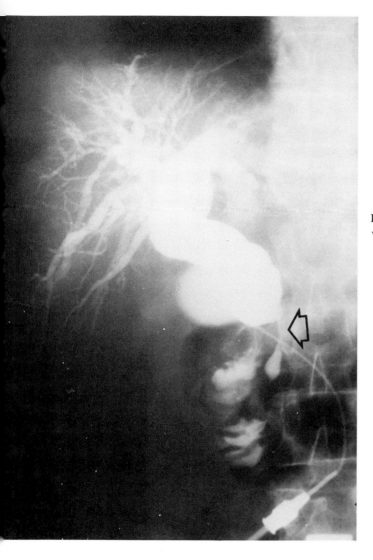

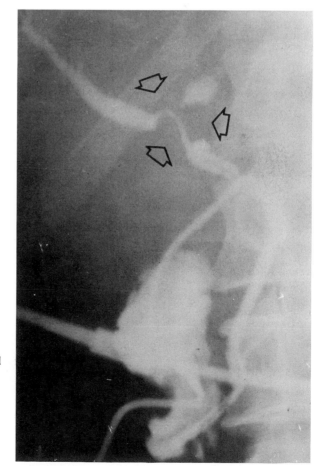

Fig. 47-62. Scirrhous carcinoma of common bile duct within the head of the pancreas (arrow).

Fig. 47-63. Scirrhous carcinoma at junction of right and left hepatic ducts.

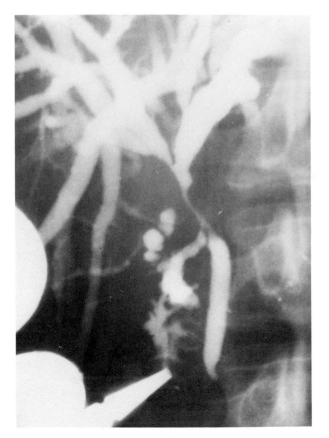

Fig. 47-64. Scirrhous carcinoma of common hepatic duct. Fistulogram demonstrates the lesion involving the common hepatic duct and extending to the distal portions of the right and left hepatic ducts. The lesion was missed at two operations prior to this examination.

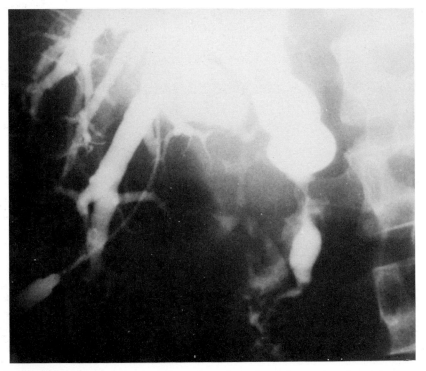

Fig. 47-65. Scirrhous carcinoma at junction of cystic and common hepatic ducts. The lesion was missed at the original operation. Jaundice recurred and a percutaneous cholangiogram revealed scirrhous carcinoma.

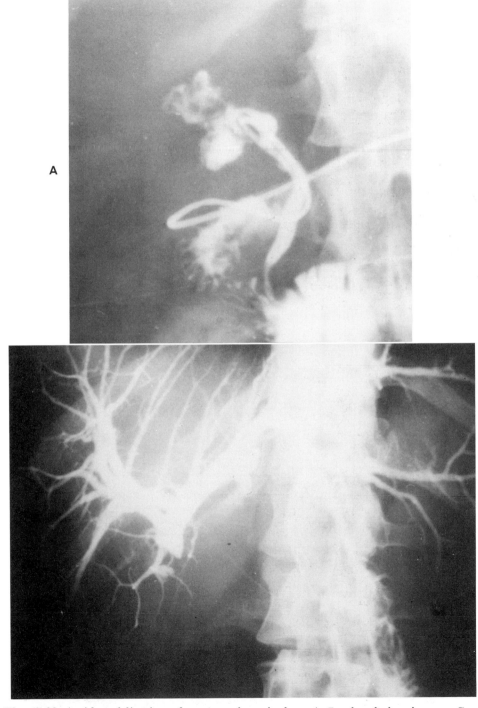

Fig. 47-66. Accidental ligation of common hepatic duct. **A, T** tube cholangiogram. Complete obstruction to retrograde flow in common hepatic duct with some extravasation of contrast. **B,** Following Longmire procedure cholangiogram reveals complete obstruction of proximal hepatic duct.

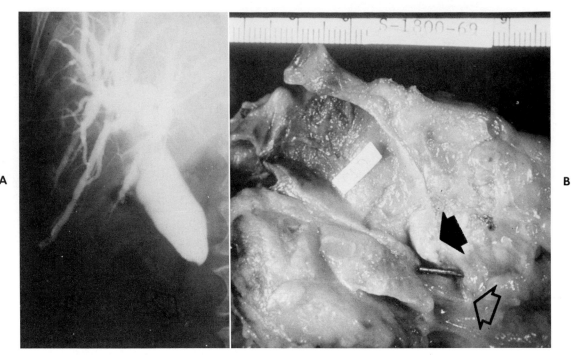

Fig. 47-67. Scirrhous carcinoma of distal common bile duct. **A,** Complete obstruction of duct about 2 cm. proximal to duodenal papilla (arrow). No evidence of mass on gastrointestinal series. **B,** One centimeter tumor (black arrow), 1.5 cm. proximal to duodenal papilla (open arrow).

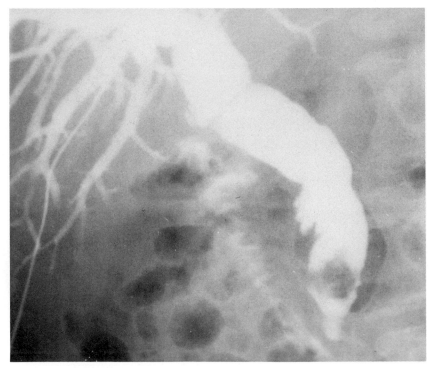

Fig. 47-68. Inflammatory polyp of the distal common duct.

For practical purposes, however, this is not a diagnostic problem because the history readily reveals the nature of the lesion. Short fibrous strictures caused by schistosomiasis have been reported from Africa, and these lesions could mimic the scirrhous tumors. Benign bile duct tumors and other primary malignant lesions such as cystoadenocarcinoma[228] and leiomyosarcoma[243] are exceedingly rare.

When there is complete obstruction of the duct problems in differential diagnosis do arise. The configuration at the site of obstruction seldom is specific unless there is an intraluminal mass. The location of the obstruction and the presence or absence of a mass on gastrointestinal studies usually provides a short, meaningful differential diagnosis. For instance, total obstruction of the intrapancreatic portion of the common duct some distance from the papilla of Vater in the absence of a mass favors the diagnosis of primary bile duct carcinoma (Fig. 47-67). Total obstruction of the common duct at the superior margin of the pancreas is, statistically, almost always caused by pancreatic carcinoma even when a mass is not demonstrated on gastrointestinal examination. Total obstruction above this level results in a differential diagnostic problem between primary bile duct carcinoma, metastatic carcinoma in the porta hepatis, or gallbladder carcinoma that has extended to involve the common hepatic duct.

BENIGN BILE DUCT TUMORS

Benign tumors of the bile duct are very rare. For example, in one report of 5,200 consecutive biliary operations, two adenomas of the extrahepatic bile ducts were found.[100] Adenoma is the most common benign tumor but many other lesions have been described including papilloma,[37] cystadenoma,[209] adenomyoma,[55] hamartoma,[55] heterotopic gastric mucosa,[245] heterotopic pancreas,[239] inflammatory pseudotumor,[88] carcinoid,[136] granular cell myoblastoma,[2,140] fibroma,[37] and neuroma.[37] Many tumors are incidental findings; but some of these lesions do cause obstructive jaundice,[83,150,239] and massive hemobilia as the result of erosion of a benign adenoma has been reported.[224] Some cholangiograms reveal nonspecific bile duct obstruction,[83,150] whereas in some others an intraluminal mass[239] or polypoid tumor[209] has been shown. With these benign tumors (Fig. 47-68) definitive diagnosis depends on histologic examination.

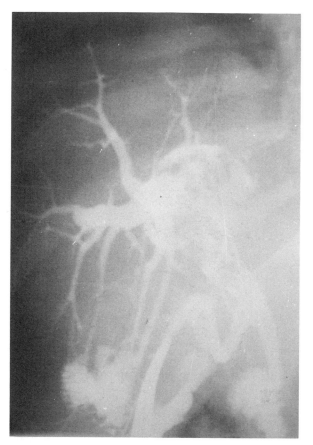

Fig. 47-69. Sarcoma botryoides. (Courtesy Dr. Jack O'Connor.)

SARCOMA BOTRYOIDES

Sarcoma botryoides is a rare bile duct tumor of late infancy or childhood.[88] The youngest patient reported was 18 months and the oldest 11 years.[88] Grossly, the tumor is a bulky intraluminal mucoid-appearing mass that distends the bile ducts. Histologically, this is a subepithelial embryonal rhabdomyosarcoma.[212] The patients usually have obstructive jaundice. Extrinsic pressure defects on the second portion of the duodenum may be found on gastrointestinal series, the same as those produced by choledochal cysts, which the lesion resembles externally. The cholangiographic findings are characteristic (Fig. 47-69) and consist of a bulky intraluminal mass in the dilated bile ducts of a child.[50,88,212] This malignant tumor may decrease in size with chemotherapy or radiation, but cure by any means has not yet been reported.[50]

REFERENCES

1. Abrams, R. M., Beranbaum, E. R., Santos, J. S., and Lipson, J.: Angiographic features of cavernous hemangioma of liver, Radiology 92:308, 1969.
2. Abt, A. B., Feinberg, E., and Kunitz, S.: Granular cell myoblastoma of the extrahepatic biliary tract, Mt. Sinai J. Med. 38:457, 1971.
3. Adam, Y. G., Huvos, A. G., and Fortner, J. G.: Giant hemangiomas of the liver, Ann. Surg. 172:239, 1970.
4. Albo, R. J., and Obata, W. G.: Radiologic diagnosis of primary sclerosing cholangitis, Radiology 81:123, 1963.
5. Alergant, C. D.: Gumma of liver with calcification, Arch. Intern. Med. 98:340, 1956.
6. Alfidi, R. J., Rastogi, H., Buonocore, E., and Brown, C. H.: Hepatic arteriography, Radiology 90:1136, 1968.
7. Allen, R. W., and Holt, A. H.: Calcification in primary liver carcinoma, Amer. J. Roentgen. 99:150, 1967.
8. Alonso-Lej, F., Rever, W. B., and Pessagno, D. J.: Congenital choledochal cyst, with a report of 2, and an analysis of 94, cases, Int. Abstr. Surg. 108:1, 1959.
9. Alpert, E., Pinn, V. W., and Isselbacher, K. J.: Alphafetoprotein in a patient with gastric carcinoma metastatic to the liver, New Eng. J. Med. 285:1058, 1971.
10. Alpert, S., Metcalf, W., Vreede, A. A., and Meng. C. H.: Right hepatectomy for hamartoma in an eleven-month-old infant, Ann. Surg. 165:286, 1967.
11. Altemeier, W. A., Gall, E. A., Zinninger, M. M., and Hoxworth, P. I.: Sclerosing carcinoma of the major intrahepatic bile ducts, Arch. Surg. 75:450, 1957.
12. Altemeier, W. A., Schowengerdt, C. G., and Whiteley, D. H.: Abscesses of the liver: surgical considerations, Arch. Surg. 101:258, 1970.
13. Alvarez, S. Z., and Fabra, R.: The clinical features of hepatobiliary tuberculosis in the Philippines. Proceedings of the fourth World Congress of Gastroenterology, Copenhagen, 1970.
14. Aronsen, K. F., Ericsson, B., Lunderquist, A., Malmbord, O., and Norden, J. G.: A case of operated focal nodular cirrhosis of the liver, Scand. J. Gastroent. 3:58, 1968.
15. Ashby, S.: Carcinoma in a choledochus cyst, Brit. J. Surg. 51:493, 1964.
16. Atkinson, A. J., and Carroll, W. W.: Sclerosing cholangitis, J.A.M.A. 188:183, 1964.
17. Azimi, P. H., Bodenbender, J. G., Hintz, R. L., and Kontras, S. B.: Chronic granulomatous disease in three female siblings, J.A.M.A. 206:2865, 1968.
18. Babbitt, D. P.: Congenital choledochal cysts: new etiological concept based on anomalous relationships of the common bile duct and pancreatic duct, Ann. Radiol. (Paris) 12:231, 1969.
19. Baker, D. H., and Harris, R. C.: Congenital absence of the intrahepatic bile ducts, Amer. J. Roentgen. 91:875, 1964.
20. Baltaxe, H. A., and Fleming, R. J.: The angiographic appearance of hydatid disease, Radiology 97:599, 1970.
21. Bartholomew, L. G., Cain, J. C., Woolner, L. B., Utz, D. C., and Ferris, D. O.: Sclerosing cholangitis, New Eng. J. Med. 269:8, 1963.
22. Beker, S. G., and Valencia-Parparcen, J.: Portal hypertension syndrome, Amer. J. Dig. Dis. 13:1047, 1968.
23. Berdon, W. E., and Baker, D. H.: Giant hepatic hemangioma with cardiac failure in the newborn intant, Radiology 92:1528, 1969.
24. Blanc, W. A., Berdon, W. E., Baker, D. H., and Wigger, H. J.: Calcified portal vein thromboemboli in newborn and stillborn infants, Radiology 88:287, 1967.
25. Block, M. A., Schuman, B. M., Eyler, W. R., Truant, J. P., and DuSault, L. A.: Surgery of liver abscesses, Arch. Surg. 88:602, 1964.
26. Boijsen, E., Gothlin, J., Hallbook, T., and Sandblom, P.: Preoperative angiographic diagnosis of bleeding aneurysms of abdominal visceral arteries, Radiology 93:781, 1969.
27. Boijsen, E., and Abrams, H. L.: Roentgenologic diagnosis of primary carcinoma of the liver, Acta Radiol. 3:257, 1965.
28. Boijsen, E., and Reuter, S. R.: Combined percutaneous transhepatic cholangiography and angiography in the evaluation of obstructive jaundice, Amer. J. Roentgen. 99:153, 1967.
29. Boyer, J. L., Sen Gupta, K. P., Biswas, S. K., Pal, N. C., Mallick, K. C. B., Iber, F. L., and Basu, A. K.: Idiopathic portal hypertension, Ann. Intern. Med. 66:41, 1967.
30. Bridges, R. A., Berendes, H., and Good, R. A.: A fatal granulomatous disease of childhood, Amer. J. Dis. Child. 97:387, 1959.
31. Bron, K. M., and Gajaraj, A.: Demonstration of hepatic aneurysms in polyarteritis nodosa by arteriography, New Eng. J. Med. 282:1024, 1970.
32. Brown, D. B., Strang, R., Gordon, J., and Hendry, E. B.: Primary carcinoma of the extrahepatic bile ducts, Brit. J. Surg. 49:22, 1961.
33. Bruwer, A. J., and Hallenbeck, G. A.: Aneurysm of hepatic artery: roentgenologic features in one case, Amer. J. Roentgen. 78:270, 1957.
34. Burke, J. F., and Scully, R. E.: Pulmonary disease associated with a disappearing abdominal mass, New Eng. J. Med. 281:1004, 1969.
35. Burnell, R. H., and Markey, G. B.: Choledochal cyst: a case report and discussion of aetiology, Arch. Dis. Child. 40:329, 1965.
36. Carson, M. J., Chadwick, D. L., Brubaker, C. A., Cleland, R. S., and Landing, B. H.: Thirteen boys with progressive septic granulomatosis, Pediatrics 35:405, 1965.
37. Chu, P. T.: Benign neoplasms of the extrahepatic biliary ducts: review of the literature and report of a case of fibroma, Arch. Path. 50:84, 1950.
38. Clain, D., and McNulty, J.: A radiological study of the lymphatics of the liver, Brit. J. Radiol. 41:662, 1968.
39. Clay, M. G., and Munro, A. I.: Bilateral diaphrag-

matic hernia from blunt injury causing a Budd-Chiari syndrome, Ann. Surg. **173**:321, 1971.

40. Clemett, A. R.: Carcinoma of the major bile ducts, Radiology **84**:894, 1965.

41. Clemett, A. R.: A technique of percutaneous transhepatic cholangiography for the seventies. Presented at the Annual Radiologic Society of North America meeting, Chicago, December, 1970.

42. Cleveland, R. J., Jackson, B. M., Newman, P. H., and Nelson, R. J.: Traumatic intrahepatic hepatic artery-portal vein fistula with associated hemobilia, Ann. Surg. **171**:451, 1970.

43. Cobo, A., Hall, R. C., Torres, E., Cuello, C. J., and Colombi, C.; Intrahepatic calculi, Arch. Surg. **89**:936, 1964.

44. Coutinho, A.: Hemodynamic studies of portal hypertension in schistosomiasis, Amer. J. Med. **44**: 547, 1968.

45. Cummack, D. H.: Gastro-intestinal x-ray diagnosis: a descriptive atlas, Baltimore, 1969, The Williams & Wilkins Co.

46. Curutchet, H. P., Terz, J. J., Kay, S., and Lawrence, W.: Primary liver cancer, Surgery **70**:467, 1971.

47. Cutler, B., and Donaldson, G. A.: Primary sclerosing cholangitis and obliterative cholangitis, Amer. J. Surg. **117**:502, 1969.

48. Cywes, S., and Krige, H.: Intravenous cholangiography and tomography in the diagnosis of biliary ascariasis, Clin. Radiol. **14**:271, 1963.

49. Dardik, H., Glotzer, P., and Silver, C.: Congenital hepatic cyst causing jaundice, Ann. Surg. **159**:585, 1964.

50. Davis, G. L., Kissane, J. M., and Ishak, K. G.: Embryonal rhabdomyosarcoma (sarcoma botryoides) of the biliary tree, Cancer **24**:333, 1969.

51. DeLorimier, A. A., Simpson, E. B., Baum, R. S., and Carlsson, E.: Hepatic-artery ligation for hepatic hemangiomatosis, New Eng. J. Med. **277**:333, 1967.

52. DeOya, J. C., Puente, J. L., Villanueva, A., and Potel, J.: Enterogenous cyst of the ampulla of Vater, Digestion **2**:201, 1969.

53. Dodd, G. D.: Lymphography in diseases of the liver and pancreas, Radiol. Clin. N. Amer. **8**:69, 1970.

54. Doehner, G. A.: The hepatic venous system, Radiology **90**:1119, 1968.

55. Dowdy, G. S., Jr., Olin, W. G., Jr., Shelton, E. L., Jr., and Walderon, G. W.: Benign tumors of the extrahepatic bile ducts: report of three cases and review of the literature, Arch. Surg. **85**:503, 1962.

56. Ecker, J. A., and Doane, W. A.: Massive cavernous hemangioma of the liver, Amer. J. Gastroent. **52**: 25, 1969.

57. Ecker, J. A., McKittrick, J. E., and Failing, R. M.: Thrombosis of the hepatic veins, Amer. J. Gastroent. **45**:429, 1966.

58. Eddleston, A. L. W., Rake, M. O., Pagaltsos, A. P., Osborn, S. B., and Williams, R.: Se-selenomethionine in the scintiscan diagnosis of primary hepatocellular carcinoma, Gut **12**:245, 1971.

59. Elmslie, R. G.: Pyogenic liver abscess associated with common duct calculi, Med. J. Aust. **1**:800, 1965.

60. Engle, J., and Salmon, P. A.: Multiple choledochal cysts, Arch. Surg. **88**:345, 1964.

61. Enjoji, M., Watanabe, H., and Nakamura, Y.: A case report: congenital biliotracheal fistula with trifurcation of bronchi, Ann. Paediat. **200**:321, 1963.

62. Evans, J. A.: Specialized technics in investigation of abdominal disease, Radiology **82**:579, 1964.

63. Feingold, M. L., Litwak, R. L., Geller, S. S., and Baron, M.: Budd-Chiari syndrome caused by a right atrial tumor, Arch. Intern. Med. **127**:292, 1971.

64. Finch, S. C., and Finch, C. H.: Idiopathic hemochromatosis, an iron storage disease, Medicine **34**: 381, 1955.

65. Fisher, M. M., Chen, S., and Dekker, A.: Congenital diaphragm of the common hepatic duct, Gastroenterology **54**:605, 1968.

66. Flemma, R. J., and Anlyan, W. G.: Tuberculous bronchobiliary fistula, J. Thorac. Cardiovasc. Surg. **49**:198, 1965.

67. Fonkalsrud, E. W., and Boles, E. T., Jr.: Choledochal cysts in infancy and childhood, Surg. Gynec. Obstet. **121**:733, 1965.

68. Foster, S. C., Schneider, B., and Seaman, W. B.: Gas-containing pyogenic intrahepatic abscesses, Radiology **94**:613, 1970.

69. Freeman, L. M., Bernstein, R. G., and Hayt, D. B.: Diagnosis of hepatic hemangioma with combined scanning technique, Radiology **95**:127, 1970.

70. Gammill, S. L., Maxfield, W. S., Font, R. G., and Sparks, R. D.: Filling defects on scintillation scans of the liver associated with dilatation of the bile ducts, Amer. J. Roentgen. **107**:37, 1969.

71. Gammill, S. L., Takahashi, M., Kawanami, M., Font, R., and Sparks, R.: Hepatic angiography in the selection of patients with hepatomas for hepatic lobectomy, Radiology **101**:549, 1971.

72. Gerson, C. D., and Schinella, R. A.: Hepatoma presenting as extrahepatic biliary obstruction, Amer. J. Dig. Dis. **14**:42, 1969.

73. Gherardi, G. J., and MacMahon, H. E.: Hypoplasia of terminal bile ducts, Amer. J. Dis. Child. **120**:151, 1970.

74. Gold, R. H., Douglas, S. D., Preger, L., Steinbach, H. L., and Fudenberg, H. H.: Roentgenographic features of the neutrophil dysfunction syndromes, Radiology **92**:1045, 1969.

75. Goswitz, J. T., and Kimmerling, R.: Perforated choledochal cyst with bile peritonitis in an infant: case report and surgical management, Surgery **59**: 878, 1966.

76. Gots, R. E., and Zuidema, G. D.: Dilatation of the intrahepatic biliary ducts in a patient with a choledochal cyst, Amer. J. Surg. **119**:726, 1970.

77. Grossman, H., Berdon, W. E., and Baker, D. H.: Gastrointestinal findings in cystic fibrosis, Amer. J. Roentgen. **97**:227, 1966.

78. Grossman, H., and Seed, W.: Congenital hepatic

fibrosis, bile duct dilatation, and renal lesion resembling medullary sponge kidney, Radiology **87:** 46, 1966.

79. Grunfeld, O., and Hinostroza, G.: Thallium poisoning, Arch. Intern. Med. **114:**132, 1964.

80. Gryboski, J. D., and Clemett, A.: Congenital hepatic artery aneurysm with superior mesenteric artery insufficiency: a steal syndrome, Pediatrics **39:**344, 1967.

81. Guida, P. M., and Moore, S. W.: Aneurysm of the hepatic artery: report of five cases with a brief review of the previously reported cases, Surgery **60:** 299, 1966.

82. Gundersen, A. E., and Green, R. M.: Traumatic hemobilia: accurate preoperative diagnosis by hepatic artery angiogram, Surgery **62:**862, 1967.

83. Haith, E. E., Kepes, J. J., and Holder, T. M.: Inflammatory pseudotumor involving the common bile duct of a six-year-old boy: successful pancreaticoduodenectomy, Surgery **56:**436, 1964.

84. Halpern, M., and Citron, B. P.: Necrotizing angiitis associated with drug abuse, Amer. J. Roentgen. **111:**663, 1971.

85. Ham, J. M., and Mackenzie, D. C.: Primary carcinoma of the extrahepatic bile ducts, Surg. Gynec. Obstet. **118:**1, 1964.

86. Hanai, H., Idriss, F., and Swenson, O.: Bile duct proliferation in atresia and related hepatic diseases, Arch. Surg. **94:**14, 1967.

87. Hawkins, P. E., Graham, F. B., and Holliday, P.: Gallbladder disease in children, Amer. J. Surg. **111:**741, 1966.

88. Hayes, M. A., Goldenberg, I. S., and Bishop, C. C.: The developmental basis for bile duct anomalies, Surg. Gynec. Obstet. **107:**447, 1958.

89. Hays, D. M., Goodman, G. N., Snyder, W. H. Jr., and Wolley, M. M.: Congenital cystic dilatation of the common bile duct, Arch. Surg. **98:**457, 1969.

90. Hays, D. M., and Snyder, W. H. Jr.: Botryoid sarcoma (Rhabdomyosarcoma) of the bile ducts, Amer. J. Dis. Child. **110:**595, 1965.

91. Held, B. T., and Clemett, A. R.: Roentgenological findings in fatal granulomatous disease of childhood. Presented at New York Roentgen Ray Society Spring Conference, April 30, 1965.

92. Hellstrom, H. R., and Perez-Stable, E. C.: Retroperitoneal fibrosis with disseminated vasculitis and intrahepatic sclerosing cholangitis, Amer. J. Med. **40:**184, 1966.

93. Hermann, R. E., and Hawk, W. A.: Congenital hepatic fibrosis as a cause of portal hypertension: report of two cases, Surgery **62:**1095, 1967.

94. Hermann, R. E., and Shafer, W. H.: Aneurysm of the portal vein and portal hypertension: first reported case, Ann. Surg. **162:**1101, 1965.

95. Hertzer, N. R., Hawk, W. A., and Hermann, R. E.: Inflammatory lesions of the liver which simulate tumor: report of two cases in children, Surgery **69:**839, 1971.

96. Hirooka, M., and Kimura, C.: Membranous obstruction of the hepatic portion of the inferior vena cava, Arch. Surg. **100:**656, 1970.

97. Hoffer, P. B., and Petasnick, J. P.: Choledochal cysts demonstrated by oral cholecystography, Radiology **93:**871, 1969.

98. Hogarth, J., and Laird, R. C.: Congenital cystic malformation of the bile ducts: report of a case and review of related literature, Canad. Med. Ass. J. **95:**57, 1966.

99. Holubitsky, I. B., and McKenzie, A. D.: Primary sclerosing cholangitis of the extrahepatic bile ducts, Canad. J. Surg. **7:**277, 1964.

100. Hulten, J., Johansson, H., and Olding, L.: Adenomas of the gallbladder and extrahepatic bile ducts, Acta. Chir. Scand. **136:**203, 1970.

101. Hunter, F. M., Akdamar, K., Sparks, R. D., Reed, R. J., and Brown, C. L.: Congenital dilation of the intrahepatic bile ducts, Amer. J. Med. **40:**188, 1966.

102. Ishak, K. G., and Glunz, P. R.: Hepatoblastoma and hepatocarcinoma in infancy and childhood, Cancer **20:**396, 1967.

103. Jackson, B. T., and Saunders, P.: Perforated choledochus cyst, Brit. J. Surg. **58:**38, 1971.

104. Jackson, F. C., and Maxwell, J. W., Jr.: Intrahepatic diverticulum—common hepatic bile duct, Arch. Surg. **89:**706, 1964.

105. Jacobson, G., and Zucherman, S. D.: Roentgenographically demonstrable splenic deposits in sickle cell anemia, Amer. J. Roentgen. **76:**47, 1956.

106. Janower, M. L., Sidel, V. W., Baker, W. H., Fitzpatrick, E. P., Guarino, F. I., and Flynn, M. J.: Late clinical and laboratory manifestations of Thorotrast administration in cerebral arteriography, New Eng. J. Med. **279:**186, 1968.

107. Jansen, W.: Intraduodenal cyst containing bile and stones: "choledochocele" in an accessory bile duct, Gastroenterology **58:**397, 1970.

108. Jarvis, L., and Hodes, P. J.: Aneurysm of the hepatic artery demonstrated roentgenographically, Amer. J. Roentgen. **72:**1037, 1954.

109. Jewel, K. L.: Primary carcinoma of the liver: clininical and radiologic manifestations, Amer. J. Roentgen. **113:**84, 1971.

110. Joffe, N.: Siderosis in the South African Bantu, Brit. J. Radiol. **37:**200, 1964.

111. Johnston, P. W.: Congenital cysts of the liver in infancy and childhood, Amer. J. Surg. **116:**184, 1968.

112. Jonasson, O., Pritchard, J., and Long, L.: Intraluminal leiomyosarcoma of the inferior vena cava, Cancer **19:**1311, 1966.

113. Jones, G. M., and Caylor, H. D.: Anomalous termination of the common duct, Amer. J. Surg. **93:**122, 1957.

114. Joseph, W. L., Fonkalsrud, E. W., and Longmire W. P.: Cystic dilatation of common bile duct in adults, Arch. Surg. **91:**468, 1965.

115. Kahn, D.: Thorotrast-induced hemangioendothelioma of liver, Conn. Med. **31:**557, 1967.

116. Kanter, D. M.: Hepatic infarction, Arch. Intern. Med. **115:**479, 1965.

117. Kanter, I. E., Schwartz, A. J., and Fleming, R. J.: Localization of bleeding point in chronic and acute

gastrointestinal hemorrhage by means of selective visceral arteriography, Amer. J. Roentgen. **103:** 386, 1968.

118. Kark, A. E.: Bile duct strictures caused by schisto-somiasis, Brit. J. Surg. **49:**419, 1962.

119. Karras, B. G., Cannon, A. H., and Zanon, B.: Hepatic calcifications, Acta. Radiol. **57:**458, 1962.

120. Kaude, J., and Rian, R.: Cholangiocarcinoma, Radiology **100:**573, 1971.

121. Kido, C., Sasaki, T., and Kaneko, M.: Angiography of primary liver cancer, Amer. J. Roentgen. **113:**70, 1971.

122. Klatskin, G.: Adenocarcinoma of the hepatic duct at its bifurcation within the porta hepatis, Amer. J. Med. **38:**241, 1965.

123. Klatskin, G.: Personal communication.

124. Koven, I. H., Golab, A., Bohnen, D. R., and Himel, H. A.: Primary sclerosing cholangitis, Canad. Med. Ass. J. **101:**103, 1969.

125. Kozower, M., Fawaz, K. A., Miller, H. M., and Kaplan, M. M.: Positive alpha-fetoglobulin in a case of gastric carcinoma. New Eng. J. Med. **285:** 1059, 1971.

126. Kreel, L., Freston, J. W., and Clain, D.: Vascular radiology in the Budd-Chiari syndrome, Brit. J. Radiol. **40:**755, 1967.

127. Krieger, J., Seaman, W. B., and Porter, M. R.: The roentgenologic appearance of sclerosing cholangitis, Radiology **95:**369, 1970.

128. Kwittken, J.: Hamartoma of liver, New York J. Med. **67:**3254, 1967.

129. Landing, B. H., and Shirkey, H. S.: A syndrome of recurrent infection and infiltration of viscera by pigmented lipid histocytes, Pediatrics **20:**431, 1957.

130. Lavender, J. P., Lowe, J., Barker, J. R., Burn, J. I., and Chaudhri, M. A.: Gallium 67 citrate scanning in neoplastic and inflammatory lesions, Brit. J. Radiol. **44:**361, 1971.

131. Lee, S. S., Chul Min, P., Kim, G. S., and Hong, P. W.: Choledochal cyst, Arch. Surg. **99:**19, 1969.

132. Legge, D. A., Carlson, H. C., Dickson, E. R., and Ludwig, J.: Cholandiographic findings in cholangiolitic hepatitis, Amer. J. Roentgen. **113:**16, 1971.

133. Legge, D. A., Carlson, H. C., and Ludwig, J.: Cholangiographic findings in diseases of the liver: a postmortem study, Amer. J. Roentgen. **113:**34, 1971.

134. Lenthall, J., Reynolds, T. B., and Donovan, A. J.: Excessive output of bile in chronic hepatic disease, Surg. Gynec. Obstet. **130:**243, 1970.

135. Lin, T.: Primary cancer of the liver, Scand. J. Gastroent. **6:**223, 1970.

136. Little, J. M., Gibson, A. A. M., and Kay, A. W.: Primary common bile-duct carcinoid, Brit. J. Surg. **55:**147, 1968.

137. Longmire, W. P., Jr.: Congenital biliary hypoplasia, Surgery **159:**335, 1964.

138. Lorenzo, G. A., Seed, R. W., and Beal, J. M.: Congenital dilatation of the biliary tract, Amer. J. Surg. **121:**510, 1971.

139. Ludwick, J. R., Markel, S. F., and Child, C. G.: Chiari's disease, Arch. Surg. **91:**697, 1965.

140. Mackay, B., Elliott, G. B., and MacDougall, J. A.: Granular cell myoblastoma of the cystic duct: report of a case with electron-microscope observations, Canad. J. Surg. **11:**44, 1968.

141. Madding, G. F., Smith, W. L., and Hershberger, L. R.: Hepatoportal arteriovenous fistula, J.A.M.A. **156:**593, 1954.

142. Maki, T., Sato, T., Yamaguchi, I., and Sato, T.: Treatment of intrahepatic gallstones, Arch. Surg. **88:**124, 1964.

143. Malt, R. A., Hershberg, R. A., and Miller, W. L.: Experience with benign tumors of the liver, Surg. Gynec. Obstet. **130:**285, 1970.

144. Mandelbaum, I., and Shumacker, H. B.: Excision of congenital hepatic cyst of bile duct origin, Amer. J. Surg. **101:**507, 1961.

145. Mandell, G. L., and Hook, E. W.: Leukocyte function in chronic granulomatous disease of childhood, Amer. J. Med. **47:**473, 1969.

146. Martin, L. W., Benzing, G., and Kaplan, S.: Congenital intrahepatic arteriovenous fistula: report of a successfully treated case, Ann. Surg. **161:**209, 1965.

147. Mattison, R. A., Gooch, W. M., Guelzow, K. W. L., and South, M. A.: Chronic granulomatous disease of childhood in a 17-year-old boy, J. Pediat. **76:**890, 1970.

148. Maynard, J. H., and Fone, D. J.: Haemochromatosis with osteogenic sarcoma in the liver, Med. J. Aust. **2:**1260, 1969.

149. McEwan-Alvarado, G., Villarreal, H. R., Broders, A. C., Best, E. B., and Broders, C. W.: Aneurysm of the hepatic artery, Amer. J. Dig. Dis. **12:**509, 1967.

150. McIntyre, J. A., and Cheng, P.: Adenoma of the common bile duct causing obstructive jaundice, Canad. J. Surg. **11:**215, 1968.

151. McLoughlin, M. J.: Angiography in cavernous hemangioma of the liver, Amer. J. Roentgen. **113:** 50, 1971.

152. McLoughlin, M. J., and Hobbs, B. B.: Selective angiography in the diagnosis of hydatid disease of the liver, Canad. Med. Ass. J. **103:**1147, 1970.

153. Mehlman, D. J., Bulkley, B. H., and Wiernik, P. H.: Serum alpha₁-fetoglobulins with gastric and prostatic carcinomas, New Eng. J. Med. **285:**1060, 1971.

154. Melhem, R. E., and Nahra, K.: Congenital diaphragm of the common hepatic duct, Brit. J. Radiol. **39:**392, 1966.

155. Melnick, P. J.: Polycystic liver: analysis of seventy cases, Arch. Path. **59:**162, 1955.

156. Meyer, J. H.: Primary sclerosing cholangitis: report of a case, Ohio S. Med. J. **58:**442, 1962.

157. Meyers, M. A.: Calcification in cholangio-carcinoma, Brit. J. Radiol. **41:**65, 1968.

158. Michels, N. A.: Newer anatomy of the liver and its variant blood supply and collateral circulation, Amer. J. Surg. **112:**337, 1966.

159. Mikkelson, W. P., Edmondson, H. A., Peters, R. L., Redeker, A. G., and Reynolds, T. B.: Extra- and intrahepatic portal hypertension without cir-

rhosis (hepatoportal sclerosis), Ann. Surg. **162**:602, 1965.

160. Mistilis, S. P., Green, J. R., and Schiff, L.: Hepatic sarcoidosis with portal hypertension, Amer. J. Med. **36**:470, 1964.

161. Mistilis, S., and Schiff, L.: A case of jaundice due to unilateral hepatic duct obstruction, Gut **4**:13, 1963.

162. Moss, A. A., Clark, R. E., Palubinskas, A. J., and Delorimier, A. A.: Angiographic appearance of benign and malignant hepatic tumors in infants and children, Amer. J. Roentgen. **113**:61, 1971.

163. Muehlbauer, M. A., and Farber, M. G.: Hemangioma of the liver—some interesting clinical and radiological observations, Amer. J. Gastroent. **44**:355, 1966.

164. Mujahed, Z., Glenn, F., and Evans, J. A.: Communicating cavernous ectasia of the intrahepatic ducts (Caroli's disease), Amer. J. Roentgen. **113**:21, 1971.

165. Myers, R. N., Cooper, J. H., and Padis, N.: Primary sclerosing cholangitis, Amer. J. Gastroent. **53**:527, 1970.

166. Nathan, M., and Batsakis, J. G.: Congenital hepatic fibrosis, Surg. Gynec. Obstet. **128**:1033, 1969.

167. Nayak, N. C., and Ramalingaswami, V.: Obliterative portal venopathy of the liver, Arch. Path. **87**:359, 1969.

168. Nayak, N. C., Malaviya, A. N., Chawla, V., and Chandra, R. K.: Fetoprotein in Indian childhood cirrhosis, Lancet **1**:68, 1972.

169. Nebesar, R. A., Tefft, M., and Colodny, A. H.: Angiography of liver abscess in granulomatous disease of childhood, Amer. J. Roentgen. **108**:628, 1970.

170. Noble, M. J. A.: Hepatic vein thrombosis complicating polycythemia vera, Arch. Intern. Med. **120**:105, 1967.

171. Okuyama, K.: Primary liver cell carcinoma associated with biliary cirrhosis due to congenital bile duct atresia, J. Pediat. **67**:89, 1965.

172. O'Mara, R. E., Brettner, A., Danieglis, J. A.: and Gould, L. V.: ^{18}F uptake within metastatic osteosarcoma of the liver, Radiology **100**:113, 1971.

173. Ostermiller, W., Jr., and Carter, R.: Hepatic abscess, Arch. Surg. **94**:353, 1967.

174. Palmer, E. D.: Budd-Chiari syndrome (occlusion of the hepatic veins): seven cases, Ann. Intern. Med. **41**:261, 1954.

175. Palubinskas, A. J., Baldwin, J., and McCormack, K. R.: Liver-cell adenoma, Radiology **89**:444, 1967.

176. Perrin, R. W.: Communicating enterogenous cyst of duodenum receiving the termination of the common bile duct demonstrated by intravenous cholangiography, Radiology **93**:675, 1969.

177. Persaud, V., Bateson, E. M., and Bankay, C. D.: Pleural mesothelioma associated with massive hepatic calcification and unusual metastases, Cancer **26**:920, 1970.

178. Pollard, J. J., Fleischli, D. J., and Nebesar, R. A.: Angiography of hepatic neoplasms, Radiol. Clin. N. Amer. **8**:31, 1970.

179. Porter, S. D., Soper, R. T., and Tidrick, R. T.: Biliary hypoplasia, Ann. Surg. **167**:602, 1968.

180. Prussin, G., and Schiffmann, A.: Solitary nonparasitic cyst of the liver, Amer. J. Gastroent. **42**:425, 1964.

181. Pyrtek, L. J., and Bartus, S. A.: Hepatic pyemia, New Eng. J. Med. **272**:551, 1965.

182. Rakov, H. L., Smalldon, T. R., and Derman, H.: Hepatic hemangioendotheliosarcoma, Arch, Intern. Med. **112**:71, 1963.

183. Ramchand, S., Suh, H. S., and Gonzalez-Crussi, F.: Focal nodular hyperplasia of the liver, Canad. J. Surg. **13**:22, 1970.

184. Ramsay, G. C., and Britton, R. C.: Intraparenchymal angiography in the diagnosis of hepatic veno-occlusive diseases, Radiology **90**:716, 1968.

185. Raney, R., Lilly, J., and McHardy, G.: Biliary calculus of roundworm origin, Ann. Intern. Med. **72**:405, 1970.

186. Rankin, J. G., Skyring, A. P., and Goulston, S. J. M.: Linver in ulcerative colitis: obstructive jaundice due to bile duct carcinoma, Gut **7**:433, 1966.

187. Reuter, S. R., Redman, H. C., and Siders, D. B.: The spectrum of angiographic findings in hepatoma, Radiology **94**:89, 1970.

188. Rizk, G. K., Tayyarah, K. A., and Chandur-Mnaymneh, L.: The angiographic changes in hydatid cysts of the liver and spleen, Radiology **99**:303, 1971.

189. Rosenquist, C. J.: Radiographic visualization of choledochal cyst by oral cholecystography, Brit. J. Radiol. **42**:61, 1969.

190. Rossi, P., and Gould, H. R.: Angiography and scanning in liver disease, Radiology **96**:553, 1970.

191. Ryan, K. G., and Lorebler, S. H.: Traumatic fistula between hepatic artery and portal vein, New Eng. J. Med. **279**:1215, 1968.

192. Sackett, J. F., Mosenthal, W. T., House, R. K., and Jeffery, R. F.: Scintillation scanning of liver cell adenoma, Amer. J. Roentgen. **113**:56, 1971.

193. Salem, S. N., and Khammash, N. F.: Amoebic liver abscess, A diagnostic problem in Kuwait with an obscure relationship to intestinal amoebiasis. Proceedings of the fourth World Congress of Gastroenterology, Copenhagen, 1970.

194. Sanders, D. M., and Garrett, J. M.: Solitary hepatic cyst, Southern Med. J. **61**:256, 1968.

195. Sane, S. M., Sieber, W. K., and Girdany, B. R.: Congenital bronchobiliary fistula, Surgery **69**:599, 1971.

196. Schaffner, F., Gadboys, H. L., Safran, A. P., Baron, M. G., and Aufses, A. H. J.: Budd-Chiari syndrome caused by a web in the inferior vena cava, Amer. J. Med. **42**:838, 1967.

197. Schapiro, R. H., and Isselbacher, K. J.: Benign recurrent intrahepatic cholestasis, New Eng. J. Med. **268**:708, 1963.

198. Schmidt, A. G.: Plain film roentgen diagnosis of amebic hepatic abscess, Amer. J. Roentgen. **107**:47, 1969.

199. Schwartz, S. I., and Dale, W. A.: Primary sclerosing

cholangitis: review and report of six cases, Arch. Surg. **77**:439, 1958.

200. Sedacca, C. M., Perrin, E., Martin, L., and Schiff, L.: Polycystic liver: an unusual cause of bleeding esophageal varices, Gastroenterology **40**:128, 1961.

201. Selke, A. C., and Cornell, S. H.: Infantile hepatic hemangioendothelioma, Amer. J. Roentgen. **106**: 200, 1969.

202. Shanbrom, E., and Zheutlin, N.: Radiologic sign in hemosiderosis, J.A.M.A. **168**:33, 1958.

203. Sharp, H. L., Carey, J. B., White, J. G., and Krivit, W.: Cholestyramine therapy in patients with a paucity of intrahepatic bile ducts, J. Pediat. **71**: 723, 1967.

204. Sherlock, S., Feldman, C. A., Moran, B., and Scheuer, P. J.: Partial nodular transformation of the liver with portal hypertension, Amer. J. Med. **40**:195, 1966.

205. Sherrick, D. W., Kincaid, O. W., and Gambill, E. E.: Calcification in the portal venous system, J.A.M.A. **187**:861, 1964.

206. Shieber, W.: Lymphangiographic demonstration of thoracic duct dilatation in portal cirrhosis, Surgery. **57**:522, 1965.

207. Shoemaker, C. P., Jr., and Baxter, J. C.: An extra-hepatic biliary tract anomaly, Amer. J. Surg. **121**: 741, 1971.

208. Shoop, J. D.: Functional hepatoma demonstrated with rose bengal scanning, Amer. J. Roentgen. **107**:51, 1969.

209. Short, W. F., Nedwich, A., Levy, H. A., and Howard, J. M.: Biliary cystadenoma, Arch. Surg. **102**: 78, 1971.

210. Smith, G. W., Westgaard, T., and Bjorn-Hansen, R.: Hepatic venous angiography in the evaluation of cirrhosis of the liver, Ann. Surg. **173**:469, 1971.

211. Snapper, I.: Clinicopathologic conference: Discussion: Hepatic failure with clonorchiasis, New York J. Med. **70**:659, 1970.

212. Soper, R. T., and Dunphy, D. L.: Sarcoma botryoides of the biliary tree, Surgery **63**:1005, 1968.

213. Staley, C. J., Valaitis, J., Trippel, O. H., and Franzblau, S. A.: Leiomyosarcoma of the inferior vena cava, Amer. J. Surg. **113**:211, 1967.

214. Sterup, K., and Mosbech, J.: Budd-Chiari syndrome after taking oral contraceptives, Brit. Med. J. **4**:660, 1967.

215. Stigol, L. C., Traversaro, J., and Trigo, E. R.: Carinal trifurcation with congenital tracheobiliary fistula, Pediatrics **37**:89, 1966.

216. Strickler, J. H., Lufkin, N., and Rice, C. O.: Hepatic portal arteriovenous fistula, Surgery **31**:583, 1952.

217. Strohl, L., Reed, W. H., Diffenbauch, W. G., and Anderson, R. E.: Carcinoma of the bile ducts, Arch. Surg. **87**:51, 1963.

218. Summerskill, W. H. J.: The syndrome of benign recurrent cholestasis, Amer. J. Med. **38**:298, 1965.

219. Sutcliffe, J., and Chrispin, A. R.: Chronic granulomatous disease, Brit. J. Radiol. **43**:110, 1970.

220. Suzuki, T., Honjo, I., Hamamoto, K., Kousaka, T., and Torizuka, K.: Positive scintiphotography of

cancer of the liver with Ga⁶⁷ citrate, Amer. J. Roentgen. **113**:92, 1971.

221. Tabrisky, J., and Pollack, E. L.: The aberrant divisional bile duct, Radiology **99**:537, 1971.

222. Talley, R. W., Poznanski, A. K., Heslin, J. H., and Brennan, M. J.: Laminagrams of the thorotrast-opacified liver in evaluation of chemotherapy for metastatic cancer, Cancer **17**:1214, 1964.

223. Talner, L. B., Boyer, J. L., and Clemett, A. R.: Intrahepatic portal vein occlusion, Radiology **92**: 1265, 1969.

224. Teter, L. F.: Massive hemorrhage from benign adenoma of biliary duct causing death, J. Mich. Med. Soc. **53**:62, 1954.

225. Tetreault, A. F., Bowen, J. R., and Sampaio, N.: Hemobilia secondary to intrahepatic aneurysm of the hepatic artery, J.A.M.A. **192**:154, 1965.

226. Thistlethwaite, J. R., and Horwitz, A.: Choledochal cyst followed by carcinoma of the hepatic duct, Southern Med. J. **60**:872, 1967.

227. Thomas, T. V.: Aneurysm of the portal vein: report of two cases, one resulting in thrombosis and spontaneous rupture, Surgery **61**:550, 1967.

228. Thompson, J. E., and Wolff, M.: Intra-hepatic cystadenoma of bile duct origin, with malignant alteration: report of a case, treated with total left hepatic lobectomy, Milit. Med. **130**:218, 1965.

229. Thorpe, M. E. C., Scheuer, P. J., and Sherlock, S.: Primary sclerosing cholangitis, the biliary tree, and ulcerative colitis, Brit. Med. Ass. **8**:435, 1967.

230. Touloukian, R. J.: Hepatic hemangioendothelioma during infancy: pathology, diagnosis and treatment with prednisone, Pediatrics **45**:71, 1970.

231. Tuttle, R. J.: Cause of recurring obstructive jaundice, New Eng. J. Med. **283**:805, 1970.

232. Urschel, H. C., Skinner, D. B., and McDermott, W. V., Jr.: Hemobilia secondary to liver abscess, J.A.M.A. **186**:797, 1963.

233. Van Heerden, J. A., Judd, E. S., and Dockerty, M. B.: Carcinoma of the extrahepatic bile ducts, Amer. J. Surg. **113**:49, 1967.

234. Viana, R. L.: Arteriographic aspects of amoebic liver abscess and hepatosplenic schistosomiasis fibrosis. Proceedings of the fourth World Congress of Gastroenterology, Copenhagen, 1970.

235. Vlachos, J., Cassinos, C., and Trigonis, G.: Choledochus cyst in a newborn, Arch. Path. **67**:395, 1959.

236. Volpe, J. A., Bergin, J. J., and Overholt, E. L.: Budd-Chiari syndrome caused by a web as a result of visceral thrombophlebitis migrans, Amer. J. Dig. Dis. **15**:469, 1970.

237. Warren, K. W., Athanassiades, S., and Monge, J. I.: Primary sclerosing cholangitis, Amer. J. Surg. **111**:23, 1966.

238. Watson, R. C., and Baltaxe, H. A.: The angiographic appearance of primary and secondary tumors of the liver, Radiology **101**:539, 1971.

239. Weber, C. M., Zito, P. F., and Becker, S. M.: Heterotopic pancreas: an unusual cause of obstruction of the common bile duct, Amer. J. Gastroent. **49**:153, 1968.

240. Wenger, J., Gingrich, G. W., and Mendeloff, J.:

Sclerosing cholangitis—a manifestation of systemic disease, Arch. Intern. Med. **116**:509, 1965.

241. Weyde, R., Galatius-Jensen, F., and Uhm, I. K.: Percutaneous transhepatic cholangiography in Korean patients, Brit. J. Radiol. **39**:833, 1966.

242. Whelton, M. J., Petrelli, M., George, P., Young, W. B., and Sherlock, S.: Carcinoma at the junction of the main hepatic ducts, Quart. J. Med. **38**:211, 1968.

243. Whitcomb, F. F., Corley, G. J., Babigian, D. N., and Colcock, B. P.: Leiomyosarcoma of the bile ducts, Gastroenterology **52**:94, 1967.

244. Whitcomb, F. F., Jr., Parikh, N. K., and Sedgwick, C. E.: Hydatid cyst disease, Amer. J. Dig. Dis. **15**: 711, 1970.

245. Whittaker, L. D., Jr., Lynn, H. B., Dockerty, M. B., and Stickler, G. B.: Heterotopic gastric mucosa in the wall of the cystic duct: report of a case, Surgery **62**:382, 1967.

246. Wilson, S. E., Braitman, H., Plested, W. G., and Longmire, W. P., Jr.: Primary leiomyosarcoma of the liver, Ann. Surg. **174**:232, 1971.

247. Wilson, T. S., and Macgregor, J. W.: Focal nodular hyperplasia of the liver, Canad. Med. Ass. J. **100**: 567, 1969.

248. Wolfson, J. J., Quie, P. G., Laxdal, S. D., and Good, R. A.: Roentgenologic manifestations in children with a genetic defect of polymorphonuclear leukocyte function, Radiology **91**:37, 1968.

249. Young, R. C.: The Budd-Chiari syndrome cause by *Aspergillus,* Arch. Intern. Med. **124**:754, 1969.

250. Zeegen, R., Stansfeld, A. G., Dawson, A. M., and Hunt, A. H.: Prolonged survival after portal decompression of patients with non-cirrhotic intrahepatic portal hypertension, Gut **11**:610, 1970.

Examination of the gallbladder | 48

Walter M. Whitehouse

HISTORICAL DEVELOPMENT OF CHOLECYSTOGRAPHY

The historical development of cholecystography is important in two major respects. First, it provided a breakthrough with the development of the concept of selective excretion of radiopaque contrast material by an organ system to aid in the evaluation of that system by roentgenographic methods. Second, it provided a tremendous contribution to roentgenologic science by two surgical investigators interested in the basic sciences of physiology and biochemistry as they pertained to their own specialty. This example of planned research is worthy of recounting in order to recall the development of biliary roentgenography that laid the groundwork for the general development of radiopaque contrast media.

As recounted recently by Dr. Warren H. Cole,[9] this step in roentgenologic history began when his chief, Dr. Evarts Graham, assigned to him a research project as part of his second year surgical residency. The project involved the excretion of phenolphthalein compounds by the liver and their concentration in the gallbladder, with the expectation that use of a halogen phenolphthalein compound might lead to the feasibility of roentgenographic demonstration of the gallbladder.

Early animal experimentation in dogs and rabbits led to demonstration of the toxicity of the available preparations of tetraiodophenolphthalein and to the extensive use of calcium tetrabromphenolphthalein. The first successful animal cholecystogram was achieved with the latter compound in a dog in November of 1923; later recall by a helper that this dog had been fasting led to a routine of administration of the compound after a fat free feeding that gave reproducible results.

Adaptation of these results to human use led to the observation of marked clinical reactions to the material, and the sodium salt of tetrabromphenolphthalein was substituted. Work with both the intravenous and oral administration of this material was then reported, with later reports on isomeric compounds; lesser doses of sodium phenoltetraiodophthalein were found satisfactory for the study of liver function and for gallbladder visualization.

Initial studies of the interpretation of the presence of stones were started when Dr. Cole placed human biliary calculi in a dog's gallbladder to study their roentgenographic appearance. The roentgenographic appearance of both opaque and lucent stones in human beings was anticipated in this fashion.

Thus the research efforts of two distinguished professors of surgery established one of the important milestones in the history of roentgenology. The basis for selective excretion of radiopaque contrast medium predominantly by one organ system had been laid, and the delineation of principles of interpretation of normal and abnormal roentgenograms of the gallbladder had been begun.

CHOLECYSTOGRAPHIC MEDIA

The use of sodium tetraiodophenolphthalein in oral cholecystography continued until the introduction of a safer diiodide compound, β-(4-hydroxy-3, 5-diiodophenyl)-α-phenylpropionic acid (Priodax). Because of its increased safety and the reliability of its results, it achieved wide use in the 1940s. The introduction of the tri-iodide compounds followed in the early 1950s. The most widely used was β-(3-amino,2,4,6-tri-iodophenyl)-α-ethylpropionic acid, known more briefly as iopanoic acid (Telepaque). It was shown to have decreased side effects and increased efficiency in demonstrating the gallbladder and its diseases.[28] Another triiodide compound, α-ethyl-β-(3-hydroxy-2,4,6-triiodophenyl) propionic acid (Teridax), was introduced; it showed no additional advantages, but some increase in side effects and prolongation of elevated protein bound iodine.[27] Better toleration is also reported with sodium tyropanoate (Bilopaque).[7] It is a derivative of iopanoic acid, but, unlike the latter, it is soluble in water.[3]

Further syntheses of appropriate compounds led to the development of sodium 3-(3-butyryl-amino-2,4,6-triiodophenyl)-2-ethylacrylate, known more briefly as sodium bunamiodyl (Orabilex). This compound was initially demonstrated to have fewer side effects, but the reports of cases of renal failure after multiple doses had been administered to patients with poor hepatorenal function[23] subsequently led to its withdrawal.

Other compounds introduced in recent years, also in the triiodide group of compounds, include the sodium 3-dimethylamino-methylene-amino)-2,4,6-triiodophenyl-propionic acid, known briefly as ipodate sodium (Oragrafin). Also available as the calcium salt in powder form, this compound has been evaluated to be a more satisfactory cholecystographic agent having a lower incidence of diarrhea than does iopanoic acid.[15]

To avoid a second day of hospitalization if the first dose of 3 gm. of iopanoic acid is unsuccessful in visualization of the gallbladder, ipodate calcium may be administered on the same morning with the iopanoic acid.[18] About one third of patients with nonvisualization or faint visualization on the initial examination with iopanoic acid will have satisfactory visualization on the second day.[5]

Burhenne and his associates have obtained good results by administering 6 gm. of iopanoic acid over a 2-day period to all outpatients for oral cholecystography. A definitive reading is given in this fashion after the first set of roentgenograms, and repeat studies with increased expense are avoided.

The continuing synthesis and evaluations of contrast media are part of a major effort of pharmaceutical companies both in the United States and abroad. Therefore, it is probable that further improvements in cholecystographic contrast media will be made. These will require extensive clinical evaluation and studies comparing them with currently used media. It is becoming increasingly apparent that such evaluation will require detailed studies of the effects of the media on liver and renal functions. The margin of safety in the use of such compounds for patients with some hepatorenal impairment will be an important factor in its acceptance.

PREPARATION OF THE PATIENT

Prior to the scheduling of cholecystography the patient should be queried regarding previous experience with contrast media and related reactions. This routine questioning should be performed by the referring physician or by the radiologist. Should any history of reaction be encountered, further consultation is indicated, and the value of the results of the examination should be balanced against the risk of further reaction. If the previous reaction was of a minor allergic nature, premedication with antihistaminic preparations may be helpful.

For optimum demonstration of the gallbladder by oral cholecystography a normal diet, including some fatty component, for several days preceding the examination is helpful. This diet assures that there has been physiologic stimulation for gallbladder emptying. For patients in whom fat induces significant discomfort, it can be omitted. The patient is asked to have a fat-free meal on the evening before the examination. A satisfactory fat-free meal easily available to outpatients consists of a small portion of lean meat, vegetables, fruit, toast or bread with jelly, and coffee or tea. The patient takes the prescribed 3 gm. dosage of contrast medium at 10:00 P.M. on the evening before the examination, with nothing thereafter to eat or drink until the examination is completed. The examination is performed in the morning. A range of 14 to 19 hours was demonstrated as giving peak opacity.[26a] This allows latitude in the scheduling of patients in the x-ray department.

DOSAGE CONSIDERATIONS

While from the accurate physiologic standpoint it might seem preferable to adjust the dosage of contrast medium to the patient's weight, from a practical standpoint iopanoic acid is effective in 3 gm. dosage in virtually all weight ranges of adults.[28] Some physicians go to 3.5 and 4 gm. for patients in the 200- to 225-pound range and above. For pediatric patients, proportionately smaller doses may be used.[12]

The use of multiple doses of cholecystographic media has been debated widely, particularly in cases with previous nonvisualization. It is my opinion that the initial evaluation of the gallbladder should be made with a single 3 gm. dose. If abnormalities suggesting filling defects are incompletely demonstrated because of poor visualization, a reenforcing dose of 3 gm. may be given for reexamination later the same day or on the following morning. If gallbladder dysfunction is suspected on the basis of faint images or nonvisualization, a repeated examination with a single dose after an interval of several days is useful for confirmation of the initial observation. If the exclusion of stones is a determining factor in surgical consultation, then a double dose might be helpful in this second evaluation. A double dose immediately after a single dose is not recommended because of possible severe reactions.

The 4-day technique of Salzman and his associates has occasionally been helpful in delineating the margins of calculi not otherwise demonstrated.[22] This repetition of 3 gm. dosage for 4 days results, in some cases, in absorption of contrast medium by the periphery of radiolucent stones otherwise missed in a nonvisualizing gallbladder or in the duct system. In using this technique one must be careful that the patient does not have impaired hepatorenal function.

Recent studies on the renal toxicity of contrast media in patients with hepatorenal damage have called attention to the danger of indiscriminate use of multiple doses of oral cholecystographic media.[23] Experiments with animals also support this warning.[11] Some conservatism in the administration of multiple doses is, therefore, indicated. If sufficient information is not obtained by a single dose examination and if repetition with a double dose is needed for more accurate delineation of radiolucent calculi, it is my conviction that intravenous cholangiography and cholecystography should then be recommended rather than the indiscriminate use of multiple doses of oral contrast medium.

TECHNICAL CONSIDERATIONS

For complete evaluation of the biliary tract by oral cholecystography, a preliminary scout film of the right upper quadrant is advisable unless prior films show this area to good advantage. This scout film is most helpful if it is taken in the same projection as the subsequent cholecystographic films, that is, with the patient in a prone left anterior oblique position. If such a scout film has not been obtained and it is suspected that contrast medium in the gallbladder is masking an opacity, the patient should be advised to return at a later time, when the gallbladder has cleared itself of contrast material. Such a scout film is also invaluable in the diagnosis of milk of calcium bile.

On the morning after the patient has taken the contrast medium prone oblique views are made. Several techniques for localization of the gallbladder are in use. A preliminary scout film of the abdomen with metallic localization markers along the spine may be used for subsequent accurate centering of the gallbladder films. In some diagnostic centers, preliminary localization by fluoroscopy is carried out. In others, initial 10 by 12 inch films are exposed covering both the upper and lower aspects of the right abdomen, and subsequent films are then centered more accurately. The initial prone oblique films are centered over the gallbladder and made with a grid technique. They should be sufficiently penetrated so that the density of the contrast medium will not obscure filling defects. Using the weight of the body of the patient on a radiolucent supporting wedge will aid by producing compression of abdominal soft tissues over the gallbladder area.

In addition to the prone oblique films, it is imperative that either upright or lateral decubitus films be obtained routinely in order to take advantage of the influence of gravity in the differentiation between fixed and movable filling defects in the gallbladder shadow. It is necessary that these films be processed promptly and inspected thoroughly before the rest of the examination is performed. If there is any question of confusion with overlying gas or incomplete delineation of calculi, fluoroscopy and compression spot films taken with the patient in the upright position are indicated. Should the patient have upper gastrointestinal examination and cholecystography on the same morning, it is helpful if the upright compression spot films are obtained routinely in the gastrointestinal suite.

Only after careful inspection of the prone oblique and decubitus films is the fat meal administered. Several preparations are available for such use.[6] A mixture of half milk and half cream is appropriate. Commercial chocolate-flavored solid "candy" bars (Colo-bar) are available. I have found a fatty diet supplement such as Lipomul-Oral, readily available in hospital pharmacies, to be effective and convenient when given in a dose of 1 tablespoonful. Repetition of the prone oblique and decubitus films 20 to 30 minutes after fat feeding, with further upright compression spot filming if deemed necessary after viewing the films, completes the examination. The routine use of cholecystagogues appears justified by the high percentage of duct demonstrations.[6] Roentgenographs taken after a fatty meal often provide better visualization of filling defects in the gallbladder, while no practical information is gained from the degree of contraction.

SIDE EFFECTS

An appreciation of the incidence of side effects with oral cholecystography is necessary primarily to enable the radiologist to recognize the possible source of any complaints that the patient may have and to offer appropriate reassurance. Table 48-1 presents the side effects my associates and I found in interviewing 400 patients after the ingestion of 3 gm. doses of iopanoic acid in various comparative studies.[29] It should be emphasized that most side effects are minimal and transient.

Table 48-1. Side effects of 3 gm. doses of iopanoic acid in 400 patients*

Side effects	Percentage of patients
None	62.5
Nausea, mild	5.8
Vomiting, mild	1.5
Diarrhea	
Mild	22.8
Severe	2.5
Dysuria	13.7
Other	2.8

*Adapted from Whitehouse, W. M., and Martin, O.: Radiology **60**:215, 1953.

COMPLICATIONS

The complications of oral cholecystography, as contrasted to transient side effects, are infrequent. Occasional progression of skin reactions to extensive hives or erythroderma is encountered. Antihistaminic medication is helpful, although occasionally dermatologic consultation is necessary for more complex therapy. The occurrence of renal shutdown as a complication of oral cholecystography has received emphasis in recent years.[23] This has been reported most frequently with multiple doses of bunamiodyl in patients with poor hepatorenal function, and much less commonly with single doses in apparently normal patients and with other contrast media. The mechanism appears to be an increase in the proportion of the contrast material excreted by the kidney, with subsequent renal damage and failure. In such instances measures to treat renal failure, including dialysis if necessary, must be employed.

It must be kept in mind that patients with poor hepatorenal function constitute a high risk group for oral cholecystography. The examination should be used only for good indication, and multiple doses should be avoided.

There is some evidence available that the combination of oral cholecystography and intravenous cholangiography on subsequent days may be dangerous.[1,26] Mild serum creatinine and urine changes have even been reported with both iopanoic acid and ipodate sodium.[25]

INTERFERENCE WITH LABORATORY DETERMINATIONS

Oral cholecystography interferes with some routine laboratory determinations. Positive results in tests for albuminuria may be obtained for 1 to 3 days after cholecystography,[14] and hence these determinations should be made before the patient is given a cholecystographic medium or be deferred for several days thereafter.

Similarly, determination of protein bound iodine should be obtained before the patient ingests cholecystographic medium, since abnormally high levels may be found for 6 months to a year after the examination.[31]

REFERENCES

1. Ansell, G.: Adverse reactions to contrast agents, Invest. Radiol. 5:374, 1970.
2. Baker, H. L., and Hodgson, J. R.: Further studies on accuracy of oral cholecystography, Radiology 74:239, 1960.

3. Benisek, G. J., and Gunn, J. A.: Preliminary clinical evaluation of a new cholecystographic medium, Bilopaque, Amer. J. Roentgen. **88**:792, 1962.

4. Berk, R. N., and Lasser, E. C.: Altered concepts of mechanism of nonvisualization of gallbladder, Radiology **82**:296, 1964.

5. Berk, R. N.: The consecutive dose phenomenon in oral cholecystography, Amer. J. Roentgen. **110**:230, 1970.

6. Burhenne, H. J.: Roentgenologic approach to a physiologic examination of the alimentary tract. In Gamble, J. R., and Wilbur, D. L., editors: Current concepts of clinical gastroenterology, Boston, 1965, Little, Brown and Company.

7. Burhenne, H. J.: Bilopaque: a new cholecystographic medium, Radiology **81**:629, 1963.

8. Cimmino, C. V.: Carcinoma in a well-functioning gallbladder, Radiology **71**:563, 1958.

9. Cole, W. H.: Historical features of cholecystography (Carman lecture), Radiology **76**:354, 1961.

10. Edinburgh, A., and Greffen, A.: Acute emphysematous cholecystitis, Amer. J. Surg. **96**:66, 1958.

11. Fink, H. E., Jr., Roenigh, W. J., and Wilson, G. P.: Experimental investigation of nephrotoxic effects of oral cholecystographic agents, Amer. J. Med. Sci. **247**:201, 1964.

12. Harris, R. C., and Caffey, J.: Cholecystography in infants, J.A.M.A. **153**:1333, 1953.

13. Hodges, F. J., and Whitehouse, W. M.: The gastrointestinal tract: a handbook of roentgen diagnosis, ed. 2, Chicago, 1965, Year Book Medical Publishers, Inc.

14. Holoubek, J. E., Carroll, W. H., Riley, G. M., and Langford, R. B.: Evaluation of pseudoalbuminuria following cholecystography in seventy-six cases, J.A.M.A. **153**:1018, 1953.

15. Juhl, J. H., Cooperman, L. R., and Crummy, A. B.: Oragrafin, a new cholecystographic medium; a double-blind comparison with Telepaque, Radiology **80**:87: 1963.

16. Marchetto, I., and Borrelli, F. J.: Pneumocholecystitis, Amer. J. Gastroent. **37**:311, 1962.

17. Netter, F. H.: The Ciba collection of medical illustrations, vol. 3, New York, 1957, Ciba Pharmaceutical Products, Inc.

18. Pogonowska, M. J., and Collins, L. C.: Immediate repeat cholecystography with Oragrafin-Calcium after initial nonvisualization of the gallbladder, Radiology **93**:179, 1969.

19. Richards, P.: Spontaneous migrations of gallstones, New Eng. J. Med. **266**:299, 1962.

20. Rous, P., and McMaster, P. D.: The concentrating activity of the gallbladder, J. Exp. Med. **34**:47, 1921.

21. Sachs, M., and Partington, P. F.: The distended gallbladder, the value of a fat meal in cholecystography, Amer. J. Roentgen. **83**:835, 1960.

22. Salzman, E., and Warden, M. R.: Telepaque opacification of radiolucent biliary calculi; the "rim sign," Radiology **71**:85, 1958.

23. Seaman, W. B., Cosgriff, S., and Wells, J.: Renal insufficiency following cholecystography, Amer. J. Roentgen. **90**:859, 1963.

24. Shehadi, W. H.: Clinical radiology of the biliary tract, New York, 1963, McGraw-Hill Book Co.

25. Tishler, J. M., and Gold, R.: A clinical trial of oral cholecystographic agents: Telepaque, Sodium Oragrafin and Calcium Oragrafin, J. Canad. Ass. Radiol. **20**:102, 1969.

26. Wangermez, A., Wangermez, J., and Debot, P.: Les risques de la cholangiographie-perfusion et les dangers des examens biliaires itératifs, J. Radiol. Electr. **51**:287, 1970.

26a. Whalen, J. P., Rizzuti, R. J., and Evans, J. A.: Time of optimal gallbladder opacification with Telepaque (iopanoic acid), Radiology **105**:523, 1972.

27. Whitehouse, W. M.: A comparative clinical study of Teridax (3 gm.) and Telepaque (2 gm.) in routine cholecystography, Radiology **65**:425, 1955.

28. Whitehouse, W. M.: Iopanoic acid, Ann. N. Y. Acad. Sci. **78**:809, 1959.

29. Whitehouse, W. M., and Martin, O.: A comparative clinical study of Priodax and Telepaque, including 1000 examinations, Radiology **60**:215, 1953.

30. Wise, R. E.: Intravenous cholangiography, Springfield, Ill., 1962, Charles C Thomas, Publisher.

31. Data supplied by Winthrop Laboratories.

32. Zboralske, F. F., and Amberg, J. R.: Cholecystocholestasis; a cause of cholecystographic error, Amer. J. Dig. Dis. **7**:339, 1962.

49 | Roentgenology of the biliary tract

Walter Frommhold
Hermann Frommhold

ANATOMY

The intrahepatic portion of the *bile duct system* starts at the cellular level where capillaries without endothelium and without wall are spaced between the liver cells (Fig. 49-1). These intracellular biliary passages radiate to the circumference of the lobule where they open into interlobular small bile ducts with shallow endothelium. Larger-caliber terminal bile ducts run from here accompanying the branches of the portal vein and hepatic artery in Glisson's capsule. These ducts then join with

others to form the ventrocranial and dorso-caudal duct in the right lobe of the liver. The confluence of these two branches into the right main radical and its junction with the single left main radical form the extrahepatic *ductus hepaticus*.[37] It is lined with cylindrical epithelium. The hepatic duct, together with a chain of lymph nodes, runs along the right border of the hepatoduodenal ligament anteriorly and to the right of the portal vein.

The 3 to 4 cm. long hepatic duct is joined by the cystic duct coming from the gallbladder to form the common bile duct or *ductus choledochus*. It is about 7 cm. long and may be divided into three parts. The first, or supraduodenal, portion of the common bile duct runs along the free margin of the hepatoduodenal ligament. The second, or retroduodenal, portion lies along the posterior wall of the duodenal bulb or the superior duodenal flexure, where an enlarged common bile duct may leave a characteristic imprint roentgenographically (Fig. 49-2). The third, or pancreatic, portion of the common duct is imbedded in the posterior surface of the head of the pancreas (common bile duct groove). A short intramural portion runs in the medial wall of the descending duodenum and forms the *papilla of Vater* with its terminal segment. The *pancreatic duct* of Wirsung joins usually with the common duct in the wall of the duodenum. This junction may also occur proximal to the duodenal wall, or the two ducts may enter the duodenum with separate orifices. The terminal segment of the common duct contains a special sphincter system with the functionally important closing apparatus of the *sphincter of Oddi*. The mucosal folds and prominences running in axial or transverse direction in the duodenum at the level of the ampulla also carry valvelike functions regulating the flow of bile and preventing the reflux of bile content.

The normal diameter of the common duct after intravenous cholangiography has been

1264

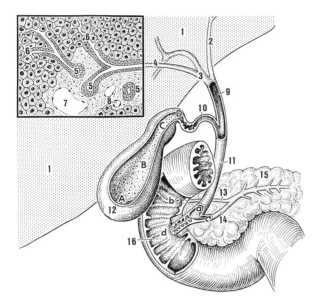

Fig. 49-1. Anatomy of the biliary system. **1,** Liver (hepar); **2,** left main hepatic duct; **3,** right hepatic duct; **4,** ventrocranial branch; **5,** bile duct (ductus interlobularis); **6,** terminal bile ducts and bile capillaries; **7,** branch of portal vein; **8,** branch of hepatic artery; **9,** hepatic duct (ductus hepaticus); **10,** cystic duct (ductus cysticus); **11,** common duct (ductus choledochus); **12,** gallbladder (vesica fellea); **A,** fundus; **B,** body; **C,** infundibulum; **D,** neck; **13,** minor pancreatic duct of Santorini; **14,** major pancreatic duct of Wirsung; **15,** pancreas; **16,** duodenum (pars descendens duodeni); **a,** pancreatic portion of common duct; **b,** minor papilla; **c,** major pancreatic duct; **d,** major papilla (sphincter of Oddi and papilla of Vater).

studied repeatedly. The majority of common ducts have an internal diameter of 3 to 6 mm., with variations at the upper and lower limits.[10] We consider an internal diameter of more than 8 mm. potentially abnormal. Mahour and co-workers found an average outer diameter of 7.4 mm. in autopsy specimens, and there was a definite increase with age but no relationship between caliber variations and body length or body weight.[26] Smith and Sherlock reviewed several studies and concluded that "it is reasonable to take 11 mm. as the upper limit of the common duct on radiographs and call 12 mm. or more dilatation."[40]

The assumption that the common duct assumes a reservoir function after cholecystectomy has not been substantiated in humans[36] but only in experimental dogs.[39] Postcholecystectomy dilatation of the common duct implies increased pressure within the duct system over some time. This postoperative dilatation of the common duct, however, must be compared with its width on early postoperative studies because the duct system may not return to a normal caliber even after the operative relief of mechanical obstruction. The poorly understood entity of fibrosis of the sphincter of Oddi may also be responsible for postcholecystectomy duct dilatation.

Most important in the roentgenographic evaluation and measurement of the common duct

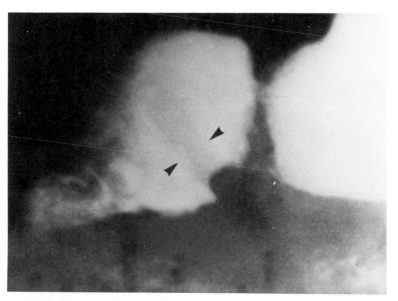

Fig. 49-2. Imprint of enlarged common bile duct on the duodenal bulb.

diameter as well as for the clinical assessment of the papilla of Vater is tomography at the time of intravenous cholangiography.

The usually pear-shaped but sometimes slender or spherical *gallbladder* (vesica fellea) is situated close to the underside of the right lobe of the liver. The gallbladder fundus extends by about 1 or 2 cm. below the lower margin of the liver. The body of the gallbladder is partially imbedded in the liver, and it is more or less adherent with its surface to the underside of the liver. Sometimes the gallbladder is quite mobile, connected to the liver bed only with a sleeve of serosa. The infundibulum of the gallbladder often shows angulation at its junction with the free neck of the gallbladder. The 3 or 4 cm. long cystic duct is connected to it in the form of a syphon. The mucosal folds of Heister protrude from both sides into the lumen in the form of spiral valves of the cystic duct close to the neck. Strong muscular fibers in the same region result in additional sphincter action. The adjacent flaccid portion of the cystic duct enters the common duct at a right angle, at a sharp angle, or spirals around the common duct and enters it posteriorly. The gallbladder is supplied

through the cystic artery. It arises from the right hepatic artery, although variations may occur. The gallbladder veins consist of several small vessels draining the blood into the right branch of the portal vein.

The topographic relationship of the gallbladder and the bile ducts is of great importance for the roentgenologic examination. The body of the gallbladder lies adjacent to the superior duodenal flexure and the transverse colon. The infundibulum and neck of the gallbladder often touch the posterior surface of the duodenal bulb. Close relationship also exists to the head of the pancreas and to the right kidney (Fig. 49-3) and pathologic processes of these neigh-

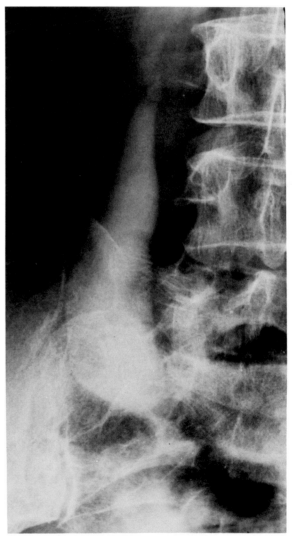

Fig. 49-4. Pendulous gallbladder.

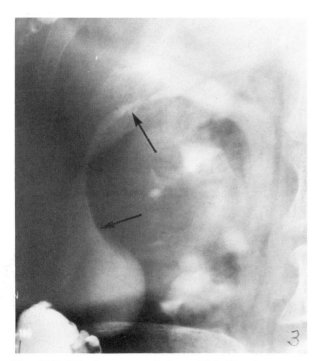

Fig. 49-3. Displacement of the gallbladder by a renal cyst.

boring organs may extend to the gallbladder or vice versa.[11]

PHYSIOLOGY

Formation of bile within the liver is a continuous process and a true energetic product of the liver cell. The secretion is characterized by its content of biliary acids, cholesterol, and bilirubin. There is a decrease in pressure from liver secretion in the direction of the gallbladder and the draining bile ducts. The normal volume of the gallbladder is about 30 to 50 ml. Water absorption in its wall may result in a tenfold bile concentration within a 24-hour period.

In response to food intake emptying of the gallbladder occurs by either an inervation reflex pathway or a humoral mechanism. The amount of bile production and the emptying mechanism depend on the type of food ingested. Meat and fat cause an increase of bile flow as contrasted to carbohydrates, which cause no increase. Maximal gallbladder contraction results from raw egg yolk, and weak contraction results from rye bread, for example.[25]

The proximal portion of the common duct exhibits only tonic activity, whereas the sphincter of Oddi has been shown to go through opening and closing phases of about 2 seconds each.[19] The frequency of these motions at the sphincter vary with the common duct pressure[4] and with different food stimuli in the duodenum. They may also be related to psychologic or autonomic regulation. Contraction and distention of the sphincter apparatus in the distal common duct occur usually synchronously with duodenal peristalsis.[33]

CONGENITAL ANOMALIES AND DEFORMITIES

Congenital anomalies and deformities are described in detail in Chapter 57. Some of the positional anomalies need further comment, since they may give rise to sometimes significant symptoms only during adulthood.

Clinically important is, for instance, the mobile, pendulous gallbladder (Fig. 49-4). It is sometimes seen in older women who have had a significant weight loss and who have an abdominal visceral ptosis. Cholelithiasis is rarely associated with a pendulous gallbladder, but a volvulus of the organ with obstruction must be clinically considered in patients with short attacks of intense pain simulating perforation of an ulcer.[24]

Transposition of the gallbladder to the left side of the abdomen is sometimes overlooked by the radiologist, particularly with the diagnosis of nonvisualization on routine right upper quadrant roentgenographs. A full film of the abdomen is needed if the gallbladder is not visualized on routine films. Transposition of the gallbladder, however, is rare in the absence of situs inversus. We have also seen herniation of the gallbladder through the foramen epiploicum into the lesser sac (Fig. 49-5).

FUNCTIONAL DISORDERS

Disorders in the dynamics of the gallbladder and the bile ducts are still labeled under "biliary dyskinesia."[34] Although in recent years we have gained some insight into the dynamics of the biliary tract, most cases of "bile duct dyskinesia" are diagnosed under this heading because some organic underlying cause is initially overlooked. We know more about the so-called dyskinesia of the gallbladder, which is caused by primary organic disease in almost all cases.[9] Hormonal and other factors, such as imbalance of the autonomic nervous system, or diseases of adjacent organs such as the pancreas and stomach may also play a role in dyskinesia. This label is often used in unexplained right upper quadrant symptoms associated with dyspepsia. Morphologic gallbladder abnormalities, such as sail-shaped membranes, septation, or prominent trabeculation, are sometimes present.[12] It has been contemplated that pressure differences occur in these cases, causing more pronounced contraction in one portion of the gallbladder than in the other. This explanation is more readily acceptable in cases with distinct circular septation resulting in two gallbladder chambers (Fig. 49-6) similar to a true diverticulum of the gallbladder fundus (Fig. 49-7). Septated gallbladders usually contain true membranes with more or less muscular components. Gallbladder septation of this type not only predisposes to stone formation but also results in inflammatory wall changes, shrinkage of the gallbladder, and even pressure necrosis by incarcerated concrements (Fig. 49-8). Single or multiple septations in the infundibulum or neck of the gallbladder suggest a possible relationship to symptoms (Fig. 49-9).

A local foreshortening in the wall of the gallbladder is present in the developmental varia-

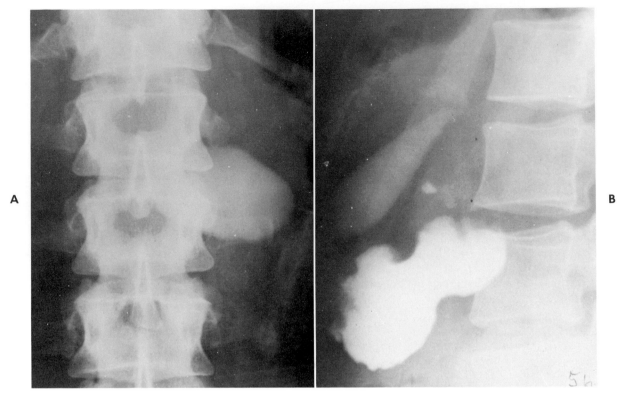

Fig. 49-5. Herniation of the gallbladder through the epiploic foramen into the lesser sac. **A,** A-P projection, displacement of the gallbladder to the left of the lumbar spine. **B,** Lateral projection, stomach outlined with barium.

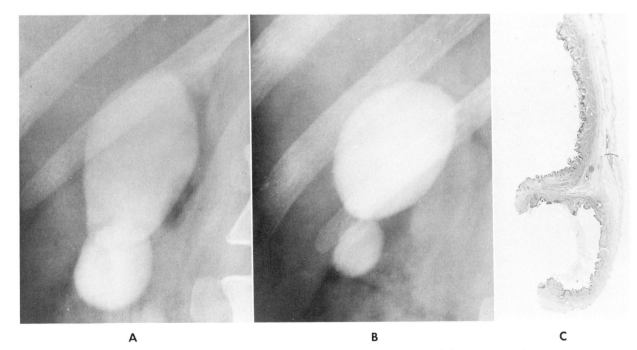

Fig. 49-6. Septation of the gallbladder. **A,** Before fatty meal. **B,** Distinct concentric septation after fatty meal. **C,** Histology of the septum.

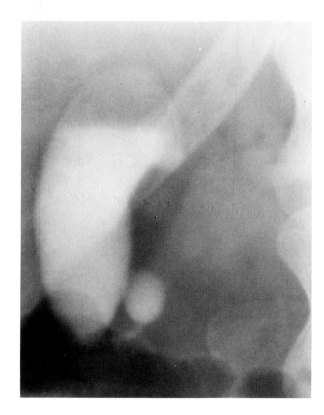

Fig. 49-7 Diverticulum of the gallbladder.

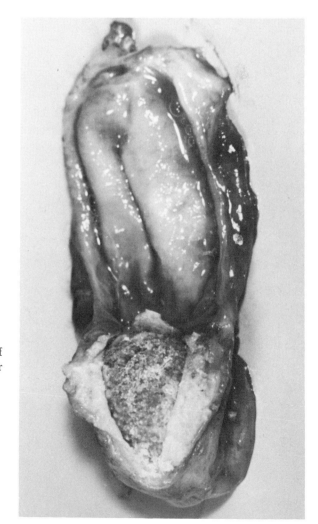

Fig. 49-8. Incarcerated gallstone and pressure necrosis of the wall with circular septation at the gallbladder fundus.

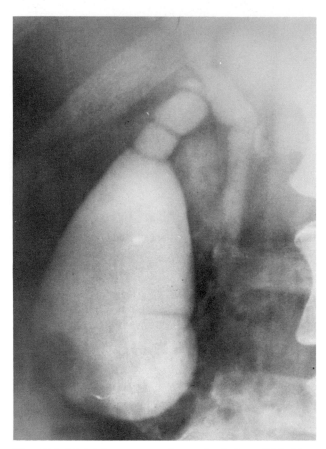

Fig. 49-9. Multiple septa at the neck of the gallbladder.

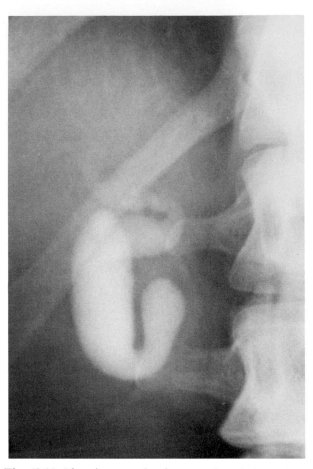

Fig. 49-10. Phrygian cap, developmental variation of the gallbladder.

tion in the so-called Phrygian cap of the gallbladder fundus (Fig. 49-10). This is thought to be caused by minor variations in the embryonal recanalization or possibly by fibrous strands.

Functional abnormalities of the biliary ducts without organic cause have little if any practical importance. One may describe the gallbladder as hypokinetic or hyperkinetic, depending on its ability to contract after the administration of a cholecystagogue. Hyperkinetic gallbladder contraction is often seen in cases of benign abnormalities of the gallbladder wall, such as hyperplastic cholecystoses. The high-fat meal ingestion after standard views are obtained is a routine method that results in better visualization of small abnormalities such as benign tumors and provides an opportunity to note the change in shape and size of the gallbladder.

In cases of suspected biliary disease with gallbladder visualization the practical roentgen-

ologic approach is the search for an organic explanation of "painful dyskinesia." This includes the investigation of neighboring organs such as pancreas, stomach, duodenum, and liver. A possible cause is abnormal motility at the neck of the gallbladder or at the sphincter of Oddi. Anatomic variations or inflammatory changes are usually responsible if symptoms occur. Various laboratory tests and the technique of pharmacoradiography with the use of Cholecystokinin[30] or morphine have helped little in the better understanding of these cases; most of these tests are no longer in use today. The symptom complex of "biliary dyskinesia" remains poorly defined.

INFLAMMATORY DISEASES
Acute cholecystitis

The majority of cases of acute cholecystitis is caused by irritation and bacterial infection with alteration in bile flow. This is the result of cystic duct obstruction by stone in about 90% of patients. The other 10% of cystic duct obstructions consists of cholecystitis in the absence of cholelithiasis.[18] Etiologic considerations have also been given to functional abnormalities at the papilla of Vater, with or without associated pancreatic or biliary reflux, to abnormalities in vascular supply, and to other causes. These include tumor, fibrosis, secondary inflammatory change from adjacent viscera, anatomic deformities, and variations in vascular development. Even infestation of the bile system with *Giardia lamblia, Ascaris,* or ameba may lead to partial obstruction favoring bacterial growth.

Acute cholecystitis is characterized by edema of the markedly reddened mucosa, which is often covered with fibrinous exudate. The ability to concentrate bile is often lessened or lost. This results in nonvisualization or poor visualization on oral cholecystography and creates a difficult diagnostic problem for the radiologist.

Animal experiments with tagged oral cholecystographic media raise the possibility of increased absorption across the gallbladder wall in the form of passive diffusion through the damaged mucosa.[5] Good visualization of the gallbladder on oral cholecystography, on the other hand, does not exclude subacute cholecystitis. A significant number of patients with acute cholecystitis show the roentgenologic sign of nonvisualization of the gallbladder with visualization of the ducts (Fig. 49-11).[17] This so-called exclusion of the gallbladder is always evidence for organic disease, which, in the majority of cases, is cystic duct obstruction caused by a stone.[8] These are usually nonopaque stones with calcification occurring only after repeated episodes of infection.

Acute cholecystitis is no contraindication to intravenous cholangiography. It is the method of choice in acute abdominal conditions to give the surgeon some information about the gallbladder and the bile ducts in a quick way that is not harmful to the patient.[17] Because there is evidence that in some cases of cholecystitis there is no real mechanical obstruction of the cystic duct, we recommend that the emergency examination be extended to 3 to 4 hours.

Drip infusions of 40 ml. iodipamide (Cholografin), ioglycamide (Bilivistan), or methylglu-

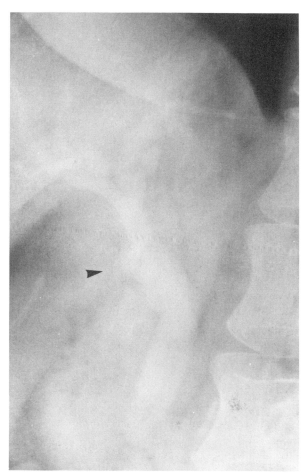

Fig. 49-11. "Exclusion of the gallbladder," clinically verified as cholecystitis, in a 62-year-old woman.

camine salt of ioglycamide (Biligram)[41] diluted in 250 ml. of double-distilled water or dextrose improve the ability to visualize lesions within the ducts or stones in the gallbladder. Side effects are statistically less frequent than with the standard method. The high amount of contrast medium given intravenously causes no increase of liver specific enzymes in patients with severe liver damage.[13,29,42]

In some cases intravenous cholangiography has resulted in satisfactory demonstration of the gallbladder and bile ducts with total serum bilirubin levels of 5 or 6 mg./100 ml., particularly if previous bilirubin levels were higher. The use of tomography or zonography shows improved results in intravenous cholangiography with better bile duct visualization.

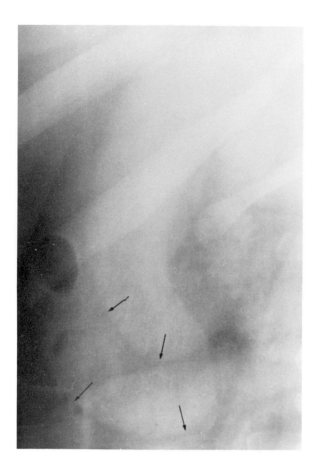

Fig. 49-12. Hydrops of the gallbladder. Plain film shows the lower pole of the right kidney (upper arrows) and the overlying fundus of the gallbladder (lower arrows).

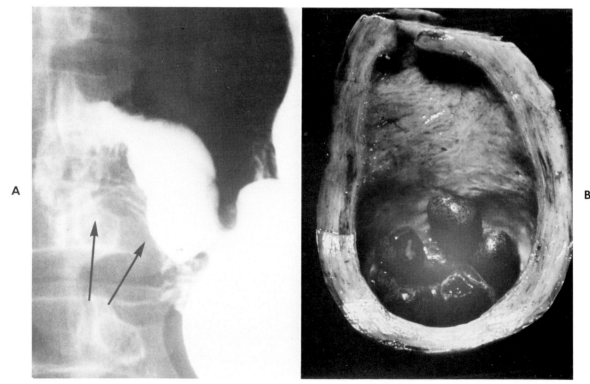

Fig. 49-13. A, Displacement of the descending duodenum by a gallbladder "tumor." **B,** Fibrous, thickened, tumor-like gallbladder with some stones and chronic cholecystitis.

Chronic cholecystitis

Chronic, usually recurring cholecystitis is the most common form of gallbladder inflammation. Fibrous thickening of the gallbladder wall with or without pericholecystic adhesions and eventual shrinkage of the viscus is usually the result of repeated inflammations. Plain roentgenographic examination may delineate the fundus of the gallbladder in some cases of hydrops. This soft tissue shadow must be differentiated from the right lower kidney pole (Fig. 49-12). Distention of the gallbladder may also lead to a flat indentation of the superior aspect of the hepatic flexure of the colon or the descending duodenum (Fig. 49-13).

Nonvisualization or poor visualization of the gallbladder suggests chronic cholecystitis even if repeated cholecystography shows no improvement in contrast outline. Again, as in acute cholecystitis, infusion cholangiography may result in satisfactory gallbladder visualization even in the presence of jaundice. Damage of the liver parenchyma by the contrast medium has not been shown.

Porcellan gallbladder

Calcium incrustation of the gallbladder wall is usually visible on plain roentgenograms. The calcium-dense opacification is characteristic in its location, outline, and size (Fig. 49-14). The term "porcellan gallbladder" was coined by Flörken. Its cause is poorly understood. Besides chronic cholecystitis as an underlying initial event, a variety of other factors has been incriminated, such as abnormalities in calcium metabolism, persistent or intermittent occlusion of the cystic duct, discrepancy between inflammatory exudation and resorption, and also difficulties in clearing of the calcium-containing bile from the gallbladder wall.

Calcium deposition in the form of plaques in the submucosa of the highly fibrotic gallbladder wall is present in porcellan gallbladder. Differential diagnostic considerations include large solitary gallstones with a calcium-containing shell and also small echinococcal cysts.[38]

Milk of calcium bile

Milk of calcium bile, limy bile, or calcium soap are synonyms for the same condition. Etiologic considerations include an increase in the saturation limit for calcium carbonate in the concentrated bile or chronic obstruction with

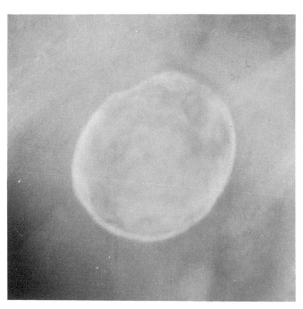

Fig. 49-14. Porcellan gallbladder.

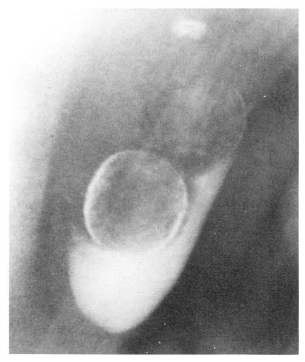

Fig. 49-15. Milk of calcium bile (plain film taken with the patient in upright position) with two large calculi and obstructing cystic duct stone.

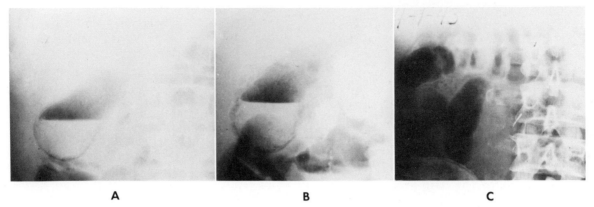

A   B   C

Fig. 49-16. Emphysematous cholecystitis.

stasis and resulting changes in the calcium level. An opaque gallstone in the region of the cystic duct is seen roentgenographically in some cases. Bile in this condition consists of a quite viscous, gray-white collection of calcium carbonate and bile soap (Fig. 49-15).

The mobile content of the gallbladder appears on plain roentgenograms as a homogeneous but very dense shadow when seen with the patient in recumbent position. The opaque matter usually levels out in the erect position. Milk of calcium bile has occasionally been seen in the common duct in patients with distal common duct stone obstruction.

The differential diagnosis of staghorn calculus in the kidney usually presents no difficulties because of its more posterior position and sometimes characteristic pelvocaliceal shape.

Emphysematous cholecystitis

Emphysematous cholecystitis is a rare condition. Gas collection in the lumen of the gallbladder or in its wall or surrounding tissue is quite characteristic on plain roentgenograms (Fig. 49-16). The gas-forming organisms primarily implicated are *Clostridium welchii, Clostridium oedematiens,* and *Escherichia coli* or *Escherichia perfringens.* Bacterial growth in the gallbladder is apparently facilitated by cystic duct occlusion by stone. Reflux from pancreatic or gastric sections and also anoxemic parts in the gallbladder wall have been implicated in this condition. Of interest is the high association of emphysematous cholecystitis with diabetes in about half of the 100 published cases.[36]

Overlying gas from the small or large bowel and gastrointestinal fistulas from the gallbladder must be differentiated. These cases usually show air in the biliary tree. Examinations of the intestine with barium sulfate are helpful in excluding fistulas between the bowel and the biliary system.

Pericholecystic adhesions with chronic cholecystitis

The inflammatory changes in chronic cholecystitis do not remain confined to the gallbladder wall. Adhesions soon extend between the gallbladder, the common duct, the duodenum, and also the hepatic flexure of the colon and adjacent ileal bowel loops. The omentum and the anterior abdominal wall are also sometimes involved. The gallbladder itself changes its outline characteristically through shrinkage. It is often impossible in such cases to separate the gallbladder from the duodenal bulb during combined cholecystography and upper gastrointestinal study even with palpation.

BILIARY PARASITES[7]

When compared to ascariasis in the intestinal tract, infestation of the biliary system is a rare event. It may present with colic-like pain in the right upper quadrant reminiscent of cholecystitis or pancreatitis. Biliary parasites are often not considered in the differential diagnosis. Infestation of the liver and bile ducts with *Clonorchis sinensis* is in its chronic stage also usually mislabeled as chronic cholecystitis and cholelithiasis. Important diagnostic indications to the

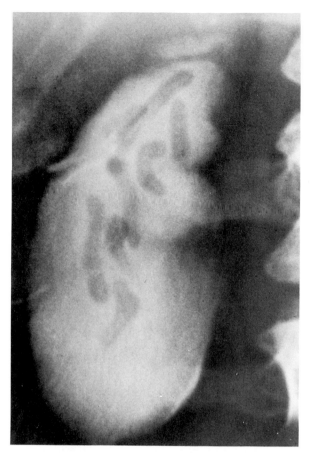

Fig. 49-17. Encrustated suture material in the gallbladder simulating parasites (55-year-old woman, 5 years after cholecystotomy for a gallstone).

correct diagnosis are diffuse urticaria, peripheral eosinophilia, or positive results of the complement fixation test.

Intravenous or operative cholangiograms may show characteristic filling defects conforming to the shape of the parasites.[27] Indurated suture material in the gallbladder after cholecystotomy because of a large stone may give a roentgenologic appearance similar to parasites (Fig. 49-17).

INFLAMMATION OF THE BILE DUCTS
Stenosing papillitis

Stenosing papillitis of the terminal segment of the common duct is seen as a secondary change with cholecystitis, cholelithiasis, choledocholithiasis, gastroduodenal ulcerations, diverticula, or pancreatic disease. Primary organic disease at the papilla is quite rare. It is also a controversial

entity for many published cases contain no adequate histologic or intraoperative roentgenologic proof. The pathologic findings include chronic atrophic inflammation with round cell infiltration, fibrosis, and glandular hyperplasia in the area of the papilla of Vater. The clinical symptoms accompanying stenosing papillitis may range from nonspecific upper abdominal complaints to colic and jaundice with cholestasis.

Serious cases of papillitis cannot be diagnosed by intravenous cholecystocholangiography because of biliary tract obstruction and altered liver function. Intravenous cholangiography is indicated in less severe cases. The diagnosis may be suspected if narrowing of the lumen in the region of the papilla is associated with delayed common duct emptying or common duct dilatation. Contrast is usually not identified in the duodenal loop on delayed roentgenograms. A small amount of contrast medium passing into the intestine with partial obstruction at the region of the papilla is best demonstrated on abdominal roentgenograms 24 hours after injection, when the contrast medium may be seen in a more concentrated form within the colon. Tomography improves bile duct visualization (Fig. 49-18). Intraoperative and postoperative cholangiography with or without radiomanometry has been used in these cases, but the final diagnosis of stenosis at the papilla is usually made at the time of operation.

Papillitis alters the normally cone shaped and tapered papillary canal with its smooth marginal outline to an elongated, stiff, and irregularly defined shape with the distal tip often distorted or distracted to one side. Serial roentgenograms show no change in this appearance even after application of spasmolytic drugs.

These changes of papillitis are seen in about 28% of patients after cholecystectomy with or without common duct exploration.[31] Papillitis may become the organic reason for the so-called postcholecystectomy syndrome.[1]

Primary sclerosing cholangitis

Primary sclerosing cholangitis is a nonspecific fibrosing, chronic, inflammatory change of the bile ducts of unknown cause.[32] It has been observed not only in the area of the papilla but also in other extrahepatic portions of the common duct and in some cases in the intrahepatic ducts. Simultaneous inflammatory and fibrosing

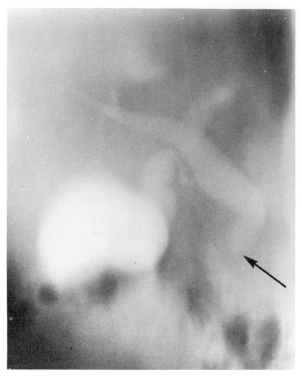

Fig. 49-18. Stenosing papillitis. Tomography shows narrowing of the distal common bile duct; no contrast medium is passing into the duodenum.

changes have been observed in these cases in other areas, such as retroperitoneal and mediastinal fibrosis, Riedel's struma, and ulcerative colitis.[3] Middle-aged men are primarily affected.

The roentgenographic appearance is that of strictures of the extrahepatic and rarely the intrahepatic biliary tract with varying length of involvement and usually without proximal dilatation and without cholelithiasis. Progressive changes eventually lead to obstructive jaundice. The differential diagnosis, therefore, includes all conditions leading to biliary tract obstruction, including carcinoma of the head of the pancreas, pancreatitis, cholelithiasis, and primary biliary cirrhosis. If preoperative intravenous cholangiography fails, the definitive diagnosis is usually made at the time of operation. Precholecystectomy operative cholangiography is indicated in order to assure optimal surgical intervention.

Strictures

Postcholecystectomy scarring of the common duct in the region of the cystic duct stump may cause strictures. Narrowing of the duct may be seen at the segment where the T tube was placed after surgery. Iatrogenic postoperative strictures are not uncommon. Strictures may be difficult to differentiate from bile duct carcinoma.

CALCULI
Cholelithiasis

Gallstone disease affects about 15% of the population in the fourth through sixth decades of life and is seen with even higher incidence after pregnancy[16] and in women with diabetes. Abnormalities in metabolism, bile stasis, precipitation on the gallbladder wall, and associated physical and chemical reactions have been implicated as a cause for primary stone crystallization. Gallbladder inflammation may be primary or secondary to gallstone formation. Increase in size of gallstones is usually continuous, although their spontaneous disappearance has been described.[28] Gallstones up to 10 mm. in size may pass through the duct system without damage; however, this phenomenon is rarely seen.

A few characteristic types may be delineated from the great variety of gallstones, but there are no fundamental differences in their chemical composition, since they are also multicrystalline mixtures with amorphous particles. Classification as homogeneous and heterogeneous calculi is useful. Heterogeneous stones may be combination stones with a macroscopic center and cortex (Fig. 49-19, *A*) or mixed stones of cholesterol and bilirubin without pattern (Fig. 49-19, *B*). Classification of gallstones according to their shape is of little practical value. There are solitary bell-shaped calculi (Fig. 49-19, *C*) and the commonly occurring multiple tetrahedral stones, which are facetted and limit each other in growth (Fig. 49-19, *D*).

The roentgenographic appearance of floating, nonopaque gallstones (Fig. 49-20, *A*) must be distinguished from the layering phenomenon of contrast medium (Fig. 49-20, *B*), the latter representing a technical artefact. Gallstones float at the interface between two immiscible bile fractions according to their specific gravity when the patient assumes the erect position.

Gallstones must be distinguished from right-sided kidney stones. This is usually possible on plain films with oblique and lateral positioning, particularly when the stones are large enough to

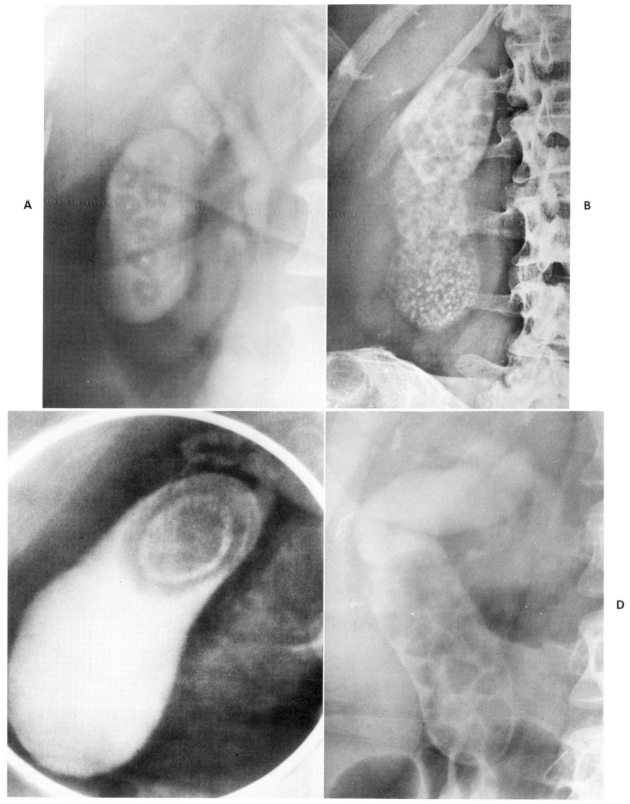

Fig. 49-19. Cholelithiasis. **A,** Combination stones with calcified center. **B,** Mixed stones. **C,** Large solitary stone showing lamination. **D,** Multiple tetrahedral stones.

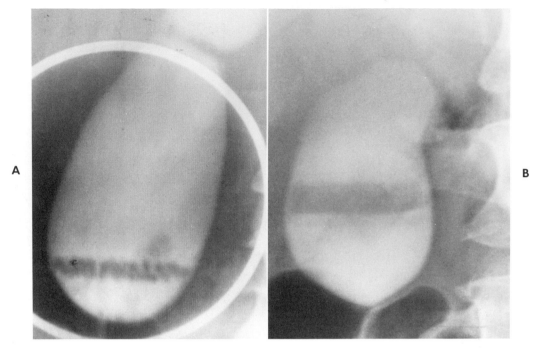

Fig. 49-20. A, Multiple small biliary calculi showing "layering phenomenon." **B,** "Layering phenomenon" of the contrast media taken with the patient in upright position is a technical artifact.

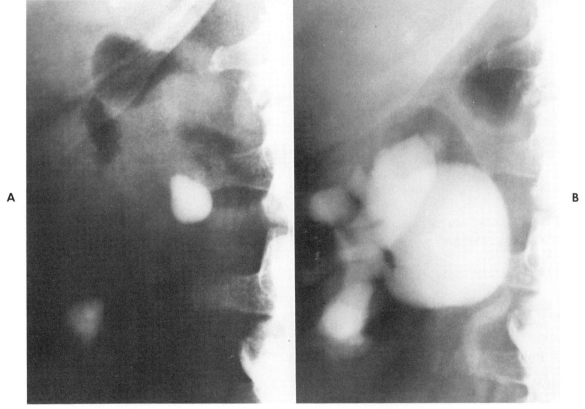

Fig. 49-21. A, Two tetrahedral-shaped calculi in the region of the gallbladder on the plain film. **B,** Intravenous pyelogram shows these stones within the renal pelvis and the lower calyx.

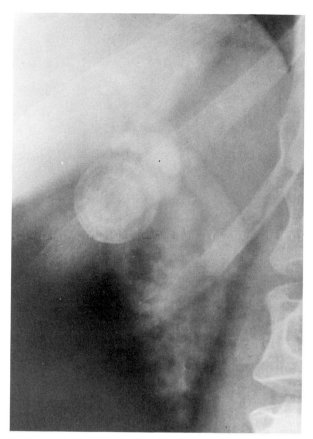

Fig. 49-22. Obstruction of the cystic duct by a large solitary stone in the infundibulum of the gallbladder.

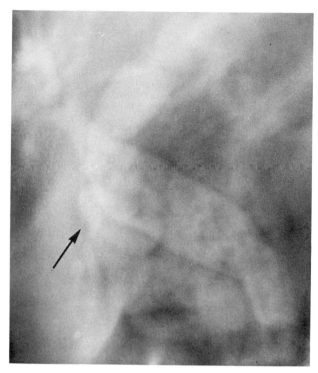

Fig. 49-23. Occlusion of the cystic duct by a nonopaque stone (arrow). Zonogram reveals multiple calculi in the enlarged common bile duct.

be visible on fluoroscopic examination. Intravenous urography or cholecystocholangiography may be necessary for diagnosis in other cases (Fig. 49-21). Rib cartilage calcification, lymph node calcification, appendicoliths, coproliths, stones in diverticula, calcifications in operative scars, calcified adrenals, and calcified *Echinococcus* cysts must be differentiated. Their roentgenographic appearance and distribution is usually characteristic enough for identification.

Cystic duct stone obstruction

The majority of gallstone carriers remain clinically asymptomatic. Thirty-five percent to 40% of patients, however, have at least one symptomatic episode. This is caused by calculus obstruction of the gallbladder in 90% of cases. Hydrops of sterile bile develops if the gallbladder continues to function in the presence of occlusion. Empyema develops with infection.

The occluding stone is usually visible on cholangiography adjacent to the common duct (Fig. 49-22). If the stone is situated in the gallbladder infundibulum, a small portion of the cystic duct will be demonstrated by contrast medium (Fig. 49-23). The sharp, convex termination of the duct stump indicates a cystic duct stone. Occlusion of the cystic duct may also occur with inflammatory stenosis or carcinoma of the gallbladder. The important roentgenologic sign is always the absence of gallbladder visualization in the presence of bile duct visualization, the sign of the "excluded gallbladder."

Bacterial chronic cholecystitis usually results with recurring episodes of partial obstruction of the gallbladder. It leads to thickening of the gallbladder wall and eventually to shrinkage of the whole viscus. This contracted gallbladder is occasionally seen late during cholecystography especially when drip infusion and tomography are used (Fig. 49-24).

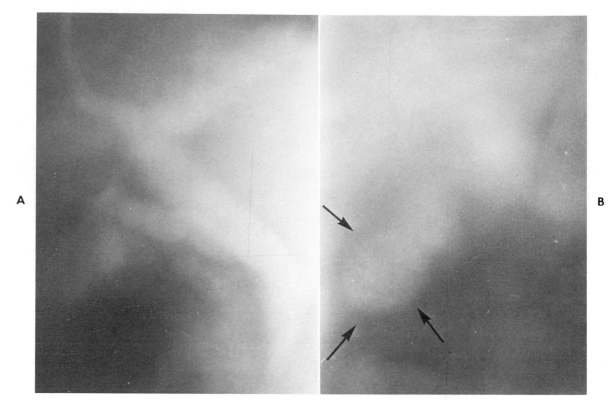

Fig. 49-24. Shrunken gallbladder demonstrated in tomograms during drip infusion cholegraphy. **A,** Tomogram at 9 cm. shows moderately enlarged bile duct system and no visualization of the gallbladder. **B,** Tomogram at 6 cm. shows faint filling of a shrunken gallbladder containing multiple small calculi.

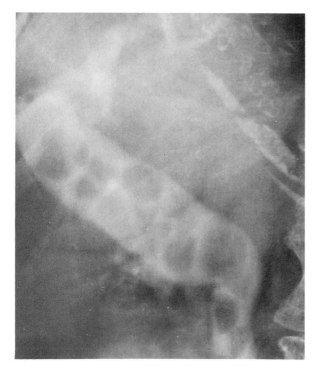

Fig. 49-25. Nonopaque calculi in the dilated common bile duct (after cholecystectomy).

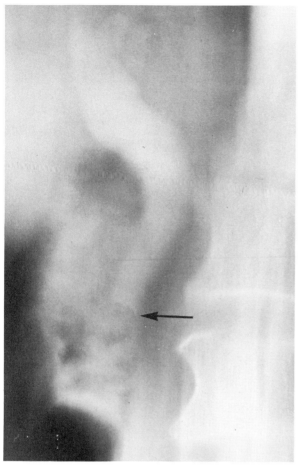

Fig. 49-26. Partial obstruction of the common bile duct by a nonopaque calculus. Tomogram shows the sharply defined filling defect near the papilla of Vater.

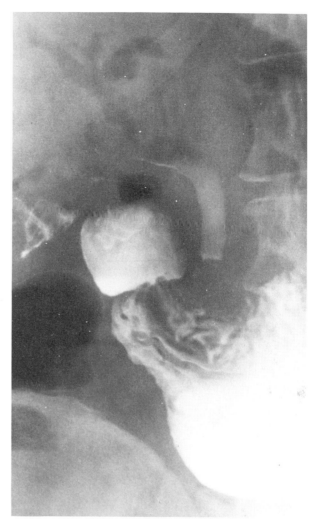

Fig. 49-27. Spontaneous fistula between duodenal bulb and common bile duct. Status after perforation of a gallstone into the duodenum.

Cholangiolithiasis

Common duct stones occur usually in combination with gallbladder stones. They may be associated with a functioning stone-free gallbladder and may be retained in the duct system after cholecystectomy. Gallbladder stones often pass into the common duct and may then be discharged into the duodenal loop without symptoms if the common duct caliber is normal and the papilla of Vater is functioning. Nonopaque bile duct stones are roentgenographically visualized as sharply defined filling defects with or without bile duct dilatation (Fig. 49-25). Tomography and zonography result in optimal roentgenographic definition and help to separate overlying gas shadows (Fig. 49-26). Choledocholithiasis occurs in about 75% of pa-

tients with chronic bile duct obstruction. This may be associated with episodes of jaundice, chills, and fever as an expression of associated cholangitis. The incomplete obstruction of the bile ducts may also lead sooner or later to intrahepatic pressure increase and damage of liver parenchyma, with the final result of cirrhosis.

Complications

In addition to the described cholecystitis or cholangitis associated with gallstone disease, perforation into adjacent viscera with spontaneous bile fistula occurs. It is quite less common but may be more serious, particularly with fistulas to the intestinal tract and subsequent gallstone

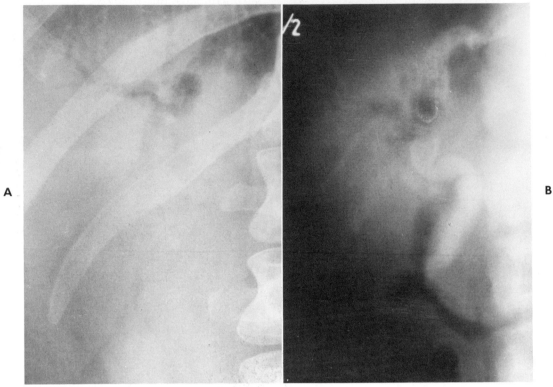

Fig. 49-28. Demonstration of a spontaneous internal biliary fistula by drip infusion cholegraphy. **A,** Plain film; air contrast in bile duct system. **B,** Sixty minutes after drip infusion visualization of the bile duct system, multiple very small calculi in the left hepatic duct ("excluded gallbladder" sign).

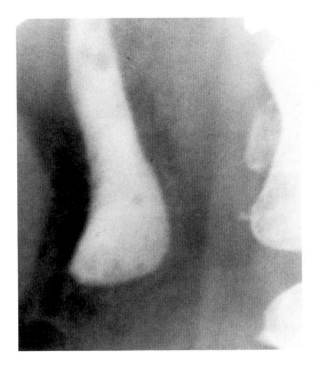

Fig. 49-29. Cholesterolosis of the gallbladder. Multiple small filling defects, fixed and varying in size.

ileus.[6] This is also unusual and accounts for only about 2% of all causes of mechanical bowel obstruction. Gallstone perforation into the duodenum is a usual occurrence (Fig. 49-27), whereas penetration to the colon or stomach is less frequently seen. Extra-abdominal gallstone perforations or spontaneous external fistulas are quite rare.

Gas in the biliary tracts or the disappearance of the previously visualized gallstones with or without their demonstration in the digestive tract are the important roentgenographic signs in the diagnosis of gallstone perforation (Fig. 49-28). It is, however, often the direct demonstration of the fistula by intravenous cholangiography or retrograde filling during gastrointestinal barium studies that clarifies the confusing clinical picture with the often nonspecific history.

HYPERPLASIA AND NEOPLASIA OF THE GALLBLADDER AND THE BILIARY DUCTS
Benign changes

In 1960 Jutras described a variety of partially degenerative and partially proliferative changes of the gallbladder wall under the general heading of "hyperplastic cholecystoses."[2,20] This term has been accepted clinically, although the definition is pathologically and anatomically insufficient. The roentgenographic appearance after all intravenous contrast studies is almost always characterized by the triad of hyperconcentration, hyperexcitability, and hyperexcretion. If this hyperkinetic function is noted, the radiologist should think of the entity of hyperplastic cholecystosis. The presence of this triad also helps in the differentiation of malignant processes.

Cholesterolosis of the gallbladder is characterized roentgenologically by multiple small filling defects (Fig. 49-29). They are caused by small polyps consisting of lipid-containing macrophages, so-called foam cells (Fig. 49-30). The generalized form of the "strawberry gallbladder" (Fig. 49-31) is not demonstrated roentgenographically. Only occasionally is this entity associated with gallstones. Stone formation around the nucleus of a separated cholesterol polyp is possible.

Adenomyoma of the gallbladder fundus is uncommon (Fig. 49-32), whereas generalized *adenomyomatosis*[14] occurs in almost 5% of all

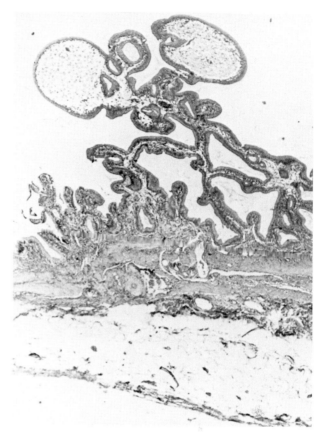

Fig. 49-30. Histology of cholesterolosis—cholesterol polyp and lipoid-storing foam cells under epithelium.

cholecystectomies according to Ten Eyck. "Cholecystitis granularis proliferans cystica" is an older designation for adenomyomatosis. It is probably less accurate because the inflammatory changes in the gallbladder wall are considered to be secondary. Filling of cystlike enlarged Rokitansky-Aschoff sinuses results in the picture of the "pearl necklace gallbladder" if most of the gallbladder wall is involved (Fig. 49-33). An "hourglass-shaped" gallbladder results in cases in which the hyperplastic area is situated in the middle of the body of the gallbladder (Fig. 49-34). If the changes are present only at the tip of the fundus, extraluminal diverticula-like formation is seen in rosette formation on cholecystography (Fig. 49-35). Muscular hypertrophy with small cavitations within it is histologically predominant (Fig. 49-36).

True *papillomas* with blood-containing stroma and epithelial surface and inflammatory polyps are extremely rare, and their differential

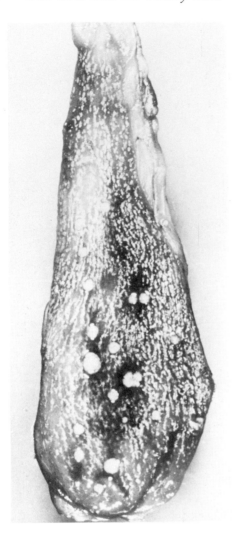

Fig. 49-31. Strawberry gallbladder. Disseminated form of cholesterolosis with multiple cholesterol polyps.

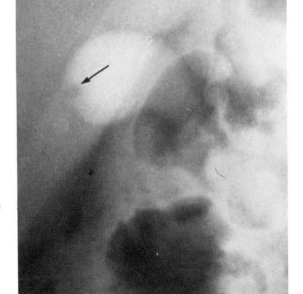

Fig. 49-32. Solitary filling defect at the fundus of the gallbladder shown histologically to be adenomyoma.

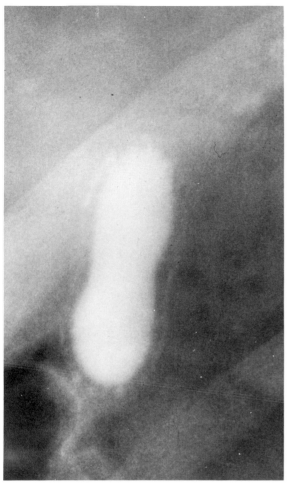

Fig. 49-33. Generalized adenomyomatosis, with Aschoff-Rokitansky sinuses.

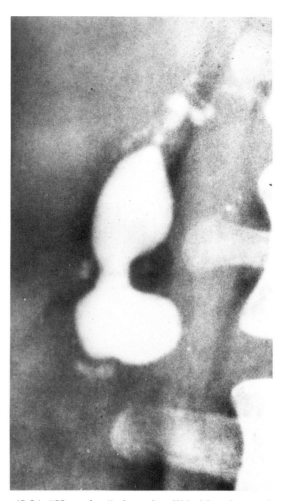

Fig. 49-34. "Hourglass" shaped gallbladder, hyperplastic area of adenomyomatosis in the middle of the gallbladder body.

diagnostic consideration is not significant. Discussion continues whether these benign papillomas or polyps (Fig. 49-37) may turn malignant. Experience has shown this to be quite unlikely. The general rule continues that good demonstration of the gallbladder with oral or intravenous method speaks for the benignancy of filling defects. Exceptions to this rule are rare.

Malignant changes

Biliary tract roentgenology is limited as a diagnostic tool in the diagnosis of malignant disease. This affects the gallbladder in about 1.25% and the extrahepatic biliary ducts in about 0.25% of autopsy material.[11] Tumors are clin-

ically silent for a long time and invade the liver parenchyma early; the roentgenographic sign of the "excluded gallbladder" may be the only help to suggest this diagnosis.

Localized papillomatous tumors are easily misinterpreted if the tumor extent is limited and the gallbladder continues to concentrate well (Fig. 49-38). Meticulous attention to good roentgenographic technique is needed to diagnose these early lesions.

In the presence of tumor of the biliary tract, contrast examination of the stomach and duodenum may be more helpful.[22] Close topographic relationship exists between the superior portion of the duodenal loop and the infundibulum and neck of the gallbladder, preferred

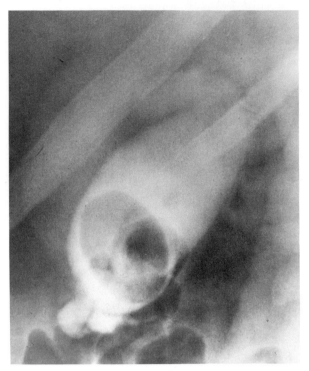

Fig. 49-35. Adenomyomatosis localized only at the fundus of the gallbladder, simulating a diverticulum.

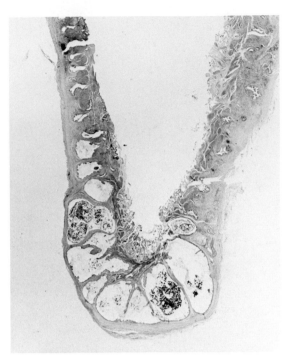

Fig. 49-36. Histology of adenomyomatosis—thickening of muscle with outpouching of mucosa into or through the muscularis.

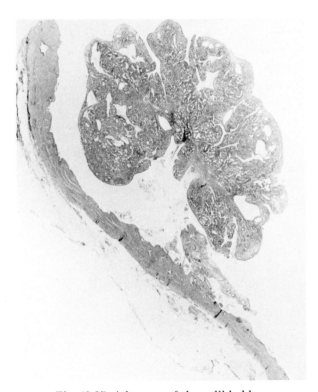

Fig. 49-37. Adenoma of the gallbladder.

sites for malignancy. The tumor may result in roentgenographically demonstrable changes ranging from shallow impressions on the upper part of duodenal loop to demonstration of direct tumor extension (Fig. 49-39). Differential diagnostic separation from extensive tumors of the head of the pancreas is usually possible.

Preoperative diagnosis of carcinoma of the bile duct is extremely rare. The major extrahepatic ducts may exhibit small indentations and irregularities of the wall or localized areas of narrowing. Confusion with strictures after cholecystectomy is likely. Selective celiac axis and superior mesenteric angiography can help to establish an early diagnosis.[21]

COMPLICATIONS OF INTRAVENOUS CHOLANGIOGRAPHY

The rate of complication in intravenous use of iodipamide (Cholografin) sodium, ioglycamide (Bilivistan), and the methylglucamine salt of ioglycamide (Biligram) is without doubt overestimated. Use of these media accounts for reactions such as nausea and vomiting in about

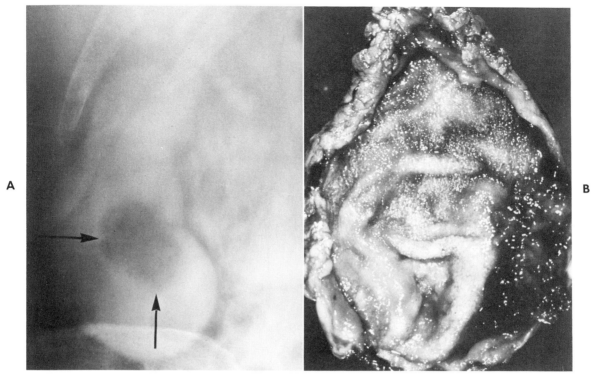

Fig. 49-38. Localized papillomatous carcinoma of the gallbladder. **A,** Filling defect in the gallbladder simulating solitary stone. **B,** Specimen of papillomatous carcinoma.

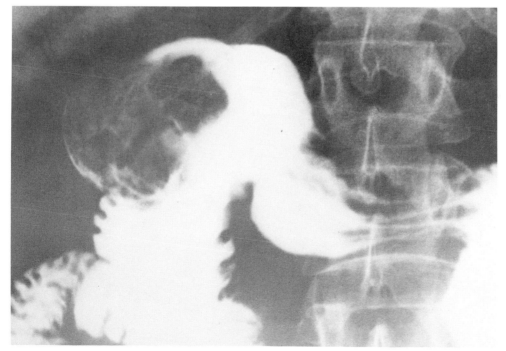

Fig. 49-39. Irregular filling defect in the lateral aspect of the duodenal bulb caused by direct extension of a carcinoma of the gallbladder.

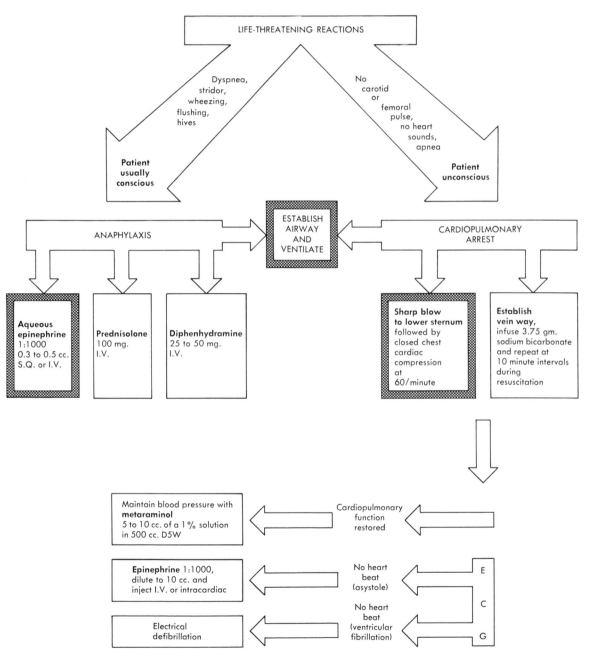

PRECAUTIONS

1. Read label on contrast bottle.

2. Elicit history of previous reactions.

3. Leave I.V. needle taped in place after injection for at least 5 to 10 minutes.

4. Epinephrine and airway in each room, other resuscitation equipment immediately available.

5. Remain readily available and know where and how to summon help (especially anesthesiologist).

6. Post this chart or one similar to it in each room.

LIFE-THREATENING REACTIONS

Dyspnea, stridor, wheezing, flushing, hives

No carotid or femoral pulse, no heart sounds, apnea

Patient usually conscious

Patient unconscious

ANAPHYLAXIS

ESTABLISH AIRWAY AND VENTILATE

CARDIOPULMONARY ARREST

Aqueous epinephrine 1:1000 0.3 to 0.5 cc. S.Q. or I.V.

Prednisolone 100 mg. I.V.

Diphenhydramine 25 to 50 mg. I.V.

Sharp blow to lower sternum followed by closed chest cardiac compression at 60/minute

Establish vein way, infuse 3.75 gm. sodium bicarbonate and repeat at 10 minute intervals during resuscitation

Maintain blood pressure with metaraminol 5 to 10 cc. of a 1% solution in 500 cc. D5W

Cardiopulmonary function restored

Epinephrine 1:1000, dilute to 10 cc. and inject I.V. or intracardiac

No heart beat (asystole)

E

C

Electrical defibrillation

No heart beat (ventricular fibrillation)

G

Fig. 49-40. Recognition and immediate management of severe reactions to contrast medium. (Adapted by Margolin, F. R.; from Barnhard, H. J., and Barnhard, F. M.: Radiology **91**:74-84, 1968; and from Nelson, J., and Carolan, J.: Personal communication.)

10% of patients, but the rate may increase to 40% or 50% if subjective indications of feeling of heat or sneezing are included. Important is the mortality of about 0.0025%, which is quite comparable to the figure of 0.0016% for intravenous urography.[15] According to general experience, the acceptance and tolerance of intravenous cholangiography has increased with the use of the infusion technique. This also has the advantage of increased diagnostic accuracy in patients with elevated total serum bilirubin levels. It also gives the examiners sufficient time to make use of the diagnostically important technique of tomography or zonography.

Selected material of hospitalized patients with clinical and laboratory evidence of biliary tract disease is, therefore, best examined by intravenous cholangiography. Oral cholecystography remains the initial diagnostic study in ambulatory patients, in the diagnostic work-up of non-specific symptoms, and for better visualization of gallstones or other filling defects in the gallbladder.

Conclusions on the so-called test injection preceding intravenous cholangiography are now permitted. A positive or negative response to a small amount of contrast medium injected intravenously has no bearing on the frequency, the severity, or the final outcome of contrast reactions. Testing of this type has no clinical meaning, and no legal implication of neglect is justified if test injections are omitted.

It is far more important that physicians and paramedical personnel are instructed in the symptoms of contrast reaction and its specific therapy. This education has to be continuous and within the radiology department. Lectures and demonstrations outside the radiology department foster a dangerously relaxed attitude of the radiology staff just as much as long intervals between incidents. The close supervision of the patient after the injection of the first milliliter of contrast medium, so-called immediate test injection, and a well-founded understanding of therapy of contrast reactions are the prerequisites for quick, efficient, and effective countermeasures in cases of contrast medium reaction (Fig. 49-40).

REFERENCES

1. Acosta, J. M., and Nardi, G. L.: Papillitis, Arch. Surg. **92**:354, 1966.
2. Aguirre, J. R., Boher, R. O., and Guraieb, S.: Hyperplastic cholecystoses: a new contribution to the unitarian theory, Amer. J. Roentgen. **107**:1, 1969.
3. Bartholomew, L. G., Cain, J. C., Woolner, L. B., Utz, D. C., and Ferris, D. O.: Sclerosing cholangitis: its possible association with Riedel's struma and fibrous retroperitonitis—report of two cases, New Eng. J. Med. **269**:3, 1963.
4. Beneventano, T., Jacobson, H. G., Hurwitt, E. S., and Schein, C. J.: Cine-cholangiomanometry: physiologic observations, Amer. J. Roentgen. **100**:673, 1967.
5. Berk, R. N., and Lasser, E. C.: Altered concepts of the mechanism of nonvisualization of the gallbladder, Radiology **82**:296, 1964.
6. Brown, D. B., Kerr, I. F., and Livingstone, D. J.: Gallstone obstruction, Brit. J. Surg. **53**:672, 1966.
7. Cremin, B. J.: Biliary parasites, Brit. J. Radiol **42**:506, 1969.
8. Eckelberg, M. E., Carlson, H. C., and McIllrath, D. C.: Intravenous cholangiography with intact gallbladder, Amer. J. Roentgen. **110**:235, 1970.
9. Fahrländer, H.: Gallenblase und Gallenwege, Bibl. Radiol. (Basel) **2**:7, 1961.
10. Frommhold, W.: Die Röntgendiagnostik der Gallenwege, Radiol. Diagn. (Berlin) **2**:185, 1961.
11. Frommhold, W.: Biliary system. In Rigler, L. G., editor: Roentgen diagnosis, Vol. V. New York, 1967, Grune & Stratton, Inc.
12. Frommhold, W., and Braband, H.: Missbildungen und Varianten der Gallenblase und der Gallenwege, Radiology **7**:33, 1967.
13. Frommhold, W.: Enzym-Untersuchungen nach Infusions-Cholegraphie bei Kranken mit Leberschaden, Deutsch. Med. Wschr. **95**:1911, 1970.
14. Frommhold, W., and Lagemann, K.: Die Adenomyomatose der Gallenblase, Fortschr. Rontgenstr. **115**:464, 1971.
15. Frommhold, W.: Die statistische Frequenz von Zwischenfällen bei Verwendung jodierter intravenöser Kontrastmittel, Röntgenblätter **21**:329, 1968.
16. Glenn, F., and McSherry, C. K.: Gallstones and pregnancy among 300 young women treated by cholecystectomy, Surg. Gynec. Obstet. **127**:1067, 1968.
17. Harrington, O. B., Beall, A. C., Noon, G., and DeBakey, M. E.: Intravenous cholangiography in acute cholecystitis, Arch. Surg. **88**:585, 1964.
18. Hoerr, S. O., and Hazard, J. B.: Acute cholecystitis without gallbladder stones, Amer. Surg. **111**:47, 1966.
19. Hornykiewytsch. T.: Zur Funktion des Ductus Choledochus und der Papille, Fortschr. Rontgenstr. **90**:323, 1959.
20. Jutras, J. A., Longtin, J. M., and Levesque, H. P.: Hyperplastic cholecystoses, Amer. J. Roentgen. **83**:795, 1960.
21. Kaude, J., and Rian, R.: Cholangiocarcinoma, Radiology **100**:573, 1971.
22. Khilnani, M. T., Wolf, B. S., and Finkel, M.: Roentgen features of carcinoma of the gallbladder on barium meal examination, Radiology **79**:264, 1962.

23. Kune, G. A.: Surgical anatomy of common bile duct, Arch. Surg. **89**:995, 1964.
24. Lal, R. B., Papper, M. ,and Puestow, C. B.: Torsion of the gallbladder, Arch. Surg. **97**:750, 1968.
25. Lindenbraten, L. D. and Krugljakow, I. O.: Röntgenphysiologie der Gallenblase, Fortschr. Röntgenstr. **101**:483, 1964.
26. Mahour, H., Wakim, K. G., and Ferris, D. O.: The common bile duct in man: its diameter and circumference, Ann. Surg. **165**:415, 1967.
27. Maida, J. W., Kratz, G., Martinez, L. O., Gassman, P., Fleming, R., and Manheimer, L.: The utilization of intravenous cholangiography in the demonstration of common duct foreign bodies, Brit. J. Radiol. **44**:388, 1971.
28. Margulies, S. I., Brogdon, B. G., Sindler, R. A., and Perilla, F. R.: Disappearing gallstones, Brit. J. Radiol. **40**:546, 1967.
29. Martinez, L. O., Viamonte, M., Gassmann, P., and Boudet, L.: Present status of intravenous cholangiography, Amer. J. Roentgen. **113**:10, 1971.
30. Nathan, M. H., Newman, A., Murray, D. J., and Camponovo, R.: Cholecystokinin cholecystography, Amer. J. Roentgen. **110**:240, 1970.
31. Niedner, F. F., and Kief, H.: Klinische und mikromorphologische Untersuchungen zur Pathogenese der Papillenstenose, Med. Welt **1**:26, 1965.
32. Olson, O. C., and Schnug, G. E.: Primary sclerosing cholangitis, Northwest. Med. **64**:26, 1965.
33. Ono, K., Watanabe, N., Suzuki, K., Tsuchida, H., Sugiyama, Y., and Abo, M.: Bile flow mechanism in man, Arch. Surg. **96**:869, 1968.
34. Pavel, I.: Die Gallenblase und die ableitenden Gallenwege. II. Die funktionellen Störungen der Gallenblase und der Gallenwege. VEB Gustav Fischer, Jena 1962.
35. Quist, C. F.: The influence of cholecystectomy on the normal common bile duct, Acta Chir. Scand. **113**:30, 1957.
36. Sarmiento, R. V.: Emphysematous cholecystitis, Arch. Surg. **93**:1009, 1966.
37. Schmidt, H., and Guttmann, E.: Schematische Anatomie der Gallengänge des Menschen—eine röntgenanatomische Studie, Acta Anat. **28**:1, 1956.
38. Shehadi, W. H.: Radiologic examination of the biliary tract: plain film of the abdomen; oral cholecystography, Radiol. Clin. N. Amer. **4**:3, 1966.
39. Shriner, W.: Studies on the common duct—pressures and mechanisms, Amer. J. Gastroent. **48**:30, 1967.
40. Smith, R., and Sherlock, S.: Surgery of the gallbladder and bile duct, London, 1964, Butterworth and Co., Ltd.
41. Strain, W. H.: Chemical composition and names of some principal water-soluble and cholecystographic contrast media, Invest. Radiol. **5**:498, 1970.
42. Taenzer, V., and Herms, H. J.: Intravenöse Cholegraphie mit Biligram, Fortschr. Rontgenstr. **114**:102, 1971.

Intravenous cholangiography | 50

Robert E. Wise

Since its introduction in 1954, intravenous cholangiography has become an accepted procedure in the diagnosis of biliary tract disease. The technique of examination and the criteria of interpretation have been developed to a high degree, and indications for performance of the examination have been established with a reasonable degree of unanimity of opinion. This chapter, which will deal with these aspects of the intravenous cholangiography examination, should begin with a discussion of the contrast medium that is used and the reactions that may occur to it.

CONTRAST MEDIUM

Sodium iodipamide, which was the contrast material used initially in intravenous cholangiography, was introduced in Germany under the trade name of Biligrafin, and shortly thereafter was marketed in the United States under the trade name of Cholografin sodium. In 1955 iodipamide methylglucamine was introduced also under the trade name of Cholografin methylglucamine. Although there may have been slight differences in reaction rates between these two, the major difference was in the volume of the dosage required—40 ml. being required for the sodium salt and 20 ml. for the methylglucamine compound. This latter product has largely replaced the original sodium salt and we at the Lahey Clinic have used it exclusively since its introduction.

Iodipamide methylglucamine is prepared in a 52% (w/v) solution. It is the methylglucamine salt of N,N'-adipyl-bis (3-amino-2, 4, 6, triiobenzoic acid). The 20 ml. dose contains approximately 5 gm. of iodine.

It has been estimated that in the normal subject approximately 90% of the compound is excreted by the liver and 10% by the kidneys. As a result, the kidneys are at least faintly opacified. This in itself is of no significance, but it should be noted that in patients with liver damage a greater proportion of the contrast medium than is usual will be excreted by the kidneys.

CONTRAST MEDIUM
  Reactions

INDICATIONS FOR EXAMINATION

VISUALIZATION

COMMON BILE DUCT
  Size
  Obstruction

DIAGNOSIS OF BILIARY TRACT DISEASE
  Choledocholithiasis
  Fibrosis of the sphincter of Oddi
  Pancreatic disease
  Chronic pancreatitis
  Stricture of the bile duct
  Cystic duct remnants and calculi

POSTULATES FOR DIAGNOSIS

Reactions

Utilizing skin, conjunctival, oral, and intravenous test doses, many attempts have been made to predict reactions to intravenously administered iodinated contrast agents. Oral and conjunctival tests have usually been discredited with other contrast agents, and we at the Lahey Clinic have not used them with this compound. We have had considerable experience with intradermal test doses of iodipamide, but have found the test to be of no value, and have therefore abandoned its use. The intravenous test, which is now employed at the Lahey Clinic, consists of the intravenous injection of 1 ml. of the contrast agent followed by a waiting period of 3 minutes. If no reaction occurs within this time, the remaining 19 ml. of the standard dose is injected at a steady rate over a 10-minute period. While we use and recommend this form of testing, it must be emphasized that it is far from reliable in predicting reactions; minor reactions such as nausea, vomiting, hypotension, or urticaria have occurred although the test result was negative. In the event of a true anaphylactic reaction, however, the intravenous test is probably of value. Although a reaction of this type from a small test dose may well be fatal, it is to be expected that reactions to the test dose would be less severe and would have a lower mortality than would reactions to the full 20 ml. dose.

In 17 years of experience with almost 10,000 injections there have been no fatal reactions at the Lahey Clinic. There have been a significant number of minor reactions, some of which have been cause for concern. Nausea and vomiting, although uncomfortable to the patient, are usually not serious. Hypotension, however, is not to be treated lightly, for prolonged hypotension could result in kidney or brain damage. To date we have not seen damage of this type.

The reaction rate at the Clinic has consistently decreased. In an initial study of 116 injections,[10] 20% of the patients had reactions. In a subsequent study in 1956, 11.3% had reactions. No further estimates of reaction rate were made until 1965, at which time we found during a controlled study of 351 consecutive injections that we were able to reduce the reaction rate to an unusually low level by using a combination of measures. A preliminary injection of 5 mg. of parabromdylamine maleate, a slow 10-minute injection of iodipamide, and examination with the patient in the hydrated and nonfasting state resulted in a reaction rate of 4.3%. Departure from our previous practice of preparation by fasting and dehydration has not resulted in a lowering of the quality of the examination.

In recent years there has been a growing trend toward the use of a double-dose (40 ml. of iodipamide) slow-infusion technique.[1,5,6,7,9] The precise methods vary somewhat, but usually the 40 ml. of iodipamide is added to 50 to 150 ml. of 5% dextrose in water. The resultant solution is then administered by slow infusion in periods varying from 20 to 240 minutes. The proponents argue that opacification is of a greater degree than is obtained with a single dose, that opacification occurs with a greater frequency despite high serum bilirubin levels, and that fewer reactions are encountered. Unfortunately, to date, there has not been a single scientifically constructed double-blind study.

There does, however, appear to be little doubt that the reaction rate is decreased with the use of the infusion technique compared with a rapid direct injection of a single or double dose. However, if a direct injection is made slowly in a patient who is not dehydrated there appears to be little difference in reaction rates.

The contention that opacification is increased in degree and frequency compared with the single dose remains unproved owing to the lack of a double-blind test and the high degree of subjectivity that frequently prevails. In our experience, similarly untested by double-blind techniques, with over one hundred double-dose infusion examinations we were unable to detect a significant increase in degree of opacification.

Despite the lack of scientific proof, however, the infusion technique is preferred by many and there appears to be little objection to its use.

INDICATIONS FOR EXAMINATION

In my opinion routine examination of the gallbladder is not an indication for intravenous cholangiography. A routine examination is best performed with the use of an oral cholecystographic agent. The oral method has a high safety factor, whereas the intravenous method has a theoretical element of danger. In a normally functioning gallbladder, opacification is usually better with an oral agent owing to the ability of the gallbladder to concentrate the oral medium. Examination with the intravenous method is indicated for patients with the gallbladder intact in whom an oral examination has failed to opacify the gallbladder.

In the event of nonvisualization of the gallbladder following a single dose of oral cholecystographic medium, we now believe that it is justifiable to immediately proceed with an intravenous cholangiogram, for rarely will opacification be obtained with a repeat single dose of oral medium. In the event of faint opacification of the gallbladder with a single dose of oral medium, a repeat single dose of oral medium is justified. Administration of ipodate (Oragrafin) calcium following the initial single dose is also justified in such a case and may result in a considerable saving of time for the patient.[8] The administration of a double dose following a single dose in the event of faint opacification or nonopacification of the gallbladder is considered unnecessary and possibly dangerous.

Although the demonstration of gallstones or

nonfunctioning gallbladder by means of oral cholecystography is usually considered adequate indication for cholecystectomy and one may legitimately proceed with surgery, it would appear that the best interests of the patient would be served if the status of the common bile duct were known before surgical intervention. Thus, in any situation when surgery appears to be indicated on the basis of evidence gained by oral cholecystography, an intravenous cholangiography should be performed in order to evaluate the bile ducts properly. This, of course, presupposes that the bile ducts were not adequately demonstrated by the oral examination. In the postcholecystectomy patient, any symptom suggestive of biliary duct disease is an indication for intravenous cholangiography.

Absolute contraindications for intravenous cholangiography are few, for there are no known conditions in which the injection of Cholografin methylglucamine would be invariably harmful. There are situations, however, in which extreme caution must be exercised and the examination performed only when unavoidable. Among these are combined severe liver and renal disease, proved sensitivity to iodine compounds, severe allergy, and any condition in which prolonged hypotension would be harmful.

VISUALIZATION

In many areas intravenous cholangiography has fallen into disrepute simply because it was attempted on many patients whose liver function status contraindicated its use. In order to obtain opacification of the bile ducts, liver function must be reasonably good. While it is never possible to predict with certainty whether or not opacification will be obtained in any given patient, the serum bilirubin levels and phenol-tetrabromphthalein sodium sulfonate (Bromsulphalein) retention values provide good criteria for the probability of opacification. With a serum bilirubin value of 1 mg. per 100 ml. or less, opacification of the ducts may be expected in 92% of injections of the contrast medium; on the other hand, if the serum bilirubin value is above 4 mg. per 100 ml., opacification of the ducts may be expected in only 9%. With a Bromsulphalein retention level below 10% after 45 minutes, opacification may be expected in 96% of injections. If the retention level is above 40%, opacification may be expected in 26%.

Recognition of these criteria will serve as a guide and eliminate many unnecessary examinations.

These values given are average and, as with any average, certain deviations are inherent. For any given level of serum bilirubin the probability of opacification is decreased if the bilirubin level is rising and increased if it is falling. The bilirubin value measures only the quantity of pigment in the serum and not the liver function at any particular time. In my experience adequate visualization occurs 90% of the time upon injection of the contrast medium when the criteria of serum bilirubin level and Bromsulphalein value are utilized and indications for visualization are favorable.

COMMON BILE DUCT
Size

With the exception of size, the anatomy of the common bile duct is well known and needs no comment. Before the advent of intravenous cholangiography, little was known concerning the size of this structure, especially in the postcholecystectomy state. It was generally accepted that after cholecystectomy, as a compensatory measure, the common bile duct dilated to act as a reservoir for bile.

Early studies at the Lahey Clinic, based upon ninety-six cases in which the gallbladder and bile ducts were found normal by intravenous cholangiography, indicated an average size of 5.5 mm. for the common bile duct, with a range of 2 to 14 mm. These findings were in agreement with those of other researchers in this field. In a later study based upon 620 cases, the average diameter was 7 mm. regardless of the presence or absence of disease of the gallbladder or bile ducts (Fig. 50-1). Thus, the earlier figure of 5.5 mm. probably more closely approximates the true average diameter in the normal subject. In patients who have had a cholecystectomy we have found unobstructed common bile ducts as large as 20 mm. This extends the range of the physiologic normal duct considerably beyond that found in the precholecystectomy state. These data indicate that the presence or absence of obstruction is a more realistic factor in the definition of the normal duct, for size alone proves nothing regarding obstruction (Fig. 50-2).

From our earliest studies we suspected that the common bile duct did not dilate simply be-

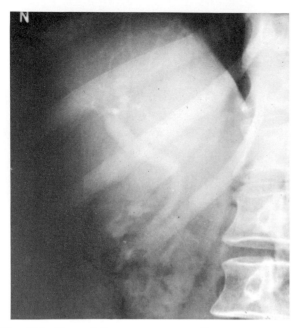

Fig. 50-1. Normal 7 mm. common bile duct. Note the tapering, undulating configuration. Relatively little opacification of the intrahepatic ducts is usually obtained in the unobstructed biliary tract.

cause the gallbladder was removed. Numerous common bile ducts with diameters below our calculated normal average of 5.5 mm. were found in patients many years after cholecystectomy had been performed. This prompted a statistical study of 1,193 patients who had had a cholecystectomy, in an attempt to evaluate the concept of postcholecystectomy dilatation of the common bile ducts. In this study the average diameter of the common bile duct was found to be 8.1 mm. Since our earlier studies indicated an average diameter before cholecystectomy of 7 mm., the new average tended to indicate a significant increase in size of the common bile duct following cholecystectomy. However, this group of 1,193 patients included a large number in whom both the gallbladder and bile ducts were considered normal. A survey of 241 examinations in which the gallbladder was present and diseased showed that the average diameter of the common bile duct was 8 mm. The insignificant difference between this figure and the 8.1 mm. diameter of post-

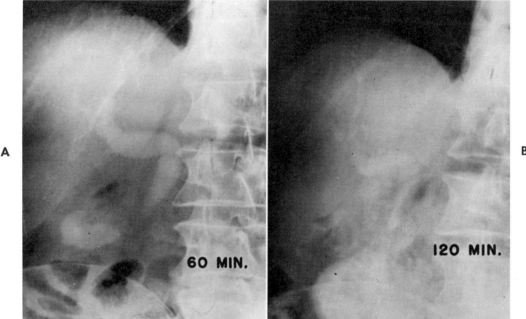

Fig. 50-2. Dilated normal common bile duct in a patient who had had a cholecystectomy previously. The common bile duct measures 17 mm. Both the 60 minute film, **A,** and the 120 minute film, **B,** demonstrate normal drainage. The duct is physiologically normal despite dilatation above average size. (From Wise, R. E.: Intravenous cholangiography, Springfield, Ill., 1962, Charles C Thomas, Publisher.)

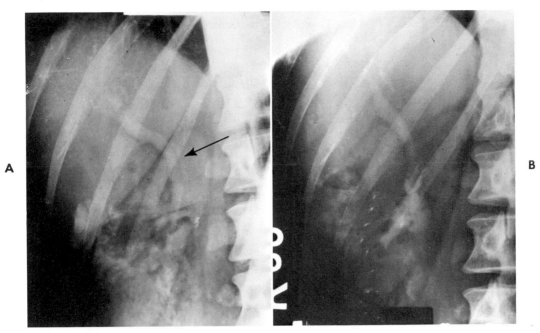

Fig. 50-3. Normal common bile duct. **A,** In a normal common bile duct before cholecystectomy nonopacification of the gallbladder is indicative of cystic duct obstruction. The arrow indicates the medial cystic duct. **B,** Thirteen months after cholecystectomy the size of the common bile duct has not increased. (From Wise, R. E.: Intravenous cholangiography, Springfield, Ill., 1962, Charles C Thomas, Publisher.)

cholecystectomy ducts casts serious doubt upon the validity of the concept that dilatation of the common bile duct occurs as a result of cholecystectomy.

Further data was obtained from a study of thirteen patients in whom intravenous cholangiography was performed before and after cholecystectomy. In nine patients in whom the diameter of the common bile duct ranged from 4 mm. to 12 mm., there was no increase in diameter during a period averaging 22.5 months. In one patient the size increased from 6 to 7 mm. (Fig. 50-3). The evidence for obstruction was considered minimal, and the duct was not explored. In three patients the size of the ducts increased from 9 to 16 mm., from 6 to 15 mm., and from 10 to 20 mm., respectively. In all three patients evidence of obstruction, stenosis of the sphincter of Oddi, or an impacted calculus was found upon operation. Since the above cases included those in which cystic duct obstruction was present, it may be said that common duct dilatation may already have taken place prior to cholecystectomy as a result of pathologic cholecystectomy, thus again casting doubt upon

the validity of the concept of postcholecystectomy dilation. In a later study, nine patients were found with opacification of the gallbladder and bile ducts, and opacification of the bile ducts after cholecystectomy. Pathologic cholecystectomy had not taken place. The intervals between surgery and the follow-up cholangiogram ranged from 1 to 68 months. In seven of the nine patients no increase in the size of the common bile ducts was observed, and in two, the increase was 1 mm.—an average increase of 0.22 mm. These data appear to support the statistical inferential data indicating that the common duct does not dilate simply because the gallbladder has been removed. Our experience also indicates that any significant increase in the size of the common duct is probably indicative of obstructive disease.

Obstruction

Whether caused by tumor, inflammation, or calculus, obstruction is the common denominator in disease of the bile ducts. It would follow, therefore, that the presence or absence of obstruction is the most important determination to be made in evaluation of the biliary ducts. Size, in itself, is relatively unimportant except as a reflection of obstruction. In our experience at the Lahey Clinic the common duct of the postcholecystectomy patient has ranged in size from 3 to 30 mm. We found that in these patients unobstructed ducts varied from 3 to 15 mm. in diameter; partially obstructed ducts ranged from 5 to 30 mm. A review of these cases suggested that when the size ranged from 15 to 30 mm. partial obstruction could be predicted on the basis of size, and when it was below 8 mm. patency of the duct could probably be predicted. Size alone appeared to be of value in the prediction of patency of the duct only 8% of the time, and in the prediction of partial obstruction 6.5%. It was of no value in the remaining 85.5% of postcholecystectomy cases, since both obstructed and unobstructed ducts were found in the group whose ducts ranged from 5 to 15 mm. in diameter.

Criteria other than size were necessary if preoperative predictions of common duct obstruction were to be accurate. In a review of our experience with common bile ducts that had been subjected to surgical exploration, several interesting facts were noted with respect to obstructed and unobstructed ducts. In a comparison of the two groups, it was found that opacification of the duct occurred slightly later in the unobstructed group than in the obstructed group, that it was not as great, and that it diminished gradually after approximately 60 minutes. In the obstructed group, the opacification tended to be maintained on a plateau, and in most instances was greater at 120 minutes than it was at 60 minutes. This finding, then, formed the basis of our time-density-retention concept, which holds that if the density of the opacified bile in the common duct is greater at 120 minutes than it was at 60 minutes, partial obstruction of the common duct may be predicted.

Utilization of the time-density-retention concept has resulted in the diagnosis of partial obstruction of the biliary tract with a high degree of accuracy, particularly in cases of common

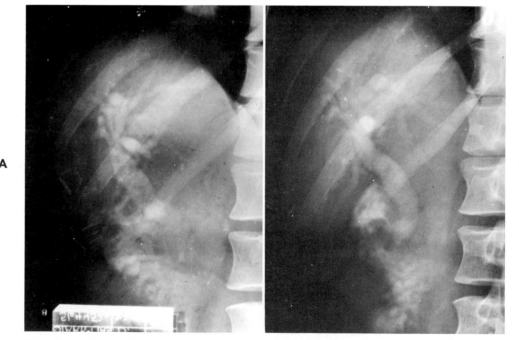

Fig. 50-4. Choledocholithiasis in a patient who had had a cholecystectomy previously. The common bile duct measures 15 mm. Opacified bile in the common duct appears less dense after 60 minutes, **A,** than after 120 minutes, **B,** indicating partial obstruction. An impacted common duct calculus was found at surgery. (From Wise, R. E.: Intravenous cholangiography, Springfield, Ill., 1962, Charles C Thomas, Publisher.)

duct calculi that would have been overlooked when the calculi were impacted and not visible by direct observation (Fig. 50-4). It must be emphasized that the concept is valid only if the gallbladder has been removed or if the cystic duct is obstructed. If the gallbladder is present and the cystic duct unobstructed, the gallbladder acts as a safety valve for the increased intraductal pressure. If the gallbladder is absent or the cystic duct obstructed, the bile ducts consist essentially of semirigid hollow tubes through which the flow of fluid is relatively constant.

In addition to size and the time-density-retention concept, structure must be considered in the diagnosis of obstruction of the common duct. The normal common bile duct pursues an undulating course and tapers from above with the distal portion being slightly narrower than the proximal or common hepatic duct portion. In the presence of obstruction, however, the structure of the duct changes considerably: the tapering characteristic is lost and the sides of the duct are approximately parallel. In addition,

one usually sees evidence of varying degrees of dilatation of the intrahepatic ducts (Fig. 50-7).

The elements of the diagnosis of obstruction of the common bile duct, then, are duct diameter, estimation of drainage, and changes in structure. Consideration of them has resulted in diagnostic accuracy with respect to obstruction of approximately 90% in surgically proved cases.

DIAGNOSIS OF BILIARY TRACT DISEASE
Choledocholithiasis

Intravenous cholangiography has been used most frequently in a search for common duct calculi, and it is in this area in which the greatest benefit has been derived.

Choledocholithiasis may be diagnosed directly or indirectly. Direct diagnosis implies that the calculus may be directly demonstrated or visualized during intravenous cholangiography as a filling defect in the common duct. In these cases

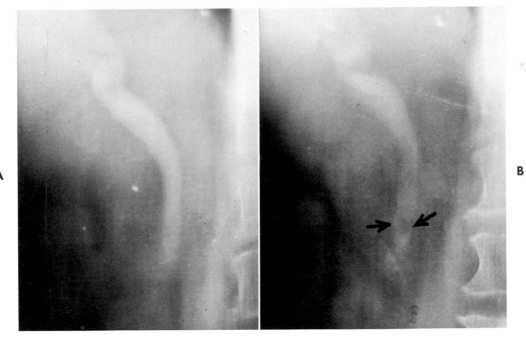

Fig. 50-5. Choledocholithiasis. **A,** The initial laminagraph at 12 cm. level demonstrates an apparently normal common bile duct without evidence of calculi. **B,** The laminagraph at 11 cm. level clearly demonstrates a large calculus in the distal duct. (From Wise, R. E.: Intravenous cholangiography, Springfield, Ill., 1962, Charles C Thomas, Publisher.)

the criteria of diagnosis are essentially the same as those used for the diagnosis of a calculus in any other contrast medium-filled structure, such as a diagnosis made using T tube cholangiography or pyelography. Since the concentration of contrast medium with the intravenous cholangiogram is relatively low, diagnosis is somewhat difficult. Laminagraphy, therefore, has been of distinct value in the demonstration of calculi, especially when the bile duct is poorly opacified (Figs. 50-5 and 50-6).

The advent of *laminagraphy* utilizing hypocycloid, circular, and elliptical motions has added a new dimension to the technique of intravenous cholangiography. There is little doubt that careful attention to details of technique with this modality will add significantly to the accuracy of diagnosis.[3]

In actual practice we subject approximately 50% of our patients to laminagraphy. While one may argue that all patients should be subjected to this procedure, it is expensive in terms of time, money, and radiation exposure. There-fore certain definite criteria for its use have been evolved. Laminagraphy is used when there are overlying gas shadows, faint opacification of the duct, dilatation of the duct, or any other factor is present that renders visualization difficult or poor.

Utilizing modern techniques of laminagraphy we have found the lateral projection to be of considerable value in improving visualization of the terminal portion of the common bile duct because of the frequent posterior inclination of the duct at this level.[15]

The indirect diagnosis of calculi is somewhat more difficult. The calculus is not visualized as a filling defect in the contrast medium-filled structure. Furthermore, calculi are frequently impacted in the ampulla of Vater and produce partial obstruction. It is in these situations that the time-density-retention concept has proved invaluable. Thus in a comparison of 120 minute films with 60 minute films, if the density is increasing on the former film, one must suspect partial obstruction of the common duct. This

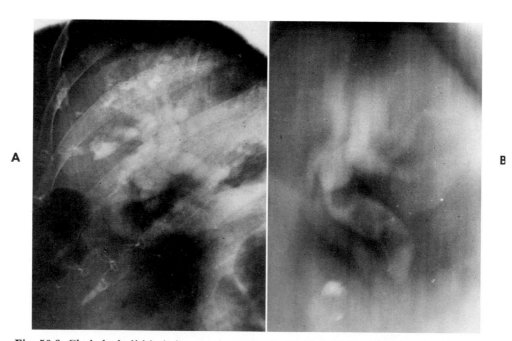

Fig. 50-6. Choledocholithiasis in a patient who had had a cholecystectomy previously. **A,** A conventional film shows evidence of obstruction with dilated intrahepatic ducts. The common bile duct is not visible. **B,** A laminagraph clearly demonstrates calculi as the cause of obstruction. The serum bilirubin level was only 0.2 mg. per 100 ml. (From Wise, R. E.: Intravenous cholangiography, Springfield, Ill., 1962, Charles C Thomas, Publisher.)

diagnosis should be supported by the other criteria previously enumerated. If a diagnosis of partial obstruction is made on the basis of these criteria, one cannot state specifically that the obstruction is the result of calculus, since it may well be produced by stenosis of the sphincter of Oddi, by tumor, or possibly by inflammation. However, since calculi are more commonly found than the other entities, we are led to suspect calculus if partial obstruction is present. In any event, definite evidence of partial obstruction is usually a justifiable indication for surgical exploration.

Our presumptive radiologic accuracy in the diagnosis of calculi has been approximately 92%. In 1,194 opacified common ducts in post-cholecystectomy patients, calculi were proved at operation in seventy-seven instances or 6.5% of the total of 1,194. Six of these were not diagnosed, resulting in a presumptive x-ray accuracy of 92%. However, of the seventy-one patients in whom the diagnosis was correct, forty-two (59%) were found by direct demonstration and twenty-nine (41%) by indirect demonstration. If the time-density-retention concept had not been used, our radiologic interpretation accuracy of calculi would have been about 50%.

The preceding figures were compiled in an era before the availability of polytome laminagraphy and very likely today would not reflect as high an incidence of diagnosis by the indirect method. Despite the use, however, of optimum laminagraphy today we not infrequently find that the diagnosis of a partially obstructing calculus impacted in the ampulla of Vater may be made with the use of the time-density-retention concept. By the same token, slow-infusion cholangiography does not preclude utilization of the principle if it is borne in mind that the principle deals with drainage of the duct and that partially obstructed ducts will not drain properly despite any technique of administration of the contrast medium that may be used.

Fibrosis of the sphincter of Oddi

The diagnosis of fibrosis of the sphincter of Oddi as a cause of obstruction of the common bile duct remains controversial and is certainly not universally accepted. At times, however, the diagnosis is valid. Utilizing the time-density-retention concept, 88% of cases later surgically proved can be diagnosed beforehand in regard

to obstruction (Fig. 50-7). This percentage compares favorably with that for the diagnosis of choledocholithiasis.

Pancreatic disease

When intravenous cholangiography became available, it was hoped that this procedure would lead to the early diagnosis of a significant number of cases of carcinoma of the head of the pancreas. We have found that the diagnosis has been made in only a few instances with any degree of certainty, and we have concluded, therefore, that intravenous cholangiography is of little value in the diagnosis of this disease. In rare instances, if a slight degree of obstruction is present, the diagnosis of partial obstruction may be made, but using only intravenous cholangiography, differentiation among the many conditions that may produce obstruction is impossible.

Chronic pancreatitis

Although intravenous cholangiography is of relatively little use in establishing the diagnosis of chronic pancreatitis, it is of considerable value in many instances after the diagnosis has been accurately established. Intravenous cholangiography has yielded valuable information concerning the degree of obstruction produced by the fibrotic pancreas, as well as information about the structure of the common duct, especially with respect to size and dilatation of intrahepatic radicles. Intravenous cholangiography is therefore recommended as an adjuvant diagnostic procedure in chronic pancreatitis despite the fact that the diagnosis may be well established.

As expected, pseudocysts and true cysts of the pancreas result in partial obstruction and displacement of the common bile duct and are readily demonstrable by intravenous cholangiography if the cyst is in a position where it may change the course or the patency of the common bile duct.

Stricture of the bile duct

Although most patients with common bile duct stricture are not subjected to intravenous cholangiography since the degree of obstruction present usually precludes visualization, this procedure, nevertheless, is of considerable value in such cases. If a stricture is suspected and liver

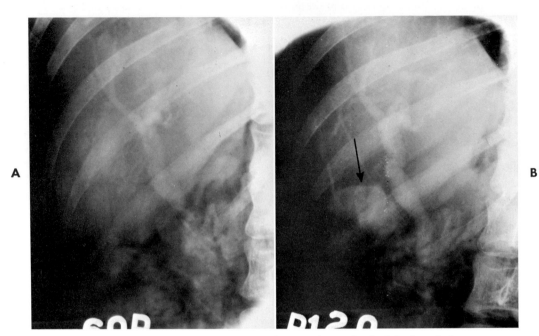

Fig. 50-7. Fibrosis of the sphincter of Oddi in a patient who had had a cholecystectomy previously. The common bile duct is slightly dilated. In a comparison of the 60 minute film, **A,** with the 120 minute film, **B,** the opacified bile appears denser after 120 minutes, indicating partial obstruction. Stenosis of the sphincter of Oddi was found during surgery. The arrow indicates contrast medium in the duodenal bulb. (From Wise, R. E.: Intravenous cholangiography, Springfield, Ill., 1962, Charles C Thomas, Publisher.)

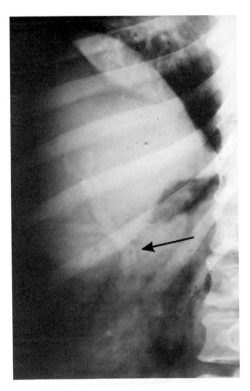

Fig. 50-8. Cystic duct remnant in a patient who had had a cholecystectomy previously. The common bile duct is normal, measuring 5 mm. The arrow indicates an anomalous medial cystic duct origin and a long remnant crossing common bile duct. Cystic ducts of this type frequently share a common wall with the main biliary tract.

function studies suggest that opacification will be obtained, considerable information may be gained by the use of intravenous cholangiography, especially when the diagnosis of stricture is in doubt. In many situations the information gained has resulted in a specific diagnosis. In addition, invaluable morphologic information, including the degree of dilatation of the common bile duct and the precise level of the stricture, may be obtained prior to surgery.

Cystic duct remnants and calculi

Although cystic duct remnants have at times been incriminated as the source of pain in the postcholecystectomy patient, we at the Lahey Clinic do not believe that a cystic duct remnant per se is of clinical significance unless it contains calculi. The search, therefore, is not primarily for cystic duct remnants, but for the presence of calculi in such remnants. The presence of a cystic duct remnant is not considered an indication for surgery.

A word of caution is necessary regarding cystic duct remnants, specifically regarding a relatively long cystic duct remnant that may be seen on the posteromedial aspect of the common bile duct (Fig. 50-8). This type of remnant usually shares a common wall with the adjacent portion of the common bile duct, and if removal is attempted, disastrous results may follow.

POSTULATES FOR DIAGNOSIS

In this chapter an attempt has been made to enunciate the principles of diagnosis in intravenous cholangiography. Specific findings and statistics are readily available in the literature, and space precludes a detailed dissertation.[1-15]

In a previous report, thirteen postulates were enunciated. They appear to have stood the test of time and are reiterated here as valid precepts in the investigation of gallbladder and biliary tract disease:

1. Increasing degrees of liver damage decrease iodipamide excretion as well as the degree and incidence of biliary duct visualization.
2. The incidence of duct visualization decreases for any given serum bilirubin level if icterus is increasing; the converse is true if icterus is decreasing.
3. Partial obstruction of the common bile duct delays visualization of the ducts sig-

nificantly, depending upon the degree of obstruction.
4. In the absence of obstructive disease of the common bile duct there is no evidence to indicate that the common duct dilates after the gallbladder is removed.
5. Dilatation of the common bile duct per se is not evidence of partial obstruction.
6. Dilatation of the common bile duct follows obstruction to the degree that obstruction is present.
7. Relief of obstruction of the common bile duct is followed by reduction in size to a degree that is not precluded by chronic thickening and fibrosis of the wall.
8. The diagnosis of obstruction may be based upon the time-density-retention concept with satisfaction of the criteria of the diagnosis of obstruction being an increasing degree of retention of contrast medium in the common duct at 120 minutes compared with retention at 60 minutes.
9. Dilatation of the common bile duct and the time-density-retention phenomenon are interrelated in the diagnosis of obstruction, being complementary in the diagnosis.
10. The structure of the bile duct responds to obstruction with loss of the tapering outline, with the dilatation of the duct, and with the blunting of intrahepatic radicles.
11. For any degree of obstruction, common duct dilatation will be lessened to the degree that the cystic duct and gallbladder are patent and expansile, as opposed to the cystic duct being occluded or the gallbladder being absent.
12. Occlusion of the cystic duct places the biliary duct system in the same status with respect to dynamics as does cholecystectomy.
13. The time-density-retention concept is valid only when the gallbladder is absent or when the cystic duct is occluded.

REFERENCES

1. Bornhorst, R. A., Heitzman, E. R., and McAfee, J. G.: Double-dose drip infusion cholangiography, J.A.M.A. **206**:1489, 1968.
2. Johnson, J. H., Jr., and Wise, R. E.: Intravenous cholangiography: a study of reactions to iodipamide

methylglucamine, Lahey Clin. Found. Bull. **13**:245, 1964.

3. Kikkawa, K., Littleton, J., and Ty, J.: Tomography and intravenous cholangiography, Guthrie Clin. Bull. **38**:35, 1968.

4. McDonough, F. E., and Wise, R. E.: Limitations to the clinical application of intravenous cholangiography in determining disease of the bile ducts after cholecystectomy, Gastroenterology **29**:771, 1955.

5. McNulty, J. G.: Drip infusion cholecystocholangiography: simultaneous visualization of the gallbladder and bile ducts, Radiology **90**:570, 1968.

6. Meyer-Burg, J., and Wilhelmi, V.: Infusion cholecystocholangiography, Fortschr. Roentgenstr. **111**:641, 1969.

7. Nolan, D. J., and Gibson, M. J.: Improvements in intravenous cholangiography, Brit. J. Radiol. **43**:652, 1970.

8. Siber, F. J., Showalter, B., and Wise, R. E.: Usefulness of calcium ipodate in the faintly opacified gallbladder, Radiology **97**:185, 1970.

9. Wax, R. E., and Crummy, A. B.: Drip infusion cholangiography, Radiology **87**:354, 1966.

10. Wise, R. E.: Intravenous cholangiography, Springfield, Ill. 1962, Charles C Thomas, Publishers.

11. Wise, R. E., and O'Brien, R. G.: Intravenous cholangiography: a preliminary report, Lahey Clin. Found. Bull. **9**:52, 1954.

12. Wise, R. E., and O'Brien, R. G.: Interpretation of the intravenous cholangiogram, J.A.M.A. **160**:819, 1956.

13. Wise, R. E., and Twaddle, J. A.: Choledocholithiasis: postcholecystectomy diagnosis by intravenous cholangiography, Surg. Clin. N. Amer. **38**:673, 1958.

14. Wise, R. E., Johnston, D. O., and Salzman, F. A.: The intravenous cholangiographic diagnosis of partial obstruction of the common bile duct, Radiology **68**:507, 1957.

15. Wise, R. E.: The lateral view in cholangiography, Radiol. Clin. Amer. **8**:139, 1970.

Operative and postoperative biliary tract | 51

H. Joachim Burhenne

GENERAL CONSIDERATIONS

We realize the importance of surgical biliary tract roentgenology when we read that over half a million patients are hospitalized for gallbladder disease in the United States each year[15] with two thirds of them undergoing surgery.[5] Cholangiography has developed into the major tool for the diagnostic evaluation of these patients before, during, and after surgery.

History

The first cholecystectomy for cholelithiasis in 1882 by Langenbuch was a milestone in biliary tract surgery.[7] Choledochotomy by Courvoiser followed in 1890. Roentgenographic visualization of the bile ducts then became possible by three important techniques: (1) Mirizzi performed direct cholangiography on the operating table in 1932.[12] (2) Transhepatic cholangiography was attempted as early as 1921[2] but did not become accepted and practical until 1952.[3] (3) Intravenous contrast medium for the third method of cholangiography became available in 1953.[6] These three techniques with their separate indications are now widely used, and surgery of the biliary tract has become unthinkable without them.

Terminology

Operative or surgical cholangiography consists of two phases with different indications.[14] *Primary cholangiography* is done before exploration of the common duct, before the biliary tract has been manipulated, and before the decision has been made concerning exploration of the biliary duct system (Fig. 51-1, *A*). This procedure is also called diagnostic, preexploratory, or precholedochotomy cholangiography. *Secondary operative cholangiography* is performed after exploration of the common duct, usually through the T tube, but before closure of the abdomen (Fig. 51-1, *B*). It is the final check on remaining pathology, and is also called control, postexploratory, or postcholedochotomy cholangiography. The *postoperative T tube cholangiogram* is usually performed through the indwelling tube within 7 to 10 days after surgery.

Radiomanometry combines pressure readings with contrast injection. It was introduced by Mallet-Guy[11] but did not receive wide application. It is primarily used by surgeons interested in dyskinesia of the biliary tracts.[1,9]

Dyskinesia of the biliary tract is an entity that has remained poorly understood, particularly since most abnormalities of intraductal pressure can be traced to morphologic and mechanical abnormalities in the biliary tract.

Cholecystocholangiography is the operative injection of the gallbladder with opacification of the biliary tree (Fig. 51-2). This technique is

1303

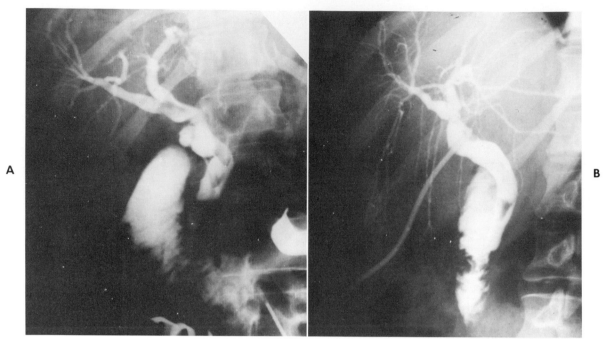

Fig. 51-1. A, Primary operative cholangiogram taken before common duct exploration was interpreted as showing four duct stones. **B,** Secondary operative cholangiogram obtained through the **T** tube after removal of four duct stones shows an additional common duct stone. This control study obtained before closure of the abdomen was followed by a second choledochotomy for removal of the fifth stone, but a second operation for retained stone was avoided by this cholangiographic practice.

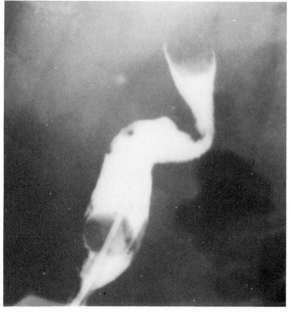

Fig. 51-2. Direct cholecystography without cholangiography. Cystic duct obstruction by a large solitary stone.

of great value in the diagnosis of congenital anomalies of the biliary tract (Fig. 51-3).

Pancreatography may be accomplished in one of three ways during surgery:[10] (1) direct puncture into a dilated duct through the parenchyma (Fig. 51-4), (2) amputation of the tail of the pancreas and injection of contrast medium through a catheter, or (3) cannulation of the pancreatic duct through the ampulla of Vater following transduodenal sphincterotomy.

Caroli's disease represents cavernous ectasia of the intrahepatic ducts.[13]

Courvoisier's syndrome is the eponym for ampulla of Vater obstruction.

The *Mirizzi syndrome* denotes partial common hepatic duct obstruction caused by pressure from a large gallstone in the adjacent cystic duct.[4]

TECHNIQUE

Calculous disease accounts for the great majority of surgery on the biliary tract. *Plain films*

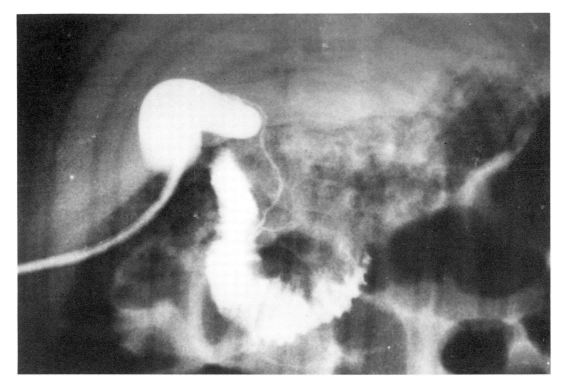

Fig. 51-3. Operative cholecystocholangiography in jaundiced infant with agenesis of the hepatic duct. Microcholedochus is apparently caused by disuse.

A 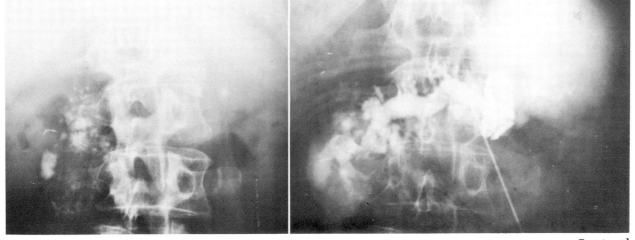 B

Continued.

Fig. 51-4. A, Extensive pancreatic calcification in chronic pancreatitis. **B,** Direct pancreatography into dilated duct in the same patient. **C,** Puestow pancreaticojejunostomy was performed. **D,** Roentgenograph obtained 6 months later shows that most of the pancreatic calcification has been passed through the anastomosis between pancreatic duct and jejunum.

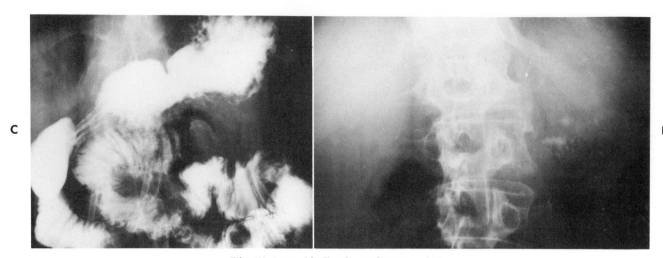

C

D

Fig. 51-4, cont'd. For legend see p. 1305.

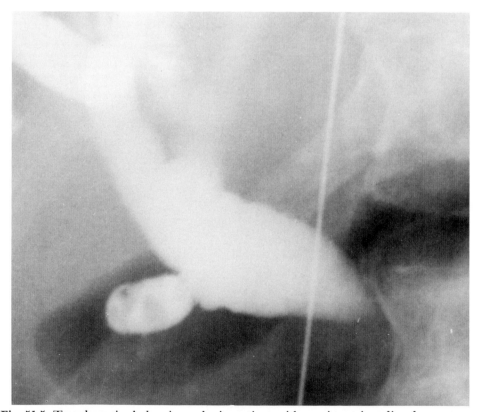

Fig. 51-5. Transhepatic cholangiography in patient with persistent jaundice demonstrates common duct obstruction caused by carcinoma of the pancreas. Incidental note is made of retained stones in cystic duct stump.

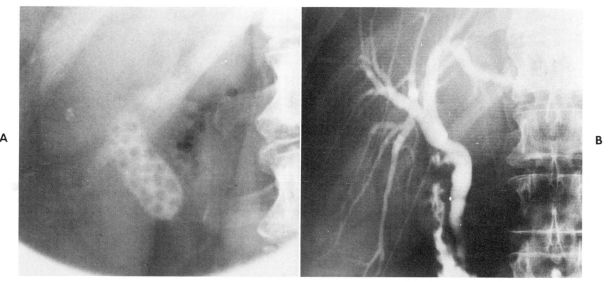

Fig. 51-6. A, Oral cholecystogram obtained 4 months before elective cholecystectomy reveals numerous small gallstones. **B,** At the time of surgery the gallbladder contained no stones and the primary operative cholangiograms were normal. Operation could have been avoided in this case of "disappearing gallstones," with a repeat oral cholecystogram obtained before surgery. Stones of this size may readily pass through the ampulla of Vater.

and oral cholecystography provide the preoperative diagnosis in almost all cases without jaundice, whereas transhepatic cholangiography may be required if persistent jaundice is present. (Fig. 51-5).

If elective cholecystectomy has been scheduled for cholelithiasis, a recent oral cholecystogram must be available (Fig. 51-6), for it has been shown that stones up to 1 cm. in size and up to thirty in number[27] can be evacuated spontaneously.[37] At least thirty such cases have been recorded.[24,31,33,36] These so-called disappearing gallstones are often seen in the postpregnancy state.[17]

Intravenous cholangiography is the preoperative method of choice in the diagnosis of duct abnormalities, particularly in the postcholecystectomy syndrome. Visualization is improved by the routine addition of tomography, but direct contrast injection into the duct system during operative cholangiography permits better diagnostic evaluation. Intravenous cholangiography should not mislead the clinician to omit the surgical cholangiogram at the time of exploration. Intravenous cholangiography is also the method of choice in acute cholecystitis, especially if the differential diagnosis of appendicitis is considered. Common duct demonstration in

the absence of gallbladder filling is diagnostic in almost all cases.[21,28]

The *primary operative cholangiogram* is the first order of business after laparotomy. The cystic duct is isolated and either a cannula[16,32] or a bulb-tipped urethral catheter[35] may be used for injection, but the cannulation of the cystic duct with a small polyethylene tube appears to be most satisfactory.[30] The cystic duct remains intubated until satisfactory roentgenograms are obtained. This interval is utilized for cholecystectomy in order to shorten the duration of anesthesia. Direct needle puncture of the common duct is also practiced (Fig. 51-7).[23,25]

Operative cholangiography can be accomplished even in the presence of acute cholecystitis.[40]

The operating table is rotated 10 to 15 degrees along the longitudinal axis to the right in order to project the distal biliary tract away from the lumbar spine. Gridlines must be across the abdomen in a right angle to the longitudinal axis of the body if a movable grid is not available.

The *contrast medium* used for direct injection during operative cholangiography must be opaque enough for marginal delineation of the bile duct, yet dilute enough to permit visualiza-

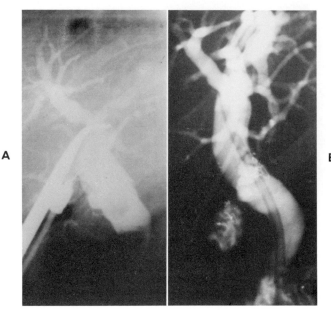

Fig. 51-7. A, Primary operative cholangiogram with injection into the markedly dilated hepatic duct with a stone obstruction. **B,** Secondary operative cholangiogram obtained after relief of obstruction shows decrease in the diameter of the hepatic duct.

tion of stones through the contrast medium. A 50% or 60% concentration of diatrizoate (Hypaque or Renografin) sodium diluted half and half with normal saline permits good visualization at a range of 80 to 90 kv. At least two films are obtained. The first injection is accomplished with 5 ml. or less of contrast medium using low injection pressure close to gravity (Fig. 51-8, *A*). The second roentgenogram is obtained after injection under mild pressure using less than 10 ml. (Fig. 51-8, *B*). An increase above normal intraductal pressure usually results in contraction of the sphincter of Oddi with retrograde filling of the intrahepatic radicals.

Barium cholangiography is practical,[34] particularly if duodenobiliary reflux occurs[22] or if a hepaticojejunal anastomosis is present (Fig. 51-9).[43]

Television monitors in the surgical suite are convenient[42] but do not match the detail seen on roentgenograms. I have found routine roentgenography in the surgical suite quite adequate. It requires less time than television fluoroscopy.

Cinefluorography may aid in the interpreta-

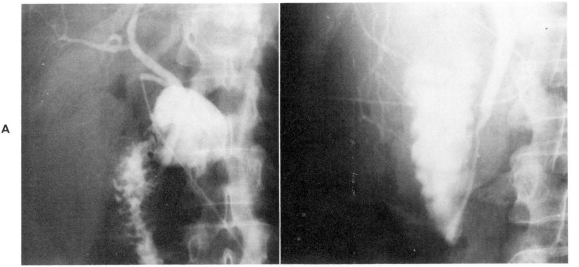

Fig. 51-8. A, The first roentgenograph of the primary operative cholangiogram was obtained too late in this patient. Also, too much contrast medium was used. The opaque medium in the duodenal bulb is obscuring the common duct. The injecting physician, furthermore, should stand on the right side of the patient. **B,** High injection pressure resulting in sphincter contraction and jet.

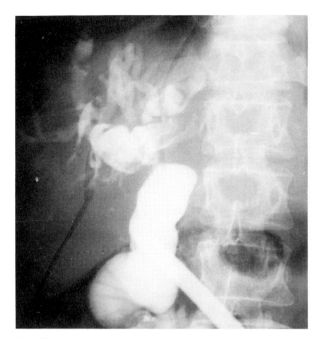

Fig. 51-9. Barium cholangiography permits evaluation of the diameter and patency of hepatojejunostomy.

tion of difficult T tube cholangiogram cases, particularly if delay occurs at the sphincter of Oddi.[38,45] Caroli used it as early as 1960 combined as cineradiomanometry.[20] This technique is ideal for scientific investigation of biliary tract physiology, but adds little to the routine roentgenographic patient examination.[18] It is useful for evaluation of pharmacoroentgenologic effects on the biliary tract and its sphincters[41] and in complicated cases (Fig. 51-10).[19]

Medication to induce spasm of the sphincter of Oddi is not needed for better visualization, but may be used to relieve spasm at the choledochoduodenal junction.[29]

The *four-day iopanoic acid* (Telepaque) *test* is useful in some cases to demonstrate retained common duct stones after removal of the T tube.[44]

Choledochoduodenostomy, choledochojejunostomy (Fig. 51-11), cholecystoduodenostomy (Fig. 51-12), or high surgical anastomoses between the hepatic ducts and the jejunum may be evaluated with a combination of intravenous

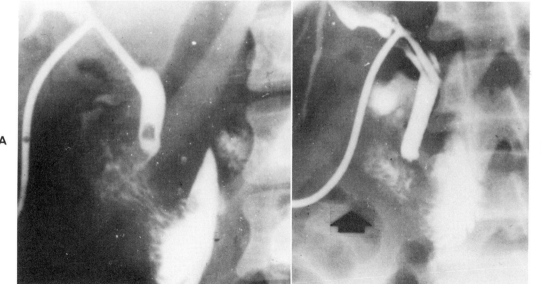

Fig. 51-10. Cinefluorography during the T tube cholangiogram was used to investigate the movement of the small common duct stone in this patient with no T tube drainage when supine, but right upper quadrant pain and prominent T tube drainage when out of bed. **A,** The small stone moved back into the common duct with the patient supine. **B,** The stone cannot be seen on spot films with the patient erect. Cinefluorographic frame analysis showed the stone to move into the intramural portion of the distal common duct, with partial duct obstruction.

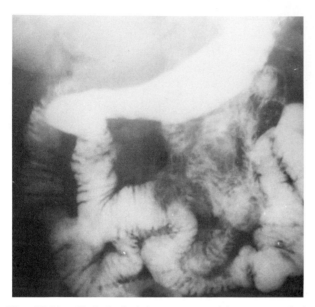

Fig. 51-11. Choledochojejunostomy with pneumocholangiogram.

cholangiography followed by upper gastrointestinal study.[39] The absence of air in the biliary ducts after anastomosis to the intestinal tract suggests anastomotic obstruction.[26]

INTERPRETATION, PITFALLS, AND MISTAKES

With good technique, the accuracy of operative cholangiography should be 90% to 95%. Duct stones of 3 mm. or smaller, however, are probably missed in half of the cases.[46] Stones may also be overlooked if their density corresponds to that of the contrast medium.[57]

Attention to details of roentgenographic technique are the obligation of the radiologist. Good films may even be obtained with portable equipment.[54] Custer analyzed the sources of error in his material of operative cholangiography and found technically unsatisfactory roentgenograms to be the leading cause.[48]

Air bubbles

Air bubbles must be eliminated by working in a closed system, using aspiration and injection with saline. This applies also to T tube cholangio-

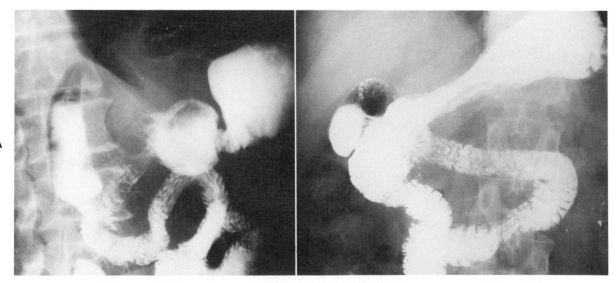

Fig. 51-12. A, Cholecystoduodenostomy and, **B,** cholecystojejunostomy with Roux-en-Y jejunojejunostomy, both cases showing barium reflux into the gallbladder. Pneumocholangiogram is less frequently present when compared with direct anastomosis of the duct system to the intestinal tract.

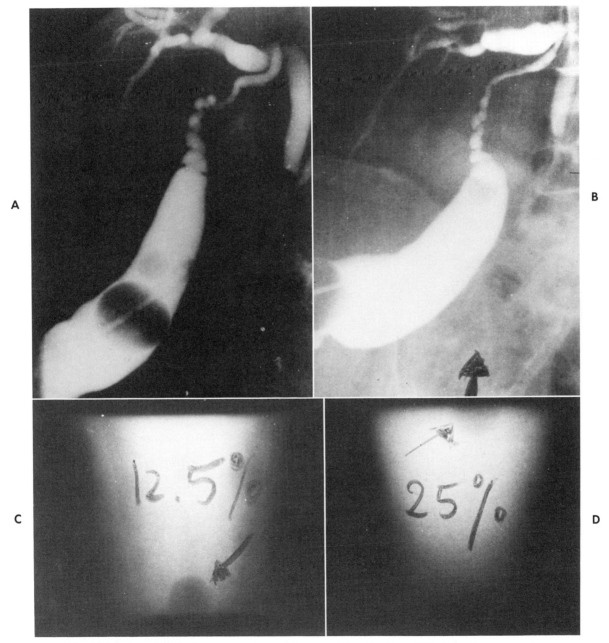

Fig. 51-13. A and **B,** Solitary, round, radiolucent defect in the gallbladder shown on cholecystocholangiography rises when the patient is turned semierect. **C** and **D,** A single cholesterol gallstone was recovered. It sinks in a 12.5% mixture of contrast medium, but floats when the contrast content is raised to 25%.

grams. The T tube is best clamped in these patients for at least 12 hours before roentgenographic examination. A needle is then introduced through the wall of the rubber catheter in order to maintain a closed-fluid system.

The differentiation between air bubbles and stones in the duct system may be solved by placing the patient in the Trendelenburg or semierect positions. But not everything that is round and rises in fluid is an air bubble, for gallstones do not have to be facetted and cholesterin stones may float in contrast medium (Fig. 51-13). Elsey has shown that the specific gravity of the lightest cholesterin stone is 1.04, which is the greatest specific gravity that native bile ever reaches.[49] This means that stones can hardly float in native bile but may float after the addition of contrast medium. Air bubbles, on the

other hand, are fortunately never facetted and never sink in bile or contrast medium.

Filling defects of the common bile duct may result from external compression, from distortion by the needle or catheter used for injection, by pressure from the hepatic artery, and by other causes. The intramural, or third, portion of the common duct may normally be narrowed where it runs in a groove posteriorly in the head of the pancreas.

Blockage at the sphincter of Oddi may be caused by spasm, particularly after manipulation of the common duct or instrumentation of the sphincter of Oddi. This contraction may even simulate stones in the distal duct. Serial films are necessary for clarification (Fig. 51-14). One must be aware of this possibility, particularly on the second operative cholangiogram, because mis-

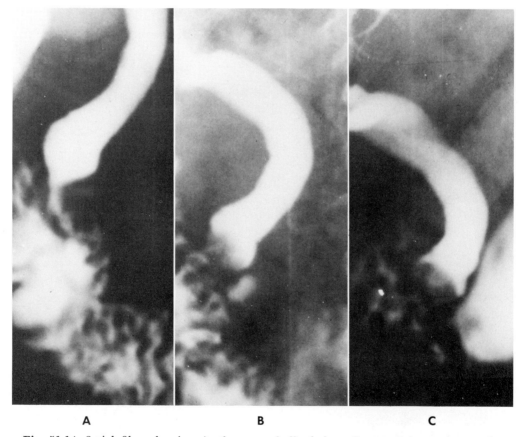

A   B   C

Fig. 51-14. Serial films showing **A,** the normal distal duct, **B,** some contraction at the sphincter, and **C,** prominent contraction at the sphincter simulating common duct stone. This "pseudocalculus sign" is frequently seen in secondary operative cholangiography following duct instrumentation.

interpretation may lead to unnecessary second exploration.[51] Obstruction of the entrance of the common duct in the duodenum can be expected in half of the cases after instrumentation.[47] If a primary cholangiogram is obtained routinely, this *"pseudocalculus"* will not be misinterpreted.[56]

The pneumocholangiogram

The presence of gas in the biliary tract may be caused by previous surgical anastomoses, by fistula from gallstone, inflammation, peptic or malignant disease, by gas-forming organisms, or by incompetence of the sphincter of Oddi from medication, tumor, adhesions, or paralytic intestinal ileus.[53] Incompetence of the sphincter of Oddi with reflux of gas and barium has also been seen in newborn infants with duodenal atresia.[50] Previous surgery on the biliary tract was responsible for air in the bile system in more than half the cases of a 10-year review done at the Mayo Clinic.[55] The pneumocholangiogram caused by gas-forming organisms must be quite unusual, whereas insufficiency of the sphincter with air reflux is more common than initially thought, particularly if we accept that patients pass gallstones spontaneously. Reflux of gas and barium occurs also in cases where the common duct enters the wall of a duodenal diverticulum (Fig. 51-15). The sphincter musculature is often deficient in these cases. An air cholangiogram is also seen as a sequel of trauma,[58] or as a complication of attempted thoracocentesis.[52]

Absence of the pneumocholangiogram sign in patients with other criteria of a gallstone ileus should raise the suspicion of a second stone in

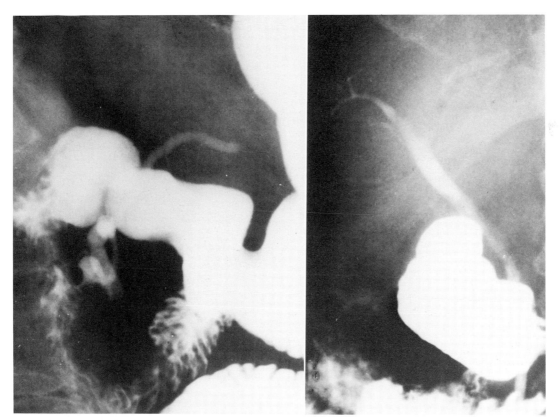

Fig. 51-15. Reflux of barium into bile duct and pancreatic duct entering a small duodenal diverticulum.

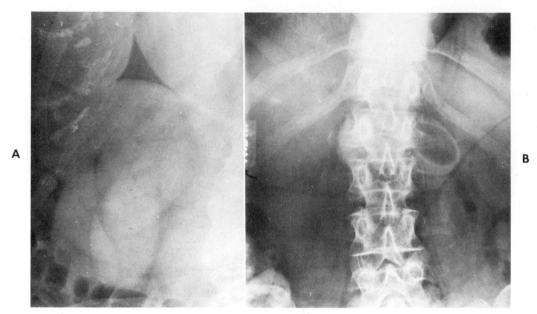

Fig. 51-16. A, Oral cholecystogram showing double gallbladder. **B,** Gallbladder containing large calculus with herniation into the lesser sac.

the duct system causing obstruction proximally to a fistula.

ANATOMIC VARIATIONS

Cholangiography may demonstrate absence of the cystic duct and gallbladder and duplication of the gallbladder with one[78] or two cystic ducts[72] entering the main duct. Guyer concludes that there are not likely to be more than 150 proved cases of double gallbladder in the world literature, and that of these only fifteen cases have been demonstrated roentgenologically and subsequently proved at operation (Fig. 51-16, *A*).[65] The gallbladder and cystic duct may be positioned anomalously on the left or in the midline. The latter is also seen with herniation of the gallbladder through the foramen of Winslow into the lesser sac (Fig. 51-16, *B*)

The common duct elongates and extends to the left of the midline after surgical procedures with mobilization of the duodenum, the so-called Kocher maneuver (Fig. 51-17).

Even triplication of the gallbladder has been described in five instances.[74]

The size of the biliary ducts can be measured quite accurately on roentgenograms. Magnification should amount to only 10% or less, the common duct having an equal distance to both the front and the back of the patient.[77]

Compensatory dilatation of the common bile duct after cholecystectomy does not occur normally. Increase in diameter after surgery is indicative of biliary tract disease.[63] The size of the common duct in asymptomatic patients remains usually the same after surgery when compared to preoperative films,[67] although normal common bile ducts show a slight but definite increase in both outer and inner circumference with age in males and females.[68] The diameter of precholecystectomy and postcholecystectomy common ducts measured the same in a study of asymptomatic patients, but proliferation of the intramural glandlike structures was noted after surgery.[69] Most authors, therefore, feel that cholangiograms in a patient with symptoms after cholecystectomy indicate an abnormality when dilatation is present on comparison to preoperative studies for when the common duct becomes larger than its normal diameter of 11 mm.[67] We have seen some immediate decrease in common duct diameter when comparing surgical cholangiograms of the same sitting just before and after relief of common duct obstruction (Fig. 51-7). This difference occurring with change in intraductal pressure is slight and appears to be caused by elastic fibers in the wall of the common duct. No true muscular contraction of the ducts is possible. The specific search

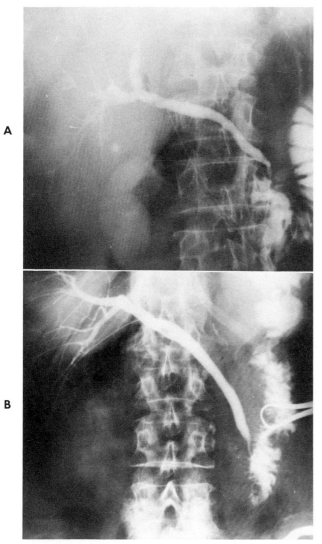

Fig. 51-17. Elongated biliary tract, **A,** with gastroduodenostomy, **B,** with gastrojejunostomy. The descending duodenum had been mobilized in both cases.

for smooth muscle in the wall of the duct revealed only scanty and disorganized fibers in twelve out of one-hundred specimens in one study[70] and thirteen out of seventy-five specimens in another.[62]

The papilla of Vater is located in the third portion of the duodenum in 8% of patients.[76]

The diameter of the largest dilators passed with ease through the *ampulla of Vater* indicates that the ampulla should be considered abnormally narrow if it does not admit at least a 3 mm. instrument.[59] The largest dilator passed in this study of normal ampullas averaged 6 mm.

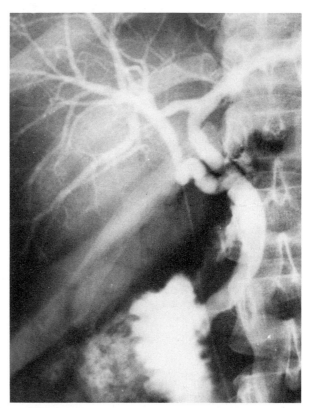

Fig. 51-18. The right hepatic duct joins the cystic duct. If this information is available from the primary operative cholangiogram, duct transsection close to the common duct can be avoided.

It is, therefore, plausible that common duct stones up to this size may pass spontaneously into the duodenum, an explanation for the entity of so-called disappearing gallstones. Passage of small gallbladder stones into the duodenum is probably more common than presently accepted.

Also more common than realized by radiologists and surgeons is the high percentage of anomalies of the major ducts of the biliary tree (Figs. 51-18 and 51-19). Schulenburg found anatomic variations of the biliary tract in 230 out of 1,093 operated cases, an incidence of 21%. Anomalies of the cystic duct were present in 13.7%, most commonly a low insertion into the common duct with portions of the distal cystic duct running in a common sheet with the major duct (Fig. 51-35). This explains the necessarily high incidence of cystic duct remnants.[75] Hayes found an even higher incidence of biliary duct anomalies.[66] He points out the risk of improperly identifying all structures and doing surgical

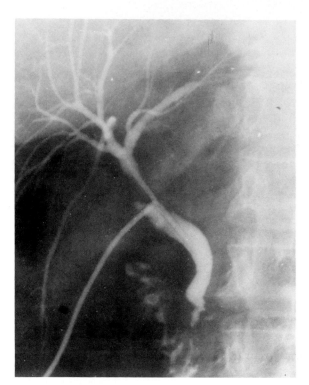

Fig. 51-19. The hypoplastic ventrocranial branch should suggest the presence of an anomaly. An accessory duct from the right lobe was found to join the cystic duct.

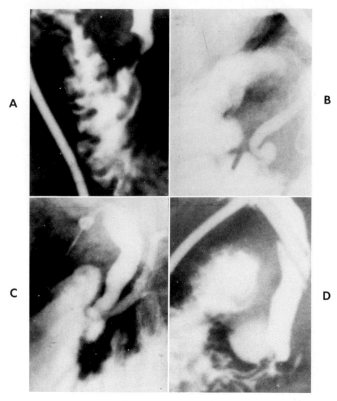

Fig. 51-20. Four different patients with entrance of the biliary tract into the wall or the neck of duodenal diverticula. Reflux is common.

damage to the biliary drainage. This emphasizes another strength of the primary operative cholangiogram—delineation of duct anomalies before exploration. The high degree of duct visualization after operative cholangiography cannot be achieved with preoperative intravenous cholangiography. Indeed, radiologists rarely identify duct anomalies by the latter method.

A third entity, which is more common than generally recognized, is the insertion of the common bile duct into duodenal diverticula (Fig. 51-20). There are now about fifty such cases described.[60,61] The diverticulum may cause duct obstruction.[71] There is also one case description of termination of the common bile duct into an enterogenous cyst of the duodenum.[73] I consider the entrance of a common bile duct and pancreatic duct into a duodenal diverticulum as a possible cause of pancreaticobiliary disease. This entity should be considered if symptoms do not improve after cholecystectomy.[79]

If the distal end of the common duct herniates into the lumen of the duodenum, it may simulate the roentgenographic appearance of the intraduodenal diverticulum.[64]

ROUTINE VS. SELECTIVE PRIMARY OPERATIVE CHOLANGIOGRAPHY

Routine primary operative cholangiography implies that all patients for cholecystectomy will undergo this procedure before common duct exploration. Surgeons advocating *selective* operative cholangiography utilize this technique only with certain indications. This practice implies that clinical indications for common duct exploration are as accurate as the roentgenologic assessment. Control studies, however, demonstrate operative cholangiography to be more accurate than any other criterion for choledochotomy and more accurate than conventional common duct exploration.[80,83,109,114]

Arguments against routine operative cholangiography

Difficulties in operating room technique are responsible for errors, but this problem should be lessened if the surgical team is accustomed to routine cholangiography. Occasional cholangiograms are more apt to give poor technical results.

The time added to the duration of operation and anesthesia in performing cholangiography has been criticized, but experienced surgeons using operative cholangiography routinely estimate the added time as 5 to 10 minutes* or no more than 10 to 20 minutes.[109,123] Furthermore, routine roentgenographic studies will decrease the incidence of exploratory choledochotomy, a procedure adding at least double that amount of time to the length of operation. Cholecystectomy is usually begun during the time the roentgenograms are developed and reviewed.

False-positive and false-negative readings are a factor. The percentage of false-positive readings is given as 4% to 7%.[83,85,104,107,122] False-negative readings may go as high as 7% to 10%.[107,109,120,125] These figures, however, must be compared with false-positive and false-negative surgical judgment relying on classical clinical criteria alone for common duct surgery. The roentgenographic accuracy is higher and is given as 78% when compared to 54% accuracy for clinical judgment.[110] Most authors using routine cholangiography have cut their number of common duct explorations to about one half.

Difficulties in cooperation between surgeon, anesthetist, and radiologist may exist. This problem is usually eliminated when all three specialists appreciate the value of routine operative cholangiography and become interested in efficient teamwork. The radiologist must be available to give immediate readings in all cases. He must also be willing to go into the surgical suite in difficult cases in order to discuss the roentgenograms and help in the direction of repeat contrast injections.

Radiation exposure to physician, personnel, and patient must be considered. The anesthetist should wear a lead apron during the injection. All other personnel should step at least 10 feet back from the table or behind a portable lead screen. Television monitoring in the surgical suite may add to the length of the procedure and to the radiation hazard.

Pancreatic reflux and postoperative pancreatitis are listed as disadvantages. Bardenheier checked his records on 840 cases and found an incidence of 4% of postoperative pancreatitis.[86] It occurred 10 times as often in cases undergoing common duct exploration as in those of 498 cases that had operative cholangiography alone. Nine percent of the roentgenographic studies showed pancreatic reflux. Pancreatic duct filling occurs frequently during operative cholangiography.[130] Beneventano observed it in 45% of cases, but found no evidence of pancreatitis.[140] Even gallstones may enter pancreatic ducts in a retrograde fashion.[84]

Incompetence of the gastric pyloric sphincter with reflux of contrast medium and duodenal contents, such as bile, into the stomach is seen in about one third of normal cases and apparently represents a further physiologic variant.[143]

Arguments in favor of routine operative cholangiography

Classical clinical indications for common duct exploration are often unreliable. Common duct stones may occur in the absence of duct dilatation and in the absence of jaundice (Fig. 51-21). Even duct palpation is unreliable for the presence or absence of common duct stones,* particularly in the distal common duct where it may be buried in the head of the pancreas posteriorly.

Precholedochotomy information is essential as to the presence of duct pathology. The surgical procedure can be tailored accordingly, particularly in regard to the large number of anomalies of the biliary tract. Warren reviewed the records on surgical repair of over 1,600 biliary strictures and showed 96% of them to be iatrogenic.[127] Walters' review of his experience with another 429 strictures of the common duct is a further reminder that this is not a rare complication.[126] Warren stresses that the surgeon identify the anatomy of the biliary tract before common duct exploration in order to avoid this dreaded complication.[127]

Cholangiography aids in the preexploratory

---

*See references 83, 98, 100, 103, 104, 111, 114, 122, and 139.

*See references 103, 105, 111, 119, 121, 122, and 129.

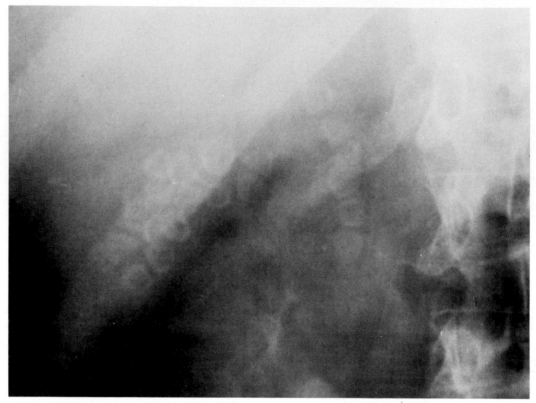

Fig. 51-21. Incidental discovery of multiple gallstones and common duct stones in patient without abdominal symptoms undergoing excretory urography prior to hysterectomy.

identification of calculi, neoplasms (Figs. 51-22 and 51-23),[113] sclerosing cholangitis (Fig. 51-24),[92,94,101,112] metastatic intrahepatic disease (Fig. 51-25), cholangitis (Fig. 51-26), liver abscess (Fig. 51-27),[82] strictures (Fig. 51-28), fibrosis of the papilla of Vater (Fig. 51-32),[81] and biliary parasites.[90]

About 15% of patients with cholelithiasis also have choledocholithiasis, and 20% of common duct stones are associated with intrahepatic stones. Madden suggests that the number of primary common duct stones is higher than we presently believe.[115] About 5% to 8% of patients with biliary tract stones show the presence of calculi limited to the common duct. Best found an incidence of 7.6% of intrahepatic calculi among 456 cases of cholelithiasis studied at autopsy.[89] Highly pigmented stones are more likely to be of intrahepatic origin than cholesterol stones.[93] Caroli's disease shows bile stasis in the cavernous ectasia of the intrahepatic ducts (Fig. 51-31), predisposing to stone formation.[117]

One case of a total bile cast of the biliary tree has been reported.[116]

Reduction in choledochotomies was accomplished with the use of routine cholangiography by several authors. Comparing their material with and without this routine roentgenographic procedure the incidence of choledochotomies was cut in half.[83,91,109,122]

Decrease in the number of retained stones and reexploration was demonstrated by Hicken and Parent.[106,119] Their comparative analysis showed that twice as many stones were missed without the use of cholangiography (Figs. 51-29 and 51-30). Reexploration for overlooked stones is accompanied by a higher morbidity and mortality than the initial surgical procedure.

The list of surgeons recommending routine operative cholangiography between the years of 1960 and 1970 is long and illustrious.* Surgeons

---

*See references 80, 83, 85, 91, 96-100, 102-104, 108, 109, 114, 118, 121, 122, 128, and 129.

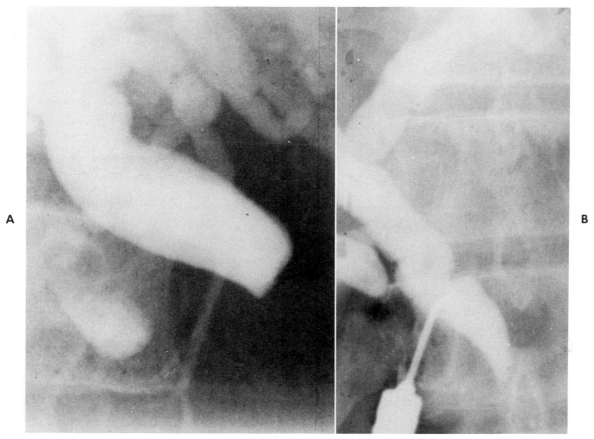

Fig. 51-22. High common duct obstruction with characteristic tapering in two patients with carcinoma of the pancreas.

practicing selective cholangiography have not published comparative studies, and they do a greater number of common duct explorations. The astonishing fact remains, however, that the majority of surgeons are still practicing selective operative cholangiography. A questionnaire sent to the American Surgical Association in 1968 with a reply of 70% from the membership showed only 18% or less of surgeons practicing routine operative cholangiography.[109]

It must be stressed that the roentgenographic cholangiogram is not competing with clinical indications for common duct explorations, for the best results are obtained if clinical judgment is combined with routine operative cholangiography.

COMPLICATIONS

Cholangiovenous reflux may occur with forced injections but requires only moderate increase above the secretion pressure of the liver in the presence of common duct obstruction (Fig. 51-32). Contrast medium (and even bacteria) enters the bloodstream through communications between the bile capillaries and the liver sinusoids[134] and is excreted with opacificaion of the kidneys. Pancreatic necrosis has been reported after cholangiography under high injection pressure.[133] The same complication has been attributed to T tube cholangiography.[132]

Bile peritonitis occurs when there is leakage of bile from the liver or the extrahepatic biliary tree into the peritoneal cavity, particularly if injuries to the main ducts or surgical transsection of aberrant divisional ducts are not recognized during surgery.[136] Soft tissue masses seen on plain abdominal roentgenograms after surgery with or without change in the flank stripe are caused by collection of bile.[137] Delay in diagnosis is common.[135] Preoperative abdominal films

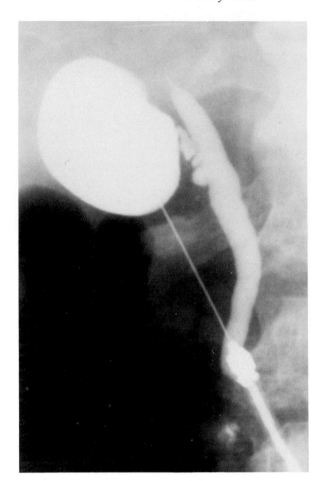

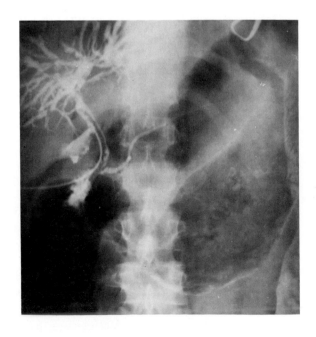

Fig. 51-23. Direct needle cholecystocholangiogram in patient with hepatic duct obstruction caused by ductal carcinoma. The rat-tail sign is present.

Fig. 51-24. Patient with sclerosing cholangitis of the extrahepatic ducts. Surgical cholangiography before common duct exploration and before cholecystectomy is mandatory to preserve the gallbladder for anastomosis.

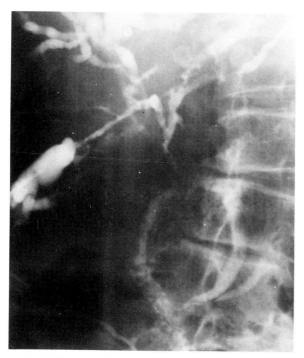

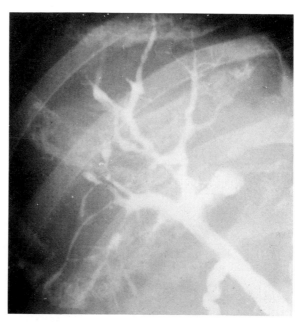

Fig. 51-25. Metastatic intrahepatic disease with distortion of intrahepatic ducts.

Fig. 51-26. Advanced intrahepatic cholangitis.

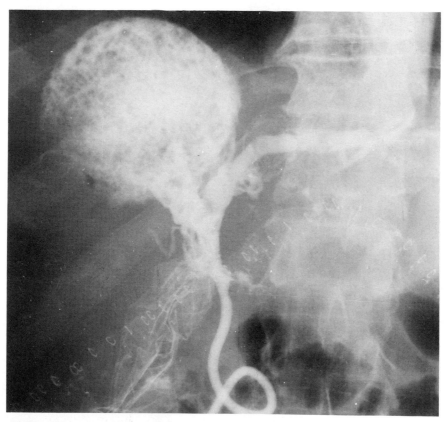

Fig. 51-27. Contrast medium enters a large liver abscess cavity during operative cholangiography.

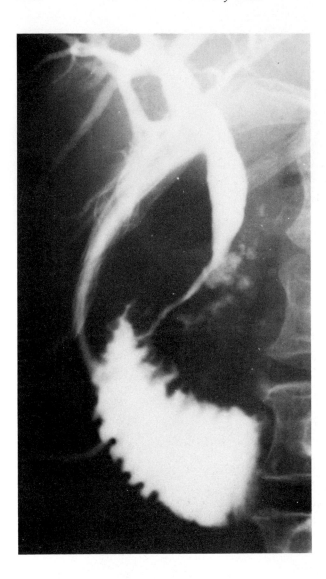

Fig. 51-28. Stricture of the distal common duct with chronic pancreatitis. If the T tube is in place, stricture dilatation may be accomplished under fluoroscopic control using instrumentation similar to stone extraction.[167] I have accomplished dilatation of bile duct strictures in seven patients, but we must await the long-term result to judge the effectiveness of this new technique.

must be compared to postoperative studies in order to recognize ill-defined masses.[131] The bile collections may be loculated, and several masses may be seen because of associated peritonitis (Fig. 51-33).

Excessive T tube drainage following cholecystectomy may be caused by distal common duct obstruction. Testing the bile for the presence of amylase will confirm the reflux of pancreatic secretions.

THE POSTCHOLECYSTECTOMY SYNDROME

If symptoms occur or persist after cholecystectomy, several of the entities under the heading of "postcholecystectomy syndrome" must be considered. They include retained duct stones, cystic duct remnants (Fig. 51-34), duct strictures or injuries, sphincter of Oddi spasm or fibrosis (Fig. 51-35), neoplastic disease, including neuroma of the cystic duct, pancreatitis, or bile peritonitis. Persistent symptoms have also been ascribed to disorders outside the biliary tract, such as hiatus hernia, peptic ulceration, abdominal angina, coronary artery disease, and spastic colon.[139]

By far the most common cause for postcholecystectomy symptoms is retained stones in the biliary tract. Intrahepatic stones overlooked at the time of surgery may have moved distally. Other abnormalities listed under the postcho-

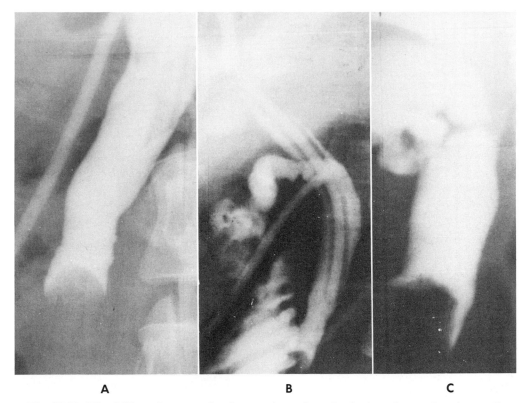

A   B   C

Fig. 51-29. The biliary duct termination at the point of calculus obstruction is usually characteristic.

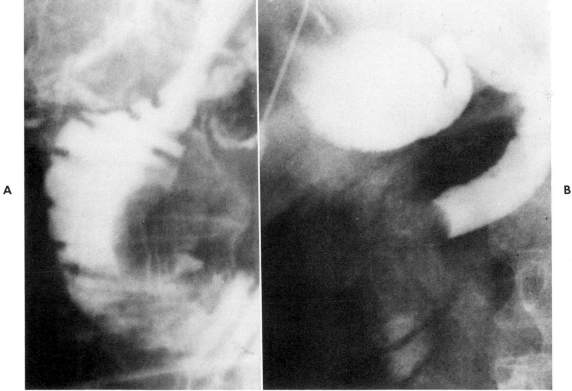

Fig. 51-30. Impacted distal common duct stone with associated surrounding edema may result in a prominent filling defect in the descending duodenum on barium examination.

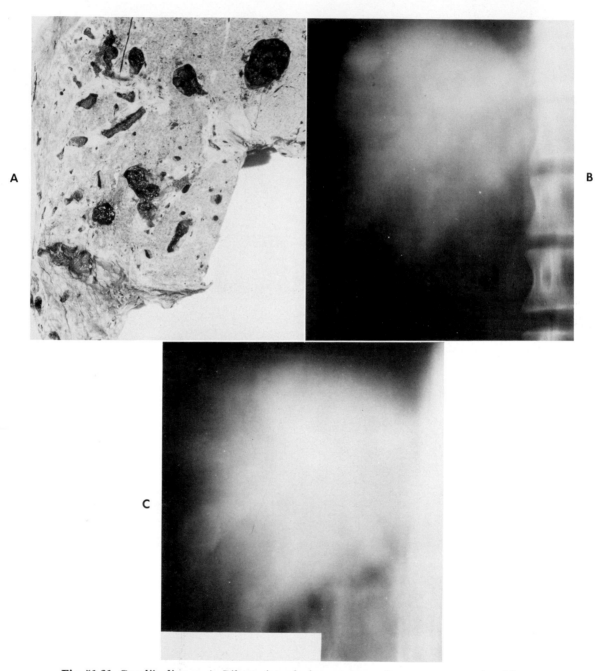

Fig. 51-31. Caroli's disease. **A,** Bile stasis and pigment stones in cavernous ectasia of intrahepatic ducts seen postmortem. **B,** Intravenous cholangiography and tomography 6 weeks before death shows contrast collection in ectatic ducts with cyst formation. **C,** Bile concrements seen within cystic dilatation. To our knowledge, this is the only case demonstrating Caroli's disease on intravenous cholangiography and diagnosed before pathologic examination. Transhepatic cholangiography or operative cholangiography is usually needed for diagnosis.

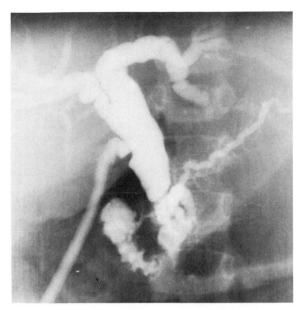

Fig. 51-32. Extensive pancreatic reflux in patient with fibrosis of the distal common duct and papilla of Vater.

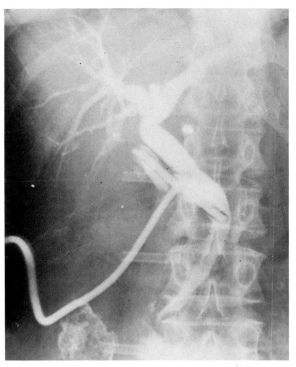

Fig. 51-34. Proximal arm of the T tube is located in a cystic duct remnant.

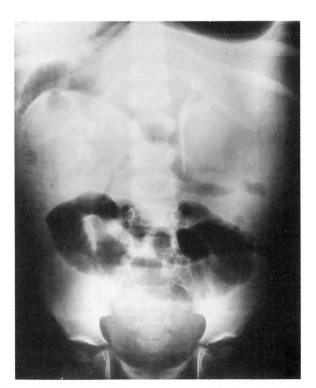

Fig. 51-33. Abdominal masses caused by loculated bile collections with peritonitis after abdominal trauma and bile duct laceration.

lecystectomy syndrome are, indeed, rare. Although retained cystic duct stumps are common, it is unlikely that this postoperative finding causes symptoms in the absence of retained stones in the cystic duct. The intramural variant of a cystic duct in apposition to the common duct and covered by a common sheath occurs in 22% of studied cadavers (Fig. 51-35).[142] Bodvall studied 500 cases postoperatively and found cystic duct remnants longer than 1 cm. in 40%.[138] When present, it occurred in the same number of patients with and without symptoms, so that the cystic duct remnant, per se, can hardly be incriminated to give symptoms. A cystic duct remnant, however, may be associated with tumors or inflammation or it may contain stones (Fig. 51-36). Resection of cystic duct remnants containing stones has relieved symptoms.[143]

Intravenous cholangiography is the method of choice for investigation of the postcholecystectomy syndrome.[140]

Fibrosis and inflammation of the sphincter of Oddi may give rise to postoperative symptoms. This probably accounts for the majority of cases previously labeled under biliary dyskinesia.

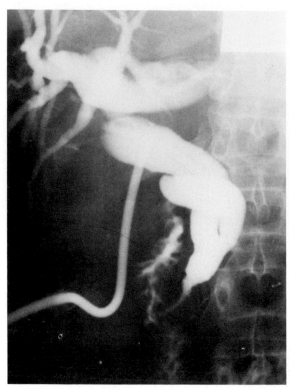

Fig. 51-35. Large cystic duct remnant in patient with fibrosis of the sphincter of Oddi. The cystic duct enters low and is in a common sheet with the major duct. This cystic duct anomaly is common and is responsible for the frequently seen cystic duct remnant.

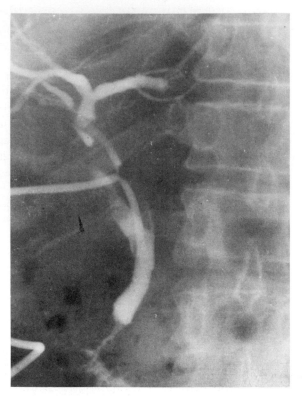

Fig. 51-36. Retained stone in cystic duct remnant.

Portorak demonstrated that normal function begins to return about 10 days after sphincterotomy and return to normal is complete in 95% of cases 6 months after surgery.[141] Barium reflux from the duodenum into the biliary tract is present only in 4% of cases after a 6-month postoperative interval. For permanent drainage, particularly in patients with recurrent and reformed biliary tract stones, choledochoduodenostomy is needed. Barium reflux persists in almost all of these cases.

BILIARY FISTULAS

Spontaneous perforation of the bile ducts has been reported in early infancy.[144] Operative cholangiography may show the point of leakage from the perforation (Fig. 51-37).[149] Biliary tract rupture has been associated with inspissated bile in the common duct. Continuous fistulas occur with avulsion or iatrogenic dissection of biliary ducts.[154]

The majority of spontaneous internal and external biliary fistulas is caused by cholelithiasis.[151] The classical roentgenographic findings of gallstone ileus are small-bowel distention, air in the biliary tract, and an abnormally located gallstone that is usually solitary, large, and laminated. Fistulas to the stomach or duodenum are demonstrated with contrast medium given by mouth.[153] One series of 819 cases of spontaneous internal biliary fistulas consisted of cholecystoduodenal fistulas in 51%, cholecystocolic fistulas in 21%, and choledochoduodenal fistulas in 19%. Rare types are cholecystogastric, choledochogastric, and cholecystocholedochal fistulas. Gallstones are associated with approximately 90% of fistulas primarily involving the gallbladder.[152] In another series the fistulas lead in 431 cases to the duodenum, in 92 cases to the colon, and in 20 cases to the duodenum and large bowel (Fig. 51-38).[145] Barium enema studies are diagnostic if the colon is involved, but cholecystograms and cholangiograms are often useless because of immediate drainage to the intestinal tract.

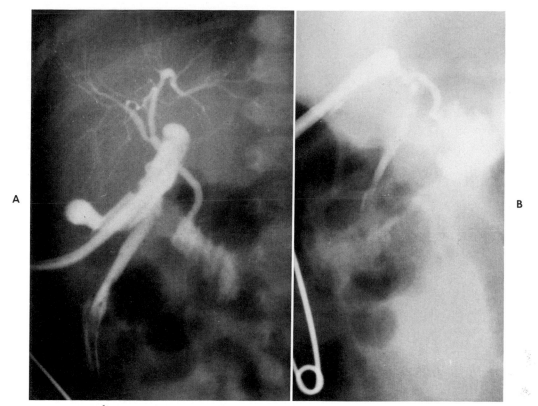

Fig. 51-37. A, Cholecystocholangiogram in child with bile duct perforation. **B,** Cholangiogram in steep oblique position is needed to identify the point of contrast extravasation from the common duct.

If the diagnosis of gallstone ileus is considered, the radiologist should always search for a second stone in the biliary tract. If the fistula is from the gallbladder to the intestinal tract, the common bile duct may not contain gas. Intravenous cholangiography aids in these cases to exclude a second stone in the common bile duct (Fig. 51-39).[155] The diagnosis of choledocholithiasis has been made by barium enema studies in cases of cholecystocolonic fistulas.[147]

Carcinoma of the biliary tract, duodenum, or colon, diverticulitis, ulcerative colitis, and decubitus erosion from cholecystostomy tubes indwelling for long periods of time[148] make up the small group of noncalculous causes of biliary fistulas. Ascending cholangitis and gastrointestinal bleeding may complicate internal biliary fistulas. Fecalent vomiting is often present with fistulas to the colon.[156]

Fistulas have also been reported between the common bile duct and the right renal pelvis,[150] between the biliary tract and the pleural space, and between the biliary and bronchial tracts.[146] The latter two have been observed after trauma, hepatic abscess, and gonococcal disease and with biliary tract obstruction.

SPECIAL TECHNIQUES AND PROCEDURES

Trans-T tube catheterization has been used to relieve postoperative biliary obstruction. Standard vascular catheters and guide wires may be employed to dislodge sediments from the indwelling T tube (Fig. 51-40).[159,162] Best described a T tube with a wider angle at the distal end of the transverse arm. This facilitates easier placement of guide wires in selected cases.[157]

Cannulation of the ampulla of Vater from the duodenum has been accomplished for direct cholangiography or pancreatography.[161] This approach is now more practical with the use of the fiberduodenoscope.[160] Cotton succeeded in can-

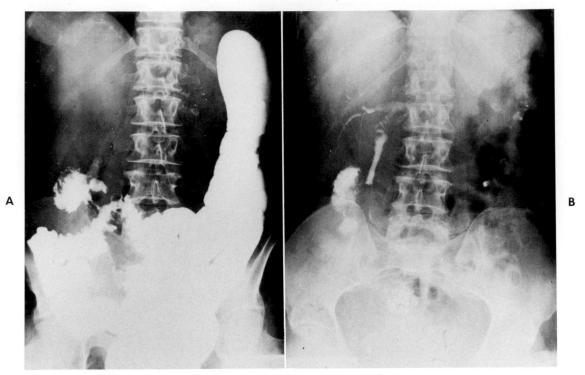

Fig. 51-38. A, Barium enema results in reflux into abscess. **B,** Delayed film shows barium reflux into biliary tract. The internal fistula was caused by gallstone perforation.

nulation of the papilla of Vater in 73% of sixty jaundiced patients.[158] Retrograde roentgenograms were then obtained of the biliary and pancreatic duct systems. This is probably the future method of choice for patients with jaundice, patients in whom transhepatic cholangiography is indicated today. Transjugular cholangiography, a more difficult technique, has been successfully used in one center.[163]

Expulsion and extraction of retained biliary duct stones

A second surgical intervention is required if postoperative T tube cholangiography demonstrates retained common duct stones. This surgical procedure carries a higher mortality and morbidity than the first operation. Even dissolution of retained stones, which has been successful in some of the small percentage of cases in which retained stones consist of cholesterol,[169] requires prolonged hospitalization. Nonsurgical removal of retained common bile duct calculi, however, has now become feasible. Mazzariello

used extraction forceps through the sinus tract of the T tube to remove stones.[174] Magarey used Desjardins forceps and the Dormia ureteral basket successfully for this purpose.[173] The use of guide wires and arteriographic catheters has been reported.[168,175] Soft rubber catheters may expel the retained stone into the duodenum,[170] particularly with the addition of saline flushes. Balloon-tipped catheters are not practical for the extraction of retained stones[164] and may result in biliary tract disruption and hematobilia.[171,172] The ureteral stone basket is more suitable mechanically (Fig. 51-41).[165]

I have developed this basket technique further in combination with the use of a remote control catheter (Fig. 51-42). It is easily steered into the distal common duct beyond the right angle turn at the point of T tube insertion. It also allows proximal catheterization into biliary radicals for retained stone extraction. The internal diameter corresponds to a No. 5 French for the passage of extraction instruments. We removed successfully one or more stones in

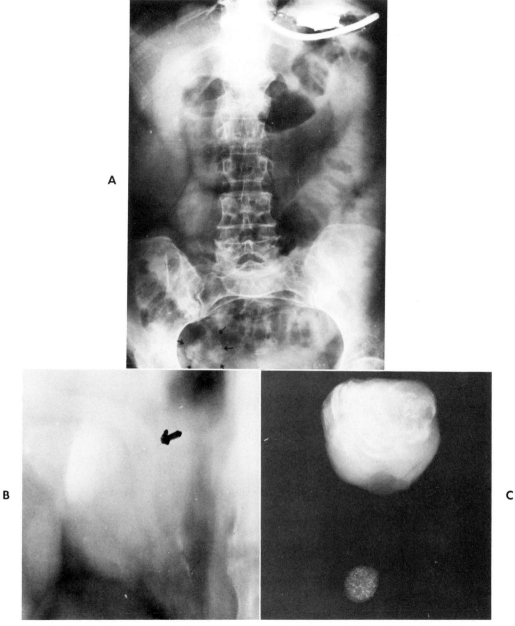

Fig. 51-39. A, Intestinal ileus with large laminated gallstone in right lower quadrant. No pneumocholangiogram is present. **B,** Intravenous cholangiogram shows filling defect in common duct. **C,** Two gallstones were removed from terminal ileum and common duct.

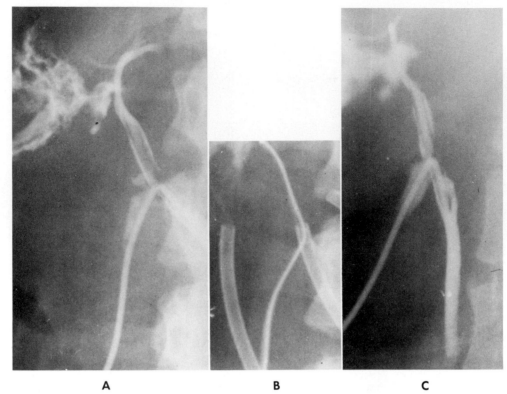

A   B   C

Fig. 51-40. **A,** Sediment blocking the proximal arm of the T tube. **B,** Introduction of guide wire. **C,** The sediment has been dislodged and the T tube is patent. Note biliary cutaneous fistula from partial hepatectomy. (From Margulis, A. R., Newton, T. H., and Najarian, J. S.: Amer. J. Roentgen. **93:**975, 1965.)

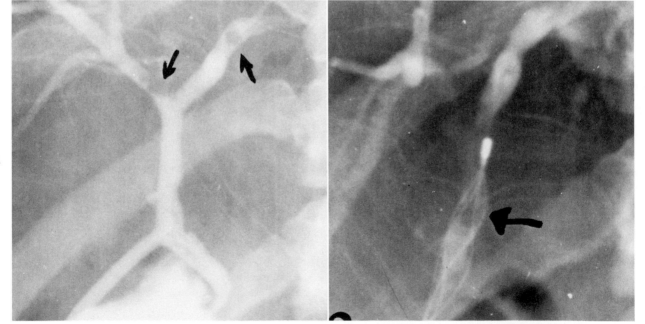

Fig. 51-41. **A,** Two retained stones in the major hepatic radicals. **B,** One hepatic stone is being extracted inside a ureteral stone basket. The second stone was also successfully extracted and surgery was avoided.

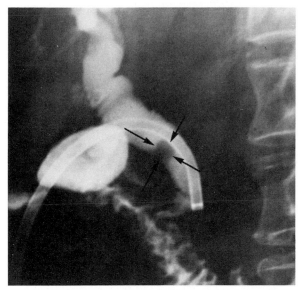

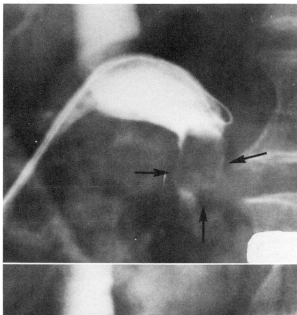

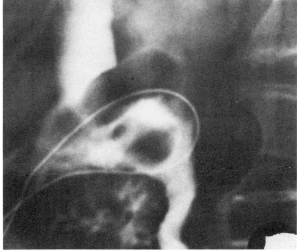

Fig. 51-42. The remote control catheter (Medi-Tech, Watertown, Mass.) has been passed beyond the common duct stone. A stone basket is then introduced through the catheter. At the present time we have used this technique in sixty-two patients, with failure in four, but avoiding surgery in the other fifty-eight patients.

thirty out of thirty-two patients.[166,167] The catheter also admits single or double wire slings (Fig. 51-43) for the removal or fragmentation of large stones. Suction may be applied through open-end tubes. The placement of small fiberoptic instruments or ultrasonic transducers for stone fragmentation may be added to this new roentgenologic procedure.

Fig. 51-43. A, After removal of the T tube a wire sling is placed through a catheter and is passed beyond the large common duct stone. **B,** The stone is extracted from the common duct. We have extracted as many as nine common duct stones in one patient.

REFERENCES

General considerations

1. Bergerhof, H. D.: Erfahrungen mit der Radiomanometrie bei 500 Gallensteinoperationen, Bruns. Beitr. Klin. Chr. **216:**602, 1968.
2. Bockhart, H., and Moller, W.: Versuche ueber die Funktion der Gallenblase und ihre Roentgendarstellung. Dtsch. Ztschr. Chir. **161:**168, 1921.
3. Carter, R. F. and Saypol, G. M.: Transabdominal cholangiography, J.A.M.A. **148:**253, 1952.
4. Clemett, A. R., and Lowman, R. M.: The roentgen features of the Mirizzi syndrome, Amer. J. Roentgen. **94:**480, 1965.
5. Ferris, D. O., and Sterling, W. A.: Surgery of the biliary tract, Surg. Clin. N. Amer. **47:**861, 1967.
6. Frommhold, W.: Cholecysto-cholangiography. In Schinz, H. R., Baensch, W. E., Frommhold, W., Glauner, R., Uehlinger, E., and Wellauer, J., editors: Roentgen diagnosis, vol. I, ed. 2, New York, 1968, Grune & Stratton, Inc., p. 378.
7. Glenn, F., and Grafe, W., Jr.: Historical events in biliary tract surgery, Arch. Surg. **93:**848, 1966.
8. Goldman, L. I., Weinberger, M., DeLaurentis, D. A., and Burnett, W. E.: Operative cholecystocholangiography, Surg. Gynec. Obstet. **128:**279, 1969.
9. Hess, W.: Surgery of the biliary passages and the pancreas, Princeton, 1965, D. Van Nostrand Co., Inc.
10. Howard, J. M., and Short, W. F.: An evaluation of pancreatography in suspected pancreatic disease, Surg. Gynec. Obstet. **129:**319, 1969.
11. Mallet-Guy, P.: L'intervention biliaire sous controle radiomanométrique, Lyon Chir. **39:**50, 1944.
12. Mirizzi, P. L.: La colangiografia durante las operaciones de las vias biliares, Bol. Trab. Soc. Buenos Aires **16:**1133, 1932.
13. Mujahed, Z., Glenn, F., and Evans, J.: Communi-

cating cavernous ectasia of the intrahepatic ducts (Caroli's disease), Amer. J. Roentgen. 113:21, 1971.

14. Schulenburg, C. A.: Operative cholangiography, London, 1966, Butterworth & Co., Ltd.

15. Statistical bulletin, Metropolitan Life Insurance Company, 46:9, 1965.

Technique

16. Aldrete, J. S., and Judd, E. S.: Metallic cannula as an aid to cysticduct operative cholangiography, Mayo Clin. Proc. 41:839, 1966.

17. Arcomano, J. P., Schwinger, H. N., and DeAngelis, J.: The spontaneous disappearance of gallstones, Amer. J. Roentgen. 99:637, 1967.

18. Beneventano, T. C., Jacobson, H. G., Hurwitt, E. S., and Schein, C .J.: Cine-cholangiomanometry: physiologic observations, Amer. J. Roentgen. 100: 673, 1967.

19. Burhenne, H. J.: Roentgenologic approach to a physiologic examination of the alimentary tract. In Gamble, J. R., and Wilbur, D. L., editors: Current concepts of clinical gastroenterology, Boston, 1965, Little, Brown, and Co.

20. Caroli, J., Porcher, P., Pequignot, G., and Delattre, M.: Contribution of cineradiography to study of the function of the human biliary tract, Amer. J. Dig. Dis. 5:677, 1960.

21. Chang, F. C.: Intravenous cholangiography in the diagnosis of acute cholecystitis, Amer. J. Surg. 120: 567, 1970.

22. Cugini, A., and Sosso, A.: Retrograde cholangiography from transpapillary duodenobiliary reflux, Ann. Radiol. Diagn. (Bologna) 35:163, 1962.

23. Ferguson, H. L., and Sampliner, J. E.: Operative needle cholangiography: a clinical evaluation, Amer. Surg. 35:476, 1969.

24. Gardner, A. M., Holden, W. S., and Monks, P. J.: Disappearing gallstones, Brit. J. Surg. 53:114, 1966.

25. Griffin, T. F., and Wild, A. A.: The case for peroperative cholangiography, Brit. J. Surg. 54:609, 1967.

26. Hafner, H. M.: Examinations following choledocho-duodenostomy, Helv. Chir. Acta 26:334, 1959.

27. Hansson, K., and Ramberg, L.: A case of spontaneous and complete disappearance of gallstones, Radiologe (Berlin) 1:97, 1961.

28. Harrington, O. B., Beall, A. C., Jr., Noon, G., and DeBakey, M. E.: Intravenous cholangiography in acute cholecystitis: use in differential diagnosis, Arch. Surg. 88:585, 1964.

29. Herman, R. E., and Hoerr, S. O.: The value of the routine use of operative cholangiography, Surg. Gynec. Obstet. 121:1015, 1965.

30. Jolly, P. C., Baker, J. W., Schmidt, H. M., and others: Operative cholangiography, Ann. Surg. 168:551, 1968.

31. Kelly, T. R., and Schlueter, T. M.: Spontaneous evacuation of gallstones, Amer. J. Surg. 111:247, 1966.

32. Kramer, S. G.: Technical aid to operative cholangiography, Surgery 64:403, 1968.

33. Kriss, N.: Disappearing and changing gallstones, Med. Radiogr. Photogr. 44:48, 1968.

34. Lucas, C. E., and Read, R. C.: Barium cholangiography, Radiology 87:1043, 1966.

35. Luttwak, E. M.: A simple method of operative cholangiography, Surg. Gynec. Obstet. 128:603, 1969.

36. Margulies, S. I., Brogdon, B. G., Sindler, R. A., and Perilla, F. R.: Disappearing gallstones, Brit. J. Radiol. 40:546, 1967.

37. Marquis, J. R., and Densler, J.: The disappearing limy bile syndrome, Radiology 94:311, 1970.

38. Myers, R. N., Haupt, G. J., Birkhead, N. C., and Deaver, J. M.: Cinecholangiography as an aid in the interpretation of T-tube cholangiogram deformities, Surg. Gynec. Obstet. 119:47, 1964.

39. Schein, C. J., Beneventano, T. C., and Jacobson, H. G.: Choledochoduodenostomy—roentgen considerations, Surgery 60:958, 1966.

40 Schulenburg, C. A.: Operative cholangiography in acute cholecystitis, Med. Proc. 16:318, 1970.

41. Stassa, G., and Grafe, W. R.: The cineradiographic evaluation of the biliary tract after drug therapy following cholecystectomy, sphincterotomy, and vagotomy, Radiology 91:297, 1968.

42. Whitaker, P. H., Parkinson, E. G., and Hughes, J. H.: Television fluoroscopy for operative cholangiography: an analysis of 150 cases, Clin. Radiol. 19:368, 1968.

43. Wise, R. E. ,and Keefe, J. P.: Radiological evaluation of hepaticojejunal anastomosis, Surg. Clin. N. Amer. 48:579, 1968.

44. Wise, R. E.: Roentgenology of the liver and biliary tract, Gastroenterology 45:644, 1963.

45. Zakl, K. S.: Cineradiographical examination of the common bile duct, Pol. Przegl. Radiol. 28:353, 1964.

Interpretation, pitfalls, and mistakes

46. Ashmore, J. D., Kane, J. J., Pettit, H. S., and Mayo, H. W., Jr.: Experimental evaluation of operative cholangiography in relation to calculus size, Surgery 40:191, 1956.

47. Beneventano, T. C., and Schein, C. J.: Pseudocalculus sign seen in cholangiography, Arch. Surg. 98:731, 1969.

48. Custer, M. D., Jr., and Clore, J. N., Jr.: Source of error in operative cholangiography, Arch. Surg. 100:664, 1970.

49. Elsey, E. C., and Jacobs, D. L.: Floating gallbladder stones, Amer. J. Roentgen. 65:73, 1951.

50. Frates, R. E.: Incompetence of the sphincter of Oddi in the newborn, Radiology 85:875, 1965.

51. Ginzburg, L., Gefen, A., and Friedman, I. H.: Pseudo-obstruction after choledochotomy, Ann. Surg. 166:83, 1967.

52. Perlin, E., Kirchner, P., Johnson, F. C., and Brackett, J. W., Jr.: The air cholangiogram as an unusual sequela to thoracocentesis, J.A.M.A. 210:2280, 1969.

53. Raknerud, N.: Gas in the biliary ducts, T. Norsk. Laegeforen. 89:1024, 1969.

54. Schulenburg, C. A.: Operative cholangiography, London, 1966, Butterworth & Co., Ltd.

55. Sedlack, R. E., Hodgson, J. R., Butt, H. R., Stobie,

G. H., and Judd, E. S.: Gas in the biliary tract, Gastroenterology 41:551, 1961.

56. Senter, K. L., and Berne, C. J.: Significance of non-passage of radiopaque media through the ampulla of Vater during operative cholangiography, Amer. J. Surg. 112:7, 1966.

57. Staple, T. W., and McAlister, W. H.: In vitro and in vivo visualization of biliary calculi, Amer. J. Roentgen. 94:495, 1965.

58. Wolfel, D. A., and Brogdon, B. G.: Intrahepatic air—a sign of trauma, Radiology 91:952, 1968.

Anatomic variations

59. Braasch, J. W., and McCann, J. C., Jr.: Choledochoduodenal junction size, Surgery 62:258, 1967.

60. Costopoulos, L. B., and Miller, J. D.: Insertion of the common bile duct and pancreatic duct into duodenal diverticula, Radiology 89:256, 1967.

61. Culver, G. J., and Pirson, H. S.: The roentgenographic findings in 3 cases of termination of the common bile duct in duodenal diverticula, Amer. J. Roentgen. 96:370, 1966.

62. Daniels, B. T., McGlone, F. B., and Shuey, H. E.: Extrahepatic bile duct motility, Amer. J. Gastroent. 48:198, 1967.

63. Edmunds, R., Katz, S., Garciano, V., and Finby, N.: The common duct after cholecystectomy, Arch. Surg. 103:79, 1971.

64. Engelholm, L., Mainguet, P., Thys, O., and others: Die intraduodenal Choledochocele, Fortschr. Roentgenstr. 108:403, 1968.

65. Guyer, P. B., and McLoughlin, M.: Congenital double gallbladder, Brit. J. Radiol. 40:214, 1967.

66. Hayes, M. A.: Biliary duct anomalies: unexpected high rate, J.A.M.A. 197:30, 1966.

67. Hughes, J., LoCurcio, S. B., Edmunds, R., and Finby, N.: The common duct after cholecystectomy: initial report of a ten-year-study, J.A.M.A. 197:89, 1966.

68. Mahour, G. H., Wakim, K. G., and Ferris, D. O.: Common bile duct in man: its diameter and circumference, Ann. Surg. 165:415, 1967.

69. Mahour, G. H., Wakim, K. G., Ferris, D. O., and Soule, E. H.: Common bile duct after cholecystectomy: comparison of common bile duct in patients who have intact biliary system with that in patients who have undergone cholecystectomy, Ann. Surg. 166:964, 1967.

70. Mahour, G. H., Wakim, K. G., Soule, E. H., and Ferris, D. O.: Structure of the common bile duct in man: presence or absence of smooth muscle, Ann. Surg. 166:91, 1967.

71. McSherry, C. K., and Glenn, F.: Biliary tract obstruction and duodenal diverticula, Surg. Gynec. Obstet. 130:829, 1970.

72. Palmisano, D. J.: Double gallbladder, Amer. J. Surg. 118:463, 1969.

73. Perrin, R. W.: Communicating enterogenous cyst of duodenum receiving the termination of the common bile duct demonstrated by intravenous cholangiography, Radiology 93:675, 1969.

74. Ross, R. J., and Sachs, M. D.: Triplication of the gallbladder, Amer. J. Roentgen. 104:656, 1968.

75. Schulenburg, C. A.: Anomalies of the biliary tract as demonstrated by operative cholangiography, Med. Proc. 16:351, 1970.

76. Schwartz, A., and Birnbaum, D.: Roentgenologic study of the topography of the choledocho-duodenal junction, Amer. J. Roentgen. 87:772, 1962.

77. Shehadi, W. H.: Clinical radiology of the biliary tract, New York, 1963, McGraw-Hill Book Co.

78. Simendinger, E. A., Krutky, T. A., and Reodica, R. E.: Double gallbladder with double cholelithiasis, J.A.M.A. 215:1823, 1971.

79. Willcox, G. L., and Costopoulos, L. B.: Entry of common duct and pancreatic duct into duodenal diverticulum, Arch. Surg. 98:447, 1969.

Routine vs. selective primary operative cholangiography

80. Acosta, J. M., Fotheringham, W. T., Ruiz, L. O., and Nardi, G. L.: Operative cholangiography, Arch. Surg. 99:29, 1969.

81. Acosta, J. M., Civantos, F., Nardi, G. L., and Castleman, B.: Fibrosis of the papilla of Vater, Surg. Gynec. Obstet. 124:787, 1967.

82. Alavi, S. M., and Keats, T. E.: Operative cholangiography in diagnosis of intrahepatic abscess: presentation of a case, J. Canad. Ass. Radiol. 20:253, 1969.

83. Allen, K. L.: Routine operative cholangiography, Amer. J. Surg. 118:573, 1969.

84. Andersson, A., Edström, C., Saltzman, G. F., and Schampi, B.: Concretions in the pancreatic duct diagnosed by cholangiography, Acta Radiol. 8:183, 1969.

85. Bardenheier, J. A., Kaminski, D. L., Willman, V. L., and Hanlon, C. R.: Ten-year experience with direct cholangiography, Amer. J. Surg. 118:900, 1969.

86. Bardenheier, J. A., Kaminski, D. L., and Willman, V. L.: Pancreatitis after biliary tract surgery, Amer. J. Surg. 116:773, 1968.

87. Beneventano, T. C., and Schein, C. J.: Pyloric sphincter incompetence in man, Gastroenterology 59:518, 1970.

88. Beneventano, T. C., Jacobson, H. G., Hurwitt, E. S., and Schein, C. J.: Cine-cholangiomanometry: physiologic observations, Amer. J. Roentgen. 100:673, 1967.

89. Best, R. B.: Incidence of liver stones associated with cholelithiasis and its clinical significance, Surg. Gynec. Obstet. 78:425, 1944.

90. Bocchi, G.: Obstruction of the common bile duct by worms, revealed radiologically (by peroperative cholangiography), Quad. Radiol. 28:437, 1963.

91. Burnett, W. E.: Jolly, and others: Operative cholangiography, Ann. Surg. 168:551, 1968.

92. Clemett, A. R.: Carcinoma of the major bile ducts, Radiology 84:894, 1965.

93. Cobo, A., Hall, R. C., Torres, E., and Cuello, C. J.: Intrahepatic calculi, Arch. Surg. 89:936, 1964.

94. Cutler, B., and Donaldson, G. A.: Primary sclerosing cholangitis and obliterative cholangitis, Amer. J. Surg. 117:502, 1969.

95. Edmunds, R., Katz, S., Garciano, V., and Finby,

N.: The common duct after cholecystectomy, Arch. Surg. **103**:79, 1971.

96. Edmunds, M. C., Jr., Emmett, J. M., and Clark, W. D.: Ten-year experience with operative cholangiography, Amer. Surg. **26**:613, 1960.

97. Edmunds, R., and Hughes, J. H.: Re-exploration of common bile duct, Arch. Surg. **90**:876, 1965.

98. Ferguson, H. L., and Sampline, J. E.: Operative needle cholangiography: a clinical evaluation, Amer. Surg. **35**:476, 1969.

99. Ferguson, W. H., and Estes, J. T.: Value of routine operative cholangiograms, Amer. J. Gastroent. **48**:311, 1967.

100. Ferris, D. O., and Sterling, W. A.: Surgery of the biliary tract, Surg. Clin. N. Amer. **47**:861, 1967.

101. Glenn, F., and Whitsell, J. C., II.: Primary sclerosing cholangitis, Surg. Gynec. Obstet. **123**:1037, 1966.

102. Goldman, L. I., Weinberger, M., DeLaurentis, D. A., and Burnett, W. E.: Operative cholecysto-cholangiography, Surg. Gynec. Obstet. **128**:279, 1969.

103. Griffin, T. F., and Wild, A. A.: The case for pre-operative cholangiography, Brit. J. Surg. **54**:609, 1967.

104. Herman, R. E., and Hoerr, S. O.: The value of the routine use of operative cholangiography, Surg. Gynec. Obstet. **121**:1015, 1965.

105. Hess, W.: Surgery of the biliary passages and the pancreas, Princeton, 1965, D. Van Nostrand Co., Inc.

106. Hicken, N. F., and McAllister, A. J.: Operative cholangiography as an aid in reducing the incidence of "overlooked" common bile duct stones, Surgery **55**:753, 1964.

107. Hight, D., Lingley, J. R., and Hurtibise, F.: An evaluation of operative cholangiography as a guide to common duct exploration, Ann. Surg. **150**:1086, 1959.

108. Isaacs, J. P., and Daves, M. L.: Technique and evaluation of operative cholangiography, Surg. Gynec. Obstet. **111**:102, 1960.

109. Jolly, P. C., Baker, J. W., Schmidt, H. M., and others: Operative cholangiography, Ann. Surg. **168**:551, 1968.

110. Jolly, P. C., Baker, J. W., Walker, J. H., and Schmidt, H. M.: Operative cholangiography, Northwest Med. **68**:639, 1969.

111. Kourias, B., and Stucke, K.: Atlas der per- und post-operativen Cholangiographie, Stuttgart, 1967, Georg Thieme Verlag.

112. Krieger, J., Seaman, W. B., and Porter, M. R.: The roentgenologic appearance of sclerosing cholangitis, Radiology **95**:369, 1970.

113. Legge, D. A., and Carlson, H. C.: Cholangiographic appearance of primary carcinoma of the bile ducts, Radiology **102**:259, 1972.

114. Letton, A. H., and Wilson, J. P.: Routine cholangiography during biliary tract operation, Ann. Surg. **163**:937, 1966.

115. Madden, J. C.: Primary and secondary common duct stones, Surg. Gynec. Obstet. **130**:1091, 1970.

116. Manier, J. W.: A total bile cast of the biliary tree, Gastroenterology **44**:682, 1963.

117. Mujahed, Z., Glenn, F., and Evans, J.: Communicating cavernous ectasia of the intrahepatic ducts (Caroli's disease), Amer. J. Roentgen. **113**:21, 1971.

118. Nienhuis, L. I.: Routine operative cholangiography, Ann. Surg. **154** (Supp.):192, 1961.

119. Parent, M., and Peloquin, A.: Peroperative cholangiography, Canad. J. Surg. **6**:129, 1963.

120. Pyrtek, L. J., and Bartus, S. H.: Critical evaluation of routine and selective operating room cholangiography, Amer. J. Surg. **103**:761, 1962.

121. Sandblom, P.: In Jolly, and others: Operative cholangiography, Ann. Surg. **168**:55, 1968.

122. Schulenburg, C. A.: Postoperative cholangiography, London, 1966, Butterworth & Co., Ltd.

123. Shehadi, W. H.: Clinical radiology of the biliary tract, New York, 1963, McGraw-Hill Book Co.

124. Shore, J. M.: The prevention of residual biliary calculi, Calif. Med. **114**:1, 1971.

125. Underberg, J. T.: Operative cholangiography, Harper Hosp. Bull. **22**:251, 1964.

126. Walters, W., Nixon, J. W. Jr., and Hodgins, T. E.: Strictures of the common duct: five to 25-year follow up of 217 operations, Ann. Surg. **149**:781, 1959.

127. Warren, K. W.: Pitfalls of gallbladder surgery, Hosp. Pract. **2**:29, 1967.

128. Whitaker, P. H., Parkinson, E. G., and Hughes, J. H.: Television fluoroscopy for operative cholangiography: an analysis of 150 cases, Clin. Radiol. **19**:368, 1968.

129. Wilkinson, L. H., Simms, A. G., and Floyd, V. T.: Operative cholangiography, Arch. Surg. **92**:677, 1966.

130. Wise, R. E.: Cholangiography and duct pancreatography in the diagnosis of pancreatic disease, Seminars Roentgen. **3**:288, 1968.

Complications

131. Babbitt, D. P., and Thatcher, D. S.: Radiographic findings in postoperative bile collections, Radiology **84**:471, 1965.

132. Boles, E. T.: Postop pancreatitis, Arch. Surg. **73**:710, 1956.

133. Hershey, J. E., and Hillman, F. J.: Fatal pancreatic necrosis following choledochotomy and cholangiography, Arch. Surg. **71**:885, 1955.

134. Hultborn, A., Jacobsson, B., and Rosengren, B.: Cholangio-venous reflux: a clinical and experimental study, Acta Chir. Scand. **123**:111-124, 1962.

135. Rosato, E. F., Berkowitz, H. D., and Roberts, B.: Bile ascites, Surg. Gynec. Obstet. **130**:494, 1970.

136. Tabrisky, J., and Pollack, E. L.: The aberrant division bile duct, Radiology **99**:537, 1971.

137. Weston, W. J.: Post-operative bile peritonitis: its radiological diagnosis, Aust. Radiol. **11**:34, 1967.

Post-cholecystectomy syndrome

138. Bodvall, B., and Overgaard, B.: Cystic duct remnant after cholecystostomy, Ann. Surg. **163**:382, 1966.

139. Dreiling, D. A.: The post-cholecystectomy syndrome, Amer. J. Dig. Dis. **7**:603, 1962.

140. Edmunds, R., Rucker, C., and Finby, N.: Intravenous cholangiography, Arch. Surg. **90**:73, 1965.

141. Portorak, J. L.: An attempt to evaluate the function of the sphincter of Oddi after sphincterotomy, Pol. Tyg. Lek. **21**:137, 1966.

142. Schwarz, E.: Die intramural cystic duct remnant, Amer J. Roentgen. **86**:930, 1961.

143. Viost, J. C.: Cystic duct remnants, Thesis, Graduate School, University of Minnesota, 1957.

Biliary fistulas

144. Colver, H. D.: Perforation of the biliary tract due to gallstones in infancy: an established clinical entity, Ann. Surg. **160**:226, 1964.

145. Dowse, J. L.: Cholecysto-duodenocolic fistulae due to gallstones, Brit. J. Surg. **50**:776, 1963.

146. Ferguson, T. B., and Burford, T. H.: Pleurobiliary and bronchobiliary fistulas, Arch. Surg. **95**:380, 1967.

147. Gudas, P. P., Haberman, G. C., and Belcher, H. V.: Cholecystocolonic fistula, Arch. Surg. **95**:228, 1967.

148. Hutchin, P., Harrison, T. S., and Halasz, N. A.: Postoperative cholecystocolic fistula, Ann. Surg. **157**:587, 1963.

149. Hyde, G. A., Jr.: Spontaneous perforation of bile ducts in early infancy, Pediatrics **35**:453, 1965.

150. Op den Orth, J. O.: A radiologically demonstrated fistula between the common bile duct and the right renal pelvis, Radiol. Clin. Biol. **38**:402, 1969.

151. Piedad, O. H., and Well, P. B.: Spontaneous internal biliary fistula: obstructive and nonobstructive types: 20-year review of 55 cases, Ann. Surg. **175**:75, 1972.

152. Pitman, R. G., and Davies, A.: The clinical and radiological features of spontaneous internal biliary fistulae, Brit. J. Surg. **50**:414, 1963.

153. Rominger, C. J., and Canino, C. W.: Internal biliary tract fistulae, Amer. J. Roentgen. **90**:835, 1963.

154. Sewell, J. A.: Avulsion of left hepatic duct, Ann. Surg. **165**:628, 1967.

155. Shehadi, W. H.: Roentgen observation in cases of fistulae of the biliary tract, J.A.M.A. **174**:2204, 1960.

156. Shocket, E., Evans, J., and Jonas, S.: Cholecysto-duodeno-colic fistula with gallstone ileus, Arch. Surg. **101**:523, 1970.

Special techniques and procedures

157. Best, R. R.: Choledochostomy—advantages of a modified T-tube, Surg. Gynec. Obstet. **90**:297, 1950.

158. Cotton, P. B., Blumgart, L. H., Davies, G. T., Pierce, J. W., Salmon, P. R., Burwood, R. J., Lawrie, B. W., and Read, A. E.: Cannulation of papilla of Vater via fiber-duodenoscope, Lancet **1**:53, 1972.

159. Margulis, A. R., Newton, T. H., and Najarian, J. S.: Removal of plug from T-tube by fluoroscopically controlled catheter: report of a case, Amer. J. Roentgen. **93**:975, 1965.

160. Oi, I., Takemoto, T., and Nakayama, K.: "Fiber-duodenoscopy"—early diagnosis of cancer of the papilla of Vater, Surgery **67**:561, 1970.

161. Rabinov, K. R., and Simon, M.: Peroral cannulation of the ampulla of Vater for direct cholangiography and pancreatography, Radiology **85**:693, 1965.

162. Short, W. F., Howard, J. M., and Diven, W. F.: Trans-T-tube catheterization, Arch. Surg. **102**:136, 1971.

163. Weiner, M., and Hanafee, W. N.: A review of transjugular cholangiography, Radiol. Clin. N. Amer. **8**:53, 1970.

Expulsion and extraction of retained biliary duct stones

164. Anderson, R. P., Leand, P. M., and Zuidema, G. D.: Balloon-tipped catheter in biliary surgery, Amer. J. Surg. **117**:55, 1969.

165. Bean, W. J., Smith, S. L., and Mahorner, H. R.: Equipment for non-operative removal of biliary tract stones, Radiology **107**:452, 1973.

166. Burhenne, H. J.: Extraktion von Residualsteinen der Gallenwege ohne Reoperation, Fortschr. Rontgenstr. **117**:62, 1972.

167. Burhenne, H. J.: Non-operative retained biliary tract stone extraction—a new roentgenologic technique, Amer. J. Roentgen. **117**:388, 1973.

168. Coyle, M. J., and Thompson, W. M.: Non-surgical removal of retained common duct stones, Alaska Med. **13**:89, 1971.

169. Danzinger, R. G., Hofmann, A. F., Schoenfield, L. J., and others: Dissolution of cholesterol gallstones by Chenodeoxycholic acid, New Eng. J. Med. **286**:1, 1972.

170. Fennessy, J. J., and You, K. D.: A method for the expulsion of stones retained in the common bile duct, Amer. J. Roentgen. **110**:256, 1970.

171. Henzel, J. H., Blessing, W. D., and DeWeese, M. S.: Intrahepatic biliary disruption, Arch. Surg. **102**:218, 1971.

172. Henzel, J. H., and DeWeese, M. S.: Common duct exploration with and without balloon-tipped biliary catheters, Arch. Surg. **103**:199, 1971.

173. Magarey, C. J.: Non-surgical removal of retained biliary calculi, Lancet **1**:7708, 1971.

174. Mazzariello, R.: Removal of residual biliary tract calculi without reoperation, Surgery **67**:566, 1970.

175. Wendth, A. J., Jr., Lieberman, R. C., and Alpert, M.: Non-surgical removal of a retained common bile duct calculus, Radiology **103**:207, 1972.

Part IX

Special procedures

Transhepatic cholangiography | 52

John A. Evans

The diagnostic differentiation between extrahepatic, or obstructive, jaundice and intrahepatic, or parenchymal, jaundice is frequently difficult despite an abundance of increasingly sophisticated laboratory procedures. Examination of the stomach and duodenum by means of the barium meal has been the standard examination in the roentgenologic evaluation of the jaundiced patient. Although simplicity and safety are the cardinal attributes of this examination, it all too often fails to provide critical diagnostic information as to the cause of the jaundice.

Obstructive lesions of the biliary system are difficult problems for the surgeon. Patients are frequently in the older age group and are generally poor surgical risks. Percutaneous transhepatic cholangiography, in my experience, has proved to be more useful in the diagnosis of lesions of extrahepatic obstruction than any of the other commonly employed methods of diagnosis. It provides the opportunity of visualizing the biliary system in the jaundiced patient, thereby permitting the differentiation between obstructive and nonobstructive jaundice. Precise information can be secured with respect to the patency, course, and appearance of the extrahepatic duct system. On the basis of the cholangiogram, a definitive diagnosis and a therapeutic judgment can be made without resort to exploratory surgery. Preoperative percutaneous cholangiograms have proved to be of far greater value than cholangiograms obtained at operation. The preoperative demonstration of an obstructive lesion of the extrahepatic duct system affords the surgeon the opportunity to formulate a specific plan of treatment and to proceed directly to his objective. The anatomic information gained by this method in problem patients with jaundice has far outweighed the risks inherent in the examination. My experience has shown percutaneous transhepatic cholangiography to be a safe procedure when it is performed under the direct visual control of television fluoroscopy and when it is followed on the same day by surgery except when

the latter is contraindicated by the cholangiographic findings.

HISTORICAL REVIEW

The history of percutaneous cholangiography predates that of oral or intravenous methods. The earliest attempt at opacifying the biliary tree occurred in 1921 when Burkhardt and Muller reported on the percutaneous injection of the gallbladder in three patients.[3] They made their injection through the eighth intercostal space, 1 cm. anterior to the midaxillary line in a horizontal direction. The needle traversed the liver substance to enter the extraperitoneal side of the gallbladder. Burkhardt and Muller were cognizant of the dangers of bile leakage if the peritoneal surface of the gallbladder was punctured. The authors nonetheless felt that with proper care and experience the technique might become a useful diagnostic tool. Interest in this method of visualizing the gallbladder and bile ducts was soon lost because of the advent of oral cholecystography.

The first report of percutaneous transhepatic cholangiography occurred in 1937 when Huard and Do-Xuan-Hop in Indo China injected iodized oil into the hepatic bile ducts in two patients with liver abscess.[12] In 1942 Lee and Royer, Solari, and Lottero-Lanari used the peritoneoscope to puncture and inject the gallbladder.[16,20] In 1952 Carter and Saypol and Leger, Zara, and Arvay stimulated further interest in the subject with their reports on the technique of transabdominal cholangiography.[4,17] Kidd in 1956 generated additional enthusiasm by reporting its successful use in a small series of patients.[15] The past 10 years has seen a large number of papers on percutaneous cholangiography published. Many of these represent reports of single cases or experience with small numbers of patients. There are, however, several reports that deal with significant numbers of patients.* Of the contemporary writers, Wiechel provides one of the most comprehensive discussions of the technique and applications of percutaneous cholangiography.[22]

PROCEDURE AND EQUIPMENT
Preparation of the patient

Blood clotting should be normal or be brought to the optimal level before the procedure is undertaken. The patient is required to fast for 8 hours prior to the examination. Selection of premedication and explanation of the objective of the procedure are of considerable importance, since apprehension and an easily reactive patient may seriously interfere with the successful outcome of the procedure. The cholangiogram is scheduled to be followed by laparotomy unless normal biliary passages are found or unless other specific findings preclude surgical exploration.

I believe that local anesthesia with sufficient premedication is to be preferred to general anesthesia. Ordinarily 0.13 gm. of phenobarbital and 100 mg. of meperidine (Demerol) is given intramuscularly 1 hour before the examination. In the geriatric patient it may be advisable to substitute chloral hydrate for the phenobarbital and meperidine. The skin over the lower chest and upper abdomen on the right side is suitably prepared and draped, and the area to be in-

jected is infiltrated with 1% procaine hydrochloride.

Puncture site and technique

Various puncture sites have been recommended. Most authors prefer introducing the needle through the anterior abdominal wall below the right costal arch and to the right of the ensiform process. When this approach is used there is the risk that the extrahepatic duct system may be punctured accidentally. In order to avoid such a complication lateral and dorsal puncture sites have been recommended. Prioton favored a dorsal puncture site because of the direct attachment of the liver to the posterior abdominal wall.[18] Because the liver in this area is without peritoneal covering, the possibility of leakage of bile or blood into the abdominal cavity is eliminated. Housset and Vantsis and Wiechel advocate a lateral intercostal approach, claiming that this site prevents accidental puncture of the gallbladder or extrahepatic ducts.[11,22] It is my opinion that the simplest, easiest, and most effective manner of performing percutaneous transhepatic cholangiography is by the anterial abdominal route.

I, like Kidd, introduce the needle approximately two fingerbreadths below the right costal arch in the mammary line.[15] The needle is introduced at an angle of about 45 degrees to the anterior abdominal wall. Its course is directed cranially and toward the hilus of the liver near the confluence of the major bile ducts (Fig. 52-1). To ensure proper placement well into the liver substance, practically the entire length of the needle is inserted. When the liver is large and easily palpable it is a simple matter to introduce the needle. The introduction and placement of the needle are facilitated by the use of the image intensifying fluoroscope and a television monitor. This permits accurate placement, particularly in those patients whose livers are small and cannot be palpated.

With needle in optimum position the stylet is removed and the needle is attached to a short length of polyethylene tubing with a syringe. In cases of obstructive jaundice with dilated ducts, bile is aspirated readily and almost immediately. The greater the obstruction and the dilatation of the biliary tree, the easier it is to enter a bile radicle. Housset and Vantsis found that in obstructive jaundice the liver

---

*See references 1, 2, 7, 10, 14, 21, and 23.

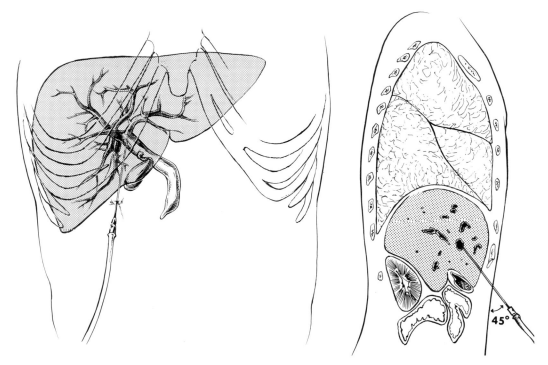

Fig. 52-1. Schematic representation of puncture site and needle placement in liver. (From Glenn, F., and others: Ann. Surg. **156**:451, 1962.)

is practically bloodless and that the arterial pressure is very low but increases as bile is withdrawn.[11] They believe that the distended bile ducts compress the other vessels in the liver and thereby make puncture of these vessels less likely. Samples of bile may be taken for culture or for microscopic or cytologic studies.

After as much bile as possible has been aspirated, the contrast agent (75% diatrizoate sodium or another iodine-containing water-soluble medium of similar contrast) is slowly injected. The filling of the bile ducts is observed on the screen of the television monitor, and once complete filling is obtained the needle is withdrawn and appropriate roentgenographs are obtained.

Hanafee and Weiner described an alternate method of reaching the biliary system.[10] They passed a catheter percutaneously via the right internal jugular vein, right atrium, and inferior vena cava. A needle was inserted through the catheter for the puncture of the biliary system inside the liver. They performed the procedure on eleven patients (Fig. 52-2).

In situations where dilated bile ducts are not immediately encountered, the position of the needle is checked by the injection of a small amount (1 to 2 ml.) of the contrast agent. It may be necessary to probe the liver under constant television monitoring, with repeated changes in position of the needle and small injections of contrast medium before a bile duct is identified. In the process of probing it is common to see transient filling of veins and lymphatics. Residual puddles of contrast medium represent small parenchymal collections. A successful examination occurs when a segment of the intrahepatic duct system becomes visible and remains so with slow filling of its companion biliary radicles.

It should be stated that failure to obtain a satisfactory cholangiogram in a jaundiced patient has a certain inferential value in that it reduces the probability of extrahepatic obstruction. However, it does not exclude such obstruction and should not of itself preclude the need for surgical exploration.

Instruments

Various types of needles and cannulas have been used to make the puncture. Fuentes, Bertoni, and Polero used a needle with multiple side perforations in its distal 6 cm. to improve

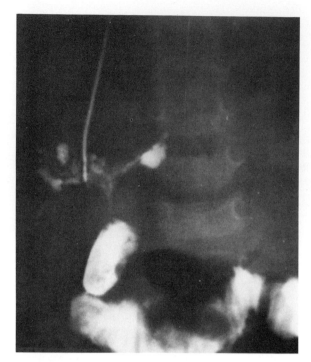

Fig. 52-2. The intrahepatic and extrahepatic bile ducts are demonstrated in this cholangiogram of a 2-year-old girl with congenital cystic hyperplasia of the bile ducts. The cholangiogram is obtained by inserting a catheter and a needle into the inferior vena cava through the jugular vein. An intrahepatic bile duct is punctured and contrast agent is injected. (Courtesy Dr. A. R. Margulis.)

the chances of entering a bile duct within the liver.[7] I have used a similar needle but found that it has no advantage over a standard 6- or 7-inch, 19- or 20-gauge needle of the type used to perform spinal punctures.

Some investigators routinely use a polyethylene catheter snugly fitted over the needle or cannula.[1,13,19,22] The introduction of this requires a small incision in the abdominal wall. Once the proper penetration into the liver has been effected, the needle is removed. The catheter is then withdrawn along the needle tract. If a bile duct is not found, another penetration with the needle is necessary. The reason for substituting a flexible catheter for the rigid needle is to minimize damage to the liver as a consequence of breathing movements. There seems to be no real evidence that the use of the catheter confers greater immunity from complications. I use the catheter only when it is deemed desirable to institute biliary decompression for

a period of time prior to definitive surgical intervention. In particular this applies to patients with longstanding jaundice in whom the cholangiogram reveals a neoplastic lesion that will require an extensive surgical procedure for its removal. It is my custom first to secure the cholangiogram by using a 7-inch, 19- or 20-gauge needle attached to a short length of polyethylene tubing to which a stopcock and syringe are fitted (Fig. 52-3).

Roentgenography

The examination is done in the radiology department, with the patient in the supine position on the fluoroscopy table. After the 7-inch, 19- or 20-gauge needle has been introduced as previously described and has successfully entered a bile duct, spot films of the cholangiogram are obtained in supine and both oblique projections. The fluoroscopy table is then raised, and spot films of the distal common duct at the level of the obstruction are obtained with the patient in the erect or semierect position. After the spot film roentgenography has been completed the fluoroscopy table is returned to the horizontal position, and conventional overhead roentgenographs with a Potter-Bucky diaphragm are obtained with a patient in the supine and oblique positions. Delayed films and films in the prone projection are taken if indicated. The roentgenologic technical factors are as follows: 16:1 grid ratio; 300 ma; 0.5 second exposure; 76 kvp for a patient 20 cm. thick.

INDICATIONS

Percutaneous cholangiography is not to be considered a substitute for the more conventional roentgenologic methods of visualizing the biliary system. It does, however, offer an alternate means of investigation in those special circumstances in which the conventional examinations fail. The primary indications for this examination are as follows:

1. To differentiate between obstructive and nonobstructive jaundice
2. To diagnose the presence, number, and location of common duct stones
3. To demonstrate intrinsic tumors of the bile ducts
4. To determine the location and character of extrinsic tumors obstructing the common duct

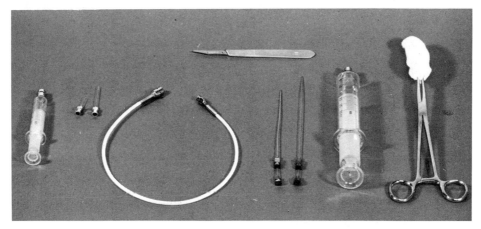

Fig. 52-3. Instrument tray for percutaneous cholangiography.

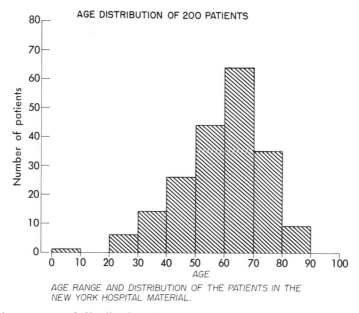

AGE DISTRIBUTION OF 200 PATIENTS

AGE RANGE AND DISTRIBUTION OF THE PATIENTS IN THE
NEW YORK HOSPITAL MATERIAL.

Fig. 52-4. Age range and distribution of 200 patients in the New York Hospital material.

5. To define the site and type of obstruction in cases of bile duct injury

THE NEW YORK HOSPITAL MATERIAL

The New York Hospital material comprises 200 patients examined by percutaneous transhepatic cholangiography because of persistent or transient jaundice thought to be secondary to biliary obstruction. In this group there were one hundred and nineteen males and eighty-one females. The age range extended from the neonatal period to the ninth decade, with the greatest number of patients in the seventh decade.

The age range and distribution is given in Fig. 52-4). A tabulation of all cases grouped by diagnostic categories is given in Table 52-1. The examination was considered successful in 71% of the cases. This is slightly lower than has been reported in some series.[6,22] The ratio of successful to unsuccessful examinations has remained essentially unchanged since my colleagues and I initially reported our experience with this technique.[5]

On further analysis of the successful cases it is apparent that the presence of a dilated biliary duct system increases the chances of a successful examination. The rate of success in patients

Table 52-1. Diseases examined by percutaneous transhepatic cholangiography

Diagnoses	Total	Successful (75%)	Unsuccessful (25%)
Calculus disease	32	18	14
Carcinoma of pancreas	67	58	9
Metastases to liver	20	15	5
Carcinoma of ampulla of Vater	9	9	0
Carcinoma of bile duct	20	19	1
Hepatitis	8	4	4
Carcinoma of gallbladder	10	6	4
Chronic pancreatitis	2	1	1
Leukemic infiltration of liver	1	0	1
Cirrhosis of liver	4	0	4
Common duct injury	20	16	4
Sclerosing cholangitis	3	2	1
Metastases to pancreas from stomach	1	1	0
Biliary atresia in a newborn	1	0	1
Stricture of choledochojejunostomy	1	0	1
Cyst of pancreas	1	1	0
Total	200	150	50

Table 52-2. Comparative value of percutaneous cholangiogram and gastrointestinal series in carcinoma of pancreas and ampulla

	Total	Correct diagnosis by cholangiogram	Diagnoses made or suspected by GI series
Carcinoma of pancreas	54	46 (85%)	20 (37%)
Carcinoma of ampulla	8	8 (100%)	4 (50%)

with a dilated ductal system is 92%. Therefore, while the overall incidence of successful examinations for the entire series was 74%, this figure was increased to 92% if only the cases with dilated bile ducts are considered. It will be observed that about half of the patients with hepatitis had a successful cholangiogram. This is about the level of success to be expected when the ducts are not dilated and there is no diffuse liver disease.

Table 52-2 compares the diagnostic value of percutaneous cholangiography with that of the conventional barium meal. There were forty-four patients with carcinoma of the pancreas in whom it was possible to compare the information obtained by the percutaneous cholangiography with that obtained from the gastroin-testinal series. The correct diagnosis was made on the cholangiographic findings in 85% of the cases, whereas in the same group of patients the results of the gastrointestinal examination were positive or suggestive in only 37% of the cases. However, the cholangiogram had the additional diagnostic advantage of providing graphic evidence of the pathologic anatomy present even in those instances where the precise diagnosis was not made. The same diagnostic advantage of the cholangiogram over the gastrointestinal series is seen to hold for the cases of carcinoma of the ampulla.

COMPLICATIONS

The two main complications of percutaneous cholangiography are hemorrhage caused by accidental perforation of a blood vessel and bile peritonitis as a result of bile seepage into the peritoneal cavity. Accidental puncture of the gallbladder or common bile duct may occur. The use of the image intensifying fluoroscope and television monitoring makes such a complication immediately recognizable.

It is not uncommon at surgical exploration after a percutaneous cholangiography to find varying amounts of bile and blood free or localized in the peritoneal cavity. This is much more likely to occur in the cases of obstruction of the extrahepatic bile ducts where multiple puncture or probing has occurred. For this reason my policy has been to follow the cholangiogram with surgery unless the examination has demonstrated a normal, unobstructed duct system or unless it is believed that surgery is not indicated or can safely be postponed.

Table 52-3 is a compilation of 901 cases collected from the literature. The four fatalities in the series represent a mortality incidence of 0.5%. In a discussion of the hazards associated with this procedure, the mortality must be viewed in the light of operative mortality figures associated with surgery of the common bile duct. Mortality figures from the best surgical clinics in the United States relative to common bile duct exploration reveal a 3% to 10% spread, depending on the age range of the groups explored. The surgical mortality in the groups with hepatocellular disease and jaundice is even higher.[8]

In the New York Hospital series one death can be attributed directly to the percutaneous cholangiogram. This was 58-year-old woman

Table 52-3. Cases collected from the world literature

Year	Authors	Number of patients	Cholangio-gram obtained	Fatalities attributed to procedure
1937	Huard and Do-Xuan-Hop	2	2	
1952	Carter and Saypol	1	1	
1952	Leger et al.	2	2	
1953	Alvarez and Jensen	12	9	
1953	Crismer	6	6	
1953	Goni Moreno	1	1	
1953	Leger et al.	14	14	1
1953	Michelini	1	1	
1953	Nurick et al.	5	5	1
1954	Fuentes et al.	4	4	
1954	Royer et al.	6	6	
1954	Sobredo et al.	20	17	
1956	Kidd	6	6	
1956	Mandl	25	15	
1956	Remolar et al.	34	20	
1956	Royer et al.	19	15	
1957	Housset and Vantsis	9	9	
1957	Redington et al.	14	13	
1958	Felci	21	19	
1958	Wilks et al.	41	38	
1959	Barbier	4	4	
1959	Halligan et al.	10	8	
1959	Marcasoli and Cetra	1	1	
1960	Santos et al.	46	38	
1960	Atkinson et al.	21	10	
1960	Zerboni et al.	100	57	
1961	Kaplan et al.	40	30	
1961	Arner; Arner et al.	80	55	1
1962	Shaldon et al.	30	22	
1963	Flemma et al.	36	30	
1963	Wiechel	60	56	
1965	Parent et al.	30	29	
1967	The New York Hospital	150	110	
1969	The New York Hospital	200	150	1
Totals		901	693	4

deeply jaundiced secondary to carcinoma of the head of the pancreas with liver metastases. The percutaneous cholangiogram established the diagnosis, which was confirmed by exploratory surgery after the cholangiogram. At operation, it was noted that the patient was bleeding from a puncture wound in the anterior surface of the liver. A cholecystojejunostomy was performed, the puncture wound of the liver was closed, and at the conclusion of surgery no bleeding site was evident. However, she showed evidence of continued bleeding in the immediate postoperative period and died on the second postoperative day. Postmortem examination demonstrated the puncture site in the liver, which had been packed with Gelfoam. The puncture tract extended deep into the liver substance, and there was evidence of a laceration of a large liver vein along the puncture tract, with hematoma formation.

ROENTGENOGRAPHIC DIAGNOSIS

The cholangiographic appearance of stone, stricture, and carcinoma of the ampulla, common bile duct, or pancreas is often highly characteristic and frequently permits a specific diagnosis to be made (Fig. 52-5).

Normal ducts

A few patients have been shown by percutaneous cholangiography to have normal-sized, unobstructed bile ducts. In the material my col-

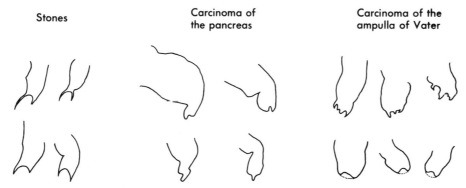

Stones   Carcinoma of the pancreas   Carcinoma of the ampulla of Vater

Fig. 52-5. The cholangiographic appearance of impacted common duct stone, carcinoma of the pancreas, and carcinoma of the ampulla. Note the difference in the type of meniscus produced by stone and that caused by carcinoma of the ampulla. Variations in the highly characteristic deformity of the distal common bile duct, seen in carcinoma of the pancreas, are also depicted. (From Evans, J. A.: Radiology 82:580, 1964.)

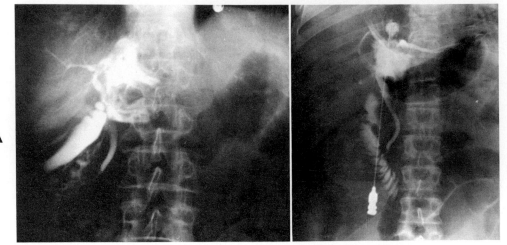

Fig. 52-6. Normal extrahepatic bile ducts. **A,** Percutaneous cholangiogram demonstrates an unobstructed extrahepatic biliary system in a patient with hepatitis. **B,** Percutaneous cholangiogram reveals patent and normal-appearing extrahepatic ducts in a jaundiced patient suspected of having cholelithiasis. The patient was dismissed from the hospital to permit the jaundice to subside. Subsequent cholecystectomy revealed cholelithiasis.

leagues and I studied there were eight patients with viral hepatitis who had percutaneous cholangiography because of the question of extrahepatic biliary obstruction. Cholangiography was successful in four patients and demonstrated normal bile ducts (Fig. 52-6, *A*). In the four patients in whom the cholangiogram was not successful there was inferential value to the negative results, in that the inability to obtain a cholangiogram made the possibility of extrahepatic obstruction less likely. In several cases this factor, together with other clinical and laboratory findings, was important in the decision not to submit the patient to exploratory laparotomy, which carries an increased risk when the patient has hepatitis.

Normal bile ducts were also demonstrated in a jaundiced patient who previously had been shown to have a nonvisualized gallbladder. The jaundice subsided and was presumably caused by a transient common duct stone. Subsequent cholecystectomy was performed for the cholelithiasis (Fig. 52-6, *B*).

Common duct stone

A stone impacted in the distal end of the common bile duct produces a deep, well-defined,

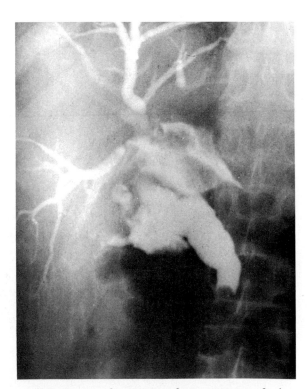

Fig. 52-7. Impacted common duct stone, producing a characteristic deep concave meniscus deformity with thin sharp margins. (From Evans, J. A.: Radiology 82:581, 1964.)

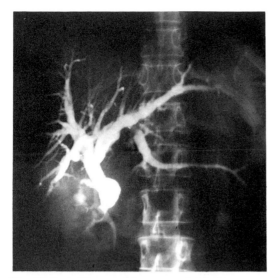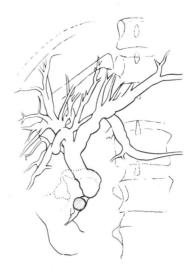

Fig. 52-8. A 54-year-old woman initially operated upon because of jaundice. The diagnosis of biliary tract malignancy was made at operation, and a palliative procedure was followed by radiation therapy. One year later she was admitted to New York Hospital for diagnostic and therapeutic evaluation. A percutaneous cholangiogram demonstrated an impacted stone in the distal common bile duct. A choledocholithotomy was performed, following which the patient made a satisfactory recovery. (From Evans, J. A.: Radiology **82:**583, 1964.)

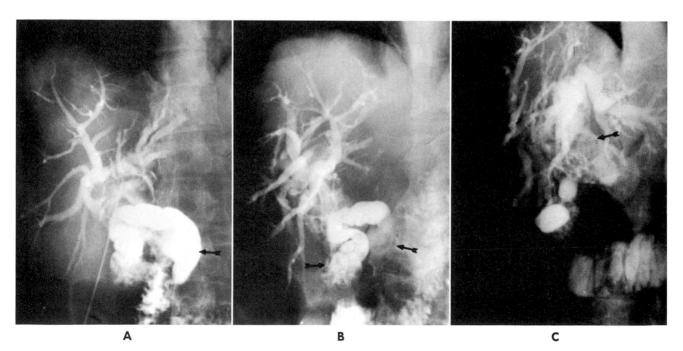

A   **B**   **C**

Fig. 52-9. A, Percutaneous cholangiogram reveals a patent but dilated common bile duct and a tortuous dilated cystic duct superimposed on the common duct. Multiple stones in the common duct are obscured by the density of the opaque medium. **B,** Delayed film taken after partial emptying shows a large stone in distal common duct (arrow) and multiple calculi in the gallbladder. **C,** Later, the common duct is seen to be packed with stones up to 2 cm. in diameter (arrow).

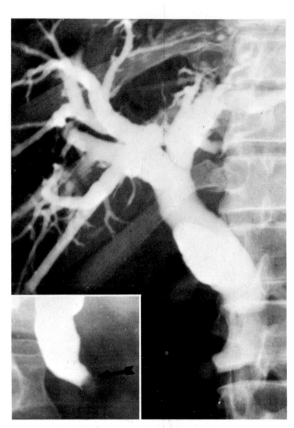

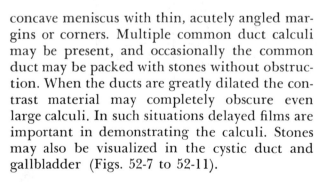

Fig. 52-10. An erect spot film accentuates the meniscus produced by a small impacted stone.

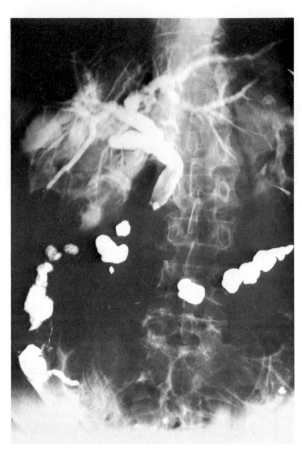

Fig. 52-11. A small stone impacted in the distal common bile duct, with sludge and debris resulting in uneven and diminished opacification.

concave meniscus with thin, acutely angled margins or corners. Multiple common duct calculi may be present, and occasionally the common duct may be packed with stones without obstruction. When the ducts are greatly dilated the contrast material may completely obscure even large calculi. In such situations delayed films are important in demonstrating the calculi. Stones may also be visualized in the cystic duct and gallbladder (Figs. 52-7 to 52-11).

Neoplasms
Carcinoma of the pancreas

The majority of patients with cancer of the pancreas seek medical aid because of the presence of clinical jaundice. Roentgenologic diagnosis of carcinoma of the pancreas has depended primarily on the barium meal examination of the duodenal loop. The level of accuracy

achieved by this method, whether conventional roentgenography or cineradiography is employed, has left something to be desired. Percutaneous cholangiography permits visualization of the biliary system of the jaundiced patient. It thus provides the means for making the diagnosis prior to surgery.

Carcinoma of the head of the pancreas is usually associated with marked dilatation of the entire biliary duct system. The large, dilated common duct may become redundant and angulated. Several cholangiographic patterns may be associated with this disease. The most common is a tapered nipple or rat-tail–like configuration of the distal obstructed margin. This cholangiographic sign, while not in itself specific for the diagnosis, is nevertheless highly characteristic, and its presence should suggest this diagnosis (Fig. 52-12). Sometimes in place of a short

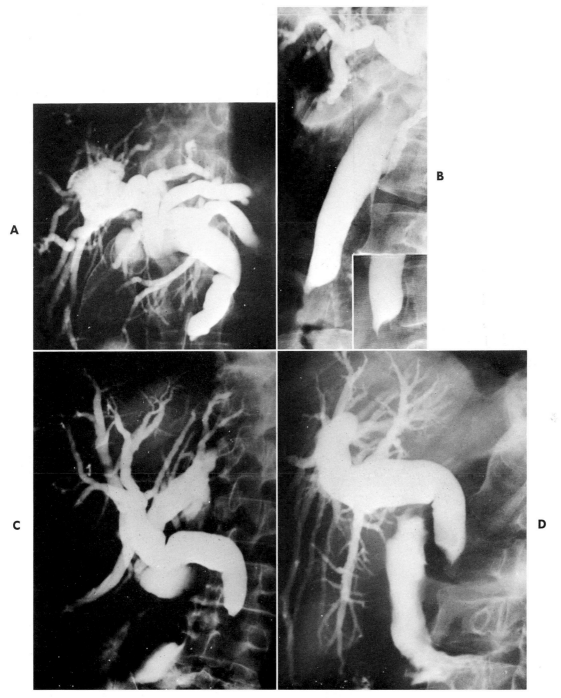

Fig. 52-12. Roentgenographic findings of carcinoma of the pancreas in four patients examined by percutaneous cholangiography. **A,** Carcinoma of the head of the pancreas. Percutaneous cholangiogram demonstrates the characteristic nipple-like deformity of the distal obstructed end of the common duct. This sign, when present, has been highly accurate for the diagnosis. **B,** Percutaneous cholangiogram illustrating obstruction of the common duct secondary to carcinoma of the pancreas. Rat-tail–like deformity of the distal margin is accentuated by an erect spot film (inset). **C,** A 68-year-old man with recent history of anorexia, fatigue, and jaundice. The differential diagnosis rested between a typical hepatitis or extrahepatic biliary obstruction. The percutaneous cholangiogram shows a stubby, nipple-like deformity of the distal common duct. The diagnosis of carcinoma of the head of the pancreas was established by operation and pathologic examination. **D,** Tapered, funnel-like deformity of the distal common duct associated with carcinoma of the head of the pancreas. Obstruction was incomplete, as evidenced by contrast medium in the duodenal loop.

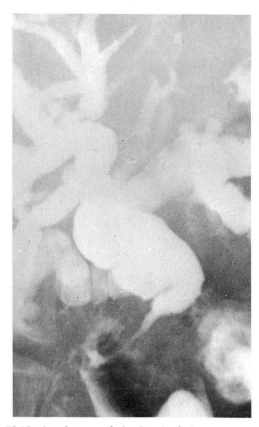

Fig. 52-13. Carcinoma of the head of the pancreas, producing a long stenotic segment of the distal common bile duct.

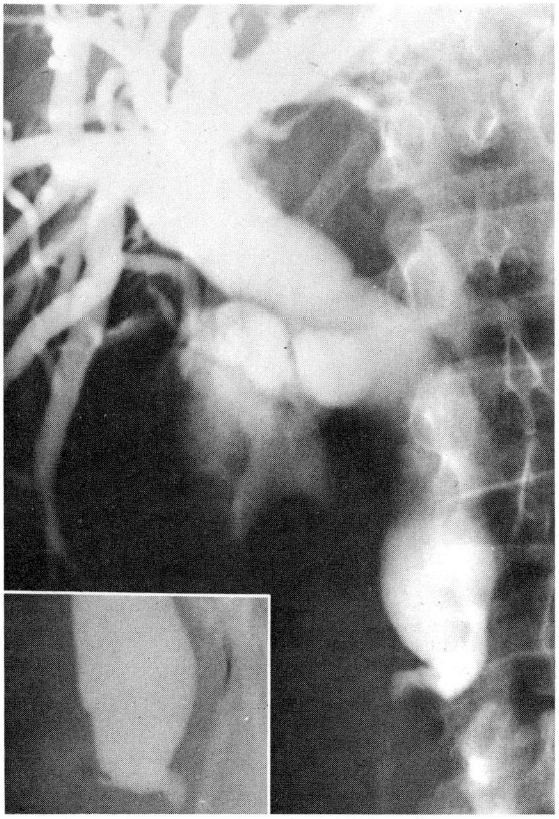

Fig. 52-14. Carcinoma of the ampulla of Vater with invasion of the pancreas, producing a rat-tail–like deformity comparable to that associated with pancreatic neoplasm.

nipple-like deformity of the distal margin there is a long, tapered segment, giving the impression that this portion of the duct is enveloped by a mass (Fig. 52-13). At times the cholangiogram does not permit differentiation of carcinoma of the pancreas from carcinoma of the papilla or from metastatic invasion of the common duct (Fig. 52-14). Occasionally it may be desirable to institute biliary decompression for a short period of time prior to definitive surgery. In particular this applies to patients with long-standing jaundice in whom the cholangiogram reveals a neoplastic lesion that will require an extensive surgical procedure for its removal. Decompression can be achieved after the cholangiogram has been secured, by the reintroduction into a hepatic bile radicle of a 20- or 21-gauge needle over which a polyethylene tube has been fitted (Fig. 52-15). Experience has shown, how-

ever, that it is difficult to maintain free bile flow for a prolonged period.

The level at which the cystic duct is inserted into the common bile duct is of considerable surgical importance in cases of extrahepatic biliary obstruction secondary to neoplasm. If the cholangiogram demonstrates a low implantation, as in Fig. 52-15, *A,* there is little possibility that a cholecystojejunostomy will provide much relief. However, if there is a high insertion of the cystic duct a surgical decompression might well provide considerable palliation.

Carcinoma of the papilla of Vater

Carcinoma of the papilla of Vater causes dilatation of the common bile duct but usually not to the extent seen in pancreatic neoplasm. Two cholangiographic patterns are highly suggestive of the diagnosis. One shows an uneven, ragged,

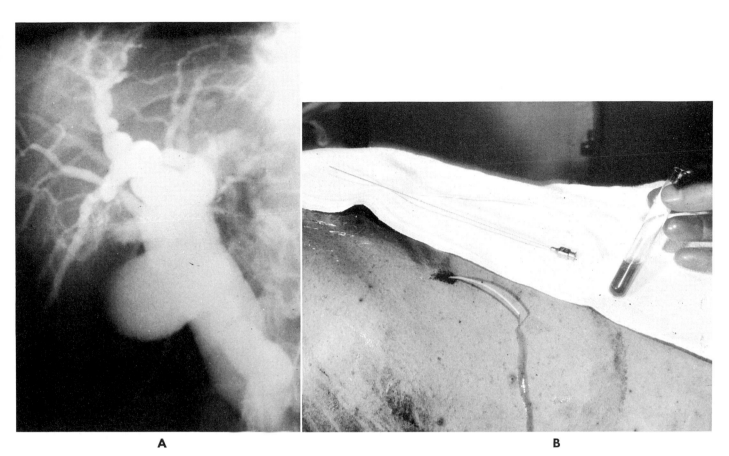

A

B

Fig. 52-15. A, Greatly dilated common duct in a patient with carcinoma of pancreas. Note the low implantation and the corresponding dilatation of the cystic duct. In such a situation a biliary intestinal shunt is unlikely to provide palliation. **B,** Percutaneous catheter decompression following the cholangiogram.

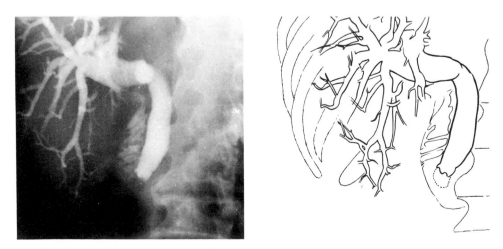

Fig. 52-16. Carcinoma of the ampulla. Note the irregular, ragged margin of the distal common duct at the ampulla. (From Evans, J. A.: Radiology 82:582, 1964.)

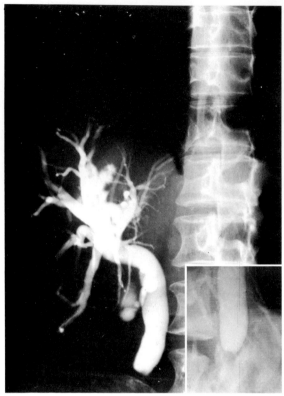

Fig. 52-17. Carcinoma of the ampulla, causing obstruction and moderate dilatation of the common bile duct. The terminal segment of the duct has a flat, rounded margin. Note the high implantation of the cystic duct. In this situation a cholecystojejunostomy might be expected to provide palliation. (From Evans, J. A.: Radiol. Clin. N. Amer. **3** (2): 305, 1965.)

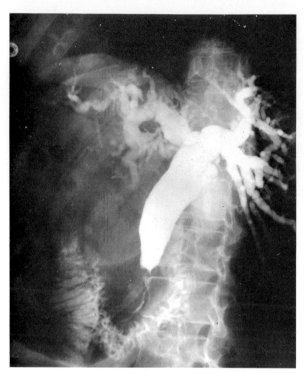

Fig. 52-18. Primary carcinoma of the distal common bile duct, resulting in a long, irregular, stenotic channel. The proximal margin has somewhat square, overhanging edges.

serrated margin at the site of obstruction (Fig. 52-16). The other pattern is that of a smooth, flat, shallow meniscus. The character of the meniscus is different from that seen in impacted common duct stone. The blunt, rounded margins and the shallowness of the concavity help to differentiate tumor meniscus from the deep, sharply marginated meniscus of impacted stone (Fig. 52-17). The ability to differentiate between carcinoma of the ampulla and carcinoma of the pancreas is of considerable practical importance. Their prognosis is not the same, and the surgical management may be quite different.

Carcinoma of the extrahepatic ducts

In the material my colleagues and I studied, eight patients with carcinoma of the extrahepatic ducts were successfully examined by per-cutaneous cholangiography. The cholangiograms in these cases showed either complete obstruction or irregular stenosis of the involved segment of the duct. In the latter instance the stenotic segment tended to be irregular and ragged as opposed to the fine, straight channel of stenosis usually seen in benign stricture (Fig. 52-18). Although no example of a discrete polypoid tumor of the main hepatic or common bile duct occurred in our series, such a case is illustrated in Wiechel's monograph.[22] The appearance may simulate that of a stone, and differentiation may not be possible.

Carcinoma of the gallbladder

It has been said that the diagnosis of carcinoma of the gallbladder is rarely made prior to exploratory laparotomy. Although it is true that

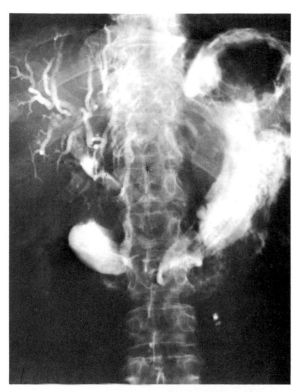

Fig. 52-19. Carcinoma of the gallbladder involving the common bile duct. The latter is somewhat displaced and demonstrates gross irregular filling defects.

a few patients with primary carcinoma of the gallbladder may present some detectable abnormality on one or more roentgenographic studies, demonstration of a malignant lesion of the gallbladder on cholecystography is very rare.

In the New York Hospital material, eight patients with carcinoma of the gallbladder were studied by percutaneous cholangiography. All were deeply jaundiced. The cholangiograms in each of the cases demonstrated infiltration, compression, and distortion of the extrahepatic bile ducts by a mass in the region of the gallbladder fossa. A diagnosis of carcinoma of the gallbladder was, therefore, inferred from the cholangiographic evidence of extrinsic pressure and displacement of a segment of the extrahepatic ducts (Fig. 52-19). Invasion of the common bile duct may also result in ragged, irregular filling and simulate the cholangiographic appearance of a primary duct neoplasm (Fig. 52-20).

Hepatic metastases

Percutaneous cholangiography is of little value in the diagnosis of liver metastases except when the metastasis occurs in the porta hepatis

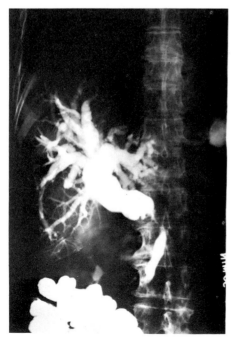
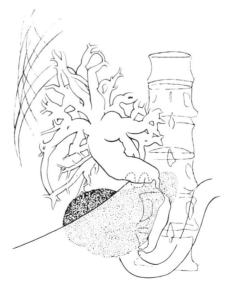

Fig. 52-20. Carcinoma of the gallbladder in an 83-year-old woman with a 2-week history of jaundice. The cholangiogram demonstrates invasion and segmental stenosis of the common bile duct. The appearance is indistinguishable from primary carcinoma of the bile duct.

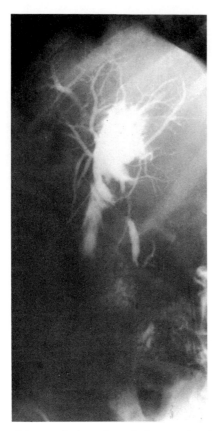

Fig. 52-21. Metastatic invasion of the proximal common bile duct from a carcinoma of the stomach. The cholangiographic appearance is similar to that of primary carcinoma of the bile duct.

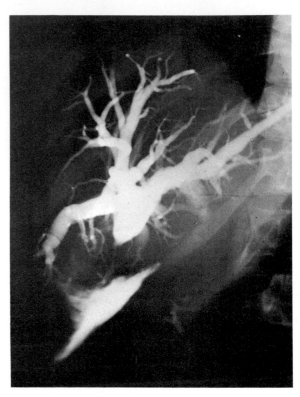

Fig. 52-22. Postoperative stricture of the common hepatic duct. The proximal margin of the stricture extends to the confluence of the right and left hepatic ducts. A small amount of contrast medium has collected beneath the liver capsule.

or results in major bile duct obstruction. Diffuse infiltration of the liver by metastatic disease usually prevents successful duct puncture. In such cases, on penetration of the liver, a certain resistance to the positioning of the needle will be detected. When this firm, hard feeling of the liver is encountered and a bile duct cannot be entered, aspiration biopsy may yield diagnostic information.

Metastases involving the extrahepatic bile ducts

Metastatic involvement of the extrahepatic ducts may result in one or more areas of stenosis of varying extent. The stenosis secondary to metastatic disease frequently cannot be distinguished from primary duct neoplasm (Fig. 52-21). Furthermore, if the stenotic segment is long and involves the distal end of the common

duct it can mimic the type of pancreatic carcinoma that produces a long stenosis.

Benign stricture of the bile ducts

In our study benign stricture of the bile ducts was seen thirteen times. In all cases the stricture was secondary to injury during a previous operation, usually for biliary tract disease. Fig. 52-22 shows an example of a stricture of the common hepatic duct at the confluence of the left and right hepatic ducts.

Sclerosing cholangitis

Sclerosing cholangitis is a rare cause of biliary tract obstruction. The lesion is a chronic inflammatory process of unknown cause, which may be diffuse and involve both the intrahepatic and extrahepatic duct systems or may be strictly segmental in distribution. It may be associated with

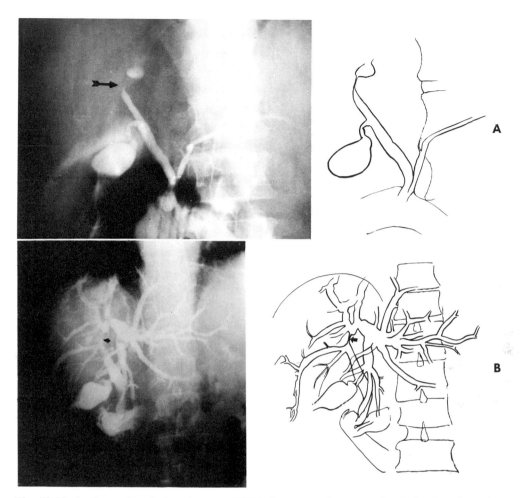

Fig. 52-23. A, Operative cholangiogram (1959) demonstrating stenosis of the intrahepatic duct. **B,** Percutaneous cholangiogram of the same patient (1962), demonstrating segmental stenosing cholangitis. It is apparent how much more information there is on the percutaneous cholangiogram than on the operative cholangiogram. (From Evans, J. A.: Radiology 82:584, 1964.)

mediastinal or retroperitoneal fibrosis, or it may occur in conjunction with granulomatous or chronic ulcerative colitis. Fig. 52-23 shows an operative cholangiogram (1956) of a 59-year-old man who was operated on because of recurrent episodes of jaundice. The cholangiogram demonstrates a short stricture of the main intrahepatic bile duct. There was no evidence of neoplasm grossly or on biopsy. A percutaneous cholangiogram (1962) was taken of the same patient when he was readmitted to the hospital because of recurrent attacks of jaundice. Reexploration again revealed no evidence of neoplasm. Biopsy of the site of the stricture showed chronic cho-

langitis. This patient died approximately a year later, and postmortem examination revealed chronic stenosing cholangitis and no evidence of neoplasm.

The cholangiogram of another patient who had ulcerative colitis and sclerosing cholangitis is shown in Fig. 52-24. The patient was a 28-year-old man. On exploration following percutaneous cholangiography his common hepatic and common bile ducts were found to be extremely narrow and fibrotic.

Patients with ulcerative colitis may develop jaundice from still another complication. Malignant degeneration in the colon may give rise

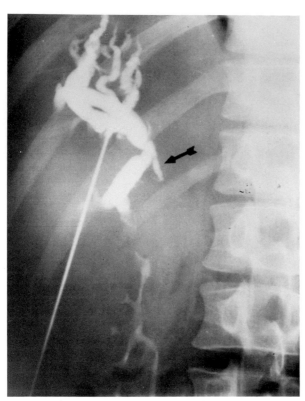

Fig. 52-24. Percutaneous cholangiogram of a 28-year-old man with ulcerative colitis and sclerosing cholangitis. Arrow points to obstructed common hepatic duct. At surgical exploration the common hepatic and common bile ducts were found to be markedly narrowed and fibrotic.

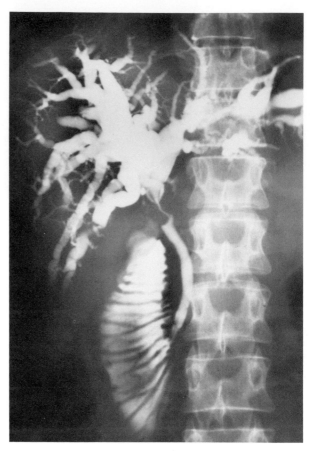

Fig. 52-25. Marked narrowing and medial displacement of the common bile duct by a metastatic mass from a carcinoma of the transverse colon complicating ulcerative colitis.

to metastases in the liver or the right upper quadrant, obstructing the flow of bile to the duodenum. Fig. 52-25 shows marked narrowing and medial displacement of the common bile duct by a metastatic mass from a carcinoma of the transverse colon complicating ulcerative colitis. The appearance of the common bile duct in this case simulates cholangitis. A close inspection, however, shows lack of uniformity in the narrowed segments and a nodularity not likely to be encountered in sclerosing cholangitis. Furthermore, the medial displacement of the duct denotes the presence of a space-occupying lesion favoring the diagnosis of metastatses over sclerosing cholangitis.

Hodgkin's disease in one of our patients (Fig. 52-26) simulated sclerosing cholangitis of the common hepatic duct. The excentricity of the narrowing, however, as well, as its abrupt termination at its lower end, suggests infiltration by a malignant disease. Segmental sclerosing cholangitis is expected to show gradual tapering at the junction of the normal with the stenosed segment. On exploration this patient was found to have Hodgkin's disease involving the common bile duct.

CONCLUSIONS

Percutaneous transhepatic cholangiography is a useful and valuable technique providing important anatomic information that can be obtained in no other way. It is particularly helpful in the presence of clinical or chemical jaundice, when conventional diagnostic x-ray examina-

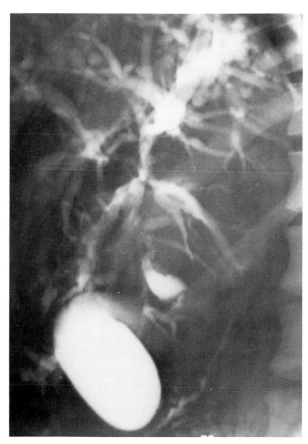

Fig. 52-26. Hodgkin's disease causing segmental narrowing of the common hepatic duct.

tion of the gallbladder and bile ducts offers no help. It permits the differentiation between obstructive and hepatocellular jaundice. It provides definitive diagnostic information in situations that might otherwise require exploratory laparotomy.

Obstructive lesions of the biliary system are difficult problems for the surgeon. Patients are frequently older and generally are poor surgical risks. A diagnostic method that provides precise information regarding the morphologic character of the disease process may well be decisive in determining the type of surgical or medical therapy indicated. When the indications are proper and the examination is done in the immediate preoperative period, percutaneous transhepatic cholangiography has distinct value.

Certain patients who have obstructive jaundice may be benefited by percutaneous catheter decompression of the biliary system at the time

of examination. In certain carefully supervised cases surgery may be advantageously postponed with the use of this procedure. Indeed, in some cases the results of the examination may well obviate the need for surgery.

REFERENCES

1. Arner, O., Hagberg, S., and Seldinger, S. I.: Transhepatisk cholangiografi, Nord. Med. **65**:730, 1961.
2. Atkinson, M., Happey, M. G., and Smiddy, F. G.: Percutaneous transhepatic cholangiography, Gut **1**: 357, 1960.
3. Burkhardt, H., and Muller, W.: Versuche über die Punktion der Gallenblade und ihre Rontgendarstellung, Deutsch. Ztschr. Chir. **161**:168, 1921.
4. Carter, F. R., and Saypol, G. M.: Transabdominal cholangiography, J.A.M.A. **148**:253, 1952.
5. Evans, J. A., Glenn, F., Thorbjarnarson, B., and Mujahed, Z.: Percutaneous transhepatic cholangiography, Radiology **78**:362, 1962.
6. Flemma, R. J., Schauble, J. F., Gardner, C. E. Jr., Anlyan, W. G., and Capp, M. P.: Percutaneous transhepatic cholangiography in the differential diagnosis of jaundice, Surg. Gynec. Obstet. **116**:559, 1963.
7. Fuentes, V., Bertoni, C., and Polero, J.: La cholangiographia per junction hepatica, Prensa Med. Argent. **44**:2873, 1957.
8. Glenn, F.: A 26 year experience in the surgical treatment of 5037 patients with non malignant biliary tract disease, Surg. Gynec. Obstet. **109**:591, 1956.
9. Glenn, F., Evans, J. A., Mujahed, Z., and Thorbjarnarson, B.: Percutaneous transhepatic cholangiography, Ann. Surg. **156**:451, 1962.
10. Hanafee, W., and Weiner, H. M.: Transjugular percutaneous cholangiography, Radiology **88**:35, 1967.
11. Housset, E., and Vantsis, G.: La cholangiographie trans-parietohepatique: a propos de 9 observations, Presse Med. **65**:772, 1957.
12. Huard, P., and Do-Xuan-Hop: La ponction transhepatique des canaux biliares, Arch. Argent. Dig. Nutr. **17**:368-382, 1942.
13. Kaplan, A. A., Brodsky, L., and Rumball, J. M.: Percutaneous transhepatic cholangiography, Amer. J. Dig. Dis. **5**:450, 1960.
14. Kaplan, A. A., Traitz, J. J., Mitchel, S. D., and Block, A. L.: Percutaneous transhepatic cholangiography, Ann. Intern. Med. **54**:856, 1961.
15. Kidd, H. A.: Percutaneous transhepatic cholangiography, Arch. Surg. (Chicago) **72**:262, 1956.
16. Lee, W. Y.: Evaluation of peritoneoscopy in intraabdominal diagnosis, Rev. Gastroent. **9**:133, 1942.
17. Leger, L., Zura, M., and Arvay, N.: Cholangiographie et drainage biliare parponction transhepatique, Presse Med. **60**:936, 1952.
18. Prioton, J. B., Vialla, M., and Pous, J. G.: Nouvelle technique de cholangiographie transparietohepatique, J. Radiol. Electr. **41**:205, 1960.
19. Remolar, J., Katz, S., Rybak, B., and Pellizari, O.:

Percutaneous transhepatic cholangiography, Gastro-enterology **31**:39, 1956.

20. Royer, M., Solari, A. V., and Lottero-Lanari, R.: La cholangiografia noquirurgica: unevo metodo de exploracion de las vias biliares, Arch. Argent. Dig. Nutr. **17**:368, 1942.

21. Shaldon, S., Barber, K. M., and Young, W. B.: Percutaneous transhepatic cholangiography, Gastroentcrology **42**:371, 1962.

22. Wiechel, K. L.: Percutaneous transhepatic cholangiography, Acta Chir. Scand. **309** (Supp.):1, 1963.

23. Zerbon, R., and Polero, R.: Cholangiographie par ponction transparietohepatique, Ann. Radiol. **3**:151, 1960.

Portography 53

Francis F. Ruzicka, Jr.

Portography may be defined as the roentgenographic visualization of the portal venous system[23,24,25,44] achieved by the introduction of contrast medium into the system by one of several approaches (Fig. 53-1). The earliest and now little-used technique employs cannulation of a tributary of the portal system at surgery and is simply called operative portal venography (Fig. 53-1, *E*).[21,32,60,83] A semischematic drawing of the anatomy of the portal system is presented in Fig. 53-2.

The first effective nonoperative approach, splenoportography, utilized a percutaneous transthoracic insertion of a needle and injection of contrast medium into the spleen (Fig. 53-1, *C*). Introduced by de Sousa-Pereira of Portugal,[50] Abeatici and Campi of Italy,[1] and Leger of France,[33] it was for approximately 15 years the most useful nonoperative means for opacification of the portal system.

With the advent of visceral[45,71] (celiac and superior mesenteric) arteriography the possibility—and later the actuality—of adequate delineation of the portal system during the venous phase of the study was realized (Fig. 53-1, *A* and *B*). This is effective in a reasonably high percentage of cases.

Somewhat concomitantly, umbilical portography was developed (Fig. 53-1, *F*).[4,19,26] This is accomplished by venous cutdown in the abdominal wall above the umbilicus, catheterization of the umbilical vein, and retrograde passage of the catheter into the splenoportal axis. This technique results in excellent roentgenologic anatomic demonstration of the portal system.

Finally, it is possible to opacify the intrahepatic portion of the portal system[66,80] and, under certain circumstances, the extrahepatic portal system to a varying extent by the retrograde wedge venogram or by an approach that is basically similar—the intrahepatic injection of contrast agent directly into the liver[33,49,63] parenchyma via a transthoracic, transhepatic catheter needle (Fig. 53-1, *D*).

INDICATIONS FOR EXAMINATION

There are several major indications for roentgenographic opacification of the portal venous system. These are as follows:

1. Determination of the presence or absence of portal venous obstruction, the location of the obstruction, and the nature of the cause of the obstruction when possible. This information is important not only in the making of a diagnosis but also for the proper planning of decompressive surgery in the presence of portal hypertension.

2. Demonstration of the hemodynamic pathophysiology of the portal system, that is, the portal venous flow patterns that have resulted from the underlying pathology. Such information is useful in preparation for shunt surgery. Furthermore, it can be of significant aid in assessing the severity and character of the disease present relative to decisions of medical therapy.

3. Investigation of gastrointestinal bleeding in patients with venous obstruction.

4. Application to the differential diagnosis of upper quadrant lesions with or without

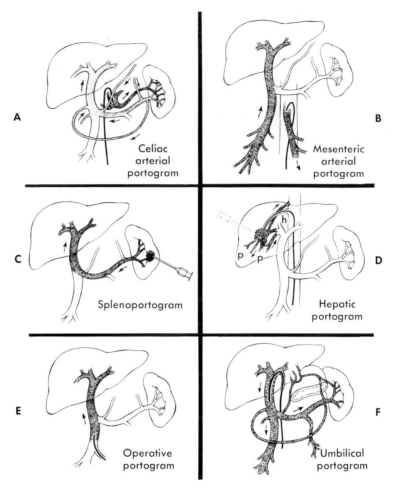

Fig. 53-1. Schematic representations of different basic approaches for roentgenographic opacification of the portal system. Arrows indicate direction of normal flow, which is hepatopetal. In **D**, both hepatic wedge technique and intrahepatic injection technique are shown. **h**, Hepatic vein; **p**, portal vein branches.

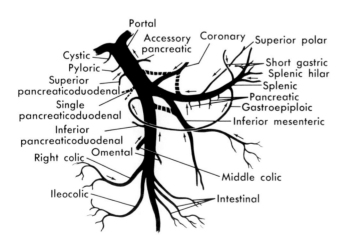

Fig. 53-2. Semidiagrammatic drawing of normal portal venous system. Arrows indicate direction of flow. (Modified from Douglas, B. E., Baggenstoss, A. H., and Hollinshead, W. H.: Anatomy of the portal vein and its tributaries, Surg. Gynec. Obstet. **91:**562-576, 1950.)

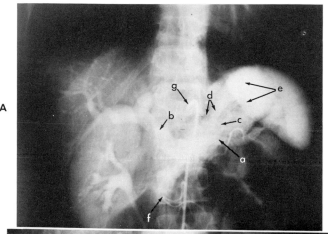

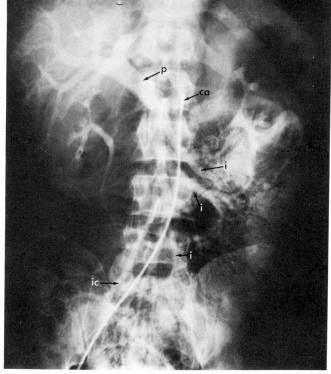

Fig. 53-3. A, Normal celiac portogram. Following injection of contrast agent into the celiac artery, the splenoportal axis becomes opacified. Splenic vein, **a,** and portal vein, **b,** are well seen. Intrahepatic portal branches are well defined. Short gastric vein, **c,** is opacified but the coronary vein is not seen in this patient. Stomach wall, **d,** is fairly densely opacified. The fundus, **e,** superimposes on the spleen. Residual arterial opacification is present at **f;** the catheter is in celiac axis at **g. B,** Different patient from **A.** Superior mesenteric portal portogram, showing various tributaries of superior mesenteric vein. Intestinal veins at **i;** ileocolic vein at **ic;** portal vein at **p.** Note absence of opacification of splenic vein and coronary vein, since flow is hepatopetal. Left tributary of middle colic vein that drains left transverse colon is not seen in this portogram but may appear normally and be confused with splenic vein. Catheter, **ca,** is in the superior mesenteric artery.

jaundice.[32] The arterial phase of arterial portography may provide information regarding the nature of the lesion and, often, the extent of the disease. Veins of the portal system are frequently obstructed, displaced, or otherwise altered by neoplasms and inflammatory lesions of the pancreas and the biliary tract.

5. Determination of the patency of a shunt postoperatively, when question of this arises.

TYPES OF PORTOGRAPHY: NORMAL ROENTGENOGRAPHIC ANATOMY
Arterial portography

Arterial portography[40,42,64] is the technique of choice for roentgenographic opacification of the portal venous system even though at the present time splenoportography provides a denser and clearer delineation of the splenoportal axis. Visualization is achieved during the venous phase of the injection of contrast medium selectively into the celiac and superior mesenteric arteries. Assuming a 4- to 8-second arterial injection, the veins are usually best seen between 14 and 20 seconds. In the presence of obstruction, filming of the venous phase should be carried to 24 to 26 seconds.

Because contrast medium is delivered to different sites of arterial distribution depending on the artery injected, different venous patterns will result (Fig. 53-1, *A* and *B*). For better visualization of the splenoportal axis, injection directly into the splenic artery is advisable, although celiac artery injection will often provide a good venous phase (Fig. 53-3, *A*). Injection into the superior mesenteric artery normally results in opacification of superior mesenteric vein tributaries, superior mesenteric vein, and portal vein (Fig. 53-3, *B*).

For several reasons it is desirable to begin the roentgenographic study of the portal venous system with arterial portography.

First, although complications of the more direct technique of splenoportography are infrequent when it is performed by experienced hands, nevertheless even the remote possibility of laceration of the spleen or subcapsular hematoma and subsequent rupture are reasons sufficient to approach the problem, initially at least, by other means.

Second, the arterial portogram provides an arterial phase—celiac, hepatic, and superior mesenteric—that affords the opportunity to assess various organs, or lesions of them (especially the liver and pancreas), in a manner not possible with a purely venous study. Thus one can evaluate liver size, the cirrhotic pattern as seen arteriographically, and any suspected or unsuspected neoplasm of the liver such as a hepatoma.[68] Arteriography may quickly show that what was thought to be a liver mass is a mass of the right adrenal gland.

Arterial portography is, at times, of aid in the differential diagnosis of jaundice. The percutaneous cholangiogram is generally the most direct approach in the assessment of such problems, but arterial portography, in spite of the relative avascularity of those lesions likely to produce obstructive jaundice (such as tumors of the gallbladder, the bile ducts, or head of the pancreas), can often show the extent of the lesion by virtue of arterial involvement and venous displacement and obstruction.

Most important, arterial portography provides a diagnostic delineation of the portal system in a high percentage of cases. Splenoportography gives sharper and often more detailed demonstration of that part of the portal system that it

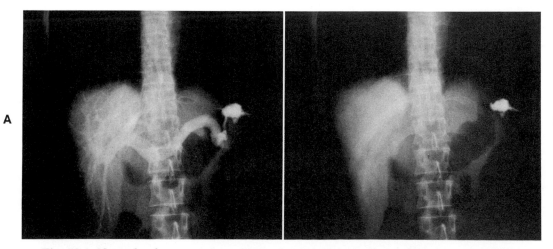

Fig. 53-4. Normal splenoportogram. Note visualization of splenoportal axis only. Right lobe of liver is elongated, being a normal variant of shape (Riedel's lobe). Vasculogram phase is seen in **A,** sinusoidal phase in **B,** Note absence of satisfactory opacification of left lobe branches in liver in **A** and practically absent density of left lobe in sinusoidal phase.

visualizes because the contrast medium being injected directly into the venous side is less diluted. Celiac and superior mesenteric arterial portography, on the other hand, provide a more complete delineation of the portal system, since contrast medium is delivered into the various territories of distribution of the arteries injected and the veins draining these territories are accordingly opacified.

Because the arterial portogram may lack sufficient density of contrast agent to produce a diagnostic study, attempts have been made with some success to improve portal venous opacification by various vasodilating drugs.[27,72] Popular among these has been tolazoline (Priscoline) hydrochloride.[53] Various experimental studies are in progress, and in the future one may expect improved opacification of the veins during arterial portography with the aid of pharmacologic agents.[75]

The greatest limitation of arterial portography is its failure at times to provide diagnostic delineation of the portal system. Some authors claim up to 90% diagnostic capacity for the method,[43] especially when large amounts of contrast medium (60 ml. or more) are employed. Much, of course, depends on the purpose and needs of the study as to what might be considered diagnostic. In my experience, injection of a volume of 60 ml. of 76% diatrizoate (Renografin) is likely to result in good opacification of the portal system in 70% of cases. Splenoportography, therefore, among other indications, is reserved for those cases in which arterial portography fails to obtain the information needed.

Technique and complications

Details of the Seldinger technique[71] employed for selective celiac and superior mesenteric artery injection may be found elsewhere. Similarly, space does not permit discussion of complications of arterial puncture[28] and catheter passage, which are carried out in arterial portography.

Splenoportography

Splenoportography, is of greatest use in defining the portal system when arterial portography has failed to do so (Fig. 53-4).[6,14,60,72] Thus it may be employed for a clearer definition of part of the portal system, such as the splenoportal axis or the coronary vein and gastric

varices. The technical failure rate at St. Vincent's Hospital and Medical Center in New York has been 5% to 6%.

In the normal patient the splenoportal axis is best seen between 2 and 10 seconds after the start of injection. In the presence of obstruction extrahepatic components of the portal system may be seen at 25 seconds and longer after the start of injection.

Splenoportography can demonstrate variceal bleeding probably with greater success than arterial portography. The direct injection of contrast medium into the venous side allows a better chance of visualizing the escape of the opaque substance in an actively bleeding patient. Therefore, when there is a high probability that variceal bleeding is the cause of upper gastrointestinal hemorrhage, splenoportography is the procedure of choice.

At times the splenoportogram may provide somewhat different information than the arterial portogram, depending on patterns of blood flow,[16,67] so that the two methods may be used to supplement one another. A major advantage of splenoportography is the opportunity to perform splenic manometry during the procedure and thereby obtain a quantitative determination of portal system pressure.

Technique

The details of performance of splenoportography are of great importance for the successful completion of the study. Since it is beyond the scope of this chapter to provide these details, reference to other sources is made.*

Complications

Complications of splenoportography are suitably discussed at this point, since they constitute a major factor in restriction of its use.[48]

Two deaths have occurred following splenic portography in more than 2,000 cases at St. Vincent's Medical Center. One patient, a woman with a subsequent diagnosis of endothelioma of the spleen, developed gas gangrene after splenic biopsy and an attempt at splenic portography in which there was no venous uptake of contrast material and no injection was made. The biopsy and attempted portogram were performed on

---

*See references 6, 7, 48, 57, 62, 70, and 73.

the same day. The source of infection, which spread rapidly from the spleen to involve the entire body, was never definitely determined but was presumably secondary to a break in aseptic technique during one of these two procedures.

The second death occurred after a successful splenic portogram in a 63-year-old cirrhotic patient with ascites. Splenic pulp pressure was elevated (40 mm. saline) and the patient had markedly decompensated liver function. He and his family refused to permit a splenectomy, which was advised when it became clear that the bleeding from the spleen could not be controlled with conservative measures. Finally, consent for operation was obtained, but the patient died during the laparotomy.

Hemorrhage following splenic puncture is the complication of greatest concern. In a series of 266 portograms performed at St. Vincent's Medical Center, bleeding requiring transfusions of 500 ml. (three cases) to 2,000 ml. (one case) occurred in 2% of the patients.[48]

In a larger series of more than 1,000 cases, three splenectomies were performed. One was done in the patient with ascites described previously. Ascites is considered a relative contraindication to splenoportography, since the free-floating spleen lacks the tamponade effect of the lateral chest wall.

The second splenectomy was performed in a 59-year-old man with normal splenic pulp pressure and a normal splenic portogram (Fig. 53-5). It was presumed that bleeding occurred secondary to a large hematoma formation and splenic rupture, which took place clinically about 18 hours after the splenoportogram. It is not understood why a tear in the splenic pulp should occur during injection, such as happened in this rare instance, when usually a simple pulp deposit of contrast takes place.

The third splenectomy was performed in a 36-year-old woman with normal splenic pulp pressure. During the first 12 hours after the procedure the patient had no unusual complaints. Over the next 4 hours, however, she developed signs of intraperitoneal bleeding with shock, and at surgery a rupture of the spleen was found. The rupture had occurred at the site of an old hematoma that presumably developed at the time of a first splenoportogram 1 year previously. During the second examination the friable tissue of the old hematoma was probably traversed by the

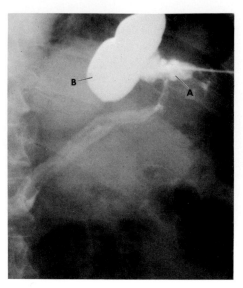

Fig. 53-5. Close-up view of spleen, selected from a serial splenoportogram showing a normal pulp deposit, **A**, and subcapsular collection of contrast at the end of injection, **B**. Since there is no preexisting subcapsular or other potential cavity within the spleen, such a sharply circumscribed pool of contrast material within the spleen indicates that a tear of the splenic pulp has occurred. Compare with appearance of pericapsular collection as seen in Fig. 53-18, *B*.

needle and constituted the basis for a new intrasplenic hematoma. In light of this case it is advocated that repeat splenoportograms be preceded by an isotope scan of the spleen to evaluate splenic integrity.

Extravasation of contrast medium may occur. A small amount of perisplenic accumulation of contrast medium, resulting from retrograde passage of the medium along the outside of the needle shaft, often occurs. It can be decreased by minimal handling of the needle and by correct positioning of the tip of the needle in the spleen. The more superficial the tip in the spleen, the greater the extravasation. The tip of the needle should be within 1 to 2 cm. of the splenic hilum, but care must be taken to avoid piercing of the medial side of the spleen.

Extravasation of contrast agent into the peritoneal cavity causes pain. Low-grade fever may accompany a localized chemical peritonitis. Such symptoms may persist for as long as 2 weeks.

False puncture is a complication that can readily be avoided by television monitoring of the needle insertion. Reports of injection into kidney, left lobe of the liver, and even the stomach wall without observable ill effect have come to my attention.

No allergic reactions have been observed in over 2,000 cases. As with any intravascular injection they may be expected, however, and due precautions should be observed, especially in patients with a history of serious allergy.

Pleuritis as a complication may occur. Since the spleen may be located very high in the left upper quadrant in close proximity to the diaphragm, the needle may traverse the lower portion of the left pleural space on occasion. Although this may be painful, merely passing the needle through the pleura is not likely to cause a serious problem; however, accidental injection of contrast medium into the pleural cavity must be avoided. Retrograde flow along the needle shaft when it traverses the pleural cavity can cause contrast to be deposited in the pleural cavity. This retrograde flow may not be noted on the test injection, but may occur only with injection of a larger amount of contrast medium. With conscious attention to the possibility of this complication it can be avoided.

Hepatic wedge venography and portography

This approach to visualization of the portal system offers certain supplementary information to arterial portography or splenoportography, or both. Further, it is useful in determining portal venous pressure, especially when splenic manometry has not been done. Either of two techniques may be employed. In one, a catheter is wedged in a hepatic vein.[30,55,66] The other is percutaneous intrahepatic needle placement.* The hepatic wedge pressure may differ from the splenic pulp pressure in a given case, and such information may permit further differential diagnosis.

With a suitably wedged catheter and an injection of sufficient volume of contrast medium rapidly enough (for example, 30 ml. of 76% diatrizoate injected at a rate of approximately 5 ml. per second), considerable retrograde flow of contrast agent into intrahepatic portal branches is possible (Fig. 53-6). In the normal patient flow of contrast medium passes in two

directions—retrograde into intrahepatic portal vein branches and antegrade into hepatic veins. At the end of injection, the contrast medium forced retrograde into portal vein branches changes direction of motion to move through sinusoids to the draining hepatic veins, following the direction of blood flow.

A method of examination that provides the same roentgenographic results as the hepatic vein wedge venogram is the intraparenchymal injection of contrast agent (Fig. 53-7).[41,52,66] The latter is technically achieved by the transthoracic, transhepatic insertion of a needle-catheter[2] to a depth of 7 to 9 cm. in a manner similar to that employed in the lateral thoracic approach for percutaneous cholangiography. Both the hepatic wedge and the intraparenchymal injection of contrast agent result, essentially, in a sinusoidal injection of contrast agent. Both also can be used to measure sinusoidal pressure. The intrahepatic, transthoracic method permits venous sampling of both hepatic and portal veins.[9,10]

Technique

Space does not permit discussion of the details of technique of these two methods of hepatic portography. Reference is made to other publications for this purpose.[41,66]

Complications

Hepatic vein wedge injections and pressure determinations cause virtually no serious complications. The hepatic wedge technique may be approached via either an antecubital vein[30,55] or the femoral vein.[66] The usual precautions of venous cutdown (antecubital fossa), or percutaneous femoral vein puncture and catheter passage must be observed. The injection into the liver is often accompanied by some pain, and a slight rise in the SGOT level[41] may be expected for 24 hours after the procedure, more so in patients with cirrhosis. A small intrahepatic hematoma develops at the site of injection. The transthoracic transhepatic catheter-needle puncture may be accompanied by some bleeding from the surface of the liver. In my experience of more than 500 such liver punctures, bleeding has never been great (50 ml. has been observed on occasion at subsequent surgery). Prothrombin time should be normal or nearly so before puncture is performed. Ascites is a relative contraindication. Passage of the needle is conducted

---

*See references 9, 10, 41, 52, 78, and 79.

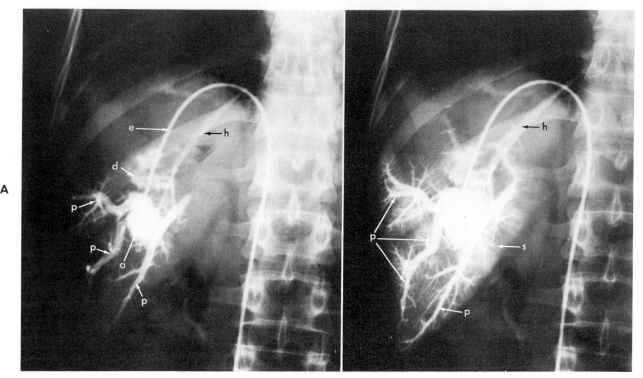

Fig. 53-6. Normal hepatic portogram. This examination, more commonly termed the "hepatic wedge venogram," will opacify the portal system to a varying degree depending on the amount of flow into liver via the portal vein. In this normal patient, only intrahepatic branches are seen. **A,** Early phase of injection. Note sinusoidal deposit at **a,** portal vein branches at **p,** and hepatic vein at **h.** Older sinusoidal deposit from transthoracic intrahepatic injection (see Fig. 53-7) seen at **d.** Catheter at **e** inserted via femoral vein. Placement into hepatic vein facilitated by Cooke deflector. **B,** Later phase of same study as **A** near end of injection of 30 ml. of 76% Renografin. Fairly extensive retrograde filling (with some subsequent orthograde flow) of normal portal vein branches achieved. Sinusoidal phase of orthograde flow beginning to visualize at **s.**

under television monitoring for proper needle placement and avoidance of important structures, including pleura, lung, and the gastrointestinal tract.

Umbilical portography

This approach to roentgenographic visualization of the portal venous system is perhaps the most satisfactory from the standpoint of clearcut delineation of the splenoportal axis and all its tributaries (Fig. 53-8).[4,19,56,76] Since a catheter is passed via the umbilical vein into the left hepatic vein or directly into the portal vein or splenic vein, the entire system can be flooded with contrast medium and excellent opacification can be achieved. An especially dense sinusoidal phase of the liver is possible with this method. Radiolucent areas, that is, space-occupying lesions as small as 1 cm. in diameter, can be demonstrated in the liver with this technique.[31] Moreover, direct portal vein pressure can be measured. The method has been used in certain centers to great advantage. Since the catheter can be left in place for some time, the technique lends itself admirably to certain continuation studies and to reasearch purposes. There are, however, three practical limitations to the method. First, it requires a cutdown performed usually in the operating room, which carries with it some risk of entering the peritoneal cavity; the patient must then be transported to the radiology department where serial camera equipment is available. Second, the umbilical vein is not always available for use, al-

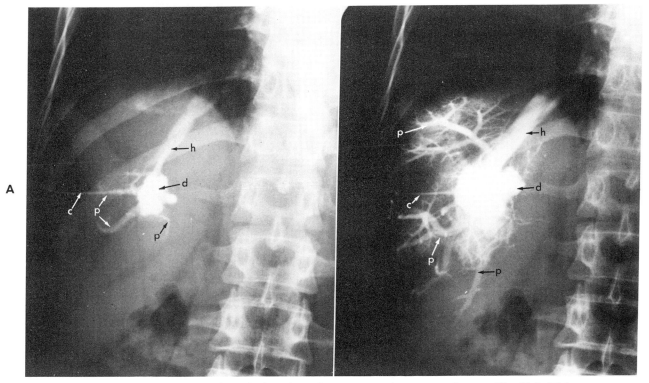

Fig. 53-7. Normal transthoracic intrahepatic portogram in same patient as Fig. 53-6. This injection immediately preceded the wedge venogram shown in Fig. 53-6 and accounts for residual parenchymal deposit shown in that figure. **A,** Early phase of injection. Note catheter at **c** (needle component has been removed). Observe intrahepatic portal branches at **p,** hepatic vein at **h,** and parenchymal deposit at **d. B,** Later phase of the same injection as **A.** More extensive retrograde filling (with some subsequent orthograde filling of portal vein branches has occurred. Differences in venous opacification between Figs. 53-6 and 53-7 are caused by different sites of sinusoidal injection.

though it can be located in a majority of cases. Third, the procedure can often be performed only once, since thrombosis of the umbilical vein is a real possibility following the procedure.

Very importantly, the umbilical portogram cannot ordinarily provide the information derived from the arterial phase of arterial portography, such as the detection of a lesion and especially lesions of organs other than the liver, best seen on the arterial side. Finally, it provides primarily anatomic information, since the force of injection alters the existing hemodynamics. However, after the end of injection, dominant flow patterns may again be reasserted and visualized to some extent.

Refer to other publications for details of technique and complications.[4,19,76]

Most suitable approach to the portal system

Basically, four different procedures are available for roentgenographic evaluation of the portal system. The choice of methods or combination of methods will vary depending upon the needs of a particular case. The most practical and generally informative approach entailing the least risk is arterial portography alone or combined with hepatic wedge venography. Hepatic wedge venography may occasionally be used alone, but is usually most helpful as a supplementary procedure. Splenoportography may be used if needed as a supplementary study or as the primary study when so indicated. Umbilical portography may be employed in special situations, as previously discussed.

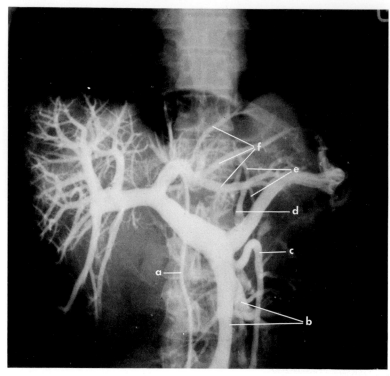

Fig. 53-8. Umbilical portal portogram executed by phlebotomy on umbilical vein and passage of catheter into portal vein by way of the left main portal branch. Note retrograde filling of various regularly occurring tributaries in this normal portal system. Vessels are densely opacified because of direct injection into portal vein and countercurrent flooding of system. **a,** Catheter; **b,** superior mesenteric vein; **c,** inferior mesenteric vein; **d,** coronary vein; **e,** short gastric vein; **f,** left intrahepatic portal branches. (Courtesy Dr. A. Legare.)

Portal manometrics

Both the techniques of splenoportography and hepatic wedge venography provide the opportunity for determination of portal venous pressure. (The direct catheterization of umbilical portography clearly affords an excellent opportunity to measure portal or splenic vein pressures or both.)

Splenic manometry

Splenic pulp pressure determination[58] is a measure of pressure of the entire portal venous system if the obstruction is intrahepatic or suprahepatic. If the portal vein is obstructed, it is still a reflection of the pressure in the remaining extrahepatic portal system. When splenic vein obliteration exists, the splenic pulp measurement indicates pressure on the splenic side of the system; that is, it then measures segmental portal hypertension. Portal vein pressure may be normal under these circumstances unless there is a coexistent intrahepatic or suprahepatic obstruction. The hepatic wedge or sinusoidal pressure will also then be normal. The celiac portogram or splenic portogram will show whether splenic vein obstruction exists.

Splenic manometry is carried out before the splenic portogram. The technique is as follows:

Following injection of 2 ml. of saline into the splenic pulp to produce a cushion effect at the needle tip, three readings are taken, using an ordinary water manometer. (A strain gauge manometer technique may, of course, be employed.) The x-ray table top serves as the base line or zero point for the position of the lower end of the manometer. To correct for this base line the figure of 12 cm. is subtracted from the average of the three readings. This figure is the average distance from the table top to the level of the anterior bodies of the first and second lumbar vertebrae, or the approximate level of the portal vein, as measured in fifty-two adult cadavers.[48] A soft, light rubber interconnecting tube is used between the needle and the manometer to avoid unnecessary drag on the needle. For injection of the contrast medium, a heavier tubing with a Luer-Lok at either end is substituted for the soft rubber tubing in order to avoid leakage of contrast medium from the force of injection.

Measurements of splenic pulp pressure below 250 mm. saline (corrected) are considered normal by this method. Pressures between 250 and 280 mm. represent either a high normal or portal venous hypertension. Any measurement over 280 mm. saline is definitely elevated.

Hepatic manometry

Hepatic vein wedge pressure and the percutaneous intrahepatic parenchymal pressure determinations have both been shown to measure sinusoidal pressure.* Either a strain gauge with electronic measurement apparatus or a simple water manometer may be used.

With the transthoracic catheter-needle method, one first measures interstitial pressure, which is apt to be quite high especially in the cirrhotic patient with attendant fibrosis. After a short time, however, by means of a drip infusion, communication is established with the sinusoids, at which time the pressure will drop to some degree and reflect true sinusoidal pressure. Vennes[78,79] describes the method in detail and correlates it with direct portal venous pressures.

For intrahepatic or hepatic vein wedge measurements the right atrium has customarily been used as the base line; that is, the strain gauge or the base of the water manometer is positioned at the level of the right atrium. In actuality, this is close to the level of the portal vein.[66] The normal wedge pressure, measured in mm. Hg, is 8 to 12 mm.[30]

The sinusoidal pressure has been shown to be a true reflection of portal vein pressure in cases of postsinusoidal obstruction. Postsinusoidal obstruction caused by cirrhosis is the most common cause of portal venous obstruction. In presinusoidal obstruction, for example, in schistosomiasis or hepatoportal fibrosis, the wedge pressures are likely to be normal although some variation is encountered. With extrahepatic portal obstruction the wedge pressure is normal.

The hepatic vein wedge pressure determination has a significant advantage over both the percutaneous, transthoracic sinusoidal pressure measurement and splenic manometry. This lies in the fact that the catheter approach through either the antecubital vein or the femoral vein permits pressure measurements not only of the liver sinusoids (normal, 8 to 12 mm. Hg.), but also of the free hepatic vein (6 to 10 mm. Hg), the cava, and the right atrium (up to 5 mm. Hg).

Cardiac failure, constrictive pericarditis, or high obstruction of the inferior vena cava can result in elevated sinusoidal pressure. In the latter case it is the gradient between the free hepatic vein and the sinusoids, or between the right atrium and the sinusoids, that becomes important in determining whether one is dealing with a sinusoidal hypertension caused by postsinusoidal cirrhosis or hypertension superimposed from a suprahepatic cause. The wedge/free hepatic vein gradient should not exceed 5 to 6 mm. Hg.[55]

The additional determination of pressures at the sites noted will aid them in differentiating between sinusoidal elevation as a result of an intrahepatic cause such as postsinusoidal obstruction and those as a result of a suprahepatic cause.

ROENTGENOLOGIC DIAGNOSIS
Hemodynamic principles and flow patterns

Basically, flow in the portal system is normally toward the liver, that is, hepatopetal (Fig. 53-2).[23,24,25,67] If injection is made into an artery, those veins draining the territory of distribution of the artery will visualize the flow proceeding toward the liver (Fig. 53-3).

If injection is made directly into the venous side, those vessels between the site of injection and the liver will be primarily opacified. For example, injection into the spleen at splenoportography will normally opacify only the splenic and portal veins (Fig. 53-4).

During umbilical portography contrast medium is forced in all directions by the pressure

*See references 30, 46, 55, 66, 78, and 79.

of injection so that the entire, or almost the entire, system is opacified. If the catheter is in the splenic vein, the smaller tributaries of the splenic vein, including the short pancreatic twigs and the short gastric veins and coronary vein, will be better visualized. If the catheter is in the superior mesenteric trunk, the tributaries of this vessel will be better seen. Once the pressure of injection has disappeared, if the portal system is normal, flow will again return to its normal direction—hepatopetal. Basically then, in contrast to arterial portography and splenoportography, the umbilical portogram is initially unphysiologic from the standpoint of blood flow; however, at the end of contrast injection, some inference on pattern of blood flow may be possible when the prevailing flow pattern again assumes predominance.

In operative portography[21,60] when usually a tributary of the superior mesenteric vein is injected, a few small vessels near the site of injection may be filled in retrograde manner by the force of injection, but otherwise, only those vessels between the liver and the site of injection will be opacified.

In the liver the portal vein shows symmetrical branching. The branches taper gradually, and a full complement of medium and small end vessels is found for each branch. Right lobe branches are ordinarily better opacified than left lobe branches regardless of the technique employed. Even with the umbilical portogram the left lobe appears less dense, possibly because of its normal thinness and fewer vessels. The intrahepatic portal tree also normally shows a right main branch larger than the left main branch (Fig. 53-3).

With the splenoportogram, the intrahepatic portal branches are best visualized between 5 and 15 seconds after injection.[63,64] The sinusoid phase of opacification of the splenoportogram (Fig. 53-4, *B*), is best observed between 10 and 25 seconds after injection. Normally, the sinusoid phase produces a homogenous opacification of the right lobe of the liver. At times, however, flow in some intrahepatic portal branches may be slower than in others. The left lobe tends to be only faintly visualized if at all. In the arterial portogram the intrahepatic portal branches appear in similar fashion but are often less well defined because of dilution after transcapillary passage.

In arterial portography two liver sinusoid phases may occur upon celiac artery injection. The first is produced by flow of contrast directly into the liver from the hepatic arteries and occurs within 3 to 6 seconds of completion of the arterial injection. It is often more dense and diagnostic than the second sinusoidal phase, which develops from contrast medium reaching the liver from the extrahepatic portal venous system. The latter is less dense because of dilution of contrast but can nevertheless sometimes be diagnostic. There may even occur some additive effect to the first sinusoidal phase.

Assuming a 4- to 8-second arterial injection, the second sinusoidal phase will be seen at about 12 to 24 seconds. In general, when obstruction of the portal system is present, flow is slowed and the sinusoidal opacification appears later.

If a selective splenic artery injection of contrast medium is made, it is obvious that only the second sinusoidal phase of liver opacification can occur.

Pathologic conditions

Various intrinsic and extrinsic disorders may affect the portal venous system.* Intrinsic lesions include vascular thrombosis and vascular anomalies such as cavernomatous transformation of the portal vein. Extrinsic lesions include cirrhosis of the liver or hepatic neoplasms, which deform and obstruct intrahepatic vessels, and extrahepatic lesions such as inflammation or neoplasms of the pancreas or other upper quadrant organs, which deform and obstruct the main splenoportal axis. The principal effect of these lesions, as manifested clinically and roentgenologically, is obstruction. When obstruction of the portal venous system exists, collateral blood flow develops.[22,24,51] Since in postuterine life the portal venous system is without valves, blood can flow in any direction. Hence, when normal or hepatopetal flow is blocked blood will flow along the course or courses of least resistance. The flow is often in a hepatofugal direction, that is, away from liver, although some hepatopetal flow may be established over bridging collaterals.

Since contrast medium is carried by the blood, the pattern encountered will depend on the location of the obstruction and the type of portogram performed, that is, the site of injection.

---

*See references 3, 5, 8, 14, 32, 39, 54, 61, 65, 68, and 73.

Collateral veins in portal venous obstruction

In intrahepatic or suprahepatic obstruction any of the tributary or developed collaterals may appear. In extrahepatic obstruction, only those collaterals hepatodistal to the obstruction will have the stimulus to appear. Moreover, only in extrahepatic obstruction will bridging collaterals carrying blood hepatopetally appear. Collaterals carrying blood in a hepatofugal direction may exist in the same patient with extrahepatic obstruction. A combination of hepatofugal and hepatopetal collaterals may exist in the same patient with extrahepatic obstruction.

Tributary collaterals. The normally occurring tributaries of the portal venous system (Fig. 53-9) are immediately available for collateral blood flow when obstruction to normal flow occurs. Those tributaries that are most important are the coronary vein (the left gastric vein), the inferior mesenteric vein, the short gastric veins, and the superior mesenteric vein. Blood passing in reverse direction over the coronary vein and short gastric veins will eventually reach the systemic circulatory system by way of the hemiazygos and the azygos systems. Blood passing over the inferior mesenteric vein in hepatofugal direction reaches the systemic system by means of various retroperitoneal communications[69] in the mesentery, which include the veins of Retzius. Other less important and less frequently opacified tributaries are the right gastric (pyloric) vein, the pancreaticoduodenal veins, and the cystic vein. For examples of tributary collaterals, see Figs. 53-14 through 53-16 and 53-17, *B.*

Developed collaterals. When obstruction of the portal venous system occurs, portal blood may seek avenues of flow in addition to those

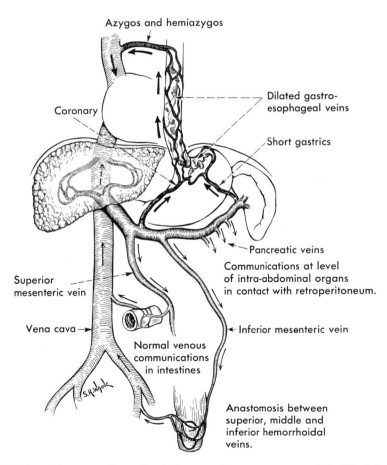

Azygos and hemiazygos

Coronary

Dilated gastro-esophageal veins

Short gastrics

Pancreatic veins

Communications at level of intra-abdominal organs in contact with retroperitoneum.

Superior mesenteric vein

Vena cava

Inferior mesenteric vein

Normal venous communications in intestines

Anastomosis between superior, middle and inferior hemorrhoidal veins.

Fig. 53-9. Major tributary collaterals of the portal venous system. (Modified from Rousselot, L. M., and others.: Ann. Surg. **150:**384, 1959.)

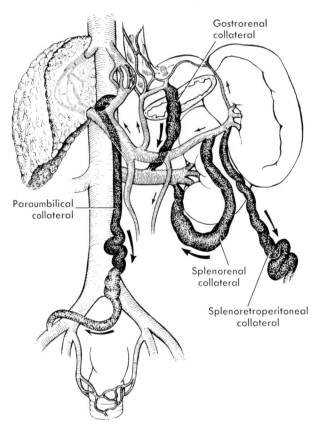

Gastrorenal
collateral

Paraumbilical
collateral

Splenorenal
collateral

Splenoretroperitoneal
collateral

Fig. 53-10. "Developed collaterals. (Modified from Rousselot, L. M., and others: Ann. Surg. **150:**384, 1959.)

offered by the normally occurring tributaries.[59] Collateral channels of varying size may develop from vessels that previously existed but did not function as main tributaries of the portal system.

The more frequently seen channels are shown in Fig. 53-10. The paraumbilical collateral arises from the left main intrahepatic branch of the portal vein or, rarely, from the right branch, and shows a variable course.[22] It seldom terminates at the umbilicus, although it not infrequently communicates with anterior abdominal wall veins. It may also terminate retroperitoneally below the level of the liver, or extend to an iliac vein or the inferior vena cava (Fig. 53-10). Its course is tortuous and lies usually to the right of the spine. Because of the variability of its course and termination, the paraumbilical collateral has also been called the transhepatic collateral.

The splenorenal collateral (Fig. 53-10) is usually a large vessel of variable length and tortuosity. It extends from the spleen or the splenic

vein to the renal vein, sometimes via the left adrenal vein. The gastric renal collateral (Fig. 53-10) is a similar type vessel, which extends from the stomach to the renal vein, often via the adrenal vein.

The splenoretroperitoneal collateral is found in the lateral portion of the abdomen, extending from the spleen to retroperitoneal vessels along the lateral abdominal wall.

The previously named vessels carry blood in a hepatofugal direction. All may appear in the presence of intrahepatic obstruction. When extrahepatic obstruction exists, the paraumbilical collateral has no stimulus to develop but the more distal collaterals may develop, depending on the site of obstruction. Examples of developed collaterals may be seen in Figs. 53-14, *C*, 53-15, *B*, 53-16, *B* and *C*, 53-17, *A*, and 53-21, *B*.

Developed collaterals that act as bridging collaterals may be seen when the portal vein is obstructed (Fig. 53-11 and 53-17, *A*). These are likely to be small but may attain fair size.

In the presence of splenic vein obstruction (Figs. 53-12, 53-17, *B*, and 53-18) a similar situation results. Bridging collaterals appear between the spleen and the portal vein. These, however, are not developed collaterals but tributary collaterals. Two major routes of blood flow are seen: (1) over the short gastric veins to the gastric veins to the coronary vein to the portal vein, and (2) over the gastroepiploic vein to the superior mesenteric vein to the portal vein. In addition to the hepatopetal flow of blood in these bridging collaterals, bridging collaterals over omental veins also may develop. These are seldom seen with present techniques. A hepatofugal flow may occur over the splenorenal collateral or the splenoretroperitoneal collateral. If the coronary vein arises from splenic vein hepatodistal to the site of obstruction it cannot, of course, act as the bridging collateral but carries blood hepatofugally to the azygos system.

Types of obstruction

There are four major types of obstruction of the portal venous system relative to location: suprahepatic, intrahepatic, extrahepatic, and combined intrahepatic and extrahepatic.

Suprahepatic obstruction. Suprahepatic obstruction frequently remains unnoticed clinically, since the degree of obstruction is seldom great and the predominant clinical interest is

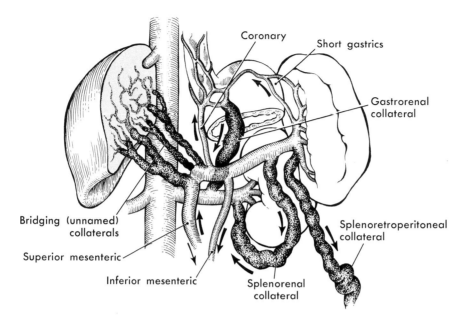

Fig. 53-11. Potential routes of blood flow when portal vein is obstructed.

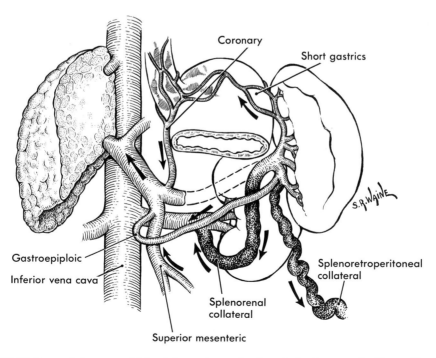

Fig. 53-12. Potential routes of blood flow when splenic vein is obstructed. (From Ruzicka, F. F., Jr.: Portal venous system, slide series, Chicago, Micro X-Ray Recorder, Inc.)

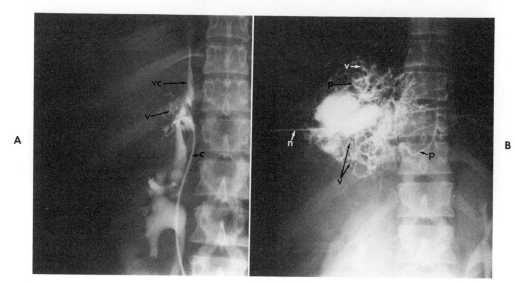

Fig. 53-13. Suprahepatic portal obstruction. Budd-Chiari syndrome in a young woman taking contraceptive medication. Patient eventually died of thrombosis of major abdominal veins. At the time of this study there was thrombosis of almost all hepatic veins In **A** a catheter has been inserted into the orifice of a partially thrombosed hepatic vein. Escape of contrast can be seen in the vena cava at **vc.** Note pattern in liver in **A** that is similar to that seen in **B,** in which percutaneous transhepatic needle has been employed for this sinusoid injection. Note interlacing network of hepatic and portal vein branches, which directly communicate. Probable portal vein branch is identified at **p.** The portal vein is thrombosed. If it were not, it would serve as an outflow tract for liver. See text for further discussion. **vc,** Vena cava; **v,** intercommunicating veins; **n,** needle; **c,** catheter.

centered elsewhere, as for example in chronic congestive heart failure or pericarditis. An exception is the Budd-Chiari syndrome. In such cases, nevertheless, it may be possible to demonstrate the presence of collateral vein development.

The intraparenchymal injection of contrast medium can be a useful procedure in hepatic vein thrombosis. With complete obstruction of all or nearly all the hepatic veins, a bizarre intercommunicating pattern of vessels may be seen (Fig. 53-13). If the portal vein is not also thrombosed, reverse flow through it may be seen with either the intraparenchymal injection or the hepatic vein wedge technique. (Such reverse flow may be sometimes seen with arterial portography under these conditions.) Wedging the catheter in a partially thrombosed hepatic vein, however, may be technically difficult and is not without the risk of dislodging a thrombus. In this situation the transthoracic intrahepatic technique is preferred to the wedge technique. Generally speaking, splenoportography and arterial portography reveal flow patterns similar to that seen with intrahepatic portal obstruction.

Intrahepatic obstruction. Intrahepatic obstruction is a common form of portal venous obstruction. Cirrhosis is by far the most frequent cause of intrahepatic portal venous obstruction.[39] On occasion primary or metastatic disease of the liver may also produce it. Laennec's is the most common form of cirrhosis that is encountered (Fig. 53-14). Postnecrotic cirrhosis secondary to hepatitis is also a frequent cause of intrahepatic obstruction. The site of obstruction in both is primarily postsinusoidal. Schistosomiasis produces a presinusoidal type of obstruction, but this cannot be seen roentgenologically.

Hepatoportal sclerosis is an unusual form of intrahepatic obstruction (5% of cases).[12,40] It is presinusoidal in location. The lesion consists of thrombosis of the larger intrahepatic portal branches, which can sometimes be readily recognized on portography. Abrupt change in diameter of larger intrahepatic portal branches occurs as a result of the multiple thromboses. A bizarre

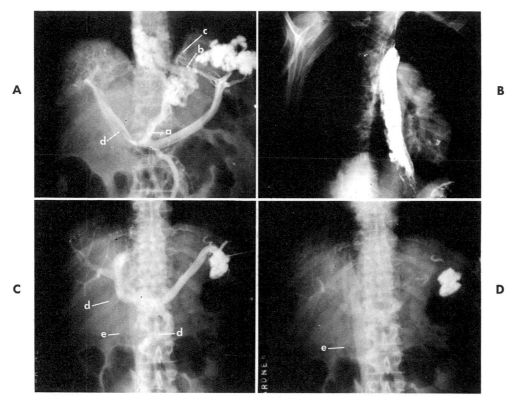

Fig. 53-14. A, Intrahepatic portal venous obstruction (cirrhosis) with large gastric and esophageal varices. Gastric varices arise primarily from coronary vein, **a.** However, a small group of gastric varices that arise from a short gastric vein, **b,** can be seen at **c.** Note huge periesophageal varices. Degree of opacification of portal vein indicates reduced blood flow, **d.** Note contracted liver and distorted hepatic vasculogram with anastomosing vessels of irregular caliber. **B,** Same case as shown in **A.** Scalloped esophageal contour with large varices, which are probably both submucosal and periesophageal. **C,** Another case showing intrahepatic obstruction due to cirrhosis. Note diminution in medium and small vessels in liver. Large paraumbilical collateral, **d,** arises from left main intrahepatic branch of portal vein and passes into the pelvis, where it empties directly into an iliac vein (not shown). Vena cava, which is opacified by this naturally occurring "developed" collateral, is seen at **e** in **C** and **D.**

intercommunicating collateral pattern of intrahepatic portal vein branches may be seen.

With celiac arterial portography or splenic artery injection (Fig. 53-15, *A*) the venous pattern in intrahepatic obstruction is likely to be very similar to that seen with splenoportography. Both the splenic and the portal vein are usually seen. Opacification of the inferior mesenteric vein is unequivocal evidence of hepatofugal blood flow by either technique. Visualization of the coronary vein on celiac artery injection in itself is not significant, since this vessel drains the area that the artery supplies. However, when gastric veins are clearly varicose or when esoph-

ageal varices are seen on celiac portography the presence of portal venous obstruction may be assumed. Visualization of the coronary vein on splenic artery injection that bypasses the left gastric artery generally means hepatofugal blood flow, but one must not be misled by greater curvature veins receiving their blood supply from short gastric arteries that arise from the splenic artery.

On both splenoportography and arterial portography, any of the tributary or developed collaterals may appear. As mentioned before, they are usually better seen on splenoportography.

Superior mesenteric artery injection generally

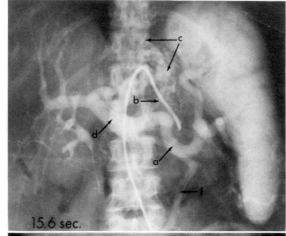

15.6 sec.

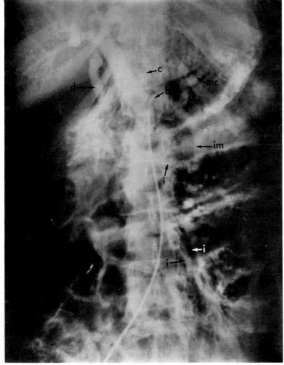

Fig. 53-15. A, Intrahepatic portal venous obstruction caused by Laennec's cirrhosis. Selective splenic arterial portogram. Note position of catheter well advanced in splenic artery. a, Splenic vein; b, short gastric vein; d, portal vein where coronary vein arises; c, gastric varices; f, inferior mesenteric vein. Opacification of the inferior mesenteric vein is unequivocal evidence of hepatofugal flow. See text for discussion. B, Superior mesenteric arterial portogram shows intrahepatic portal venous obstruction and cirrhosis. Catheter, b, is in trunk of superior mesenteric artery. Hepatofugal flow demonstrated over coronary vein at c, paraumbilical vein at d, inferior mesenteric vein at im. i, Intestinal veins$_1$; mc, left branch of middle colic. The tortuosity and relative size distinguish the left branch of the middle colic from the splenic vein. (A from Ruzicka, F. F., and Rossi, P.: Arterial portography: patterns of venous flow, Radiology **92:**777-787, 1969.)

results in some demonstration of hepatofugal flow when intrahepatic obstruction exists (Fig. 53-15, *B*). Depending on the degree of reduction of flow toward the liver in the portal vein, contrast medium may flow hepatofugally through the inferior mesenteric vein, splenic vein, and even up into the coronary-gastric-esophageal system. Even the "developed" collaterals may occasionally be opacified with superior mesenteric artery injection.

The superior mesenteric portogram has been

a useful means of demonstrating a patent portal vein that does not appear during splenoportography (Fig. 53-16, *C*)[13,16] or during the spleno-portal phase of the celiac portogram because of flow patterns.

If the superior mesenteric portogram fails to show a patent portal vein, a wedge venogram or intrahepatic injection is usually successful (Fig. 53-16, *A* and *B*).

It should be mentioned that the hepatic wedge technique or the intrahepatic injection

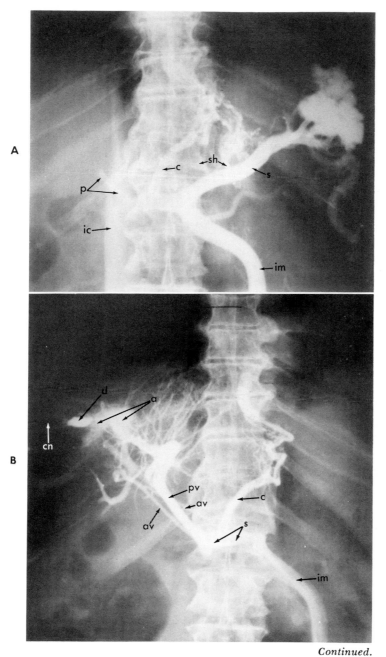

Continued.

Fig. 53-16. Intrahepatic portal obstruction caused by cirrhosis. **A,** Splenic portogram shows dilated splenic vein, **s,** partial opacification of portal vein, **p,** heavy hepatofugal flow to pelvis over inferior mesenteric vein, **im,** and visualization of inferior cava, **ic,** via rectal-hypogastric route in pelvis. Coronary vein, **c,** and short gastric veins, **sh,** carry contrast hepatofugally to gastric and esophageal varices. From this study question of patency of portal vein cannot be determined. **B,** Same patient as **A.** Intrahepatic portogram. Injection of 30 ml. or 76% Renografin into a sinusoid liver site, **a.** Transthoracic transhepatic catheter component of catheter needle faintly seen at **cn.** Sharply circumscribed deposit at **cd** is interstitial or periportal in contrast to parenchymal or sinusoid deposit at **a.** Retrograde flow of contrast is seen over portal vein, **pv,** and accessory veins, **av.** Once contrast reaches splenic vein, **s,** it is carried by predominant portal current over inferior mesenteric vein, **im,** and coronary vein, **c.**

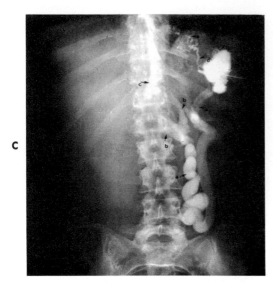

Fig. 53-16, cont'd. C, Patent splenic and portal veins that are not opacified during splenoportography, **a,** Spleno-renal "developed" collateral; **b,** renal vein; **c,** vena cava displaced to left by enlarged right lobe of liver; **d,** short gastric vein; **e,** gastric varices; **f,** esophageal varices. (**C** from Rousselot, L. M., and others: Ann. Surg. **150:**3, 1959.)

are also useful in delineating the portal outflow tract (the hepatoproximal segment of portal vein) after a side-to-side portocaval shunt. Common hepatic artery injection may accomplish the same.

The portal vein may also be opacified because of reverse flow, with injection of the common hepatic artery in the presence of hepatoma. The latter is caused by arteriovenous communications in the tumor.

Extrahepatic obstruction. Extrahepatic obstruction results from a variety of diseases that affect the splenoportal axis.[3,5,65] Inflammatory and neoplastic processes in both upper quadrants may cause narrowing, flattening, or obliteration of portal or splenic veins or both. Among the more common inflammatory lesions related to extrahepatic obstruction is pancreatitis (Fig. 53-17, *B*),[38] which is an important cause of splenic vein thrombosis. Cysts of the pancreas resulting from pancreatitis may compress and obliterate the splenic vein.[77] Carcinoma arising in the left upper quadrant, especially of the tail or body of the pancreas, may also destroy the splenic vein (Fig. 53-18).

Similarly, inflammatory and neoplastic processes in the right upper quadrant may obstruct the portal vein (Figs. 53-17, *A,* and 53-20) by thrombosis or constriction. Omphalitis in the newborn and sometimes trauma in children may be the cause of portal vein thrombosis.[57] Neoplasms of the gallbladder, the biliary tract, the head of the pancreas, and even the retroperitoneal tissues may obliterate the portal vein.

Thrombosis of the portal vein may occur as a result of phlebitis caused by septic processes in the draining territory of the portal system or as a result of stasis of blood flow caused by intrahepatic obstruction as happens in cirrhosis. Bland thrombosis of the portal vein is said to develop in approximately 10% of cirrhotic patients.[26]

Complete or incomplete thrombosis of the portal vein may be encountered. When thrombosis is complete (Fig. 53-20, *A* and *B*), the vein is effectively obliterated and no opacification of it occurs except on the rare occasion when recanalization develops. If this does happen the vein appears as an irregular channel with a septum-like radiolucent line extending along its longitudinal axis. Bridging collaterals from splenic vein and superior mesenteric vein frequently develop to span the obliterated portal vein, although inadequately. Incomplete thrombosis of the portal vein may be recognized by the dilated, densely opacified splenic vein with a narrowed irregular contour and sometimes by a filling defect of the portal vein. The streaming phenomenon that produces a streaked filling defect in the portal vein (Fig. 53-14, *A*), caused by the presence of nonopacified blood from the superior mesenteric vein, does not exhibit the other characteristics of incomplete thrombosis. Tumor thrombus may develop in the portal vein by retrograde extension from hepatoma in the liver and is readily recognized as a filling defect.

When the thrombosis of both the portal and splenic veins occurs (Fig. 53-20, *C*), the main splenoportal axis is obliterated. Bridging collaterals from the spleen to the liver appear. These communicate freely among themselves, and bizarre arrangements of veins are found spanning the obliterated main channels. The thrombosis may extend to involve the tributaries.

Early in their development, various tumors may narrow the portal or splenic veins or dis-

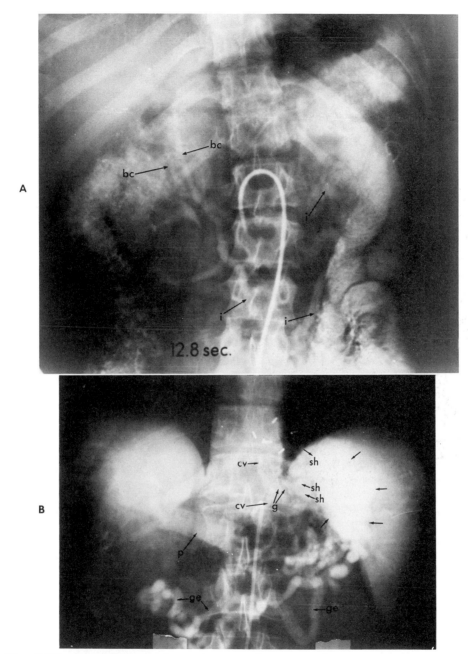

Fig. 53-17. A, Extrahepatic obstruction; superior mesenteric arterial portogram in post-splenectomy patient with portal vein thrombosis. Tip of the catheter is in the superior mesenteric artery. Return flow opacifies intestinal veins, **i,** and bridging collaterals, **bc,** from superior mesenteric system to liver. **B,** Celiac portogram. Obstructed splenic vein followed subtotal gastrectomy. Spleen is enlarged. Flow from spleen reaches portal vein, **p,** via short gastrics, **sh,** to gastric, **g,** to coronary vein route, **cv,** and gastroepiploic route, **ge.** Catheter tip in celiac axis. Dense area (arrows) represents opacified fundus (vessels and mucous membrane blush), which superimpose on spleen. (Courtesy Dr. Eduardo Reynoso.)

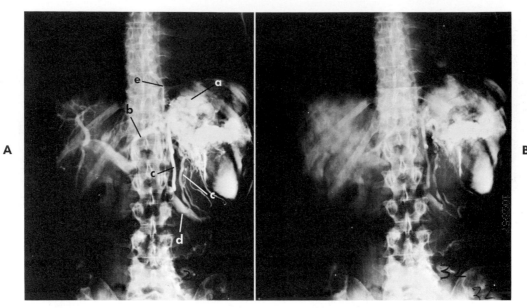

Fig. 53-18. Extrahepatic obstruction caused by carcinoma of body and tail of pancreas. Splenic vein is entirely obliterated. Contrast medium passes from the spleen to varicose gastric veins, **a,** thence over coronary vein, **b,** to portal vein. Veins, **c,** extend from gastric region and splenic hilum to communicate with a left renal vein. Film seen in **A** made at 20 seconds. Film in **B** made at 32 seconds in sinusoidal phase of liver opacification (delayed because of splenic vein obstruction) shows multiple rounded areas of radiolucency caused by metastatic carcinoma. Vein visualized at **e** is mediastinal vein. No esophageal varices are demonstrated. Note perisplenic extravasation of contrast medium, best seen in **B.** (Modified from Ruzicka, F. F., Jr., Gould, H. R., Bradley, E. G., and Rousselot, L. M.: Amer J. Med. **29:**434, 1960.)

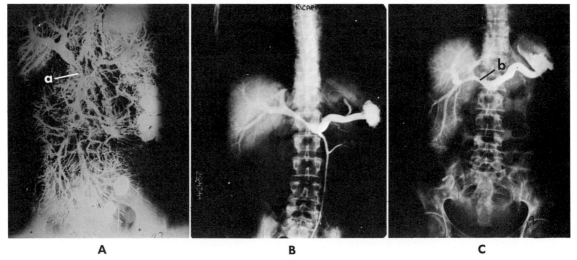

Fig. 53-19. Carcinoma involving portal vein in three different patients. **A,** Postmortem portogram performed at autopsy. Note constriction of portal vein at **a** because of carcinoma arising in the gallbladder. **B,** Narrowing of portal vein is caused by carcinoma of the head of the pancreas. Note collateral vein appearance (inferior mesenteric vein) although splenic pulp pressure was normal. **C,** Constricting deformity of portal vein, **b,** caused by recurrent carcinoma of the gallbladder. (Modified from Ruzicka, F. F., Jr., Gould, H. R., Bradley, E. G., and Rousselot, L. M.: Amer. J. Med. **29:**434, 1960.)

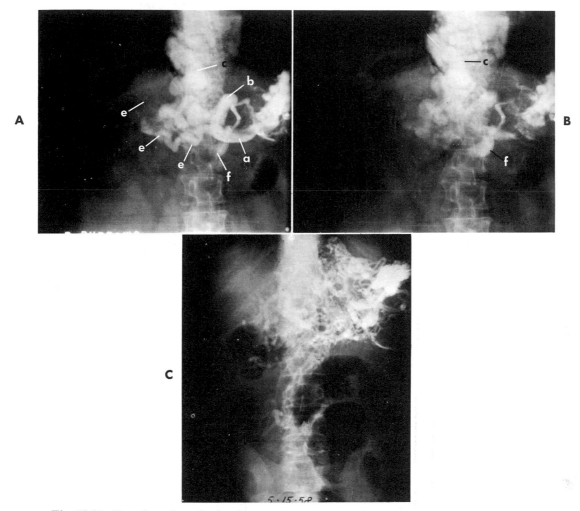

Fig. 53-20. Complete thrombosis of portal vein is shown in **A** and **B**. Liver is markedly contracted (advanced cirrhosis); **a,** splenic vein; **b,** dilated coronary vein; **c,** esophageal varices; **e,** bridging collaterals from splenic vein to liver; **f,** probable splenorenal collateral. Film in **B** was exposed 4 seconds after **A**. **C,** Complete thrombosis of both splenic and portal veins. A mass of tortuous bridging collaterals attempts to carry contrast material from spleen to liver. Gastric varices are present.

place them with obstruction (Fig. 53-19, *C*). Sooner or later, however, obstruction to blood flow becomes great enough to produce portal hypertension. This same process applies to intrahepatic lesions. Thus, cirrhosis may be present for sometime before the degree of obstruction reaches a stage sufficient to result in portal hypertension.

In the demonstration of extrahepatic portal vein obstruction, the venous pattern is similar whether celiac artery injection, splenic artery injection or splenoportography is performed;

that is, one may expect nonopacification of the portal vein. If the latter is accompanied by bridging collaterals between splenic vein and liver, the diagnosis can be quite definite (Fig. 53-20, *A* and *B*). If no bridging collaterals are visualized, the nonopacification could be caused by flow phenomena. Usually, tributary or developed collaterals, or both, are seen carrying hepatofugal flow. Superior mesenteric artery injection may also show similar bridging collaterals (Fig. 53-17, *A*). If the splenic vein is patent, flow is likely to pass into it and its tributaries.

When the splenic vein is obstructed, celiac or splenic artery injection and splenoportography will again be quite similar, showing bridging collaterals as demonstrated in Figs. 53-17, *B*, and 53-18. Hepatofugal flow, especially over splenorenal or splenoretroperitoneal collaterals, also may develop. When the splenic vein is obstructed, the superior mesenteric artery injection will show a normal venous phase; that is, those tributaries draining the territory supplied by the superior mesenteric artery, the superior mesenteric vein, and the portal vein will be opacified.

Hyperkinetic hypertension. Occasionally one encounters a patient with bleeding esophageal varices and portal hypertension in the absence of demonstrable suprahepatic, intrahepatic, or extrahepatic venous obstruction and with normal liver biopsy. Collateral vein opacification may be seen by splenoportography. According to Tisdale and his colleagues, cases of this type may be explained by the factors of vascular resistance and the volume of blood flow. Thus, an increase in the volume of blood passing through the portal vein raises the portal pressure if there is no accompanying change in vascular resistance. The latter condition could be present with a traumatic arteriovenous fistula involving the portal system. There is evidence that capillary shunts exist within the spleen that may permit rapid inflow of blood into the portal bed. Some investigators have postulated abnormal arteriovenous anastomoses within the liver, which might permit increased blood flow into the portal system. Increased venous tone of the portal trunk and its intrahepatic branches might cause increased vascular resistance that could result in portal hypertension.

In a few cases we have encountered an elevated splenic pulp pressure with visualization of the splenoportal axis but no collateral flow. The opposite, a normal splenic pulp pressure with the appearance of collaterals, including varices, has been seen.[42,47] These occurrences are rare. No suitable explanation for them can be offered.

Combined intrahepatic and extrahepatic obstruction. Combined intrahepatic and extrahepatic obstruction may occur. In cirrhosis there may be accompanying pancreatitis or pancreatic cyst formation, and thus two factors may play a role in the obstruction of the portal venous system. Carcinoma of the pancreas may produce both intrahepatic and extrahepatic obstruction—the former by virtue of multiple metastatic nodules, and the latter by direct involvement of the splenoportal axis. A hepatoma may obstruct intrahepatically as a result of a tumor thrombus of the portal vein. Bland thrombosis of the portal vein in a cirrhotic patient also results in a combined type of obstruction.

In the usual course of events it would be difficult to determine the respective components of the intrahepatic and the extrahepatic contributions to the total obstruction. In the case of the bland thrombosis of the portal vein, the thrombosis would not be expected to occur without severe obstruction within the liver and greatly reduced blood flow. In this situation then, one may safely assume that both factors exist. On the other hand, in a carcinoma of the pancreas with multiple metastases to the liver it may be difficult to determine whether or not the intrahepatic lesions are contributing to the obstruction. Elevated splenic pulp pressure would simply indicate portal venous obstruction with the site of obstruction undetermined. The appearance of a hepatofugal collateral between the two sites of obstruction would, however, indicate that the intrahepatic obstruction was significant, and the hepatic wedge pressure determination would be useful.

Varices

Umbilical portography and splenoportography (Figs. 53-14, *A,* and 53-21) are the best roentgenographic modalities for the demonstration of varices.[18]

The effectiveness of splenoportography was studied at St. Vincent's Medical Center in 124 patients who had splenoportograms performed and who also had a diagnosis of gastric or esophageal varices, or both, based on one or more of the following: (1) postmortem findings, (2) endoscopy, (3) recorded observations during portacaval surgery, (4) a clearly diagnostic barium examination, and (5) a clinical diagnosis based on an episode of severe hematemesis with the cessation of gastric bleeding after the insertion of a Sengstaken balloon, and an adequate barium meal examination that failed to demonstrate a peptic ulcer or other reason for bleeding.

It was assumed in this study that if lower esophageal varices were proved to be present, gastric varices were also present. If gastric var-

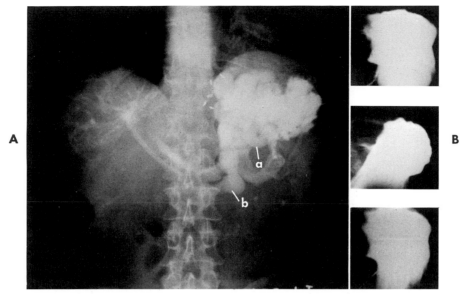

Fig. 53-21. A, Huge gastric varices in the region of the cardia that arise from the short gastric vein, **a,** and probably from the coronary vein, which is not definitely identified. Note the gastrorenal collateral, **b,** and absence of esophageal varices in presence of heavy run-off over gastrorenal collateral. **B,** Filling defect at the cardia of a barium-filled stomach caused by these gastric varices.

ices were proved to be present it was assumed that esophageal varices were present unless a large gastrorenal collateral was found (Fig. 53-21). In the 124 cases so studied, the portograms of 112 patients revealed unequivocally the presence of gastric varices (90.2%). In six cases (4.9%) the portogram revealed the presence of vessels in the region of the stomach but it could not be determined whether these represented gastric varices or retroperitoneal collaterals arising from the splenic vein.

In two of the cases a Sengstaken balloon was inflated at the time of portography. Despite the use of the balloon, there was partial opacification of the coronary or short gastric veins, or both. However, the pressure from the balloon resulted in collapse of the gastric veins, which accordingly did not opacify. Partial opacification of the coronary or short gastric veins, or both, under these circumstances may be considered reasonable evidence of the existence of varices of the gastroesophageal system, but these two cases were still rated as equivocal in this study. (The pressure in the Sengstaken balloon may temporarily be released during the injection to improve the results of the study.)

In six other cases (4.9%) no collateral vein

opacification occurred and therefore no demonstration of varices was possible. Four of the six cases were technically unsatisfactory as a result of a large pericapsular extravasation. In one case a Sengstaken balloon was inflated, and in another case no reason for the failure to visualize collaterals was determined.

Splenoportography was somewhat less accurate in determining the presence of esophageal varices. Thus, in this group of 124 cases, ninety patients (73%) showed unequivocal evidence of esophageal varices. In an additional fifteen cases (12%) the findings by portography were compatible with varices. Thus, in 85% of the cases where esophageal varices were proved to be present according to the criteria previously mentioned, they were demonstrated or suggested by portography.

The accuracy of arterial portography in the demonstration of gastric and esophageal varices is not as high as with splenoportography because of the dilution of contrast agent following arterial injection. Nevertheless, the accuracy is probably good and will certainly improve as techniques for increasing the contrast concentration on the venous side improve.

Umbilical portography is an excellent method

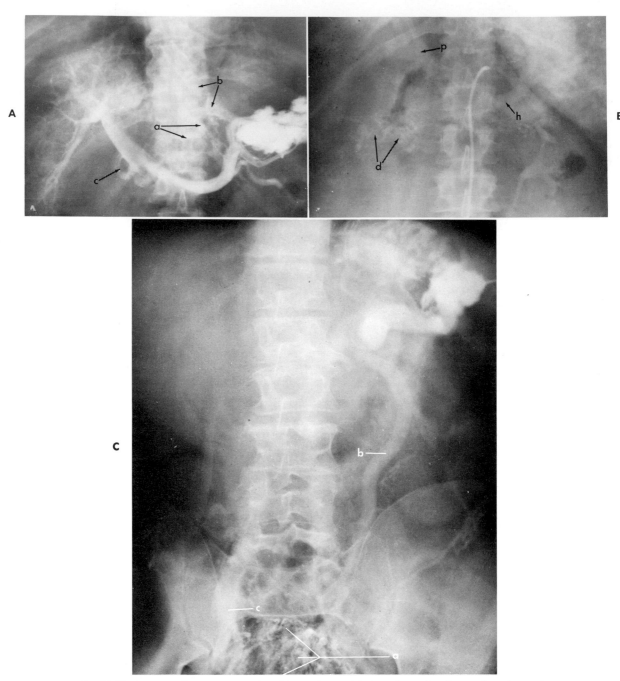

Fig. 53-22. A, On splenoportography this patient with intrahepatic obstruction shows hepatofugal flow into gastroepiploic vein at **c,** coronary vein at **a,** and gastric varices at **b. B,** On celiac arterial portography (in same patient), pancreaticoduodenal varices are visible at **d.** Splenic vein is faintly visible at **h,** and portal vein at **p.** Arterial portography is generally superior to splenoportography in demonstration of pancreaticoduodenal and intestinal varices. **C,** Example of sigmoidorectal varices, **a,** arising from inferior mesenteric vein, **b.** A direct communication between the varices and the systemic system (right common iliac vein), **c,** is demonstrated. (**A** and **B** from Ruzicka, F. F., and Rossi, P.: Arterial portography: patterns of venous flow, Radiology **92:**777-787, 1969.)

for the demonstration of both gastric and esophageal varices. The accuracy should be close to 100%, especially for gastric varices in the technically successful cases.

Varices occur in other portions of the gastrointestinal tract. After the stomach and esophagus the next most common locations are the sigmoid and the rectum (Fig. 53-22, C). Varices in these locations are produced by heavy blood flow over the inferior mesenteric vein. Such varices may bleed, causing the discharge of red blood through the rectum. When large enough, they may, on barium enema examination, cause a filling defect in the sigmoid. An instance of such a filling defect, which simulated carcinoma of the sigmoid, has been reported.[20]

Sigmoidal and rectal varices may be demonstrated by both splenoportography (Fig. 53-22, C) and arterial portography. Injection into the splenic or superior mesenteric arteries would show flow hepatofugally through the inferior mesenteric vein to the varices. Injection into the inferior mesenteric artery would also show a flow reversal in an inferior direction (hepatofugal) in the inferior mesenteric vein and varices.

In addition to the sigmoidorectal location bleeding varices have been reported in the duodenum,[49,82] in the cecum,[36] and in the jejunum[37] near a jejunoesophageal anastomosis following a total gastrectomy. On rare occasions varices, which may bleed, also occur on either the thoracic or the abdominal surface of the diaphragm and in the root of the mesentery.[37] Liebowitz reports rupture of a varix in the mesentery with the accumulation of 2,400 ml. of clotted blood in the peritoneal cavity.[37]

Arterial portography is more useful in demonstrating varices of small and large bowel, including pancreaticoduodenal varices (Fig. 53-22, A and B) than splenoportography. Similarly, varices of mesentery and diaphragm would probably be better seen with arterial portography.

Acute gastrointestinal bleeding

Acute gastrointestinal bleeding may occur as a complication of portal hypertension.[11,17,29,36,49] Massive bleeding from a ruptured varix is a grave problem. It has been stated that the first hemorrhage has a fatal issue in from 30% to 50% of cases.[38] At the St. Vincent's Hospital and

Medical Center, endoscopy is the method of choice for the detection of the bleeding site in acute upper gastrointestinal bleeding. Certain patients, for various reasons, however, cannot be endoscoped or the endoscopist may require confirmation of his findings.

If the patient is to be examined roentgenologically, emergency splenoportography should be performed when clinical findings weigh heavily in favor of the possibility of bleeding from a ruptured varix. It is possible with splenoportography to both show the varices and pinpoint the venous bleeding site by demonstration of a leak of contrast medium into the lumen of esophagus or stomach (Fig. 53-23).

It is also possible to show venous bleeding during the venous phase of an arterial portogram, but because of the dilution factor it would be more difficult than with splenoportography, in which the contrast medium is injected directly into the venous side. Generally speaking, bleeding may be considered to be venous in origin if varices are shown to be present and arteriography, performed during active bleeding, fails to show evidence of a leak of contrast during the arterial phase.

Alcoholic patients not infrequently bleed from causes other than a ruptured varix. In a study at St. Vincent's Hospital and Medical Center acute upper gastrointestinal bleeding in alcoholic patients occurred in a significant number of cases.[35] Often there is question as to whether such a patient, even one with known varices, is bleeding from a Mallory-Weiss tear or from an ulcer or erosive gastritis or esophagitis. A patient actively bleeding under these circumstances (providing endoscopy has not been performed) may be best examined first with selective celiac and superior mesenteric arteriography and arterial portography. At times superselective left gastric or gastroduodenal artery injection may be of value. It is well to be prepared to do both arterial portography and splenic portography at the same investigative session, as required by the needs of the particular case.

Anomalies

Major anomalies that produce problems in roentgenologic interpretation of the portogram are relatively rare. In 2,000 splenoportograms at St. Vincent's Medical Center, there have been

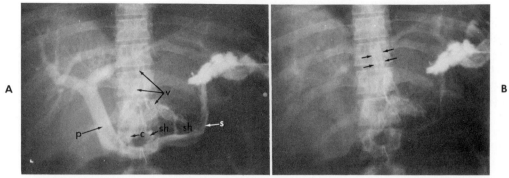

Fig. 53-23. A, Splenoportogram in cirrhotic patient with acute massive gastrointestinal bleeding. **s,** Splenic vein; **p,** portal vein; **c,** coronary vein; **sh,** short gastric vein; **v,** gastric and esophageal varices. **B,** Later phase of same splenoportogram showing leak of contrast medium caused by ruptured varix in lumen of esophagus at arrows. This appearance can usually be differentiated from large or closely approximated varices, since the latter maintain the varicose outline (see Fig. 53-16, *B*) as opposed to the homogenous character of the opacity and outline of the esophageal wall as in the present instance.

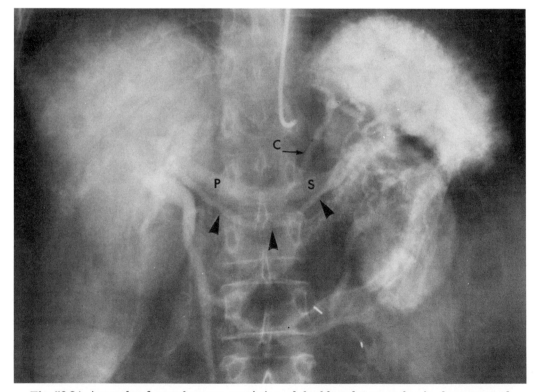

Fig. 53-24. Anomaly of portal system consisting of double splenoportal axis, demonstrated during venous phase of celiac portogram. **c,** Coronary vein; **p,** portal vein; **s,** splenic vein. The anomalous axis (arrowheads) arises from a confluence of short gastric veins and splenic hilar radicles and passes inferiorly to the main splenic and portal veins to enter the liver separately. (From Ruzicka, F. F., and Rossi, P.: Normal vascular anatomy of the abdominal viscera, Radiol. Clin. N. Amer. **8:**3-29, 1970.)

instances of agenesis of the portal vein, cavernomatous transformation of the portal vein, and aneurysm of the portal vein.

Agenesis itself is difficult to establish in any given case, although it probably occurs. The problem of identification lies in the fact that in a child thrombosis of portal vein may occur without an antecedent history suggestive of or compatible with thrombosis. Consequently, when the child is seen only the effects of portal vein obliteration are found. The cause of portal vein absence is thus difficult to prove.

The most plausible explanation for the development of congenital atresia, stricture, or stenosis is that variations in the involutional process that affect the umbilical vein and the ductus venosus extend to involve the entire portal vein or a short segment of it, completely or incompletely. Most cases reported show a local stenosis or atresia of portal vein near the hilum of the liver. In any event, the result is an extrahepatic obstruction that behaves like extrahepatic obstruction from any other cause.

Cavernomatous transformation of the portal vein is sometimes encountered. The true congenital malformation of the portal vein or its major branches, however, is quite rare. One such case showed a normal portal vein that abruptly terminated after 1 to 2 cm. into a racemose angiomatous structure that effectively obstructed the portal vein.[57] Pseudocavernomatous transformation is not infrequently seen as a result of portal vein obstruction from any cause. It consists of a mass of tortuous bridging collaterals that simulate a cavernoma but that represent the result of an attempt to span the defect in the portal vein.

Aneurysm of the portal vein has been seen in this series. It was an incidental finding in a patient with cirrhosis and portal hypertension. At surgery the aneurysm was found to consist of an extremely thin-walled sac about 5 cm. in diameter. Its relationship to the portal hypertension, if any, could not be determined.

There are other rare congenital anomalies of the portal vein.[25,44] The portal vein may lie anterior to the head of the pancreas and the duodenum. A double portal vein may occur (Fig. 53-24). The portal vein may enter into the inferior vena cava; the hepatic artery is then considerably enlarged. Very rarely the total pulmonary venous drainage may empty through a common channel into the portal vein.

Intrahepatic lesions

Portography itself is not the method of choice for demonstration of intrahepatic lesions. Radioisotope scanning and selective hepatic or celiac arteriography (which may be readily made a part of arterial portography) generally constitute a more effective radiologic approach for study of lesions of the liver.

Nevertheless, the portographic method, and in particular splenoportography,[63,64] because it brings more contrast medium in greater concentration to the liver than the venous phase of arterial portography, can provide diagnostic information of certain pathologic changes in the liver. With umbilical portography, in which sinusoids can be literally flooded with contrast medium, nodules as small as 1 cm. can readily be demonstrated in the sinusoidal phase.[31]

Certain information regarding intrahepatic lesions can be derived from portography. Thus, when the extrahepatic portal venous system is being evaluated by any of the techniques of portography, the additional information discovered regarding the liver may be significant for diagnosis, treatment, or prognosis. For example, in a patient with carcinoma of the body or tail of the pancreas, not only obliteration of the splenic vein by the carcinoma but also metastatic deposits in the liver may be demonstrated (Fig. 53-18).

In cirrhosis of the liver the vasculogram phase of portography shows alterations of the intrahepatic portal branches, which vary with the stage of the disease (Figs. 53-14, 53-15, *A*, and 53-16, *B*). In the earlier stages when the liver may be swollen and enlarged, attenuation and spreading of the branches occurs. Later, as the diffuse inflammatory process produces fibrosis and nodular hyperplasia, the larger portal branches become gnarled and distorted and the medium and small-sized branches diminish in number. Tapering of the branches becomes less gradual and is often abrupt. In advanced cirrhosis, when the liver is small and contracted, the deformity of the intrahepatic vasculature is excessive and interlacing of the anastomotic channels may prolong the vasculogram phase beyond its normal range of 2 to 16 seconds. The vasculogram phase is definitely abnormal in 65% of cirrhotic patients and shows changes suggestive of cirrhosis in an additional 20%. Indeed, the positive vasculogram may be the only evidence of cirrhosis in certain cases in which the liver function tests are normal. This is the result of the compensatory capacity of the liver and the fact that the secondary effects of intrahepatic obstruction have not yet become obvious.

The sinusoid phase of splenoportography in cirrhosis generally shows a uniformly diminished density compared to normal, which is caused by the run-off of contrast medium over hepatofugal collaterals and also by shunting via venovenous shunts within the liver itself. One may encounter, however, a mottled density pattern that may vary from moderately coarse to patchy. This appearance is probably related to the degree of fibrosis and nodular hyperplasia within the liver.

Neoplasms or other space-occupying lesions[15,65] produce only flattening and displacement of veins in the vasculogram phase, since the portal vein does not supply them. In the sinusoid phase space-occupying lesions[15,64] appear as radiolucent defects (Fig. 53-18, *B*). Single lesions as small as 1.5 cm. in diameter can, under good conditions, be demonstrated by splenoportography. Lesions as small as 1 cm. in diameter, if they are multiple and form a pattern, may be detected. Thus, whereas the vasculogram phase is more informative for cirrhosis, the sinusoid phase is more helpful in the detection of neoplasm. As already mentioned, umbilical portography provides the clearest sinusoid phase.

A limitation of the splenoportographic examination for evaluation of intrahepatic lesions is the frequent poor opacification of the left lobe.[6] This is not a serious drawback in cirrhosis, which is a diffuse and widespread inflammatory process, but it may be of considerable importance when neoplasm is present only in the left lobe of the liver.

Umbilical portography is more successful in delineation of the left lobe, Even with this technique, because of the usual thinness of the left lobe, detection of lesions may be difficult.

An important differential point to be considered in the evaluation of the vasculogram phase is that in the presence of portal vein obstruction and the development of multiple bridging collaterals to the liver (pseudocavernomatous transformation), the intrahepatic portal branches lack the symmetrical appearance resultive from single trunk origin. Instead, they present a somewhat disorganized arrangement caused by the entry of multiple veins and the anastomotic pattern among portal vein branches.

The vasculogram and sinusoidal phases of the liver that occur during the venous phase following arterial injection are sometimes fairly diagnostic but are generally inferior to the splenic portogram because of dilution. If the studies are of good quality, the same principles of diagnostic interpretation are applied.

REFERENCES

1. Abeatici, S., and Campi, L.: La visualizzazione radiologica della porta per via splenica (nota preventiva), Minerva Med. 1:593, 1951.
2. Amplatz, K.: The catheter needle. In Schobinger, R., and Ruzicka, F. F., Jr., editors: Vascular roentgenology, arteriography, phlebography, lymphography, New York, 1964, The Macmillan Co.
3. Basu, A. K.: Use of splenoportal venography in the diagnosis of extrahepatic venous obstruction, J. Roy. Coll. Surg. Edinb. 4:19, 1958.
4. Bayly, J. H., and Carbalhaes, O. G.: The umbilical vein in the adult: diagnosis, treatment and research, Amer. Surg. 30:56, 1964.
5. Bergstrand, I.: The localization of portal obstruction by splenoportography, Amer. J. Roentgen. 85:1111, 1961.
6. Bergstrand, I.: Splenoportography. In Abrams, H. L., editor: Angiography, Boston, 1961, Little, Brown and Co.
7. Bergstrand, I., and Ekman, C. A.: Lieno-portal venography in the study of portal circulation in the dog, Acta Radiol. (Stockholm) 47:257, 1957.
8. Bergstrand, I., and Ekman, C. A.: Portal circulation in portal hypertension, Acta Radiol. (Stockholm) 47:1, 1957.
9. Bierman, H. R., Kelly, K. H., Coblents, A., and Fischer, A.: Transhepatic venous catheterization and venography, J.A.M.A. 158:1331, 1955.
10. Bierman, H. R., White, L. P., Kelly, K. H., and Steinbach, H. L.: Biochemical and hematological characteristics of blood from the hepatic portal vein in man, J. Appl. Physiol. 5:567, 1953.
11. Blackburn, C. R. B.: The management of portal hypertension with special reference to bleeding esophageal varices, Med. J. Aust. 1:921, 1956.
12. Boyer, J. L., Sen Gupta, K. P., Gismus, S. K., Pal, N. P., Mallick, K. C., Basu, I. F. and Basu, A. K.: Idiopathic portal hypertension, Amer. J. Med. 66:41, 1967.
13. Bron, K. M., Jackson, F. C., Haller, J., Perez-Stable, E., Eisen, H. B., and Poller, S.: The value of selective arteriography in demonstrating portal and splenic vein patency following nonvisualization by splenoportography, Radiology 85:448, 1965.
14. Bruwer, A., and Hallenbeck, G. A.: Roentgenologic findings in splenic portography, Amer. J. Roentgen. 7:324, 1957.
15. Bunnag, T. S., Koaparisuthi, V., Arthachinta, S.,

Chienpradit, K., and Binbakaya L.: Percutaneous splenic portography in amebic liver abscess, Amer. J. Roentgen **80**:324, 1958.

16. Burchell, A. R., Moreno, A. H., Panke, W. F., and Rousselot, L. M.: Some limitations of splenic portography. 1, Incidence, hemodynamics and surgical implications of the nonvisualized portal vein, Ann. Surg. **162**:981, 1965.
17. Butler, H.: Gastro-esophageal haemorrhage in hepatic cirrhosis, Thorax **7**:159, 1952.
18. Butler, H.: Veins of oesophagus, Thorax **6**:276, 1951.
19. Carbalhaes, O. G.: Portography: a preliminary report of a new technique via the umbilical vein, Clin. Proc. Child. Hosp. **15**:120, 1959.
20. Case reports: Mass. Gen. Hosp. No. 40102, New Eng. J. Med. **150**:434, 1954.
21. Child, C. G., Ill., O'Sullivan, W. D., Payne, M. A., and McClure, R. D., Jr.: Portal venography, preliminary report, Radiology **57**:691, 1951.
22. Doehner, G. A., Ruzicka, F. F., Jr., Rousselot, L. M., and Hoffman, G.: The portal venous system: on its pathological roentgen anatomy, Radiology **66**:206, 1956.
23. Douglas, B. E., Baggenstoss, A. H., and Hollinshead, W. H.: The anatomy of the portal vein and its tributaries, Surg. Gynec. Obstet. **9**:562, 1950.
24. Edwards, E. A.: Functional anatomy of the portal systemic communications, Arch. Intern. Med. **88**:137, 1951.
25. Gilfillan, R. S.: Anatomic study of the portal vein and its main branches, Arch. Surg. (Chicago) **61**:449, 1950.
26. Hunt, A. H., and Whittard, B. R.: Thrombosis of the portal vein in cirrhosis hepatitis, Lancet **1**:281, 1954.
27. Kahn, P. C., O'Halloran, J. F., and Paul, R. E.: Improved portography by delayed post-epinephrine celiac and mesenteric arteriography, **92**:86, 1969.
28. Jacobsson, B., and Schlossman, D.: Thromboembolism of leg following percutaneous catheterization of femoral artery for angiography, Acta Radiol. **8**:109, 1969.
29. Learmouth, J. R., and MacPherson, A. J. S.: Surgery of portal hypertension: an account of 16 cases, Lancet **2**:882, 1948.
30. Leevey, C., and Gliedman, M.: Practical and research value of hepatic vein catheterization, New Eng. J. Med. **258**:696, 1958.
31. Legare, A.: Personal communication.
32. Leger, L.: Indications, contraindications, limitations: portal phlebography. In Schobinger, R., and Ruzicka, F. F., Jr., editors: Vascular roentgenology, arteriography, phlebography, lymphography. New York, 1964, The Macmillan Co.
33. Leger, L.: La phlebographie portale par injection splenique intraparenchymatunse, Mem. Acad. Chir. (Paris) **77**:712, 1951.
34. LeMaire, A., and Housset, E.: La Mesure de la pression portale par punction du Foie, Presse Med. **63**:1063, 1955.
35. Lepore, M. J.: Personal communication.

36. Levy, J. S., Hardin, J. H., Schipp, H., and Kelling, J. H.: Varices of the cecum as an unusual cause of gastrointestinal bleeding, Gastroenterology **33**:637, 1957.
37. Liebowitz, H. R.: Bleeding esophageal varices: portal hypertension, Springfield, Ill., 1959, Charles C Thomas, Publisher.
38. McDermott, W. J., Jr.: Portal hypertension secondary to pancreatic disease, Ann. Surg. **152**:147, 1960.
39. McMichael, J.: The pathology of hepato-lineal fibrosis, J. Path. Bact. **39**:481, 1934.
40. Mikkelsen, M. P., Edmundson, H. A., Peters, R. L., Redeker, A. G., and Reynolds, T. B.: Extra-Intrahepatic portal hypertension without cirrhosis (hepatoportal sclerosis), Amer. Surg. **162**:602, 1965.
41. Moreno, A. H., Ruzicka, F. F., Jr., Rousselot, L. M., Burchell, A. R., Bono, R. F., Slafsky, S. F., and Burke, J. H.: Functional hepatography: a study of the hemodynamics of the outflow tracts of the human liver by intraparenchymal deposition of contrast medium, with attempts at functional evaluation of the outflow block concept of cirrhotic ascites and the accessory outflow role of the portal vein, Radiology **81**:65, 1963.
42. Morton, J. H., and Whalen, T. J.: Esophageal varices without portal hypertension, Surgery **36**:1135, 1954.
43. Nebesar, R. A., and Pollard, J. J.: Portal venography by selective arterial catheterization, Amer. J. Roentgen. **97**:477, 1966.
44. Netter, F. H.: The Ciba collection of medical illustrations, Summit, N. J. 1957, Ciba Pharmaceutical Products, Inc.
45. Odman, P.: Percutaneous selective angiography of the celiac artery, Acta Radiol. (Supp. 159), 1958.
46. Orrego-Matte, H., Amenabar, E., Lara, G., Barona, E., Palma, R., and Massad, F.: Measurement of intrahepatic pressure as index of portal pressure, Amer. J. Med. **247**:278, 1964.
47. Palmer, E. D., and Brick, I. B. Varices of distal esophagus without portal hypertension, Amer. J. Med. Sci. **230**:515, 1955.
48. Panke, W., Bradley, E. G., Moreno, A. H., Ruzicka, F. F., Jr., and Rousselot, L. M.: Techniques, hazards and usefulness of percutaneous splenic portography, J.A.M.A. **169**:1032, 1959.
49. Perchik, L., and Max, T. C.: Massive hemorrhage from varices of the duodenal loop in a cirrhotic patient. Radiology **80**:641, 1963.
50. de Sousa Pereira, A.: La méthode phlébographique dans l'étude des troubles de la circulation de systeme porte, Communications of the I World Congress of Cardiology, Paris, 1950, vol. 13, Paris, 1952, J. B. Bailliere and Sons.
51. Pick, L.: Ueber totale haemangiomatose obliteration des Pfortaderstammes und ueber hepatopetale Kollateralbahnen, Virchow. Arch. Path. Anat. **197**:490, 1909.
52. Ramsey, G. C., and Britton, R. C.: Intraparenchymal angiography in the diagnosis of hepatic veno-occlusive diseases, Radiology **90**:716, 1968.
53. Redman, H., and Reuter, S. R.: Angiographic dem-

onstration of portacaval and other decompressive liver shunts, Radiology **92**:778, 1969.

54. Resh, I., Bret, I., and Khirurygal, L. M.: Transportal splenoportography in the diagnosis of epigastric tumors, J. Roy. Coll. Surg. Edinb. **35**:10, 1959.

55. Reynold, T., Redeker, A., and Geller, H.: Wedged hepatic venous pressure, Amer. J. Med. **22**:341, 1957.

56. Roberti, G., D'Agnolo, B., Servello, M., and others: L'onfaloportografia: un nuovo mezzo di indagine del sistema portale, Minerva Med. **56**:334, 1965.

57. Rosch, J.: Splenoportography in childhood, Fortschr. Rontgenstr. **96**:61, 1962.

58. Rousselot, L. M., and Burchell, A. R.: Portal venography and manometry. In Schiff, L., II, editor: Diseases of the liver, Philadelphia, 1963, J. B. Lippincott Co.

59. Rousselot, L. M., Moreno, A. R., and Panke, W. F.: Studies on portal hypertension IV. The clinical and physiopathologic significance of self-established (non-surgical) portal systemic venous shunts, Ann. Surg. **150**:384, 1959.

60. Rousselot, L. M., Ruzicka, F. F., Jr., and Doehner, G. A.: Portography in portal hypertension: its application in diagnosis and surgical planning, Surg. Clin. N. Amer. **36**:361, 1956.

61. Ruzicka, F. F., Jr.: Radiologic methods in liver disease. In Popper, H., and Schaffner, F., editors: Progress in liver disease, vol. 2, New York, 1965, Grune & Stratton, Inc.

62. Ruzicka, F. F., Jr.: Technique (percutaneous splenoportography). In Schobinger, R., and Ruzicka, F. F., Jr., editors: Vascular roentgenology: arteriography, phlebography, lymphography, New York, 1964, The Macmillan Co.

63. Ruzicka, F. F., Jr., Bradley, E. G., and Rousselot, L. M.: The intrahepatic vasculogram and hepatogram in cirrhosis following percutaneous splenic injection, Radiology **71**:175, 1958.

64. Ruzicka, F. F., Jr., Bradley, E. G., and Rousselot, L. M.: Two-phase opacification of the liver in cirrhosis, Ann. N. Y. Acad. Sci. **78**:819, 1959.

65. Ruzicka, F. F., Jr., Gould, H. R., Bradley, E. G., and Rousselot, L. M.: Value of splenic portography in the diagnosis of intrahepatic and extrahepatic neoplasm, Amer. J. Med. **29**:434 1960.

66. Ruzicka, F. F., Jr., Carillo, F. J., D'Alessandro, D., and Rossi, P.: The hepatic wedge pressure and venogram and the intraparenchymal liver pressure and venogram: a comparative study, Radiology. In press.

67. Ruzicka, F. F., Jr., and Rossi, P.: Arterial portography: patterns of venous flow, Radiology **92**:777, 1969.

68. Ruzicka, F. F., Jr., and Rossi, P.: The hepatic circulation and portal hypertension: radiologic evaluation, Ann. N. Y. Acad. Sci. **170**:148, 1970.

69. Sappey, C.: Memoir sur les veines portes accessoires, J. de l'anat. et physiol. (Paris) **19**:517, 1883.

70. Seldinger, S. I.: A simple method of catheterization of the spleen and liver, Acta Radiol. (Stockholm) **48**:93, 1957.

71. Seldinger, S. I.: Catheter replacement of the needle in percutaneous arteriography, Acta Radiol. **39**:368, 1953.

72. Steckel, R. J., and Grottman, J. H., Jr.: Pharmacologic enhancement in selective visceral angiography, editorial, Radiology **91**:583, 1968.

73. Steiner, R. E., Sherlock, S., and Turner, M.: Percutaneous splenic portal portography, J. Fac. Radiol. **8**:185, 1957.

74. Tisdale, W. A., Klatskin, G., and Glenn, W. W. L.: Portal hypertension and bleeding esophageal varices: their occurrence in the absence of both intrahepatic and extrahepatic obstruction of the portal vein, New Eng. J. Med. **261**:109, 1959.

75. VanHeertum, R. L., Cioffi, C. M., and Ruzicka, F. F., Jr.: The use of alpha blocking and beta stimulating drugs in combination to improve opacification of the portal venous system, Radiology **100**:679-682, 1971.

76. Viallet, A., Legare, A., and Lavoie, P.: Hepatic and umbilicoportal catheterization in portal hypertension, Ann. N. Y. Acad. Sci. **170**:177, 1970.

77. Varriale, P., Bonanno, C. A., and Grace, W. J.: Portal hypertension secondary to pancreatic pseudocysts, Arch. Intern. Med. **112**:191, 1963.

78. Vennes, J.: Intrahepatic pressure: an accurate reflection of portal pressure, Medicine **45**:445, 1966.

79. Vennes, J.: Transhepatic pressure measurements, Ann. N. Y. Acad. Sci. **170**:193, 1970.

80. Viamonte, M. Jr., Warren, W. D., and Fomon, J. J.: Liver angiography in the assessment of portal hypertension in liver cirrhosis, Radiol. Clin. N. Amer. **1**:147, 1970.

81. Viamonte, M., Jr., Donner, P., Warren, W. D., and Fomon, J.: A new technique for the assessment of hyperkinetic portal hypertension, Radiology **96**:539, 1970.

82. Wheeler, H. B., and Warren, R.: Duodenal varices due to portal hypertension from arterio-venous aneurysm, Ann. Surg. **146**:229, 1957.

83. Whipple, A. O.: The problem of portal hypertension in relation to the hepatosplenopathies, Ann. Surg. **122**:449, 1945.

Arteriography of the alimentary tract | 54

Mordecai Halpern

Modern selective arteriography of the alimentary tract adds a new parameter to the study of diseases of the abdominal viscera.* Its purpose is to complement routine clinical, laboratory, and roentgenographic examinations in order that the most thorough and accurate evaluation of patients may be obtained prior to the institution of therapy. Alimentary arteriography yields detailed study of vascular anatomy and pathology in vivo. This information is subjected to critical appraisal in serving its prime purposes: (1) to improve the accuracy of diagnosis and (2) to demonstrate vascular anatomy and variant normal anatomy.

Arteriographic examination can be applied to a wide range of diseases of the gastrointestinal tract to derive valuable information that is not obtainable in any other way. Maximum benefit is derived when the study is directed toward specific problems. The indiscriminate use of this procedure produces little information that is of either academic or practical value. Angiographic investigations have greatly broadened the knowledge of pathologic vascular anatomy and provided significant advances in the understanding of various disease states. It is this knowledge that is to be applied to practical diagnosis. The following general outline, encompassing the full scope of alimentary arteriography, serves as a guide to the indications for its performance:

1. Demonstration of vascular anatomy (Preoperative knowledge of the nature and extent of anatomic disturbances is valuable to the surgeon.)
2. Diagnosis of vascular diseases of the alimentary tract, including aneurysms and arteriovenous fistulas
3. Demonstration of the splenoportal venous system
4. Diagnostic study of abdominal mass lesions
5. Angiographic diagnosis of specific lesions

*See references 2, 13, 14, 19, 45, and 49.

PERCUTANEOUS CATHETER REPLACEMENT TECHNIQUE

NORMAL ROENTGENOGRAPHIC ANATOMY

DIAGNOSTIC ROENTGENOGRAPHIC CRITERIA

PATHOLOGIC ANATOMY
The liver
The spleen
The pancreas
The stomach
The intestines

PRIMARY VASCULAR DISEASE OF THE ALIMENTARY TRACT

ABDOMINAL MASS LESIONS

CONCLUSIONS

of various abdominal organs (primary liver carcinoma, islet cell tumor of the pancreas, carcinoid tumors of the bowel, visceral trauma)
6. Academic angiographic investigation to ensure the accuracy and validity of observations made

PERCUTANEOUS CATHETER REPLACEMENT TECHNIQUE

The percutaneous catheter replacement technique of selective arteriography is the basic method for accurate demonstration of the vascular anatomy and pathology of the abdominal viscera in vivo.[50,63] The femoral artery is the preferred site of entrance into the arterial system, since it provides the shortest and simplest path for the catheter to the orifices of the three important branch arteries of the aorta: the celiac axis (Fig. 54-1), the superior mesenteric artery (Fig. 54-2), and the inferior mesenteric artery (Fig. 54-3). The insertion of two catheters for simultaneous opacification of the celiac axis and the superior mesenteric artery has been em-

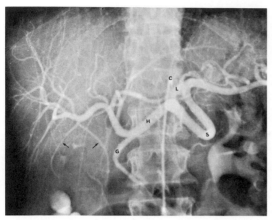

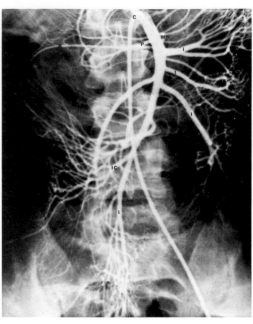

Fig. 54-1. Selective celiac arteriogram in acute chole-cystitis. **C,** Catheter in orifice of celiac axis; **S,** splenic artery; **H,** common hepatic artery; **L,** left gastric artery; **G,** gastroduodenal artery. Observe the abnormal blood flow resulting in nonopacification of the distal portion of this artery and its branch vessels. Delayed filling showed normal structure. It is difficult to positively es-tablish the cause of this hemodynamic alteration. The arrows point to cystic artery branches that are bowed and slightly dilated. The diagnosis of emphysematous cholecystitis was established at operation.

Fig. 54-2. Normal selective superior mesenteric arterio-gram. **C,** Catheter in orifice of superior mesenteric ar-tery; **M,** middle colic artery; **R,** right branch of middle colic artery; **P,** inferior pancreaticoduodenal artery; **I,** intestinal branches; **IC,** ileocolic artery.

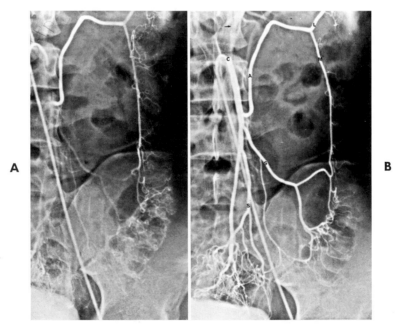

Fig. 54-3. Normal selective inferior mesenteric arteriogram. Arterial phase (**A,** early; **B,** late). *C,* Catheter in inferior mesenteric artery; *A,* left colic branch; *S* sigmoid branches; *M,* part of marginal artery of Drummond; *L,* segment of left colic branch, which anastomoses with left branch of the middle colic artery in the region of the splenic flexure of the colon. Arrow indicates a small amount of reflux into the superior mesenteric artery, which has occurred through the anastomotic branch.

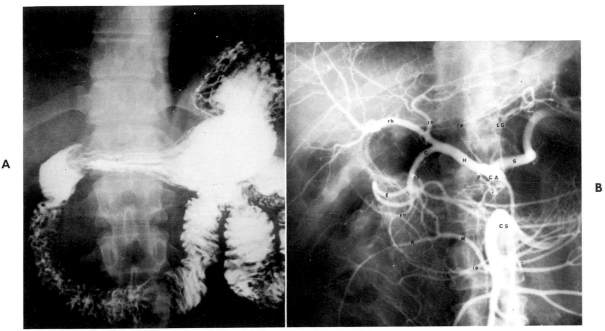

Fig. 54-4. Double catheter visceral arteriography (hepatitis). **A,** Gastrointestinal series—patient had jaundice of obscure cause. **B,** Visceral arteriogram: *CA,* catheter in orifice of celiac axis; *CS,* catheter in orifice of superior mesenteric artery. Branches derived from celiac axis: *LG,* left gastric artery; *S,* splenic artery; *H,* common hepatic artery; *G,* gastroduodenal artery; *E,* right gastroepiploic artery; *rg,* right gastric artery; *rh,* right hepatic artery; *lh,* left hepatic artery; *P,* dorsal pancreatic artery; *sp,* superior pancreaticoduodenal artery. Branches derived from superior mesenteric artery: *M,* middle colic artery; *R,* right branch of middle colic artery; *L,* left branch of middle colic artery; *p,* inferior pancreaticoduodenal artery. Observe the slight spreading and attenuation of the intrahepatic branch arteries. The diagnosis of hepatitis was established by repeat laboratory studies and full recovery of the patient on conservative therapy. (Courtesy Department of Radiology, The New York Hospital—Cornell Medical Center.)

ployed for complete visualization of the blood supply to the pancreas (Figs. 54-14, 54-26, 54-28, and 54-32). Visualization of both the superior pancreaticoduodenal artery, arising from the gastroduodenal branch of the hepatic artery, and the inferior pancreaticoduodenal artery, arising as a branch of the superior mesenteric artery, is necessary for complete visualization of the pancreatic arterial supply. The origin of either a minor or a major right hepatic artery from the superior mesenteric artery is a frequent variation in the hepatic arterial supply (Figs. 54-5 and 54-18). Double catheter hepatic arteriography may be employed in such situations. For this purpose, cannulization of both femoral arteries is preferred, though the two catheters may be inserted through one femoral artery. It should be emphasized

that simple abdominal aortography may be an indispensable part of the complete vascular study (Fig. 54-25).

An automatic pressure injector adjusted to deliver contrast medium (75% sodium diatrizoate) at a flow rate of 12 to 15 ml. per second provides excellent opacification of the arterial system. The amount of contrast medium per catheter varies between 25 and 50 ml., depending in part on the estimated size and pathologic state of the vascular bed. Larger amounts properly delivered seem to result in superior diagnostic studies. A **Y** connector permits halving of the total dose for double catheter examination.

Seriographic filming is necessary in angiographic studies of the abdominal viscera. Finely detailed, high contrast roentgenographs that

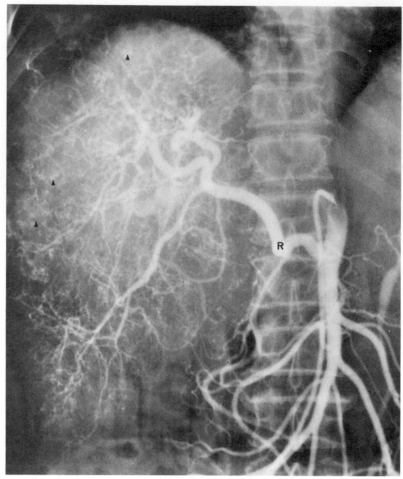

Fig. 54-5. Superior mesenteric arteriogram, showing replaced right hepatic artery and **primary hepatoma. The** right hepatic artery, **R,** arises in the first branch of the superior mesenteric artery. Irregular tumor vessels are present throughout the enlarged right lobe of the liver. Patchy areas of tumor stain are scattered about the periphery (arrowheads).

Fig. 54-6. Hepatic arteriogram of a primary hepatoma. **A,** Gastrointestinal series, anteroposterior projection. Arrowheads show displacement and narrowing of second portion of the duodenum. **B,** Gastrointestinal series, lateral projection. Line identifies anterior margin of lumbar spine. Arrowheads show marked degree of anterior displacement of the duodenum. **C,** Arteriogram, anteroposterior projection. *C,* Catheter in celiac axis; *S,* catheter in superior mesenteric artery (not employed during this phase of the examination); *AH,* accessory right hepatic artery; *R,* right hepatic artery displaced by tumor mass. Arrows point to some of the innumerable pathologic vessels which produce tumor stain. **D,** Arteriogram, lateral projection. *C,* Catheter in celiac axis; *S,* catheter in superior mesenteric artery; *AH,* accessory hepatic artery arising from the superior mesenteric artery; *R,* right hepatic artery. Note the degree of posterior displacement. Selective arteriogram of accessory hepatic artery arterial, *E,* and capillary, *F,* phases demonstrate pathologic vessels and tumor stain. Arteriogram performed by directing catheter in the superior mesenteric artery into the orifice of the accessory hepatic artery. NOTE: This tumor was associated with severe hypoglycemia. Diagnosis was confirmed through open biopsy of the liver.

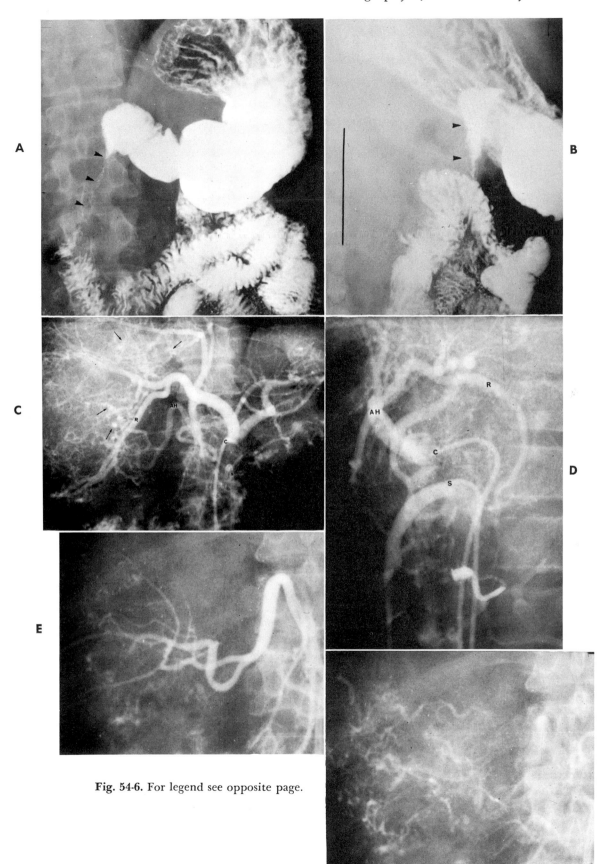

Fig. 54-6. For legend see opposite page.

cover the arterial, capillary, and venous phases of such studies must be obtained. A basic programming consists of four films per second for 3 seconds, one film per second for 3 seconds, and then one film every other second for 14 seconds. A 20-second time interval can be filmed with a total of twenty-two roentgenographs in this fashion.

The anteroposterior position is basic and is supplemented by a right prone oblique study for hepatic and pancreatic arteriography. Lateral projections are employed, when indicated, as a separate examination or as part of a biplane anteroposterior-lateral study. Through the simple expedient of gaseous distention of the stomach, the recognition of arterial anatomy is eased (Figs. 54-23, 54-24, 54-41, and 54-42). Similarly, an air-filled colon at the time of arteriography is an asset to its study.

More recently gastric distention has been accomplished by ingestion of 240 ml. of liquid nutrient supplement by the patient about 5 to 10 minutes prior to the filming procedure. This has been well tolerated. The arterial dilatation produced enhances the quality of the angiogram (Fig. 54-45). Marked improvement in the demonstration of the arterial supply to the stomach and its venous drainage has benefited gastric arteriography.[15] A preliminary injection of 15 ml. of contrast medium into the celiac catheter has also been effectively used to create vasodilatation.

The common hepatic and splenic arteries are often accessible to selective catheterization by the original catheter (Figs. 54-41 and 54-57), but selective study of the dorsal pancreatic, the gastroduodenal, and similar vessels usually requires a more elaborate catheter manipulation (Fig. 54-28). When selective examination of such branch vessels of the major arterial trunks may be expected to add valuable arteriographic information, a catheter may be directed through the lumen of the original diagnostic catheter, passing beyond its tip so that it can be guided into the major arterial channel and then directed to the orifice of the branch artery (Fig. 54-6, *E* and *F*).

Superselective arteriography is now more often used to delineate additional detail of a specific vascular bed. For this purpose the original catheter is replaced by a selected preformed catheter that is manipulatd into the

artery to be studied (Figs. 54-22, 54-28, and 54-36). In superselective studies the quantity of contrast is reduced in proportion to the vessel size, and flow rate is decreased to 2 to 4 ml. per second. While the potential value of the superselective arteriogram is considerable, it is accomplished in a limited number of instances and the total time for the angiographic evaluation of the patient may be significantly prolonged.

When conditions warrant, the axillary artery can be used as a secondary but convenient point of access into the arterial system (Fig. 54-56). It is generally preferable to the brachial artery for visceral angiography. The optimum shape of a preformed selective catheter is determined by the anatomic vascular relationship, the chosen site of puncture, and the prime organ of interest. The addition of ancillary pharmacophysiologic devices to enhance the detailed roentgenographic visualization of various organs is under investigation. The results have been disappointing. Magnification arteriography has also not significantly improved the diagnostic detail of the visceral angiogram. It is quite impossible at this time to assess the potential diagnostic value of combining angiography with isotope scanning techniques.

NORMAL ROENTGENOGRAPHIC ANATOMY

The interpretation and production of visceral arteriograms requires a thorough knowledge of normal and variant anatomy. Recognition of the fact that in vivo arteriographic anatomy may have important differences from classic postmortem study is equally important. Reference to standard anatomy texts should be supplemented by detailed works that have evolved from investigations of arteriographic anatomy.[40,42]

The celiac axis arises from the anterior aspect of the aorta, usualy at the level of the twelfth thoracic vertebra. Its length varies between 1 and 2.5 cm., and its normal luminal diameter approaches 10 mm. The angle of juncture of the celiac trunk with the aorta is approximately a 120-degree obtuse angle when approached in an antegrade manner or is an acute angle of about 60 degrees when catheter arteriography is performed as a retrograde transfemoral study. Trifurcation of this vessel gives origin to the common hepatic, splenic, and left gastric arteries. Variations are not uncommon in the main trunk and may consist of absence of one or more of the branches. An independent origin of the common hepatic artery, or its origin, wholly or in part, from the superior mesenteric artery has obvious technical significance. A common origin of the entire celiac and superior mesenteric trunks is also seen occasionally. Absence of the tripod of Haller with separate orifices for the gastric, hepatic, and splenic arteries is an unusual anatomic variant (Fig. 54-37).

The splenic artery is large and commonly tortuous in its course toward the left, paralleling the superior aspect of the pancreas. Its pancreatic branches are an important supply to the body and tail of this organ. The pancreatica magna artery and the caudal pancreatic artery may be visualized as prominent vessels supplying the body and tail of the pancreas. The dorsal pancreatic artery is a short vessel that usually takes origin from the proximal portion of the splenic artery, though in 14% of cases it comes from the superior mesenteric trunk and may arise from the hepatic artery. It has a straight caudad course to the pancreas, where it produces the transverse pancreatic artery and a branch toward the head of the pancreas. Direct anastomosis between elements of the pancreatic blood supply are common. Additional significant branches of the splenic artery are the short gastric vessels and the left gastroepiploic artery to the stomach and the posterior epiploic arteries to the mesentery and retroperitoneal space.

The common hepatic artery is a long arterial trunk that characteristically divides into the left and right hepatic arteries after giving origin to the gastroduodenal artery. The cystic artery and the right gastric artery are branches of it that are somewhat inconsistently seen. Opacification of the latter artery is increased fourfold by use of nutrient supplement prior to gastric arteriography.[15] The gastroduodenal artery gives branches to the descending duodenum, produces the important superior pancreaticoduodenal arteries, and terminates as the right gastroepiploic vessel.

The superior mesenteric artery has a level of origin related to the twelfth thoracic interspace and the upper third of the body the first lumbar vertebra. Like the celiac axis, it has an acute angle of juncture with the aorta. Its luminal diameter is slightly smaller. Origin of some portion of the right hepatic arterial supply may be expected to come from the superior mesenteric artery about 26% of the time (Figs. 54-5 and 54-18). The origin of the dorsal pancreatic artery as a branch has been mentioned. The inferior pancreaticoduodenal artery is a constant branch, occasionally appearing as a double trunk. The remaining divisions of the superior mesenteric artery are small bowel branches, the middle colic, the right colic, and the ileocolic vessels. The open anastomosis between the celiac axis and the superior mesenteric artery by way of the gastroduodenal vessel is important. The potential colic anastomosis through the middle colic artery to the inferior mesenteric artery is also of considerable significance.

The inferior mesenteric artery is a much smaller vessel arising at the level of the third lumbar vertebra in 80% of cases (Fig. 54-3). Its major divisions are the sigmoid and hemorrhoidal vessels and the superior left colic artery, which courses toward the splenic flexure of the colon to anastomose with the left branch of the middle colic artery to complete this portion of the marginal artery of Drummond. There is a second anastomosis between the middle colic vessel of the superior mesenteric artery and the superior left colic vessel of the inferior mesenteric artery through the arch of Riolan.

These simple facts of vascular anatomy determine the manner of arteriographic investigation, the preferred site of entry into the arterial system, and the shape of the catheter that is molded in advance to make selective catheterization of the arterial trunk possible. All of the features of the technique of visceral arteriography have been devised to produce complete and accurate reproduction of the vascular anatomy that can be critically analyzed for diagnostic purposes.

DIAGNOSTIC ROENTGENOGRAPHIC CRITERIA

The vascular alterations that are studied in the interpretation of visceral arteriograms are those common to all forms of arteriography. They are as follows:

1. Displacement of vessels (Figs. 54-6, *C,* 54-7, 54-20, and 54-29)
2. Distortion of vessels, that is, pathologic vessels and inflammatory and tumor neo-

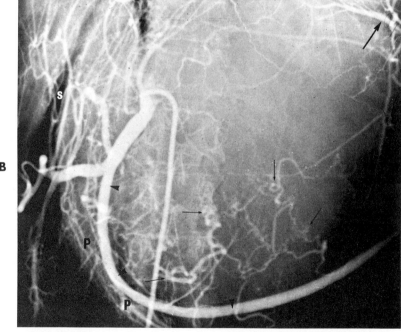

Fig. 54-7. Celiac arteriogram showing displacement of splenic artery caused by adrenal carcinoma. **A,** Gastrointestinal series, lateral projection. There is marked posterior displacement of the stomach. The viscus was also displaced to the right. **B,** Arteriogram. **S,** Displaced and compressed stomach; **P,** displaced pancreas. Large arrow points to displaced spleen. Small arrows point to pathologic vessels. Arrowheads point to displaced and stretched splenic artery. NOTE: Suprarenal arteries were not defined at the time of aortography. The tumor was totally extirpated. (Courtesy Department of Radiology, The New York Hospital—Cornell Medical Center.)

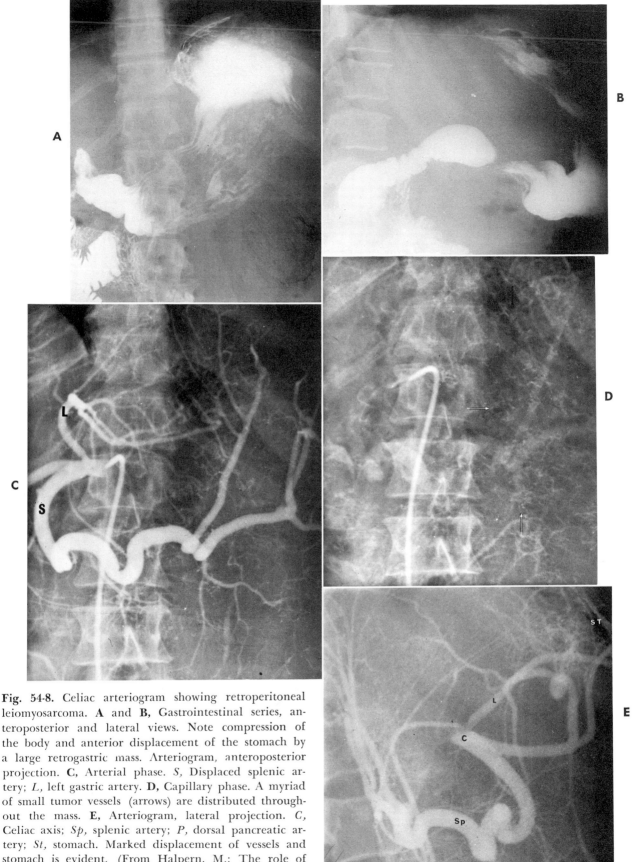

Fig. 54-8. Celiac arteriogram showing retroperitoneal leiomyosarcoma. **A** and **B,** Gastrointestinal series, anteroposterior and lateral views. Note compression of the body and anterior displacement of the stomach by a large retrogastric mass. Arteriogram, anteroposterior projection. **C,** Arterial phase. *S,* Displaced splenic artery; *L,* left gastric artery. **D,** Capillary phase. A myriad of small tumor vessels (arrows) are distributed throughout the mass. **E,** Arteriogram, lateral projection. *C,* Celiac axis; *Sp,* splenic artery; *P,* dorsal pancreatic artery; *St,* stomach. Marked displacement of vessels and stomach is evident. (From Halpern, M.: The role of angiography in diagnosis of cancer. In Recent advances in the diagnosis of cancer, Chicago, 1966, Year Book Medical Publishers, Inc.)

vascularization (Figs. 54-5, 54-8, 54-10, and 54-44)

3. Tissue staining (Figs. 54-17, 54-44, and 54-48)

4. Abrupt termination of vessels because of inflammatory or neoplastic obstruction or thrombosis (Figs. 54-14 and 54-42)

5. Arteriovenous shunting and disturbances of normal hemodynamics (Figs. 54-9, 54-10, and 54-21)

Intrinsic vascular disease results in varying degrees of irregularity of the lumina of vessels, occlusion, and secondary mural changes such as aneurysm and stenosis. Perforation may be demonstrated through extravasation of contrast material (Fig. 54-43). Areas of necrosis, cyst, or abscess are revealed as generally well-demarcated areas of decreased tissue density associated with the displacement of vessels around the area (Figs. 54-18 and 54-20).

Diagnostic restrictions result from the technical inability to define vessels of small caliber as distinct structures. Few malignant lesions of the intestinal tract are vascular, so that diagnosis often rests upon the indirect features of displacement and thrombosis rather than being made by visualizing the intrinsic vascular character of the tumor. The fact that there is frequently no vivid line of separation between inflammatory changes and tumor alterations also presents a diagnostic dilemma, and, of course, the two pathologic conditions may coexist to present an almost insurmountable problem.

PATHOLOGIC ANATOMY
The liver
Neoplasms

Primary and secondary neoplasms of the liver produce displacement and deformity of the intrahepatic vasculature (Figs. 54-5, 54-6, and 54-10). The disordered patterns characteristic of malignancy appear to involve larger branches and to be more prominent in hepatoma than in secondary metastases. Primary hepatoma usually demonstrates a moderate to high degree of neovascularity. The pathologic tumor vessels are ectatic and disordered. Pooling of contrast medium within the abnormal vascular bed is common (Fig. 54-10). The tumor tends to invade the portal venous system directly, permitting angiographic visualization of these venous radicles in time sequence different from that present in

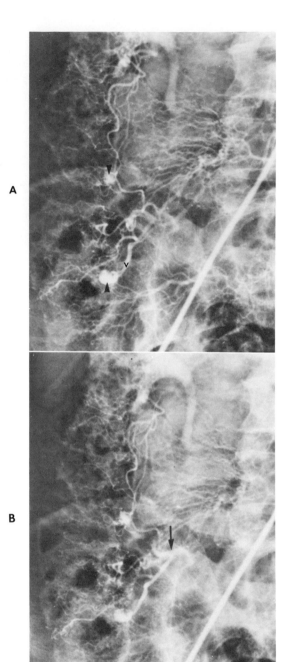

Fig. 54-9. Superior mesenteric angiogram showing arteriovenous fistulas of the right colon. The diagnosis is hereditary hemorrhagic telangiectasia. **A**, Arterial phase. Two conglomerate masses of angiectasis are present (arrowheads). The lower lesion is close to the ileocecal valve. Early opacification of the draining vein is present, **v. B,** Late arterial-capillary phase. There is early, dense opacification of a dilated ileocolic vein (arrow). (From Halpern, M., Turner, A. F., and Citron, B. P.: Hereditary hemorrhagic telangiectasia, an angiographic study of abdominal visceral angiodysplasias associated with gastrointestinal hemorrhage, Radiology **90:**1143, 1968.)

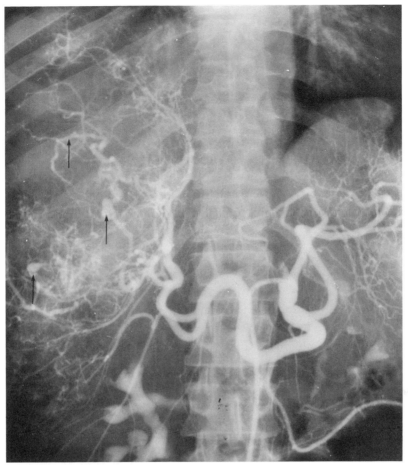

Fig. 54-10. Celiac arteriogram of a primary hepatoma. There is displacement of the major intrahepatic arterial branches that ramify into pathologic tumor vessels. These have an erratic course through the liver. Large, ectatic channels are readily recognizable (arrows).

the normal celiac angiogram. In metastases a peripheral blood supply of the metastatic focus, with central necrosis of the lesion, is common. Such globular masses of tumor tissue may be well defined during the capillary and venous phases (Fig. 54-11). The diagnostic limitations are distracting. Small lesions may not be recognizable, either because they do not produce sufficient vascular change or because the minimal alterations produced are beyond the acuity of our interpretation. The opposite extreme can also present a problem. Diffuse invasion of the liver by a tumor may cause so much necrosis and tissue reaction that visible abnormal vessels and tumor staining are not manifest and the resultant vessel displacements appear throughout the substance of the liver without presenting

recognizable contrast with normal areas (Fig. 54-12). The correct diagnosis can be easily overlooked in these circumstances. Certainly neoplasia is the most important lesion to be accurately diagnosed. The ultimate role of hepatic arteriography will be determined by the degree of improved diagnostic accuracy that will result from future technologic advances and an increase in knowledge, experience, and observer accuracy.

Abscesses

Abscesses of the liver are readily detectable on arteriograms. Such cavities are demarcated as well-defined areas of decreased radiodensity. The intrahepatic arteries and veins are displaced

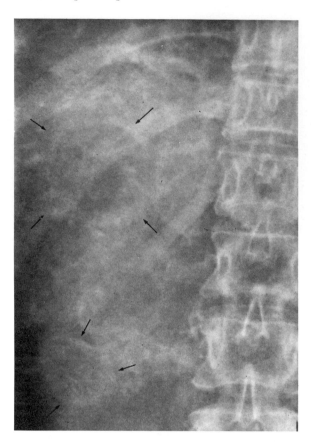

Fig. 54-11. Hepatic arteriogram of a liver metastases. The hepatogram (capillary phase of arteriogram) is distorted by nodules of tumor tissue. Arrows outline the necrotic lucent centers. (Courtesy Department of Radiology, The New York Hospital–Cornell Medical Center.)

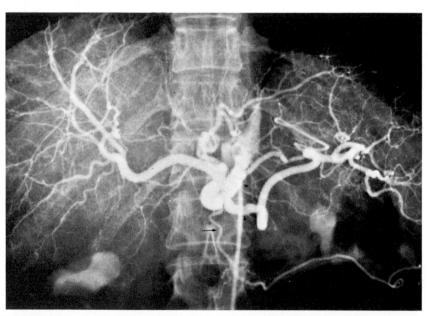

Fig. 54-12. Hepatic arteriogram of diffuse metastases. The liver was diffusely involved by metastatic carcinoma, yet no significant vascular displacements are present in the right lobe of the liver. Observe the avascularity of the medial portion of the left lobe. The gastroduodenal artery (arrow) is displaced toward the left and is small. Slight contour irregularities (arrowheads) in the celiac axis and proximal splenic artery are present.

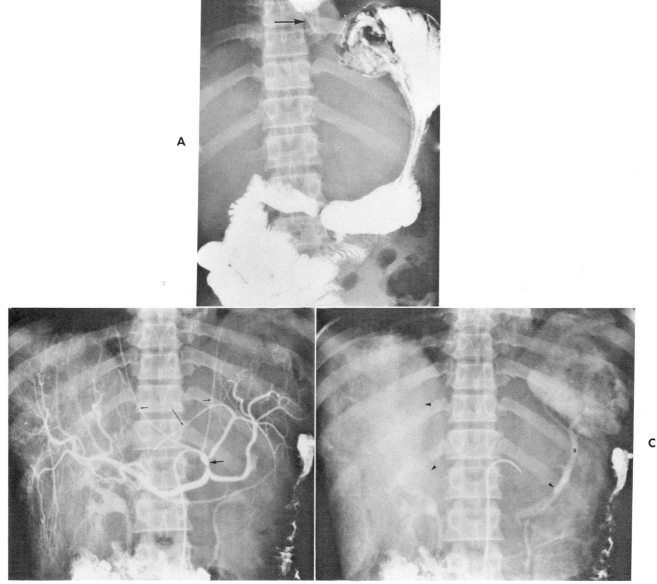

Fig. 54-13. Celiac angiogram of an amebic abscess in the left lobe of the liver. **A,** Gastrointestinal series. Lateral displacement of the stomach and mass imprint on the lesser curvature are present. Note the partial obstruction at the distal end of the esophagus (arrow). **B,** Arterial phase. Stretching and displacement of branches of the celiac axis, which is displaced (large arrow; note segmental narrowing caused by catheter spasm) involves the inferior phrenic arteries (short, thin arrows). A replaced left hepatic artery (long, thin arrow) is also stretched and shows smooth segmental narrowing caused by surrounding inflammation. **C,** Venous phase. The margins of the avascular abscess (arrowheads) are readily visible. Displacement and narrowing of the splenic vein is present, **s.**

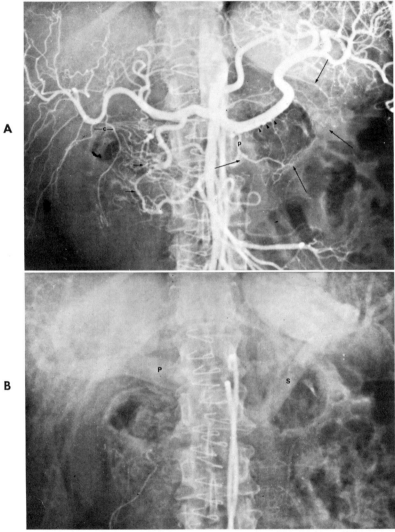

Fig. 54-14. Pancreatic arteriogram showing pancreatitis (double catheter arteriography). **A,** Arterial phase. *C,* Cystic artery branches; *P,* dorsal pancreatic artery. Long arrows demarcate the area of the body and tail of the pancreas. The walls of the vessels in this area show irregular contour deformities. There are abrupt terminations of some vessels, probably caused by inflammatory thrombosis. Short arrows point to some vascular deformities in the region of the head of the pancreas. This may, in part, be an effect of prior surgery for pancreatic pseudocyst. Arrowheads indicate irregularities of the wall of the splenic artery secondary to the inflammatory process. Observe the slight coiling of the intrahepatic branches. This finding is consistent with a diagnosis of early cirrhosis. **B,** Venous phase. *P,* Portal vein; *S,* splenic vein. The two catheters are readily visible. The upper one lies in the celiac axis, the lower in the superior mesenteric artery.

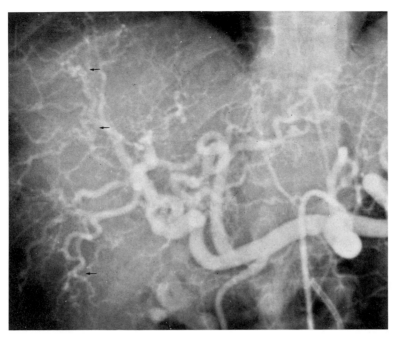

Fig. 54-15. Hepatic arteriogram showing biliary cirrhosis. The dilated, coiled intrahepatic arteries (arrows) are characteristic of moderately advanced cirrhosis. (Courtesy Department of Radiology, The New York Hospital—Cornell Medical Center.)

around the area of disease (Fig. 54-13). Active inflammation in the tissues contiguous to the lesion may produce tissue staining, but tumor vessels are absent. The angiographic presentation of hepatic cysts and localized areas of necrosis and hematoma following trauma is identical (Fig. 54-18). Hydatid disease often causes fibrosis and calcification of the wall of the lesion. Thrombosis and obliteration of vessels in the periphery of such a lesion may be recognizable as additional evidence of the inflammatory nature of the disease.

Inflammatory disease

Diffuse inflammatory disease of the liver has been encountered in hepatic arteriography performed during the investigation of patients with jaundice (Fig. 54-4). This hepatic vascular pattern is common to hepatitis, intrahepatic obliterative cholangitis, and sclerosing cholangitis. There is attenuation, spreading, and sparsity of the intrahepatic vessels, and the capillary hepatogram is "thin," which is to say that its density is considerably diminished from the normal level. To establish such a diagnosis is to obviate the need for hazardous exploratory laporotomy.

Cirrhosis

Cirrhosis of the liver presents a gradation of vascular changes that can be correlated with the state of the disease.[59] Fatty infiltration of the liver with early cirrhosis shows minimal degrees of coiling and tortuosity of the intrahepatic arterial tree (Fig. 54-14). With progression of the disease the vessels become larger and are more serpentine (Fig. 54-15). The shrunken, nodular, cirrhotic liver reveals a reduction of the caliber of the vessels, which course in disarray through the liver parenchyma (Fig. 54-16). Local arterial displacement may reveal interspersion of hypertrophied liver lobules. The development of hepatoma is diagnosed by the presence of arteriographic signs of malignancy.

Hepatic trauma

The judicious use of angiography applied to hepatic trauma can be quite informative.[5,39] In most instances the clinical situation of liver trauma precludes preoperative angiography. With resolution of the acute situation arteriographic evaluation can be of value in demonstrating the extent of an intrahepatic injury that was not apparent at the time of exploratory

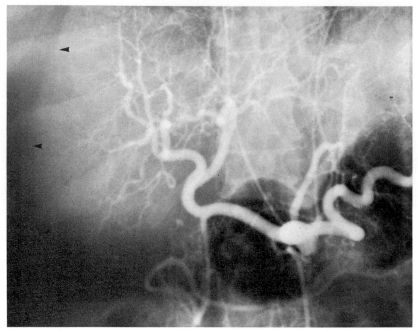

Fig. 54-16. Hepatic arteriogram showing advanced cirrhosis with ascites and esophageal varices. The lateral margin of the liver (arrowheads) is displaced away from the abdominal wall because of ascites. The primary intrahepatic branches are disproportionate in size compared to the peripheral branches, which show some degree of tortuosity. There is minimal evidence of vascular displacement suggesting nodular cirrhosis. (Courtesy Department of Radiology, The New York Hospital—Cornell Medical Center.)

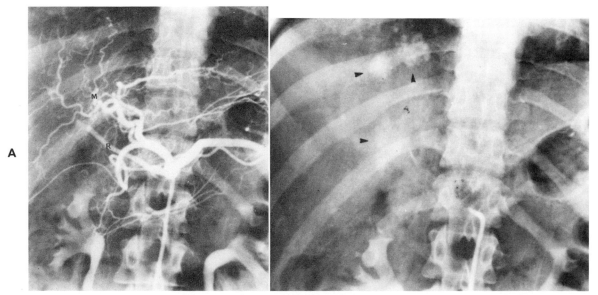

Fig. 54-17. Celiac angiogram showing intrahepatic trauma. **A,** Arterial phase. Slight tortuosity of the branches of the middle hepatic artery is present, **M.** Part of the blood supply to the right lobe of the liver arises as an independent branch of the celiac trunk, **R. B,** Capillary-venous phase. Ill-defined areas of extravasation show the extent of the intrahepatic injury.

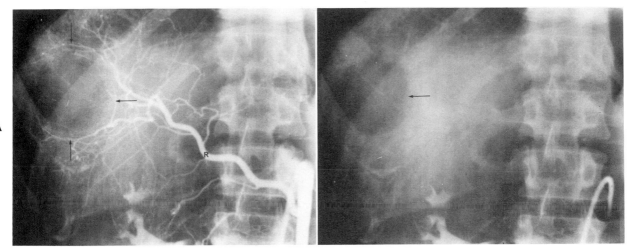

Fig. 54-18. Superior mesenteric arteriogram, of a replaced right hepatic artery showing hepatic trauma. **A.** Arterial phase. Peripheral intrahepatic branches are displaced about an area of avascularity (arrows). Replaced right hepatic artery, **R,** is present. **B,** Venous phase. Intrahepatic veins are displaced by the area of necrosis and hematoma in the right lobe of the liver (arrow). (From Meyers, H. I., and Halpern, M.: Modern trends in accident surgery and medicine. In London, P. S., editor: Radiology of blunt abdominal trauma, London, 1970, Butterworth and Co., Ltd.)

surgery. Areas of significant intrahepatic contusion allow extravasation of contrast medium and produce areas of pooling of contrast medium and tissue staining (Fig. 54-17). The common types of hepatic injury, subcapsular and intraparenchymal hematoma are readily defined. Hepatic hematoma or a localized area of necrosis is defined as a well-demarcated area of avascular radiolucency causing displacement of vascular structures about the periphery of the lesion (Fig. 54-18).

The spleen
Cysts and tumors

Indications for splenic arteriography are infrequent. The organ has an easily definable vasculature, which is orderly and extensive. Neoplasms, either primary or secondary, are manifested by the appearance of abnormal arterial patterns and displacement of vessels. In splenomegaly, considerable increase in the size of the main vessels occurs, with spreading and attenuation of the intrasplenic branches (Fig. 54-19). During the capillary phase, homogenous opacification of the parenchyma is seen. The existence of microaneurysms has been noted in splenomegaly (Figs. 54-19 and 54-56). It is believed that they represent a response to the en-

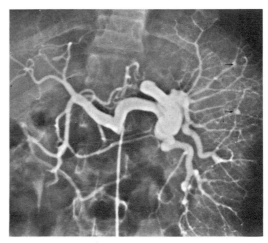

Fig. 54-19. Celiac arteriogram showing splenomegaly. The intrasplenic arterial branches are spread. Small microaneurysms (arrows) are present. (Courtesy Department of Radiology, The New York Hospital—Cornell Medical Center.)

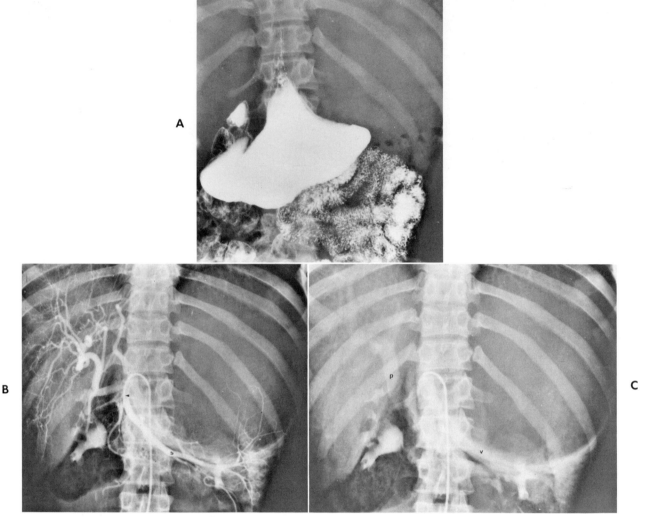

Fig. 54-20. Angiogram of a splenic cyst. **A,** Gastrointestinal series. A large, left upper quadrant mass has caused downward and medial displacement of the stomach. **B,** Arterial phase. The catheter has been selectively placed into the splenic artery (arrowhead). There has been considerable reflux of contrast medium into the common hepatic artery. There is gross downward displacement and stretching of the splenic artery, *S.* **C,** Venous phase. The large avascular cyst is sharply demarcated from the deformed but normal splenic parenchyma. The splenic vein, *V,* is displaced along the inferior circumference of the cyst. The portal vein is slightly displaced to the right, *P.*

largement of the spleen and the demand for increased blood flow rather than a feature of intrinsic vascular disease. Splenic cysts and abscesses appear as well-defined areas of avascularity and, therefore, as radiolucent defects in the splenogram (Fig. 54-20). Wedge-shaped marginal defects and contour irregularities are produced by infarcts and by invasion from extrasplenic disease.

Trauma

Arteriography may be used in the diagnosis of splenic trauma.[1,28,46,54,73] Rupture of the splenic pulp permits the extravasation of contrast material, and injury to the arterial trunks can be recognized. Defects and disruption of the splenogram provide further evidence of the extent of the injury. Subcapsular and perisplenic hematoma present as avascular masses associ-

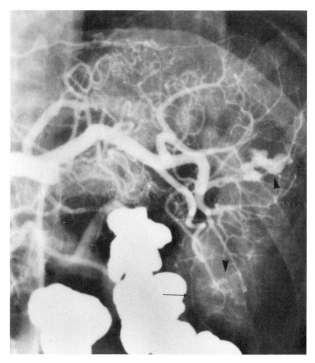

Fig. 54-21. Splenic arteriogram showing splenic trauma. A multilocular pseudoaneurysm is present (upper arrowhead). The inferior tip of the spleen is tense and distended. Medial bowing of a small vessel is present (arrow). An area of contrast extravasation into the traumatized splenic pulp is evident (lower arrowhead).

ated with displacement of vessels and pressure distortion of the splenic artery. The injured spleen may be contracted rather than enlarged. Stretching and straightening of the splenic artery may result from extensive retroperitoneal bleeding. The splenic artery may also evidence spasm, narrowing, and, at times, shortening with increased tortuosity. The direct signs of splenic trauma are areas of contrast extravasation in the splenic pulp, arteriovenous shunting, and pseudoaneurysm formation (Fig. 54-21). While the application of arteriography in trauma has not been common, there has been some increase in its use as an emergency diagnostic procedure to augment the preoperative evaluation of critically ill patients. Arteriographic assessment of the traumatized spleen provides a basis for anticipating delayed rupture and has been used to demonstrate that spontaneous healing of intrasplenic parenchymal and vascular injuries can occur (Fig. 54-22).

Splenoportal venography

The venous phase of splenic arteriography is perhaps its most important practical attribute. Excellent visualization of the splenoportal venous system is obtainable[3,53] (Fig. 54-23). The double catheter technique of visceral arteriography is often employed to enhance the venogram (Fig. 54-14). This means of opacifying the mesenteric venous blood prevents the dilution of the portal venogram by nonopacified blood entering the system through the inferior and superior mesenteric veins. This technique has generally been superseded by selective splenic arteriography using large volumes of contrast material (40 to 80 ml.). Splenoportography performed in this manner opacifies the normal coronary vein in contradistinction to splenotography performed by percutaneous puncture of the spleen, during which only the abnormal coronary vein is seen. Study of the splenectomized patient can be accomplished in this fashion.

The contour and course of the splenic artery and vein are important in the diagnosis of retroperitoneal lesions. Straightening, narrowing, and displacement (Fig. 54-7) of the main vessels can be caused by invasion of the area by carcinoma of the stomach (Fig. 54-24) or by carcinoma of the pancreas (Figs. 54-25 and 54-28), they may result from primary retroperitoneal sarcomas (Fig. 54-8), or they may be caused by inflammatory lesions of the pancreas (Fig. 54-36). The posterior epiploic branches of the splenic artery may be an important source of blood supply to such tumors, providing them with characteristic pathologic vessels (Figs. 54-26 and 54-57).

The pancreas

Selective pancreatic arteriography is an established method for the study of diseases of the pancreas.[14,29,37,38,48] The early and accurate diagnosis of such neoplasms remains a challenge. The anatomic relationships of the pancreas are such that diseases of this organ are usually advanced before they become manifest through routine diagnostic procedures. Similarly, function is maintained until a large amount of parenchymal destruction occurs. Arteriography reproduces the vascular alterations caused by pancreatic disease and thereby enables earlier diagnosis. The clinical findings that suggest the presence of a pancreatic malignancy and indi-

Text continued on p. 1414.

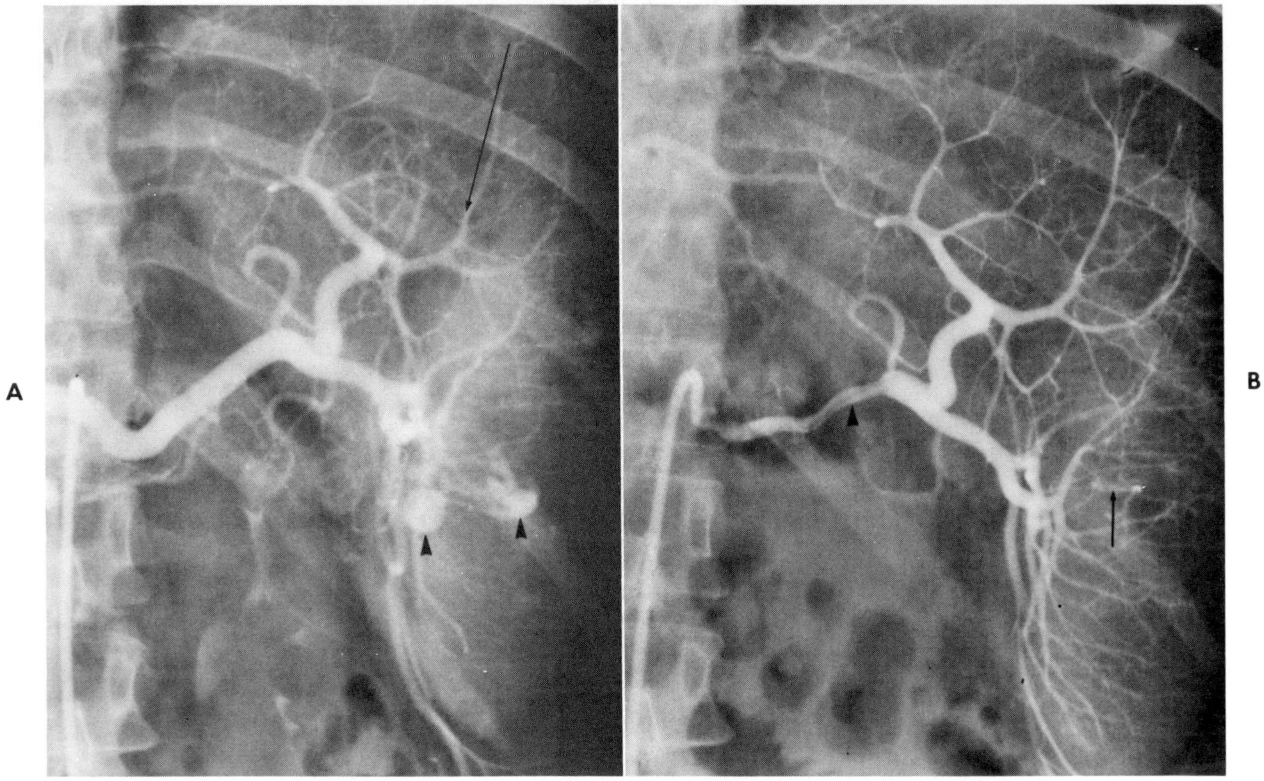

Fig. 54-22. Splenic arteriogram of a splenic trauma with spontaneous healing. **A,** Arteriogram taken shortly after trauma. Large pseudoaneurysms (arrowheads) are the major finding. An oblique fracture line through the splenic hilum is also present (arrow). Splenomegaly is secondary to chronic alcoholism. Patient also manifested hepatomegaly, ascites, and recurrent jaundice. **B,** Arteriogram taken after 3 weeks of conservative management. There has been almost total regression of the lesions. The remaining vascular deformity (arrow) is minimal. There is marked narrowing of the main splenic artery (arrowhead). The linear line of lucency may represent thrombus. A long-term follow up of this patient has revealed no complication of the splenic trauma.

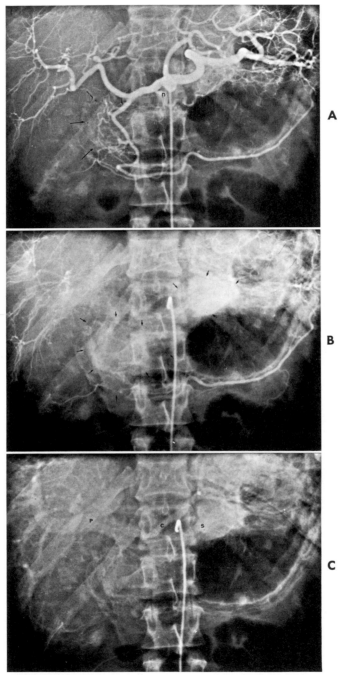

Fig. 54-23. Celiac arteriogram showing normal portal venous system. **A,** Arterial phase. Arrows point to hypervascularity and mild dilatation of the vessels in the head of the pancreas and of the vessels supplying the descending duodenum. *D,* Dorsal pancreatic artery. **B,** Capillary phase. Arrows show capillary staining of the pancreas. There is increased tissue staining in the head of the pancreas adjacent to descending duodenum. **C,** Venous phase. *P,* Portal vein; *C,* coronary vein; *S,* splenic vein.

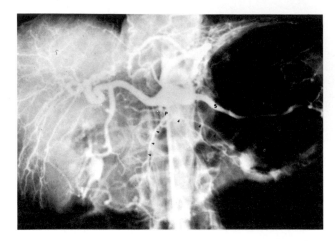

Fig. 54-24. Celiac arteriogram showing carcinoma of the stomach invading the pancreas and retroperitoneal space. Splenic artery, **S,** is stretched. Its midportion is slightly narrowed. Arrowheads demonstrate bowing of the right branch and transverse pancreatic division of the dorsal pancreatic artery, **P.** Vascular changes indicating the gastric origin of the carcinoma are not identified. Stomach is distended with gas. (Courtesy Department of Radiology, The New York Hospital—Cornell Medical Center.)

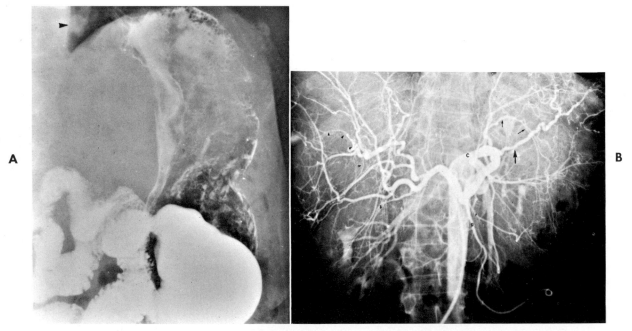

Fig. 54-25. Celiac arteriogram showing carcinoma of the pancreas with extensive metastases and gastric invasion. **A,** Gastrointestinal series; the gastric deformity is evident. **B,** Arteriogram, arterial phase. The celiac axis, *C,* is deformed and the vascular anatomy is difficult to analyze. The gastroduodenal artery, *g,* is displaced toward the left. The terminal radicles of the right gastric artery, *r,* are slightly irregular. The splenic artery (large arrow) is irregular in outline, narrowed and stretched due to encasement by tumor. Involvement and displacement of the left gastric artery (small **arrows) is also present.** Displacement of vessels within the liver (arrowheads) designates a metastatic focus.

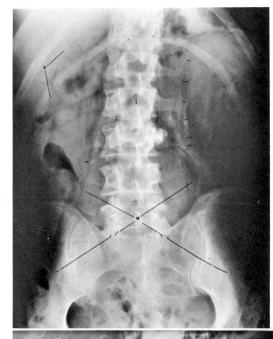

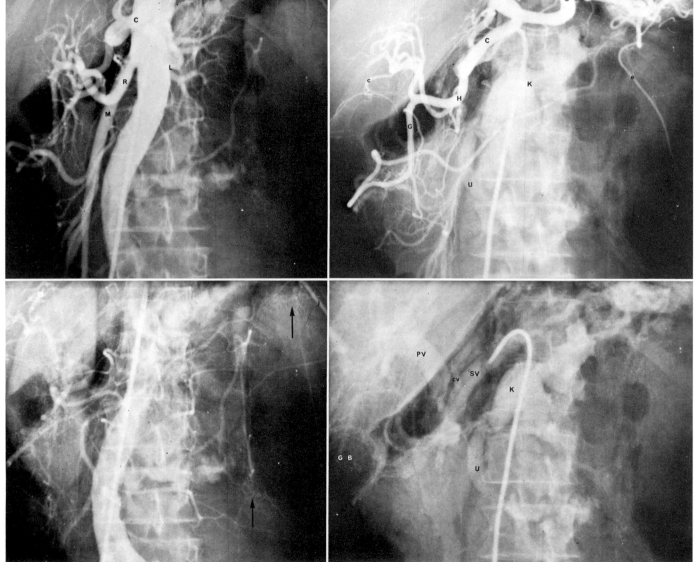

Fig. 54-26. Celiac arteriogram and aortogram showing retroperitoneal sarcoma. **A,** Plain film of the abdomen. *R,* Right kidney; the left renal shadow is not identified; *M,* lower abdominal component of the large mass containing many calcifications (small arrows); short lines in upper right indicate laminated medial border of the left upper quadrant portion of the mass. **B,** Abdominal aortogram, early phase. *C,* Celiac axis; *L,* displaced left renal artery; *R,* right renal artery is superimposed on the superior mesenteric artery, *M.* The left 11th intercostal artery, *i,* provides some supply to the tumor and is dilated. The distal abdominal aorta is displaced to the right. **C,** Abdominal aortogram, late phase. There are only two areas (arrows) of the large tumor in which definable tumor vessels are present. This blood supply arises from the intercostal vessel and a lumbar artery. The importance of abdominal aortography is well demonstrated. **D,** Celiac arteriogram; there is no evidence of tumor supply from the celiac axis. *C,* Celiac axis displaced superiorly and to the right; *S,* splenic artery is displaced superiorly; *H,* hepatic artery; *G,* gastroduodenal artery; *c,* cystic artery; *e,* postepiploic artery arising from the splenic artery; *K,* displaced left kidney; *U,* displaced left ureter. **E,** Celiac arteriogram, venous phase. *PV,* Portal vein; *SV,* displaced splenic vein; *CV,* coronary vein; *GB,* lumen of gallbladder; *K,* left kidney; *U,* left ureter.

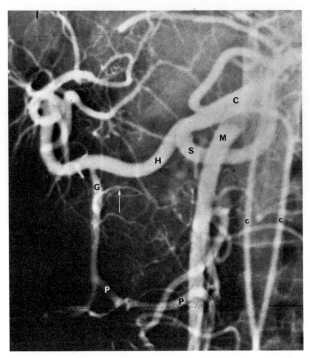

Fig. 54-27. Pancreatic arteriogram showing carcinoma of the head of the pancreas. Double catheter arteriogram, right posterior oblique projection. **C,** Celiac axis; **S,** splenic artery; **H,** hepatic artery; **G,** gastroduodenal artery; **M,** superior mesenteric artery; **c,** catheters. There is superior bowing of the posterior superior pancreaticoduodenal artery (arrow) due to the mass in the head of the pancreas. A large direct communication is present between the anterior superior pancreaticoduodenal and inferior pancreaticoduodenal arteries, **P—P.** (Courtesy Department of Radiology. The New York Hospital—Cornell Medical Center.)

cate the need for arteriography tend to be subtle and appear relatively late in the course of the disease. This detracts from the potential value of the study.

The complex vascular supply of the pancreas stems from multiple arterial sources. The splenic artery commonly provides the dorsal pancreatic artery, small rami to the pancreas, the pancreatica magna, and the caudal pancreatic arteries to the body and tail of the pancreas. The primary supply to the head of the pancreas is an elaborate anastomosis from the anterior and posterior pancreaticoduodenal divisions of the gastroduodenal branch of the common hepatic artery and the anterior and posterior pancreaticoduodenal divisions of the inferior pancre-

aticoduodenal branch of the superior mesenteric artery. There is considerable variability in the role played by each of these arteries. It is, therefore, important to opacify all these structures. This concept underlies the dual catheterization technique of pancreatic arteriography and the superselective study of specific pancreatic vessels (Fig. 54-28).

It is apparent that diagnosis that is to rest on arterial changes requires complete definition of the arteries. In addition to frequent anatomic variations, the response of the pancreatic blood supply to disease presents problems in obtaining such definition. Vessels become obliterated both by inflammatory and neoplastic processes and are then not demonstrable roentgenographically. There are few lesions that produce increased vasculature to simplify their recognition. Since it is believed that function equilibrates with blood flow, it has been hoped that stimulation of the pancreas would enhance its arteriographic visualization. To date pharmacoangiographic attempts to improve the diagnostic value of pancreatic arteriography have not proved effective. Though research involving the iatrogenic stimulus of the pancreas has not measurably increased the ability to opacify this organ, it is proper that such investigation continue.

The demonstration of the details of the entire vascular bed is the important feature of the examination. Arterial dislocation, irregular stenosis, thrombosis, and the occasional appearance of tumor vessels and tumor stain permit the arteriographic diagnosis of carcinoma of the pancreas. Cystadenoma of the pancreas presents a distinctly abnormal vascular pattern similar to that shown by its malignant counterpart[70] (Fig. 54-29). Insulinomas are usually demonstrable by virtue of hypervascularity that produces a distinct area of tumor stain within the pancreas in about two thirds of the cases.[1,51]

While opacification of the pancreatic parenchyma does occur during the capillary-venous phase, this portion of the angiogram is generally not diagnostically significant because detail is restricted and reproducibility is inconstant. Indeed, it is the normal pancreas that is most often visible on a pancreaticogram. The presence of a large dorsal pancreatic artery, a transverse pancreatic artery, and a dominant pancreatica magna artery favor capillary opacification of the pancreas. Selective catheterization

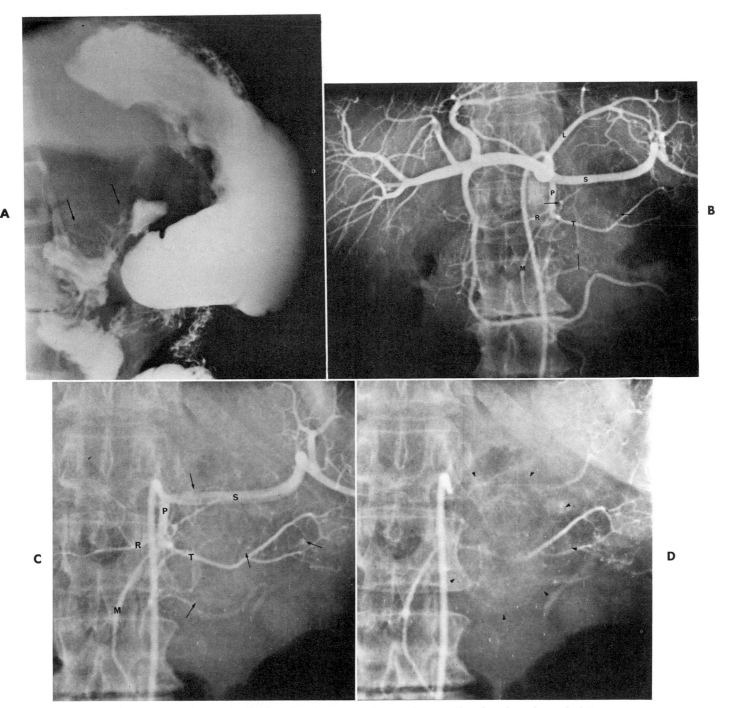

Fig. 54-28. Celiac and selective dorsal pancreatic arteriogram showing invasion of the pancreas by malignant lymphoma. **A,** Gastrointestinal series, lateral projection. The retrogastric mass involving the posterior portion of the lesser curvature of the stomach is apparent. Note impingement on the postbulbar portion of the duodenum (arrows). **B,** Celiac arteriogram, anteroposterior projection. The splenic, *S,* and left gastric, *L,* arteries are stretched. A large dorsal pancreatic artery, *P,* gives origin to a right branch, *R,* and transverse pancreatic branch, *T,* both of which show some contour irregularities. The middle colic branch, *M,* arising from the dorsal pancreatic appears to be encased by tumor. A few pathologic vessels are faintly discernible (arrows). Selective dorsal pancreatic arteriogram, early, **C,** and late, **D,** arterial phases. The catheter is in the orifice of the dorsal pancreatic artery. Observe that vascular details are clearer and small tumor vessels (arrows) more evident. Tumor stain outlines the main bulk of the tumor (arrowheads). Partial filling of the splenic artery, *S,* is caused by overflow.

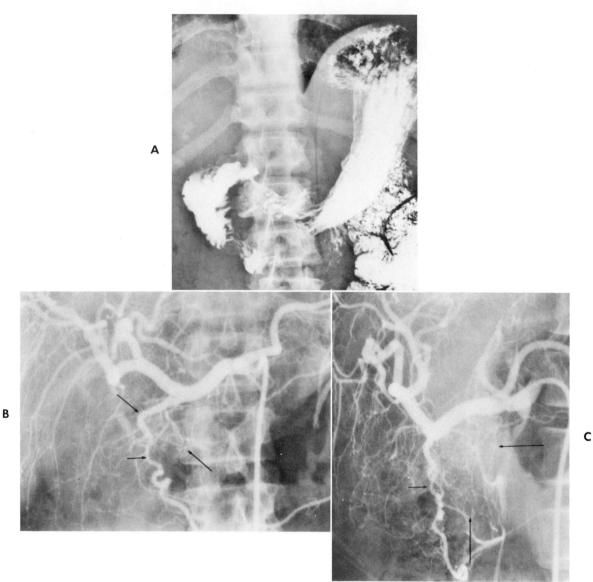

Fig. 54-29. Pancreatic arteriogram showing cystadenocarcinoma of the pancreas. **A,** Gastrointestinal series demonstrates changes in the gastric antrum and duodenal loop in a patient with epigastric pain, weight loss, and jaundice. **B,** Arteriogram taken in the anteroposterior position. The area of disease is designated by arrows. There is more vascularity present than is usually seen with carcinoma of the pancreas. Segmental narrowing of the gastroduodenal artery is present (short arrow). **C,** Arteriogram taken in the right posterior oblique position. Moderate tumor vascularity in the head of the pancreas is present.

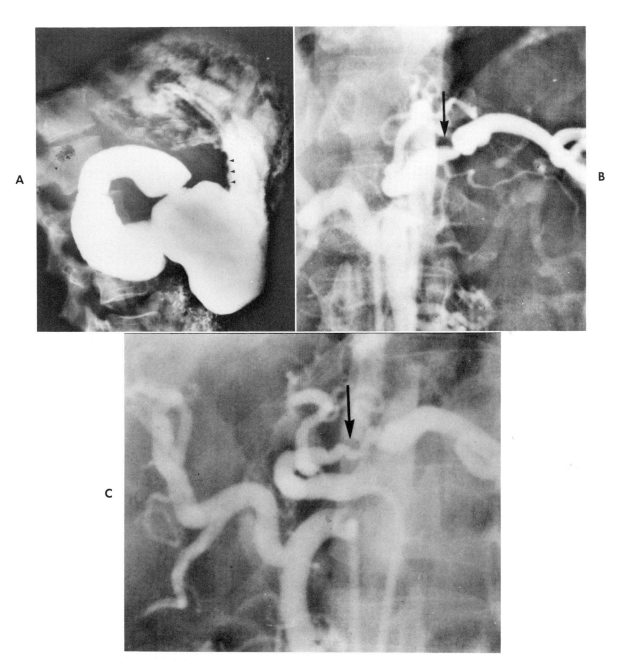

Fig. 54-30. Pancreatic arteriogram showing carcinoma of the pancreas. **A,** Gastrointestinal series. There is some irregularity along the lesser curvature aspect of the stomach (arrowheads). **B,** Arteriogram taken in the anteroposterior position. Double catheter technique has been employed. Arrow designates irregular stenosis of the splenic artery. **C,** Arteriogram taken in the right posterior oblique position. The full extent of the irregular stenosis (encasement) of the splenic artery is shown (arrow).

of an individual arterial trunk yields superior vascular detail of the portion of the organ supplied by the vessel (Figs. 54-28 and 54-36). Angiographic establishment of diagnosis and location of functioning tumors within the pancreas is a significant contribution that obviates blind exploration and pancreatic resection.

Tumors

Pancreatic angiography is an important adjunct in the diagnosis of carcinoma of the pancreas. The angiographic criteria that provide the basis for diagnosis in order of importance are (1) irregular stenosis of major arteries providing blood supply to the pancreas (Figs. 54-30 to 54-32); (2) pathologic tumor vessels and neovascularization (Figs. 54-28 and 54-29); (3) dislocation of vessels (Fig. 54-31); and (4) tumor stain. Only irregular stenosis or pathologic vessels, or both, are sufficiently specific for objective angiographic diagnosis. The gastroduodenal artery and its branches, the anterior and posterior superior pancreaticoduodenal arteries, and the supraduodenal and retroduodenal arteries are involved in carcinoma of the head of the pancreas (Fig. 54-32). The splenic artery, individual pancreatic rami, pancreatica magna, dorsal pancreatic, transverse pancreatic, and caudal pancreatic arteries are involved in carcinoma of the body and tail of the pancreas (Fig. 54-31). Involvement of the celiac axis, hepatic, gastric, and superior mesenteric arteries may be seen in association with the arteries mentioned as evidence of spread of the lesion (Fig. 54-32). Although invasion of venous radicles is a feature of the histopathology of this carcinoma and is responsible for certain clinical manifestations, splenic vein involvement or obstruction is not a prominent angiographic finding. Other histologic features that explain the angiographic presentation are the tendency of the carcinoma to fuse with the surrounding parenchyma, the frequent occurrence of pseudopodial projections of the tumor, and the tumor's abundant fibrous stroma. These features result in obliteration of pancreatic arteries and in the formation of irregular stenosis (that is, encasement) of vessels. Pancreatic carcinoma is most often a sparsely vascular or avascular lesion. Although many of the arteriographic features are also seen in pancreatitis, angiographic separation of the two entities is possible in most instances. When irregu-

lar stenoses appear in pancreatitis, the magnitude of arterial involvement is less (Figs. 54-33 and 54-34), arterial displacement is greater (Figs. 54-35 and 54-36), pathologic vessels do not occur, tissue staining is more prominent, and splenic vein involvement is more common.

Marked irregular stenosis of the main vessels always seems to be a sign of pancreatic carcinoma, though unfortunately it is inoperable. Diagnosis of early lesions is not as yet within the scope of angiography even when the special techniques of pharmacoangiography, magnification arteriography, and superselective angiography are applied.

Cysts

The angiographic manifestation of a pancreatic cyst is identical to that of cysts of other organs. There is displacement of vessels about a well-demarcated area of avascularity[48] (Figs. 54-29 and 54-37). The status of the neighboring extrapancreatic vessels assists in the determination of the size of the lesion and its relation to adjacent structures. While simple displacement is compatible with the presence of a benign noninvasive lesion, vascular contour distortions and vascular rigidity are used as evidence of encasement of the vessel by malignant tissue; however, diffuse inflammatory disease and primary vascular disease produce changes that may be indistinguishable.

Pancreatitis

Inflammatory disease of the pancreas results in an irregularity of arterial radicles and produces evidence of inflammatory obstruction and hyperemia (Fig. 54-14). Coarse mottling of the capillary pancreaticogram may be visible. Gross enlargement of the pancreas may be a feature of pancreatitis in the absence of pseudocyst formation. There are angiographic characteristics of this chronic inflammatory process that reliably identify the mass as a benign lesion. Medial displacement of the gastroduodenal artery may be quite pronounced and may be associated with upward displacement of the common hepatic artery (Figs. 54-33 and 54-36). Minimal contour irregularity of the gastroduodenal artery is often noted, with similar involvement of branches to the descending duodenum and head of the pancreas. Inflammatory thrombosis is recognized by the abrupt termination of the involved vessel.

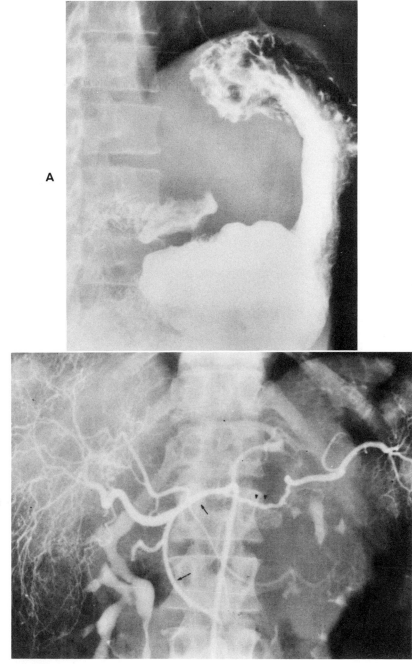

Fig. 54-31. Pancreatic arteriogram showing carcinoma of the pancreas. **A,** Gastrointestinal series. There are changes involving the posterior aspect of the lesser curvature of the stomach. **B,** Arterial phase. Mass displacement of the common hepatic and gastroduodenal arteries is present (arrows). Irregular stenosis and narrowing of the proximal segment of the splenic artery are shown (arrowheads). Note the marked degree of avascularity of the tumor.

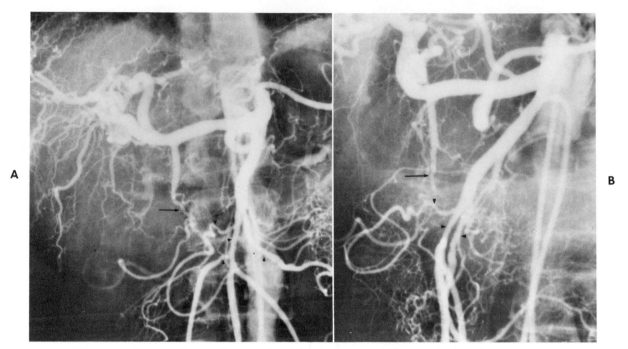

Fig. 54-32. Pancreatic arteriogram showing carcinoma of the pancreas with invasion of the mesentery. **A,** Arteriogram taken in the anteroposterior position. Double catheter technique has been employed. There is marked irregular stenosis of the distal portion of the gastroduodenal artery (arrow). Irregular stenosis of intestinal branches of the superior mesenteric artery is evidence of local invasion (arrowheads) into the mesentery. **B,** Arteriogram taken in the right posterior oblique position. Irregular stenoses of the gastroduodenal artery (arrow), the superior mesenteric artery, and its intestinal branches are present (arrowheads).

Vessels may become stretched over the mass lesion and demonstrate segmental narrowing and irregularity (Figs. 54-33, 54-34, and 54-36). These inflammatory vascular changes are somewhat similar to the irregular stenosis of carcinoma. However, pathologic tumor vessels are not seen (Fig. 54-34). Tissue staining of the inflamed pancreas can be quite marked. The pancreaticoduodenal arteries and the vascular arcade in the head of the pancreas may be opacified in detail in pancreatitis. Arterial displacement indicates the presence of a mass lesion in the head of the pancreas. This combination of angiographic findings seems to be inconsistent with the diagnosis of carcinoma of the pancreas and reasonably characteristic of inflammatory mass lesion (Fig. 54-38). Straightening, narrowing, and obstruction of the splenic vein is more often a feature of pancreatitis than of carcinoma.

These changes are reasonably distinct from the alterations caused by a primary vasculitis. In the later instance, subtle contour irregularities and segmental alterations in the luminal diameters of intrapancreatic vessels are discernible (Fig. 54-39). Since the clinical symptom complex caused by arteritis often mimics conditions that require operative intervention rather than medical therapy, recognition and proper interpretation of the arteriographic features of a vascular disease are important (Figs. 54-39, 54-40, and 54-55).

Objectivity is important in the assessment of pancreatic arteriography. Technical modifications and improvements may be expected to permit a broader application of the procedure. At this time, when specific indications for the examination exist, the angiographic information obtained is often invaluable.[16,17]

The stomach

Conventional diagnostic studies of the stomach have a high degree of accuracy in recogni-

Text continued on p. 1429.

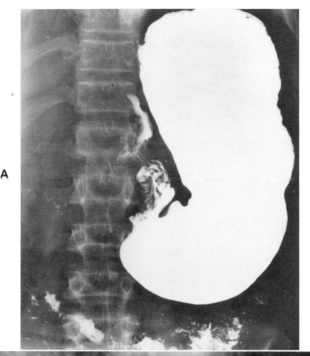

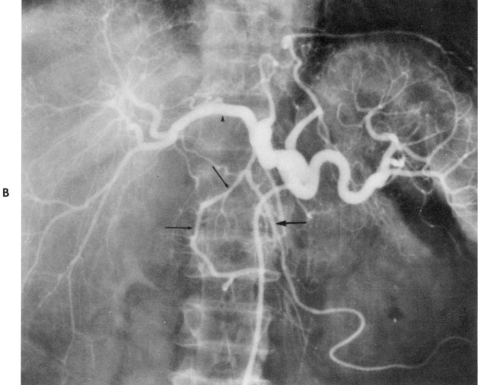

Fig. 54-33. Pancreatic arteriogram showing pancreatitis. **A,** Gastrointestinal series. There is a partial obstruction of the outlet of the stomach. **B,** Arteriogram. Medial displacement of the gastroduodenal artery is present (large arrow). The superior pancreaticoduodenal artery (small arrows) is large and shows scattered segmental areas of minimal luminal narrowing. There is upward displacement of the common hepatic artery (arrowhead).

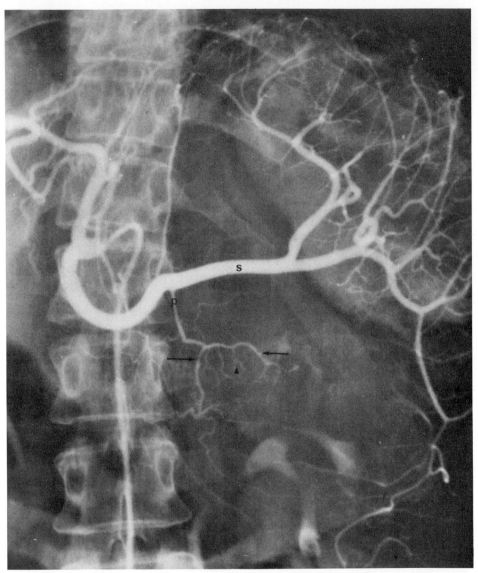

Fig. 54-34. Pancreatic arteriogram showing pancreatitis with pseudocyst. The splenic artery, **S,** is straightened. There are irregular, segmental narrowings involving the pancreatic magna, **P,** and its branches (arrows). Some of the small arteries have an appearance similar to that of tumor neovascularization (arrowhead).

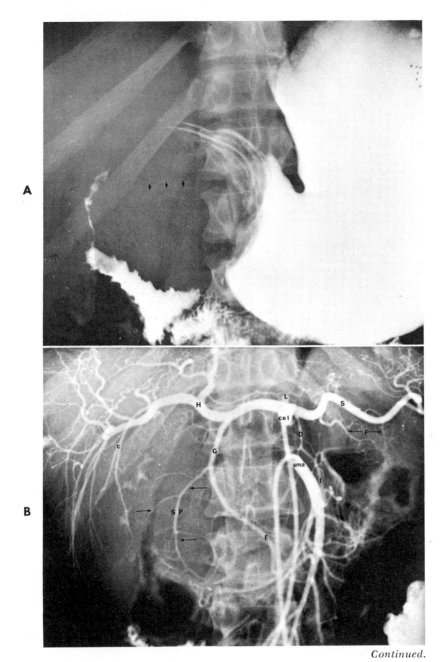

Continued.

Fig. 54-35. Double catheter pancreatic arteriogram; pseudocyst of pancreas. **A,** Gastrointestinal series; duodenal compression and distortion of duodenal loop caused by a mass are evident. Small calcifications are present (arrows). **B,** Arteriogram, anteroposterior projection. Displacement of vessels due to mass which is avascular is the dominant feature. *cel,* Celiac axis; *sma,* superior mesenteric artery; *L,* left gastric artery, partially opacified; *S,* splenic artery; *H,* hepatic artery; *G,* gastroduodenal artery; *E,* right gastroepiploic artery; *SP,* with arrows, indicates superior pancreaticoduodenal artery and branches; *I,* inferior pancreaticoduodenal artery; *D,* dorsal pancreatic artery; *P,* with arrows, indicates pancreatic rami from splenic artery; *C,* cystic artery (gallbladder is not enlarged). **C,** Arteriogram, right posterior oblique projection. This view aids in the anatomic definition in lesions of the head of the pancreas. Displacement of the hepatic, *H,* and gastroduodenal arteries, *G,* is vivid. *cel,* Celiac axis; *sma,* superior mesenteric artery; *L,* left gastric artery; *S,* splenic artery; *E,* right gastroepiploic artery; *D,* dorsal pancreatic artery; *I,* inferior pancreaticoduodenal artery. **D,** Arteriogram, capillary-venous phase. The large avascular pseudocyst is clearly shown. The portal vein, *PV,* is displaced superiorly. *SV* is the splenic vein.

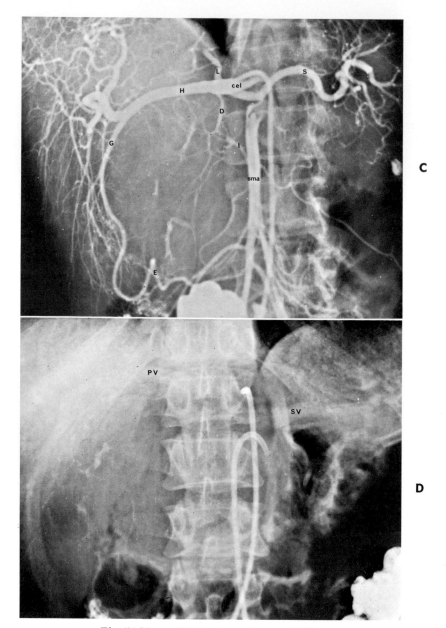

Fig. 54-35, cont'd. For legend see p. 1423.

Fig. 54-36. Pancreatic arteriogram showing pancreatitis with pseudocyst. **A,** Gastrointestinal series. Gross changes involve the distal stomach and duodenal loop. **B,** Arteriogram. Medial displacement of the distal gastroduodenal artery is present, **G.** Its contours are normal. There is displacement and minimal contour irregularity of branches of the gastroduodenal artery (oblique arrows) due to the inflammatory mass in the head of the pancreas. There is an abrupt irregular narrowing of the pancreatic magna artery (vertical arrow) indicating involvement of the body and tail of the pancreas.

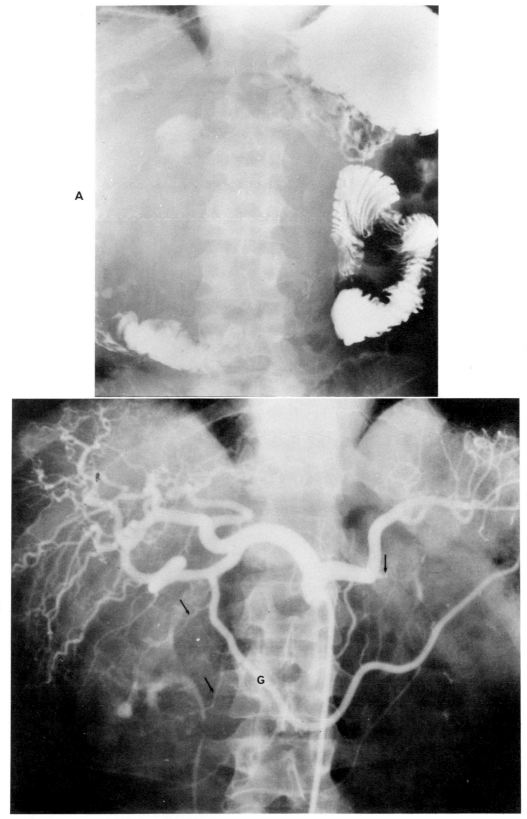

Fig. 54-36. For legend see opposite page.

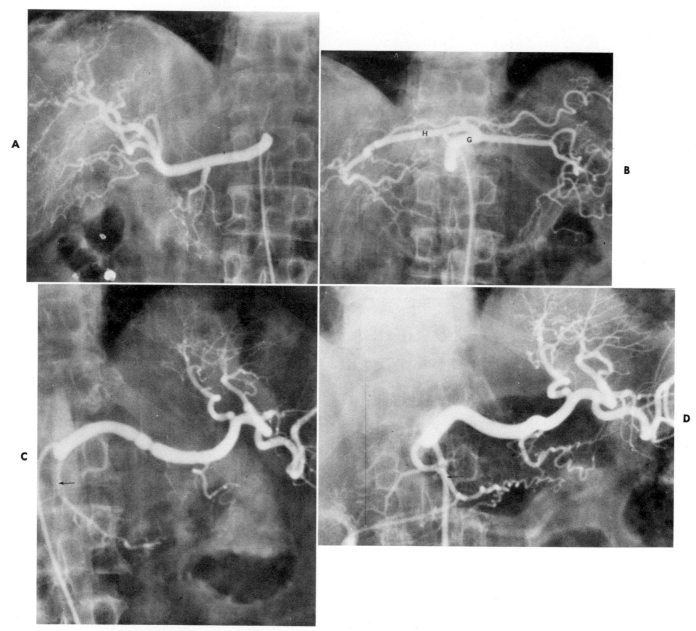

Fig. 54-37. Pancreatic arteriogram showing pseudocyst of the pancreas. The celiac axis has been replaced by individual orifices for the hepatic artery, the gastric artery, and the splenic artery. **A,** Hepatic arteriogram. **B,** Gastric arteriogram. The left hepatic artery, *H,* is a branch of the left gastric artery, *G.* **C,** Splenic arteriogram. There is medial bowing of the dorsal pancreatic artery caused by pressure from an avascular pseudocyst (arrow). **D,** Splenic arteriogram performed postoperatively shows that the course of the dorsal pancreatic artery has returned to normal (arrow).

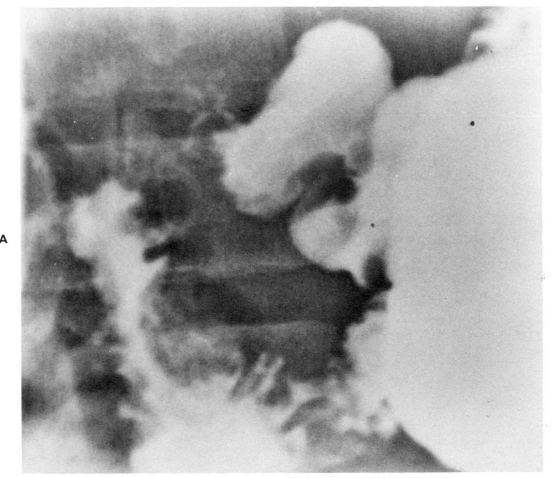

Continued.

Fig. 54-38. Pancreatic arteriogram showing impacted common duct stone. **A,** Gastrointestinal series. There is a mass imprint on the medial aspect of the second portion of the duodenum. **B,** Arteriogram taken in the anteroposterior position. There is lateral displacement of the gastroduodenal artery (arrow). Note the excellent visualization of the details of the vascular arcade in the head of the pancreas and the opacification of inferior pancreaticoduodenal artery through anastomotic channels, I. **C,** Arteriogram taken in the right posterior oblique position. The mass lesion is outlined by displacement of the gastroduodenal artery and downward bowing of the anterior superior pancreaticoduodenal artery (arrows). NOTE: This type of vascular pattern seems to be inconsistent with a diagnosis of carcinoma of the pancreas.

B
C

Fig. 54-38, cont'd. For legend see p. 1427.

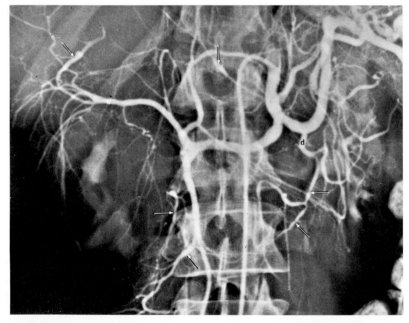

Fig. 54-39. Celiac arteriogram showing arteritis. Many of the branch vessels of the celiac axis show localized areas of irregularity and ectasia (arrows). Special attention should be directed to the branches of the dorsal pancreatic artery, **d.** This female patient presented a differential diagnostic problem of an acute abdomen involving the diagnostic possibilities of acute cholecystitis and acute pancreatitis. (Courtesy Department of Radiology, The New York Hospital—Cornell Medical Center.)

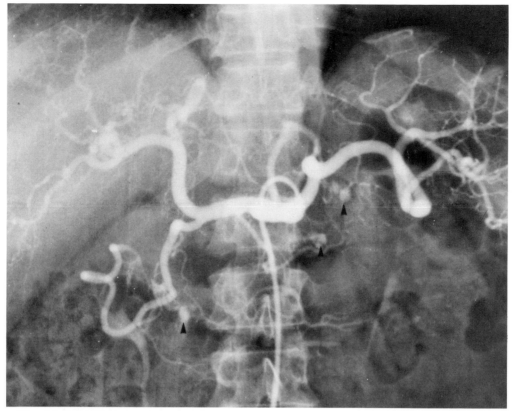

Fig. 54-40. Celiac arteriogram showing hereditary hemorrhagic telangiectasia. Several angiectatic masses in the pancreas (arrowheads) are demonstrated.

tion of organic disease and in the differentiation of benign from malignant lesions. The diagnostic potential of arteriography is so great that academic investigation of its possible role in study of lesions of the stomach was anticipated. It was necessary first to determine whether or not angiography could provide positive information that would enhance the preoperative diagnosis of gastric lesions. With a background knowledge of pathologic vascular anatomy the resolution of special problems might then be accomplished through angiographic study. It is reasonable to presume that analysis of gastric vascular patterns can (1) assist in establishing the presence of the questionable mass lesion of the fundus of the stomach; (2) establish the precise location of a mass lesion, showing whether it is extragastric or gastric in origin; and (3) assist in understanding and handling the problem of gastric bleeding[25,47,57] (Fig. 54-43). What then is the character of the morbid anatomy depicted on a gastric arteriogram, and what is the positive in-

formation that will enhance the accuracy of diagnosis?

Clear depiction of the blood supply to the stomach and capillary opacification of the wall of this viscus requires selective catheterization of the celiac axis. Artificial distention of the stomach at the time of arteriography by having the patient drink soda water, soda bicarbonate and water, or a nutrient supplement assists in the recognition of the branch vessels to the stomach and produces clear visualization of the gastric wall.

Gastric angiographic diagnosis is a complex problem. Microarteriographic studies of the vascular patterns of gastric lesions have revealed distinct changes involving branch vessels of small caliber.[32,36,66] The vascular alterations caused by inflammatory and malignant processes are not profound in the majority of instances, and their demonstration, recognition, and analysis is difficult. Indeed, the diagnostic changes often involve vessels of such small caliber that

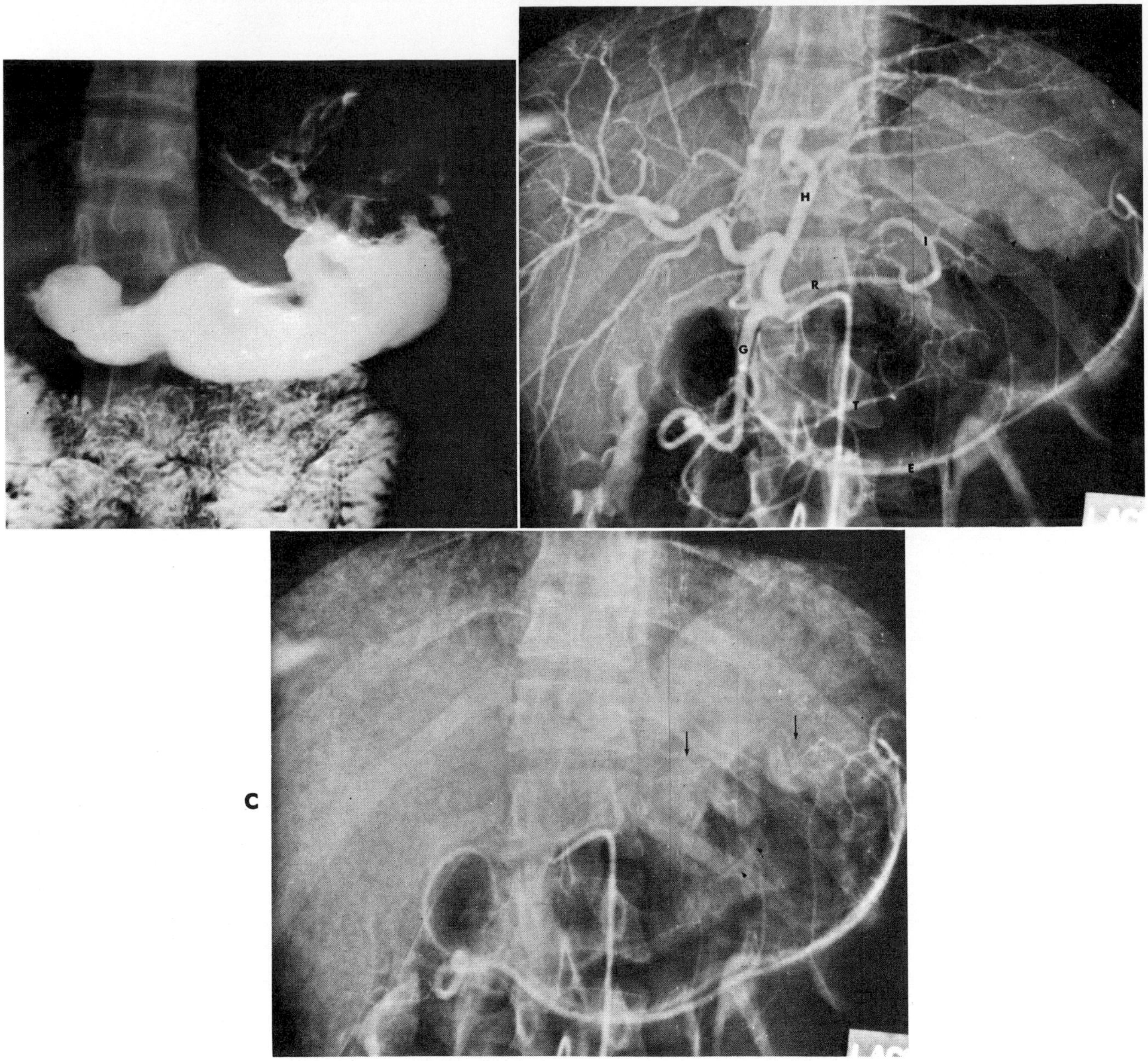

Fig. 54-41. Celiac arteriogram; recticulum cell sarcoma of the stomach. **A,** Gastrointestinal series, lobular masses of tumor and mucosal involvement are present in the fundus and body of the stomach. **B,** Arteriogram, arterial phase. The tip of the catheter is in the common hepatic artery distal to the origin of the left gastric and splenic divisions of the celiac axis. Opacified blood flows through the right gastric artery, *R,* into the left gastric artery, *l.* Abrupt termination of filling of the proximal part of the left gastric artery is due to a nonopacified jet of blood. *H,* Left hepatic artery; *G,* gastroduodenal artery; *T,* transverse pancreatic artery; *E,* right gastroepiploic artery. Tumor tissue perfused by small branches of the left gastric artery and branches of the left gastro-epiploic artery show minimal irregularity of form. **C,** Arteriogram, capillary phase. Only a few pathologic vessels and minimal tumor stain are present (arrows). Early venous shunting is seen in the gastric wall (arrowheads).

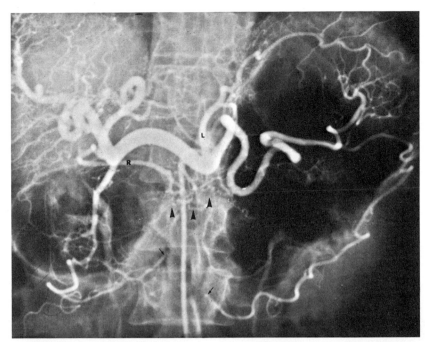

Fig. 54-42. Celiac arteriogram showing ulcerating carcinoma of the stomach. Coiled and dilated tumor vessels are present in the gastric mass (arrowheads). Thrombosis of the gastroepiploic vessels is present on the greater curvature of the stomach (arrows). **R,** Right gastric artery. (Courtesy Department of Radiology, The New York Hospital—Cornell Medical Center.)

these structures are not recognized as discrete entities on an arteriogram. Study of the vascular histopathology of inflammatory and neoplastic lesions of the stomach reveals that many of the malignant lesions are sparsely vascular (Fig. 54-41). Inflammatory tissue changes and areas of avascularity secondary to fibrotic changes are frequently associated with both benign and malignant processes. It is difficult to elicit the differential diagnostic criteria and discouraging to find that even bulky, ulcerating carcinomas produce only subtle angiographic changes (Fig. 54-42).

Locally invasive lesions cause more easily recognizable displacement and distortion of neighboring arteries and veins. It is important to recall that primary gastric malignancies, primary pancreatic malignancies, and primary retroperitoneal sarcomas all may encase and deform a structure such as the splenic artery. In such situations the presence of the mass is readily discernible, but its character and site of origin may remain obscure. That pancreatitis and intrinsic vascular disease may produce

changes indistinguishable from those of perivascular invasion has previously been noted.

At this time it is difficult to be enthusiastic about arteriography of the stomach since the degree to which the arteriogram complements routine diagnostic studies appears to be restricted and of controversial value.

The localization of the site of upper gastrointestinal hemorrhage can be accomplished by angiography. This examination is indicated in the actively bleeding patient when the diagnosis is not determined by conventional methods such as a gastrointestinal study performed with water-soluble contrast media or when the magnitude of the bleeding obscures the gastroscopist's field. It is generally accepted that a rate of active bleeding of at least 0.5 ml. per minute must be present for angiography to be successful. Leakage or pooling of contrast material identifies the bleeding site (Fig. 54-43). Arteriovenous malformations and angiomas are most often shown in patients with hereditary hemorrhagic telangiectasia. Their presence does not necessarily identify the bleeding site.[21,22]

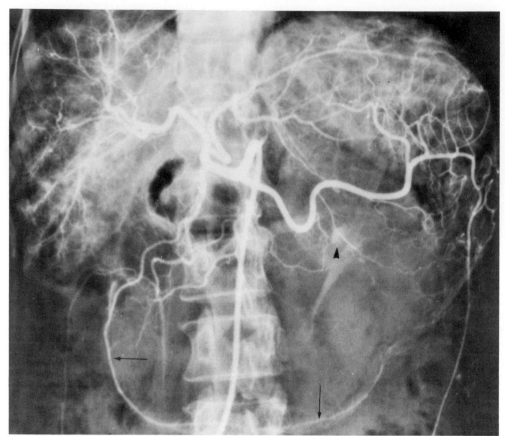

Fig. 54-43. Celiac arteriogram showing bleeding gastric ulcer. The stomach is distended with blood (arrows identify the right gastroepiploic artery coursing along the greater curvature). The bleeding lesser curvature gastric ulcer is demonstrated as a pool of extravasated contrast (arrowhead).

The intestines

Selective catheter angiography of the superior and inferior mesenteric arteries produces finely detailed reproduction of the vascular anatomy of both the small and the large intestines.[20,69] Capillary opacification of the bowel wall and visualization of its venous drainage are also obtained by multifilm programming. While the clinical problem seldom warrants such a specialized approach, the therapeutic importance of resolving specific differential diagnostic problems has motivated academic and practical study of intestinal angiography. It is an indicated study when a mass deforms the duodenal loop in a nonjaundiced patient. An uncommon lesion is apt to be the cause (Fig. 54-44).

Microarteriographic studies of specimens have shown that different vascular patterns are pres-

ent in inflammatory and neoplastic disease and have resulted in the use of operative intestinal arteriography to assist formulation of proper surgical therapy.[36,60] These investigations vividly point out the problems encountered in diagnostic mesenteric angiography: (1) many of the vascular changes present in intestinal diseases affect small-caliber vessels that are not angiographically visualized in the living patient; (2) many bowel tumors do not have a distinctive increased vascularity; and (3) differentiation of tumor vessels from distortions resulting from inflammatory hyperemia is extremely difficult. It should be borne in mind that the intestinal branches of the major sources of blood supply to the bowel first bifurcate to form intestinal arterial arcades that give rise to vasa recta to the bowel wall and that these in turn

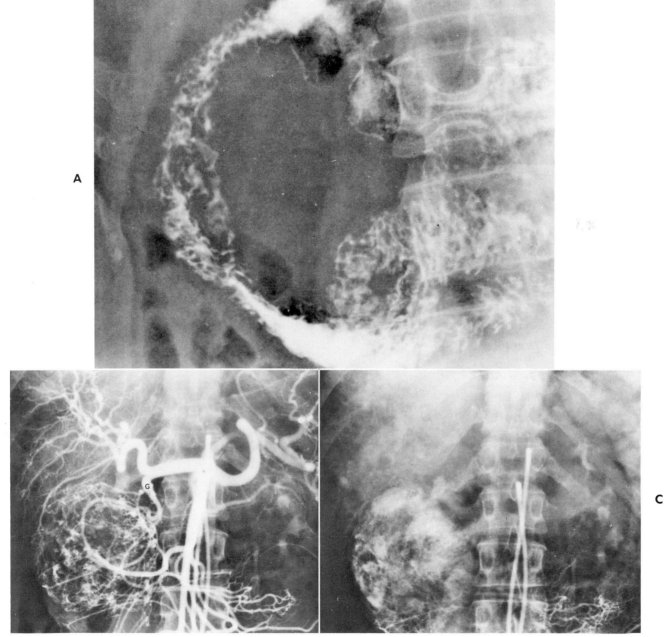

Fig. 54-44. Celiac arteriogram showing leiomyosarcoma of the duodenum. **A,** Gastrointestinal series. A large mass causes a pressure imprint and displacement of the second portion of the duodenum. Jaundice was not present. **B,** Arterial phase. Branches of the gastroduodenal artery, **G,** show extensive tumor neovascularization throughout the mass. **C,** Capillary phase. There is intense staining of the well-marginated tumor.

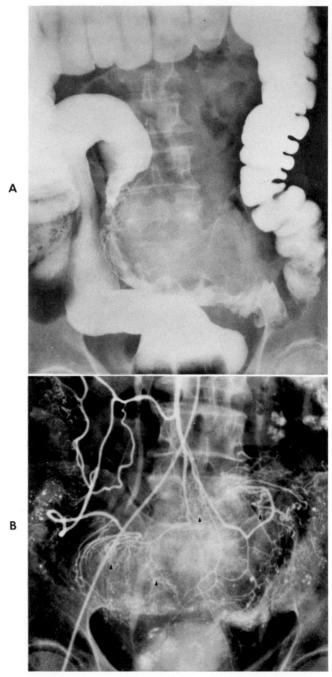

Fig. 54-45. Inferior mesenteric arteriogram showing lymphosarcoma of the colon. **A,** Barium enema demonstrates the large exophytic lesion involving the sigmoid colon. **B,** There is obvious displacement of the sigmoid and superior hemorrhoidal divisions of the inferior mesenteric artery. A few, irregularly ectatic vessels can be identified (arrowheads). There are scattered flecks of residual barium in the colon.

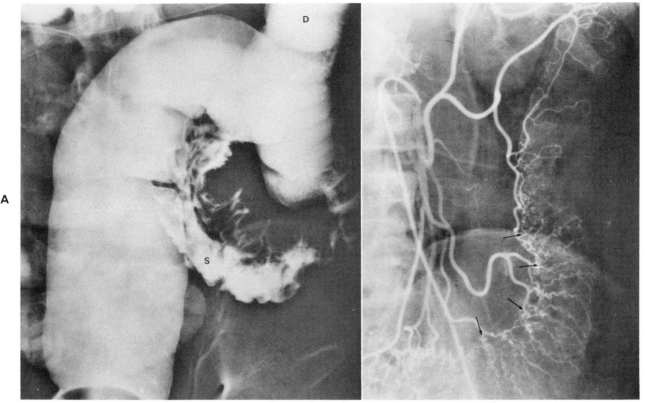

Fig. 54-46. Inferior mesenteric arteriogram showing mucus-secreting adenocarcinoma of the colon. **A,** Barium enema demonstrates an exophytic mass lesion involving the distal descending sigmoid, *S,* portions of the colon. The middescending colon, *D,* appears normal. **B,** Arteriogram demonstrates an unusual "corkscrew" change involving the colonic end arteries (arrows) in the area of the mass lesion. These spiral-like arterial changes extend into the middescending colon almost to the splenic flexure. This vascular change is thought to have resulted from the scirrhous nature of this tumor, which caused marked narrowing of the lumen of the colon with thickening of the colonic wall.

bifurcate to enter the mesenteric border as small vascular channels that finally ramify into a diffuse submucosal anastomosis. It becomes evident then that the vessels of diagnostic importance may be extremely small and, as mentioned, too minute for discrete angiographic visualization. Vascular occlusions result from the direct pressure of tumor mass or are secondary to thrombosis. In either instance, the evidence from which diagnoses are derived is incomplete.

The capillary phase of intestinal angiography that produces tissue staining does not commonly become a usable diagnostic criterion, but the value of the venous phase is retained. An increased rate of blood flow through arteriovenous shunting in neoplastic tissues provides earlier opacification of the draining veins than is found in normal tissue.[69] When this feature is combined with a chaotic arrangement of distorted arterial channels, sufficient evidence to establish a diagnosis of malignancy is obtained (Fig. 54-44). It is unfortunate that the more common intestinal malignancies, such a lymphosarcoma (Fig. 54-46) and adenocarcinoma (Fig. 54-45), do not seem to have a highly vascular matrix. The marked vascularity of the carcinoid tumor permits recognition of that lesion.[71] There are angiographic features of this lesion that may be distinctive[56] (Fig. 54-47). The arteries at the tumor site tend to be arranged in a stellate pattern, the deep mesenteric branches are narrow, staining of the tumor tissue is not

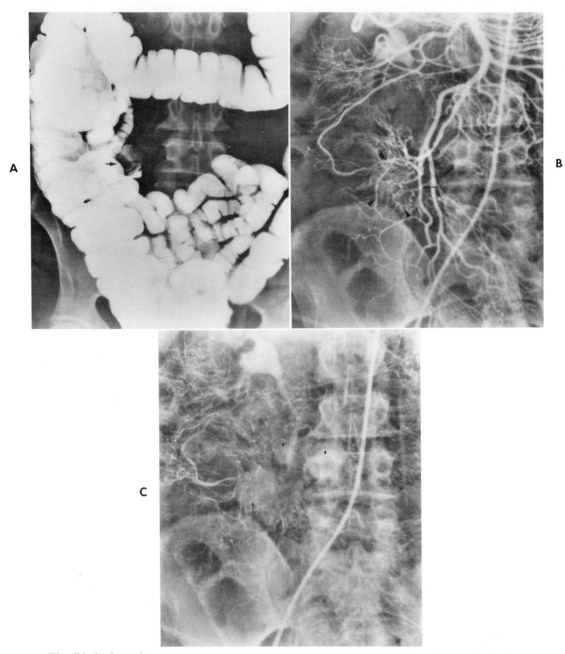

Fig. 54-47. Superior mesenteric arteriogram showing carcinoid of the ileum. **A,** Barium enema shows reflux into the ileum and a filling defect in the distal ileum (arrow). **B,** The ileocolic artery (arrow) is the prime supply to the carcinoid tumor (arrowheads). **C,** Late arterial phase. Tumor blush is present (arrow). Metastatic involvement of regional nodes (arrowheads) is demonstrated. Draining veins are absent.

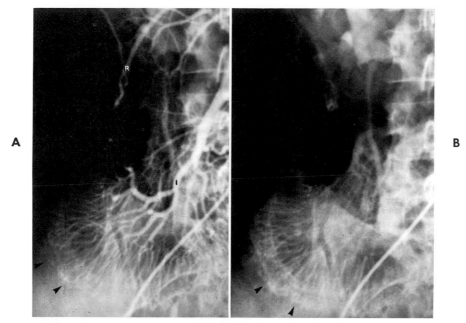

Fig. 54-48. Superior mesenteric arteriogram; regional ileitis. **A,** Arteriogram, arterial phase. Observe the hypervascularity and dilatation of the blood vessels supplying the terminal ileum (arrowheads). *I,* Ileocolic artery; *R,* right colic artery. **B,** Arteriogram, capillary-venous phase. Dilated veins drain the terminal ileum. Observe the thickening of the wall of the ileum (arrowheads). (Courtesy Department of Radiology, The New York Hospital—Cornell Medical Center.)

marked, and the draining veins are not visualized.

Inflammatory conditions of the small and large bowel produce changes in the vascular bed similar to those found in other organs of the body. In inflammation the blood supply to the area is increased primarily through an increase in number and dilatation of vessels. The arteries so affected reveal an increased tortuosity, but they ramify and attenuate in an orderly fashion unlike the bizarre course and luminal changes presented by tumor vessels. The increase in caliber and number of regional vessels intensifies the capillary tissue staining and increases the rate of blood flow. This hemodynamic alteration results in earlier opacification of veins than exists in healthy tissue, but the change is less extreme than that found in neoplastic tissue. It is important to recognize that these vascular responses enable roentgenographic visualization of arterial structures not seen under normal conditions.

Various vascular patterns dissimilar to those of bowel malignancy, and apparently specific

enough to allow the nature of a given lesion to be determined, have been defined. Interest in the angiographic patterns of ileitis, colitis, and diverticulitis stems from the instances when the clinical problem warrants a specialized approach because routine investigative studies have failed to provide a definitive diagnosis.[4,7,30,31] This interest has been furthered by recent recognition that vascular disease may have a significant etiologic role in some of these conditions. The vascular architecture of the involved segment of gut reveals some degree of dilatation and tortuosity of individual arteries, an increase in the number of regional vessels, and areas of intensified tissue staining in response to the increased blood flow demands of the inflamed tissues. There is recognizable thickening of the bowel wall in regional ileitis (Fig. 54-48), granulomatous colitis (Fig. 54-49), chronic ulcerative colitis (Fig. 54-50), and reversible vascular occlusion (Fig. 54-51). Each of these entities may reveal a degree of increased arteriovenous transit time and mild dilatation and tortuosity of the draining veins. The magnitude of the various

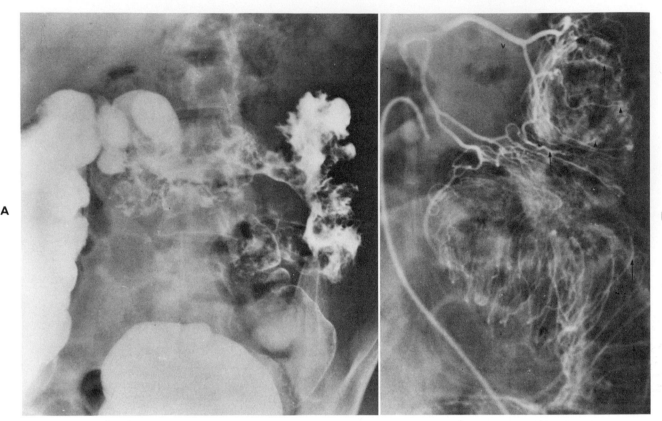

Fig. 54-49. Inferior mesenteric arteriogram showing granulomatous colitis. **A,** Barium enema shows asymmetrical areas of narrowing with deformity of the distal transverse and descending colon. Normal mucosa is absent; nodular mucosal remnants were present on the postevacuation film. **B,** Late arterial phase. The colonic end arteries are slightly tortuous (arrowheads). Some arterial ectasia (arrows) on the antimesenteric side of the colon is present. The bowel wall is thickened. Early opacification of a draining vein is seen, **V.**

angiographic alterations is generally proportional to the activity of the disease. Experience seems to indicate an inability to determine specific diagnosis by an objective evaluation of intestinal angiography. Barium studies remain the diagnostic procedure of choice.

It is unfortunate that selective arteriography does not seem to visualize the important abnormal intramural vessels that have been shown on microarteriographic studies to arise at right angles to the bifurcating vasa recta and to course parallel to the long axis of the bowel. These structures characterize inflammatory disease and are in sharp contrast to the disordered patterns of malignancy (Figs. 54-44 and 54-45). Primary vascular disease will be considered separately.

Localized abscesses, usually subacute or chronic in nature, may be difficult to evaluate

preoperatively, but accurate knowledge of the nature of such a lesion may bear on the therapeutic approach. Arteriography reveals displacement of regional vessels around the abscess while the lesion itself remains avascular. Ancillary signs of inflammation other than thrombotic obliteration of some regional vessels are generally not seen.

PRIMARY VASCULAR DISEASE OF THE ALIMENTARY TRACT

In the past, it has been possible to recognize the presence of mesenteric vascular disease through the manifestations present on routine roentgenologic studies of the bowel.[72] However, even when there was acute massive disruption of blood flow to the bowel, occasioned by superior mesenteric occlusion, the classic roentgenologic

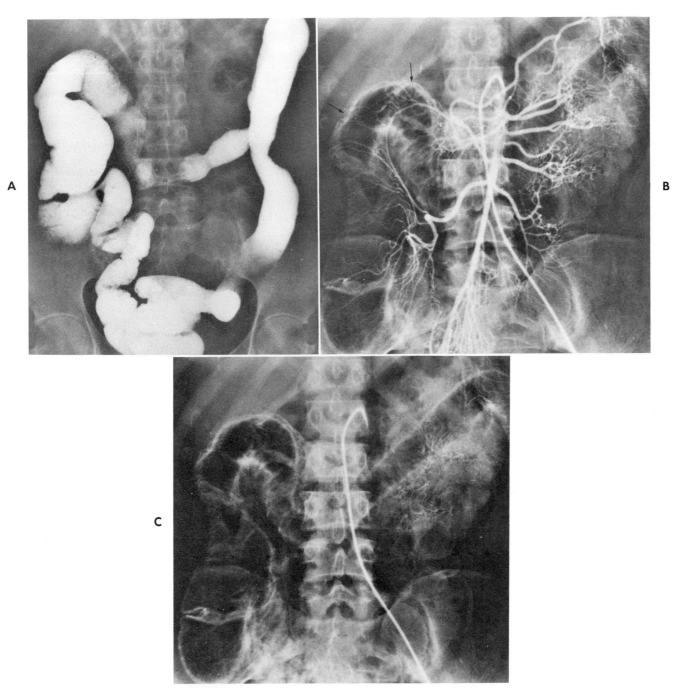

Fig. 54-50. Superior mesenteric arteriogram showing chronic ulcerative colitis. **A,** Barium enema. **B,** Arterial phase. The colonic end arteries appear to be slightly ectatic on the antimesenteric side of the bowel (arrows). **C,** Capillary phase. Diffuse thickening of the bowel wall is present.

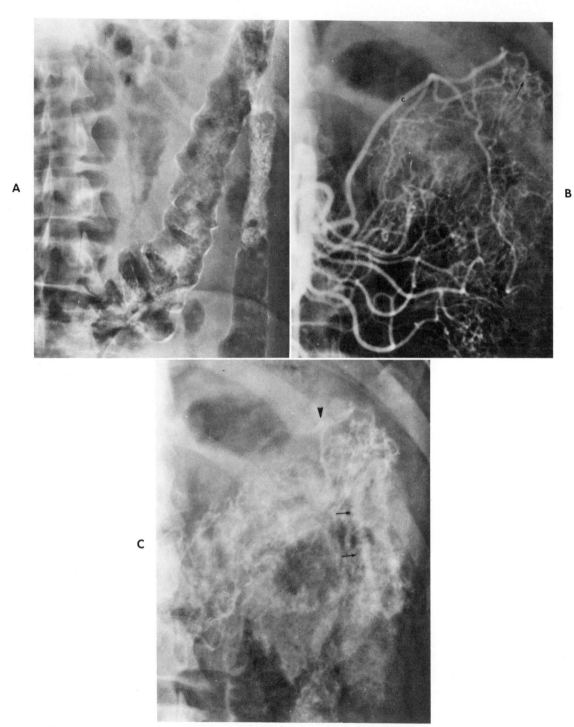

Fig. 54-51. Superior mesenteric arteriogram showing vascular insufficiency of the colon.
A, Barium enema. The distal transverse colon reveals mucosal swelling, loss of mucosal
folds, and "thumbprinting." **B,** Arterial phase. The left branch of the middle colic
artery, *C,* is dilated. There is slight tortuosity of the colonic end arteries (arrow). **C,**
Capillary-venous phase. The small draining veins are tortuous and ectatic and the middle
colonic vein has an increased density (arrowhead). The bowel wall is thickened (arrow).

features were often lacking. The clinical picture also presented a variety of patterns, and the clinical management of patients with abdominal vascular disease became more confused when it became evident that the correlation between symptoms and roentgenologic and pathologic findings was inconstant. The grave prognosis of this condition has been discouraging, but the possibility of altering the picture exists with recent improvement in techniques of vascular surgery.[11,43,44] Exact diagnosis is a necessity and is invaluable to proper therapy. It should be a truism that if the underlying disease is vascular, angiography is the means by which the diagnosis can be made.

The syndrome of abdominal angina represents a response of the gastrointestinal tract to ischemia. Both acute and chronic forms of occlusive vascular disease of the celiac and mesenteric arterial systems have been recognized. Partial and segmental occlusions and primary venous thrombosis exist. The symptoms are abdominal pain, disturbed intestinal peristalsis, malabsorption, fatty diarrhea, and weight loss. The presence of an abdominal bruit strongly suggests a significant vascular abnormality. While a variety of disorders can be present, the clinical manifestations of mesenteric insufficiency can also exist when no organic cause can be uncovered.[18] Indeed, infarction of the gastrointestinal tract does occur without vascular occlusion.[9]

In an acute situation, emergency arteriography is indicated whenever consideration is given to the diagnosis in the evaluation of the patient. Angiographic study of the patient with chronic abdominal angina is dictated by the need to establish the cause of the patient's symptoms and by the need to define the abnormal vascular anatomy prior to the surgical attempts to revascularize the bowel. The lateral projection can become a dominant part of the serial filming procedure.

Although arteriosclerosis is characteristically the underlying cause of the occlusive process, additional causes are being recognized. Idiopathic fibromuscular dysplasia of the celiac axis has been reported,[52] as has anatomic variation of the medial arcuate ligament of the diaphragm. In this latter instance, a portion of the diaphragmatic crura is so placed as to compress the proximal part of the celiac axis[12] (Fig. 54-52).

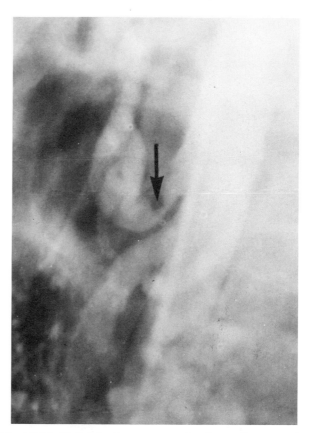

Fig. 54-52. Abdominal aortogram showing celiac stenosis. Lateral projection of the aortogram demonstrates celiac stenosis (arrow) secondary to displacement of the medial crura of the diaphragm. Poststenotic dilatation is present.

The exact role that vascular disease plays in the origin of several clinical conditions of the gut is not clear.[33] Intestinal arteriography has seldom been applied to their study. The etiology of segmental infarction of the bowel is, of course, a vascular process.[26] Vascular studies can establish an accurate diagnosis in such cases and provide an important contribution to the understanding of the process and the course of therapy.[64]

ISCHEMIA OF THE COLON

It is well recognized that ischemia of the colon may cause roentgenologic changes closely resembling ulcerative and granulomatous colitis. Prior investigations demonstrated that obliteration of the terminal portions of colonic end arteries does produce local mucosal changes that progress to superficial ulceration of the

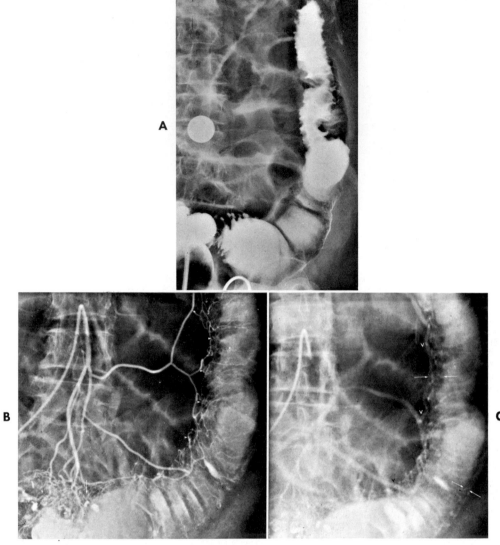

Fig. 54-53. Inferior mesenteric arteriogram; reversible vascular occlusion? **A,** Barium enema—"thumbprinting" of descending colon is demonstrated. Diverticulosis is present in the sigmoid colon. **B,** Arteriogram, arterial phase. There is hypervascularity along the mesenteric border of the descending colon. Arrows designate increased vascularity in the area of diverticulosis. **C,** Arteriogram, venous phase. An increased draining venous plexus is present. **V,** Major veins. Residual contrast density in the colon permits an estimation of the thickening of the bowel wall (arrows).

mucosa.[6,55,58,61,62] The tissue changes cause pseudotumors of the bowel wall to become visible on barium enema examination. These changes have been shown to be reversible when treated conservatively. Arteriographic study can show inflammatory alteration of the regional vessels with thickening of the bowel wall (Figs. 54-51, 54-53, and 54-54). The healing process occurs because a satisfactory level of tissue perfusion has been maintained.

Insufficiency of the blood supply to the bowel may also result in gangrene with necrosis of the entire thickness of the bowel wall and subsequent slough of the mucosa. With less extensive vascular compromise mucosal sloughing occurs, but the colonic blood supply is sufficiently intact to maintain the integrity of the wall of the colon. Fibrosis and stricture may be the end result.

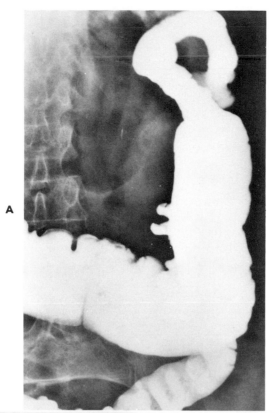

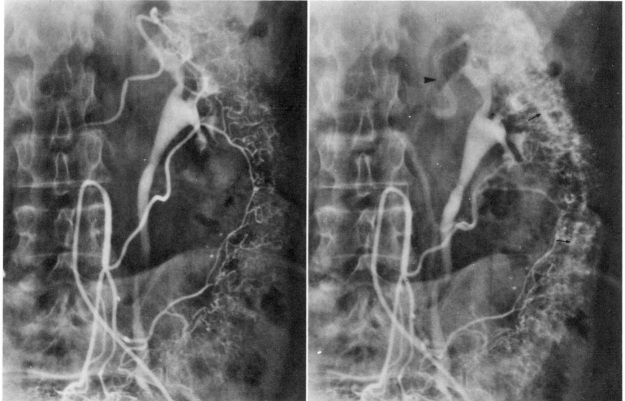

Fig. 54-54. Inferior mesenteric arteriogram showing ischemic colitis. **A,** Barium enema shows absence of mucosal folds and narrowing of the splenic flexure. **B,** Early arterial phase. The major vessels are normal. There is minimal tortuosity of the colonic end arteries. **C,** Late arterial phase. Small draining veins are irregular and ectatic. The bowel wall is thickened (arrows) and its lumen narrowed. Increased arteriovenous transit time is present. The draining middle colonic vein (arrowhead) shows early opacification.

Demonstration of a major vascular occlusion that produces gangrene of the colon is uncommon. It must be recognized that normal angiography does not rule out colonic infarction.

Angiography of reversible vascular disease usually reveals a normal or slightly attenuated arterial supply without dilatation. Mild acceleration of the arteriovenous transit time and thickening of the bowel wall may be recognized during the capillary phase. Small, tortuous, ectatic draining veins present increased density in the venous phase. The angiographic features of ischemic colitis are quite similar to those of inflammatory disease. The demonstration of a distinct pattern of dilatation, tortuosity, and crowding of end arteries in regional ileitis (Fig. 54-48) in comparison to the regional hypervascularity with tortuosity, irregular coursing of serosal vessels, and bowel thickening in vascular colonic disease, is believed to be only a reflection of the severity of the process (Figs. 54-53 and 54-54).

Aneurysms of the visceral arteries are not common but in specific instances are of major diagnostic importance.[27,34,65] An extremely high mortality has been associated with the crisis of a ruptured splenic artery aneurysm in the third trimester of pregnancy. In contrast, the presence of a calcified splenic artery aneurysm in the older patient is probably of little or no clinical significance. Serendipity has played a role in definition of aneurysms of such vessels as the hepatic artery and gastroduodenal artery. The clinical course is not too well known, but the possibility of rupture and thrombosis of these structures generally dictates surgical intervention when the diagnosis has been made.

Arteriovenous fistulas are often of iatrogenic origin, but congenital and spontaneous fistulas have been recognized.[24,67] Such lesions may mimic the symptoms of abdominal angina and may present dramatic bruits on physical examination. The systemic effects of such arteriovenous fistulas are well recognized although the lesion is uncommon. After their angiographic demonstration, surgical intervention may be advisable.

A variety of angiodysplastic lesions including angioma, aneurysms, arteriovenous fistulas (Figs. 54-9, 54-40, and 54-56), and phlebectasia have been shown to be a hallmark of hereditary hemorrhagic telangiectasia.[21,22] Widespread visceral involvement precludes surgical eradica-

tion. However, angiographic demonstration of the site of dominant lesions may be vital for proper therapy of uncontrolled bleeding in this disease. That spontaneous closure of arteriovenous fistulas and thrombotic obliteration of telangiectasia and angiomas can occur is also of considerable import in the treatment of these patients.[68] This has become a major therapeutic consideration since the spontaneous eradication of fistulas has been shown to occur in splenic (Fig. 54-22), renal, and peripheral arterial lesions.

Angiography has also brought to light the presence of diffuse arteriosclerotic disease of many vessels of the abdominal viscera and, at times, their involvement by some form of diffuse angiitis. The specific form of arteritis is not known, since its demonstration precludes operative intervention. Severe abdominal pain similar to that of acute pancreatitis may be a prominent clinical feature. A specific etiology for a necrotizing vasculitis of the abdominal viscera has been described in association with drug abuse[8,23] (Fig. 54-55). Its potential for severe involvement of the liver, stomach, pancreas, and mesentery of the intestine in addition to renal involvement results in a clinical symptom complex encompassing many systems of the body.

The possibility of a vascular etiology must be considered in patients who have vague abdominal pain, diarrhea, or any of the several features of the syndrome of abdominal angina. It would seem advisable to consider the vascular origin of disease far more often than now occurs in this differential diagnosis of gastrointestinal complaints of obscure origin. The serious prognosis of acute superior mesenteric occlusion can today be altered through modern vascular surgery. Prompt arteriographic investigation can result in the institution of therapy before irreparable damage to the bowel has resulted. At the other extreme, hazardous exploratory laparotomy in the patient with diffuse mesenteric arterial disease can be avoided through angiographic diagnosis. A more vigorous application of angiography of the alimentary tract appears to be indicated whenever the differential diagnosis includes disease conditions in which vascular abnormalities may be the cause.

Angiography for localization of an undetected site of intestinal bleeding may be performed by means of abdominal aortography,[25,35,57] but

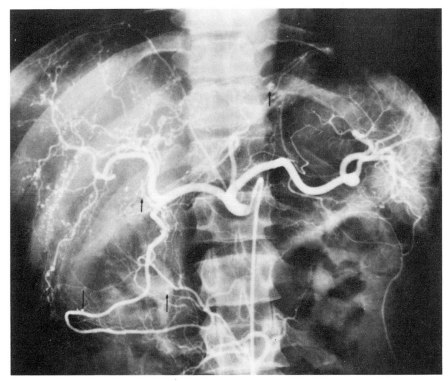

Fig. 54-55. Celiac arteriogram showing necrotizing angiitis of drug abuse. Many small aneurysms are present throughout the liver. A few of the less conspicuous aneurysms are designated by arrows.

selective superior and inferior mesenteric arteriography is generally preferred. As in the upper gastrointestinal hemorrhage, vigorous active bleeding is usually a prerequisite for successful angiography. Diffuse arterial and arteriovenous malformations may be demonstrable (Fig. 54-56). Hematobilia may be seen. Preoperative localization of these lesions is extremely important. Pooling of contrast in a bleeding diverticulum of the colon is identical in appearance to a bleeding gastric ulcer. Neovascularization with tissue stain in an undiagnosed tumor of the gut may be diagnosed in this manner. Conversely, complete selective arteriography of the intestine may fail to designate the bleeding site. Exploratory surgery may also fail to detect the source of hemorrhage, while in other instances its success has served to point up the deficiency of angiography. Nonetheless, specific problem cases merit angiographic investigation.

ABDOMINAL MASS LESIONS

Abdominal mass lesions represent one of the prime indications for exploratory laparotomy.

In a significant number of cases, precise diagnosis cannot be made prior to the operative procedure. However, arteriography is a valuable method for securing important information not otherwise available to the surgeon. It may provide additional clarification of the diagnostic problem and may diagram crucial anatomic information that can have considerable bearing on the operative management of the case.[10,20]

An abnormal increase in blood supply and distortion and displacement of large vessels can be readily demonstrated. These findings direct attention both to the organ of origin of the mass and to its growth potential. Many new growths, however, are poorly vascularized, and in many inflammatory thrombosis supervenes to reduce vascularity. Large masses also tend to compress and obscure vascular changes adjacent to the mass. Arteriographic diagnosis is also made more complex when a tumor obliterates its primary supply and borrows from contiguous structures in a parasitic fashion (Fig. 54-7). It may become impossible to determine from what tissues the neoplasm actually originated. The therapeutic

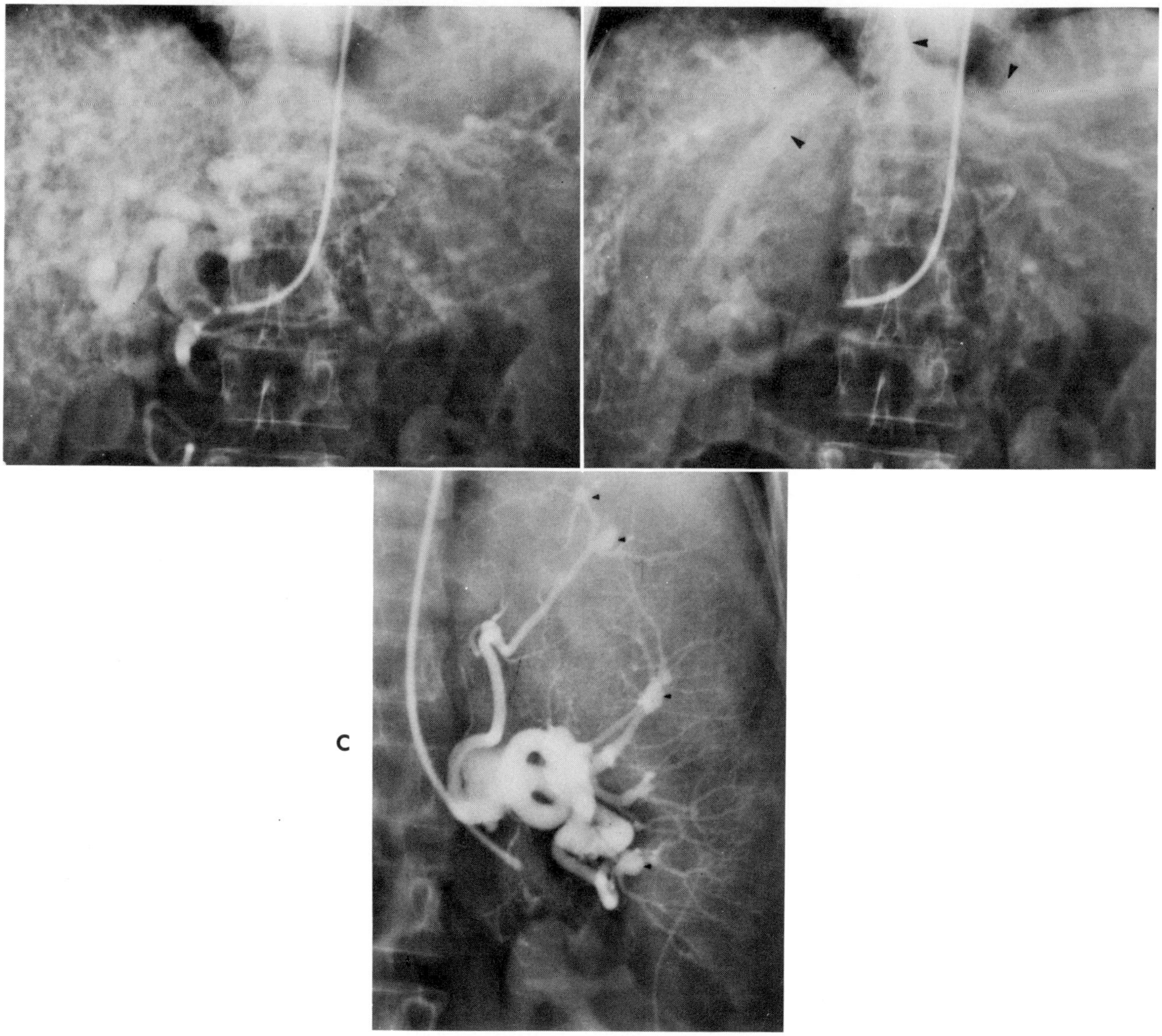

Fig. 54-56. Transaxillary visceral angiogram showing hereditary hemorrhagic telangiectasia. **A,** Arterial phase of selective hepatic angiogram. Angiodysplasia involves the entire intrahepatic vascular bed. There is marked dilatation and tortuosity of the vessels. Peripheral ramifications are represented by blotchy, conglomerate masses. **B,** Venous phase of selective hepatic angiogram. Dense opacification of the hepatic veins (arrowheads) and inferior vena cava (upper arrowhead) is a distinctive feature of the hepatic artery–hepatic vein shunts present in this disease. **C,** Selective splenic arteriogram. Spreading of the intrasplenic vessels is caused by splenomegaly. Several intrasplenic aneurysms are present (arrowheads).

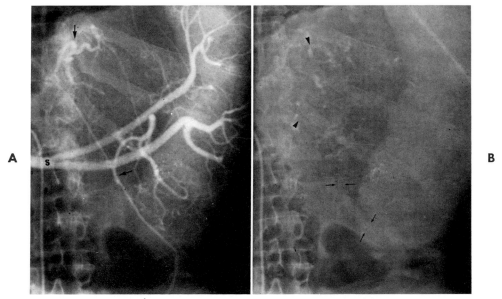

Fig. 54-57. Splenic arteriogram showing retroperitoneal liposarcoma. **A,** Arteriogram, arterial phase. The catheter has been placed in the orifice of the splenic artery, **S.** The lower arrow points to an epiploic branch, which gives rise to irregular, ectatic tumor vessels (upper arrow). **B,** Arteriogram, venous phase. Arrows show the course of the perisplenic vein, indicating obstruction. This was confirmed by phlebograms. Vascular "tumor lakes" are present (arrowheads). (Courtesy Department of Radiology, The New York Hospital—Cornell Medical Center.)

importance of the information obtained angiographically should not be underestimated in spite of these problems. The vascular anatomy of the retroperitoneal space and mesentery affords additional insight into the problem. Intercostal and lumbar arteries and their branches and the various epiploic vessels must be identified since they may play a major role in the tumor's vascularity (Figs. 54-8, 54-26, and 54-57).

Regardless of the problems involved in the angiographic diagnosis of abdominal mass lesions, the need for explicit preoperative evaluation represents a specific indication for the angiographic procedure as a study complementary to other means of investigation. The greatest use of the examination is obtained when there has been careful consideration of the entire problem, both diagnostic and therapeutic. There are many examples to attest to the fact that the surgical management of patients with ambiguous abdominal masses receives valuable assistance from angiographic studies.

CONCLUSIONS

A considerable fund of knowledge has been obtained through study of the vascular patterns present in diseases of the alimentary tract. Its correlation with clinical and laboratory evidence has provided more complete preoperative diagnostic evaluation of patients with known and obscure lesions of the abdominal viscera. In this way, visceral arteriography has become a valuable adjunct to routine diagnostic techniques. In selected instances, angiography has yielded pertinent information not obtained in any other way, thereby influencing both the interpretation of other diagnostic studies and the choice of therapy.

Many reasons for careful restraint in appraising visceral arteriography have been given. The future would seem to hold much of interest with the incorporation of pharmacologic agents into the protocol of angiography and the complementary use of intra-arterial radioisotope technique. The superb in vivo demonstration of angiographic anatomy and physiology provided by selective arteriography must, of necessity, achieve for it a significant role in the future of organ transplantation.

It is therefore necessary to be vigorous in research investigations but to carefully reflect upon the accomplishments and the depth of experience and to recognize failures and limitations. It is certainly not prudent to draw broad and positive conclusions from limited experience; it is far wiser to remember that truth is the daughter of time.

REFERENCES

1. Baum, S., Roy, R., Finkelstein, A. K., and Blakemore, W. S.: Clinical application of selective celiac and superior mesenteric arteriography, Radiology **84**:279, 1965.
2. Boijsen, E., and Bron, K. M.: Visceral arteriography, Ann. Rev. Med. **15**:273, 1964.
3. Boijsen, E., Ekman, C. A., and Olin, T.: Celiac and superior mesenteric angiography in portal hypertension, Acta Chir. Scand. **126**:315, 1963.
4. Boijsen, E., and Reuter, S. R.: Mesenteric angiography in evaluation of inflammatory and neoplastic disease of the intestine, Radiology **87**:1028, 1966.
5. Boijsen, E., Judkins, M. P., and Simay, A.: Angiographic diagnosis of hepatic rupture, Radiology **86**:66, 1966.
6. Boley, S. J., Schwartz, S., Lash, J., and Sternhill, V.: Reversible vascular occlusion of the colon, Surg. Gynec. Obstet. **116**:53, 1963.
7. Brahme, F.: Mesenteric angiography in regional enterocolitis, Radiology **87**:1037, 1966.
8. Citron, B. P., Halpern, M., McCarron, M., Lundberg, G., McCormick, R., Pincus, I. J., Tatter, D., and Haverback, B. J.: Necrotizing angiitis in drug addicts, New Eng. J. Med. **283**:1003, 1970.
9. Corday, E., and Vyden, J. K.: Splanchnic vascular syndromes, Mod. Concepts Cardiovasc. Dis. **39**:85, 1970.
10. Crosta, C.: Diagnostic value of abdominal aortography in clinically obscure extraperitoneal tumors, Panminerva Med. **5**:167, 1963.
11. Dardik, H., Seidenberg, B., Parker, J. G., and Hurwitt, E. S.: Intestinal angina with malabsorption treated by elective revascularization; case report and review of the literature with emphasis on absorption studies, J.A.M.A. **194**:1206, 1965.
12. Dunbar, J. D., Molnar, W., Beman, F., and Marable, S. A.: Compression of the celiac trunk and abdominal angina—preliminary report of 15 cases, Amer. J. Roentgen. **95**:731, 1965.
13. Evans, J. A.: Specialized roentgen diagnostic techniques in the investigation of abdominal disease; Annual oration in memory of Clarence Elton Hufford, Radiology **82**:579, 1964.
14. Evans, J. A., and Halpern, M.: Celiac and superior mesenteric arteriography. In Schobinger, R. A., and Ruzika, F. F., Jr., editors: Vascular roentgenology, New York, 1964, The Macmillan Company.
15. Finck, E., and Halpern, M.: The nutrient supplement enhanced celiac angiogram, Radiology **101**:79, 1973.
16. Glenn, F., Evans, J. A., Halpern, M., and Thorbjarnarson, B.: Selective celiac and superior mesenteric arteriography, Surg. Gynec. Obstet. **118**:93, 1964.
17. Glenn, F., and Halpern, M.: Celiac and superior mesenteric arteriography, Rev. Int. Heptat. **15**:337, 1965.
18. Gooding, R. A., and Couch, R. D.: Mesenteric ischemia without vascular occlusion, Arch. Surg. (Chicago) **85**:186, 1962.
19. Halpern, M.: The role of angiography in the diagnosis of cancer. In IX Clinical Conference on Cancer, Anderson Hospital and Tumor Institute, 1964, Chicago, 1966, Year Book Medical Publishers, Inc.
20. Halpern, M.: Selective inferior mesenteric arteriography; clinical implications, Vasc. Dis. **1**:294, 1964.
21. Halpern, M., Turner, A. F., and Citron, B. P.: Hereditary hemorrhagic telangiectasia. An angiographic study of abdominal visceral angiodysplasias associated with gastrointestinal hemorrhage, Radiology **90**:1143, 1968.
22. Halpern, M., Turner, A. F., and Citron, B. P.: Angiodysplasias of the abdominal viscera associated with hereditary hemorrhagic telangiectasia, Amer. J. Roentgen. **102**:783, 1968.
23. Halpern, M., and Citron, B. P.: Necrotizing angiitis associated with drug abuse, Amer. J. Roentgen. **111**:663, 1971.
24. Hufnagel, C. A., and Conrad, P.: Abdominal arteriovenous fistulas, Surg. Gynec. Obstet. **114**:470, 1962.
25. Koehler, P. R., and Salmon, R. B.: Angiographic localization of unknown acute gastrointestinal bleeding, Radiology **89**:244, 1967.
26. Kradjian, R. M.: Ischemic stenosis of small intestine, Arch. Surg. (Chicago) **91**:829, 1965.
27. Kraft, R. O., and Fry, W. J.: Aneurysms of celiac axis, Surg. Gynec. Obstet. **117**:563, 1963.
28. Love, L., Greenfield, G. B., Braun, T. W., Moncada, R., Freeark, R. J., and Baker, R. J.: Arteriography of splenic trauma, Radiology **91**:96, 1968.
29. Lunderquist, A.: Angiography in carcinoma of the pancreas, Acta Radiol. (Stockholm) Suppl. **235**, 1965.
30. Lunderquist, A., and Lunderquist, A.: Angiography in ulcerative colitis, Amer. J. Roentgen. **99**:18, 1967.
31. Lunderquist, A., Lunderquist, A., and Knutsson, H.: Angiography in Crohn's disease of the small bowel and colon, Amer. J. Roentgen. **101**:338, 1967.
32. McAlister, W. H., Margulis, A. R., Heinbecker, D., and Spjut, H.: Arteriography and microangiography of gastric and colonic lesions, Radiology **79**:769, 1962.
33. McCombs, R. P.: Systemic "allergic" vasculitis; clinical and pathological relationships, J.A.M.A. **194**:1059, 1965.
34. McCorriston, J. R., Allin, G. E., and Crowell, D. E.: Splenohepatic arterial anastomosis for aneurysms of hepatic artery, Surgery **47**:636, 1960.
35. Margulis, A. R., Heinbecker, P., and Bernard, H. R.: Operative mesenteric arteriography in the search for the site of bleeding in unexplained gastrointestinal hemorrhage, Surgery **48**:534, 1960.
36. Margulis, A. R., and Heinbecker, P.: Mesenteric arteriography, Amer. J. Roentgen. **86**:103, 1961.
37. Meaney, T. F., and Buonocore, E.: Arteriographic manifestations of pancreatic neoplasm, Amer. J. Roentgen. **95**:720, 1965.

38. Meaney, T. F. Winkelman, E. I., Sullivan, B. H., and Brown, C. H.: Selective splanchnic arteriography in the diagnosis of pancreatic tumors, Cleveland Clin. Quart. **30**:193, 1963.

39. Meyers, H. I., and Halpern, M.: Radiology of blunt abdominal trauma. In London, P. S., editor: Modern trends in accident surgery and medicine, London, 1970, Butterworth & Co. (Publishers) Ltd., p. 71.

40. Michels, N. A.: Blood supply and anatomy of the upper abdominal organs with a descriptive atlas, Philadelphia, 1955, J. B. Lippincott Co.

41. Michels, N. A.: Collateral arterial pathways to liver after ligation of hepatic artery and removal of celiac axis, Cancer **6**:708, 1953.

42. Michels, N. A., Siddharth, P., Kornblith, P. L., and Parke, W. W.: The variant blood supply to the descending colon, rectosigmoid and rectum based on 400 dissections; its importance in regional resections; a review of medical literature, Dis. Colon Rectum **8**:251, 1965.

43. Morris, G. C., Jr., Crawford, E. S., Cooley, D. A., and DeBakey, M. E.: Revascularization of the celiac and superior mesenteric arteries, Arch. Surg. (Chicago) **84**:113, 1962.

44. Morris, G. C., Jr., and DeBakey, M. E.: Abdominal angina—diagnosis and surgical treatment, J.A.M.A. **176**:89, 1961.

45. Nebesar, R. A., Pollard, J., Edmunds, L. H., Jr., McKhann, C. F.: Indication for selective celiac and superior mesenteric angiography—experience with 128 cases, Amer. J. Roentgen **92**:1100, 1964.

46. Norell, H. G.: Traumatic rupture of the spleen diagnosed by abdominal aortography; report of a case, Acta Radiol. (Stockholm) **48**:449, 1957.

47. Nusbaum, M., Baum, S., Blakemore, W. S., and Finkelstein, A. K.: Demonstration of intra-abdominal bleeding by selective arteriography; Visualization of celiac and superior mesenteric arteries, J.A.M.A. **191**:389, 1965.

48. Odman, P.: Pancreatic arteriography. In Abrams, H. L., editor: Angiography, Boston, 1961, Little, Brown and Company.

49. Odman, P.: Percutaneous selective angiography of the celiac artery, Acta Radiol. (Stockholm) **159** (Suppl.):1, 1959.

50. Odman, P.: Percutaneous selective angiography of the main branches of the aorta, Acta Radiol. (Stockholm) **45**:1, 1956.

51. Olsson, O.: Angiographic diagnosis of an islet-cell tumor of the pancreas, Acta Chir. Scand. **126**:346, **1963**.

52. Palubinskas, A. J., and Ripley, H. R.: Fibromuscular hyperplasia in extrarenal arteries, Radiology **82**:451, 1964.

53. Pollard, J. J., and Nebesar, R. A.: Catheterization of the splenic artery for portal venography, New Eng. J. Med. **271**:234, 1964.

54. Redman, H. C., Reuter, S. R., and Bookstein, J. J.: Angiography of abdominal trauma, Ann. Surg. **169**: 57, 1969.

55. Reeves, J. D., and Wang, C. C.: The stages of mesenteric artery disease, Southern Med. J. **54**:541, 1961.

56. Reuter, S. R., and Boijsen, E.: Angiographic findings in two ileal carcinoid tumors, Radiology **87**:836, 1966.

57. Reuter, S. R., and Bookstein, J. J.: Angiography for localization of gastrointestinal bleeding, Gastroenterology **54**:876, 1968.

58. Reuter, S. R., Kanter, I. E., and Redman, H. C.: Angiography in reversible colonic ischemia, Radiology **97**:371, 1970.

59. Rossi, P.: Selective celiac arteriography in hepatic cirrhosis (transfemoral approach). In Schobinger, R. A., and Ruzicka, F. F., Jr., editors: Vascular roentgenology, New York, 1964, The Macmillan Company.

60. Schobinger, R.: Operative intestinal arteriography in diagnosis of diverticulitis of the colon, Acta Radiol. (Stockholm) **52**:28, 1959.

61. Schwartz, S., Boley, S., Lash, J., and Sternhill, V.: Roentgenologic aspects of reversible vascular occlusion of colon and its relationship to ulcerative colitis, Radiology **80**:625, 1963.

62. Schwartz, S., Boley, S. S., Robinson, K., Krieger, H., Schultz, L., and Allen, A. C.: Roentgenologic features of vascular disorders of intestines, Radiol. Clin. N. Amer. **3**:71, 1964.

63. Seldinger, S. I.: Catheter replacement of needle in percutaneous arteriography, Acta Radiol. (Stockholm) **39**:368, 1953.

64. Shippey, S. H., Jr., and Acker, J. J.: Segmental infarction of the colon demonstrated by selective inferior mesenteric arteriography, Amer. J. Surg. **109**:671, 1965.

65. Spittel, J. A., Jr., Fairbairn, J. F., II, Kincaid, O. W., and ReMine, W. H.: Aneurysm of the splenic artery, J.A.M.A. **175**:452, 1961.

66. Spjut, H., Margulis, A. R., and McAlister, W. H.: Microangiographic study of gastrointestinal lesions, Amer. J. Roentgen. **92**:1173, 1964.

67. Steinberg, I., Tillotson, P. M., and Halpern, M.: Roentgenography of systemic (congenital and traumatic) arteriovenous fistulas, Amer. J. Roentgen. **89**:343, 1963.

68. Stocks, L. O., Halpern, M., and Turner, A. F.: Spontaneous closure of an arteriovenous fistula. Report of a case in hereditary hemorrhagic telangiectasia, Radiology **92**:1499, 1969.

69. Strom, B. G., and Winberg, T.: Percutaneous selective angiography of the inferior mesenteric artery, Acta Radiol. (Stockholm) **47**:401, 1962.

70. Swanson, G. E.: A case of cystadenoma of the pancreas studied by selective angiographty, Radiology **81**:592, 1963.

71. Viamonte, M., Jr., and Stevens, R. C.: Guided angiography, Amer. J. Roentgen. **94**:30, 1965.

72. Wang, C. C., and Reeves, J. D.: Mesenteric vascular disease, Amer. J. Roentgen. **83**:895, 1960.

73. Woodruff, J. H., Ottoman, B. E., Simonton, J. H., and Averbook, B. D.: The radiologic differential diagnosis of abdominal trauma, Radiology **72**:641, 1959.

55 | Endoscopic camera correlation

Shoichi Yamagata
Makoto Ishikawa

Recent advances in the endoscopic apparatus include a gastrocamera and fiberoptics with an automatic exposure mechanism and a cold-light source.[9,13] This apparatus permits observation of the interior of the digestive tract in color.[7] Furthermore, cytologic and biopsy studies are performed under direct visualization. Endoscopic examination is an important supplement to increasing roentgenologic accuracy. Whereas with roentgenography lesions at the cardia, antrum, and anterior wall of the stomach may be overlooked, with endoscopy the common "blind spots" are in the upper part of the body, especially on the posterior wall and in the pyloric region.[2]

ENDOSCOPIC EQUIPMENT

A gastrocamera, type V or type PA, serves for routine endoscopic examination, and a GTF-A fiberscope with a gastrocamera in its tip is employed for further examination. The best photographs are obtained by a type V or PA gastrocamera. We consider the type PA gastrocamera to be a perfect instrument because its wide photographic angle of 108 degrees and wide bending angle of 200 degrees eliminate most "blind spots" on the gastric mucosa. The slender flexible tube, 7-mm. diameter, permits a U-shaped turn of the distal end for complete visual survey. An automatic exposure mechanism with an electric eye produces clear pictures and shortens the time of examination. Routinely, outpatients are examined roentgenographically on the first visit and by gastrocamera on the next day.

EARLY CANCER OF THE STOMACH

The term "early cancer" is applied to all carcinomas of the stomach that are grossly confined to the mucosa and submucosa (Figs. 55-2 and 55-3). A macroscopic classification for early cancer of the stomach was proposed by the Japanese Gastroenterological Endoscopy Society in 1962 (Fig. 55-1). The classification has been widely adopted by Japanese investigators, including radiologists, endoscopists, surgeons, and pathologists. It has contributed greatly to the recent progress in this field.[4,10,12] In our hands, 76.2% of 122 early cancers of the stomach were diagnosed correctly, an additional 12.3% were suspected on the initial and subsequent roentgenologic examinations, 4.9% were misdiagnosed as polyp, ulcer, or other benign lesions, and 6.6% of early malignant neoplasms were overlooked. Conversely, 74.3% of 140 early cancers of the stomach were correctly diagnosed as cancer by endoscopic examination, 17.1% were suspected of being cancer, 5.7% were mistaken as benign polyps, and 2.9% were missed.

BENIGN ULCER DISEASE

Murakami[5] classified four groups according to depth of mucosal ulceration, defect of mucous membrane, or erosion; defect of submucosal tissue with penetration of muscularis mucosae; defect reaching but not penetrating muscular layers; and deep ulceration penetrating all layers of the stomach wall. The last two groups were designated as being classic ulcers. Oi[8] noted that 97.0% of 855 ulcers were situated adjacent to mucosal boundaries and on the side of the boundary opposite the area of the fundic gland.

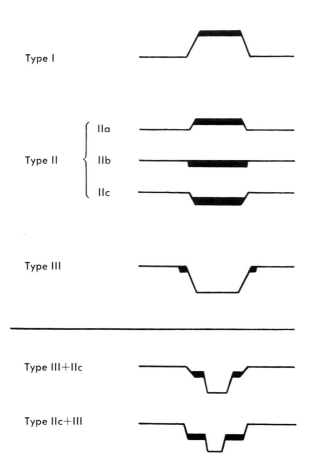

Fig. 55-1. Macroscopic classification of early gastric carcinoma. In applying this classification, the histogenesis of carcinomas should not be considered. The difference between type IIc and type III is that the depression of the latter is limited beyond the submucosa.

Type I. (Protruded type)
Protrusion into the gastric lumen is eminent.

Type II. (Superficial type)
Unevenness of the surface is inconspicuous. This is further divided into 3 subtypes:

Type IIa. (Elevated type)
The surface is slightly elevated.

Type IIb. (Flat type)
Almost no recognizable elevation or depression from the surrounding mucosa.

Type IIc. (Depressed type)
The surface is slightly depressed.

Type III. (Excavated type)
An excavation in the gastric wall is prominent.

When a carcinoma shows diverse morphologic patterns, two or more types are described together, for example, type III+IIc or IIc+III. The first Roman numeral indicates the predominant pattern.

This position might explain the frequent occurrence of ulcers at the angulus of the lesser curvature and the presence of linear ulcers usually vertical to the longitudinal axis of the stomach.

Even duodenal ulcers are now within reach of the endoscope (Fig. 55-4).

Linear ulcer

Shirakabe and associates[12] diagnosed linear ulcers regardless of the size, although Murakami[5] originally designated the linear ulcer as one more than 3 cm. in length (Fig. 55-5).

Linear ulcers, including kissing ulcers, are also called symmetrical ulcers. They are situated on both the anterior and the posterior walls, mounting the lesser curvature. About 50% of linear ulcers are found within 3 cm. of the pyloric ring. Antral linear ulcers parallel to the horizontal axis of the stomach cause shortening of the lesser curvature.

Although a shortened lesser curvature is easily seen in roentgenograms, demonstration of the entire linear niche may be difficult. Only about half the linear ulcers are diagnosed by means of barium filling. They are best demonstrated in supine views obtained with double contrast and compression. Endoscopic examination, however, demonstrates these ulcers more readily than does roentgenographic examination.

Multiple ulcers

Multiple ulcers are best demonstrated by an air-contrast study and compression.[3] These ulcers characteristically produce a pronounced deformity of the stomach, particularly on the lesser curvature (Fig. 55-6).

Small and shallow ulcers are not uncommonly multiple and are easily overlooked.

Ulcer scars

The roentgenographic features of the ulcer scar are convergence or interruption of the mucosal folds around the lesion and an irregular, reticulated, nodular pattern. A scar from a benign ulcer may be difficult to differentiate from an early cancer of the superficial depressed type, which is diagnosed more readily by endoscopic examination, biopsy, and cytologic study.

Erosive gastritis

Abel[1] described two types of gastritis seen radiologically: the erosive type, which disap-

Text continued on p. 1462.

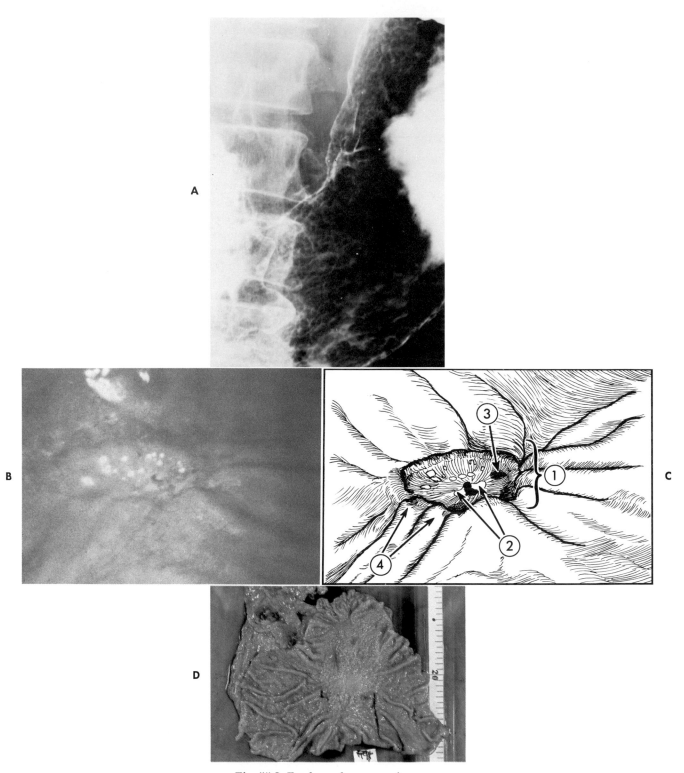

Fig. 55-2. For legend see opposite page.

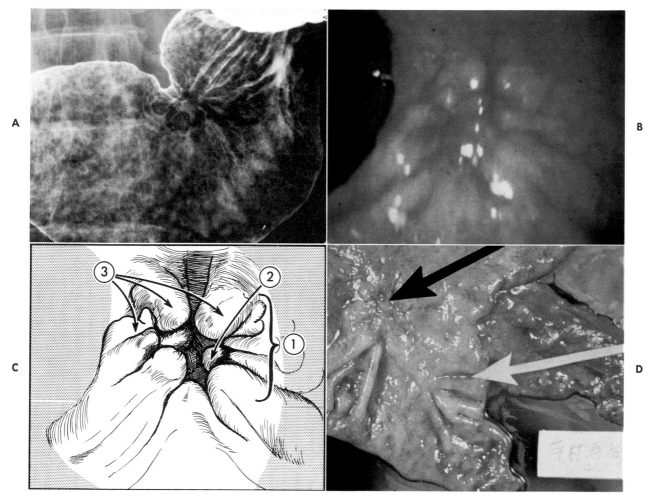

Fig. 55-3. A, Air-contrast roentgenograph taken with the patient in prone position shows folds converging to a nodular area close to the incisura. **B,** The endoscopic view shows the irregular shallow ulceration surrounded by mucosal protuberance. **C,** Illustration of **B** with 1, irregular erosion; 2, islands of remaining mucosa; 3, nodularity of club-shaped converging mucosa. (Light reflections not shown.) **D,** The surgical specimen showed an early gastric adenocarcinoma with invasion confined to the mucosa and submucosa, mixed Types IIc and IIa.

Fig. 55-2. A, Roentgenographic air-contrast study shows a small area of irregular and stiffened mucosal folds on the lesser curvature above the inciscura. Folds converge toward a flattened area with increased barium collection. **B,** The endoscopic view shows a mucosal depression with blanching of the mucosa. Folds stop at the clearly demarcated, but irregular margin of the flat crater. **C,** Illustration of **B** with 1, flat irregular crater; 2, mucosal debris; 3, punctate hemorrhage; 4, converging folds with club-shaped termination. Some adjacent folds are fusing. **D,** The resected specimen of a 15 by 7 mm. Type IIc, early gastric carcinoma.

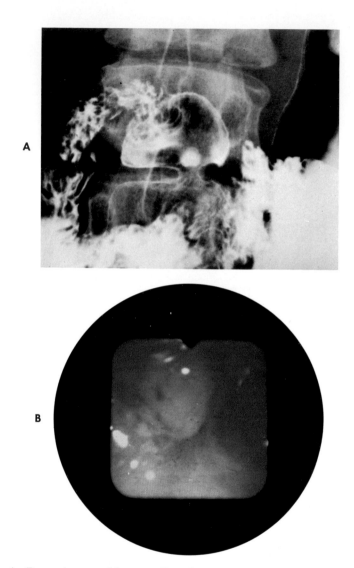

Fig. 55-4. A, Roentgenographic spot film shows ulcer crater on the posterior wall of the base of the duodenal bulb just beyond the pylorus. **B,** Endoscopic view of the duodenal ulcer faintly seen through the pylorus.

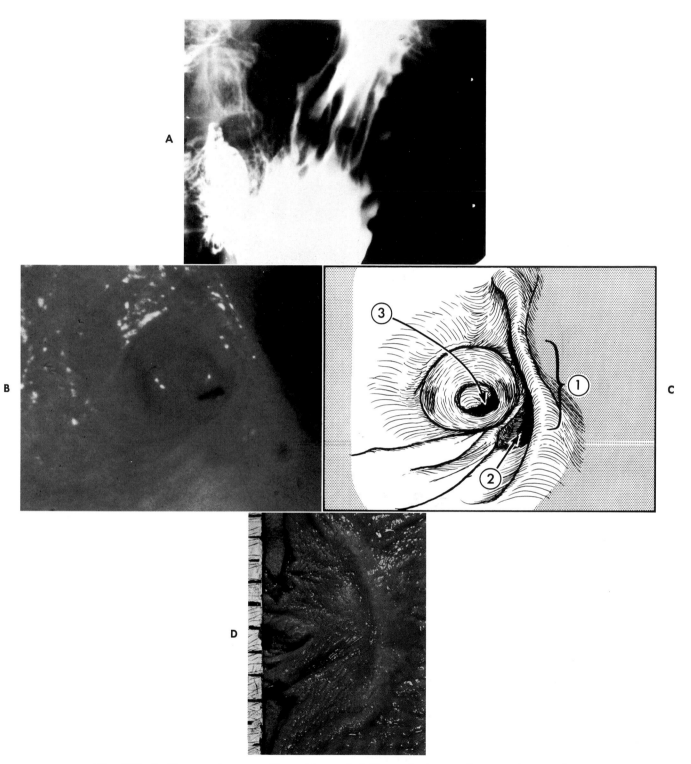

Fig. 55-5. A, Compression spot film with vertical linear barium stripe running to the lesser curvature. **B,** Shallow stripe of erosion on the lesser curvature of the antrum. These lesions are best detected endoscopically, but are difficult to differentiate from Type IIc early cancer. **C,** Illustration of the endoscopic view in **B** with 1, angulus of the stomach; 2, shallow linear erosion surrounded by injected mucosa; 3, pylorus. (Light reflections are deleted.) **D,** The surgical specimen revealed a linear benign ulcer in the antrum vertically to the longitudinal axis of the resected stomach.

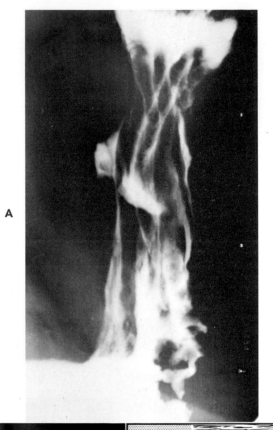

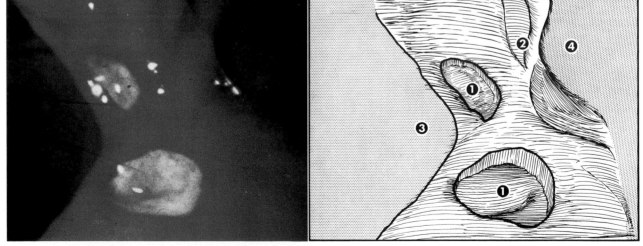

Fig. 55-6. A, Two benign-appearing ulcer craters in the midportion of the body of the stomach. **B,** Endoscopic view shows two ulcer niches with clear-cut margins, covered with **mucus and debris. C,** Illustration of the endoscopic view with **1,** two sharply demarcated **benign ulcer craters; 2,** tapering and interruption of mucosal folds; **3,** gastric antrum; **4,** body of the stomach.

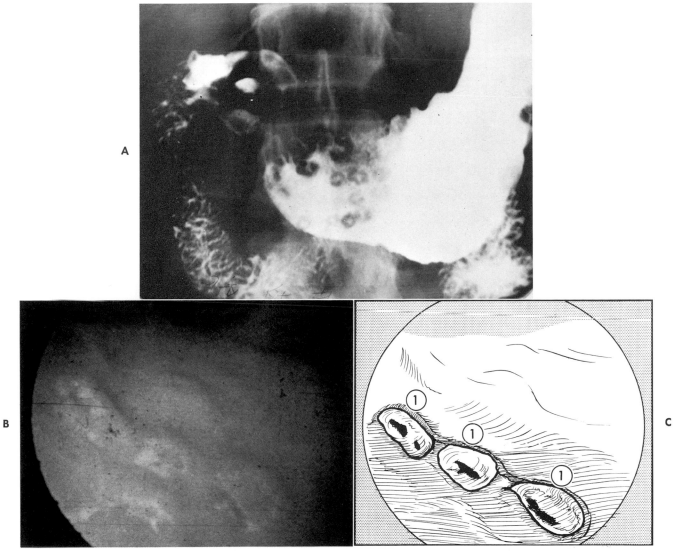

Fig. 55-7. A, Roentgenograph showing multiple polypoid protuberances in the antrum with small central barium collections. A duodenal ulcer crater is present in the center of the bulb. **B,** Endoscopic view of varioliform erosive gastritis on the greater curvature side of the antrum. The ischemic mucosa is blanched. **C,** Illustration of **B** with 1, multiple varioliform mucosa protuberances with small central craters and erosions.

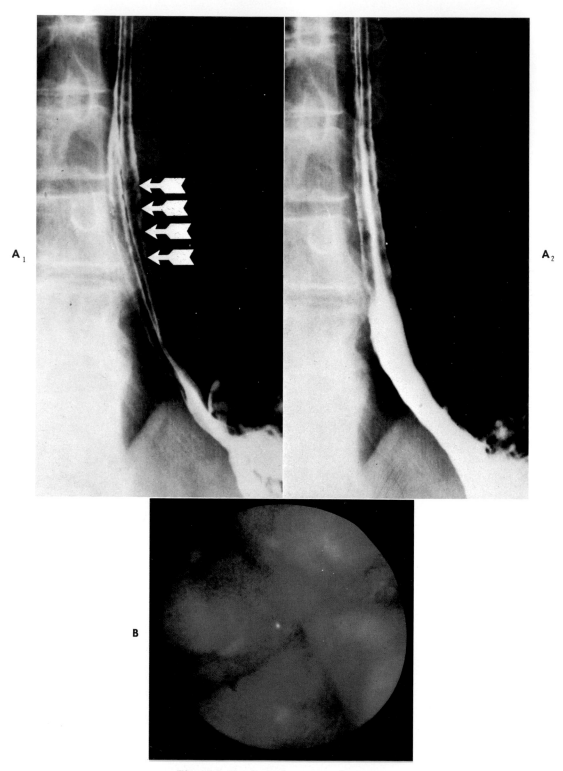

Fig. 55-8. For legend see opposite page.

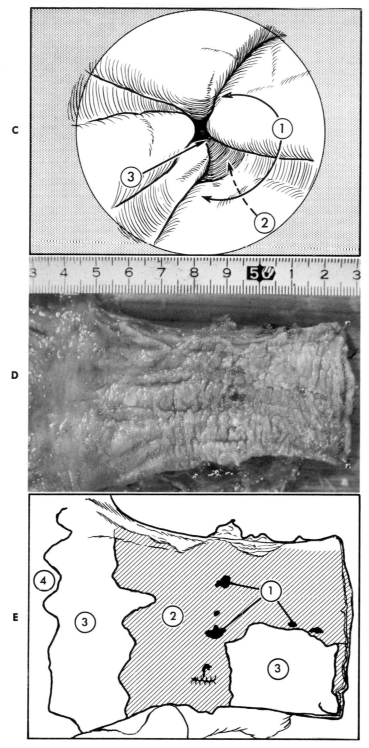

Fig. 55-8. A, Esophageal roentgenographs taken with the patient in supine R-A-O position. Note the minimal irregularity on the lateral margin (arrows) with zig zag of the mucosal line. The uneven barium density indicates irregular mucosal surface. There was no hiatus hernia and no reflux. **B,** Endoscopic view with injected mucosa and some erosion. **C,** Illustration of endoscopic view, **B,** with **1,** diminishing caliber of mucosal folds; **2,** extensive erosion; **3,** esophageal lumen. Malignancy suspected. Biopsy showed squamous cell carcinoma. **D,** Surgical specimen of the same esophagus with erosions extending from the lower to the middle esophagus. Carcinoma was limited to the squamous epithelium. **E,** Illustration of **D** with **1,** erosions; **2,** decolorated mucosa; **3,** esophageal mucosa; **4,** gastric mucosa.

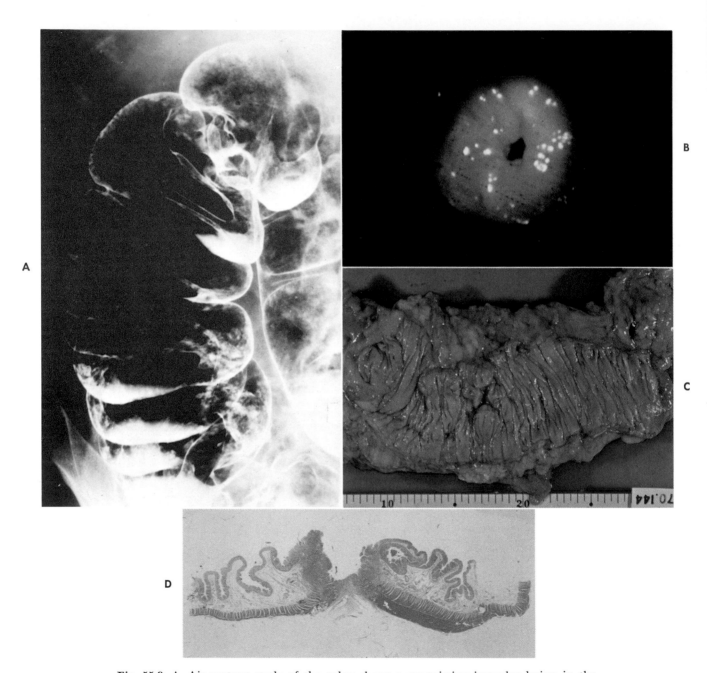

Fig. 55-9. A, Air-contrast study of the colon shows a constricting irregular lesion in the hepatic flexure. **B,** Endoscopic view through the colonofiberscope. Distal view of the stenosing carcinoma. **C,** Surgical specimen with small malignant ulcerating tumor. **D,** Histology section shows the infiltrating and ulcerating adenocarcinoma of the hepatic flexure extending to the serosa.

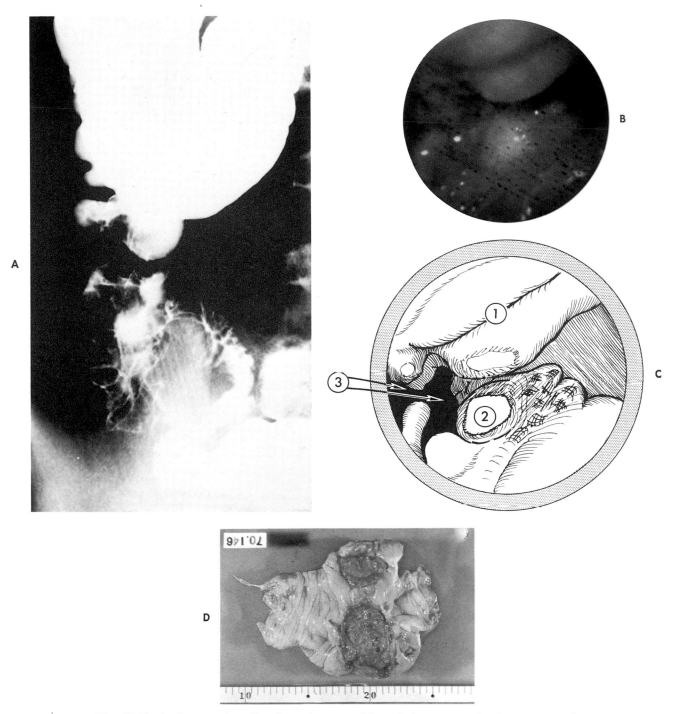

Fig. 55-10. A, Compression film shows honeycombing of the mucosa in the cecum and barium collection in two ulcerations. **B,** Colonofiberscopic view of the cecal ulcerations. **C,** Illustration of **B** with **1,** normal mucosa of the ascending colon; **2,** ulcer in the cecum (the second ulcer above the ileocecal valve is faintly seen); **3,** hemorrhage. **D,** Surgical specimen showing two colonic ulcerations, nonspecific, apparently arteriosclerotic in this 76-year-old patient.

pears within a few months, and the invasive form, which may persist for up to a few years. The invasive form is caused by hyperplasia. Walk[14] originally classified gastric erosions on endoscopic examination into three types, according to their marginal appearances: varioliform,[11] punctiform, and mixed.

Hyperacidity, which is common in varioliform erosive gastritis, was complicated by gastric and duodenal ulcers in 32% of our patients (Fig. 55-7).

EARLY CANCER OF THE ESOPHAGUS

Early cancer of the esophagus is defined as an infiltration limited to the submucosal layer, whether or not lymph nodes are involved.[6] Between 1966 and 1970 twenty-eight cases of early esophageal carcinoma were reported in Japan. Preoperative biopsy and cytologic studies in twenty-one patients undergoing endoscopy and roentgenologic study showed a correct diagnosis of carcinoma in all but one, which was diagnosed as a benign tumor. These results illustrate the high accuracy of diagnosis by this combined method (Fig. 55-8).

COLONIC ENDOSCOPY

Early experience with the colonic fiberscope indicates great future importance of this new endoscopic technique (Fig. 55-9). A sufficiently experienced physician is able to advance the endoscope into the cecum of some patients under fluoroscopic control (Fig. 55-10). The colon can be irrigated through the instrument.

REFERENCES

1. Abel, W.: Die Röntgendiagnose der gastritis erosiva, Fortschr. Röntgenstr. **80**:39, 1954.
2. Ashizawa, S., and Kidokoro, T.: Endoscopic color atlas of gastric diseases, New York, 1970, Intercontinental Medical Book Cooperation.
3. Ichikawa, H.: Practice of the x-ray diagnosis for diseases of the stomach, Tokyo, 1964, Bunkodo.
4. Kuru, M., editor: Atlas of early carcinoma of the stomach, Tokyo, 1967, Nakayama-Shoten.
5. Murakami, T.: A new concept for an ulcer-cancer, Juntendo Med. J. **13**:159, 1967.
6. Nabeya, K.: Early carcinoma of the esophagus, Stomach Intestine **5**:1213, 1970.
7. Nelson, R. S.: Gastroscopic photography, Chicago, 1966, Year Book Medical Publishers, Inc.
8. Oi, M., and others: A possible dual control mechanism in the origin of peptic ulcer, Gastroenterology **57**:280, 1969.
9. Oshima, H., editor: Gastrokamera-Untersuchung, Berlin, 1971, Walter De Cruyter.
10. Sakita, T., and others: Observations on the healing ulcerations in early cancer, the life cycle of the malignant ulcer, Gastroenterology **60**:835, 1971.
11. Sata, H., and others: Endoscopic observations and bioptic findings of varioliform erosion of the stomach, Stomach Intestine **6**:1141, 1971.
12. Shirakabe, H., and others: Atlas of x-ray diagnosis of early gastric cancer, Tokyo, 1966, Igaku-Shoin.
13. Yamagata, S.: An atlas of endoscopic diagnosis, Tokyo, 1969, Nakayama-Shoten.
14. Walk, L.: Erosive gastritis, Gastroenterologia **84**:88, 1955.

Part X

Pediatric roentgenology

The gastrointestinal tract in children | 56

Edward B. Singleton

The roentgenologic investigation of the alimentary tract of the pediatric patient requires a knowledge of many conditions found only in this age group as well as an appreciation of technical differences in the method of examination as compared with the adult patient. Careful fluoroscopic examination and adequate roentgenographic studies are as essential in children as in adults. The inconvenience of examining an uncooperative infant or child should never serve as an excuse for foregoing a complete roentgenologic study. The gonadal areas of the patient should be protected, the field size should be made as small as possible consistent with adequate visualization, and, when possible, image amplification should be used. Equipment capable of rapid exposure time, utilizing a generator capacity of at least 300 ma, is essential for good quality roentgenograms of children.

A detailed roentgenologic description of all pediatric alimentary tract abnormalities is beyond the scope of this chapter. Other publications provide this information.[3,9,35] The purpose of this chapter is to provide the radiologist with information regarding some of the differences between pediatric and adult roentgenology, particularly in the methods of patient preparation and in the technique of examination, and to discuss the roentgenologic findings in the more common diseases affecting the alimentary tract of infants and children.

SYMPTOMS REQUIRING ROENTGENOLOGIC EXAMINATION

Because routine upper gastrointestinal tract and colon examinations are neither advisable nor necessary in the pediatric patient, the order in which the various portions of the alimentary tract are to be examined depends upon careful clinical evaluation, particularly in the infant, who is unable to describe his condition in terms of localization of pain or other symptoms. The major symptoms and signs of alimentary tract disease that require roentgenologic investigation are abdominal pain, vomiting, constipation or diarrhea, blood in the stools, and abdominal distention. The presence of one of these presenting signs or symptoms indicates the logical site of disease and directs the radiologist to that portion of the alimentary tract that is to be studied.

Abdominal pain

Abdominal pain in infants is difficult to evaluate, but intermittent crying accompanied by flexion of the thighs and defecation suggests pain of bowel origin. A preliminary scout roentgenogram of the abdomen is mandatory in such cases to determine whether or not intestinal obstruction is present. This may be followed by barium enema studies if there is evidence of low bowel obstruction. Upper gastrointestinal tract examination is seldom of value in determining the cause of this symptom.

Abdominal pain in the older child is the most common symptom requiring roentgenologic evaluation of the intestinal tract. The symptom is variable in location, time of appearance, and severity. The child usually points to the periumbilical or epigastric regions when asked where the pain is. Upper gastrointestinal tract examination is usually performed first, and the barium meal may be observed as it moves into the colon without subjecting the patient to an unnecessary and usually uninformative separate colon examination. Intravenous pyelograms and electroencephalograms are frequently more rewarding than upper gastrointestinal and colon studies. Peptic ulcer is, in spite of several reports, an uncommonly demonstrable lesion in this age group.[36]

Vomiting

Vomiting is the most common sign requiring roentgenologic study of the infant's gastrointestinal tract. In the newborn, one must consider the various types of congenital obstruction. A preliminary abdominal scout film is mandatory for the proper evaluation of such cases and should always precede any studies using contrast media. If there is roentgenographic evidence of high small bowel obstruction, the use of ingested contrast media is unnecessary, since air is usually present in sufficient amount to identify the location of the obstruction. If the obstruction is obviously in the colon or if it is impossible to differentiate the level of the obstruction, barium enema studies are commonly required. Oral contrast media should not be given if there is a questionable colonic obstruction, and they are usually unnecessary in the roentgenologic evaluation of small bowel obstruction. In the young infant physiologic disturbances of deglutition and of the gastroesophageal region, as well as pyloric obstruction, are of foremost consideration.

In older infants and young children vomiting may be secondary to esophageal stricture or reflux esophagitis. A foreign body in the esophagus is a common cause for unexplained vomiting in this age group.

Constipation or diarrhea

Either constipation or diarrhea should direct attention to the colon or anorectal area. If the patient is an infant, aganglionosis or inflammatory disease of the colon should be considered. Habit or functional constipation is more common in the postinfantile age group.

Bleeding

Melena in the infant or child usually is the result of bleeding in the upper gastrointestinal tracts; therefore, examination of this area should precede colon studies. Hematochezia usually indicates bleeding from the colon or from a Meckel's diverticulum. Because low rectal lesions are more common than colonic polyps or inflammatory lesions of the colon, protoscopy to exclude anal fissures should precede roentgenographic studies of the colon.

There are many causes of gastrointestinal bleeding (Table 56-1), and the site may be impossible to determine by roentgenologic methods. A scout film of the abdomen is indicated in all infants with abdominal distention. The results will determine whether or not additional contrast studies of the upper gastrointestinal tract or colon are to follow.

Malabsorption and abnormal motility

The roentgenographic evaluation of malabsorption syndromes and disorders of bowel motility is very difficult and frequently impossible to make in the infant but is more informative in the ambulatory child.

In all instances a logical approach toward identifying the suspected disease is required,

Table 56-1. Etiology of gastrointestinal bleeding

Chart I—dark blood	Chart II—dark and/or bright blood	Chart III—bright blood
Swallowed blood	*Hepatobiliary disease*	*Tumors*
Maternal	Hematobilia	Colonic polyps
Bleeding in utero	Hepatitis	Inflammatory
Bleeding nipples	Posttraumatic	Adenomatous
Oral blood	Cholelithiasis	Familial
Respiratory bleeding	Hypoprothrombinemia	Intestinal polyps
		Peutz-Jeghers syndrome
Mucosal ulceration	*Aberrant gastric and pancreatic tissue*	(melanin spots)
Stress	Duplications	Carcinoma
Anoxia	Meckel's diverticulum	Lymphosarcoma
Trauma		Neuroblastoma
Head injury	*Volvulus*	Teratoma
Burns	Mesenteric thrombosis	Sacrococcygeal
Endocrine lesion		Ovarian
Adrenal	*Intussusception*	Gastric
Pheochromocytoma	Acute	Rhabdomyosarcoma
Corticoma	Chronic	
Cushing tumor	Postoperative	*Enterocolitis*
Aldosteroma	Rectal	Infectious
Parathyroidoma		Specific
Pancreatic	*Systemic disease*	Pseudomembranous
Hypothalamic—pituitary	Allergy	Granulomatous
Peptic ulcers	Milk	Ulcerative
Esophagitis	Schönlein-Henoch purpura	Idiopathic
Gastroduodenal	Glomerulonephritis	Amebic
Marginal	(purpuras)	Renal insufficiency
Obstructive		
Esophageal	*Trauma*	*Anorectal*
Pyloric	External	Proctitis
Intestinal	Blunt	Fissures
Drugs	Penetrating	Fistula
Aspirin	Internal	Hemorrhoids
Antibiotics	Gastrointestinal suction	Impactions
Steroids	Swallow—foreign body	Stercorium ulcers
Nitrogen mustard	Suppositories	
Numerous poisons	Anal—foreign body	
Varices	*Tumors*	
Gastric	Hemangioma	
Esophageal	Telangiectasia	
Intestinal		

(Bracket annotations in table: "Pain" beside Peptic ulcers group in Chart I; "Pain" beside Duplications through Rectal group in Chart II; "Pain at some stage of disease" beside Carcinoma through Rhabdomyosarcoma group, and "Pain" beside Enterocolitis through Anorectal group in Chart III.)

avoiding unnecessary examinations and preparatory procedures, particularly in the critically ill or dehydrated infant. Delaying roentgenographic examinations should not be made when surgical exploration is imperative.

METHOD OF ROENTGENOLOGIC INVESTIGATION
Contrast media

Barium is the contrast medium of choice in the examination of the upper gastrointestinal tract and the esophagus and in the evaluation of swallowing disorders. Oily preparations of iodide materials have no place in the examination of the alimentary tract. Because of their high viscosity they are extremely difficult for an infant to swallow without aspirating. The use of water-soluble iodide materials is also unneces-

sary, and they may, if given in sufficient amounts, produce severe hypovolemia and even death.[20,24] Barium-water mixture and flavored barium mixtures provide palatable contrast media that are readily ingested and safe.

Preparation of patient

The method of preparation used for an examination of the upper alimentary tract depends upon the age of the patient. Most infants undergoing examination of the upper gastrointestinal tract should be kept without a feeding for 3 to 4 hours before fluoroscopic examination. This is also advisable in the evaluation of swallowing difficulties and of questionable abnormalities of the esophagus. One of the hazards in the examination of a young infant who is vomiting is aspiration. This danger is considerably lessened by examination of the infant when the stomach is empty. Older infants and children who are not on a night feeding schedule may be prepared in a manner similar to that for the adult: they are not permitted to eat or drink after going to sleep the evening before the examination. Needless to say, with this preparation the earlier the fluoroscopic procedure is carried out the easier it is on the patient and the more appreciative are the parents.

There is a certain amount of disagreement regarding the method in which contrast medium should reach the esophagus and stomach of the infant patient. A number of experienced pediatric radiologists prefer, mainly for the sake of expediency, to inject contrast medium into a catheter that has been passed through the infant's nose and into the upper alimentary tract. It is my feeling, as well as of the majority of pediatric radiologists, that the barium can be administered more effectively and just as efficiently with a nursing bottle if there is an adequate hole in the nipple to allow a sufficient amount of barium to be swallowed. At this age the patient hungrily takes the contrast medium, particularly if a flavoring agent has been added. The fluoroscopist has the advantage of studying the infant's ability to suck and to swallow, and these are important physiologic observations in

this age group. Esophageal movements are also more easily studied by this method, and the hazard of the infant's gagging and aspirating contrast medium is less than when the medium is administered by a tube.

Examination

The roentgenologic examination of the upper intestinal tract in ambulatory children is similar to that in the adult patient. In the infant, contrast material is observed passing down the esophagus with the patient in a supine right anterior oblique position. When this method is used the esophagus is clear of the spine and can be carefully studied, with particular attention to the gastroesophageal junction (Fig. 56-1). This position also allows contrast medium to pool in the fundus and prevents it from filling the antrum and the pyloric canal before these areas can be studied. The patient is then turned slowly to his right, into a left posterior oblique position while the contour of the stomach and filling of the duodenum are observed fluoroscopically.

In the examination of the infant's or child's colon, the use of Foley or other types of balloon catheters is not only unnecessary but also uncomfortable; it may also obscure the rectal area and damage the rectal mucosa. Disposable in-

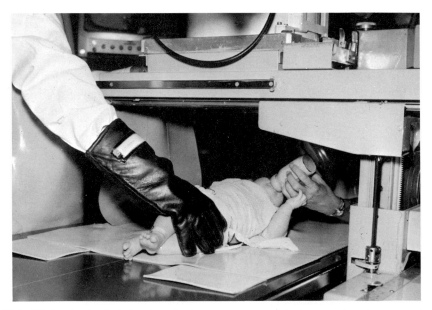

Fig. 56-1. Method of administering barium to a young infant undergoing examination of the upper gastrointestinal tract.

fants' and children's enema tips are preferable. The small tip is necessary in the neonatal period in order to prevent injury to the rectal mucosa. Adult tips are suitable for children. In each case the tip is secured by taping the buttocks together (Fig. 56-2).

Adequate cleansing of the colon is not as necessary in the pediatric patient as in the adult. Barium is the contrast medium of choice even in the evaluation of megacolon of Hirschsprung's disease, provided one is careful to examine only the lower portion of the colon and avoids filling the dilated segment with contrast material. The use of isotonic saline as the vehicle is also unnecessary in such cases if one carefully avoids filling the distended portion of the bowel. No preparation is necessary if the examination is for the evaluation of chronic constipation or intussusception.[32]

Only in the examination of the colon for suspected polyps is thorough cleansing necessary.

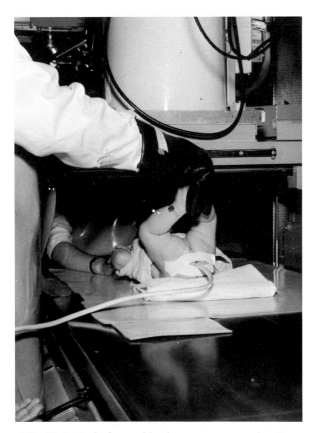

Fig. 56-2. Technique of barium enema examination.

In such cases a cathartic may be given the evening before, and cleansing enemas given prior to, the examination. In addition, one may use preliminary barium filling of the colon as a cleansing enema if fecal material is encountered.[14]

Air contrast studies are seldom utilized but may occasionally be of value in demonstrating a polyp. The use of tannic acid has been prohibited but was perhaps of value in demonstrating the mucosal pattern of the colon. Table 56-2 gives the types of preparation that have been used successfully in the Department of Radiology at Texas Children's Hospital.

CONGENITAL LESIONS OF THE ESOPHAGUS

The frequency of dysphagia in the newborn infant was not appreciated until cinegraphic methods and videotape recordings were incorporated within the radiologist's armamentarium.

Pharyngeal incoordination

Pharyngeal incoordination occurs most commonly in premature infants and in babies who have brain damage, but it may be seen in normal infants, presumably resulting from incoordination of the swallowing mechanism. Careful fluoroscopic observations of swallowing should be made in infants with dysphagia and in infants with chronic pneumonitis, particularly if the pneumonia involves the right upper lobe. Frequently these infants show an inability to suck normally, and once contrast medium passes into their mouths their swallowing movements are unsuccessful in propelling the bolus into the esophagus. Instead, the medium may pass into the nasopharynx or be aspirated into the trachea. Pharyngonasal reflux frequently extends into the eustachian tubes and may be responsible for recurrent otitis media.[40] Occasionally a deficient gag reflex appears to be present as determined by the accumulation of contrast media in the hypopharynx. Incoordinated movements of the esophagus may also be observed in these infants, with secondary peristaltic waves beginning in the mid- or lower portion of the esophagus and passing cephalad. Pharyngeal and esophageal incoordination may be so severe that feeding by gastrostomy is necessary. As the infant grows and becomes older, the condition usually improves, and after several

Table 56-2. Preparations used at Texas Children's Hospital

Procedure	Preparation	Special notes
Esophagus	No preparation if it is the only examination	
Upper gastrointestinal	Nothing by mouth after midnight	Babies accustomed to scheduled feedings may have a bottle as late as 5 hours before the study.
Colon or barium enema	Under 5 years: Cleansing enemas prior to examination 5 years and over: 1 ounce of castor oil at 4:00 P.M. day preceding examination and enemas preceding examination	1. If done for evaluation of constipation, megacolon, or intussusception *no* preparation or enemas should be given. 2. Liquid supper and breakfast may be given.

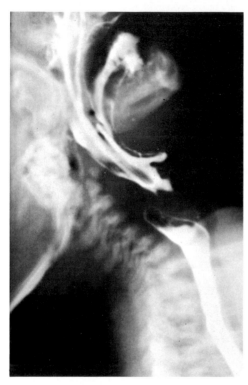

Fig. 56-3. Cephalic diverticulum of the esophagus. There is communication of the hypopharynx with the cervical portion of the esophagus, but there is abnormal extension of the proximal portion of the esophagus into the retrohypopharyngeal space. Pharyngonasal reflux is also pronounced. (Courtesy Dr. John Fawcitt.)

weeks or a few months deglutition may occur normally.

Cephalic diverticulum

Cephalic diverticulium of the esophagus is a rare cause of dysphagia. It apparently represents an anomalous communication of the stomodeum with the cephalic portion of the primitive esophagus (Fig. 56-3).

Esophageal atresia and fistula

Esophageal atresia with or without tracheoesophageal fistula, or tracheoesophageal fistula alone, should be suspected in an infant who has an increased amount of mucus and salivation or who strangles during attempted feedings. If esophageal atresia is suspected, preliminary roentgenograms of the chest and abdomen in both frontal and lateral projections are necessary. If atresia is present the blind upper esophageal pouch may be distended with air (Fig. 56-4).

The most common form of esophageal atresia and tracheoesophageal fistula is that in which the lower esophageal segment communicates with the tracheobronchial tree. Consequently there is air, usually in large amounts, in the gastrointestinal tract. If esophageal atresia alone is present there is an absence of gas in the stomach.

After a preliminary roentgenogram of the chest and abdomen has been made, an opaque catheter should be passed, under fluoroscopic observation, through the infant's nose, and the point at which the passage of the catheter is obstructed should be observed. Unless this is done under fluoroscopic control the catheter may coil upon itself and give the erroneous impression that it is passing into the stomach. Once the catheter has met obstruction in the upper blind esophageal pouch, a small amount (1 ml. or less) of contrast material may be injected to delineate more accurately the lower limit of the obstruction (Fig. 56-5). After this, the contrast medium should be aspirated and the nasal tube removed. It is advisable to place the infant in the partially prone position prior to the removal of the contrast medium in an effort to determine whether there is an additional fistula between the upper esophageal pouch and the trachea.

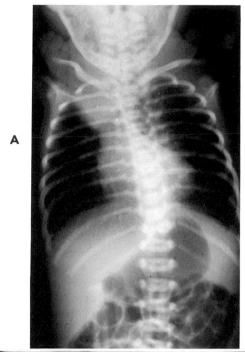

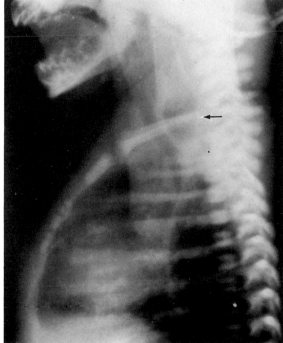

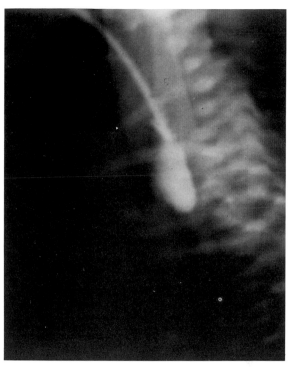

Fig. 56-5. Esophageal atresia. A minimal amount of contrast media has been injected into the catheter in the lower section to identify the point of atresia.

Fig. 56-4. Esophageal atresia with tracheoesophageal fistula. **A,** Anteroposterior roentgenograph of the chest shows atelectasis and pneumonia of the right upper lobe, the most common site for aspiration pneumonia. **B,** Lateral chest roentgenograph shows air within the blind upper esophageal pouch (arrow).

Many surgeons prefer to perform a gastrostomy on an infant with esophageal atresia prior to repair of the defect. If this is done, barium may be instilled into the stomach to identify the lower esophageal segment and provide a clearer picture of the length of the atresia (Fig. 56-6). If reflux into the lower esophageal segment does not occur, purposely making the infant gag will usually accomplish this.

Postoperative fluoroscopic and roentgenographic examination of the esophagus following repair of esophageal atresia is of value in determining the patency of the anastomosis and in determining whether or not dilatations are necessary. Alteration in the physiologic activity of the esophagus below the anastomosis is invariably present. Segmental contractions may occur, but a progressive peristaltic wave from the upper segment through the area of anastomosis into the lower esophagus does not occur.[13]

Solitary tracheoesophageal fistula

The identification of a solitary tracheoesophageal fistula without esophageal atresia may be

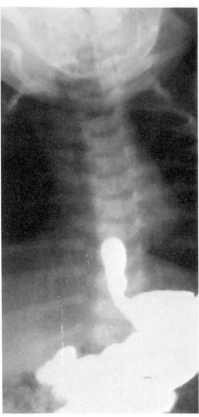

Fig. 56-6. Esophageal atresia. Barium has been introduced through gastrostomy, and reflux into the lower esophageal segment outlines the length of this segment.

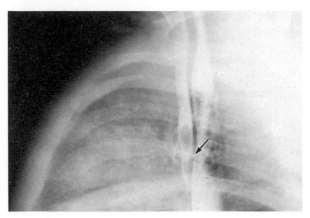

Fig. 56-7. Tracheoesophageal fistula. Contrast medium has been forcefully injected into the upper portion of the esophagus, and communication between this structure and the opacified trachea can be identified (arrow).

very difficult, especially if the communication between the two structures involved is small. Infants with this condition commonly show chronic pneumonia and atelectasis involving the right upper lobe, but any infant with chronic recurring pneumonia should be investigated for the possibility of a tracheoesophageal fistula. The presence of air distending the esophagus and stomach is a common finding.[1] The use of ciné studies or videotape recordings is of particular value in these cases in order to determine whether contrast medium reaches the tracheobronchial tree through a fistula or is aspirated over the larynx.

After the swallowing mechanism has been studied a catheter is passed through the nose into the upper portion of the esophagus, and with the patient in a semiprone position with his left side slightly elevated, contrast medium is injected. Forceful distention of the esophagus is often necessary to force contrast medium through the

fistula into the trachea. However, this must be done under careful fluoroscopic control in order to avoid overfilling the esophagus and causing aspiration into the trachea.

If a tracheoesophageal fistula is present the fistula may be identified, but more commonly contrast material can be seen extending cephalad in the trachea from the site of the communication (Fig. 56-7). A small fistula may be extremely difficult to identify; several attempts are frequently necessary. Positioning the infant in the prone position with his left side slightly elevated and his head down is preferable because the fistula is directed cephalad from the esophagus. This is presumably the result of the esophagus growing at a greater rate than the trachea during intrauterine life, thereby putting the esophageal end of the fistula at a slightly lower level than the tracheal opening.

Stenosis or congenital stricture

Stenosis or congenital stricture of the esophagus is probably secondary to unrecognized intrauterine anoxia with resulting capillary damage, focal necrosis, cicatricial changes, and stricture formation. Although this process is hypothetical, it offers a better explanation than does failure of recanalization of the esophagus after the solid stage of embryonic development. Esophageal stenosis of this type is usually located in the midportion of the esophagus; the lower portion, including the gastroesophageal area, is

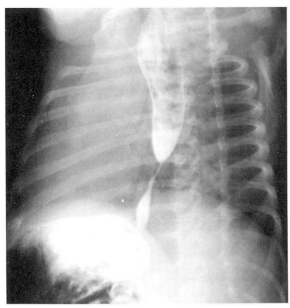

Fig. 56-8. Congenital esophageal stricture. There is a stricture of the lower third of the esophagus with dilatation proximal to this. The gastroesophageal junction is normal, and there was no evidence of gastroesophageal reflux at fluoroscopy.

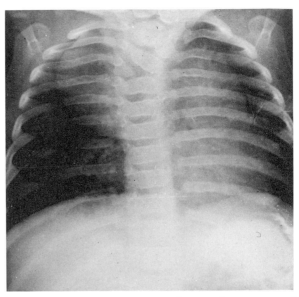

Fig. 56-9. Mediastinal neurenteric cyst in a 1-year-old infant. A large mass was seen in the right posterior mediastinum. Associated anomalies of the upper dorsal spine are present.

normal (Fig. 56-8). The possibility that ectopic gastric mucosa in the esophagus produces the stricture is also to be considered but is unlikely. Congenital stenosis of this type is usually not recognized until the infant begins taking solid food, at which time a bolus of meat or a swallowed foreign body becomes lodged at the stricture.

Neurenteric cysts

Neurenteric cysts represent remnants of one of the accessory canals of Kovalevsky that embryologically connects the primitive alimentary tube with the notochord.[25] Pressure of these lesions upon the esophagus produces vomiting, and chest roentgenographs show a posterior mediastinal mass, commonly associated with anomalies of the spine (Fig. 56-9). Duplications of the esophagus and gastroenteric cysts probably have a similar embryonic origin.

Chalasia

Abnormalities of the gastroesophageal junction of young infants are of particular interest. In spite of many theories regarding the valvular mechanism in this area, it is obvious that the gastroesophageal area (the gastroesophageal vestibule) is in a tonic or closed state except when forced open by the weight of ingested material or by an esophageal peristaltic wave (Fig. 56-10). If this normal tonicity is not present gastroesophageal reflux or chalasia (Fig. 56-11) occurs. This is apparently normal to a small degree in many infants, but when severe and persistent it may lead to esophagitis and cicatricial changes with resulting retraction of the cardia into the thorax. Measurements of sphincteric pressure have shown that abnormal neuromuscular tone at the sphincter in young infants results in gastroesophageal reflux.[38]

The most common reason for gastrointestinal tract examination of the young infant is a complaint by the mother that the infant regurgitates most or part of the feedings. In many cases this is exaggerated by the parent, who confuses the normal "spitting up" with an abnormal condition. A negative fluoroscopic examination in such cases usually indicates that mild but insignificant chalasia is present. However, some form of milk allergy or milk incompatibility may be

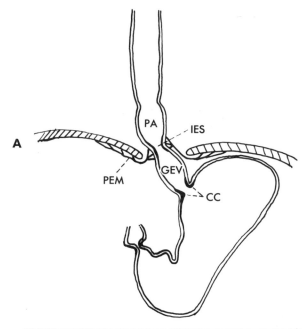

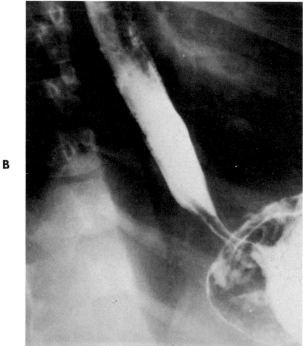

Fig. 56-10. A, Anatomy of the lower esophagus. **PA,** Phrenic ampulla; **IES,** inferior esophageal sphincter; **PEM,** phrenoesophageal membrane; **CC,** constrictor cardiae; **GEV,** gastroesophageal vestibule. **B,** Normal gastroesophageal vestibule. Spot film shows tonic constriction of the gastroesophageal vestibule during the resting phase. (**A** from Singleton, E. B.: X-ray diagnosis of the alimentary tract in infants and children, Chicago, 1959, Year Book Publishers, Inc.)

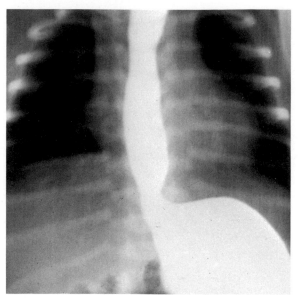

Fig. 56-11. Chalasia in a 3-month-old infant. Pressure was applied to the abdomen, resulting in the reflux of barium from the stomach into the esophagus.

responsible, and improvement in such cases will occur if the infant is placed on milk substitutes.

Chalasia in a severe form may occur in premature babies or babies with brain damage and is occasionally seen in normal term infants. Keeping the infant in an upright position after feeding, keeping him in a prone position, or thickening the feedings will lead to improvement in most cases, but all too frequently the infant reappears some months later with a shortened esophagus and a hiatus hernia (Fig. 56-12). Once this occurs, persistent reflux is common,[11] and eventual surgical correction, often by colon substitutes, is necessary.[15]

Achalasia

The opposite condition is achalasia. It is characterized by an unusually tonic gastroesophageal vestibule and by failure of the normal esophageal peristaltic waves or weight of ingested food to open it (Fig. 56-13). This may be a condition different from that seen in older patients, in whom the primary disturbance appears to result from absence of normal primary peristaltic activity of the esophagus. After a period of time dilatation of the esophagus develops, and surgical correction may be necessary. This condition may also be transient and may improve as the infant becomes older.

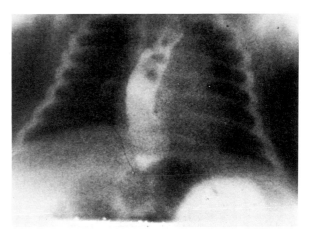

Fig. 56-13. Achalasia in a 2-week-old infant (ciné study). The gastroesophageal vestibule was abnormally tonic and the esophagus dilated, but showed adequate peristaltic movement. Reexamination in 2 months showed no abnormality.

ACQUIRED LESIONS OF THE ESOPHAGUS
Caustic strictures

Acquired inflammatory lesions of the esophagus are uncommon in older children, but the ingestion of caustic material is a common cause of acute esophagitis and esophageal stricture in the younger age group. One cannot predict the severity of the cicatricial changes that will occur in caustic strictures, but careful roentgenologic studies during the healing phase and afterward are of value in treatment either by dilatation or by resection. Such strictures usually occur in the upper half of the esophagus and may produce severe dysphagia (Fig. 56-14). If the ingested material is acid rather than a base, cicatricial changes of the stomach may also develop.

Foreign bodies

Foreign bodies become lodged at the thoracic inlet but may also stop at the gastroesophageal vestibule or, less likely, in the upper third of the esophagus, where they pass behind the left main bronchus. The foreign bodies include any objects that the infant can put in his mouth. This is frequently unsuspected until roentgenologic examination of the esophagus is performed because of the infant's failure to eat and because of excess salivation (Fig. 56-15).

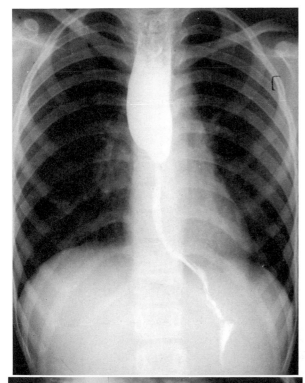

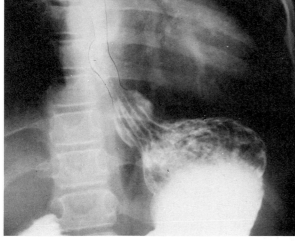

Fig. 56-12. Acquired esophageal stricture secondary to gastroesophageal reflux. The patient had a history of vomiting from birth. **A,** Esophagram shows constriction of the lower half of the esophagus. Gastroesophageal reflux was demonstrated at the time of fluoroscopy. **B,** Two years later marked shortening of the esophagus has occurred with resulting hiatus hernia.

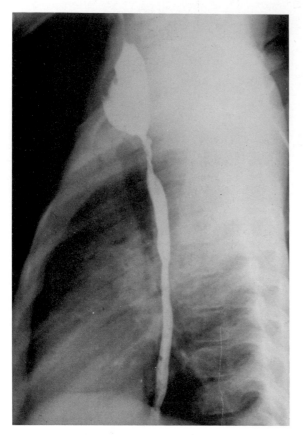

Fig. 56-14. Caustic stricture following ingestion of lye. Localized stricture is identified in the proximal portion of the thoracic esophagus.

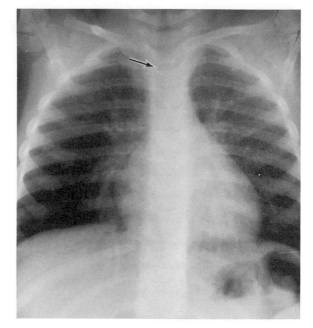

Fig. 56-15. Foreign body in a 3-year-old child. The wire segment of a Christmas tree ornament can be faintly identified in the upper portion of the esophagus (arrow).

Esophageal varices

Esophageal varices are rare in infants but are not uncommon in children with portal hypertension. The roentgenographic appearance is similar to that seen in the adult patient. Splenoportograms are of value in determining the extent of the varices and the location of the venous obstruction. Excretory pyelography is advised to exclude renal tubular ectasia, which may accompany congenital cirrhosis.[19]

Colon substitutes are becoming more and more common for the treatment of esophageal strictures and esophageal varices.[21] Long-term followups are not yet available to determine the ultimate efficacy of this type of replacement. However, in the majority of those children who have had this type of procedure, the overall clinical result is good. The roentgenographic findings are unusual in their appearance. Actual peristaltic waves such as one associates with a normal esophagus are not seen (Fig. 56-16). Although segmental contractions do occur, most of the ingested food reaches the stomach as a result of gravity. I have seen one case of a colon substitute with obstruction caused by a colonic polyp.

DIAPHRAGMATIC HERNIAS

Diaphragmatic hernias are not uncommon in infants. Acquired esophageal hiatus hernia as the result of gastroesophageal reflux and esophagitis is the most common form. Herniation of bowel through the foramen of Bochdalek, or pleuroperitoneal hiatus, is the most common form of congenital diaphragmatic hernia. The hernia is usually on the left, and the left hemithorax is filled with multiple radiolucent blebs, some of which may show fluid levels. Although

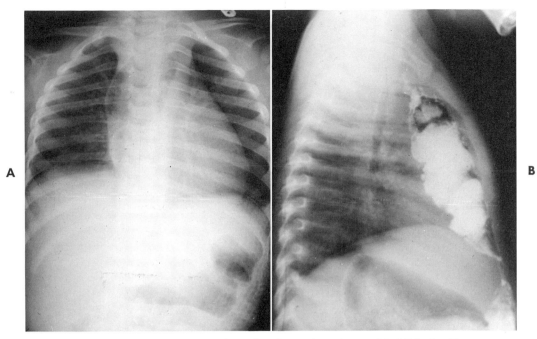

Fig. 56-16. Colon substitute for esophageal stricture in a 6-year-old child. **A,** Chest roentgenograph shows air and fluid level in the colon transplant. **B,** Barium outlines the transplant and shows characteristic colonic haustrations.

the roentgenographic appearance may suggest cystic disease of the lung, the absence of normal bowel pattern in the abdomen indicates that a hernia is present (Fig. 56-17). Although the condition is usually diagnosed in young infants, it may not be discovered until the child is older (Fig. 56-18). Unusual forms of *foramen of Bochdalek hernia* may occur in which only the spleen or a portion of the stomach may be herniated (Fig. 56-19). Paraesophageal and foramen of Monro hernias are less common (Fig. 56-20).

CONGENITAL INTESTINAL OBSTRUCTION

Obstructive lesions of the gastrointestinal tract in the newborn infant are common anomalies, and early recognition is necessary for survival. The clinical findings consist of vomiting, abdominal distention, and obstipation. The higher the level of the obstruction the earlier the onset of vomiting. If the obstruction is in the lower part of the alimentary tract, abdominal distention and obstipation are the presenting signs. In cases of gastrointestinal tract obstruction the radiologist is faced with three questions:

Is obstruction present? What is the location of the obstruction? What is its etiology?

An accurate diagnosis of intestinal obstruction in the newborn may be difficult if one is not familiar with the many variations of normal gas pattern in this age group.[33] The cardinal signs of intestinal obstruction in the adult, such as dilated loops of small bowel, air-fluid levels, continuity of loops, and hairpin turns, may be normal variations in the infant. During infancy and before the ambulatory age is reached, one expects to see gas within the stomach, small bowel, and colon. The honeycomb appearance of gas scattered throughout loops of small bowel in a young infant is a normal finding (Fig. 56-21) and is very reassuring in an infant who clinically may be suspected of having an obstructive lesion. However, a large amount of air can be swallowed by a crying infant, and the Mueller effect of sobbing against a closed glottis may force great quantities of air into the stomach (Fig. 56-22). Also, any infant with a disturbance in respiration will commonly show an abundance of gas in the stomach and scattered through the intestinal tract. Distention of loops

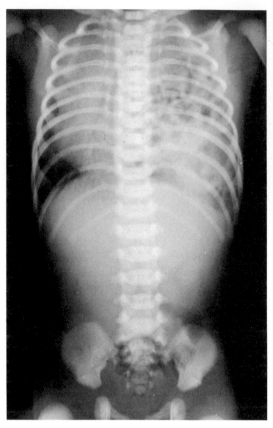

Fig. 56-17. Congenital pleuroperitoneal hiatus hernia. There is absence of gas within the abdomen, and multiple gas-filled loops of bowel are seen in the left hemithorax with displacement of the mediastinum to the right.

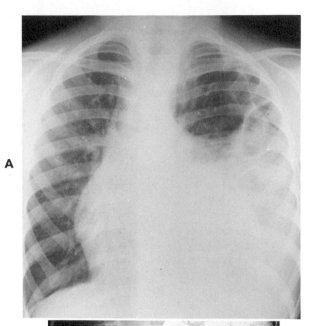

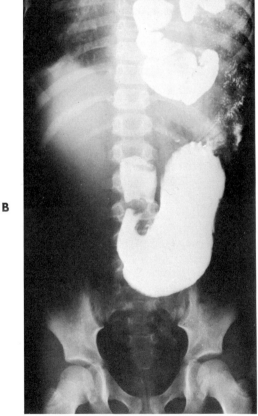

of small bowel commonly occurs in such conditions, and if films are made with the infant in the upright position air-fluid levels may be identified. These are variations of normal (Fig. 56-23) and are also identical to the roentgenographic findings of acute enteritis. Consequently, it is extremely important that the roentgenologic findings be carefully correlated with the clinical story in order to avoid a misdiagnosis of intestinal obstruction in this age group.

Most cases of small intestinal obstruction in the newborn are characterized by a deficiency in the intestinal gas pattern rather than by the accumulation of a large amount of gas. Air usually enters the stomach during the first few minutes of life, and as a rule, an abdominal scout film of a newborn infant will show gas within the stomach. After approximately 30 min-

Fig. 56-18. Pleuroperitoneal hiatus hernia in a 7-year-old boy. **A,** Roentgenographs of the chest suggest empyema, but the patient was asymptomatic. **B,** Fluoroscopic examination demonstrated all of the small bowel and most of the colon in the left hemithorax.

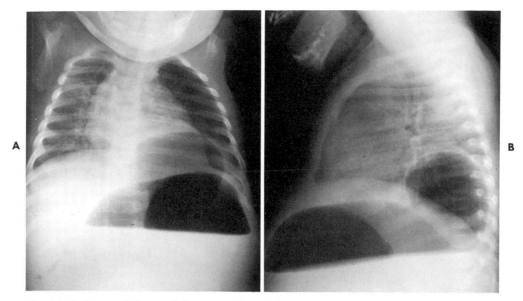

Fig. 56-19. Unusual form of foramen of Bochdalek hernia in a young infant. **A,** Chest roentgenograph shows air-fluid level in the stomach as well as a collection of air above the left hemidiaphragm. **B,** Lateral view shows the herniated segment of the fundus through the pleuroperitoneal foramen to better advantage.

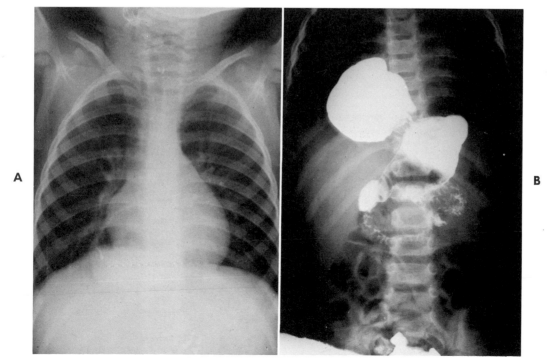

Fig. 56-20. Paraesophageal hiatus hernia in 2-year-old infant. **A,** Air-fluid level is seen in the lower medial hemithorax. **B,** Gastrointestinal tract examination shows herniation of the proximal half of the stomach in the paraesophageal region.

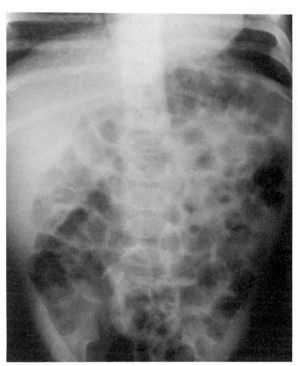

Fig. 56-21. Normal intestinal gas pattern of an infant.

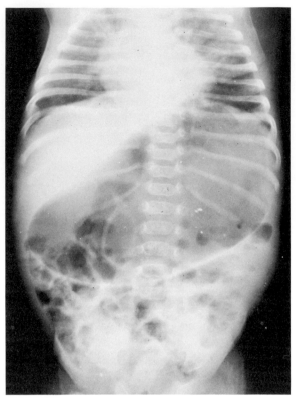

Fig. 56-22. Distention of the stomach in a young infant secondary to prolonged crying.

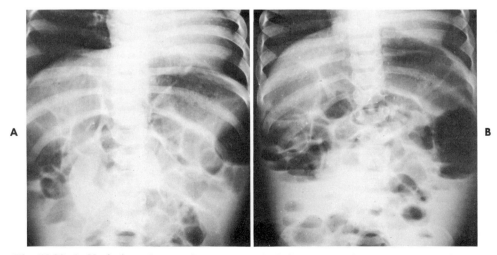

Fig. 56-23. **A,** Variation of normal gas pattern in infant. **B,** Supine roentgenograph shows normal honeycombed appearance. Upright film shows multiple air-fluid levels. (From Singleton, E. B.: X-ray diagnosis of alimentary tract in infants and children, Chicago, 1959, Year Book Medical Publishers, Inc.)

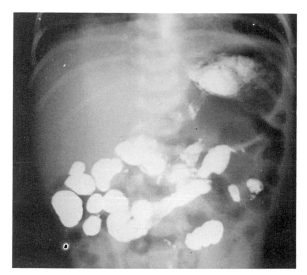

Fig. 56-24. Delay in transient time of contrast medium through small bowel in a baby with brain damage. Abdominal roentgenograph made 10 hours after ingestion of medium shows barium within proximal small bowel.

utes air can be identified in the proximal small bowel, and after 3 to 4 hours air usually has reached the colon. As a rule, at 6 to 7 hours gas has reached the distal colon and rectum. A delay in this progression of gas within the intestinal tract may occur in babies who have brain damage (Fig. 56-24), in babies who are born of overly sedated mothers, or in infants who for other reasons do not cry and respond vigorously during the neonatal period. Consequently, a delay in the extension of gas into the distal portions of the small bowel and colon is frequently more informative in the evaluation of obstruction than is the amount of intestinal gas.

Obstruction in the duodenum

The roentgenologic identification of duodenal or proximal small-bowel obstruction is relatively easy. Air is present in the bowel proximal to the obstruction, and there is a deficiency of gas distal to the obstructed area. There are several forms of duodenal obstruction, including atresia, duodenal diaphragm with a small diaphragmatic opening, stenosis, annular pancreas, and volvulus. The frequent occurence of duodenal obstructions with mongolism should alert the radiologist to look for osseous changes of mongolism in all infants with congenital duodenal obstructions.[10]

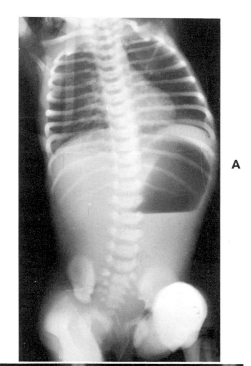

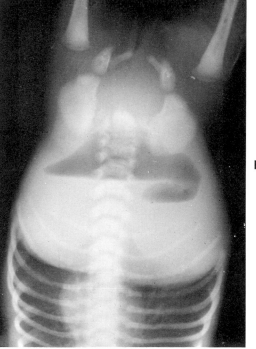

Fig. 56-25. Duodenal atresia. **A,** Upright film shows air within the fundus of the stomach, but the duodenum is not visualized. **B,** Abdominal roentgenograph, made with the infant inverted, outlines the duodenal bulb and pyloric canal.

The contrast medium of choice for the identification of these lesions is air. If there is insufficient air in the stomach and duodenum to accurately locate the obstruction, a small catheter may be passed into the stomach and fluid removed and replaced with air. There is no need to use liquid contrast media in such cases. The danger of aspiration is a considerable hazard in the lives of infants with proximal bowel obstruction; consequently, the use of air as a contrast medium is preferable.

Abdominal roentgenographs of infants with duodenal obstruction will usually show the so-called *double bubble sign*, representing air within the duodenal bulb and the gastric fundus and a deficiency of gas distal to the duodenum. If there is dilatation of the duodenal bulb the most likely diagnosis is duodenal atresia, duodenal diaphragm, or annular pancreas (Fig. 56-25). A smaller duodenum is more often associated with volvulus or peritoneal band (Fig. 56-26). Presumably, in the former conditions the obstruction has been present for a longer period of time, with resulting greater dilatation of the duodenum.

Obstruction in the jejunum or ileum

Obstructions of the jejunum or proximal ileum will show distention of the proximal small bowel. In these cases, as in duodenal obstruction, air is the only contrast medium necessary. Etiologic considerations include peritoneal bands, atresia and stenosis, herniation of bowel through mesenteric defects (Fig. 56-27), and volvulus. Extrinsic masses may also obstruct the bowel (Fig. 56-28).

Even though the scout films show obvious high intestinal obstruction, barium enema studies are frequently helpful in alerting the surgeon to the probability that lower small-bowel obstruction may also be present. The identification of an abnormally small colon associated with a high small bowel obstruction usually indicates that additional bowel obstructions are present. The intrauterine development of the colon depends to some extent upon the succus entericus produced by the intestinal tract and passed into the colon during its development. Consequently in low small-bowel obstruction there will be less succus entericus entering the colon. Therefore, if the scout film shows a high small-bowel obstruction with microcolon, there is a high prob-

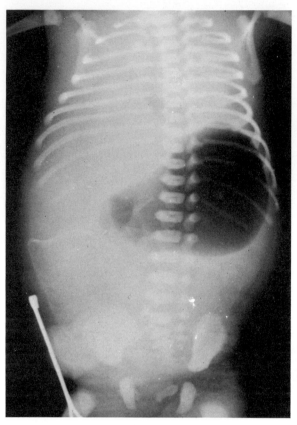

Fig. 56-26. Volvulus obstructing the duodenum. The duodenal bulb is identified within the air-filled antrum and is not appreciably dilated. Absence of gas distal to the duodenum indicates complete obstruction. There is associated meconium peritonitis as determined by the calcification within the peritoneal cavity.

ability that an additional lower obstructive lesion is present.[8]

Lower obstruction

Localization of the obstruction becomes more difficult when the obstruction is lower. It may be impossible to determine on abdominal scout films whether the obstruction is in the small bowel or colon. In such cases, barium enema studies are informative. If the colon fills completely and appears normal or if the entire colon is patent but has an unusually small lumen (microcolon), the obstruction is obviously in the terminal portion of the small bowel. Differential diagnoses include ileal atresia, volvulus, peritoneal bands, meconium ileus, or agangliosis (Fig. 56-29). If the cecum is abnormally movable by palpation or is in an abnormal position, one

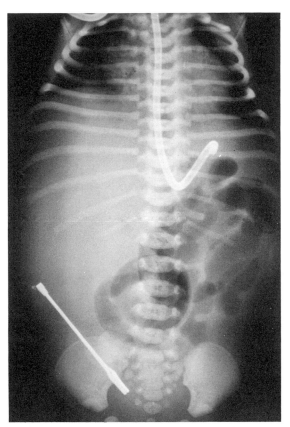

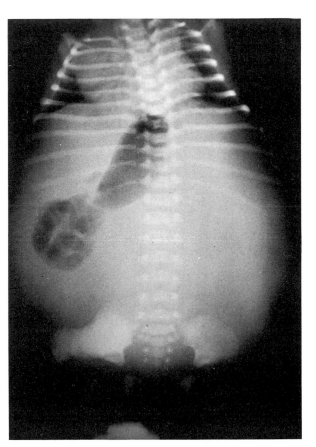

Fig. 56-27. Congenital obstruction caused by volvulus of bowel, which was found at surgery to be incarcerated within a mesenteric defect.

Fig. 56-28. Obstruction of the proximal jejunum in a newborn infant with large solitary left renal cyst.

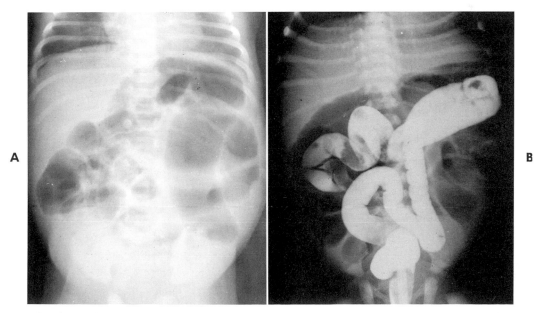

Fig. 56-29. Ileal atresia. **A,** Dilated loops of small bowel are present but without definite gas in the colon. **B,** Barium enema shows a small colon with obstruction in the terminal ileum.

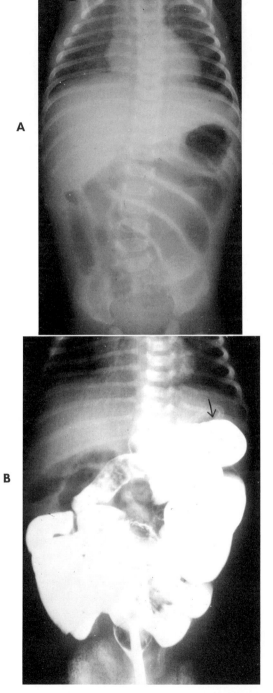

Fig. 56-30. Malrotation with small-bowel obstruction. **A,** Abdominal roentgenograph shows dilated loops of small bowel. **B,** Barium enema study shows cecum in the left upper quadrant (arrow).

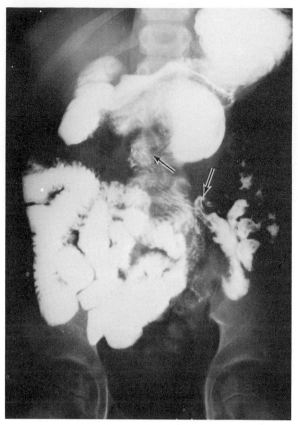

Fig. 56-31. Peritoneal band obstructing the proximal jejunum in a 6-year-old boy. Cecum and appendix are identified in the left midabdomen.

may assume that *malrotation* and volvulus are present (Fig. 56-30). The embryonic development of the bowel and its relationship to a variety of anomalies, including omphalocele, nonrotation of the foregut, and peritoneal bands, are extremely interesting. Frequently, obstruction does not develop until later in life (Fig. 56-31).

Because of the variety of complications resulting from failure of normal rotation and fixation of the fetal intestinal tract, an understanding of the embryology of normal midgut rotation is necessary. Beginning at approximately the sixth week of intrauterine life, the alimentary tube undergoes rapid increase in length and protrudes into the umbilical cord as a single loop, having the superior mesenteric artery as its axis. With further elongation of the loop, possibly initiated by the growth of the liver and by unequal growth of the duodenal wall associated with development of the pancreas, an initial 90-degree rotation occurs in a counterclockwise direction around the axis of the superior mesenteric artery. Following this there is continued counterclockwise rotation of the midintestine with return of the prearterial segment to the left upper quadrant of the abdomen beneath the axis of the superior mesenteric artery. The subsequent complete 270-degree rotation and packing of the bowel into the coelomic cavity with the last of the midintestine, including the ascending colon and cecum, returning to the right side of the abdomen completes the rotation process. The final, or third, stage, which lasts from approximately the eleventh or twelfth week of intrauterine life, is characterized by fixation of the normal retroperitoneal structures (the duodenum, cecum, and ascending colon) and the fusion of the midgut and the mesentery to the posterior parietal peritoneum on a broad base extending from the duodenojejunal junction to the ileocecal junction.

If the normal herniation of the midgut into the umbilical cord occurs without return to the abdominal cavity, an omphalocele results. If the return of the intestine occurs after the initial 90-degree first stage of rotation, the jejunum returns to the right upper portion of the abdomen and the cecum usually lies in the midline or to the left lower quadrant. There are many additional variations of the rotation process, but in all instances the major complication is obstruction, which, if not present at birth, may develop later in life. This is caused by the fact that in all of these situations there is a narrow mesenteric pedicle rather than the normal broad pedicle, and volvulus with resulting obstruction may easily occur. In addition to this, peritoneal bands, usually extending from the cecum to the posterior portion of the upper peritoneum, are frequently formed and pass across the duodenum, obstructing it.

Volvulus is an extremely common cause of intestinal obstruction during the first few weeks of life. As mentioned previously, it should be suspected if there are plain film indications of bowel obstruction associated with an abnormally positioned or abnormally movable cecum. In milder forms where the peritoneal bands (Ladd's bands) produce duodenal obstruction, upper gastrointestinal tract studies may be informative by showing the duodenal dilatation, malposi-

tioned ligament of Treitz, and active peristalsis of the duodenum associated with obstruction near the duodenojejunal junction.[7]

Meconium ileus

Meconium ileus deserves special consideration. This is the earliest clinical and roentgenographic manifestation of *fibrocystic disease*. Any newborn infant having evidence of intestinal obstruction should have upright films of the abdomen.

If intestinal obstruction is present, absence of air-fluid levels within the colon and distal small bowel suggests the presence of meconium ileus (Fig. 56-32).[39] In this condition the meconium is so tenacious and thick that air-fluid levels are usually absent or less prominent than in other forms of mechanical obstruction. The "soap bubble" appearance of gas and meconium within the small bowel is seen in conditions other than meconium ileus. It is not uncommonly seen in ileal atresia or total colonic aganglionosis.

Obstruction of the colon

In obstructions of the colon one expects to find distention of the entire small bowel as well as of the colon proximal to the obstruction. Barium enema studies are of value in confirming this. Colonic atresias (Fig. 56-33) and stenoses may be identified by such a procedure, but more common causes of obstruction are the meconium plug syndrome and aganglionosis.

Meconium plug syndrome

The meconium plug syndrome may be responsible for obstipation during the neonatal period. Barium enema studies will identify the site of the obstruction. Differentiation of this condition from Hirschsprung's disease may be difficult, but if the plug can be expelled as a result of the barium enema or hypertonic water-soluble iodide enema, the resulting clinical course is usually that of a healthy infant. Obstructions produced by meconium plug may also be present in Hirschsprung's disease.[16]

In any condition in which there has been an obstruction to the passage of meconium into and through the colon during intrauterine life, whether the cause be ileal atresia, atresia of the proximal portion of the colon, meconium ileus, or meconium plug syndrome, barium enema

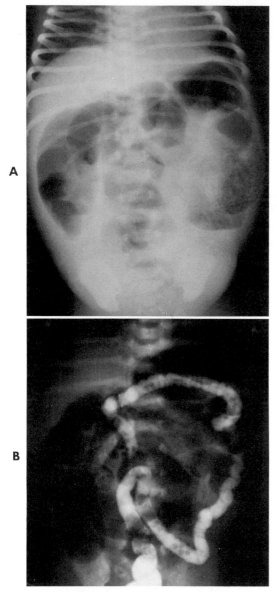

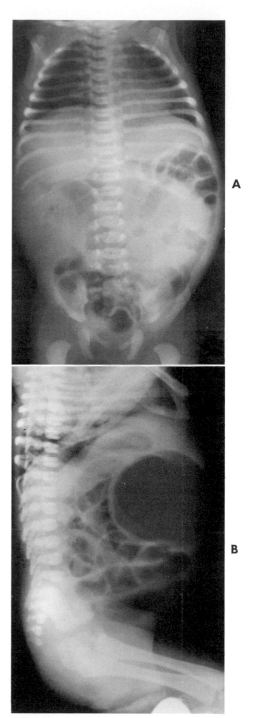

Fig. 56-32. Meconium ileus. **A,** Upright film of the abdomen shows "soap bubble" appearance of meconium and air within small bowel. There is an absence of the usual air-fluid level within small bowel, suggestive of meconium ileus. **B,** Barium enema study shows very small colon with obstruction in the proximal portion.

Fig. 56-33. Atresia of the colon. **A,** Abdominal scout film shows ill-defined area of radiolucency in midabdomen representing distention of the colon proximal to the site of atresia. **B,** Lateral view shows the dilated transverse portion of the colon to better advantage. (Courtesy Dr. Z. Petrany.)

studies will show an abnormally small colonic lumen, the so-called microcolon. This should not be misinterpreted as a primary defect of the colon; it simply represents underdevelopment of the colon because of its failure to serve as a conduit for the movement of meconium into the distal bowel during intrauterine life.

Aganglionosis

Aganglionosis or Hirschsprung's disease of the colon may be difficult to diagnose during the neonatal period or during early infancy because there has been insufficient time for megacolon to develop. Constipation is usually the presenting complaint, although later in infancy recurrent episodes of diarrhea and constipation may occur because of associated colitis. In the absence of large bowel dilatation the transition area between normal rectum and megacolon cannot be identified, and one must rely upon the infant's failure to evacuate the enema after 24 to 48 hours.[35] Retention of the enema after this period of time is presumptive evidence of aganglionosis, and biopsy of the rectal mucosa and muscularis

is necessary for confirmation. However, if associated colitis is present, evacuation may occur quickly (Fig. 56-34).

The bowel proximal to the aganglionotic area is distended with air, the degree depending on the severity of the obstruction. In total colonic aganglionosis, the small bowel may be markedly distended, far exceeding the diameter of the colon. In the older infant and occasionally in the neonatal period, the transition zone between a small rectum and dilated sigmoid can be identified and the diagnosis readily made during fluoroscopy (Fig. 56-35). In such cases, no attempt should be made to fill the entire colon with barium. The examination should be discontinued after the transition zone has been identified. Carrying the examination beyond this point may cause water intoxication and may add to the obstruction.

Imperforate anus

Imperforate anus and rectal atresia are common causes of low alimentary tract obstruction in the newborn. The diagnosis of imperforate

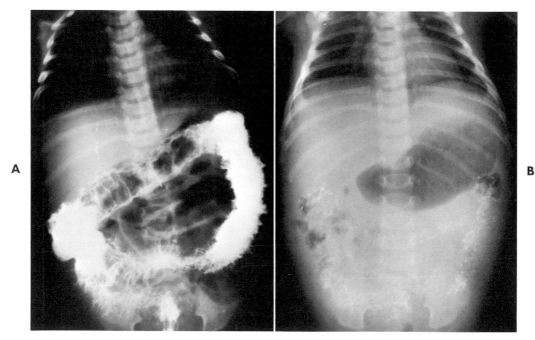

Fig. 56-34. Hirschsprung's disease in 3-week-old infant who had recurrent episodes of diarrhea. **A,** There is marked irregularity of the rectosigmoid and descending portions of the colon with evidence of extensive ulceration. **B,** Postevacuation film made after the barium enema study shows nearly complete evacuation. Biopsy confirmed the presence of aganglionosis of the rectum.

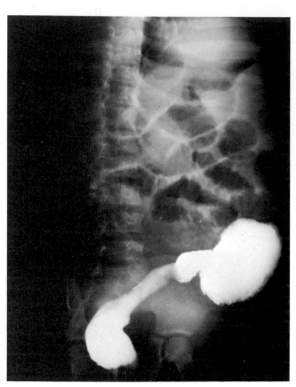

Fig. 56-35. Hirschsprung's disease in a 5-year-old child. The rectum is small, and the transition zone to the dilated sigmoid is identified.

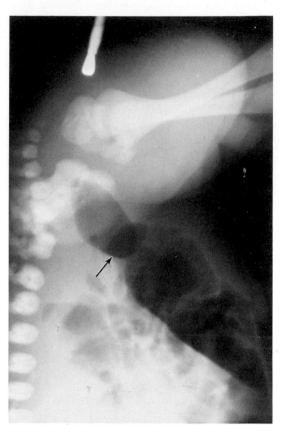

Fig. 56-36. Imperforate anus. Inverted film shows distance between gas in the distal rectal segment and the anal dimple marked by a thermometer. The descending and sigmoid portions of the colon are dilated compared to the size of the rectum, suggesting Hirschsprung's disease, which was later confirmed. (Arrow at transitional zone.)

anus is readily made by inspection of the infant, and in both conditions there is, of course, an absence of meconium stools.

Roentgenographs made with the infant in the inverted lateral position are of value in determining the distance between the distal rectal segment and the cutaneous anal region (Fig. 56-36). Because at least 6 hours are usually necessary for swallowed air to reach the rectum of a newborn infant, examination prior to this time is usually uninformative. It is important to remember that the apparent distance between the gas in the colon and the anocutaneous region is subject to inaccuracies, depending upon the length of time the infant has been kept in an inverted position prior to filming and upon the amount of meconium that may be packed into the distal rectal segment. Lateral views are far more reliable than anteroposterior views in assisting the radiologist to judge the length of the atretic seg-

ment. Aganglionosis of the rectum may also be present and frequently can be suspected from an examination of the inverted lateral roentgenograph. Direct needle puncture of the perineum and injection of sterile water-soluble iodide contrast medium into the rectal pouch under fluoroscopic control may give more accurate information.

Associated anomalies, particularly of the genitourinary tract, are extremely common in anorectal malformations, and excretory urograms are advised. Approximately 70% of male infants with rectal atresia have an associated rectovesical fistula. Consequently, the radiologist should carefully observe the vesical area for the presence of air. In females, rectovaginal

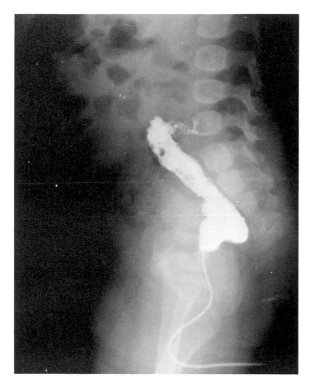

Fig. 56-37. Rectovaginal fistula with imperforate anus. Catheter has been passed into the vagina and contrast medium fills the rectum through a rectovaginal fistula.

communication may be present. The anomaly may be visualized by filling the vagina with contrast material (Fig. 56-37). A dilated air-fluid–filled vagina may be associated with rectovaginal vesical fistulas.

MISCELLANEOUS ABNORMALITIES OF THE ALIMENTARY TRACT
Necrotizing enterocolitis

There is a miscellaneous group of alimentary tract abnormalities in the neonate, both congenital and acquired, with which the radiologist should be familiar. One of these is necrotizing or noninfectious enterocolitis, a condition that is being recognized more frequently and probably is secondary to some form of prenatal stress phenomenon or anoxia. The clinical findings are abdominal distention and vomiting. Roentgenographs of the abdomen show distention of the intestinal tract (Fig. 56-38), and if perforation has occurred pneumoperitoneum is present. Associated pneumatosis intestinalis and gas within the portal vein have been reported.[6]

Although Tannler's theory of intestinal tract atresia based upon the failure of recanalization of the solid cell stage of alimentary tract devel-

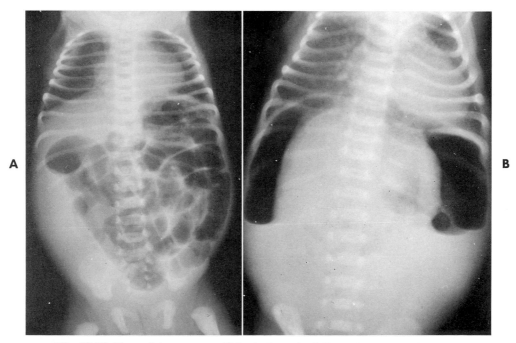

Fig. 56-38. Necrotizing enterocolitis. **A,** Intestinal distention; **B,** perforation.

opment has been an accepted hypothesis for bowel atresia, it now appears that vascular injury to an area of the fetal or embryonic gut with resulting necrosis and cicatrization may account for many forms of atresia.[5,37] This may be a condition similar to that of necrotizing enterocolitis in newborn infants but having occurred at an earlier stage of intrauterine development.[28] This explanation for bowel atresia is especially attractive when one considers the number of cases of atresia in which meconium containing bile and epithelial cells is distal to the obstruction. Because the canalization of the alimentary tract occurs prior to the formation of bile, the presence of this substance within the colon distal to the obstruction would not be possible on this basis; consequently the obstruction must develop at a later period of intrauterine life.

Bowel obstruction caused by hernias

Obstruction of the bowel caused by umbilical and inguinal hernias may develop suddenly. Roentgenographic studies are of value in demonstrating the degree of bowel distention and

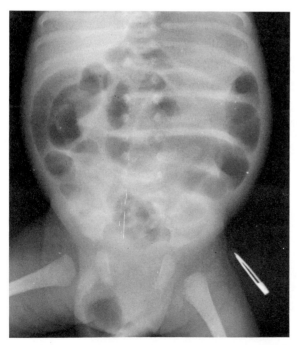

Fig. 56-39. Incarcerated inguinal hernia in a young infant. Dilated loops of small bowel are identified as well as gas in the right side of the scrotum.

the location of the obstruction (Fig. 56-39). If reduction can be accomplished the bowel pattern quickly returns to normal. Persistence of abdominal distention suggests the possibility of nonviable bowel.

Duplication of the ileum

Duplication of the ileum and Meckel's diverticulum may present identical roentgenologic findings. Gastrointestinal bleeding and abdominal pain may be the clinical findings in either case. Roentgenographic demonstration is frequently impossible unless barium enters the duplication sac and careful small bowel studies are obtained (Fig. 56-40). Positive differentiation is made at the time of laparotomy. A Meckel's diverticulum is on the antimesenteric side of the ileum, and the duplication is within the mesentery.

Dilatation of a segment of small bowel following an end-to-side anastomosis for the treatment of an obstructive lesion may produce marked dilatation of the blind segment and lead to signs of a malabsorption syndrome or chronic macrocytic anemia. The latter is the result of chronic enteritis (Fig. 56-41) and bacterial overgrowth.

Pneumatosis intestinalis

Although pneumatosis intestinalis (Fig. 56-42) is commonly a benign condition in adults, it represents a serious complication in infants who have chronic enteritis, various forms of intestinal obstruction, infantile diarrhea, and necrotizing enteritis.[26] Although the pathogenesis has never been satisfactorily explained, in all probability there is a passage of gas and gas-forming bacteria through an abrasion of the intestinal mucosa as a result of increased intestinal intraluminal pressure accompanying increased peristalsis. Roentgenographically, multiple collections of small gas bubbles or linear areas of radiolucent paralleling loops of small bowel and colon can be identified. A serious complication signifying a grave prognosis is the presence of gas in the portal system.

Functional obstruction

Functional intestinal obstruction[31] is a rare neonate condition in which there is clinical and roentgenographic evidence of intestinal obstruction, but contrast studies of the colon show no evidence of obstruction and reflux into the ter-

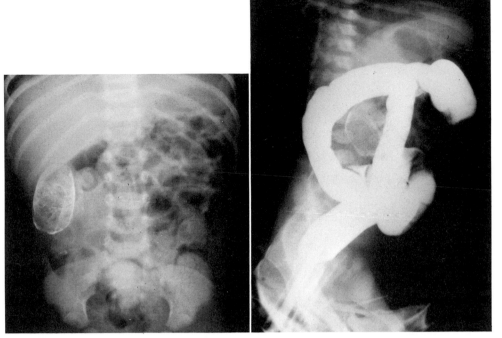

Fig. 56-40. Duplication of the ileum in a 2-month-old infant with melena. **A,** Residual barium is seen in a cystic structure in the right side of the abdomen following upper gastrointestinal examination. **B,** Colon examination shows fill of terminal ileum, which is obstructed by the extraluminal cyst. Laparotomy disclosed duplication of the ileum.

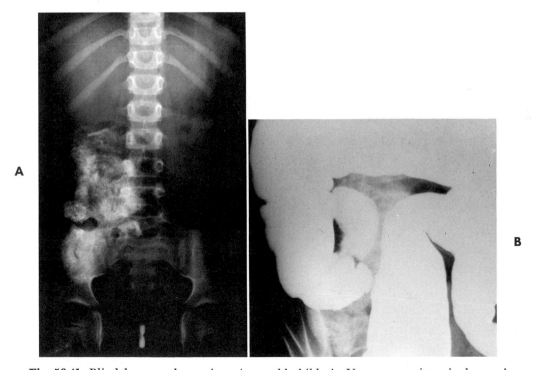

Fig. 56-41. Blind loop syndrome in a 4-year-old child. **A,** Upper gastrointestinal examination shows collection of contrast media in a structure having the appearance of ascending colon and cecum. **B,** Barium enema study shows no abnormality of the cecum or terminal ileum. At operation a blind ileal loop was discovered incident to end-to-side anastomosis for treatment of ileal atresia at birth.

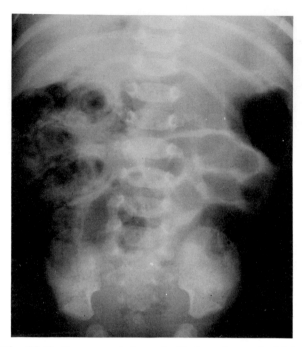

Fig. 56-42. Pneumotosis intestinalis in a 3-month-old infant. Radiolucent air shadows are identified within the wall of the terminal ileum.

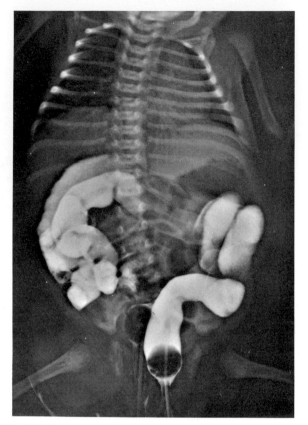

Fig. 56-43. Duplication of the entire colon in a newborn infant. In addition, there were two vaginal openings as well as two anal orifices.

minal ileum may be accomplished. Surgical exploration shows the bowel to be patent without definite evidence of organic obstruction or aganglionosis. The possibility of this condition being associated with some form of altered physiologic activity of the small bowel and colon secondary to fetal or neonatal stress is a consideration.

Duplication of the colon

Duplication of the colon is a rare anomaly that may be accompanied by duplication of other pelvic structures (Fig. 56-43).

Hypertrophic pyloric stenosis

Hypertrophic pyloric stenosis is the most common form of acquired alimentary tract obstruction in infants. Although the clinical picture of a palpable olive-sized mass in the epigastrium of a 3- to 6-week old male infant who has projectile vomiting is usually diagnostic of this condition,

all too frequently the clinical findings are atypical. In such cases the roentgenologic examination is confirmatory. The condition was once thought to be congenital. However, the development of pyloric stenosis in many infants who have previously had normal gastrointestinal tract examinations indicates that it is an acquired lesion of unknown cause.

A presumptive diagnosis of hypertrophic pyloric stenosis may be made by a preliminary scout film of the abdomen, which will show distention of the stomach with a decrease in the amount of gas distal to the pyloric area. Fluoroscopy is mandatory in order to determine the true length of the pyloric canal. All too frequently roentgenographs made during contraction of the gastric antrum will simulate an abnormally elongated pyloric canal. Only by observing where gastric waves stop can the radiologist identify the proximal portion of the pyloric canal.

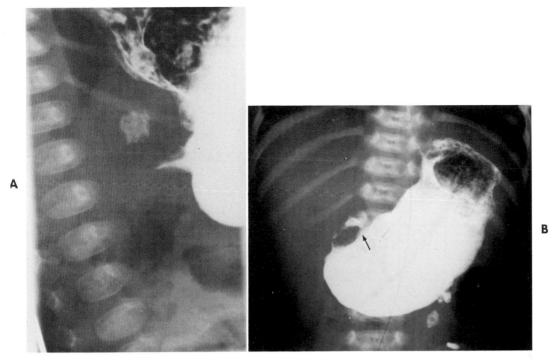

Fig. 56-44. Hypertrophic pyloric stenosis. **A,** Pyloric beak is identified and represents extension of contrast medium into the compressed distal antrum and narrowed pyloric canal. **B,** The elongated and angulated pyloric canal is opacified, and in addition the "shoulder sign" is demonstrated (arrow).

Besides the well-known "string sign" there are other additional pathognomonic signs of hypertrophic pyloric stenosis. The most common of these is the pyloric beak, which is the extension of contrast medium into the compressed portion of the distal antrum (Fig. 56-43). In severe cases of hypertrophic pyloric stenosis the contrast medium will not enter the pyloric canal. If the beak can be observed, there is no necessity for prolonging the fluoroscopic observation for the sake of identifying the pyloric canal. The "shoulder sign"[12] and pyloric tit[30] are additional features of hypertrophic pyloric stenosis (Fig. 56-44).

Chalasia occurs in approximately 10% of the infants with pyloric stenosis; when it is present it is of value in explaining the postoperative vomiting that some of these infants have. Delay in gastric emptying is invariably present, and although postoperative examination may show persistence of the defect of the pyloric canal for a period of weeks or months, the emptying time after surgical correction is normal.

Intussusception

Intussusception offers the radiologist the opportunity of diagnosis as well as treatment. The hydrostatic reduction of an ileocolic or colocolic intussusception should not be considered as a form of treatment competitive with surgical reduction; there are indications for both forms of treatment.

The feasibility of hydrostatic reduction can be accurately predicted by an abdominal scout film of infants with this condition (Fig. 56-45). If there is no evidence, or if there is only minimal evidence, of intestinal obstructon as determined by abdominal roentgenographs, hydrostatic reduction may be accomplished with ease.[32] If there is roentgenographic evidence of moderate obstruction, with distention of the terminal ileum and with a relative decrease in the amount of gas in the colon, reduction may be attempted but is frequently unsuccessful. Even so, partial reduction will be accomplished, and this in turn will facilitate surgical reduction. If there is evidence of significant obstruc-

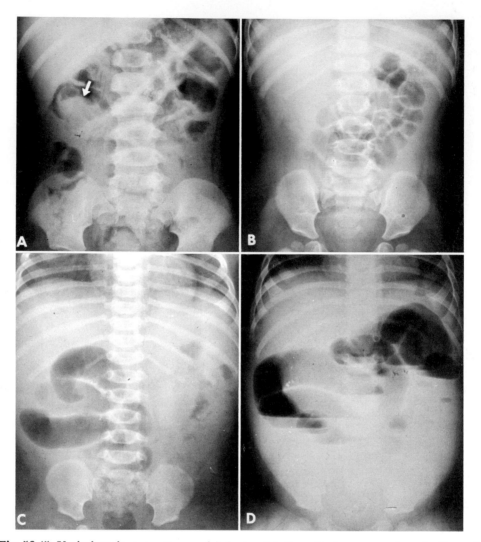

Fig. 56-45. Variations in gas patterns of infants with ileocolic intussusception. **A,** Normal gas pattern with gas in the colon and small intestine in normal amounts (arrow denotes location of intussusception). **B,** Nearly complete absence of gas in the colon with beginning distention of the small bowel. Reduction by hydrostatic pressure should be anticipated but with more difficulty than in **A. C,** Complete absence of colonic gas with distention of the terminal ileum. Reduction by hydrostatic method is doubtful. **D,** Marked obstruction with free peritoneal fluid. Attempts at hydrostatic reduction were contraindicated. (From Singleton, E. B.: Pediat. Clin. N. Amer. **10:**571, 1963.)

tion with dilatation of the terminal ileum, hydrostatic reduction is not feasible, and prolonged attempts to reduce the intussusception should be avoided. If the patient has evidence of peritonitis, including leukocytosis, abdominal tenderness, and rigidity, even a diagnostic barium enema is contraindicated because perforation of the bowel has probably occurred.

The age of the patient is also a factor in se-

lecting patients for hydrostatic reduction. The cause of an intussusception in infancy is usually unknown, and direct causes such as Meckel's diverticulum or hypertrophied Peyer's patch are rare in this age group, occurring only in 2%.[17] Direct causes are much more common after infancy, and consequently candidates for hydrostatic reduction do not include this older age group.

The case for hydrostatic reduction

Opponents of hydrostatic reduction claim that: (1) the reduction or perforation of devitalized bowel may result from the hydrostatic pressure, (2) the method creates an additional hardship to the patient, and (3) it results in needless x-ray exposure. These are not valid arguments. If the hydrostatic pressure is limited to no more than 3 feet above the table top, neither reduction of devitalized bowel or perforation of bowel will occur.[26] Also, this method of reduction is less hazardous to the patient than is surgical reduction. Supportive measures and intravenous fluids should be instituted if needed, whether the child is to have surgery or a barium enema. Unnecessary x-ray exposure is also not a valid argument, because hydrostatic reduction, when feasible, requires little more fluoroscopic time than that required for a diagnostic colon study. In addition, the fluoroscopic shutters should be kept at a small size, consistent with adequate visualization of the intussusception, and the fluoroscopist should limit his observations to split-second glances until the reduction is completed.

The technique of hydrostatic reduction

The technique of hydrostatic reduction is somewhat different from that required in a routine barium enema study. This is the only examination in which a catheter with an inflated bag can be used with good advantage. It is preferable to begin the study after the infant has been sedated. A barbiturate given in an intravenous infusion allows the infant to rest during the examination and makes hydrostatic reduction much easier than if the infant is awake and struggling. Once the catheter is inserted and inflated, the buttocks should be taped together. Then with the level of the barium in the container held no more than 3 feet above the table top, contrast material is allowed to flow into the rectum.

The advancing column of barium should be observed carefully. If intussusception is present, a convex meniscus defect will be observed. This is usually encountered in the splenic or transverse portion of the colon but may be identified at wherever the intussusception is located. With sustained hydrostatic pressure, the contrast medium is seen to flow around the intussusceptum and gradually to displace it proximally.

The retrograde displacement of the intussusceptum is occasionally delayed at the hepatic flexure and invariably in the region of the cecum. It may be necessary on occasion to lessen the hydrostatic pressure by lowering the enema reservoir and allowing the colon to evacuate. Resumption of the hydrostatic pressure, in such instances, is usually successful in producing further reduction. The appendix often fills with barium as reduction into the ileocecal region occurs. However, with persistent and sustained hydrostatic pressure, complete reduction may be anticipated, and it may be confirmed when contrast medium is seen entering the terminal ileum (Fig. 56-46). It is necessary to fill several inches of terminal ileum in order to be certain that ileoileal intussusception is not also present.

Even if complete reduction is impossible by hydrostatic means, partial reduction invariably occurs, and this in turn facilitates surgical reduction. One should keep in mind that intussusception in children past the age of infancy is commonly associated with a direct cause such as Meckel's diverticulum, hypertrophied Peyer's patch, aberrant pancreatic tissue, or ileal duplication. Consequently, surgical reduction in this older group is preferable. Recurrence of intussusception after hydrostatic reduction should be considered as being the result of a definite etiologic lead point, and no attempt should be made to repeat the hydrostatic reduction.

The advantages of hydrostatic reduction are obvious. Laparotomy is avoided and the hazards, even though remote, of a general anesthetic are obviated. Consequently, if the patient is an infant and if the abdominal scout film shows slight or only a moderate degree of mechanical obstruction, an attempt at hydrostatic reduction should be made. If this is unsuccessful, partial reduction will at least be accomplished, and this facilitates the surgical reduction.

Inflammatory lesions

Inflammatory lesions of the gastrointestinal tract are rare in infants. Infectious diarrhea of gastroenteritis in a young infant or child is commonly seen, and the roentgenographic findings are similar to those seen in a severe adynamic ileus. Air is present in all portions of the intestinal tract, and upright films show multiple fluid levels in the small bowel and colon.

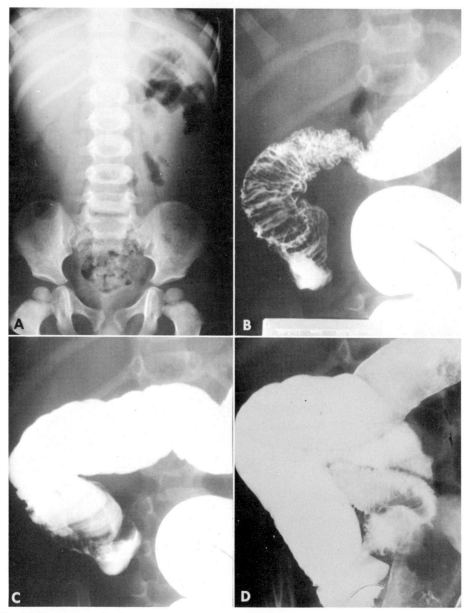

Fig. 56-46. Steps in hydrostatic reduction of intussusception. **A,** A rather common scout film shows no evidence of significant obstruction. **B,** Intussusception has been reduced to the hepatic flexure. **C,** Reduction has been accomplished to the region of the cecum. **D,** Extensive fill of terminal ileum has occurred, indicative of complete reduction. (From Singleton, E. B.: Pediat. Clin. N. Amer. **10**:571, 1963.)

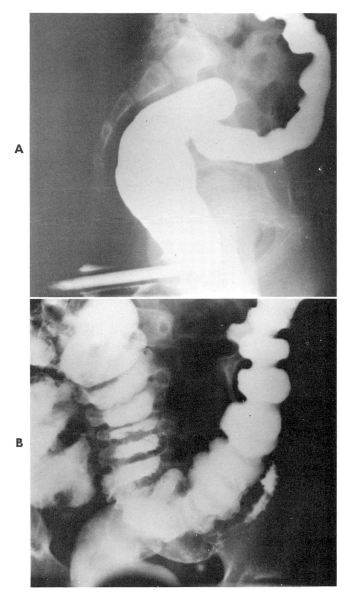

Fig. 56-47. Bacterial colitis in an 8-year-old child. **A,** Lateral view of the rectosigmoid shows minute areas of ulceration involving the rectum and sigmoid. **B,** Post-evacuation film shows area of spasm and ulceration in the sigmoid.

Acute ulcerative colitis

Acute ulcerative colitis as the result of *Shigella, Salmonella,* or other virulent organisms is occasionally seen in an infant or young child and may mimic the early changes of chronic ulcerative colitis. Roentgenologic examination shows areas of ulceration in the rectosigmoid region, with evidence of distinct irritability of the bowel

(Fig. 56-47). Appropriate bacteriologic studies and followup roentgenologic examinations will serve to establish this condition as acute colitis rather than a chronic ulcerative form.

Regional enteritis and chronic ulcerative colitis

More chronic forms of enteritis are occasionally encountered in young children. Regional enteritis, granulomatous colitis,[27] and chronic ulcerative colitis are conditions that may affect the pediatric patient. The roentgenographic features are similar to those seen in the adult (Fig. 56-48). Chronic ulcerative colitis may make its appearance in infancy but is more commonly seen in young children. The onset is frequently acute, and progression of the condition may be rapid, with roentgenographic evidence of denudation of the mucous membrane, multiple areas of ulceration, cicatricial changes, and resulting shortening of the colon. This disease in a young child presents many problems in regard to the type of treatment, and all too frequently extensive resection of the colon with permanent colostomy is necessary.

Ascariasis

Chronic bacterial and parasitic infections of the bowel are very rare in the United States and when present are similar to the same conditions seen in the adult patient. The roentgenologic identification of *Ascaris* in the bowel is common in many indigent children, and the roentgenographic findings are typical. The Ascaris may appear as radiolucent filling defects in the bowel or may be coated by the barium meal; the barium may even outline the linear alimentary tube of the *Ascaris* (Fig. 56-49).

Acute appendicitis

Acute appendicitis commonly results in rather specific roentgenographic findings. This is particularly true if perforation of the appendix has occurred. In such instances one may expect to see on the abdominal scout films distention of the terminal ileum similar to that seen in mechanical obstruction of this structure. Whether this is the result of localized paralytic ileus adjacent to periappendiceal abscess or whether there is actual mechanical obstruction of the terminal ileum by the pericecal infection is

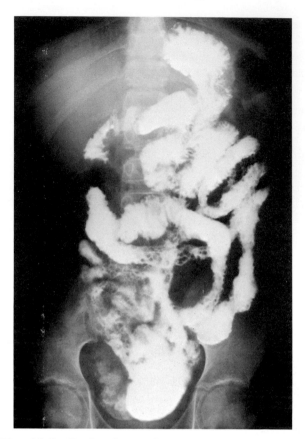

Fig. 56-48. Regional enteritis in an 8-year-old boy. There is loss of normal small-bowel mucosa as well as multiple granulomatous polyps.

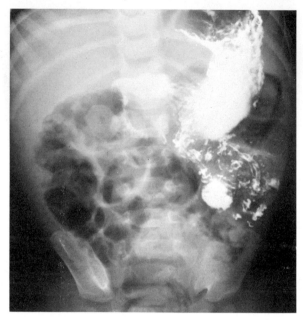

Fig. 56-49. *Ascaris lumbricoides.* Linear filling defects in the proximal jejunum represent the ascaris worm.

difficult to determine. Free gas within the peritoneal cavity may be identified, particularly in the form of scattered areas of radiolucency in the pericecal region. The peritoneal fat line in such instances is usually obliterated adjacent to the infection.

Commonly an appendicolith, with its characteristic laminated appearance, can be seen and when present is pathognomonic evidence that appendicitis is present. The identification of an appendicolith prior to the clinical onset of appendicitis is considered by most authorities to justify prophylactic appendectomy. In any event, the identification of an appendiceal stone should serve as a warning that acute appendicitis with perforation may occur.

Peptic ulcer

Peptic ulcer involving the stomach or duodenum is uncommon in the pediatric patient.

Anoxic ulcers of the stomach or duodenum may be cause for severe bleeding or even bowel perforation in the newborn; however, these lesions, because of their small size, are extremely difficult to identify by fluoroscopy. In spite of numerous reports suggesting that peptic ulcer is a common finding in the pediatric patient, the experience of most pediatric radiologists would indicate that it is rare.[34] When it is present, the roentgenologic features are similar to those seen in the adult patient.

Pneumoperitoneum as a result of perforating peptic ulcer in older children or as a result from any cause leading to perforation of the intestinal tract is easily identified in upright films. If films are made with the patient supine, the radiolucency produced by the air about the falciform ligament produces a sign that has been compared to the appearance of a football[23] (Fig. 56-50).

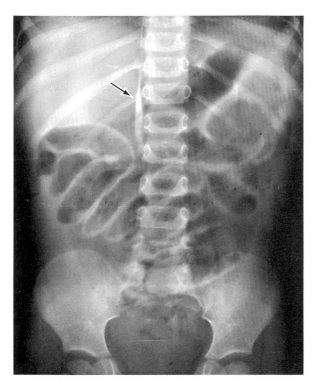

Fig. 56-50. Pneumoperitoneum in a child. The general radiolucency represents air in the peritoneal cavity and the arrow denotes the falciform ligament. At operation a perforated duodenal ulcer was identified.

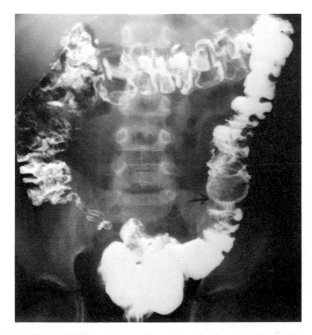

Fig. 56-51. Solitary juvenile polyp in lower descending colon of a 5-year-old child.

Traumatic lesions

Traumatic lesions of the gastrointestinal tract should be suspected in any ambulatory infant or child if obstruction of the small bowel develops. This is particularly true in obstructive lesions of the third portion of the duodenum. Trauma in this area commonly leads to duodenal hematoma with distention of the duodenum proximal to the lesion. Hemorrhage in the intestinal tract may also occur in patients with Schönlein-Henoch purpura with or without a history of trauma. The roentgenographic findings in these patients are highly suggestive by virtue of the thumbprint deformity involving the wall of the affected bowel.[18]

Benign polyps

Benign polyps of the colon in young infants are common and are usually identified at the time of proctoscopy or roentgenologic studies of the colon following the appearance of blood in the stool. These juvenile polyps of the colon are benign lesions, and their roentgenologic identification is not as important as finding a polyp in an adult patient (Fig. 56-51). In most instances the polylp, after outgrowing its blood supply, will be passed spontaneously; the only indication for surgical removal is severe bleeding.

Familial polyposis represents a more serious condition, in which there is potential malignancy. Consequently, accurate identification of the polyps in this condition is very important so that surgical removal can be accomplished.

Peutz-Jeghers syndrome is another form of polyposis involving the small bowel and also occasionally the stomach and colon. Children with this syndrome show characteristic melanin deposits on their lips, as well as on the buccal mucosa (Fig. 56-52). These polyps may produce intestinal obstruction either as a result of their mass or because of resulting intussusception. Their localization by roentgenologic methods is important for surgical removal. Although these lesions are pathologically hamartomas, there are reports of malignant change.[2]

Neoplasms

Malignant neoplasms of the gastrointestinal tract are extremely rare in infants but become more common during the later years of childhood. Lymphomas of various forms are the most common malignant neoplasms in this age group

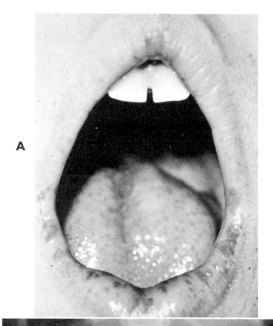

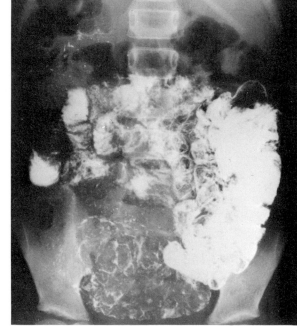

Fig. 56-52. Peutz-Jeghers syndrome. **A,** Pigmentation of the lips; **B,** multiple polyps scattered throughout the small intestine with massive collection of the tumors in the terminal ileum.

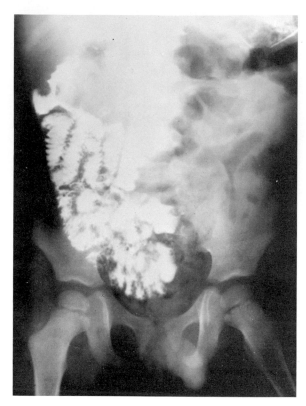

Fig. 56-53. Reticulum cell sarcoma of the duodenum in a 4-year-old boy. There is loss of normal mucosal pattern. Location of jejunum on right indicates associated nonrotation of the bowel.

and show changes similar to identical lesions in the adult patient (Fig. 56-53). The lesion, however, is usually localized and obstructive.

Tumors of the pancreas are extremely rare in children but may occur. Consequently, the radiologist should not discount the possibility of an "adult type" of lesion even in a child (Fig. 56-54).

Malabsorption

There are numerous malabsorption syndromes, including celiac disease, fibrocystic disease (Fig. 56-55), collagen diseases, agammaglobulinemia, parasitic diseases, chronic enteritis, intestinal lymphangiectasis (Fig. 56-56), hereditary fructose intolerance, disturbance of intestinal hydrolysis of lactose or maltose, and exudative enteropathy, to mention only a few.[22] The roentgenographic findings are similar. There is coarsening of mucosal folds of the small bowel, with segmentation and puddling of the barium columns. In the evaluation of the small bowel

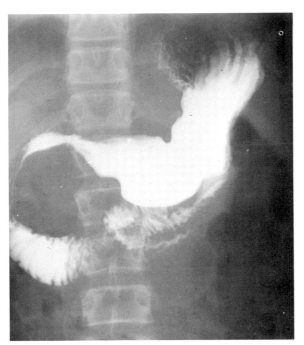

Fig. 56-54. Pancreatic adenoma in a 14-year-old boy. There is compression of the duodenal loop.

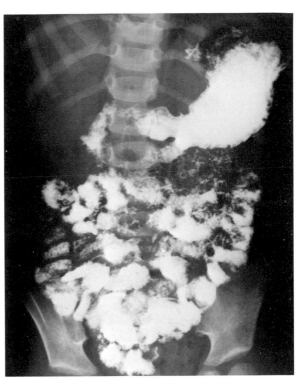

Fig. 56-55. Malabsorption syndrome secondary to fibrocystic disease. There is puddling and segmentation of barium within the small bowel as well as coarsening of the mucosal pattern.

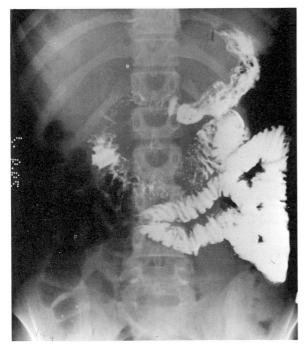

Fig. 56-56. Malabsorption syndrome secondary to intestinal lymphangiectasia (exudative enteropathy). There is thickening of the mucosal folds. (Courtesy Dr. J. Dorst and Dr. W. Schubert.)

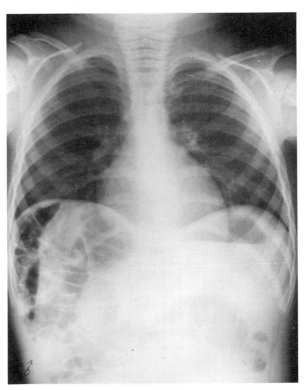

Fig. 56-57. Chiliaditis syndrome. There is interposition of the hepatic flexure between diaphragm and liver.

pattern, one must appreciate the fact that in infants segmentation and irregularity of the small bowel patern is commonly a normal finding.

The mucosal pattern of the colon may be altered in a child with fibrocystic disease. There is coarsening of the mucosal folds as well as multiple cobblestone-like filling defects seen most commonly in the descending and sigmoid portions.

Chiliaditis syndrome

Chiliaditis syndrome consists of interposition of the hepatic flexure between the liver and diaphragm. Clinically, it is characterized by abdominal pain that becomes increasingly worse during the day and is often accentuated by deep breathing. Roentgenographic studies show gas within the hepatic flexure interposed between liver and diaphragm[4] (Fig. 56-57). The validity of this as a true clinical syndrome is openly questioned, in that interposition of the bowel between liver and diaphragm is occasionally seen in normal and asymptomatic individuals.

Functional constipation

Functional constipation in the young infant is a common complaint, and it is the most common cause for colon examination in this age group. The clinical history is usually diagnostic, and differentiation from Hirschsprung's disease can frequently be made on clinical information alone. Children with functional constipation are well until late infancy or until toilet training age, when for some unexplained reason their bowel difficulty begins. This is due in many cases to anal fissure, with resulting pain on defecation. In contrast, Hirschsprung's disease has a history of constipation dating from birth. A child with functional constipation usually constantly soils his underclothes, and when bowel movements occur they are frequently of enormous size. On the other hand, the child with Hirschsprung's disease does not as a rule have a history of soiling, and bowel movements are small.

Roentgenographic studies are helpful in differentiating these conditions.[35] The child with functional constipation has a large rectum, and the dilated colon is accompanied by marked elongation and redundancy of the rectosigmoid area (Fig. 56-58). It is difficult to determine

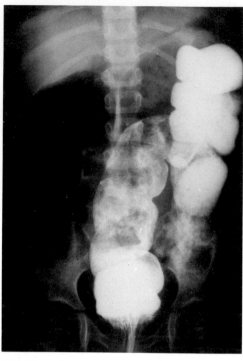

Fig. 56-58. Functional constipation with associated dilatation of the rectosigmoid and descending portions of the colon.

whether this increased length of the colon is secondary to chronic constipation or whether it is present initially and plays an important factor in the patient's symptoms. In all probability, children with functional constipation have an excessively long colon initially. In the roentgenologic examination one should not attempt to fill the colon completely but simply allow enough barium to enter the distal colon to establish the diagnosis.

REFERENCES

1. Able, L.: Tracheoesophageal fistula without esophageal atresia, Texas J. Med. **61**:22, 1965.
2. Achord, J. J., and Proctor, H. D.: Malignant degeneration and metastasis in Peutz-Jeghers syndrome, Arch. Intern. Med. **111**:498, 1963.
3. Astley, R.: Radiology of the alimentary tract in infancy, London, 1956, Edward Arnold, Publishers.
4. Behlke, F. M.: Hepatodiaphragmatic interposition in children, Amer. J. Roentgen. **91**:669, 1964.
5. Berdon, W. E., and others: Necrotizing enterocolitis in the premature infant, Radiology **83**:879, 1964.
6. Berdon, W. E., and Baker, D. H.: Roentgenographic diagnosis of Hirschsprung's disease in infancy, Amer. J. Roentgen. **93**:432, 1965.

7. Berdon, W. E., Baker, D. H., Bull, S., and Santulli, T. V.: Midgut malrotation and volvulus, Radiology **96**:375, 1970.

8. Berdonu, W. E., Baker, D. H., Santulli, T. V., Amoury, R. A., and Blanc, W. A.: Microcolon in newborn infants with intestinal obstruction: Its correlation with the level and time of onset of obstruction, Radiology **90**:878, 1968.

9. Caffey, J.: Pediatric x-ray diagnosis, ed. 3, Chicago, 1956, Year Book Medical Publishers, Inc.

10. Caffey, J., and Ross, S.: Mongolism (mongoloid deficiency) during early infancy—some newly recognized diagnostic changes in the pelvic bones, Pediatrics **17**:642, 1956.

11. Carre, I. J., and Astley, R.: Fate of partial thoracic stomach (hiatus hernia) in children, Arch. Dis. Child. **35**:484, 1960.

12. Currarino, G.: The value of double contrast examination of the stomach with pressure spots in the diagnosis of infantile hypertrophic pyloric stenosis, Radiology **83**:873, 1964.

13. Desjardins, J. G., Stephens, C. A., and Moes, C. A. F.: Results of surgical treatment of congenital tracheoesophageal fistula with note on cinefluorographic findings, Ann. Surg. **160**:141, 1964.

14. Dunbar, S.: Personal communication.

15. Filler, R. M., Randolph, J. G., and Gross, R. E.: Esophageal hiatus hernia in infants and children, J. Thorac. Cardiov. Surg. **4**:551, 1964.

16. Gillis, D. A., and Grantmyre, E. B.: Meconium plug syndrome and Hirschsprung's disease, Canadian M.A.J. **92**:225, 1965.

17. Gross, R. E.: The surgery of infancy and childhood, Philadelphia, 1953, W. B. Saunders Co.

18. Grossman, H., Berdon, W. E., and Baker, D. H.: Reversible gastrointestinal signs of hemorrhage and edema in the pediatric age group, Radiology **84**:33, 1965.

19. Grossman, H., Winchester, P. H., and Chisari, F. V.: Roentgenographic classification of renal cystic disease, Amer. J. Roentgen. **104**:319, 1968.

20. Harris, P. D., Neuhauser, E. B. D., and Gerth, R.: The osmotic effect of water soluble contrast media on circulating plasma volume, Amer. J. Roentgen. **91**:694, 1964.

21. Koop, C. E., and Kavianian, A.: Reappraisal of colonic replacement of distal esophagus and proximal stomach in management of bleeding varices in children, Surgery **57**:454, 1965.

22. Marshak, R. H., and Lindner, A. E.: Malabsorption syndrome, Seminars Roentgen. **1** (2):138, 1966.

23. Miller, R. E.: Perforated viscus in infants; a new roentgen sign, Radiology **74**:65, 1960.

24. Nelson, S. W., Christoforidis, A. J., and Roenigk, W. J.: Dangers and fallibilities of iodinated radiopaque mediums in obstruction of small bowel, Amer. J. Surg. **109**:546, 1965.

25. Neuhauser, E. B. D., Harris, G. D., and Berrett, A.: Roentgenographic features of neurenteric cysts, Amer. J. Roentgen. **79**:235, 1956.

26. Ravitch, M.: Nonoperative treatment of intussusception—hydrostatic pressure reduction by barium enema, Surg. Clin. N. Amer. **36**:1495, 1956.

27. Rudhe, U., and Keats, T. E.: Granulomatous colitis in children, Radiology **84**:24, 1965.

28. Santulli, T. V., and Blanc, W. A.: Congenital atresia of the intestines, pathogenesis and treatment, Ann. Surg. **154**:939, 1961.

29. Seaman, W. B., Fleming, R. J., and Baker, D. H.: Pneumatosis intestinalis of the small bowel, Seminars Roentgen. **1** (2):234, 1966.

30. Shopfner, C. E.: The pyloric tit in hypertrophic pyloric stenosis, Amer. J. Roentgen. **91**:674, 1964.

31. Sieber, W. K., and Girdany, B.: Functional intestinal obstruction in the newborn infant with morphologically normal gastrointestinal tract, Surgery **53**:357, 1963.

32. Singleton, E. B.: Hydrostatic reduction of intussusception, Pediat. Clin. N. Amer. **10**:175, 1963.

33. Singleton, E. B.: Radiologic evaluation of intestinal obstruction in the newborn, Radiol. Clin. N. Amer. **1**:571, 1963.

34. Singleton, E. B.: The radiologic incidence of peptic ulcer in infants and children, Radiology **84**:956, 1965.

35. Singleton, E. B.: X-ray diagnosis of the alimentary tract in infants and children, Chicago, 1959, Year Book Medical Publishers, Inc.

36. Singleton, E. B., and Faykus, M. H.: Incidence of of peptic ulcer as determined by radiologic examinations in the pediatric age group, J. Pediat. **65**:858, 1964.

37. Singleton, E. B., Rosenburg, H. M., and Samper, L.: Radiologic considerations of the perinatal distress syndrome, Radiology **76**:200, 1961.

38. Strawczynski, H., Beck, I. T., McKenna, R. D., and Nickerson, G. H.: Behavior of lower esophageal sphincter in infants and its relationship to gastroesophageal regurgitation, J. Pediat. **64**:17, 1964.

39. White, H.: Meconium ileus; new roentgen sign, Radiology **66**:567, 1956.

40. Wittenborg, M. H., and Neuhauser, E. B. D.: Simple roentgenographic demonstration of eustachian tubes and abnormalities, Amer. J. Roentgen. **89**:1194, 1963.

57 | The biliary tract in children

Hooshang Taybi

Although diseases of the biliary tract are relatively rare in infancy and childhood, roentgenologic examination plays an important part in their diagnosis and management.

The position of the gallbladder varies in infancy. In some infants the gallbladder is deeply embedded in the liver substance, its lower end lying above the liver edge.[205] In others, it may protrude below the liver margin and, on a plain roentgenogram of the abdomen, appear to be outlined by the gas-filled colon.

TECHNIQUE OF EXAMINATION
Oral cholecystography

Satisfactory opacification of the gallbladder does not occur with the same regularity in early infancy as in older children and adults. The dose of iopanoic acid (Telepaque) recommended by Harris and Caffey is 0.15 gm./kg. of body weight.[113] In only six of twelve infants less than 6 months of age was a satisfactory demonstration of gallbladder achieved by these au-

thors. The dosage of iopanoic acid I routinely use is as follows:

0.15 gm./kg. of body weight for children under 13 kg.

2 gm. for children 13 kg. to 23 kg.

3 gm. for children over 23 kg.

In thirty-eight examinations, Bétoulieres and co-workers used Solubiloptine* in infants younger than 1 month of age.[25] They recommend a dose of 0.45 gm./kg. of body weight in this age group. The dosage of 0.90 gm./kg. of body weight was used in those patients in whom the opacification of the gallbladder was not obtained with the above dose. With this contrast medium, roentgenograms are obtained 7 to 8 hours after its ingestion.[25]

Intravenous cholecystography

Iodipamide sodium (Cholografin) given in a dose of 0.6 to 1.2 ml./kg. of body weight resulted in satisfactory cholecystograms in nine of twelve infants younger than 8 months, as reported by Reichelderfer and Van Hartesveldt.[215] The bound iodine content of this preparation is about 13%, whereas the bound iodine content of iodipamide methylglucamine is about 26%, and the recommended dose is 0.3 to 0.6 ml./kg. of body weight. Visualization of the biliary system takes place 30 minutes to 4 hours after the injection of the contrast medium.

Operative cholangiography

Operative cholangiography is used primarily in the evaluation of biliary atresia, biliary stenosis, or choledochal cyst in infants.[70,112,197,250] A catheter is inserted into the gallbladder during laparotomy. One-half strength solution of a contrast medium usually used for excretory urography is injected through the catheter. The film is exposed at about the time the injection ends. Respiration should be suspended by the

*Solubiloptine, or SH 550 (calcium-bisn-β-[3-dimethyl-amino-methyleneamino-2, 4, 6-triiodophenyl]-propionate) known in the United States as ipodate calcium (Oragrafin).

anesthesiologist at the time the exposure is being made. The amount of the contrast medium depends on the size of the gallbladder and visible portion of the bile duct and varies from 5 to 15 ml. If the contrast medium drains into the duodenum but does not pass in a retrograde direction into the hepatic duct, then the distal common bile duct may be temporarily obstructed during a second injection of the contrast medium.[197]

When an extrahepatic system is not found at surgical exploration, the presence of a dilated intrahepatic duct may be sought. A 19-gauge needle is then inserted into the liver and aspiration is done in a systematic manner at several sites. If bile is aspirated, 5 ml. of a diluted contrast medium is injected and the roentgenogram is obtained.[249]

CONGENITAL ANOMALIES
Hepatic and common bile ducts

The recognition of the high incidence of anomalies of the biliary tract is of utmost importance to surgeons. In a review of 1,000 consecutive patients undergoing surgery for cholelithiasis or its complications, Hayes and his colleagues reported 47.7% had duct structures that departed from the anatomic ideal.[116] Anomalous length of common hepatic duct and accessory ducts constituted 93.4% of the malformations. Operative cholangiography, before exploration of the ducts, is recommended to prevent the occurrence of complications at operation.[117]

Biliary atresia

Biliary atresia is the cause in 75% of the instances of obstructive jaundice in young infants.[164]

The extrahepatic tract may be completely absent, or a fibrous cord may be the only structure present.[70,197] More than 80% of the patients are inoperable. In rare instance, a familial occurrence of the disease has been reported.[151] An anatomic classification suggested by Hasse shows the range of these anomalies (Fig. 57-1).[115]

Anomalies associated with biliary atresia have been reported. These consist of malrotation of the bowel,[124,240] duodenal atresia,[166] tracheo-

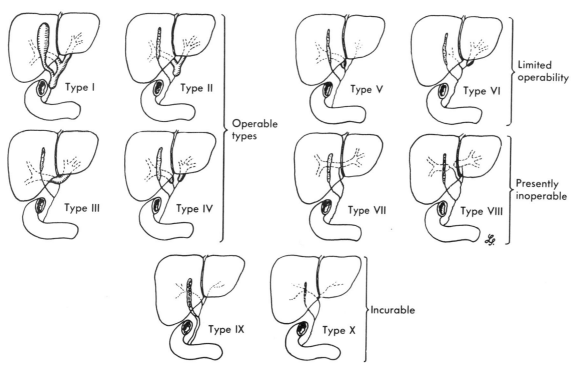

Fig. 57-1. Types of atresia of the bile ducts. (From Hasse, W.: Arch. Dis. Child. 40:162, 1965.)

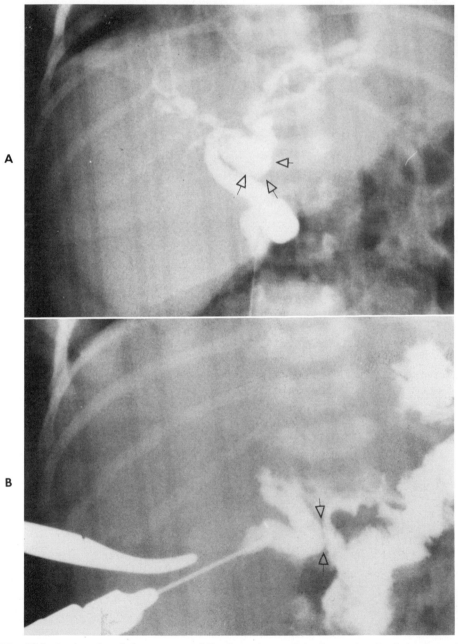

Fig. 57-2. A, Atresia of the common bile duct (arrows) is shown by the injection of the contrast medium into the gallbladder in a 4-week-old male infant. Note the nonuniform dilatation of the intrahepatic bile ducts. **B,** A second injection after choledochoduodenostomy shows the free passage of contrast medium into the duodenum.

esophageal fistula, imperforate anus, congenital heart disease, and polycystic kidney.[243] Still others reported are choledochal cyst,[22,207] anencephaly, mongolism, syndactyly,[243] congenital amputation, and trisomy 17-18.[5,262,269] Primary hepatic carcinoma associated with biliary cirrhosis resulting from congenital atresia of the bile duct has also been reported.[196]

Isotope studies, in particular demonstration of low fecal excretion of I^{131} rose bengal, are helpful in the detection of obstructive jaundice of newborn infants.[265] A normal excretion is 70% in 72 hours. Patients with biliary atresia excrete less than 5%.[92]

Operative cholangiography is necessary to demonstrate biliary atresia (Fig. 57-2).* The procedure may be misleading in some patients, since the collapsed duct may fail to fill. In such

*See references 70, 112, 127, 187, 197, and 250.

cases the roentgenologic appearance may simulate that of biliary atresia.[197]

In congenital absence of intralobular bile duct (MacMahon-Tannhauser syndrome) the liver biopsy is necessary for a definite diagnosis.[15,167,187] Postmortem injection of contrast medium has shown an absence of the fine intrahepatic ramifications of the hepatic ducts.[76] Operative cholangiography in such cases may be misleading because the extrahepatic ducts may appear normal.[76,152]

Rickets and esophageal varices may result from biliary atresia.[158] Digital clubbing, joint effusion, skeletal demineralization, failure of funnelization and cylindrization, periosteal elevation, and subperiosteal new bone formation are some of the manifestations of hepatic osteoarthropathy in older children with biliary atresia or absence of the intralobular bile ducts (Fig. 57-3).[15]

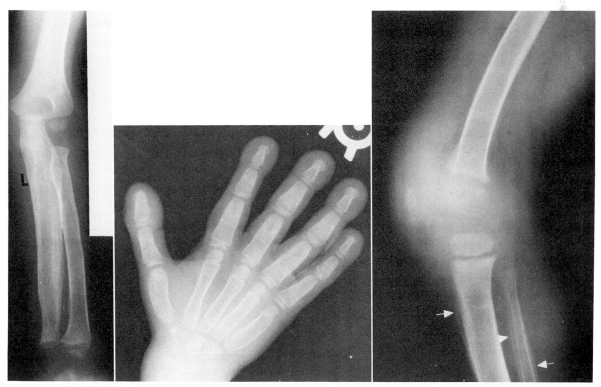

Fig. 57-3. Osteoarthropathy in a 4-year-old girl with biliary atresia. Surgical exploration at 6 months of age revealed a small gallbladder. The liver biopsy showed very early biliary type cirrhosis. Note osteoporosis, digital clubbing, and joint effusion in the knee. Periosteal elevation and subperiosteal new bone formation of the long bones are present (arrows).

Biliary hypoplasia

A reduction in the lumen of the hepatic duct intrahepatically, extrahepatically, or both, may result in an inadequate biliary drainage.[164,201] The degree of hepatic damage depends on the severity of the hypoplasia.

Biliary tract stenosis

Localized narrowing of the intrahepatic or extrahepatic ducts is demonstrable by intravenous or operative cholangiography.[98,111] The stenosis may be single or multiple.[187] Congenital diaphragm of the common hepatic duct has been reported as a cause of biliary cirrhosis.[80] Stenosis of the ampulla of Vater may be complicated by the presence of pancreatitis.[120]

Cystic dilatation of bile ducts

Common bile duct. Localized globular dilatation of the common duct, or fusiform enlargement, which may also involve the hepatic and cystic ducts, has been divided in four different anatomic types (Fig. 57-4).

Type I. Choledochal cyst—a sharply defined dilatation of the common duct. Frequently the duct is narrow distal to the cyst and is mildly dilated proximally.[14,28,226] Usually the gallbladder is small or of normal size.[124]

Type II. Diverticulum cyst—arises from the common bile duct.

Type III. Choledochocele—a cystic dilatation of the intramural portion of the duct in the duodenal wall.[137,225] Through a small opening, the "cyst" communicates with the duodenal lumen. The pancreatic duct enters the "cyst."

Type IV. Multiple hepatocholedochal cysts. These may be in the form of dilatation of the duct or in the form of a diverticulum.[10,68,72]

A total of 403 authentic and sixteen questionable cases of cystic dilatation of bile ducts were collected and reported by Alonso-Lej in 1959.[4] The anomaly has been described in all age groups. Only one fourth of the patients, however, are less than 14 years of age[256] and 5% less than 7 months.[124] The disease is preponderant in females except in those of Asiatic race. About one third of the patients reported have been Japanese.

The cause of the disease is not known.[14] A localized weakness of the ductal wall with or without a congenital or acquired obstruction of the duct or of the sphincter of Oddi has been suggested.[144,169,216,230] Neuromuscular disturbance has also been suggested as a possible etiologic factor.[136]

The wall is composed of fibrous tissue and smooth muscle, and its thickness may vary from 2 to 10 mm. The cysts are of various sizes. Browne reported a patient in whom needle aspiration was done on four occasions; 10 liters of fluid were removed preoperatively.[40] At operation another 11 liters of bile were aspirated from the cyst.

The triad of abdominal pain, mass, and jaundice is present in about 60% of patients with cystic dilatation of the bile duct. The intermittence of symptoms is a significant clinical feature of the disease. In the newborn infant and in early infancy, obstructive jaundice is usually the presenting symptom of this anomaly (Fig. 57-5).[82,108] Some of the clinical symptoms may represent complications. These may be cholangitis, biliary cirrhosis,[186] cholecystitis,[102] and bleeding esophageal varices, probably from portal ob-

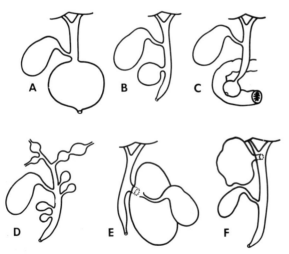

Fig. 57-4. Types of cystic dilatation of bile ducts: **A,** Type I—choledochal cyst; **B,** Type II—diverticulum cyst; **C,** Type III—choledochocele; **D,** Type IV—multiple hepatocholedochal cysts; **E,** Type V—cystic duct cyst seen in oblique projection; **F,** Type VI—hepatic duct cyst, diverticulum type. (Redrawn from Arthur, G. W., and Stewart, J. O.: Brit. J. Surg. **51:**671, 1964; Eisen, H. B., and others: Radiology **81:**276, 1963; Silberman, E. L., and Glaessner, T. S.: Radiology **82:**470, 1964; Weinstein, C.: Arch. Intern. Med. **115:**339, 1965.)

struction by the cyst.[94] Other complications are spontaneous or traumatic rupture,[26,28] pancreatitis,[14,120] and stone formation.[216] Malignant degeneration has been reported in three of the patients reviewed by Alonso-Lej.[4]

Associated reported anomalies are accessory hepatic duct,[168] double common bile duct,[247] double gallbladder,[143] bifid gallbladder,[256] absence of gallbladder,[216] biliary atresia,[22,207] polycystic kidney, and megaureter.[4]

Roentgenologic features. The digestive system should always be examined roentgenologically if a cyst is suspected. This examination may demonstrate esophageal varices and a round, soft tissue mass contiguous with the liver that displaces the stomach downward and to the left (Fig. 57-6).[212] The duodenum is commonly displaced anteriorly, inferiorly, and to the left (Fig.

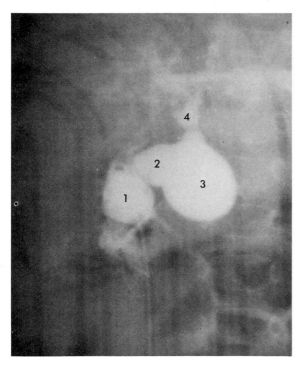

Fig. 57-5. Cystic dilatation of common bile duct with complete obstruction in a 6-week-old girl with persistent jaundice. Operative cholangiography with the injection of contrast medium into the gallbladder, **1**, reveals the dilatation of the common duct, **3**, with a complete blockage between the choledochal cyst and the duodenum. The blockage may be the result of atresia or severe stenosis with inspissation of bile at the site of the stenosis. The cystic duct, **2**, and the common hepatic duct, **4**, are also dilated.

57-7).[160] With a large cyst, the hepatic flexure of the colon may become displaced downward and anteriorly. In type III the major roentgenologic abnormality is a filling defect in the duodenum. In type IV reflux of barium from the duodenum into the cystic biliary tree has been reported.

Displacement of the right kidney, hydronephrosis, and hydroureter are rarely caused by choledochal cysts.

In some patients oral cholecystography performed between the attacks of jaundice may show opacification of the cyst.[58,109,126,230] Hoffer and Petasnick's review of the literature revealed six cases of cystic dilatation of the bile duct demonstrated by oral cholecystography, to which they added two new cases.[126] Also shown by oral cholecystography were multiple diverticular cystic dilatations of the common and hepatic ducts in a patient reported by Eguerra-Gomez.[72] Multiple doses of contrast medium increase the likelihood of visualization of the cyst.

The intravenous method of cholangiography (Fig. 57-7) has resulted in more satisfactory demonstration of the cyst than has the oral method.[160,225] It permits study of the sequence of filling of the duct, gallbladder, and the cyst. Intravenous cholangiography may be combined with an upper gastrointestinal series for better evaluation of the anomaly.[137]

Percutaneous aspiration and injection of contrast medium have been performed by some workers[136,147]; others consider the procedure unsafe.[212]

Operative cholangiography should always be performed for a detailed evaluation of the anomaly (Figs. 57-5, 57-6, and 57-8).[14] It may demonstrate absence of the passage of the contrast medium into the duodenum and thus reveal complete obstruction.

Ultrasonic study may be of some help in the preoperative diagnosis of the choledochal cyst.[93]

Hepatic duct cysts. Saccular cystic dilatation of the subcortical branches of the biliary duct, with diffuse dilatation of the hepatic and common ducts (Caroli's disease) has been demonstrated by intravenous cholangiography.[20,49,131,187] In several of these patients elevation of serum alkaline phosphatase has been reported. Multiple intrahepatic stone formation and hepatic fibrosis are other findings in some of the patients with this disease.

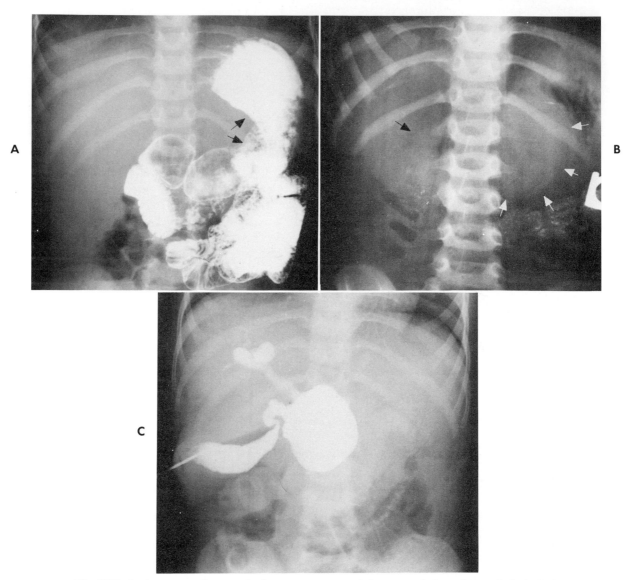

Fig. 57-6. A, A compression on the lesser curvature of the stomach by a large choledochal cyst (arrows) in a 3½-year-old girl. **B,** Oral cholecystography showing a vaguely opacified gallbladder on the right side and choledochal cyst on the left side (arrows). **C,** Operative cholangiography revealed cystic dilation of the common bile duct and the branches of the hepatic duct.

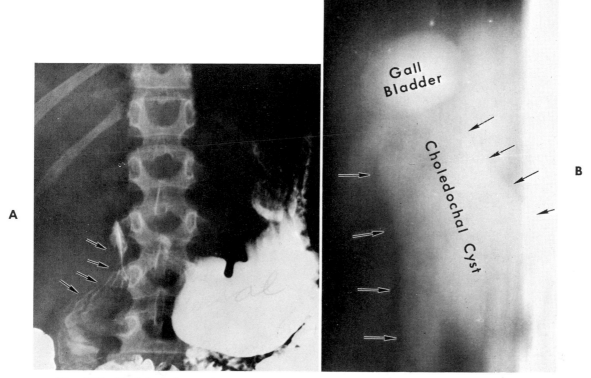

Fig. 57-7. Choledochal cyst in a 7-year-old girl with a history of recurrent jaundice. **A,** Downward and medial displacement of duodenum by the mass (preoperative). **B,** Postoperative intravenous cholangiography and tomography demonstrate a small gallbladder and the large choledochal cyst. Choledochoduodenostomy had been performed.

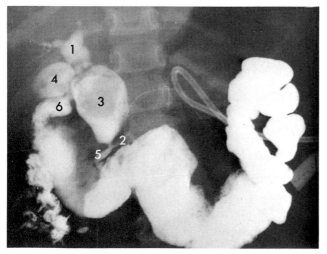

Fig. 57-8. Choledochal cyst with a diverticulum of the cyst in a 6-year-old girl who has undergone two previous operations. In the first operation, a choledochoduo-

denostomy was performed. Because of the persistence of symptoms, at the second operation, this anastomosis was taken down, the gallbladder was removed, and choledochojejunostomy was performed. The patient still remained symptomatic and clinical manifestations of pancreatitis were present. At the third operation, a fine catheter was introduced into the pancreatic duct, **2,** and contrast medium was injected. An anomalous entrance of the common bile duct into the pancreatic duct, **5,** was demonstrated. In addition to a cystic dilatation of the common bile duct, **3,** another cystic lesion, **4,** was opacified. On direct inspection this was found to be an outpouching (diverticulum) of the choledochal cyst. The previous jejunal anastomosis was to this diverticulum, **6.** Dilatation of hepatic duct, **1,** and branches are also shown. Some barium remains in the colon from an upper gastrointestinal study performed on the previous day. A pancreaticojejunostomy was performed and an anastomosis between the cyst, **3,** and duodenum was created.

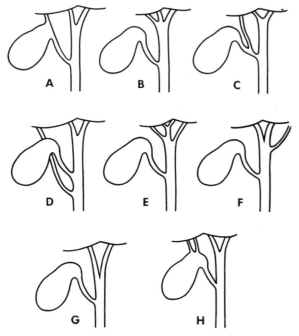

Fig. 57-9. Variations of hepatic ducts. **A,** Hepatocystic duct; **B,** accessory right hepatic duct terminating into common hepatic duct; **C,** accessory hepatic duct terminating into cystic duct; **D,** accessory right hepatic duct terminating into the common bile duct; **E,** right and left accessory hepatic ducts; **F,** accessory left hepatic duct; **G,** deep bifurcation of the hepatic duct; **H,** two accessory ducts form the right lobe entering the gallbladder. (Redrawn from Hess, W.: Surgery of biliary passages and the pancreas, Princeton, N. J., 1965, D. Van Nostrand Co., Inc.; Williams, C., and Williams, A. M.: Ann. Surg. **141:**598, 1955.)

Cystic duct cyst. A single case of this anomaly has been reported by Weinstein (Fig. 57-4).[263]

Accessory ducts

Accessory ducts are of special importance to surgeons because of their possible injury during cholecystectomy.[84] Their occurrence in the general population has been estimated at from 2% to 5%.[162] The duct may extend from the parenchyma of the liver to the gallbladder, hepatic duct, or cystic or common bile duct (Fig. 57-9).[85,124,228] Most hepatocystic ducts are less than 1 mm. in caliber. Operative cholangiography may demonstrate the larger accessory ducts.[124]

Anomalous termination of bile ducts

Anomalous termination of hepatic ducts into the gallbladder[267] and termination of the common bile duct into the pylorus, the stomach,[34] or pancreatic duct[14,139] are rare (Fig. 57-8). A case of reflux of contrast medium into a duplicated common bile duct has been reported. One of the branches terminated into the stomach and the other into the duodenum.[74] A communicating enterogenous cyst of duodenum receiving the termination of the common bile duct has been demonstrated by intravenous cholangiography.[199] Nahum and associates have reported a case of biliopancreatic cyst into which the common bile duct opened.[187]

Duplication

When the common duct is duplicated, both ducts may enter the duodenum or one may empty into the stomach and the other into the duodenum. A case of duplication of the cystic and common hepatic duct containing gastric mucosa has been reported.[154]

Anomalous communication with respiratory system

Anomalous tract that connects the tracheobronchial tree and the biliary tract is a rare disease, the presenting symptoms of which may be a foamy bile-stained sputum. Bronchography may demonstrate the anomalous tract.[69,191,241,258] A communication of the right bronchial tree and duodenum via the pancreatic duct has been noted by Astley.[12]

Gallbladder and cystic duct
Congenital absence of gallbladder

From the results of necropsies, the incidence of this anomaly has been estimated at about 0.04%.[173] The frequency was higher in necropsies in the pediatric age group. In one report it was estimated at 0.37%.[182]

The anomaly may range from one of complete absence of the gallbladder and cystic duct to that of presence of a cystic duct alone.[16,79]

In two thirds of the patients with this anomaly other malformations are present, 25% of which are in the biliary tract or pancreas.[124] The gallbladder has been reported to be absent in one sixth of the infants with atresia of the extrahepatic bile duct.[102] Absence of gallbladder is one of the manifestations of the polysplenia syndrome. Other unusual associated anomalies have been aberrant hepatic ducts, which emptied separately into the duodenum,[202] and dupli-

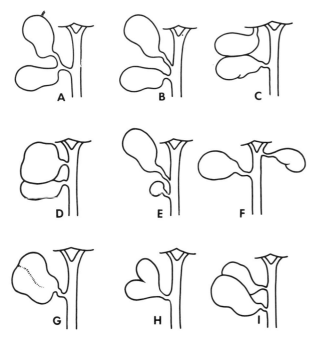

Fig. 57-10. Types of double gallbladder: **A,** Double gall-bladder with a single cystic duct; **B,** double gallbladder, each with a separate cystic duct; **C,** double gallbladder, one with a hepatocystic duct; **D,** double gallbladder, one dilated; **E,** rudimentary gallbladder in addition to a normal gallbladder; **F,** double gallbladder, one terminating into the left hepatic duct; **G,** septate gallbladder with a common gallbladder neck and common cystic duct; **H,** cleft-type double gallbladder; **I,** two gallbladders fused externally but with two cystic ducts. (Redrawn from Hess, W.: Surgery of the biliary passages and the pancreas, Princeton, N. J., 1965, D. Van Nostrand Co., Inc.; Anderson, R. E., and Ross, W. T.: Arch. Surg. 76:7, 1958.)

cation of the common bile duct, one branch emptying into the duodenum and the other into the stomach.[74]

Surgical exploration without operative cholangiography may be misleading.[47,91] A left-sided gallbladder, an intrahepatic gallbladder, an atrophic gallbladder, or a gallbladder surrounded by fibrous adhesions may be mistaken for an absence of this organ.[79,81]

Multiple gallbladder and cystic duct

Double gallbladder. The various types of double gallbladder (Fig. 57-10) are rare anomalies occurring at the rate of 1:3,000 to 1:4,000 of the population.[7,33,95,101,133] Shehadi reported an incidence of 1:12,000 in roentgenologic ex-

amination of the biliary tract.[228] In a review of the literature only 10% of 150 proved cases of double gallbladder has been demonstrated roentgenographically.[104] Such gallbladders are more prone to be affected with associated diseases.[104]

Triple gallbladder. This anomaly is extremely rare.[32,219,233] Each gallbladder may have its own separate cystic duct, demonstrable by intravenous cholecystography. Milk of calcium bile has been reported in two of the three gallbladders in one patient.[32]

Double cystic duct with single gallbladder. Two cystic ducts, one primary and the other rudimentary, in the presence of a single gallbladder is a most uncommon congenital anomaly.[198,227]

Abnormal position of gallbladder

Usually, a left-sided gallbladder in the absence of situs inversus is located under the left lobe of the liver (Fig. 57-11).[27,73,102] When aberrant, the cystic duct often terminates in the right hepatic duct and less often in the left.[124] The routine roentgenologic examination in the absence of opacification of the gallbladder should include a roentgenogram of the entire upper abdomen to exclude the possibility of malposition of the gallbladder.[73]

A most unusual anomaly is that of isolated left-sided liver and gallbladder without situs inversus abnormalities. With this anomaly, the stomach, spleen, and pancreas have been reported to be in their normal positions directly behind the liver.[153]

The gallbladder, without associated situs inversus abdominalis, may also be located in the midline.[228] Midline gallbladder is very often present in asplenia syndrome. A careful search should always be made for superimposition of the gallbladder over the shadow of the vertebral column.

An intrahepatic type of gallbladder may be missed by routine study when the abnormal position of the organ is not included on the roentgenogram. Surgical exploration may give the impression that the gallbladder is absent.[79] A high incidence of biliary stone has been reported in patients with partial or total intrahepatic position of the gallbladder.[81]

A free floating (pendulous) gallbladder has been seen in 4% of patients during the operative

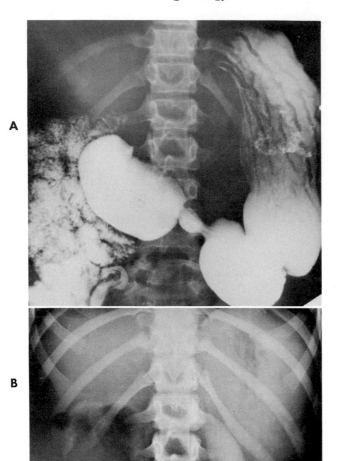

Fig. 57-11. Left-sided gallbladder, malrotation of bowel, and incomplete obstruction of duodenum by the anomalous course of the common bile duct. Eleven-year-old girl with the history of intermittent abdominal pain of several years' duration. A gastrointestinal study at 5 years of age revealed a partial obstruction of the duodenum and malrotation of the bowel. Division of periduodenal bands and an appendectomy were performed. The bands were considered to be producing the obstruction. The small bowel was located in the right side of the abdomen and the large bowel on the left side. After surgery, the patient remained mildly symptomatic. Repeat upper gastrointestinal study at 11 years of age, **A**, again revealed a partial obstruction of duodenum. At the second operation two lobes of the liver were noted, one in the right upper and the other in the left upper quadrants of abdomen, connected in the midline. The gallbladder was attached to the left lobe of the liver with a long common duct which went across the midline of the abdomen and across the first portion of the duodenum to enter the duodenum at approximately the junction of the second and third portion. The spleen was located high up in the left upper quadrant. A duodenoduodenostomy was performed, to bypass the site of obstruction, which corresponded to the position of the crossing of the common duct over the first portion of the duodenum. An intravenous cholangiogram at 12½ years of age, **B**, demonstrates the position of the gallbladder in the left upper abdomen. A phrygian cap deformity of gallbladder is also present.

procedure.[124,142] Torsion and gangrene of a pendulous gallbladder have been reported in children and in adults with a clinically acute condition within the abdomen. Some of the patients may complain of recurrent right upper abdominal pain.

Other unusual locations of the gallbladder are in the abdominal wall,[45] in the suprahepatic region,[6,214] in the falciform ligament,[190] and in the retroperitoneal area.[209] The gallbladder may rarely assume a transverse position.[46,101]

Anomalous shape of gallbladder

Various anomalous forms of the gallbladder have been described, some clinically significant.*

---

*See references 81, 124, 142, 208, 209, and 228.

These include phrygian cap, vestigeal, diverticulum-like, hourglass, trilocular, fish-hook, syphon-type, and transversely septated gallbladder.

In the phrygian cap gallbladder, the fundus is folded and a septum may be present at the site of the kink (Fig. 57-11).[35] The frequency of the occurrence of this anomaly has been estimated at from 2% to 6% of all cholecystographies.[81]

A diverticulum-like gallbladder with complete absence of the cystic duct may simulate a diverticulum of the common bile duct.[208]

A transverse septum is usually close to the fundus of the gallbladder and divides the gallbladder into two compartments.[124] Multiseptate gallbladders have been reported.[149,231] The septa are usually demonstrated on roentgenographic examination, where they are more prominent than on the examination of surgical specimen.[142] The congenital folds, as demonstrated in roentgenograms, remain unchanged with postural change and respiration, and their form remains the same before and after fatty meals.[125]

Diverticulum of gallbladder

True congenital diverticulum of the gallbladder is rare. It retains all the histologic features of the gallbaldder. Arcomano and Barnett reported three cases that, they stated, constituted approximately 10% of those with this anomaly reported in the literature.[8] Most of the diverticula are located near the gallbladder neck, although they may occur anywhere along the body of the gallbladder.[101]

Anomalous junction of cystic duct and hepatic ducts

The cystic duct joins the hepatic duct at various angles. The variations in site and the form of their junction are many (Fig. 57-12).*

Intramural cystic duct

In this anomaly, the length of the inclusion of the cystic duct into the wall of the common bile duct may vary. At cholecystectomy, this segment may be left intact and be demonstrable by tube cholangiography.[223]

Another reported unusual anomaly was a cystic duct with its origin at the fundus of the gallbladder and then extended submucosally to the neck of the gallbladder. It then joined the hepatic duct in the pancreas.[232] The gallbladder neck was only a blind pouch.

Congenital stenosis of cystic duct

This extremely rare anomaly may be complicated by the presence of cholelithiasis.[260]

Ectopic tissue in wall of gallbladder

Heterotopic gastrointestinal mucosa in the wall of a nonfunctioning gallbladder and the common bile duct causing partial obstruction has been reported.[200,264] Aberrant pancreatic tissue arising in the wall of the gallbladder is usually of no clinical significance.[135,254]

---

*See references 36, 117, 124, 228, 267, and 268.

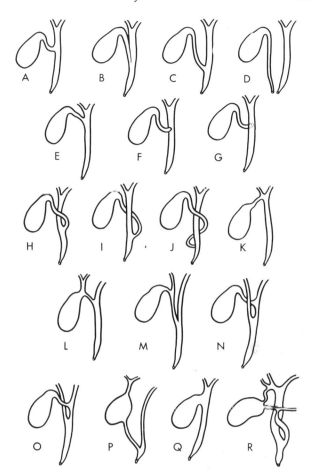

Fig. 57-12. Cyst duct variants: **A,** Normal; **B,** low junction with septum; **C,** long cystic duct with low junction; **D,** direct entrance of cystic duct into duodenum; **E,** high junction of cystic duct at bifurcation; **F,** anterior implantation of cystic duct; **G,** posterior implantation of cystic duct; **H,** anterior spiral course; **I,** posterior spiral course; **J,** double spiral course; **K,** cystic duct junction with right hepatic duct; **L,** termination of the right hepatic duct into the infundibulum; **M,** low junction of hepatic ducts, with cystic duct joining the right hepatic duct; **N,** junction of the cystic and left hepatic ducts with cystic duct passing posterior to right hepatic duct; **O,** junction of the cystic and left hepatic ducts with cystic duct passing anterior to right hepatic duct; **P,** absence of cystic duct with wide opening of gallbladder into the right hepatic duct; **Q,** absent, or wide and short cystic duct; **R,** accessory cystic duct from a right hepatic duct to gallbladder. "Maine" cystic duct crosses the large right hepatic duct (common hepatic duct?), joins a small left hepatic duct, the latter then joins the right hepatic duct at a low point resulting in a short common bile duct. (Redrawn from Hess, W., Surgery of the biliary passages and the pancreas, Princeton, N. J., 1965, D. Van Nostrand Co., Inc.; Shehadi, W. H.: Amer. J. Roentgenol. **76:**7, 1956.)

Liver

Accessory lobes and ectopia

Accessory lobes originating from the undersurface of the liver may compress the neighboring viscera and present diagnostic problems.[64] The lobe may depress the hepatic flexure, compress the greater or lesser curvature of the stomach, displace the distal stomach and proximal duodenum anteriorly, and displace and distort the duodenal loop.[178] The accessory lobes are attached directly to the liver by either hepatic tissue or mesentery.[86] The pedicle of an accessory lobe may become twisted and cause strangulation and gangrene.[57]

Partial ectopia of the liver may occur in the supradiaphragmatic region.[77,129,157,211] An unusual form of this anomaly is that of a liver mass in the right costophrenic sulcus of the pleural cavity. The pedicle, which contains vessels and bile duct, reaches the main substance of the liver by passing through the diaphragm.[110]

An accessory lobe, or partial ectopia of the liver, projecting through a hiatus in the upper abdominal wall, has been reported.[138] The accessory lobe may also be attached to the gallbladder,[18,41] be located in the splenic capsule,[119] or in the suprarenal gland,[57] or it may be herniated through the umbilical cord.[194]

Of help in the diagnosis of some of these anomalies may be isotope studies and diagnostic pneumoperitoneum.[77]

Hypoplasia or aplasia of right lobe

Portal hypertension and gastroesophageal bleeding may prompt the patient to consult a physician. The roentgenologic manifestations of this anomaly are a small hepatic shadow, high position of the hepatic flexure, and esophageal varices. An ectopic gallbladder is demonstrated on cholecystogram and a lack of hepatic venous obstruction by splenoportography.[23] The gallbladder is high and to the right[31,185]; it may even be in contact with the right abdominal wall.

Absence of left lobe

Absence of the left lobe is not as rare as that of the right; it may remain unrecognized for a long time. It may result in an intermittent organoaxial volvulus of the stomach.[24,176,177,178,213]

The clinical symptoms of this anomaly may be abdominal pain, nausea, and vomiting. On roentgenologic examination the right lobe of the liver is more or less vertical, with the gallbladder situated on the medial surface of the liver. A scanogram or arteriogram may satisfactorily show the abnormal anatomy.[224]

Congenital hepatic fibrosis

Proliferation of fibrous tissues and cystic dilatation of the small bile ducts in the portal spaces are the primary pathologic findings in congenital hepatic fibrosis.* Tubular ectasia of the kidneys resembling medullary sponge kidney has been frequently reported.[54,103] Portal hypertension may be the major presenting clinical manifestation of the disease.[103] The relationship of the disease to that of hepatorenal polycystic disease has not been satisfactorily determined.[146,188]

CHOLECYSTITIS AND CHOLELITHIASIS

These diseases occur rarely in infancy and childhood. Wilenius noted cholelithiasis in 0.28% of necropsies of children younger than 15 years.[266] This figure compared with 11.6% in persons older than 20 years, as reported by Lieber,[159] demonstrates the relative rarity of this condition in childhood. Cholecystitis and cholelithiasis appear to be more common in some communities than others.[184,187,245]

In a review of the literature in 1938, Potter found 432 cases of biliary disease reported in children.[204] Ulin and coauthors reviewed the literature from 1938 to 1949 and added another 43 cases.[257] They expressed the belief that of these 475 cases, 326 could be accepted as proved cases of cholecystitis, of which only nineteen were associated with cholelithiasis. Brenner and Stewart have recently reviewed reports of 244 patients.[37] Calculi were present in 170, but only twenty-one had hemolytic anemia. Nearly all of the children with inherited hemolytic anemia had stone without cholecystitis. There is a higher incidence of calculi formation in hereditary spherocytosis as compared with that of thalassemia major and sickle cell disease.[63,180]

Most of the patients with cholecystitis and cholelithiasis are in the age group of 6 to 16 years.[236] These diseases have been reported also, however, in early infancy[9,235] and biliary stones have been seen in the stillborn.[37] Milk of cal-

---

*See references 19, 54, 75, 103, 145, 146, and 248.

cium bile has very rarely been reported in children.[17,171]

The possible causes of cholecystitis in children are the same as in adults.[42,83,195] Acute cholecystitis in children, more often than in adults, is associated with systemic infection.[96,238] Obstructive lesions such as congenital stenosis of the biliary ducts or enlargement of the lymph nodes may contribute to the development of cholecystitis in some cases.[259,260]

Abdominal pain, nausea, vomiting, constipation, intolerance of fatty foods, fever, and jaundice may be the presenting symptoms. Perforation of the biliary tract and pancreatitis may complicate cholelithiasis or cholecystitis.[55]

In children, particularly in girls older than 10 years of age, cholecystography has been recommended as a part of the general workup for indefinite abdominal pain.[236] Cholecystography results in an accurate diagnosis in a high percentage of children with cholelithiasis. The indication for operative cholangiography in cases of cholelithiasis is the same in pediatric patients as in adults.[55]

ACUTE HYDROPS OF GALLBLADDER

The cause of acute and usually transient distention of the gallbladder is not very often known.[51] Inspissated bile and enlargement of lymph nodes have been considered to be two of the etiologic possibilities.[29,163,210] The cause of hydrops of the gallbladder in scarlet fever remains uncertain.[244] In patients with amebic hepatic abscess an "ileus" has been suggested to be the cause of distention of the gallbladder (Fig. 57-13).[222]

Abdominal pain, vomiting, right upper quadrant tenderness, and palpable mass are the major clinical manifestations.[51]

The roentgenologic examination may reveal a mass in the upper abdomen that displaces neighboring viscera and even causes obstruction of the pylorus.[99,107,155]

RUPTURE OF THE BILIARY SYSTEM

In early infancy spontaneous rupture may occur on the anterior aspect of the common duct or at the junction of gallbladder and cystic duct. Less often the perforation occurs in the hepatic duct.[55,235] Clinically, the condition may be acute or subacute.[132] Failure to thrive, vomiting, jaundice, dark urine, acholic stools, and bile

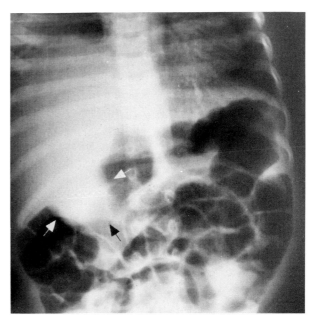

Fig. 57-13. One and one-half-year-old male patient with multiple amebic abscesses of the liver and amebic encephalitis involving the basal ganglia, cerebellum, pons, and medulla. Note the distended gallbladder. At the postmortem study the gallbladder was found to have a thin wall. It contained a clear green, slightly viscous bile. Adhesions seemed to account for the dilatation of the gallbladder in this case.

staining of the abdominal wall may be presenting symptoms. A sudden rupture of a localized bile collection into the peritoneal cavity may cause acute symptoms.

The cause of the spontaneous rupture remains unsettled in most cases. Plugging of the bile, stones, and stenosis of the duct have been reported in some infants.

Roentgenologic examination of the abdomen may reveal generalized ascites. An ill-defined mass may represent the loculated bile collection, most often in the region of the porta hepatica. Displacement of the stomach, duodenum, and colon may be detected on the plain roentgenogram and by studies with a contrast medium. Operative cholangiography usually shows the site of the rupture (Fig. 57-14) and, if present, the obstruction.[71,132,187]

Traumatic and postoperative collection of bile in the abdominal cavity may remain unrecognized for weeks.[13,48] Ascites, single or multiple abdominal masses (Fig. 57-15), pseudocholedo-

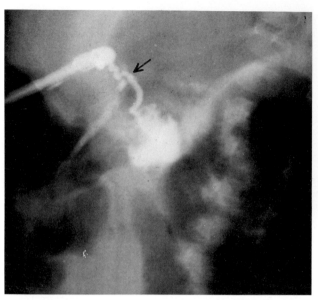

Fig. 57-14. Spontaneous rupture of common bile duct. This 2½-week-old male infant was admitted with a history of vomiting and abdominal distention of about 18 hours' duration. At surgery cloudy bile-stained ascites and a perforation of less than 1 mm. in diameter of the common bile duct was found. Tube cholangiography performed 2 weeks after surgery revealed a persistent leak from perforation site (arrow). A repeat cholangiogram one week later showed that the perforation had sealed. (From G. A. Hyde, Jr.: Pediatrics 35:453, 1965.)

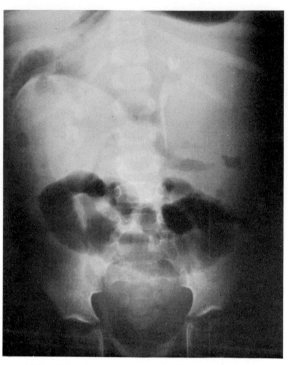

Fig. 57-15. Traumatic rupture of common bile duct. Five-year-old male patient with a history of development of abdominal swelling and jaundice, following trauma to abdomen one month earlier. At surgery loculated thick bile-stained fluid was found. A large collection was in the left abdomen, another in the right lower abdomen, and a third in the subhepatic region. At one point about 1 cm. from the estimated point at which the common duct descended into the duodenum, a small leak of bile was noted. The upper abdominal masses and distortions of gastrointestinal system are seen on this roentgenogram taken during the course of an excretory urography.

chal cyst,[234] displacement of neighboring viscera, pleural effusion, and impaired diaphragmatic motion are the roentgenographic manifestations of the disease. Traumatic rupture may occur in the hepatic duct, common bile duct, or gallbladder.[114] Bile peritonitis without demonstrable site of rupture has also been reported in infancy.[128,179]

TUMORS, CYSTS, AND TUMOR-LIKE LESIONS
Tumors of the biliary tract
Gallbladder tumors

Primary tumors of the gallbladder are extremely rare in childhood. Brown and Brown stated in a report on hamartoma of gallbladder that only three cases of carcinoma of the gallbladder in children were noted in the literature.[39]

Rhabdomyosarcoma of bile ducts

Botryoid sarcoma of bile ducts is a rare tumor, occurring only in late infancy and in childhood. This type of tumor has been reported in the literature in twenty-three instances.[60,118] The tumors cause obstructive jaundice. A mass in the right upper abdomen with displacement of the stomach and duodenum may be found on roentgenologic examination.[237]

At laparotomy, the lesion may be mistaken for a choledochal cyst. Operative cholecystography demonstrates the obstruction and distortion of the bile ducts.[60,187] Biopsy is necessary for the correct diagnosis.[60]

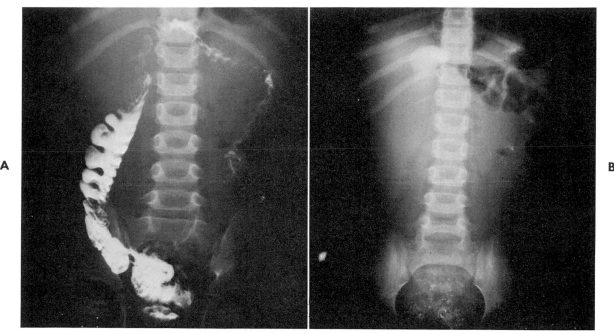

Fig. 57-16. Hepatic cysts. Five-year-old boy with history of intermittent diarrhea of about 4 years and a protuberant abdomen of 2 years' duration. Inferomedial displacement of the hepatic flexure of colon, **A,** and upward displacement and distortion of gallbladder, **B,** by the cystic lesion are demonstrated. The specimen consisted of 6 to 8 cysts separated by liver tissue. The microscopic examination was reported as diffuse lymphangiectasia (hamartoma).

Tumors, cysts, and tumor-like lesions of the liver

Hepatic tumors during infancy and childhood are rare, and those that have been reported were more often in children of less than 2 years of age.[3,53] Congenital cysts, teratoma, focal nodular hyperplasia, adenoma, adrenal rest tumor, mesenchymal hamartoma, cavernous hemangioma, infantile hemangioendothelioma, hepatoma and sarcoma are the primary hepatic tumors reported in infancy and childhood.[53,66,239,246]

Roentgenologic examination of the chest and abdomen in patients with a hepatic mass may reveal an elevation or a localized bulge of the right hemidiaphragm.[43] Calcification in the cyst wall[183] and calcification or ossification in the neoplastic lesions have been reported.[150,170,239]

Masses originating from the right lobe of the liver cause displacement of the stomach to the left and depress the hepatic flexure of the colon. Downward displacement of the right kidney may occur. The transverse colon may be wrapped around the mass or be displaced downward[170,192] The second portion of the duodenum and duodenojejunal junction remain undisplaced. The enlargement of the left lobe of the liver displaces the splenic flexure of the colon, the duodenojejunal flexure, and the left kidney downward. The stomach is displaced to the left. The transverse colon is often displaced anteriorly, wrapped around the mass.[52,170,192] This displacement may be in a superior or inferior direction.

Displacement of the gallbladder (Fig. 57-16) and a concave extrinsic defect may be demonstrable roentgenographically. In rare instances, the involvement of the extrahepatic biliary tract by the invasive neoplastic lesion of the liver result in an obstruction.[65]

Radioisotopic scanning of the liver has been helpful in the recognition, localization, and differentiation of the intrahepatic space-occupying lesions.[1,251]

Angiography is very often of help in the determination of the benign or malignant nature

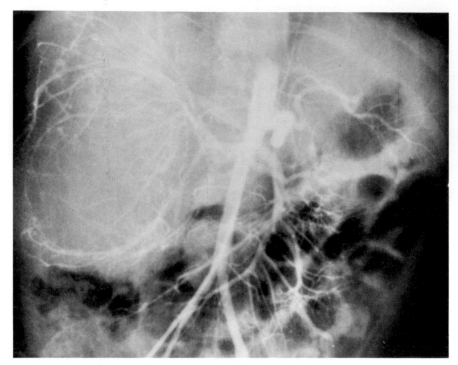

Fig. 57-17. Hepatoblastoma of the right lobe of the liver in an 11-month-old infant, discovered on routine physical examination. Bone survey revealed general osteoporosis. Note on arteriography the displacement and stretching of the branches of the hepatic artery and pathologic circulation within the tumor.

of the mass, the vascular supply to the tumor and normal portion of the liver and the plan for the surgical management (Fig. 57-17).[61,88,172,189,203]

Osteoporosis of mild to severe degree is one of the manifestations of benign and malignant hepatic neoplasms (Fig. 57-18).[172,239,252,253] In severe osteoporosis collapse of vertebrae and fracture from minor trauma may occur.[172,239] This demineralization has been considered as a compensatory reaction to a systemic deficit of protein as a result of hepatic dysfunction.[252,253] Subsidence of osteoporosis after resection of the hepatic tumor has been reported in several patients.[239,252,253]

Hepatic cysts

Cysts and cystic tumors of the liver may originate from the bile ducts, lymphatics, mucous gland, or the ligamentum teres.[97] The exact origin is not always possible to identify since, for example, flattened bile duct epithelium may simulate lymphatic endothelium.[100]

Cysts may be classified into the following types: congenital unilocular or polycystic, cystic hamartoma, traumatic, inflammatory (specific and nonspecific), cystadenoma, cystic teratoma, lymphangioma, biliary angioma, mucous gland, and hydatid.[49,100,121,140] The polycystic is the most common form.[121] Rosenberg estimated that nearly 250 cases of solitary nonparasitic cysts of liver, mostly multilocular, had been reported in the literature.[218]

Subacute or chronic clinical symptoms may be the result of pressure on the stomach, duodenum, colon, or common bile duct. Acute abdominal symptoms may also develop as a result of torsion of the pedicle, intracystic hemorrhage, or rupture of a cyst of the liver into the peritoneal cavity.[122] Rarely, carcinoma may complicate a hepatic cyst.[100]

Roentgenologic studies, such as barium examinations of the digestive tract,[62] cholecystography,[90,220] cholangiography, liver isotope studies, angiography,[44,203] hepatotomography,[165,174] and injection of contrast medium into the cyst, have been used to evaluate hepatic cysts. Distortion and irregularity of a gallbladder shadow from extrinsic pressure by hepatic cyst

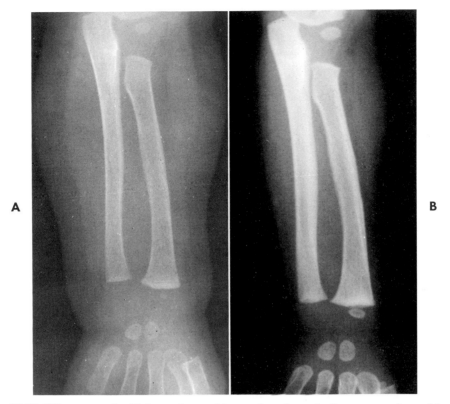

Fig. 57-18. Fifteen-month-old boy who at 14 months of age had an operation with the removal of the left lobe of the liver that was involved with an embryonal carcinoma. At 15 months of age an enlargement of the right lobe of the liver was noted. Bone survey, **A**, shows demineralization. The patient was treated with a course of Actinomycin D. At 21 months of age, the liver is only slightly enlarged and demineralization has subsided, **B**.

may suggest the correct diagnosis.[38,89,220] Feldman, in a review of 374 collected cases of polycystic disease of the liver reported that 51.6% of the patients also had polycystic kidney.[78] In necropsies of 173 cases of polycystic disease of kidneys, Dalgaard found sixty-four with liver cysts.[59] Accompanying cystic disease may involve other organs, including the pancreas, spleen, lungs, and ovaries.[123,175]

Cavernous hemangioma and hemangioendothelioma

Cavernous hemangioma and hemangioendothelioma of the liver have been reported in infants with increasing frequency.[172,193,255] Hemangiomatosis may be diffuse throughout the hepatic parenchyma[2] or may be localized to one lobe.[242] Hemangioendothelioma is generally considered to be a benign vascular tumor that is almost exclusively a lesion of the first 6 months of life.[193,255] The histology of the tumor is that of blood-containing sinusoidal channels lined by proliferating endothelial cells.

The presence of a large liver in conjunction with hemangioma of the skin is almost diagnostic of these tumors.[66] A pulsation may be felt and a blowing sound may be heard over the liver.[2] Thrombocytopenia, intraperitoneal hemorrhage from the tumor, and high output cardiac failure are complicating factors and may cause death.[2,21,242]

Plain film of the abdomen in some cases has shown calcific densities within the liver.[88] High dose excretory urography with total body opacification may suggest the diagnosis.[21] Arteriography demonstrates the enlarged arteries entering the liver and characteristic angiomatous blush within the liver and usually determines

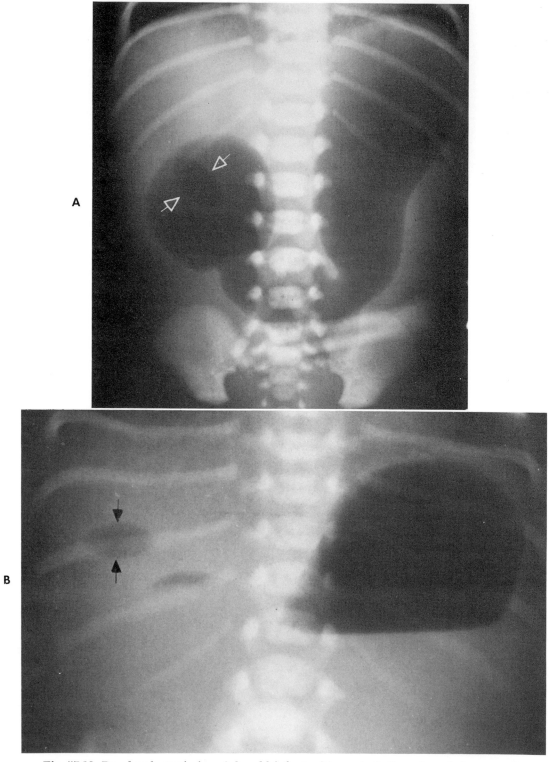

Fig. 57-19. Duodenal atresia in a 2-day-old infant with marked distention of the stomach and duodenum. Note the presence of gas in the gallbladder (arrows).

the nature and the extent of the vascular anomalies.[21,88,255]

Primary hepatic cell carcinoma

Primary hepatic cell carcinoma is the most common malignant tumor of the liver in infancy and childhood.* It occurs more often in males younger than 2 years.[134,229,261] An interesting report is that of primary hepatocarcinoma in three male siblings.[106] In 1962 Alcalde and co-workers noted reports of 139 cases of primary carcinoma of the liver in children 1 day to 16 years of age.[3] Of the 139, 59% were liver cell carcinoma; 12.1% bile duct carcinoma; 7.8% mixed type, and 21.1% unclassified. Only eight of these patients also had cirrhosis of the liver. The rare combined occurrence of cirrhosis and hepatoma in children as compared with adults has also been noted by others.[88,148,206,239] The tumors diagnosed before 3 years of age are usually a mixture of embryonal hepatic parenchymal tissue and neoplastic mesenchymal tissue (hepatoblastoma). Those occurring in children older than 6 years are characterized by hepatic parenchymal elements alone (hepatocarcinoma).[134,150,181]

Abdominal swelling, weight loss, and fever are the major presenting symptoms.[134] Jaundice is uncommon in this disease. One of the rare manifestations of hepatoma is precocious puberty.[130] Hypercholesterolemia, which rarely occurs in adult hepatoma, has been reported in about two thirds of the pediatric patients.[161]

In one fourth to one third of cases of primary carcinoma of the liver in children calcification within the tumor is detectable on the plain film of the abdomen.[170,193,239] Aortography or selective arteriography reveals the displacement and stretching of the branches of the hepatic artery and typical pathologic circulation within the tumor mass (Fig. 57-17).[88,172,189]

MISCELLANEOUS BILIARY MALADIES
Metachromatic leukodystrophy

An accumulation of sulfatides (sulfuric acid esters of cerebrosides), metachromatic substance, in different organs is called metachromatic leukodystrophy.[105] The central nervous system is usually involved, and in the late stage of the disease a decerebrate rigidity is present. Often

---

*See references 3, 134, 148, 161, 170, 181, 193, and 239.

the disease also involves the parenchymal liver cells and macrophages of the mucous folds of the gallbladder.

A progressive inability of the gallbladder to concentrate bile is one of the roentgenographic manifestations of this disease. In advanced cases, air studies may show cerebral atrophy.

Incompetence of the sphincter of Oddi in the newborn

Two cases of incompetence of the sphincter, both associated with duodenal atresia and annular pancreas, have been reported by Frates.[87] Reflux of gas and barium into the biliary tree was found on roentgenographic examination. In some such cases the gas may be trapped in the gallbladder (Fig. 57-19). Gas may also by-pass the site of a complete duodenal obstruction via the hepatopancreatic duct. In these cases the duct has been reported to have a double termination with one orifice on each side of the atresia.[11]

Inspissated bile syndrome

The majority of the cases formerly diagnosed as neonatal obstructive jaundice caused by inspissated bile have been more recently considered to be examples of hepatitis.[217] However, operative cholangiography in exceptional cases has shown the obstructing bile plug.[201,217]

Biliary tract in cystic fibrosis of pancreas

In over one third of children with cystic fibrosis, anatomic and functional abnormalities of the biliary tract have been reported.[221] Small gallbladder and "nonfunctioning" gallbladder have been noted as the roentgenographic manifestations of the disease.[141,187,221]

REFERENCES

1. Ackerman, N. B., and McFee, A. S.: Radioisotope liver scanning in children as a diagnostic aid to the surgeon, Surg. Gynec. Obstet. **117:**41, 1963.
2. Aicardi, J., and Nezelof, C.: L'hemangiomatose multinodulaire du foie du nourrisson: commentaires anatomo-cliniques a propos de quatre observations, Arch. Franc. Pediat. **20:**933, 1963.
3. Alcalde, V. M., Traisman, H. S., and Baffes, T.: Primary carcinoma of the liver in infancy and childhood, Amer. J. Dis. Child. **104:**245, 1962.
4. Alonso-Lej, F., Rever, W. B., Jr., and Pessagno, D. J.: Congenital choledochal cyst with a report of 2, and an analysis of 94, cases, Surg. Gynec. Obstet. **108:**1, 1959.
5. Alpert, L. I., Strauss, L., and Hirschhorn, K.: Ne-

onatal hepatitis and biliary atresia associated with trisomy 17-18 syndrome, New Eng. J. Med. **280**:16, 1969.

6. Anderson, R. D., Cornnell, T. H., and Lowman, R. M.: Inversion of the liver and suprahepatic gallbladder associated with eventration of the diaphragm, Radiology **97**:87, 1970.

7. Anderson, R. E., and Ross, W. T.: Congenital bilobed gallbladder, A.M.A. Arch. Surg. (Chicago) **76**:7, 1958.

8. Arcomano, J. P., and Barnett, J. C.: Diverticulum of the gallbladder; report of three cases and a review of the literature, Amer. J. Digt. Dis. **4**:556, 1959.

9. Arnspiger, L. A., Martin, J. G., Krempin, H. O.: Acute noncalculous cholecystitis in children; report of a case in a seventeen day old infant, Amer. J. Surg. **100**:103, 1960.

10. Arthur, G. W., and Stewart, J. O.: Biliary cysts, Brit. J. Surg. **51**:671, 1964.

11. Astley, R.: Duodenal atresia with gas below the obstruction, Brit. J. Radiol. **42**:351, 1969.

12. Astley, R.: Personal communication, 1970.

13. Babbitt, D. P., Keller, T. A., and Thatcher, D. S.: Radiographic findings in postoperative bile collections, Radiology **84**:471, 1965.

14. Babbitt, D. P.: Congenital choledochal cyst: new etiological concept based on anomalous relationships of the common bile duct and pancreatic duct, Ann. Radiol. **12**:231, 1969.

15. Baker, D. H., and Harris, R. C.: Congenital absence of the intrahepatic bile ducts, Amer. J. Roentgen. **91**:875, 1964.

16. Bartone, N. F., and Grieco, R. V.: Absent gallbladder and cystic duct, Amer. J. Roentgen. **110**:252, 1970.

17. Bass, H. N.: Gallbladder disease in childhood: report of four cases including one with "milk of calcium bile," Clin. Pediat. **9**:229, 1970.

18. Bassis, M. L., and Izenstark, J. L.: Ectopic liver; its occurrence in gall bladder, A.M.A. Arch Surg. (Chicago) **73**:204, 1956.

19. Benhamon, J. P., Antoine, B., Debray, C., Nezelof, C., Roux, M., Watchi, J. M., and Pequignot, H.: La fibrose hepatique congenitale (Confrontations de l'Hopital Necker), Presse Med. **77**:167, 1969.

20. Bennet, J., Fortier-Beaulieu, M., and Nahum, H.: Dilatation anevrysmale des voies bilaires intrahepatiques de l'enfant, Ann. Radiol. **13**:321, 1970.

21. Berdon, W. E., and Baker, D. H.: Giant hepatic hemangioma with cardiac failure in the newborn infant: value of high-dosage intra-venous urography and umbilical angiography, Radiology **92**:1523, 1969.

22. Bernheim, M., Marion, P., Roux, J. A., Lanternier, J., and Bethenod, M.: Les kystes congenitaux du choledoque chez le nourrisson, Pediatrie **42** (n.s.8): 677, 1953.

23. Bertrand, L., Betoulieres, P., and Jaumes, F.: Diagnostic radiologique de l'hypoplasie du lobe droit du foie, J. Radiol. Electr. **45**:171, 1964.

24. Bertrand, L., Marchal, G., and Jaumes, F.: Diag-

nostic radiologique de l'absence du lobe gauche du foie, J. Radiol. Electr. **45**:175, 1964.

25. Bétoulieres, P., Balmès, J., Loustanu, J. A., and Balmès, J. L.: La cholécystographie chez le nourrisson et l'enfant en bas age, J. Radiol. Electr. **45**:364, 1964.

26. Blegen, H. M., and Boyer, E. L.: Perforation of choledochus cyst with biliary peritonitis; report of case submitted to 3-stage operation, Lancet **66**:177, 1946.

27. Bleich, A. R., Hamblin, D. O., and Martin, D.: Left-upper quadrant gallbladder, J.A.M.A. **147**:849, 1951.

28. Blocker, T. G., Jr., Williams, H., and Williams, J. E.: Traumatic rupture of congenital cyst of choledochus, Arch. Surg. (Chicago) **34**:695, 1937.

29. Bobek, D. W.: Hydrops of the gallbladder in a three-year old girl, J. Okla, Med. Ass. **55**:125, 1962.

30. Bogle, J. H.: Gangrene of gallbladder due to torsion in 9-year-old child, Amer. J. Dis. Child. **89**:484, 1955.

31. Bohan, E. M.: Aplasia of right lived lobe with cholelithiasis, Delaware Med. J. **28**:291, 1956.

32. Boni, R.: Cistifiellea tripla e bile calcarea, Radiol. Med. (Torino) **44**:833, 1958.

33. Boyden, E. A.: Accessory gallbladder; embryological and comparative study of aberrant biliary vesicles occurring in man and domestic mammals, Amer. J. Anat. **38**:177, 1926.

34. Boyden, E. A.: The problem of double ductus choledochus (an interpretation of accessory bile duct found attached to pars superior of duodenum), Anat. Rec. **55**:71, 1932.

35. Boyden, E. A.: "Phrygian cap" in cholecystography; a congenital anomaly of ballbladder, Amer. J. Roentgen. **33**:589, 1935.

36. Braasch, J. W.: Congenital anomalies of the gallbladder and bile ducts, Surg. Clin. N. Amer. **38**:627, 1958.

37. Brenner, R. W., and Stewart, C. F.: Cholecystitis in children, Rev. Surg. **21**:327, 1964.

38. Bret, P., and Duquesnel, C.: Polykystose hépatorenale, Ann. Radiol. **7**:665, 1964.

39. Brown, R. C., and Brown, R. J.: Hamartoma of the gallbladder in a child, J. Pediat. **52**:319, 1958.

40. Browne, H. J.: Choledochal (bile duct) cysts, J. Irish Med. Ass. **37**:208, 1955.

41. Brownlee, H. F.: Accessory lobe of liver attached only to gallbladder, J.A.M.A. **86**:193, 1926.

42. Brunet, G., Jacques, G., and Tremblay, R.: La cholecystite et la cholélithiase chez l'enfant, Canad. Med. Ass. J. **91**:1354, 1964.

43. Brust, R. W., Jr., and Conlon, P. C.: Roentgenologic manifestations of primary hepatoma with particular reference to some unusual cholecystographic findings, Amer. J. Roentgen. **87**:777, 1962.

44. Buchet, R., and Leblanc, J.: Maladie polykystique du foie et des reins (a propos de deux cas): aspect radiologique du problème, J. Radiol. Electr. **43**:12, 1962.

45. Bullard, R. W., Jr.: Subcutaneous or extraperi-

toneal gallbladder (a report of an unusual case), J.A.M.A. **129**:949, 1945.

46. Burke, J.: An anomaly in the position of the gallbladder, J.A.M.A. **177**:508, 1961.

47. Carnevali, J. F., and Kunath, C. A.: Congenital absence of the gallbladder, Arch. Surg. (Chicago) **78**: 440, 1959.

48. Caro, A. M., and Losa, J.M.O.: Complete avulsion of the common bile duct as a result of blunt abdominal trauma—case report of a child, J. Pediat. Surg. **5**:60, 1970.

49. Caroli, J., and Corcos, V.: La dilatation congenitale des voies biliaires intrahepatiques, Rev. Medicochir, Mal Foie, **39**:1, 1964.

50. Case records of the Massachusetts General Hospital, case 45211 New Eng. J. Med. **260**:1080, 1959.

51. Chamberlain, J. W., and Hight, D. W.: Acute hydrops of the gallbladder in childhood, Surgery **68**:899, 1970.

52. Clatworthy, H. W., Jr., Boles, E. T., Jr., and Newton, W. A.: Primary tumours of the liver in infants and children, Arch. Dis. Child. **35**:22, 1960.

53. Clatworthy, H. W., Jr., Boles, E. T., Jr., and Kottmeier, P. K.: Liver tumors in infancy and childhood, Ann. Surg. **154**:475, 1961.

54. Clermont, R. J., Maillard, J.-N., Benhamon, J.-P., and Fauvert, R.: Fibrose hepatique congenitale. Canad. Med. Ass. J. **97**:1272, 1967.

55. Colver, H. D.: Perforation of the biliary tract due to gallstones in infancy; an established clinical entity, Ann. Surg. **160**:226, 1964.

56. Cooper, W. H., and Martin, J. F.: Hemangioma of the liver with thrombocytopenia, Amer. J. Roentgen. **88**:751, 1962.

57. Cullen, T. S.: Accessory lobes of liver; accessory hepatic lobe springing from surface of gallbladder, Arch. Surg. (Chicago) **11**:718, 1925.

58. Culver, G. J., and Ehrlich, M.: Choledochal cyst; report of a case with contrast visualization, Amer. J. Roentgen. **86**:934, 1961.

59. Dalgaard, O. Z.: Bilateral polycystic disease of the kidneys; a follow-up of two-hundred and eighty-four patients and their families, Acta Med. Scand. **158** (Suppl.):1, 1957.

60. Davis, G. L., Kissane, J., and Ishak, K. G.: Embryonal rhabdomyosarcoma (sarcoma botroyoides of the biliary tree: report of five cases and a review of the literature, Cancer **24**:333, 1969.

61. Debrun, G., and Gasquet, C.: Explorations vasculaires des tumeurs abdominales de l'enfant, Les monographies des Ann. de Radiol., Expansion Scientifique Francaise, 1970.

62. Desser, P. L., and Smith, S.: Nonparasitic liver cysts in children, J. Pediat. **49**:297, 1956.

63. Dewey, K. W., Grossman, H., and Canale, V. C.: Cholelithiasis in the thalassemia major, Radiology **96**:385, 1970.

64. Dick, J.: Riedel's lobe and related partial hepatic enlargements, Guy's Hosp. Rep. **100**:270, 1951.

65. Dickinson, S. J., and Santulli, T. V.: Obstruction of common bile ducts by hepatoma, Surgery **52**: 800, 1962.

66. Edmondson, H. A.: Differential diagnosis of tumors and tumorlike lesions of liver in infancy and childhood, Amer. J. Dis. Child. **91**:168, 1956.

67. Eisen, H. B., Poller, S., Maxwell, J. W., Jr., and Jackson, F. C.: Hepatodochal diverticulum: a difficult roentgen diagnosis, Radiology **81**:276, 1963.

68. Engle, J., and Salmon, P. A.: Multiple choledochal cysts: report of a case, Arch. Surg. (Chicago) **88**: 345, 1964.

69. Enjoji, M., Watanabe, H., and Nakamura, Y.: A case report: congenital biliotracheal fistula with trifurcation of bronchi, Ann. Paediat. (Basel) **200**: 321, 1963.

70. Ericsson, N. O., and Rudhe, U.: Cholangiography in infancy as an aid in the operative diagnosis of the biliary obstruction, Acta Chir. Scand. **107**:275, 1954.

71. Ericsson, N. O., and Rudhe, U.: Spontaneous perforation of the bile ducts in infants: presentation of a case and review of the literature, Acta Chir. Scand. **118**:439, 1960.

72. Esguerra-Gomez, G., and Riveros-Gamboa, E.: A case of multidiverticular cystic dilatation of the common and hepatic ducts, Amer. J. Roentgen. **94**:177, 1965.

73. Etter, L. E.: Left-sided gallbladder; necessity for films of entire abdomen in cholecystography, Amer. J. Roentgen. **70**:987, 1953.

74. Everett, C., and Macumber, H. E.: Anomalous distribution of extrahepatic biliary ducts; report of case, Ann. Surg. **115**:472, 1942.

75. Farmer, R. G., Hermann, R. E., and Sullivan, B. H.: Congenital hepatic fibrosis of Riedel's lobe causing portal hypertension, Cleveland Clin. Quart. **36**:143, 1969.

76. Farriaux, J.-P., Hollinghausen-Colle, J., Saint-Aubert, P., Dupont, A., and Fontaine, C.: L'agenesie des voies biliares intra-hepatiques: a propos d'une observation, Ann. Pediat. **13**:706, 1966.

77. Feist, J. H., and Lasser, E. C.: Identification of uncommon liner lobulations, J.A.M.A. **169**:1859, 1959.

78. Feldman, M.: Polycystic disease of the liver, Amer. J. Gastroent. **29**:83, 1958.

79. Ferris, D. O., and Glazer, I. M.: Congenital absence of gallbladder: four surgical cases, Arch. Surg. (Chicago) **91**:359, 1965.

80. Fisher, M. M., Chen, S., and Dekker, A.: Congenital diaphragm of the common hepatic duct, Gastroenterology **54**:605, 1968.

81. Flannery, M. G., and Caster, M. P.: Collective reviews; congenital abnormalities of gallbladder; 101 cases, Surg. Gynec. Obstet. **103**:439, 1956.

82. Fonkalsrud, E. W., and Boles, E. T., Jr.: Choledochal cysts in infancy and childhood, Surg. Gynec. Obstet. **121**:733, 1965.

83. Forshall, I., and Rickham, P. P.: Cholecystitis and cholelithiasis in childhood, Brit. J. Surg. **42**:161, 1954.

84. Foster, J. H., and Wayson, E. E.: Surgical significance of aberrant bile ducts, Amer. J. Surg. **104**:14, 1962.

85. Franke, W.: Beitrag zur röntgenologischen Darstellung einer seltenen Anomalie der Gallenwege und zum Problem der postoperativen Cholangitis, Chirurg 32:14, 1961.
86. Fraser, C. G.: Accessory lobes of liver, Ann. Surg. 135:127, 1952.
87. Frates, R. E.: Incompetence of the sphincter of Oddi in the newborn, Radiology 85:875, 1965.
88. Fredens, M.: Angiography in primary hepatic tumours in children, Acta Radiol. [Diagn.] 8:193, 1969.
89. Gambill, E. E., and Hodgson, J. R.: Polycystic disease of the liver, with unusual cholecystographic manifestations: report of a case, Gastroenterology 38:1003, 1960.
90. Geist, D. C.: Solitary nonparasitic cyst of liver; review of literature and report of 2 patients, Arch. Surg. (Chicago) 71:867, 1955.
91. Geraci, C. L.: Congenital absence of the gallbladder; diagnosis by operative cholangiography, Arch. Surg. (Chicago) 78:437, 1959.
92. Ghadimi, H., and Sass-Kortsak, A.: Evaluation of radioactive rose-bengal test for the differential diagnosis of obstructive jaundice in infants, New Eng. J. Med. 265:351, 1961.
93. Gilday, D. L., Brown, R., and Macpherson, R. I.: Choledochal cyst—a case diagnosed by radiographic and ultrasonic collaboration, J. Canad. Ass. Radiol. 20:25, 1969.
94. Gillis, D. A., and Sergeant, C. K.: Prolonged biliary obstruction and massive gastrointestinal bleeding secondary to choledochal cyst, Surgery 52:391, 1962.
95. Glay, A.: Double gallbladder: report of one asymptomatic case demonstrated roentgenologically, J. Canad. Ass. Radiol. 10:1, 1959.
96. Glenn, F., and Hill, M. R., Jr.: Primary gallbladder disease in children, Ann. Surg. 139:302, 1954.
97. Gondring, W. H.: Solitary cyst of the falciform ligament of the liver: report of a case and review of the literature, Amer. J. Surg. 109:526, 1965.
98. Grayer, S. P.: Congenital stenosis of the common duct as a cause of abdominal pain and emesis, Surgery 66:398, 1969.
99. Greenstein, N. M., and Wesson, H.: Hydrops of gallbladder in 14-month-old infant, Amer. J. Dis. Child. 87:208, 1954.
100. Grime, R. T., Moore, T., Nicholson, A., and Whitehead, R.: Cystic hamartomas and polycystic disease of the liver, Brit. J. Surg. 47:307, 1959.
101. Gross, R. E.: Congenital anomalies of the gallbladder; review of 148 cases with report of a double gallbladder, Arch. Surg. (Chicago) 32:131, 1936.
102. Gross, R. E.: Surgery of infancy and childhood: its principles and techniques, Philadelphia, 1953, W. B. Saunders Co.
103. Grossman, H., and Seed, W.: Congenital hepatic fibrosis, bile duct dilatation and renal lesion resembling medullary sponge kidney (congenital "cystic" disease of the liver and kidneys), Radiology 87:46, 1966.
104. Guyer, P. B., and McLoughlin, M.: Congenital double gallbladder: a review and report of two cases, Brit. J. Radiol. 40:214, 1967.
105. Hagberg, B., Sourander, P., and Svennerholm, L.: Clinical and laboratory diagnosis of metachromatic leukodystrophy, Cereb. Palsy Bull. 3:438, 1961.
106. Hagstrom, R. M., and Baker, T. D.: Primary hepatocarcinoma in three male siblings, Cancer 22:142, 1968.
107. Haith, E. E., Kepes, J. J., and Holder, T. M.: Inflammatory pseudotumor involving the common bile duct of a six-year-old boy: successful pancreatico-duodenectomy, Surgery 56:436, 1964.
108. Han, S. Y., Collins, L. C., and Wright, R. M.: Choledochal cyst: report of five cases, Clin. Radiol. 20:332, 1969.
109. Hankamp, L. J.: Congenital choledochal cyst; demonstration by oral cholecytography, Amer. J. Dis. Child. 97:97, 1959.
110. Hansbrough, E. T., and Lipin, R. J.: Intrathoracic accessory lobe of the liver, Ann. Surg. 145:564, 1957.
111. Hardy, J. D.: Congential bile duct stenosis. Intrahepatic cholangiocholecystojejunostomy (Roux Y) with removal of intrahepatic stones, J. Pediat. 59:265, 1961.
112. Harris, J. H., Jr., O'Hara, A. E., and Koop, C. E.: Operative cholangiography in the diagnosis of prolonged jaundice in infancy, Radiology 71:806, 1958.
113. Harris, R. C., and Caffey, J.: Cholecystography in infants, J.A.M.A. 153:1333, 1953.
114. Hartman, S. W., and Greaney, E. M., Jr.: Traumatic injuries to the biliary system in children, Amer. J. Surg. 108:150, 1964.
115. Hasse, W.: Intrahepatic vascular and bile-duct system as related to operative treatment of bile-duct atresia, Arch. Dis. Child. 40:162, 1965.
116. Hayes, M. A.: (Medical News Section) J.A.M.A. 197:30, 1966.
117. Hayes, M. A., Goldenberg, I. S., and Bishop, C. C.: Developmental basis for bile duct anomalies, Surg. Gynec. Obstet. 107:447, 1958.
118. Hays, D. M., and Snyder, W. H., Jr.: Botryoid sarcoma (rhabdomyosarcoma) of the bile ducts, Amer. J. Dis. Child. 110:595, 1965.
119. Heid, G. J., Jr., and von Haam, E.: Hepatic heterotopy in the splenic capsule, Arch. Path. (Chicago) 46:377, 1948.
120. Hendren, W. H., Greep, J. M., and Patton, A. S.: Pancreatitis in childhood: experience with 15 cases, Arch. Dis. Child. 40:32, 1965.
121. Henson, S. W., Jr., Gray, H. K., and Dockerty, M. B.: Benign tumors of the liver; adenomas, Surg. Gynec. Obstet. 103:23, 1956.
122. Henson, S. W., Jr., Gray, H. K., and Dockerty, M. B.: Benign tumors of the liver; solitary cysts, Surg. Gynec. Obstet. 103:607, 1956.
123. Henson, S. W., Jr., Gray, H. K., and Dockerty, M. B.: Benign tumors of the liver; polycystic disease of surgical significance, Surg. Gynec. Obstet. 104:63, 1957.

124. Hess, W.: Surgery of the biliary passages and the pancreas, Princeton, N. J., 1965, D. Van Nostrand Co., Inc.

125. Hodes, P. J.: Diagnostic studies in affections of gallbladder and bile ducts. In Bockus, H. L., editor: Gastroenterology, vol. 3, ed. 2, Philadelphia, 1965, W. B. Saunders Co.

126. Hoffer, P. B., and Petasnick, J. P.: Choledochal cysts demonstrated by oral cholecystography, Radiology **93**:871, 1969.

127. Holder, T. M.: Atresia of the extrahepatic bile duct, Amer. J. Surg. **107**:458, 1964.

128. Hoofer, W. D.: Idiopathic infantile bile peritonitis, J. Pediat. **67**:1202, 1965.

129. Hudson, T. R., and Brown, H. N.: Ectopic (supradiaphragmatic) liver, J. Thorac. Cardiovasc. Surg. **43**:552, 1962.

130. Hung, W., Blizzard, R. M., Migeon, C. J., Camacho, A. M., and Nyhan, W. L.: Precocious puberty in a boy with hepatoma and circulating gonadotropin, J. Pediat. **63**:895, 1963.

131. Hunter, F. M., Akdamar, K., Sparks, R. D., Reed, R. J., and Brown, C. L., Jr.: Congenital dilatation of the intrahepatic bile ducts, Amer. J. Med. **40**:188, 1966.

132. Hyde, G. A., Jr.: Spontaneous perforation of bile ducts in early infancy, Pediatrics **35**:453, 1965.

133. Ingegno, A. P., and D'Albora, J. B.: Double gallbladder; roentgenographic demonstration of case of "Y" type; classification of accessory gallbladder, Amer. J. Roentgen. **61**:671, 1949.

134. Ishak, K., and Glunz, P. R.: Hepatoblastoma and hepatocarcinoma in infancy and childhood: report of 47 cases, Cancer **20**:396, 1967.

135. Jacobson, A. S.: Accessory pancreas in wall of gallbladder, Arch. Path. (Chicago) **30**:908, 1940.

136. Jamis-Muvdi, A.: Giant cyst of the common bile duct: preoperative visualization by transhepatic cholangiography in 2 cases, Amer. J. Dig. Dis. **5**:935, 1960.

137. Jesseman, W. C., and Treasure, R. I.: Choledochal cyst with emphasis on preoperative diagnosis, Arch. Surg. (Chicago) **83**:689, 1961.

138. Johnstone, G.: Accessory lobe of liver presenting through a congenital deficiency of anterior abdominal wall, Arch. Dis. Child. **40**:541, 1965.

139. Jones, G. M., and Caylor, H. D.: Anomalous termination of the common duct, Amer. J. Surg. **93**:122, 1957.

140. Jones, J. F.: Removal of retention cyst from liver, Ann. Surg. **77**:68, 1923.

141. Jones, M., Sakai, H., and Rogerson, A.: Intravenous cholangiography in children with fibrocystic disease of the pancreas, J. Pediat. **59**:172, 1958.

142. Kaiser, E.: Congenital and acquired changes in gallbladder form, Amer. J. Dig. Dis. **6**:938, 1961.

143. Kazar, G.: Kettos epeholyag es choledochyscysta, Magyar Sebeszet **3**:298, 1950; abstract in Excerpta Med. (Sect. IX, Surgery) **5**:733, 1951.

144. Keith, L. M., Jr., Rini, J. M., and Martin, L. H.: Congenital cystic dilatation of the common duct (choledochal cyst); report of two cases, Arch. Surg. (Chicago) **75**:143, 1957.

145. Kerr, D. N., Harrison, C. V., Sherlock, S., and Walker, R. M.: Congenital hepatic fibrosis, Quart. J. Med. **30**:91, 1961.

146. Kerr, D. N., Warrick, C. K., and Hart-Mercer, J.: A lesion resembling medullary sponge kidney in patients with congenital hepatic fibrosis, Clin. Radiol. **13**:85, 1962.

147. Kjellberg, S. R.: Water soluble contrast medium for precise roentgenological diagnosis of cysts of common bile duct, Acta Radiol. (Stockholm) **29**:307, 1948.

148. Kkeda, K., Oogami, H., Hiyama, T., and Tsuchiya, S.: Clinical observation of hepatoma of infancy in Japan, Operation **19**:829, 1965.

149. Knetsch, A.: Beitrag zu den sog. Septengallenblasen, Fortschr. Geb. Rontgenstr. **77**:587, 1952.

150. Koch, K., and Bradford, J.: Primary carcinoma of liver in infancy, Amer. J. Dis. Child. **98**:86, 1959.

151. Krauss, A. N.: Familial extrahepatic biliary atresia, J. Pediat. **65**:933, 1964.

152. Krovetz, L. J.: Intrahepatic biliary atresia, Lancet **79**:228, 1959.

153. Large, A. M.: Left-sided gallbladder and liver without situs inversus, Arch. Surg. (Chicago) **87**:982, 1963.

154. Lee, C. M., Jr.: Duplication of the cystic and common hepatic ducts, lined with gastric mucosa: a rare congenital anomaly, New Eng. J. Med. **256**:927, 1957.

155. Lee, C. M., Jr., and Englender, G. S.: Massive hydrops of gallbladder producing pyloric obstruction in 7 year old boy, Pediatrics **11**:449, 1953.

156. Leeming, B. W. A.: Metastatic hepatoblastoma present at birth, Clin. Radiol. **15**:279, 1964.

157. Le Roux, B. T.: Heterotopic intrathoracic liver, Thorax **16**:68, 1961.

158. Levin, E. J.: Congenital biliary atresia with emphasis on skeletal abnormalities, Radiology **67**:714, 1956.

159. Lieber, M. M.: Incidence of gallstones and their correlation with other diseases, Ann. Surg. **135**:394, 1952.

160. Liebner, E. J.: Roentgenographic study of congenital choledochal cysts; pre- and postoperative analysis of five cases, Amer. J. Roentgen. **80**:950, 1958.

161. Lin, T.-Y., Chen, C.-C., and Liu, W.-P.: Primary carcinoma of the liver in infancy and childhood: report of 21 cases, with resection in 6 cases, Surgery **60**:1275, 1966.

162. Lindner, H. H., and Green, R. B.: Embryology and surgical anatomy of the extrahepatic biliary tract, Surg. Clin. N. Amer. **44**:1273, 1964.

163. Longino, L. A., and Martin, L. W.: Abdominal masses in the newborn infant, Pediatrics **21**:596, 1958.

164. Longmire, W. P., Jr.: Congenital biliary hypoplasia, Ann. Surg. **159**:335, 1964.

165. Lowman, R. M., and Haber, S.: Hepatonephro-

tomography: its value in the diagnosis of polycystic kidney and liver disease, Angiology 12:583, 1961.

166. MacKenzie, W. C., Lang, A., Friedman, M. H., and Calder, J.: Congenital atresia of the second portion of the duodenum with associated obstruction of the biliary tract, Surg. Gynec. Obstet. 110: 755, 1960.

167. MacMahon, H. E., and Thannhauser, S. J.: Congenital dysplasia of the intralobular bile duct with extensive skin xanthoma: congenital acholangic biliary cirrhosis, Gastroenterology 21:488, 1952.

168. Macpherson, C. R.: Congenital cystic dilatation of common bile duct associated with accessory hepatic ducts, S. Afr. Med. J. 25:965, 1951.

169. Mallet-Guy, P., Rebouillat, J., and Rosowski, F.: La dilatation congenitale du choledoque: a propos de 6 cas operes en huit ans, sous controle manometrique et radiographique, Lyon Chir. 57:15, 1961.

170. Margulis, A. R., Nice, C. M., Jr., and Rigler, L. G.: Roentgen findings in primary hepatoma in infants and children: analysis of eleven cases, Radiology 66:809, 1956.

171. Marquis, J. R., and Densler, J.: The disappearing limy bile syndrome, Radiology 94:311, 1970.

172. McDonald, P.: Hepatic tumor in childhood, Clin. Radiol. 18:74, 1967.

173. McIlrath, D. C., ReMine, W. H., and Baggenstoss, A. H.: Congenital absence of the gallbladder and cystic duct: report of ten cases found at necropsy, J.A.M.A. 180:782, 1962.

174. Melnick, G. S.: Roentgenographic demonstration of a giant congenital cyst of the liver, Amer. J. Gastroent. 40:154, 1963.

175. Melnick, P. J.: Polycystic Liver; analysis of 70 cases, Arch. Path. (Chicago) 59:162, 1955.

176. Merrill, G. G.: Complete absence of left lobe of liver. Arch. Path. (Chicago) 42:232, 1946.

177. Messing, A., and Ashley-Montagu, M. F.: A note on case of complete absence of left lobe of liver in man, Anat. Rec. 53:169, 1932.

178. Meyers, H. I., and Jacobson, G.: Displacements of stomach and duodenum by anomalous lobes of the liver, Amer. J. Roentgen. 79:789, 1958.

179. Meynadier, A., Guillaud, R., Barret, C., Pous, J.-G., and Adrey, J.: Peritonites biliaires neo-natales: formes calcifiantes et form necrosantes, Ann. Pediat. 17:504, 1970.

180. Mintz, A. A., Gaylord, C., and Adams, E. D.: Cholelithiasis in sickle cell anemia, J. Pediat. 47: 171, 1955.

181. Misugi, K., Okajima, H., Misugi, N., and Newton, W. A., Jr.: Classification of primary malignant tumors of liver in infancy and childhood, Cancer 20:1760, 1967.

182. Monroe, S. E., and Ragan, F. J.: Congenital absence of gallbladder, California Med. 85:422, 1956.

183. Montgomery, A. H.: Solitary nonparasitic cysts of liver in children, Arch. Surg. (Chicago) 41:422, 1940.

184. Morales, L., Taboada, E., Toledo, L., and Radri-

gan, W.: Cholecystitis and cholelithiasis in children, J. Pediat. Surg. 2:565, 1967.

185. Morgenstern, L., and Mazur, M.: Hypoplasia of the right hepatic lobe, Amer. J. Surg. 98:628, 1959.

186. Moseley, J. E.: Radiographic demonstration of choledochal cyst by oral cholecystography, Radiology 68:849, 1957.

187. Nahum, H., Poree, C., and Sauvegrain, J.: The study of the gallbladder and biliary ducts, Progr. Pediat. Radiol., 2:65, 1969.

188. Nathan, M., and Batsakis, J. G.: Congenital hepatic fibrosis, Surg. Gynec. Obstet. 128:1033, 1969.

189. Nebesar, R. A., Pollard, J. J., and Stone, D. L.: Angiographic diagnosis of malignant disease of the liver, Radiology 86:284, 1966.

190. Nelson, P. A., Schmitz, R. L., and Perutsea, S.: Anomalous position of gallbladder within falciform ligament, Arch. Surg. (Chicago) 66:679, 1953.

191. Neuhauser, E. B. D., Elkin, M., and Landing, B. H.: Congenital direct communication between biliary system and respiratory tract, Amer. J. Dis. Child. 83:654, 1952.

192. Nice, C. M., Jr., Margulis, A. R., and Rigler, L.: Roentgen diagnosis of abdominal tumors in childhood, Springfield, Ill. 1957, Charles C Thomas, Publisher.

193. Nikaidoh, H., Boggs, J., and Swenson, O.: Liver tumors in infants and children: clinical and pathological analysis of 22 cases, Arch. Surg. 101:245, 1970.

194. Nora, E., and Carr, C. E.: Umbilical accessory liver, Amer. J. Obstet. Gynec. 52:330, 1946.

195. Oates, G. D.: Perforated empyema of the gallbladder in an infant, Brit. J. Surg. 48:686, 1961.

196. Okuyama, K.: Primary liver cell carcinoma associated with biliary cirrhosis due to congenital bile duct atresia; first report of a case, J. Pediat. 67:89, 1965.

197. Pellerin, D., Aicardi, J., and Nezelof, C.: Les icterese de type retentionnels du nourrisson (104 observations receuillies a la Clinique Chirurgicale des Enfants-Malades, Ann. Pediat. 13:684, 1966.

198. Perelman, H.: Cystic duct reduplication, J.A.M.A. 175:710, 1961.

199. Perrin, R. W.: Communicating enterogenous cyst of duodenum receiving the termination of the common bile duct demonstrated by intravenous cholangiography, Radiology 93:675, 1969.

200. Pessel, J. F., Beairsto, E. B., Wise, J. S., Greeley, J. P., and Rathmell, T. K.: Gastro-intestinal mucosa in wall of human gallbladder, Gastroenterology, 15:533, 1950.

201. Pickett, L. K.: Obstructive jaundice. In Mustard, W. T., Ravitch, M. M., Snyder, W. H., Jr., Welch, K. J., and Benson, C. D.: Pediatric Surgery, ed. 2, Chicago, 1969, Year Book Medical Publishers, pp. 732-740.

202. Pines, B., and Grayzel, D. M.: Congenital absence of the gallbladder and cystic duct, Arch. Surg. (Chicago) 77:171, 1958.

203. Pollard, J. J., Nebesar, R. A., and Mattoso, L. F.:

Angiographic diagnosis of benign diseases of the liver, Radiology **86**:276, 1965.

204. Potter, A. H.: Biliary disease in young subjects, Surg. Gynec. Obstet. **66**:604, 1938.

205. Potter, E. L.: Pathology of the fetus and infant, Chicago, 1961, Year Book Medical Publishers, p. 413.

206. Potter, J. F.: Cirrhosis and hepatoma in a child, Amer. J. Surg. **111**:764, 1966.

207. Prochiantz, A.: Les icteres par retention de la periode neonatale et du nourrisson (essai de synthese), Ann. Chir. Infant. **3**:159, 1962.

208. Rabinovitch, J., Rabinovitch, P., Rosenblatt, P., and Pines, G.: Congenital anomalies of the gallbladder, Ann. Surg. **148**:161, 1958.

209. Rachlin, S. A.: Congenital anomalies of gallbladder and ducts, Milit. Surg. **109**:20, 1951.

210. Rankin, W.: Acute distention of gallbladder in children, Arch. Dis. Child. **30**:60, 1955.

211. Ravitch, M., and Handelsman, J. C.: Defects in right diaphragm of infants and children with herniation of liver, Arch. Surg. (Chicago) **64**:794, 1952.

212. Ravitch, M. M., and Snyder, G. B.: Congenital cystic dilatation of the common bile duct; with special reference to radiographic studies, Surgery **44**:752, 1958.

213. Reddy, D. J.: Complete absence of left lobe of liver, J. Indian Med. Ass. **23**:405, 1954.

214. Regen, J. F., and Poindexter, A.: Suprahepatic position of the gallbladder; a report of an unusual case, Arch. Surg. (Chicago) **90**:175, 1965.

215. Reichelderfer, T. E., and Van Hartesveldt, J.: Intravenous cholecystography with cholografin in infants, Amer. J. Dis. Child. **89**:591, 1955.

216. Rheinlander, H. F., and Bowens, O. L., Jr.: Congenital absence of the gall bladder with cystic dilatation of the common bile duct, New Eng. J. Med. **256**:557, 1957.

217. Rickham, P. P., and Lee, E. Y. C.: Neonatal jaundice: surgical aspects, Clin. Pediat. **3**:197, 1964.

218. Rosenberg, G. V.: Solitary non-parasitic cysts of liver, Amer. J. Surg. **91**:441, 1956.

219. Ross, R. J., and Sachs, M. D.: Triplication of the gallbladder, Amer. J. Roentgen. **104**:656, 1968.

220. Sandy, R. E.: Cholecystography in presence of polycystic disease of liver; report of case and review of literature, Radiology **85**:895, 1965.

221. Sauvegrain, J., and Feigelson, J.: La cholecystographie dans la mucoviscidose, Ann. Radiol. **13**:311, 1970.

222. Schmidt, A. G.: Plain film roentgen diagnosis of amebic hepatic abscess, Amer. J. Roentgen. **107**:47, 1969.

223. Schwarz, E.: The intramural cystic duct remnant, Amer. J. Roentgen. **86**:930, 1961.

224. Semat, P., and Chapiro, E.: Agenesie du lobe gauche du foie et arteriographie selective, J. Radiol. Electr. **51**:507, 1970.

225. Serfas, L. S., and Lyter, C. S.: Choledochal cyst, with a report of an intraduodenal choledochal cyst, Amer. J. Surg. **93**:979, 1957.

226. Shallow, T. A., Eger, S. A., and Wagner, F. B., Jr.: Congenital cystic dilatation of common bile duct; case report and review of literature, Ann. Surg. **117**:355, 1943.

227. Shehadi, W. H.: Cholografin; new intravenously administered contrast medium for visualization of gallbladder and bile ducts (intravenous cholecystocholangiography) with report on 104 cases, Amer. J. Roentgen. **76**:7, 1956.

228. Shehadi, W. H., and Jacox, H. W.: Clinical radiology of the biliary tract, New York, 1963, McGraw-Hill Book Co.

229. Shorter, R. G., Baggenstoss, A. H., Logan, G. B., and Hallenbeck, G. A.: Primary carcinoma of the liver in infancy and childhood: report of 11 cases and review of the literature, Pediatrics **25**:191, 1960.

230. Silberman, E. L., and Glaessner, T. S.: Roentgen features of congenital cystic dilatation of the common bile duct; a report of two cases, Radiology **82**:470, 1964.

231. Simon, M., and Tandon, B. N.: Multiseptate gallbladder: a case report, Radiology **80**:84, 1963.

232. Sinner, B. L.: Unusual anomaly of gallbladder and bile duct, J. Missouri Med. Ass. **45**:265, 1948.

233. Skielboe, B.: Anomalies of the gallbladder; vesica fellea triplex; report of a case, Amer. J. Clin. Path. **30**:252, 1958.

234. Smith, A. G., and Seeley, S. F.: Pseudocholedochal cyst, Pediatrics **12**:536, 1953.

235. Snyder, W. H., Jr., Chaffin, L., and Oettinger, L., Jr.: Cholelithiasis and perforation of gallbladder in infant, with recovery, J.A.M.A. **149**:1645, 1952.

236. Soderlund, S., and Zetterstrom, B.: Cholecystitis and cholelithiasis in children, Arch. Dis. Child. **37**:174, 1962.

237. Soper, R. T., and Dunphy, D. L.: Sarcoma botryoides of the biliary tree, Surgery **63**:1005, 1968.

238. Sorge, D. V.: Cholecystitis and cholelithiasis in children: report of four cases, Pediatrics **29**:46, 1962.

239. Sorsdahl, O. A., and Gay, B. B., Jr.: Roentgenologic features of a primary carcinoma of the liver in infants and children, Amer. J. Roentgen. **100**:117, 1967.

240. Sterling, J. A., and Lowenburg, H.: Observations of infants with hepatic duct atresia and use of artificial duct prosthesis, Pediat. Clin. N. Amer. **9**:485, 1962.

241. Stigol, L. C., Traversaro, J., and Trigo, E. R.: Carinal trifurcation with congenital tracheobiliary fistula, Pediatrics **37**:89, 1966.

242. Stone, H. H., and Nielson, I. C.: Hemangioma of the liver in the newborn; report of a successful outcome following hepatic lobectomy, Arch. Surg. (Chicago) **90**:319, 1965.

243. Stowens, D.: Congenital biliary atresia, Amer. J. Gastroent. **32**:577, 1959.

244. Strauss, R. G.: Scarlet fever with hydrops of the gallbladder, Pediatrics **44**:741, 1969.

245. Strauss, R. G.: Cholelithiasis in childhood, Amer. J. Dis. Child. **117**:689, 1969.

246. Sutton, C. A., and Eller, J. L.: Mesenchymal hamartoma of the liver, Cancer 22:29, 1968.

247. Swartley, W. B., and Weeder, S. D.: Choledochus cyst with double common bile duct, Ann. Surg. 101:912, 1935.

248. Sweetnam, W. P., and Sykes, C. G.: Congenital fibrosis of the liver as a familial defect, Lancet 1:374, 1961.

249. Swenson, O.: Pediatric surgery, New York, 1958, Appleton-Century-Crofts.

250. Swenson, O., and Fisher, J. H.: Utilization of cholangiogram during exploration for biliary atresia, New Eng. J. Med. 247:247, 1952.

251. Tefft, M.: Radioisotope liver scans in pediatrics, Amer. J. Roentgen. 101:570, 1967.

252. Teng, C. T., Daeschner, C. W., Jr., Singleton, E. B., and Rosenberg, H. S.: Liver diseases and osteopororis in children; etiological considerations, J. Pediat. 59:703, 1961.

253. Teng, C. T., Daeschner, C. W., Jr., Singleton, E. B., Rosenberg, H. S., Cole, V. W., Hill, L. L., and Brennan, J. C.: Liver disease and osteoporosis in children; clinical observations, J. Pediat. 59:684, 1961.

254. Thorsness, E. T.: Aberrant pancreatic nodule arising on neck of human gallbladder from multiple outgrowths of mucosa, Anat. Rec. 77:319, 1940.

255. Touloukian, R. J.: Hepatic hemangioendothelioma during infancy: pathology, diagnosis and treatment with prednisone, Pediatrics 45:71, 1970.

256. Tran Ngoc Ninh, Pham Bieu Tam, Feroldi, J., and Lichtenberger, R. P.: La dilatation kystique congenitale du choledoque chez l'enfant: remarques anatomiques et chirirgicales a propos de six cas personnels, Ann. Chir. Infant. 5:245, 1964.

257. Ulin, A. W., Nosal, J. L., and Martin, W. L.: Cholecystitis in childhood: associated obstructive jaundice, Surgery 31:312, 1952.

258. Wagget, J., Stool, S., Bishop, H. C., and Kurtz, M. B.: Congenital broncho-biliary fistula, J. Pediat. Surg. 5:566, 1970.

259. Walker, C. H.: Aetiology of cholelithiasis in childhood, Arch. Dis. Child. 32:293, 1957.

260. Walker, G. R., Field, P., and Conen, P. E.: Cholelithiasis associated with congenital malformation of the cystic duct in a young child, Brit. J. Surg. 48:78, 1960.

261. Watkins, G. L.: Primary carcinoma of the liver in an infant: right lobectomy with six-year survival, Ann. Surg. 162:264, 1965.

262. Weichsel, M. E., Jr., and Luzzatti, L.: Trisomy 17-18 syndrome with congenital extrahepatic biliary atresia and congenital amputation of left foot, J. Pediat. 67:324, 1965.

263. Weinstein, C.: Choledochal cyst, Arch. Intern. Med. 115:339, 1965.

264. Welling, R. E., Krause, R. J., and Alamin, K.: Heterotopic gastric mucosa in the common bile duct, Arch. Surg. 101:626, 1970.

265. White, W. E., Welsh, J. S., Darrow, D. C., and Holder, T. M.: Pediatric application of the radioiodine (I 131) rose bengal method in hepatic and biliary system disease, Pediatrics 32:239, 1963.

266. Wilenius, R.: Cholecystitis and cholelithiasis in childhood, Ann. Chir. Gynaec. Fenn. 40:135, 1951.

267. Williams, C., and Williams, A. M.: Abnormalities of bile ducts, Ann. Surg. 141:598, 1955.

268. Williams, J. E.: The anomalous cystic duct: a surgical and radiological problem, Clin. Radiol. 13:333, 1962.

269. Windmiller, J., Marks, J. F., Reimold, E. W., Costales, F., and Peake, C.: Trisomy 18 with biliary atresia, J. Pediat. 67:327, 1965.

Systemic diseases affecting the alimentary tract

58

J. Scott Dunbar and
Barry D. Fletcher

CYSTIC FIBROSIS OF THE PANCREAS

Cystic fibrosis, a genetic disorder of children that is transmitted as an autosomal recessive trait, is one of the most important causes of morbidity and mortality in children. Although chronic illness and eventual death are largely attributable to pulmonary disease and resultant cor pulmonale, numerous gastrointestinal and hepatic abnormalities result from the pancreatic exocrine dysfunction and generalized mucous obstruction of organ passages that are the hallmarks of the disease.[30] The diagnosis is made by the finding of elevated sweat electrolytes.

Neonatal manifestations
Meconium ileus

Meconium ileus occurs in 10% to 15% of neonates with cystic fibrosis.[27] In addition to pancreatic insufficiency, these infants have abnormally tenacious mucus in the intestine in larger than normal amounts. Of these two factors, tenacious mucus seems to be the more important in the pathogenesis of meconium ileus.[32,111] The inspissated meconium causes obstruction, usually at the level of the distal ileum but occasionally more proximally in the small bowel or even more distally, resulting in obturation of the proximal colon.[59]

Failure to pass meconium in the first days of life, together with progressive abdominal distention and possible vomiting, suggests the diagnosis of bowel obstruction. Roentgenologic examination at this stage is of extreme importance. Just as in other causes of suspected obstruction, anteroposterior supine views of the abdomen should be supplemented by erect or, more simply, horizontal beam lateral projections. Roentgenographic examination of the chest should be included in the abdominal series, since a number of patients may already have pulmonary abnormalities, caused either by cystic fibrosis or by aspiration of gastric contents.

The inspissated meconium pellets lead to the roentgenologic findings of obstruction in which classically a "bubbly" appearance of the intestines[88] and a paucity or absence of air fluid levels is seen.[117] However, these signs are frequently absent even in "uncomplicated" meconium ileus (Fig. 58-1).[73] Another difficulty is determination of the level of obstruction by

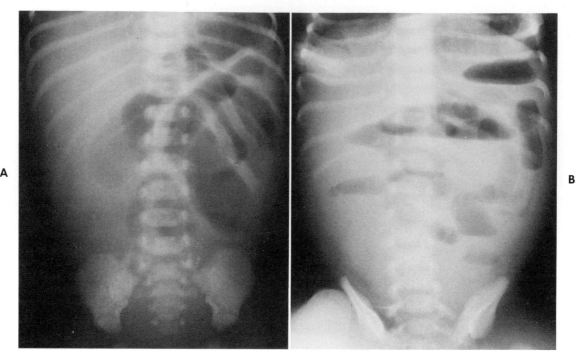

Fig. 58-1. Newborn infant with meconium ileus. **A,** Dilatation of the bowel is seen on the supine view of the abdomen. **B,** The erect view shows a number of air fluid levels. Note the variation in caliber of the air-containing bowel. There is no evidence of the classical "soap-bubble" appearance. No atresia or other complications of meconium ileus was found at operation.

plain films alone, since it is often difficult to distinguish between the large and small bowel in newborn infants. On occasion, obstructions involving the colon, such as Hirschsprung's disease and meconium plug syndrome, result in roentgenologic findings that are easily confused with the "classical" picture of meconium ileus.

Contrast examination of the colon is extremely helpful in these patients in order to rule out colonic obstructions. We have recently begun to use water-soluble contrast medium (meglumine diatrizoate) diluted to a 30% solution with water in order to avoid barium inspissation if colonic obstruction should be present. The contrast medium can be gently instilled into the colon by means of a syringe and small rectal tube.

The finding of a "microcolon," in which the large bowel is of diminished caliber but normal length, indicates the presence of a distal small-bowel obstruction that would be expected in meconium ileus or ileal atresia.[12] A distal ileal

filling defect caused by inspissated meconium has also been demonstrated on a barium enema examination in which the barium refluxed into the small bowel.[17] The distal ileum was noted to be "telescoped" over the meconium mass. More recently, the ability to obtain reflux into the distal ileum in uncomplicated meconium ileus has resulted in several successful attempts to relieve meconium ileus by means of small-bowel enemas using diacetylaminotriiodobenzoate or diatrizoate.[43,89,113] A nonoperative procedure has obvious advantages over surgical interference in patients who are already at risk because of pulmonary disease. However, the unsuspected presence of complications and the as yet slight experience with this technique necessitate great caution. Perforations of the colon apparently occur easily in these infants.[32] Very little is known about the reaction of the peritoneum to the various contrast media.

The complications of meconium ileus are atresia of the small intestine, perforation, volvulus, and meconium peritonitis. Except for meconium peritonitis, the complications may be difficult to recognize roentgenologically.[73]

Intestinal atresia

Ileal atresia is the result of meconium inspissation, which can lead to obliteration of the intestinal lumen and is a frequent complication of meconium ileus.[90,124] Discontinuity of the bowel may also result from adhesions associated with meconium peritonitis or from antenatal volvulus.[14] It is also important to recognize that intestinal atresia can occur because of mechanical and vascular abnormalities of the fetal bowel in the absence of cystic fibrosis.[75,97]

The only consistent roentgenologic findings on plain films in patients with intestinal atresia with meconium ileus are those of small-bowel obstruction.[14] Leonidas and associates[73] have suggested that the presence of prominent intestinal air fluid levels is unusual in the presence of uncomplicated meconium ileus.[73]

Volvulus

If volvulus occurs during fetal life, ischemic necrosis and resorption of intestinal loops may occur, resulting in a "pseudocyst."[54] The roentgenologic appearance may be that of an intra-abdominal mass in association with what appears to be a high intestinal obstruction.[73]

Meconium peritonitis

Intraperitoneal meconium may calcify within 24 hours,[87] and although intraluminal[67] and intramural[112] calcifications are sometimes seen, the presence of calcifications on abdominal roentgenograms usually indicates the presence of meconium peritonitis that is caused by spillage of sterile fetal meconium into the peritoneal cavity. Although meconium peritonitis may be the result of other causes of fetal intestinal obstruction, meconium ileus is responsible for this finding in 50% of cases.[29] Meconium peritonitis is often associated with obstructive phenomena, volvulus, or gangrene, but bowel obstruction or even a site of perforation may not always be found. The presence of meconium peritonitis in a patient with cystic fibrosis is a grave prognostic sign.[104] The survival rate in meconium ileus is considerably lowered in the presence of peritonitis, perforation, or gangrene.[62]

Perforation of the small bowel may also result

in massive ascites caused by peritonitis. Intra-abdominal calcifications may be absent.[9] This finding has also been reported in patients in whom there was also pneumoperitoneum apparently caused by perforation of the colon.[73]

In the presence of a patent processus vaginalis in male infants, scrotal meconium calcifications may be visible roentgenologically.[61] The resulting hydroceles may become hard, calcified scrotal masses by 4 weeks of age.[15]

Meconium plug syndrome

The meconium plug syndrome[23] is an uncommon cause of low-grade intestinal obstruction in the newborn period in which the obstruction can frequently be relieved spontaneously or by means of water-soluble contrast enemas. This may be related to a transient abnormality of mucolytic enzymes during the first days of life but has not been found to be associated with cystic fibrosis.[34] Hirschsprung's disease however, has been demonstrated in patients with this syndrome.[48]

Later manifestations
Meconium ileus equivalent

Even if meconium ileus was absent in the newborn period, some patients with cystic fibrosis are subject to episodes of low-grade obstruction later in life, which has been called "meconium ileus equivalent" (Fig. 58-2). Abdominal roentgenograms usually show generalized intestinal dilatation with "bubbly" appearing semisolid material in the small bowel and ascending colon. Infants and older children can be affected. The presence of meconium ileus equivalent is not necessarily related to the severity of pulmonary or hepatic disease.[25] Numerous factors such as abnormal intestinal mucous secretion, dehydration, and inadequate therapy with pancreatic enzymes have been implicated. The symptoms usually respond to medical therapy.[39] A diagnostic barium enema may also have a therapeutic effect (Fig. 58-3). Abnormalities of propulsion of inspissated stool can also lead to intussusception. Asymptomatic cecal masses and volvulus of the sigmoid and small intestine have also been reported.[85,106]

Duodenal ulcers

Because of increased acidity of the duodenal juices in cystic fibrosis, duodenal ulceration

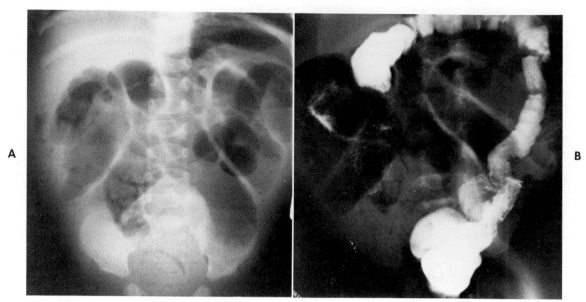

Fig. 58-2. Meconium ileus equivalent in a 3-month-old infant with cystic fibrosis. **A,** The dilatation affects mainly the small bowel. **B,** There was some difficulty in filling the cecum with barium.

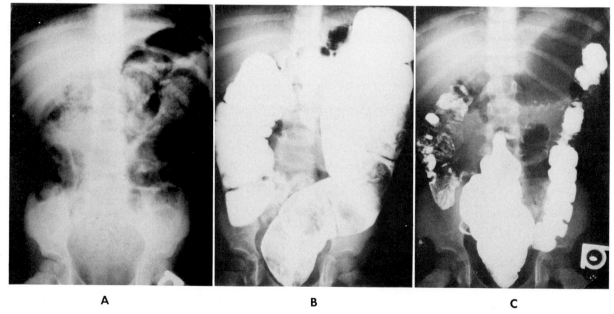

Fig. 58-3. Meconium ileus equivalent in a 4-year-old cystic fibrosis patient, with mild respiratory involvement and recent onset of crampy abdominal pain. The abdominal roentgenograph, **A,** shows a large collection of fecal material, which was thought to be in the colon. A barium enema was performed, **B,** which confirmed that a large mass of fecal material was present in the colon. After evacuation of the barium and the fecal material, **C,** no other abnormality was demonstrated. The symptoms were relieved by the barium enema.

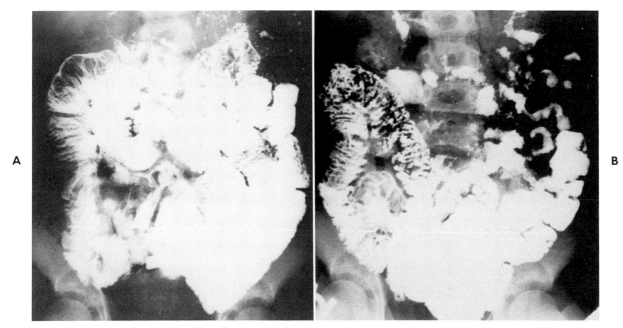

Fig. 58-4. A, Mildly disordered small-bowel pattern in a 10-year-old girl with cystic fibrosis and abdominal pain of unknown origin. **B,** After further transit of barium, nodular mucosal defects of the small bowel are seen, which are probably caused by dilated intestinal mucosal glands.

might be expected more frequently. In spite of this, duodenal ulcers have been reported infrequently.[7]

Small-bowel abnormalities

Patients with cystic fibrosis have steatorrhea and faulty digestion of proteins. Contrast examination of the nonobstructed small bowel may show nonspecific disordering of its pattern.[88] The presence of true celiac disease, that is, gluten enteropathy, in association with cystic fibrosis is, however, extremely rare.[60] A mild dilatation of small-bowel loops with thickened and "smudged" duodenal folds and thickened valvulae conniventes is sometimes seen.[54,116] A more specific finding is that of marginal small-bowel filling defects that are probably caused by mucus distention of mucosal glands (Fig. 58-4).[10]

Colonic abnormalities

The colonic manifestations of cystic fibrosis include a cobblestone appearance of the colon as seen on postevacuation barium enema films.[50] Redundant, hyperplastic mucosal folds and small marginal polypoid defects have also been described, which are possibly caused by distended crypt goblet cells (Fig. 58-5).[116]

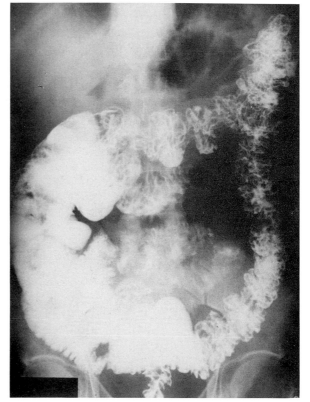

Fig. 58-5. Redundant, hyperplastic, mucosal folds of the colon are demonstrated on a postevacuation barium enema film of an adult patient with cystic fibrosis.

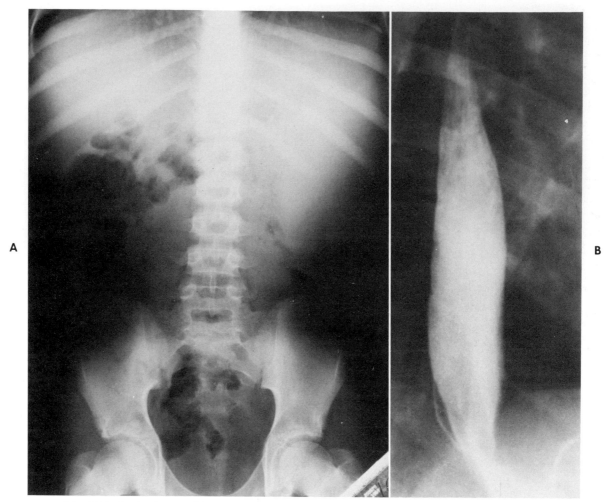

Fig. 58-6. A, A 12-year-old cystic fibrosis patient with splenic enlargement caused by portal hypertension and biliary cirrhosis. **B,** A varix is also present in the lower esophagus.

White and Rowley have also seen cases of pneumatosis cystoides intestinalis that they feel are most likely caused by associated chronic pulmonary overdistention.[118] Rectal prolapse is also a fairly common clinical finding that most often occurs between the ages of 6 months and 3 years in children with untreated cystic fibrosis.[72]

Pancreatic abnormalities

In spite of the marked pancreatic fibrosis and fatty infiltration that eventually occurs,[3] diabetes mellitus has been a relatively uncommon finding in cystic fibrosis.[95] Its incidence however, may be expected to increase as the life expectancy of these patients also improves. However, the roentgenologic finding of pancreatic calcifi-

cation associated with diabetes caused by cystic fibrosis is extremely rare.[29,95,118]

Hepatic abnormalities

Cystic fibrosis accounts for one third of all cases of cirrhosis of the liver in pediatric patients.[28] However, only a small number of patients with cystic fibrosis have symptomatic cirrhosis. At autospy, focal biliary cirrhosis with concretions in the cholangioles and bile ducts caused by inspissation of bile is a constant finding. A more advanced stage is multilobular biliary cirrhosis with concretions in which there is coalescence of these foci and increased fibrosis. This can result in portal hypertension with hepatosplenomegaly, hypersplenism, gastrointesti-

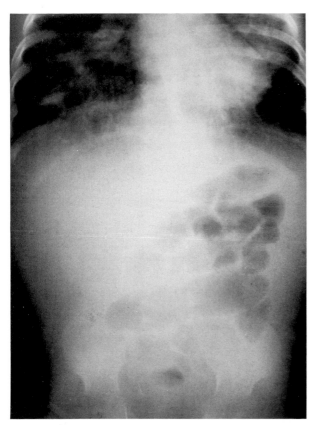

Fig. 58-7. Rare finding of a fatty, hyperlucent liver in an infant with cystic fibrosis. This may have resulted from an inability to utilize dietary protein.

nal bleeding with esophageal varices, and ascites (Fig. 58-6).[28] Hepatic abnormalities seem to be more common in patients who have had meconium ileus in the neonatal period.[90] Fatty metamorphosis of the liver[108] is rare in the presence of better nutrition (Fig. 58-7). In infants, a substitution of soybean feedings or even human milk for cow's milk leads to hypoproteinemia because of improper utilization of the substituted proteins.[42] This may lead to generalized edema and ascites, which may be demonstrable roentgenologically.[54]

Biliary abnormalities

Abnormalities of the gallbladder have been noted in 33% of autopsy cases of cystic fibrosis.[36] These consist of mucus-containing cysts in the wall of the gallbladder and mucoid material in the lumina. The gallbladder and cystic duct may be hypoplastic and a "microgallbladder" with

irregular contours may be demonstrated roentgenologically in some patients.[98] The eventual formation of calculi might be expected and has been described by White and Rowley.[118] Gallbladder disease, however, is not common and does not usually coincide with the abdominal pain frequently experienced by many patients with cystic fibrosis.

EXOCRINE PANCREATIC INSUFFICIENCY, BLOOD DISORDERS, AND METAPHYSEAL DYSOSTOSIS

Recently, a hereditary disorder of exocrine pancreatic insufficiency associated with bone marrow dysfunction with neutropenia, anemia, and thrombocytopenia has been described (Fig. 58-8).[100] Patients with this disorder, in whom failure to thrive is noted during infancy, have diarrhea but no gross steatorrhea. One patient with this syndrome whom we have seen has a disordered small-bowel pattern resembling celiac disease. These patients are often thought to have cystic fibrosis, and the pancreatic acinar tissue is atrophic, but sweat electrolytes are normal and pulmonary disease is absent.

Of prime importance in correctly diagnosing these patients is the fact that metaphyseal dysostosis may be an associated roentgenographic abnormality.[110]

HEMATOLOGIC DISEASE
Leukemia

The effects of leukemia on the alimentary tract are often present at autopsy and abdominal symptoms and signs such as pain and hemorrhage may be present clinically. Necrotizing enteropathy is a frequent complication.[2] Specific gastrointestinal abnormalities are less frequently recognized roentgenologically. Leukemia may involve any portion of the alimentary tract. The pathologic findings are those of hemorrhagic necrosis, leukemic infiltration, agranulocytic necrosis, and mycotic lesions.[92] The roentgenologic features of the associated necrotizing enteropathy include paralytic ileus and obstruction caused by inflammatory masses resulting from gangrene and perforation of the distal ileum, appendix, cecum, and ascending colon.[47] Acute appendicitis in childhood leukemia may be related to cytotoxic drug therapy.[66] Wagner and co-workers suggest that typhlitis in terminally ill leukemic patients with agranulocytosis can be

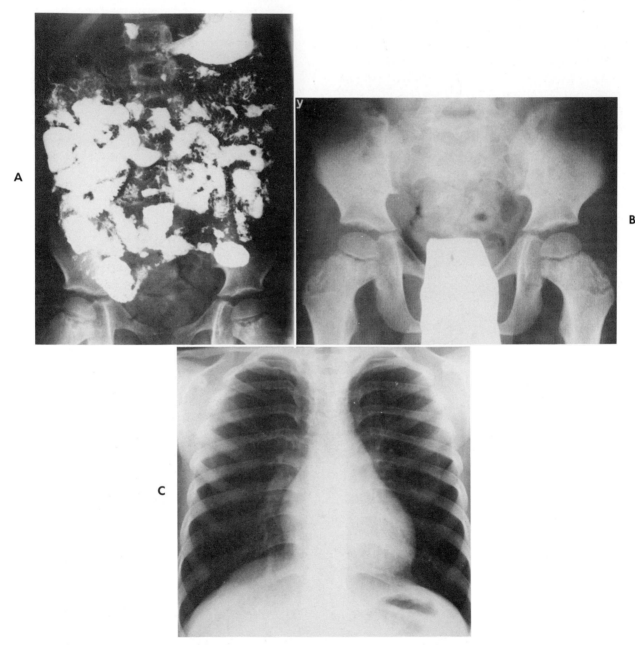

Fig. 58-8. A 7-year-old boy with probable syndrome of pancreatic insufficiency, bone marrow dysfunction, and metaphyseal dysostosis. **A,** The small-bowel study shows a disordered pattern consistent with malabsorption. **B,** There is irregularity of the metaphyses of the proximal femora. The distal femoral metaphyses were also similar in appearance but showed less marked abnormalities. **C,** Chest roentgenogram taken at age 10 years shows none of the chronic pulmonary disease usually associated with cystic fibrosis.

diagnosed roentgenologically, since the hemorrhagic necrosis of the cecum causes plain film findings similar to appendicitis with the addition of a right-sided mass thought to be a fluid-filled, atonic ascending colon.[114] Khilnani and associates cite leukemia as a cause of intramural intestinal hemorrhage.[70]

Leukemic infiltrates may be seen as localized submucosal nodules of the stomach and intestines.[102] Multiple small nodular defects similar to those seen in lymphososarcoma within a short segment of small bowel have also been described.[79] Lower esophageal filling defects caused by leukemia have been reported in a child who had dysphagia.[1]

Candida esophagitis

If infection with *Candida albicans* is present, esophagrams may show a more diffuse "cobblestone pattern" of multiple nodular defects resulting from inflammatory changes of the esophageal wall.[51] Decreased esophageal motility is also a feature of this condition and deep ulcers may be present, particularly in the lower esophagus. It is not uncommon in children who are being treated with corticosteroids, antimetabolites, and antimicrobial drugs for a malignant disease.[68]

Another possible complication of corticosteroid treatment of leukemia is pneumatosis intestinalis.[63]

Lymphosarcoma

The most common intestinal malignancy of childhood is lymphosarcoma.[86] The disease is most frequently encountered between the ages of 3 and 8 years but also may occur in early infancy. Clinically, there may be a palpable mass and findings suggestive of appendicitis or appendiceal abscess.[80] Some patients may have hepatosplenomegaly or ascites.[99]

The sarcomas arise from submucosal lymphoid collections, and therefore the ileum is the most common site of involvement.[80] However, the stomach,[79] duodenum,[99] jejunum,[80] and colon[79] are also sites of involvement.

Several roentgenographic presentations of intestinal lymphosarcoma have been described.[78,79] These include multiple nodular defects, an infiltrating form, a polypoid form, an endoexocentric form, and mesenteric invasion resulting in extramural masses or a sprue pattern. Of

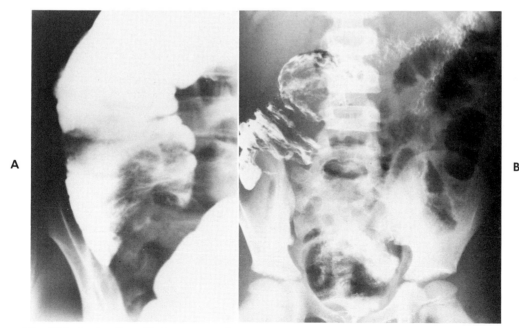

Fig. 58-9. A, An ileocolic intussusception caused by localized lymphosarcoma in a 6-year-old boy. **B,** The postevacuation barium enema film shows an intraluminal tumor mass remaining in the area of the hepatic flexure.

these, the most frequent presentation in childhood is the polypoid form, which presents as a distal ileal intraluminal mass causing intussusception (Fig. 58-9).[41,99] Felson and Wiot state that after the first 6 months of life lymphoma is a more common cause of intussusception than polyp.[41]

Hodgkin's disease

Hodgkin's disease is said to produce findings similar to lymphosarcoma except that increased fibrosis and luminal narrowing as present.[79] However, intestinal Hodgkin's disease in children is not frequently encountered.

Reticuloendotheliosis

Autopsy examination in patients with Letterer-Siwe and Hand-Schüller-Christian diseases may reveal evidence of intestinal involvement.[8] Histiocytic infiltration of Peyer's patches and intestinal submucosa, which is sometimes seen pathologically,[21] might reasonably be expected to be visible on barium examination. Occasionally, these patients have symptoms relating to the gastrointestinal tract. Feinberg and Lester demonstrated a coarse pebble-like appearance in the small bowel of one infant who had vomiting and symptoms of obstruction.[38] Another patient who lacked gastrointestinal symptoms nevertheless had a mildly disordered small-bowel pattern. Extensive visceral involvement in reticuloendotheliosis is frequently manifested by hepatosplenomegaly and mesenteric node involvement.

Burkitt's tumor

Burkitt's tumor is a lymphoma-like disease of childhood that is common in Africa but is only occasionally seen in North America.[26] Numerous skeletal and visceral abnormalities may be caused by the tumor, perhaps the best known of which are deposits that cause swelling of the mandible or maxilla. Lesions of the gastrointestinal tract are frequently silent, but multiple, rounded, well-circumscribed deposits have been described in the stomach and intestines similar to the findings in the Peutz-Jeghers syndrome (Figs. 58-12 and 58-13). Cecal and appendiceal deposits may result in appendicitis.[24] An elongated, irregular descending colonic stricture caused by Burkitt's tumor was recorded in a North American patient.[26]

Hemophilia

Hemophilia is a cause of intramural intestinal bleeding that can be either spontaneous or the result of minor trauma. Although numerous

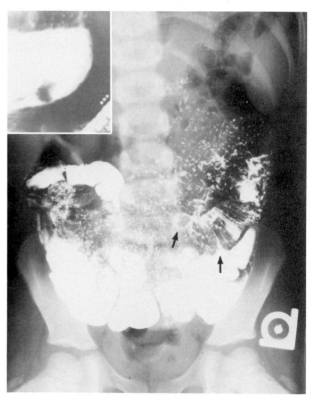

Fig. 58-11. Intestinal (arrows) and gastric polyps (inset) in a young child with Peutz-Jeghers syndrome.

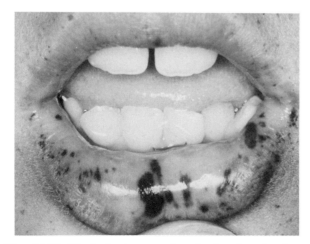

Fig. 58-10. Typical circumoral melanin deposits in a patient with Peutz-Jeghers syndrome.

cases of intramural hematoma have been reported since the description by Felson and Levin in 1954,[40] surprisingly few of these have been described in patients with hemophilia.[49,81,84] In the duodenum, the resultant intramural mass is sharply marginated and the valvulae conniventes are crowded into a coil spring pattern similar to that seen in intussusception.[40] The hematoma may result in intestinal obstruction (Fig. 58-14).

Khilnani and co-workers have described a characteristic thickening of the folds of the small intestine with a parallel spiked appearance of their margins that resemble stacked coins.[70] This is particularly noticeable in the jejunum. Multiple lucent filling defects or "thumb-printing," which has been shown to be caused by mucosal hemorrhage,[74] has also been described in this disease.[70,120] Wiot suggests that spontaneous intramural hemorrhage is more infiltrative and

less likely to cause a mass than is hemorrhage caused by trauma.[120] Intussusception is also a possible complication of hemorrhage in children with hemophilia.[82]

Besides the duodenum, intramural bleeding caused by hemophilia has also been demonstrated roentgenologically in the jejunum,[31] distal ileum and ileocecal valve area,[31,121,146] and distal descending colon.[31] When this phenomenon occurs in the stomach, very large obstructing hemorrhagic masses may result.[53,123]

Christmas disease causes findings similar to hemophilia.[82] An early case of duodenal hematoma was reported in a baby with an undetermined type of hemorrhagic disease of the newborn, possibly hemophilia.[49] It is quite reasonable, therefore, to expect intramural hemorrhage in neonates with bleeding diatheses of other causes.

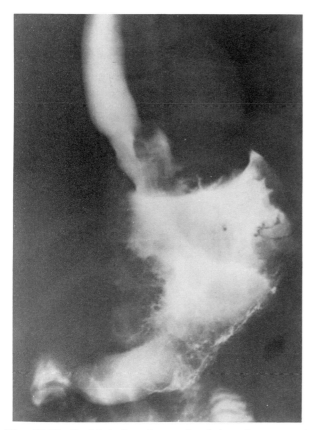

Fig. 58-12. Burkitt's lymphoma involving the stomach in an African child. (Courtesy Prof. P. Cockshott.)

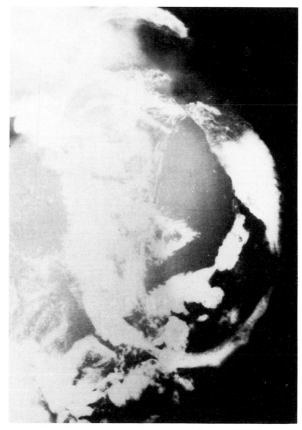

Fig. 58-13. Massive involvement of the stomach and small bowel by Burkitt's lymphoma in an African child. Note incidental infestation with *Ascaris*. (Courtesy Prof. P. Cockshott.)

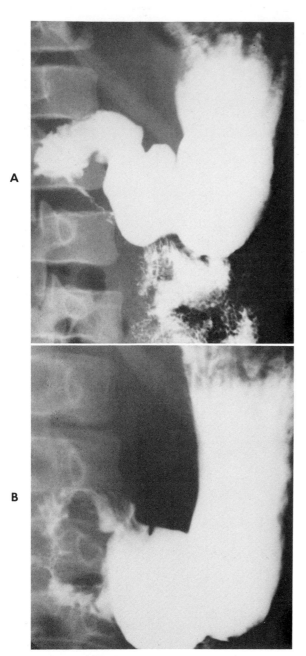

Fig. 58-14. A, Duodenal obstruction caused by an intramural hematoma in a 15-year-old hemophilia patient who was involved in an automobile accident. **B,** Nine days later the duodenum is normal with the exception of slight thickening of the mucosal folds.

Since surgery is hazardous in patients with coagulation defects, the roentgenologic recognition of the effects of hemophilia on the intestine is of extreme importance. Eventual spontaneous disappearance of the clinical and roentgenological abnormalities is to be expected.[31]

Schönlein-Henoch purpura (nonthrombocytopenic purpura)

Schönlein-Henoch purpura is also a disorder frequently encountered in childhood, which enters the differential diagnosis of spontaneous intramural hemorrhage.[120] Abdominal pain may be associated with the finding of dilated, separated loops of small bowel with marginal defects or "thumb-printing" caused by submucosal hemorrhage.[53] These findings, as well as the clinical manifestations of purpura, abdominal pain, and arthralgia, are reversible. However, we have seen a patient with this condition who required surgical relief of an ileocolic intussusception. Schönlein-Henoch purpura has been discussed in detail elsewhere in this book.

Lymphoid hyperplasia

Polypoid filling defects of the colon caused by lymphoid hyperplasia have been demonstrated on air-contrast barium enemas in children by Capitanio and Kirkpatrick.[20] The presence of apical umbilication of the nodules indicates the benign nature of these lesions. Similar lymphoid colonic polyps have been demonstrated in a mother and four siblings all of whom had café-au-lait spots.

Lymphoid hyperplasia of both the colon and small bowel may be associated with dysgammaglobulinemia (Fig. 58-15).[122]

TRISOMY SYNDROMES
Trisomy 21 (Down's syndrome, mongolism)

In patients with Down's syndrome there is a high incidence of clinically significant anomalies of the intestine.[91] Duodenal intrinsic stenosis and duodenal atresia are most frequently encountered, and indeed the demonstration or suspicion of duodenal obstruction in a newborn infant should alert the radiologist to the possibility that the patient may have Down's syndrome.[16,37,57] Esophageal atresia and Hirschsprung's disease[35] also have a disproportionately high incidence in patients with trisomy 21 but are not as frequent in this syndrome as are duo-

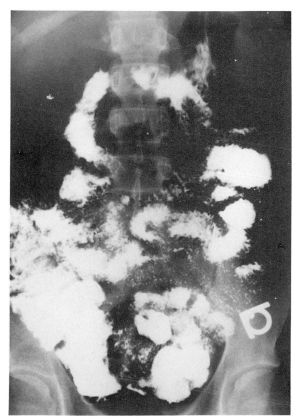

Fig. 58-15. Small-bowel examination of a patient with severe hypogammaglobulinemia. The roentgenographs show innumerable, small nodular lesions scattered throughout the small bowel and moderate disordering of the small-bowel pattern consistent with malabsorption. Autopsy confirmed that the nodular lesions were caused by lymphoid hyperplasia.

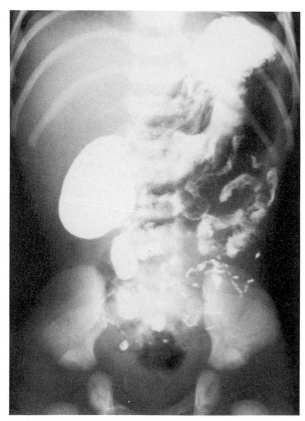

Fig. 58-16. A partial duodenal obstruction is present in this newborn infant with mongolism. The pelvis shows widening of the iliac wings and horizontally disposed acetabular roofs, characteristic of Down's syndrome.

denal anomalies. The recognition of Down's syndrome from the contours of the pelvis is well established since the work of Caffey.[19] It is thus frequently possible to recognize that the patient is suffering from this syndrome when he is being investigated for intestinal obstruction (Fig. 58-16).

The pathologic characteristics and physiologic derangements caused by the intestinal anomalies found in patients with Down's syndrome do not differ from those that are discovered in otherwise normal children or in association with other syndromes. The diagnostic roentgenographic methods to detect and assess the obstruction and its cause are likewise similar to those used in other groups of patients. In view of the known high association of congenital heart disease with Down's syndrome, however, the heart and lungs on chest films obtained in such patients should be examined with particular attention.[91] Similarly, when a patient with Down's syndrome is found to have one gastrointestinal anomaly such as esophageal atresia, other anomalies should be anticipated and sought.

Trisomy 13-15(D) and 18(E)

In trisomy 13 syndrome and in the trisomy 18 syndrome, there is an increased incidence of Meckel's diverticulum and intestinal malrotation.[105] It is uncommon, however, for such anomalies to be presenting or predominating findings in terms of signs and symptoms. Rather, infants with trisomy syndrome tend to be feeble and fail to thrive.[45] Aggressive investigations to discover and treat gastrointestinal anomalies are not appropriate for such patients, since the prog-

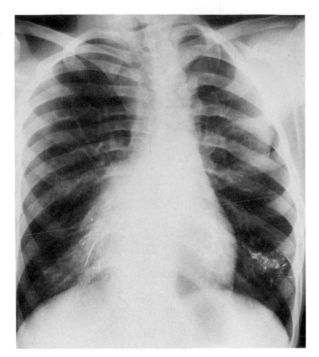

Fig. 58-17. Characteristic findings in a patient with familial dysautonomia. Chronic pneumonia is shown in the lower lungs, and there is barium in the bronchi bilaterally following its aspiration in the course of a recent contrast examination of the pharynx and esophagus. Scoliosis of moderate degree is present and is also characteristic of this disorder.

nosis is extremely poor and the incidence of brain malformations, particularly in trisomy 13 syndrome, is high.[64,65,115]

DISORDERS ASSOCIATED WITH PHARYNGEAL AND ESOPHAGEAL ABNORMALITIES
Familial dysautonomia (Riley-Day syndrome)

The gastrointestinal tract is regularly involved in patients with familial dysautonomia in that there is almost always impaired pharyngeal and esophageal coordination; the incoordination is most severe and most symptomatically important at the pharyngoesophageal junction because it is responsible for a tendency to aspirate swallowed fluid into the tracheobronchial tree.[56,77] This chronic or repeated aspiration of swallowed fluid may be the cause of chronic, recurrent, or resistant pneumonia (Fig. 58-17). In such a case, the abnormal pharyngeal function can readily be demonstrated by fluoroscopic study of swallowing in lateral projection (preferably

with videotape or cinerecording for detailed and slow-motion analysis). Disturbance of motility throughout the esophagus and improper relaxation of the lower esophageal sphincter are also frequently present; they probably account for the frequent finding of feeding difficulty in early infancy and the symptom of dysphagia in childhood.

In childhood the syndrome of familial dysautonomia is so characteristic that it seldom escapes recognition if the patient is seen by an experienced pediatrician; but in infancy, failure to thrive and recurrent respiratory infection may go unexplained until the diagnosis is suspected. Familial dysautonomia's clinical features are numerous and characteristic, including mental retardation, absent or hypoactive tendon and corneal reflexes, postural hypotension, emotional lability, relative indifference to pain, and absence of fungiform papillae on the tongue. A simple diagnostic test of great value is the intradermal injection of histamine, which in normal patients produces a skin flare but in patients with familial dysautonomia elicits no reaction.[94]

Roentgenologically, in addition to chronic or recurrent pneumonia and the pharyngoesophageal motility disturbances, scoliosis is a common finding.

Sandifer's syndrome

Sandifer described patients having a peculiar and often severe tic, with repeated hyperextension of the head and neck in a jerking movement. Vomiting is a common symptom and hematemesis occasionally occurs. In a few of such patients, diaphragmatic hiatus hernia with or without gastroesophageal reflux has been found by roentgenologic examination, and the repair of the hernia and prevention of reflux is reported to result in great improvement or disappearance of the tic.[71,101,109] Others have found that the tic is not invariably relieved by repair of the hernia,[103] and it may be that the symptom complex is one that awaits confirmation by further experience.

Rumination

Rumination has long been regarded as a manifestation or complication of emotional deprivation. Emotionally deprived children characteristically induce regurgitation of stomach contents into the pharynx and mouth, usually by inserting their fingers into the throat.[44] Regurgitated gastric contents are then manipulated and reswallowed in the mouth and pharynx, and this recycling of stomach content can be so severe as to prevent or reduce normal ingestion of food. The clinical behavior of these infants or young children is so named because of the strong resemblance to the behavior of ruminant animals in which recycling of the gastric contents is part of normal digestion. The clinical management of such patients has until recently consisted of "tender, loving care," predicated upon the impression that the rumination is a source of satisfaction to the emotionally deprived child. Recently, it has been suggested that the vomiting is not so much self-induced as spontaneous and caused by gastroesophageal incompetence with reflux.[58]

The roentgenographic demonstration of rumination in the pediatric patient has usually been felt to be of interest to the radiologist and pediatrician but of little clinical importance, since this syndrome is clinically characteristic. It now appears that such children should be carefully examined for gastroesophageal junction incompetence, with or without hiatus hernia. In addition, other causes of regurgitation, such as esophageal stricture, cardiospasm, and pyloric and duodenal lesions should be excluded by appropriate roentgenographic examination. Untreated rumination is a cause of severe malnutrition and even death, and thus thorough roentgenologic evaluation should precede treatment.

Epidermolysis bullosa

Epidermolysis bullosa is a rare hereditary skin disease in which slight trauma disrupts the cohesion between the epidermis and the dermis, resulting in the formation of vesicles, bullae, and ulcers. Of the three types that have been described, the third, or hypoplastic dystrophic type, is an autosomal recessive trait, with its onset at or slightly after birth. Widespread bullae follow minor trauma, affecting both the skin and mucosa, and heal with excessive scarring. Although most of the cases with roentgenologic changes have been described in adults. Becker and Swinyard have reported four cases in the pediatric age group.[11] Segmental areas of the esophagus are involved with stenotic changes, the upper third being more frequently affected

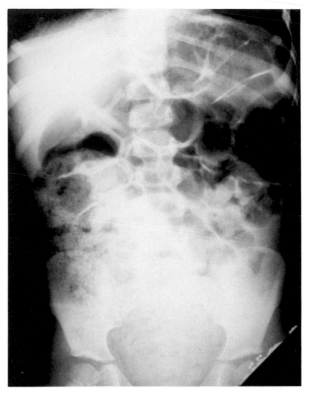

Fig. 58-18. Typical functional megacolon with a large amount of retained feces shown by a plain film of the abdomen of a 4-year-old boy.

then the lower third. Ulcers, vesicles, and bullae may be demonstrated endoscopically, but esophageal stenosis and its complications are recognized roentgenologically.[33] The complications include retention or impaction of swallowed food, osteoporosis, distal soft tissue atrophy, and acquired webbing.

PSYCHOGENIC DISORDERS
Functional megacolon (chronic constipation)

Chronic constipation in the pediatric age group is a common problem and is frequently difficult to manage. Many authorities feel that it is the result of psychogenic causes, often associated with parental overanxiety or stress. The problem as it is presented to the radiologist is one of assessing the degree of fecal retention and of demonstrating its cause.

The severity of fecal retention can be evaluated by a plain film of the abdomen made without any preparation of the patient (Fig. 58-18). It is important, however, to recognize that no roentgenologic criteria for chronic constipation have ever been defined and that there is an understandable tendency on the part of surgeons, pediatricians, and radiologists to accept as constipation findings that are in no way different from the fecal content of the normal child's intestine. This tendency is explained by the fact that the specialists concerned are looking for an explanation for the child's symptoms, and in the characteristically difficult psychosomatic setting in which the symptoms present, overdiagnosis is possible. In addition, the radiologist is accustomed to examining the urinary and gastrointestinal tract after colonic cleansing; unexpelled feces are a visual impediment to diagnosis and are likely to be perceived as abnormal.

In the search for a cause of chronic constipation the emphasis should be on the diagnosis or elimination of Hirschsprung's disease. If the rectum, clinically or roentgenologically, is filled or distended with feces, Hirschsprung's disease becomes highly unlikely, and in many such cases no further roentgenographic evaluation is necessary. The impression of a feces-filled or distended rectum can sometimes be confirmed by a lateral projection of the pelvis without the use of contrast medium.

If, however, it is decided that contrast examination should be done, it is best not to prepare the patient with cleansing enemas beforehand. The colon should be examined in the unprepared state so that the roentgenologic findings represent and hopefully explain the clinical problem. It is of great importance that only enough barium suspension be introduced to outline the rectum and the distal colon sufficiently to appreciate the contours of this terminal part of the large bowel. If a large amount of barium is used, it may become inspissated and aggravate the problem of constipation or even convert constipation to obstruction. Indeed, the patient who is examined by barium enema for constipation should not be discharged from the radiology department until sufficient evacuation has been obtained to assure that the barium will not be a cause of trouble.

The lateral projection of the rectum, preferably before and after evacuation (Fig. 58-19), is essential in the evaluation of all such problems and should take precedence over anteroposterior projections.

If a patient does present for roentgenographic evaluation of chronic constipation and if the colon has been emptied before or during the barium enema, the chronically distended rectum, when collapsed, may give a picture of large mucosal folds that resemble those found in

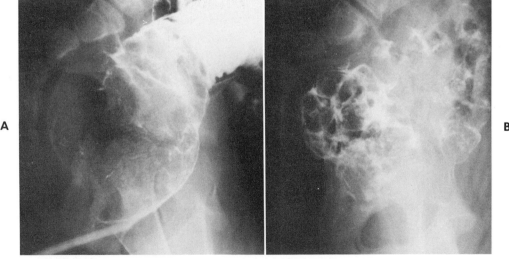

Fig. 58-19. Lateral roentgenographs of the distal sigmoid and rectum in a child with chronic constipation. **A,** Before evacuation the rectum is distended with a large fecal mass. **B,** After evacuation the rectum is almost completely evacuated. The mucosa appears moderately redundant after discharge of the large rectal fecal mass.

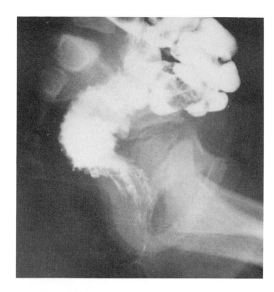

Fig. 58-20. A lateral film of the sigmoid, rectum, and anal canal following cleansing of the bowel in a patient with chronic constipation. The previously distended rectum is now almost completely empty and the redundant mucosa and wide retrorectal space simulates inflammatory change.

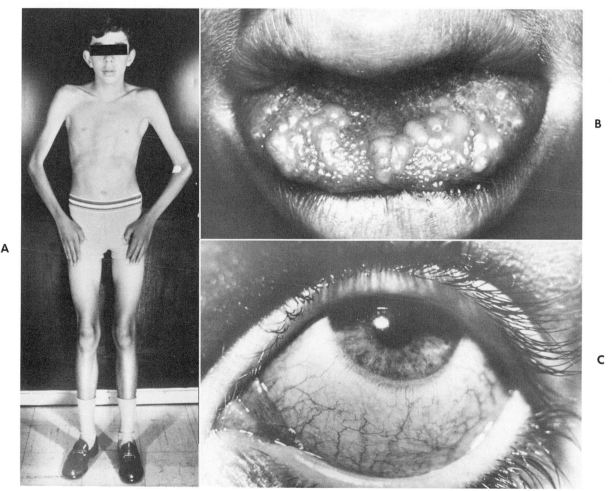

Fig. 58-21. The mucosal neuroma syndrome. A, Marfanoid changes. The patient also has a high palate, slight kyphosis, and pes cavus, which are not seen. B, Close-up view demonstrates prominent lips and the fleshy neuromas on the anterior third of the tongue. C, Whitish neuromatous tissue can be seen heaped up along the limbus of the cornea. (From Anderson, T. E., Spackman, T. J., and Schwartz, S. S.: Roentgen findings in intestinal ganglioneuromatosis, Radiology 101:93-96, 1971.)

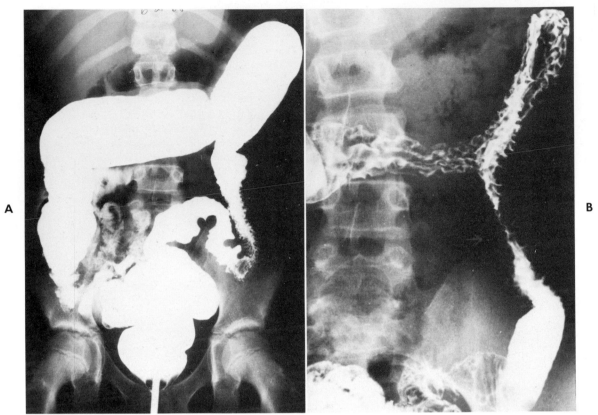

Fig. 58-22. A, The barium-filled colon has unusual haustral markings and a segmental area of spasm. **B,** Evacuation film demonstrates thick mucosal folds without ulceration or exudate. A diverticulum may be seen in the descending colon. (From Anderson, T. E., Spackman, T. J., and Schwartz, S. S.: Roentgen findings in intestinal ganglioneuromatosis, Radiology **101:**93-96, 1971.)

fibrocystic disease of the pancreas or that may even suggest hypertrophic or inflamed mucosa (Fig. 58-20).

MISCELLANEOUS
Neurofibromatosis

The protean manifestations of neurofibromatosis occasionally include intra-abdominal masses and gastrointestinal abnormalities.[46] Nodular tumors of the bowel wall may be present and can cause mucosal ulceration and gastrointestinal bleeding. Intussusception and perforation may also occur. An unusual manifestation of plexiform neurofibromatosis has been reported in which involvement of the wall of the distal colon and rectum resulted in a lesion that simulated Hirschsprung's disease.[107]

Mucosal neuroma syndrome

The recently described and still rare mucosal neuroma syndrome includes intestinal ganglio-

neuromatosis, long slender extremities, and other features similar to Marfan's syndrome, such as prominent lips and nodular deformity of the tongue caused by multiple neuromas, corneal limbus thickening, and a high association with medullary thyroid carcinoma and pheochromocytoma. Barium examination of the colon is said to demonstrate a distinctive triad as follows:

1. An abnormal haustral pattern in the barium-filled colon
2. Thickened mucosal folds on postevacuation films
3. Colonic diverticula

Such roentgenographic findings, particularly when encountered in a young patient with diarrhea, should suggest the diagnosis of intestinal and adrenal tumors (Figs. 58-21 and 58-22).

Zollinger-Ellison syndrome

The Zollinger-Ellison syndrome may be said to be a general one with gastrointestinal involve-

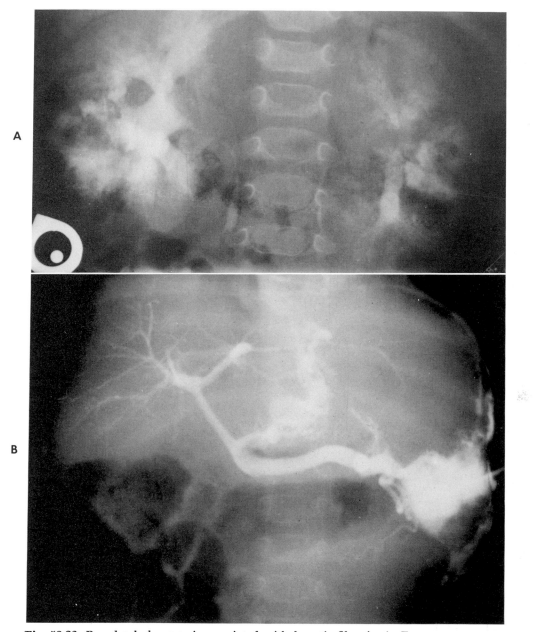

Fig. 58-23. Renal tubular ectasia associated with hepatic fibrosis. **A,** Excretory urogram, showing characteristic changes of renal tubular ectasia. **B,** Splenoportogram, showing changes caused by portal hypertension, with gastric and esophageal varices.

ment, since in addition to the well-known findings of peptic ulcers, which are severe, recurrent, or resistant to therapy and frequently postbulbar in distribution, such patients may have multiple endocrinopathies. The incidence of this syndrome is much lower in childhood than in the adult, but the findings are essentially similar. The discovery of a postbulbar ulcer in a child or of peptic ulceration that is unusually severe or resistant to therapy should alert the radiologist to the possibility of this disease.[18,96] Gastric mucosal fold (rugal) hypertrophy, duodenal dilatation caused by hypersecretion, and small-bowel findings consistent with the malabsorption syndrome may also be shown. Clinical and biochemical diagnosis requires the identification of gastric hypersecretion and high levels of free and total gastric acidity. Final diagnosis depends on surgical and pathologic confirmation of a nonbeta islet cell tumor, usually located in the pancreas but sometimes located ectopically in the duodenal wall or as a metastatic lesion elsewhere, such as the liver.

Renal tubular ectasia and hepatic fibrosis

As pointed out by Reilly and Neuhauser,[93] and subsequently emphasized by others, the patient with renal tubular ectasia characteristically first presents because of manifestations of portal hypertension and in particular hematemesis. Abdominal enlargement or swelling, and hepatosplenomegaly are other but less common presenting signs.[55,69] In such patients the renal tubular ectasia, which can be shown by excretory urography, is similar to, but likely distinct from, medullary sponge kidney. Renal function is usually little impaired, but the associated congenital hepatic fibrosis is responsible for portal hypertension, which in turn characteristically gives rise to esophageal varices and symptoms of hematemesis or melena. Thus the patient who is discovered to have esophageal varices as the cause of hematemesis or melena should have an excretory urogram in the course of his roentgenologic investigation (Fig. 58-23). The same policy should apply to children who are discovered to have "cirrhosis" of the liver, causing abdominal swelling of liver and spleen enlargement.

Congenital hepatic fibrosis with renal tubular ectasia is a familial disease likely having an autosomal recessive mode of inheritance.

REFERENCES

1. Al-Rashid, R. A., and Harned, R. K.: Dysphagia due to leukemic involvement of the esophagus, Amer. J. Dis. Child. **121**:75, 1971.
2. Amromin, G. D., and Solomon, R. D.: Necrotizing enteropathy; a complication of treated leukemia or lymphoma patients, J.A.M.A. **182**:23, 1962.
3. Anderson, D. H.: Pathology of cystic fibrosis, Ann. N. Y. Acad. Sci. **93**:500, 1962.
4. Anderson, T. E., Spackman, T. J., and Schwartz, S. S.: Roentgen findings in intestinal ganglioneuromatosis, Radiology **101**:93, 1971.
5. Andrén, L., and Frieberg, S.: Spontaneous regression of polyps of the colon in children, Acta Radiol. **46**:507, 1956.
6. Astley, R.: Trisomy 17/18, Brit. J. Radiol. **39**:86, 1966.
7. Aterman, K.: Duodenal ulceration and fibrocystic pancreas disease, Amer. J. Dis. Child. **101**:210, 1961.
8. Avery, M. E., McAfee, J. G., and Guild, H. G.: The course and prognosis of reticuloendotheliosis (eosinophilia granuloma, Schüller-Christian disease and Letterer-Siwe disease), Amer. J. Med. **22**:636, 1957.
9. Baghdassarian, O. M., Koehler, P. R., and Schultze, C.: Massive neonatal ascites, Radiology **76**:586, 1961.
10. Bartram, C. I., and Small, E.: The intestinal radiological changes in older people with pancreatic cystic fibrosis, Brit. J. Radiol. **44**:195, 1971.
11. Becker, M. H., and Swinyard, C. A.: Epidermolysis bullosa dystrophica in children: radiologic manifestations, Radiology **90**:124, 1968.
12. Berdon, W. E., Baker, D. H., Santulli, T. V., Amoury, R. A., and Blanc, W. A.: Microcolon in newborn infants with intestinal obstruction, Radiology **90**:878, 1968.
13. Berdon, W. E., Baker, D. H., Becker, J., and de Sanctis, P.: Scrotal masses in healed meconium peritonitis, New Eng. J. Med. **277**:585, 1967.
14. Bernstein, J., Vawter, G., Harris, G. B. C., Young, V., and Hillman, L. S.: The occurrence of intestinal atresia in newborns with meconium ileus, Amer. J. Dis. Child. **99**:804, 1960.
15. Blanc, W. A., Santulli, T. V., and Anderson, D. H.: Pathogenesis of jejunoileal atresia, Amer. J. Dis. Child. **98**:564, 1959.
16. Bodian, M., White, L. L. R., Carter, C. O., and Louw, J. H.: Congenital duodenal obstruction and mongolism, Brit. Med. J. **1**:77, 1952.
17. Bryk, D.: Meconium ileus: demonstration of the meconium mass on barium enema study, Amer. J. Roentgen. **95**:214, 1965.
18. Burmester, H. B. C., Hall, R., and Munawer, N.: The Zollinger-Ellison syndrome in a child, Gut **10**:800, 1969.
19. Caffey, J., and Ross, S.: Mongolism (mongoloid deficiency) during early infance—Some newly recognized diagnostic changes in the pelvic bones, Pediatrics **17**:642, 1956.
20. Capitanio, M. A., and Kirkpatrick, J. A.: Lymphoid hyperplasia of the colon in children: Roentgen observations, Radiology **94**:323, 1970.
21. Case Records of the Massachusetts General Hospital, No. 17-1970, New Eng. J. Med. **282**:917, 1970.
22. Chalkley, T., and Bruce, J. W.: Neurofibromatosis of the colon, small intestine, and mesentery in a child, Amer. J. Dis. Child. **64**:888, 1942.
23. Clatworthy, H. W., Howard, W. H. R., and Loyd, J.: The meconium plug syndrome, Surgery **39**:131, 1956.
24. Cockshott, W. P.: Radiological aspects of Burkitt's tumor, Brit. J. Radiol. **38**:172, 1965.
25. Cordonnier, J. K., and Izant, R. J., Jr.: Meconium ileus equivalent, Surgery **54**:667, 1963.
26. Davidson, J. W., and Renouf, J. H. P.: Radiographic findings in "Burkitt type" lymphoma, J. Canad. Ass. Radiol. **19**:121, 1968.
27. di Sant'Agnese, P. A.: Cystic fibrosis of the pancreas, Amer. J. Med. **21**:406, 1956.

28. di Sant'Agnese, P. A., and Blanc, W. A.: A distinctive type of biliary cirrhosis of the liver associated with cystic fibrosis of the pancreas: recognition through signs of portal hypertension, Pediatrics **18**:387, 1956.

29. di Sant'Agnese, P. A., and Lepore, M. J.: Involvement of abdominal organs in cystic fibrosis of the pancreas, Gastroenterology **40**:64, 1961.

30. di Sant'Agnese, P. A., and Talamo, R. C.: Pathogenesis and physiopathology of cystic fibrosis of the pancreas, New Eng. J. Med. **277**:1287, 1967.

31. Dodds, W. J., Spitzer, R. M., and Friedland, G. W.: Gastrointestinal roentgenographic manifestations of hemophilia, Amer. J. Roentgen. **110**:413, 1970.

32. Donnison, A. B., Shwachman, H., and Gross, R. E.: A review of 164 children with meconium ileus seen at Children's Hospital Medical Center, Boston, Pediatrics **37**:833, 1966.

33. Dupree, E., Hodges, F., Jr., and Simon, J. L.: Epidermolysis bullosa of the esophagus, Amer. J. Dis. Child. **117**:349, 1969.

34. Ellis, D. G., and Clatworthy, H. W., Jr.: The meconium plug syndrome revisited, J. Pediat. Surg. **1**:54, 1966.

35. Emanuel, B., Padorr, M. P., and Swenson, O.: Mongolism associated with Hirschsprung's disease, J. Pediat. **66**:437, 1965.

36. Esterly, J. R., and Oppenheimer, E. H.: Observations in cystic fibrosis of the pancreas. I The gall bladder, Bull. Johns Hopkins Hosp. **110**:247, 1962.

37. Federman, D. D.: Down's syndrome, Clin. Pediat. **4**:331, 1965.

38. Feinberg, S. B., and Lester, R. G.: Roentgen examination of the gastrointestinal tract as an aid in the diagnosis of acute and subacute reticuloendotheliosis, Radiology **71**:525, 1958.

39. Feldman, W., and Belmonte, M. M.: The inspissated stool syndrome: an unusual mode of presentation of cystic fibrosis beyond the newborn period, Canad. Med. Ass. J. **96**:158, 1967.

40. Felson, B., and Levin, E. J.: Intramural hematoma of the duodenum: a diagnostic roentgen sign, Radiology **63**:823, 1954.

41. Felson, B., and Wiot, J. F.: Some interesting right lower quadrant entities, Radiol. Clin. N. Amer. **7**:83, 1969.

42. Fleisher, D. S., DiGeorge, A. M., Barness, L. A., and Cornfeld, D.: Hypoproteinemia and edema in infants with cystic fibrosis of the pancreas, J. Pediat. **64**:341, 1964.

43. Frech, R. S., McAlister, W. H., Ternberg, J., and Strominger, D.: Meconium ileus relieved by 40 per cent water soluble contrast enemas, Radiology **94**:341, 1970.

44. Geffen, N.: Rumination in man: report of a case, Amer. J. Dig. Dis. **11**:963, 1966.

45. Gellis, S. S., and Feingold, M.: Atlas of mental retardation syndromes: visual diagnosis of facies and physical findings, Washington, 1968, U. S. Government Printing Office.

46. Ghrist, T. D.: Gastrointestinal involvement in neurofibromatosis, Arch. Intern. Med. **112**:357, 1963.

47. Gildenhorn, H. L., Springer, E. B., and Amromin, G. D.: Necrotizing enteropathy: roentgenographic features, Amer. J. Roentgen. **88**:942, 1962.

48. Gillis, D. A., and Grantmyre, E. B.: The meconium-plug syndrome and Hirschsprung's disease, Canad. Med. Ass. J. **92**:225, 1965.

49. Glass, G. C.: Hemorrhage in a newly born infant, causing intestinal and biliary obstruction: report of a case with necropsy, Amer. J. Dis. Child. **54**:1052, 1937.

50. Glazer, J.: Personal communication. Cited in White, H., and Rowley, W. F.: Cystic fibrosis of the pancreas: clinical and roentgenographic manifestations, Radiol. Clin. N. Amer. **1**:539, 1961.

51. Goldberg, H. I., and Dodds, W. J.: Cobblestone esophagus due to monilial infection, Amer. J. Roentgen. **104**:608, 1968.

52. Gorlin, R. J., Sedano, H. O., Vickers, R. A., and others: Multiple mucosal neuromas, pheochromocytoma and medullary carcinoma of the thyroid-a syndrome, Cancer **22**:293, 479, 1968.

53. Grossman, H., Berdon, W. E., and Baker, D. H.: Reversible gastrointestinal signs of hemorrhage and edema in the pediatric age group, Radiology **84**:33, 1965.

54. Grossman, H., Berdon, W. E., Baker, D. H.: Gastrointestinal findings in cystic fibrosis, Amer. J. Roentgen. **97**:227, 1966.

55. Grossman, H., and Seed, W., Congenital hepatic fibrosis, bile duct dilatation, and renal lesion resembling medullary sponge kidney (congenital "cystic" disease of the liver and kidneys), Radiology **87**:46, 1966.

56. Gyepes, M. T., and Linde, L. M.: Familial dysautonomia: the mechanism of aspiration, Radiology **91**:471, 1968.

57. Hall, B.: Mongolism in newborn infants, Clin. Pediat. **5**:4, 1966.

58. Herbst, J., Friedland, G. W., and Zboralske, F. F.: Hiatal hernia and "rumination" in infants and children, J. Pediat. **78**:261, 1971.

59. Herson, R. E.: Meconium ileus, Radiology **68**:568, 1957.

60. Hide, D. W., and Burman, D.: An infant with both cystic fibrosis and coeliac disease, Arch. Dis. Child. **44**:533, 1969.

61. Holland, J. M., Haslam, R. A. H., and King, L. R.: Meconium in the processus vaginalis of infants, J. Urol. **92**:140, 1964.

62. Holsclaw, D. S., Eckstein, H. B., and Nixon, H. H.: Meconium ileus: a 20-year review of 109 cases, Amer. J. Dis. Child. **109**:101, 1965.

63. Jaffe, N., and Griscom, N. T.: Personal communication.

64. James, A. E., Jr., Belcourt, C. L., Atkins, L., and Janower, M. L.: Trisomy 18, Radiology **92**:37, 1969.

65. James, A. E., Jr., Belcourt, C. L., Atkins, L., and Janower, M. L.: Trisomy 13-15, Radiology **92**:44, 1969.

66. Johnson, W., and Borella, L.: Acute appendicitis in childhood leukemia, J. Pediat. **67**:595, 1965.

67. Kasmersky, C. T., and Howard, W. H. R.: The significance of intra-abdominal calcification in the newborn infant, Amer. J. Roentgen. **68**:395, 1952.

68. Kaufmann, H. J.: Candida oesophagitis in children with malignant disorders, Ann. Radiol. **13**:157, 1970.

69. Kerr, D. N. S., Warrick, C. K., and Hart-Mercer, J.: A lesion resembling medullary sponge kidney in patients with congenital hepatic fibrosis, Clin. Radiol. **13**:85, 1962.

70. Khilnani, M. T., Marshak, R. H., Eliasoph, J., and Wolf, B. S.: Intramural intestinal hemorrhage, Amer. J. Roentgen. **92**:1061, 1964.

71. Kinsbourne, M.: Hiatus hernia with contortions of the neck, Lancet **1**:1058, 1964.

72. Kulczycki, L. L., and Shwachman, H.: Studies in cystic fibrosis of the pancreas: occurrence of rectal prolapse, New. Eng. J. Med. **259**:409, 1958.

73. Leonidas, J. C., Berdon, W. E., Baker, D. H., and Santulli, T. V.: Meconium ileus and its complications: a reappraisal of plain film roentgen diagnostic criteria, Amer. J. Roentgen. **108**:598, 1970.

74. Littman, L., Boley, S. J., and Schwartz, S.: Sigmoidoscopic diagnosis of a reversible vascular occlusion of the colon, Dis. Colon Rectum **6**:142, 1963.

75. Louw, J. H., and Barnard, C. N.: Congenital intestinal atresia: observations of its origin, Lancet **2**:1065, 1955.

76. Ljungberg, O., Cederquist, E., and Studnitz, W. von: Medullary thyroid carcinoma and phaeochromocytoma: a familial chromaffinomatosis, Brit. Med. J. **1**:279, 1967.

77. Margulies, S. I., Brunt, P. W., Donner, M. W., and Silbiger, M. L.: Familial dysautonomia: a cineradiographic study of the swallowing mechanism, Radiology **90**:107, 1968.

78. Marshak, R. H., and Lindner, A. E.: Radiology of the small intestine, Philadelphia, 1970, W. B. Saunders Co.

79. Marshak, R. H., Wolf, B. S., and Eliasoph, J.: The roentgen findings in lymphosarcoma of the small intestine, Amer. J. Roentgen. **86**:682, 1961.

80. Mestel, A. L.: Lymphosarcoma of the small intestine in infancy and childhood, Ann. Surg. **149**:87, 1959.

81. Mestel, A. L., Trusler, G. A., Thompson, S. A., and Moes, C. A. F.: Acute obstruction of small intestine secondary to hematoma in children, Arch. Surg. **78**:25, 1959.

82. Middlemiss, J. H.: Hemophilia and Christmas disease, Clin. Radiol. **11**:40, 1960.

83. Miekle, J. E., Becker, K. L., and Gross, J. B.: Diverticulitis of the colon in a young man with Marfan's syndrome associated with carcinoma of the thyroid gland and neurofibromas of the tongue and lips, Gastroenterology **48**:379, 1965.

84. Moore, S. W., and Erlandson, M. E.: Intramural hematoma of the duodenum, Ann. Surg. **157**:798, 1963.

85. Mullins, F., Talamo, R., and di Sant'Agnese, P. A.: Late intestinal complications of cystic fibrosis, J.A.M.A. **192**:741, 1965.

86. Nelson, W. E., Vaughan, V. C., and McKay, R. J.: Textbook of pediatrics, ed. 9, Philadelphia, 1969, W. B. Saunders Co.

87. Neuhauser, E. B. D.: The roentgen diagnosis of fetal meconium peritonitis, Amer. J. Roentgen. **51**:421, 1944.

88. Neuhauser, E. B. D.: Roentgen changes associated with pancreatic insufficiency in early life, Radiology **46**:319, 1946.

89. Noblett, H. R.: Treatment of uncomplicated meconium ileus by gastrografin enema: a preliminary report, J. Pediat. Surg. **4**:190, 1969.

90. Oppenheimer, E. H., and Esterly, J. R.: Observations in cystic fibrosis of the pancreas. II Neonatal intestinal obstruction, Bull. Johns Hopkins Hosp. **3**:1, 1962.

91. Penrose, L. S., and Smith, G. F.: Down's anomaly, Boston, 1966, Little, Brown & Co.

92. Prolla, J. C., and Kirsner, J. B.: The gastrointestinal lesions and complications of the leukemias, Ann. Intern. Med. **61**:1084, 1964.

93. Reilly, B. J., Neuhauser, E. B. D.: Renal tubular ectasia in cystic disease of the kidneys and liver, Amer. J. Roentgen. **84**:546, 1960.

94. Riley, C. M., and Moore, R. H.: Familial dysautonomia differentiated from related disorders: case reports and discussions of current concepts, Pediatrics **37**:435, 1966.

95. Rosan, R. C., Shwachman, H., and Kulczycki, L. L.: Diabetes mellitus and cystic fibrosis of the pancreas, Amer. J. Dis. Child. **104**:625, 1962.

96. Rosenlung, M. L., Crean, G. P., Johnson, D. G., Holtzapple, P. D., and Brooks, F. P.: The Zollinger Ellison syndrome in a 10 year old boy, J. Pediat. **75**:443, 1969.

97. Santulli, T. V., and Blanc, W. A.: Congenital atresia of intestine: pathogenesis and treatment, Ann. Surg. **154**:939, 1961.

98. Sauvegrain, J., and Feigelson, J.: La cholécystographie dans la mucoviscidose, Ann. Radiol. **13**:311, 1970.

99. Sherman, R. S., and Wolfson, S. L.: Roentgen diagnosis of lymphosarcoma and reticulum cell sarcoma in infancy and childhood, Amer. J. Roentgen. **86**:693, 1961.

100. Shwachman, H., Diamond, L. K., Oski, F. A., and Khaw K-T.: The syndrome of pancreatic insufficiency and bone marrow dysfunction, J. Pediat. **65**:645, 1964.

101. Sidaway, M. D.: Torsion spasm and hiatus hernia, Ann. Radiol. **8**:15, 1965.

102. Siegal, D. L., and Bernstein, W. C.: Gastrointestinal complications of leukemias, Dis. Colon Rectum **8**:377, 1965.

103. Siegel, N. J., Margolis, C. Z., Long, J. J., and Spackman, T. J.: Syndrome of hiatus hernia with torsion spasms and abnormal posturing (Sandifer's syndrome), Amer. J. Dis. Child. **121**:53, 1971.

104. Smith, B., and Clatworthy, H. W., Jr.: Meconium peritonitis; prognostic significance, Pediatrics **27:** 967, 1961.

105. Smith, D. W.: Recognizable patterns of human malformation: genetic, embryologic, and clinical aspects, vol. 7, In major problems in clinical pediatrics, Philadelphia, 1970, W. B. Saunders Co.

106. Snyder, W. H., Gwinn, J. L., Landing, B. H., and Asay, L. D.: Fecal retention in children with cystic fibrosis: report of 3 cases, Pediatrics **34:**72, 1964.

107. Staple, T. W., McAlister, W. H., and Anderson, M. S.: Plexiform neurofibromatosis of the colon simulating Hirschsprung's disease, Amer. J. Roentgen. **91:**840, 1964.

108. Steinbach, H. L., Crane, J. T., and Bruyn, H. B.: The roentgen demonstration of cirrhosis of the liver with fatty metamorphosis: report of a case due to congenital fibrocystic disease, Radiology **62:**858, 1954.

109. Sutcliffe, J.: Torsion spasms and abnormal postures in children with hiatus hernia: Sandifer's syndrome, Progr. Pediat. Radiol. **2:**190, 1969.

110. Taybi, H., Mitchell, A. D., and Friedman, G. D.: Metaphyseal dysostosis and the associated syndrome of pancreatic insufficiency and blood disorders, Radiology **93:**563, 1969.

111. Thomaidis, T. S., Arey, J. B.: The intestinal lesions in cystic fibrosis of the pancreas, J. Pediat. **63:**444, 1963.

112. Van Buskirk, R. W., Kurlander, G. J., and Samter, T. G.: Intramural jejunal atresia and cystic fibrosis, Amer. J. Dis. Child. **110:**329, 1965.

113. Wagget, J., Johnson, D. G., Borns, P., and Bishop, H. C.: The nonoperative treatment of meconium ileus by gastrografin enema, J. Pediat. **77:**407, 1970.

114. Wagner, M. L., Rosenberg, H. S., Fernbach, D. J., and Singleton, E. B.: Typhlitis: a complication of leukemia in childhood, Amer. J. Roentgen. **109:** 341; 1970.

115. Warkany, J., Passarge, E., Smith, L. B.: Congenital malformations in autosomal trisomy syndromes, Amer. J. Dis. Child. **112:**502, 1966.

116. Weinstein, L. D., Clemett, A. R., and Herskovic, T.: Morphologic and radiologic findings in the intestines in cystic fibrosis, Gastroenterology **54:**1282, 1968.

117. White, H.: Meconium ileus: a new roentgen sign, Radiology **66:**567, 1956.

118. White, H., and Rowley, W. F.: Cystic fibrosis of the pancreas: clinical and roentgenographic manifestations, Radiol. Clin. N. Amer. **1:**539, 1963.

119. Williams, E. D., and Pollock, D. J.: Multiple mucosal neuromata with endocrine tumours: A syndrome allied to von Recklinghausen's disease, J. Path. Bact. **91:**71, 1966.

120. Wiot, J. F.: Intramural small intestinal hemorrhage:—a differential diagnosis, Seminars Roentgen. **1:**219, 1966.

121. Wolf, B. S.: Case #29 intramural hematoma of terminal ileum and ileocecal valve due to hemophilia, J. Mt. Sinai Hosp. **25:**89, 1958.

122. Wolfson, J. J., Goldstein, G., Krivit, W., and Hong, R.: Lymphoid hyperplasia of the large intestine associated with dysgammaglobulinemia: report of a case, Amer. J. Roentgen. **108:**610, 1970.

123. Wright, F. W., and Matthews, J. M.: Hemophilic pseudotumor of the stomach, Radiology **98:**547, 1971.

124. Zuelzer, W. W., Newton, W. A.: Pathogenesis of fibrocystic disease of the pancreas: a study of 36 cases with special reference to the pulmonary lesions, Pediatrics **4:**53, 1949.

Part XI

Infectious and vascular diseases

Gastrointestinal parasites | 59

J. Howard Middlemiss

Abu Ali al Hussein ibn Abdullah ibn Sina, more familiarly known as Avicenna (A.D. 980-1037), in his treatise *Kitab al Qanun* described for the first time with meticulous care the symptoms produced by tapeworms, roundworms, and threadworms. Not only was he the first physician to appreciate the connection between these helminths and the symptoms they produced, but he also first differentiated between anthelmintics, which killed the worms, and purgatives, which merely promoted their evacuation, and first realized the importance of administering a purgative after an anthelmintic drug in order to eliminate the dead worms and avert systemic toxemia caused by their disintegration within the bowel.

However, Avicenna was by no means the first to be aware of the presence of parasitic worms in the alimentary tract. In the Ebers Papyrus, inscribed 2,500 years earlier in ancient Egypt (circa 1550 B.C.), there are recognizable descriptions of tapeworm and roundworm infection, as well as of infection with *Schistosoma haematobium*. Ancient Hebrew writings contain many passages that, in the light of modern knowledge, may be interpreted as referring to parasitic infections. The description of the plague of fiery serpents given in the Book of Numbers undoubtedly refers to the guinea worm; the method of extraction recommended, winding the worm around a piece of stick, is not only still used in indigenous areas but also forms the symbol by which the medical profession is known throughout the world.

Parasitism can be defined as a physiologic association between two organisms belonging to different species, one of which (the parasite) is smaller and weaker and lives within or on the surface of the body of the larger and stronger one (the host), from which it obtains its food and on which it generally inflicts some degree of injury. There are many forms of parasite, and in particular of intestinal parasites, to which man is heir—a state of affairs that cannot provoke great wonder. The anthropoid ancestors of man handed down a considerable legacy of parasites, as we know from modern geologic and veterinary studies, and to this, succeeding ages have added. As man moved to a terrestrial habitat from his arboreal ancestors, contact with swamp and river waters brought schistosomiasis; the habit of walking on ground led to increasing frequency of infection with *Strongyloides* and hookworms. The invention of primitive weapons, which enabled him to kill animals, brought with it such meat-borne infections as tapeworms. The domestication of animals brought as a consequence animal infections like hydatid cyst. The habit of eating fish brought liver fluke to man. Thus evolution towards civilization brought with it many forms of parasitism that inevitably affected the health of man.

Some parasites are favored by warm climates, either in general or by the presence of appropriate intermediate hosts in those climates, and so many of the diseases ascribed to the presence of parasitism are most common in tropical and subtropical zones of the world. However, in modern circumstances, where education, hygiene, and sanitation may be ideal or if not ideal are at least controlled, incidence of these conditions has in many instances been reduced or even eliminated. The incidence rate can thus be related to geography, social status, cultural practices, education, hygiene, and public facilities such as water supply and sanitation.

In general, of the principal parasitic infections affecting man the highest world incidence is that of ascariasis (roundworm), followed by ankylostomiasis (hookworm), trichuriasis (whipworm), enterobiasis (threadworm), and infection with *Wuchereria bancrofti* (the filarial infection that may cause lymphedema or elephantiasis). Not all of these infections involve the alimentary tract, and not all produce changes that are of roentgenologic significance. They are, however, all caused by helminths, or parasitic worms. The helminths are classified according to their zoologic characteristics. Those that can cause diseases in man that may be of roentgenologic significance fall within the classes of nematodes (roundworms), trematodes (flukes), cestodes (segmented worms), and pentastomides (tongue worms).

In addition to infection with parasitic worms, the condition of amebiasis may occur, arising in the first instance from intestinal infection by the protozoan parasite, *Entamoeba histolytica*. Similarly, an intestinal flagellate, *Giardia lamblia*, can cause the condition of giardiasis.

HELMINTHIC INFECTIONS
Roundworms (nematodes)
Ankylostomiasis (hookworm disease)

Hookworm infection may be a transitory and relatively unimportant event to an otherwise healthy person, but chronic or frequent massive infection, as occurs in epidemic form among many malnourished peoples in developing countries, is associated with a debilitating clinical syndrome called hookworm disease. The effects of hookworm disease depend upon a number of factors, such as the extent of the infection, the type of worm, and the nutritional status of the patient.

The common features are pallor, fatigue, weakness, dizziness, varied gastrointestinal disturbances, malnutrition, retarded growth, and anemia; the latter, which results from intestinal bleeding, may be of such severity that cardiac function is impaired. The parasite enters the body through the skin, probably the skin of the feet in many communities where the people are unshod, and passes through the lung on its way to the duodenojejunal region, where the females

rapidly mature. The worm attaches itself to the mucosa of the duodenum and small intestine and sucks the blood of the host, passing it through its own lumen into the lumen of the intestine. In addition, there is oozing of blood from the sites of attachment of the worm.

Many patients have hookworm ova in the stool but show no roentgenologic abnormality on barium examination of the upper alimentary tract. Early workers stated that thick mucosal folds may be shown in the duodenum and upper jejunum,[18] but this feature alone is a notoriously difficult roentgenologic sign to evaluate. More recently it has been shown that a malabsorption pattern with steatorrhea may occur.[31,32] This pattern has been variously described as consisting of mucosal folds in the jejunum that are thickened and irregular, with "cog-wheel irregularities," a moderate degree of flocculation, "puddling," and segmentation. Intestinal hurry has also been described. It is also worthy of note that in a large series reported from West Africa there was no evidence of malabsorption.[13]

Strongyloidiasis

Infection with *Strongyloides stercoralis*, a helminthic parasite entering the body by the skin and passing through the lung on its way to the duodenum and upper jejunum, is widespread in tropical countries. Although in the majority of instances the infection is asymptomatic, serious disease and even death may ensue.[4] In fact, the condition carries a relatively high mortality. Symptoms may occur in the skin or the lungs, where there may be a pneumonitis, but the most common complaints are related to the alimentary tract. Infection with this parasite should be borne in mind in examining any undernourished patient, especially if he has severe malnutrition, who complains of abdominal symptoms. The parasite is cosmopolitan, occurring in many parts of the world, but since its free-living stages are favored by warmth it is more abundant in the tropics and subtropics than in temperate climates. Its distribution approximately parallels that of hookworm, and since its ova and larvae resemble very closely those of hookworm (though there are several points of specific difference) it is possible that this parasite may have been underdiagnosed in the past.

It has been shown[24] that infection with *Strongyloides* may produce duodenitis and je-

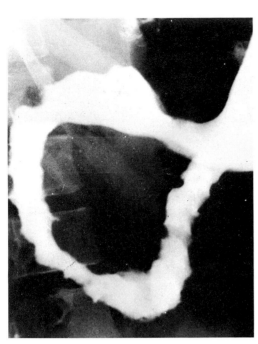

Fig. 59-1. Duodenal loop in a gross case of strongyloidiasis showing pipestem rigidity. (Courtesy Dr. J. Barton.)

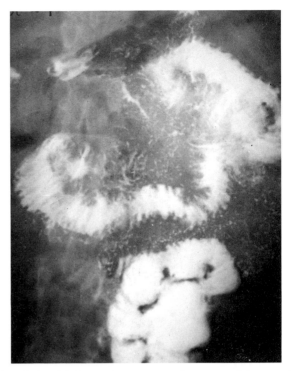

Fig. 59-2. Malabsorption pattern in upper jejunum in strongyloidiasis. (Courtesy Prof. P. Cockshott.)

junitis and that this can lead to intestinal malabsorption and steatorrhea (Fig. 59-1). Whereas hookworms are merely attached to the mucosa, in strongyloidiasis the worms, particularly the larvae, invade the mucosa, causing edema and inflammation of the intestinal walls. This can lead to a stenosis, resulting in persistent vomiting and consequent malnutrition. Paralytic ileus as the result of massive invasion of the bowel wall has been described.[27] Duodenal biopsy has shown the lesions to consist of flattening of villi, with infiltration by inflammatory cells and invasion by worms and with ova in the mucosal crypts, and has also shown the condition to be reversible after successful treatment.[24]

The roentgenologic appearances are characteristic enough to arouse suspicion of duodenal infection, although they are not specific to the disease. Plain film examination of the abdomen may show distention of the stomach and duodenum or even of the whole upper alimentary tract. Barium examination may show dilatation of the proximal two thirds of the duodenum, edematous mucosal folds, delay in the third part

of the loop (even amounting to duodenal ileus), or stenosis, usually in the third or fourth part of the duodenum. Cineradiographic studies have demonstrated abnormal motility of the duodenum, and a completely aperistaltic duodenal loop with obliteration of mucosal folds, producing a rigid pipestem appearance with irregular narrowing, has been described.[24] Similarly, extensive ulceration throughout the duodenal loop has been demonstrated.

The appearances in the duodenum may be reversible under treatment. But in severe cases, though treatment may rid the patient of the infection with no worms, larvae, or eggs detectable in the stool, there may be no change in the roentgenologic pattern. This is particularly so when an apparent stenosis has been demonstrated.

In severe cases there may be delay in gastric emptying and dilatation of the upper jejunal loops, with swelling of mucosal folds. In long-standing cases with malnutrition, a malabsorption steatorrhea pattern in the small bowel may be demonstrated (Fig. 59-2).

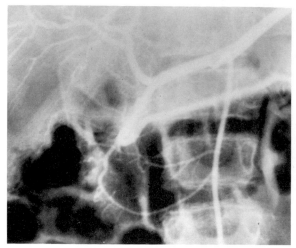

Fig. 59-3. Celiac axis arteriogram in a case of strongyloidiasis, showing dilatation of the pancreaticoduodenal artery.

Ascariasis (roundworm disease)

Ascaris lumbricoides infection is cosmopolitan in distribution, occurring in all parts of the world. Naturally it is most common where education and hygiene are of a low order. According to Watson it affects approximately 30% of the world population, and in some parts of the Caribbean, the Far East, and the Middle East the incidence may be as high as 50% to 80% of the population.[35] Man is infected by ingesting ova from contaminated vegetables, water, or soil. An ovum passed in the excreta undergoes a molt within its capsule and then becomes infective to man. On being swallowed the ova hatch in the small bowel; then the larvae penetrate the intestinal wall and enter venules or lymphatics, migrating to the lungs by way of either the liver or the thoracic duct. In the pulmonary capillaries they become arrested and emerge into the alveoli. This migration takes about a week. From the alveoli they voyage by the branchioles, bronchi, trachea, glottis, and esophagus to the jejunum, where they mature in 2 to 2½ months.

The mature roundworm, varying in length from 15 to 35 cm., is capable of producing 200,000 eggs daily. Once it is established, ascariasis is readily diagnosed by microscopic examination of the stools, for the eggs have a well-recognized appearance.

The clinical severity of any symptoms or signs ascribed to ascariasis depends upon the density

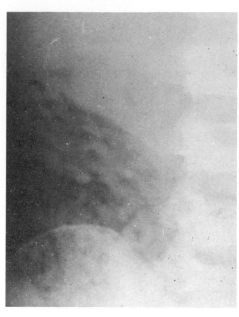

Fig. 59-4. Soft tissue film of abdomen of a child showing multiple ascarides in a loop of bowel.

of the infection. The effect of such an infection results from hypersensitivity and from the mechanical presence of large numbers of worms.

During maturation and passage through the lungs ascaris pneumonitis may occur, often heralded by hemoptysis. Small areas of consolidation in the lungs may be seen roentgenologically at this period. However, this feature is rarely demonstrated conclusively, since the examination and diagnosis presuppose a high degree of suspicion and clinical awareness by the physician.

The adult worms inhabit the jejunum and in the less sophisticated parts of the world are frequently noted in barium examination of the gastrointestinal tract. The clinical significance of sporadic findings of this sort is difficult to assess.

Makidino states that 99% of the worms reside in the jejunum and ileum, mostly in the mid-jejunum.[19] They may, however, be seen in the duodenum or stomach and have been reported in the common bile and pancreatic ducts.[16] Jaundice may occur if the biliary tract has been entered, and pseudocysts of the pancreas have been described following penetration of the pancreatic duct.[11]

On plain film examination of the abdomen a single adult ascaris may be seen as a long, slen-

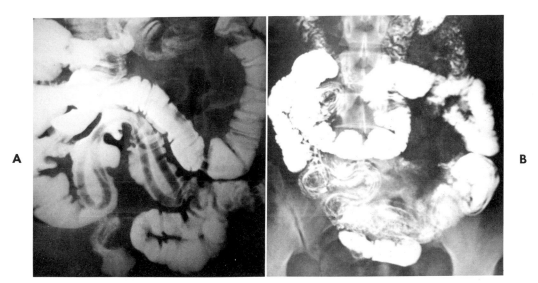

Fig. 59-5. **A,** *Ascaris* in the mid small bowel outlined with barium. **B,** *Ascaris* in the small bowel with the alimentary tract of the *ascaris* demonstrated. (Courtesy Dr. J. P. Balikian.)

der, curved shadow within an intestinal gas shadow. In children in areas where endemicity is high, such as Nigeria or Southeast Asia, a common cause of intestinal obstruction is massive infection by roundworms, a bolus of worms actually plugging the lumen of the intestine and causing partial obstruction. Plain film examination of suspected cases of intestinal obstruction may therefore reveal masses of coiled worms contrasted against intestinal gas (Fig. 59-4). Obstruction should be attributed to the worms only if large numbers are clearly revealed. Diatrizoate methylglucamine (Gastrografin) has been given in cases of doubt and establishes the diagnosis.

At barium examination of the small bowel the barium coats the body of the ascaris, which appears as two radiopaque parallel lines within the lumen of the bowel. The apposing surfaces, 3 to 5 mm. apart, are smooth, and the radiolucent filling defect represents the cylindric body of the ascaris (Fig. 59-5, *A*). If the patient has been fasting for more than 12 hours often the barium may be ingested by the worm, and its alimentary tract appears as a longitudinally bisecting thin line along the length of the worm, usually wider at its anterior end (Fig. 59-5, *B*). After evacuation of the barium by the patient the barium may remain in the alimentary tract

of the worm and appear as a thin, curved "string" line. If there are multiple worms they appear as a tangled mass of filling defects, some with barium coating them and some with barium in their alimentary tracts.

In the biliary tract the presence of an ascaris in the common bile duct may be shown at intravenous cholangiography and such demonstrations are improved and the diagnosis is made more certain by tomography.[8]

Oesophagostomum apiostomum and Oesophagostomum stephanostomum

Oesophagostomum apiostomum and *Oesophagostomum stephanostomum* are nematode worms normally parasitic in various species of apes and monkeys in Africa, India, the Philippines, and China and are occasionally found in man. It has been stated that *Oesophagostomum apiostomum* has been found in 4% of prisoners in jails in Northern Nigeria.[20] The adult worm is about 2 cm. long.

Infection is by the oral route; the larvae, on reaching the cecum or colon, penetrate the bowel wall, where they give rise to nodule formation. Histologically these lesions show extensive edema with chronic inflammation and fibrosis involving the submucosa, muscularis, and pericolonic fatty tissues. Rupture of these

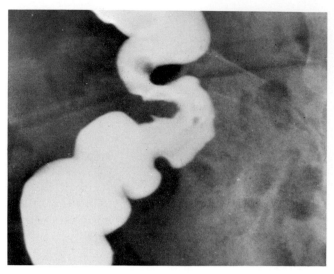

Fig. 59-6. A crypt in a narrow segment of colon in a patient infected with *Oesophagostomum apiostomum*. (Courtesy Dr. M. Welchman.)

nodules may give rise to ulcer formation, hemorrhage, and dysenteric symptoms and paves the way for secondary infection with pyogenic organisms. Helminthic abscess, or helminthoma, thus formed may be seen at barium enema examination with characteristic though not diagnostic appearances.[36] The nodular stage may appear as a filling defect, most commonly in the cecum but possibly elsewhere in the bowel. If rupture of the nodule has taken place the worm track may be seen as an ulcer or spiky projection from the bowel lumen, almost certainly in a segment of colon that will not distend normally because of the surrounding inflammatory reaction or granulomatous mass (Fig. 59-6). Occasionally the parasites may become entombed in the granulomatous and fibrous mass, and the cretified worm may be seen as a calcified spiral or crescentic shadow within the abdomen.

Dracunculus medinensis (guinea worm disease)

A nematode worm infection that is widespread throughout a belt stretching across Africa and Asia and now the Caribbean, is caused by the *Dracunculus medinensis*, commonly known as guinea worm. This does not cause alimentary tract disease, but since the alimentary tract is the portal of entry the disease merits brief mention here.

The female worm, lying in the subcutaneous tissues of the infected person, discharges mobile larvae into water through a blister ulcer. These larvae are ingested by a species of water flea *(Cyclops),* where they ungergo metamorphosis. The infected water flea is later ingested with water by man (the condition only occurs after a person drinks polluted water and disappears when a locality obtains a good piped water supply). The larvae emerge from the *Cyclops* to pass through the intestinal wall and migrate into the subcutaneous tissues of the host. After fertilization the female worm seeks to come to the surface of the body, preferably in a part of the body that comes into contact with water, such as the legs, and there discharges her eggs. Having done so she dies, and after necrosis the body of the worm becomes calcified. A calcified worm is of no clinical significance; it is merely a manifestation of the entombed, cretified past event.

Roentgenologically these calcified worms have a characteristic appearance. They may show as tangled, whorled opacities or as stringlike curvilinear calcifications. They may occur anywhere in the muscle tissue planes, neck, thorax, trunk, or pelvis, but most commonly in the lower limb (Fig. 59-7).[22]

Flukes (trematodes)

The flukes consist of four main groups classified by the site or system that the parasite chooses as its habitat in man: the intestinal, the liver, the lung, and the circulatory flukes.

Intestinal flukes (Busk's fluke)

Of the intestinal flukes, Busk's fluke *(Fasciolopsis buski)* is the most important and probably the most widely disseminated, occurring throughout Southeast Asia, especially South China, Formosa, Indochina, Assam, Bengal, Siam, Borneo, Sumatra, and the Malay Peninsula. The intermediate host is a snail from which cercariae emerge to encyst on aquatic vegetation. The latter is ingested by man, and the parasite excysts and attaches itself to the wall of the duodenum. It is a worm 2 to 7 cm. long and ranging from 1 to 2 cm. wide. At present I know of no roentgenologic case report of the demonstration of this worm, but in view of its extensive distribution, its size, its traumatic effect on the duodenal and jejunal mucosa, where deep inflammatory ulcerations occur, and

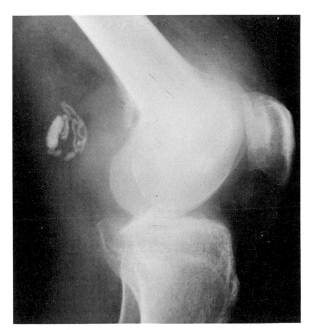

Fig. 59-7. Calcified guinea worm lying behind the knee joint.

its severe clinical manifestations, there can be no doubt that roentgenologic literature on the subject is merely a question of time.

Liver flukes

Of the liver flukes there are two main species that affect man. The sheep liver fluke *(Fasciola hepatica)* occurs in Europe, the U.S.S.R., the Middle East, Asia, Africa, Australia, and Central and South America. Its life cycle and the mode of infection of man are similar to those of Busk's fluke, but the adult worms, measuring 2 to 3 cm. in length, live in the bile ducts. The Chinese liver fluke *(Clonorchis sinensis)* occurs throughout East Asia in Japan, Korea, Central and South China, Formosa, and Indochina. This parasite has two intermediate hosts, a snail followed by fresh-water fish of which about forty different species have been incriminated. Man becomes infected by eating the raw or only partially cooked fish. These parasites also measure 2 to 3 cm. in length and live in the bile ducts.[15]

In liver fluke disease the cercariae migrate from the alimentary tract to the liver in the portal venous circulation, where they mature to become worms. The migration of the young worms through the liver parenchyma to the bile ducts damages and destroys hepatic tissue, caus-

ing inflammation, necrosis, and fibrosis. Liver abscess is a not uncommon event in such infections.[12] Also, the flukes may crowd together and plug a smaller duct, thereby causing remittent and incomplete obstruction. Biliary stasis then sets in, and the portion of the duct proximal to the block may become dilated. Stagnation of bile favors bacterial infection and leads to cholangitis.

At operative cholangiography the flukes may be demonstrated. They have a characteristic crescentic shape, appearing either as a filling defect within the filled bile duct or as a semilunar mound attached to the wall of a duct (Fig. 59-8).

Lung flukes

There is only one form of lung fluke, the *Paragonimus westermani,* the cause of paragonimiasis, which is endemic in the Far East and also is known to occur in West Africa and South America. The definitive host, man, acquires the infection by ingesting raw crab or crayfish containing infective cercariae that excyst in the duodenum and migrate through the intestinal wall, abdominal cavity, diaphragm, and pleural cavity to reach the lungs. The nature of the migration route by the young worms gives abundant opportunity for aberration and consequent development of adults in ectopic foci. Therefore, in addition to the typical pulmonary form of the disease other clinical types are occasionally recognized, of which the abdominal type is one. In this condition lesions resulting from the presence of worms in the liver, pancreas, peritoneum or intestinal wall may occur.

I know of no specific alimentary tract roentgenologic changes attributed to this fluke, but it seems likely that its presence in an ectopic site, causing the symptoms it is known to cause, and with its wide geographic distribution in the Far East, will in the not too distant future be found to produce demonstrable roentgenologic changes.

Circulatory flukes (Schistosoma)

The circulatory flukes comprise the schistosomes, of which there are three main forms infective to man and which are responsible for the disease known as schistosomiasis or bilharzia. The three forms are *Schistosoma haematobium,* occurring throughout Africa, the Mediterranean and Southwest Asia; *Schistosoma mansoni, oc-*

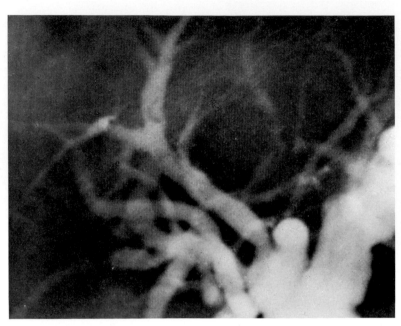

Fig. 59-8. *Clonorchis sinensis* showing as a crescentic filling defect in a hepatic duct. (Courtesy Dr. H. C. Ho.)

curring in parts of Africa, Arabia, the West Indies, and the northern part of South America; and *Schistosoma japonicum,* occurring in the coastal area of China, Japan, Formosa, the Philippines, and Celebes. Owing to their overlapping distribution, *Schistosoma haematobium* and *Schistosoma mansoni* infections not infrequently occur in the same patient.

The worms live in pairs in copula in the portal vein and tributaries of the definitive host. The female leaves the male and swims against the direction of the blood flow to reach the capillaries and venules in the wall of either the urinary bladder *(Schistosoma haematobium)* or the intestine and rectum *(Schistosoma mansoni* and *Schistosoma japonicum)* and there deposits its eggs. Occasionally *Schistosoma haematobium* reaches and deposits its eggs in the intestinal wall.

The eggs leave the host in the urine or feces by rupturing the enclosing blood vessels and so are accompanied by the passage of blood and often by disturbance of bowel habit. The eggs, on reaching water, hatch to release miracidia, which penetrate the suitable snail hosts that inhabit slow-moving streams, irrigation canals, paddy fields, and lakes. After about a month of maturation in the snail, cercariae emerge into

the water, many thousands from each miracidium. The cercaria then penetrates the unbroken human skin or buccal mucous membrane (it is destroyed in the stomach by gastric acidity) to enter the definitive host, enters the lymphatics, and is carried through the lymph nodes, thoracic duct, lungs, and left heart to the mesenteric capillaries and thence to the portal system and liver. The larvae do not break through into the lung air spaces as do the juveniles of *Ascaris.* They mature in the liver and then return in pairs to the portal system, where they may continue to live for 10 to 15 years. With such a complicated migration it is not surprising that some worms mature in other organs or that some go astray causing small hemorrhages and are destroyed, producing fibrosis.

The main clinical manifestations occur during the period of oviposition and are mainly caused by the presence of eggs in the tissues and by the irritation and reaction caused by them.

When *Schistosoma* eggs ulcerate through the mucous membrane of the rectum and colon, healing takes place by fibrosis. Because many hundreds of eggs are being passed a considerable fibrotic reaction occurs, and as subsequent crops of eggs reach the terminal capillaries their

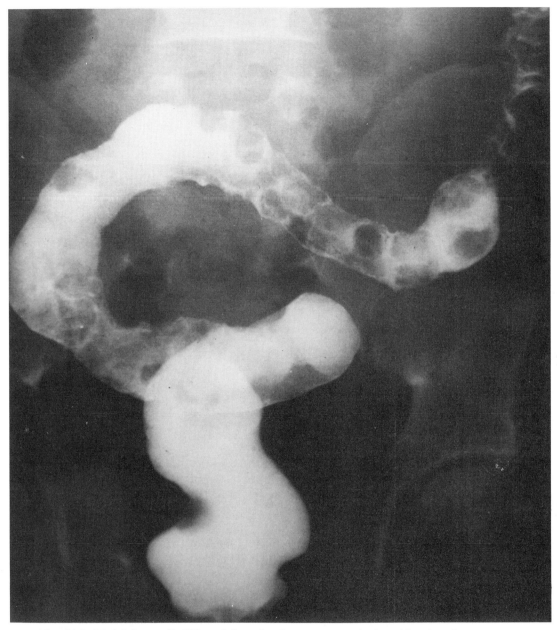

Fig. 59-9. Multiple small filling defects in the rectum and sigmoid colon in a patient infected with *Schistosoma mansoni*.

way to ulceration is barred and they become entombed, although some may be carried back with the venous flow to become lodged in the portal system where they produce a periportal cirrhosis. In the wall of the bowel the irritative action of the ova may produce a further tissue reaction, with granulomas forming around them.

As a result of the periportal fibrosis, hepatomegaly usually occurs, and the liver may reach a very considerable size. Since portal hypertension often develops secondarily, there may be great splenomegaly, and the roentgenologic features of portal hypertension, that is, gastric varices and esophageal varices may be demonstrated as the collateral circulation develops. These are late features of the disease but are common in long-standing cases of *Schistosoma mansoni* and *Schistosoma japonicum* infections.

Plain x-ray examination of the abdomen may therefore reveal hepatomegaly and splenomegaly, either with or without elevation of the right dome of the diaphragm, and displacement of the stomach gas shadow.

Barium enema examination may show alteration in the bowel lumen or in its mucosal surface. Polypoid masses may appear as multiple small filling defects, most profuse in the sigmoid colon, or they may appear singly or with a lobulated surface (Fig. 59-9). Ragheb first showed this in Egypt, where there is mixed *Schistosoma mansoni* and *Schistosoma haematobium* infection,[29] and subsequently in Egypt Dimmette and his colleagues confirmed these findings.[9]

The lesions are best seen after evacuation and preferably with air insufflation. More recently Medina and colleagues have shown that in Puerto Rico, where the infection is pure *Schistosoma mansoni*, polyps, though they occur, are less frequent and that diffuse induration with extensive pericolonic infiltration is more common.[21] Thus in their experience granulomatous colitis, strictures, and polyps are the chief roentgenologic manifestations. Occasionally these parasitic granulomas assume large proportions projecting into the bowel, narrowing the lumen, and producing obstructive symptoms. These lesions have been reported from Brazil in *Schistosoma mansoni* infection[33] and from China in *Schistosoma japonicum* infection.[6] Roentgenologically they are indistinguishable from carcinoma, and even after excision may appear to have the features of neoplasm; only histologic examination shows their true nature.

Ileus has been known to occur in *Schistosomiasis mansoni* infections, and Tesluk described the pathologic findings in such a case.[34] The schistosomiasis was limited to the distal 6 cm. of ileum, and there was intense edema with lymphangitic and endophlebitic lesions, resembling regional enteritis. Medina and his colleagues have also published what looks like the classic appearances of regional enteritis occurring in a case of *Schistosomiasis mansoni* infection.[21] It has been known for some time that eggs may be passed in very large numbers from the small bowel, and it would indeed be surprising if no accompanying roentgenologic changes were to occur. It seems reasonable, in conditions where the eggs being passed are known to produce a hypersensitivity to this foreign protein, to expect that the local tissue reaction may be of this nature. Similarly it might be expected that some effect on absorption might take place, producing a malabsorption pattern. Recently in Uganda Briers has shown this very feature in some few cases of uncomplaining subjects with proved *Schistosoma mansoni* infection. As yet it is too early to state that the schistosomiasis can be incriminated for the condition. In a disease so widespread over the earth's surface—almost 200 million people in the world have one form or another of schistosomiasis—much more work remains to be done.[4a]

Segmented worms or tapeworms (cestodes)

The two common tapeworms to occur in man are the beef tapeworm (*Taenia saginata*) and the pork tape worm (*Taenia solium*). The life cycle is identical in both, only the intermediate host (cattle or pig) differing. The adult worm lives in the alimentary tract of man, attached by its scolex to the mucosal surface usually of the mid small bowel. The worms vary from 6 to 30 feet in length. They have no alimentary tract and absorb their nutrition from the contents of the intestine through their surfaces. Eggs are passed with the stool of the definitive host and are ingested by grazing cattle or pigs. The egg hatches in the intestine of the intermediate host, and the oncosphere bores through the intestinal wall to reach a blood vessel or lymph channel, whence it is carried to striated muscle. There the larva develops into cysticercus bovis in cattle and cysticercus cellulosae in the pig, and finally the life cycle is completed by man's eating raw or insufficiently cooked meat from the relevant animal. The pork tapeworm is cosmopolitan in distribution, whereas the beef tapeworm is commonest in Moslem countries and in the Far East. They usually occur only singly in an individual.

There are frequently no clinical manifestations of this infection, but there may be abdominal discomfort, anorexia, chronic indigestion, or diarrhea. There is usually an eosinophilia. More severe complications such as appendicitis caused by the presence of proglottides in the lumen of the appendix have been reported.

Reports of roentgenologic demonstration of the worm have been few.[14,25] It is usually shown in the lower ileum. This parasite broadens in shape from its neck, where it is 1 to 2 mm. wide, to its distal end, where it may be 12 mm. wide. The appearance within the barium-filled small bowel, therefore, is of a translucent line that is broader more distally. Its point of attachment is rarely shown since it is so narrow. Because it is so long, it may become folded and reduplicated upon itself, but it nevertheless appears mainly as a continuous structure. Since it has no alimentary tract no barium is seen within it. Its great length, its site in the lower ileum, its gradual broadening, and the absence of barium from within it help to distinguish it from ascaris infection.

In the case of the pork tapeworm man may also act as the intermediate host, in places where sanitation is poor, by ingesting the eggs. When this happens the individual develops cysticercosis. The cysticercus cellulosae cyst is irritant to the host and becomes encapsulated with fibrous tissue and eventually calcifies following the death of the parasite. Calcification takes about 5 years to occur. The effect on man, of course, depends on the number and location of the cysts. In muscle they may not give rise to symptoms. In the brain they can give rise to epileptiform attacks. The calcification tends to be patchy, and the densest area corresponds to the scolex.

Tongue worms (pentastomides)

Only one of the tongue worms is of medical significance, and it is not strictly a gastrointestinal parasite, though it gains entry into man through the alimentary tract.

Armillifer armillatus, which along with *Armillifer moniliformis* is responsible for the condition known as porocephaliasis, falls into this category. The tongue worms are degenerate wormlike arthropods. They are parasites living in the trachea and bronchi of snakes, *Armillifer armillatus* being found in African pythons and *Armillifer moniliformis* is snakes in India, Malaya, and the East Indies. The eggs of the adult worms reach the outside world in the saliva and excreta of the snake and are then ingested with contaminated water or food by rats, monkeys, and other wild animals. Man may become the host in a similar fashion. When the eggs have reached the intestinal tract of the host, the larvae are liberated, penetrate the intestine, and come to lie under the peritoneum, there molting to become nymphs. Some may migrate across the diaphragm to lie in the pleural cavity. For the cycle to be repeated it is necessary for the snake to eat the animal containing the encysted nymphs.

In many individuals there are probably no symptoms attributable to the presence of nymphs; however, a heavy infection of worms may simulate an acute abdominal emergency with peritoneal irritation. At laparotomy live nymphs have been found wriggling beneath the peritoneum. If they do not appear thus, the worms die, become necrotic, and calcify.

Roentgenologically, the phase of active invasion has not been described. Most cases have occurred in out-of-the-way places as acute abdominal emergencies. However, when the nymphs become necrotic and calcify they may be demonstrated. They are always multiple and may be seen in the abdomen and thorax. The

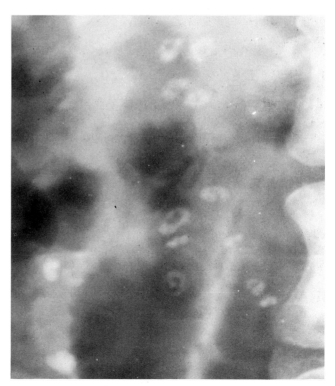

Fig. 59-10. Calcified *Armillifer armillatus* in the peritoneum.

calcified shadow outlines the coiled nymph and is crescentic.[2] Its characteristic shape and its absence from muscle distinguish it from cysticercosis (Fig. 59-10).

OTHER INTESTINAL PARASITIC DISEASES
Amebic dysentery (amebiasis)

Amebic dysentery and its complications are caused primarily by infection of the large bowel with the protozoan parasite *Entamoeba histolytica.* The mode of infection is by ingestion of contaminated water and foodstuffs. Flies are probably a potent source of spread. The distribution of the disease is worldwide, but it is most common in warm climates and where sanitation is poor. In the tropics the parasite can live as a commensal in intestinal contents, but in circumstances not yet fully understood it can eat its way into the mucosa and submucosa. During dysenteric attacks amebas are swept out to the exterior in loose stools; during intermissions cysts are passed in the formed stools. Diagnosis is established by recovery and identification of the parasite. Amebic infection can travel from the large intestine either by direct extension to surrounding tissues or by embolism in the portal circulation, thus giving rise to amebic hepatitis and liver abscess; this in turn may cause involvement of the diaphragm, pleura, and lung. Other ectopic sites such as the brain or other organs may be affected by hematogenous spread. In the event of direct extension from the large intestine, hard tumors, called amebomas, caused by amebic infection together with a secondary bacterial infection, form in, on, or adjacent to the bowel. These are often mistaken for neoplasms and treated surgically; a colostomy leaking ameba-laden matter is followed by amebic infection of the wound tissues, with a spreading area of cutaneous amebiasis.

Clinically the bowel infection may manifest itself as an acute attack of diarrhea with loose, mucoid, blood-stained stools. The attack may subside spontaneously after a few days or may persist for weeks. Periods of remission alternate with subsequent attacks, and this pattern may continue for years. This pattern of remission and exacerbation is the picture of chronic amebic dysentery. In the primary infection of the bowel the lesions are most plentiful at points of stasis, the cecum and the hepatic and splenic flexures. The pathologic process is an amebic invasion of the mucosa and submucosa, causing local necrosis with much cell debris and mucosal sloughing. Secondary bacterial infection of these lesions produces a true inflammatory reaction.

The diagnosis of amebiasis rests on identification of the parasite. However, examination of specimens is not always entirely satisfactory, and the diagnosis of chronic amebic dysentery or of liver or pulmonary complications may first be suspected roentgenologically. Despite this fact, the real function of roentgenologic examinations in suspected cases is probably not so much as a diagnostic tool in the first instance, as a means of demonstrating the extent of the disease in known cases.

The roentgenologic changes are described best as those affecting the bowel and those affecting the liver and thorax.

Changes affecting the bowel

At barium enema examination there may be changes in contour or in mucosal pattern, strictures, amebomas, or fistula formations. Each of these is discussed in the following paragraphs.

Changes in contour. The normal saclike shape of the cecum may disappear and be replaced by a narrow funnel shape. The cecum is said to be less distensible and to be shaggy in appearance. Obviously a fecal residue may cause similar appearances. Air insufflation after evacuation may clear any doubts, but in the presence of severe disease demonstrable elsewhere in the colon during the examination it may be wise to avoid air insufflation. There may be associated apparent shortening of the ascending colon, presumably resulting from spasm.

Changes in mucosal pattern. Changes in mucosal pattern are not specific for amebic dysentery, since they may occur in any ulcerating form of colitis. They consist of loss of normal mucosal pattern, replacement by a granular appearance, fine irregularities of the bowel margin, and distortion of the mucosa by segmental spasm.

Strictures. In long-standing chronic amebic dysentery, stenosis of the lumen of the bowel may occur. During the acute phase when mucosal ulceration occurs, the superimposed secondary bacterial inflammatory reaction that takes place

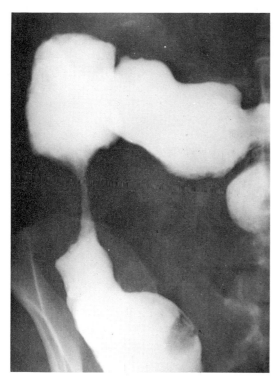

Fig. 59-11. Stricture in the ascending colon with severe alteration in the mucosal pattern of the right half of the colon in a patient with amebiasis.

may involve the muscle layer of the bowel wall. Subsequent healing takes place by fibrosis, and this results in stricture formation. The stenosed segments, most common in the transverse colon and at the hepatic and splenic flexures, are often several inches in length and often multiple (Figs. 59-11 and 59-12). The mucosal pattern in such cases may be distorted throughout the colon. However, a significant feature of these long stenoses is that sometimes they are so long and yet at either end may merge into bowel of normal caliber and with a normal mucosa.

Ameboma. The granulomatous reactions that may occur around areas of secondarily infected amebic infection often produce large, hard masses. They are usually fixed and tender to palpation. They may appear as filling defects within the lumen of the bowel, or they may merely show as a stenosed segment of bowel in relation to a palpable mass (Fig. 59-13). Occasionally, if the ameboma has formed after the direct extension of the amebic process through the bowel wall, the mass may be seen to have a cavity continuous with the lumen of the bowel (Fig. 59-14). If it is possible in these cases to

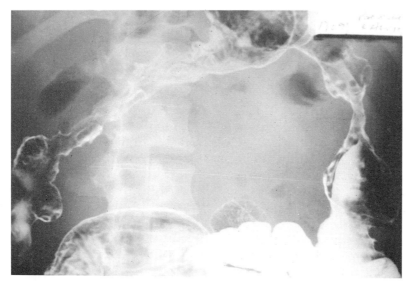

Fig. 59-12. Multiple strictures and complete distortion of the mucosal pattern in the ascending, transverse, and descending colon in a patient with amebiasis.

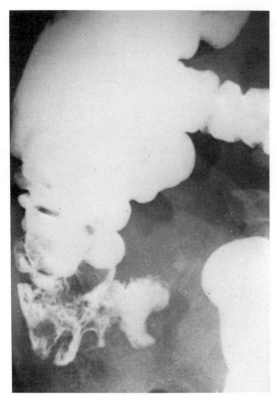

Fig. 59-13. Ameboma in the cecum. (Courtesy Dr. H. E. Engelbrecht.)

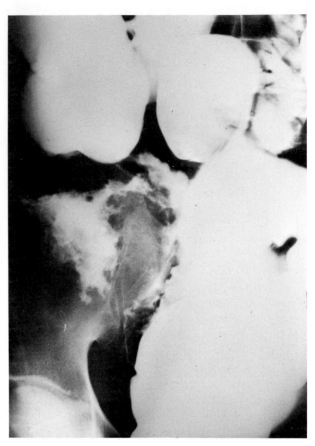

Fig. 59-14. Ameboma adjacent to the cecum having a cavity connecting with the lumen of the bowel.

obtain satisfactory mucosal pattern studies it is always seen to be distorted. The lesions may be multiple.

The differentiation of solitary ameboma from neoplasm, especially if there is an intraluminal filling defect, may be impossible; it may not even be in the patient's best interest to attempt such a differential diagnosis on roentgenologic grounds alone. Nevertheless, it is an important distinction to establish, because in the case of ameboma surgery is contraindicated.

The inflammatory reaction around an ameboma may be so intense as actually to occlude the bowel lumen and cause a clinical presentation of intestinal obstruction. Amebomas diminish in size and resolve with anti-amebic therapy. Roentgenologic demonstration of this feature can be of value in the clinical management and assessment of a case.

Fistula formation. Perforation of the bowel with fistula formation may occur, and such fistulas may be demonstrated at barium enema examination. All the varieties of fistula—colo-

vesical, rectovesical, rectovaginal, enterocolic, fistulas into the retroperitoneal space, and external fistulas—have been described and demonstrated in this condition.[3]

Changes affecting the liver and thorax

Hepatitis and liver abscess. When the diaphragmatic surface of the liver is involved there is usually complete immobilization of the dome of diaphragm on the affected side during respiration seen at fluoroscopy. There may, however, only be restriction of respiratory movement. In liver abscess the affected lobe is grossly enlarged, and this often produces marked elevation of the diaphragm. If the left lobe of the liver is affected the stomach is usually displaced anteriorly or laterally. The abscess cavity is not visible roentgenologically unless air or gas replacement takes place during aspiration or perforation into a gas-containing viscus. In those regions where liver abscess is common the differentiation of a subphrenic source from primary pulmonary disease in the right lower zone of the chest is a frequent problem in diagnosis.

At necropsy, it has been noted that extension of amebic liver abscess into the thorax results in adhesions forming between the superior surface of the liver and the diaphragm. Ellman and co-workers recommend the technique of pneumoperitoneum for the demonstration of such adhesions when inadequate or equivocal information has been provided by the clinical findings and simpler roentgenologic techniques.[10]

Intrathoracic complications. Rowland pointed out that in a series in West Africa, of all the clinical and laboratory criteria suggesting a diagnosis of amebic liver abscess roentgenologic abnormality in the thorax on chest roentgenography was encountered as frequently as any other feature.[30] A small pleural effusion is a common finding, even when the abscess is still restricted within the liver. Larger effusions may occur, especially as the amebic process spreads across the diaphragm. Pulmonary collapse in the lung adjacent to the liver is a common finding. It is most common in the right lung but may occur on the left side if there is an abscess in the left lobe of the liver. Lung abscess may occur, usually in the portion of lung adjacent to the diaphragm. Consolidation usually does not occur except in the presence of lung abscess. Sometimes these patients present an illness primarily respiratory, occasionally without liver enlargement.[23] There is usually pleural effusion present along with lung abscess.

Giardiasis

Giardia lamblia is an intestinal flagellate that can cause symptoms, especially in children. The duodenum and upper small bowel are the common sites of infection, the parasite attaching itself to the mucosa. It is a minute organism and in severe infections may be present in very large numbers; Jassinowsky found a million per square centimeter in the intestines of rabbits.[17] Examination of the stools may fail to demonstrate the *Giardia* cysts, but duodenal aspiration will always demonstrate the parasite, and it is important to emphasize the necessity of examining the duodenal aspirate to rule out this condition. Powell and Cortner showed reduced fat absorption in children with giardiasis,[7,28] and in

some the absorption of fat is so low as to simulate celiac disease. Amini showed that in some adults with giardiasis steatorrhea also occurs.[1] Petersen showed roentgenologic changes in the intestinal pattern in adults similar to those associated with nutritional disorders and also showed that following elimination of the parasites the intestinal pattern can return to normal.[26] Giardiasis may frequently be encountered in patients with dysgammaglobulinemia, accounting in many of these cases for intestinal malabsorption.[37]

ECHINOCOCCUS DISEASE

Echinococcus infections are caused by two types of larvae: (1) *Echinococcus granulosus*, which is more common, and rarely (2) *Echinococcus multilocularis*. *E. multilocularis* produces destructive invasive lesions indistinguishable from malignancy. *E. granulosus* produces cystic expanding lesions that are frequently calcified and most often involve the liver and lungs.[20] This discussion will deal entirely with *E. granulosus*.

Man, cattle, sheep, horses, and hogs are the main intermediate hosts for *E. granulosus*. The infection is contracted by ingestion of eggs that are present in the feces of the dog, the principal definitive host. Following ingestion, the embryos escape from the eggs and penetrate the intestinal mucosa, entering venous and lymphatic channels. Hydatid cysts develop in the organs where the embryos become lodged. Budding from the wall of the cyst is always endogenous. Transmission to the definitive host, the dog, occurs following ingestion of hydatid cysts containing scolices.

Roentgenologic appearance

Echinococcus cysts in the liver very frequently calcify (Fig. 59-15). The liver is by far the most common site, with the lung second. The cysts in the lung are usually not calcified. In the liver, the cysts can show polycyclic calcification, with the mother and daughter cysts showing calcified walls or a single curvilinear outline that may just be segmentally calcified. The differential diagnosis includes calcified old liver abscess, calcification of metastatic pseudomyxoma peritonei, adrenal or renal cysts, and calcified aneurysm of the hepatic artery.

The cyst may rupture into the pleural or

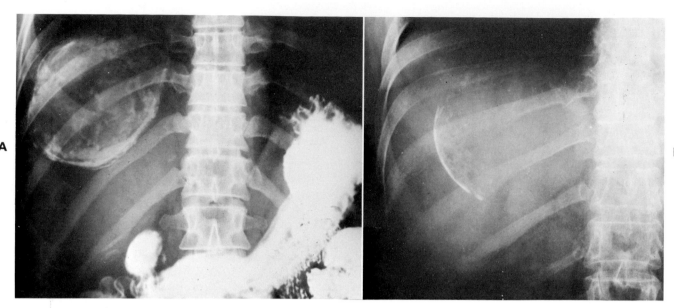

Fig. 59-15. Calcified *echinococcus* cysts in the liver. **A,** Calcified cyst containing multiple daughter cysts in a 37-year-old Basque woman. **B,** Segmentally calcified *echinococcus* cyst in a young Greek woman.

peritoneal cavity or into the biliary tract. Polycyclic or fine eggshell-type calcifications may be seen as a result of previous rupture.

Although the liver and lungs are the most common locations for hydatid cysts, they have been described in the peritoneal cavity, spleen, kidney, bone, brain, and spinal canal. Isolated cases of hydatid cysts can occur almost anywhere in the body.

CONCLUSIONS

In conclusion, it can be seen that the roentgenology of gastrointestinal parasites falls naturally into a few quite separate clearly defined groupings.

First, there is the direct demonstration of the parasite itself. The one of major significance because of its worldwide distribution and its high incidence in many communities, is the roundworm, *Ascaris lumbricoides.* The demonstration of a parasite is of course dependent on its size, and this particular one is large. The liver fluke *(Clonorchis sinensis)* and the tapeworm *(Taenia saginata)* may also be shown, and some other less common round worms, like the *Oesophagostome apiostomum.* Others inhabiting the alimentary tract are small and rarely seen roentgenologically, though some of those

that gain entrance by the alimentary tract, though not strictly gastrointestinal parasites, may be seen on roentgenographs when they are dead, cretified, and no longer of clinical significance. Their importance is of course that they should be recognized for what they are and should not mislead radiologists and clinicians into attaching a significance to them that does not exist.

Next the effect of parasitism on the alimentary tract must be considered, and here there may be demonstrated changes in function or changes in structure.

Changes in function all relate to the small bowel, and fall into what is today called the "malabsorption" pattern. It is not the purpose of this chapter to deal with malabsorption. It is sufficient to say here that the roentgenologic appearances themselves cannot be labeled as "malabsorption." Absorption is a function of the alimentary tract and the particular roentgenologic pattern demonstrated is one that may be associated with disorders of absorption—some of known cause, others unknown. Radiologists know that these features may be associated with other factors, some of them artifacts, and thus the greatest attention to technical detail is essential at all times when one is investigating this type of problem. Experienced radiologists are thus often in a position to evaluate the significance of such findings. The parasites that may be associated with this type of appearance are two of the smaller roundworms (nematodes), namely *Strongyloides* and the hookworm, and the intestinal flagellate, *Giardia lamblia*.

Structural changes in the alimentary tract may be caused either by the tissue reaction to the presence of the parasite or its eggs or by the effect of the parasite in a remote system of the body. An example of the latter is that of the detectable roentgenologic changes resulting from esophageal or gastric varices secondary to portal hypertension, one of the causes of which may be bilharziasis as a result either of *Schistosoma mansoni* or *Schistosoma japonicum* infection. There are, of course, many other causes of portal hypertension, and the roentgenologic features give no indication whatsoever of the cause.

On the other hand tissue reactions may be necrotic, inflammatory or reparative, or result from hypersensitivity, and in some cases probably more than one factor is involved.

Granulomatous lesions in the large bowel are caused by a combination of necrosis and inflammation in amebiasis and by a combination of hypersensitivity and inflammation in *Schistosoma mansoni* infections. This may also be the case with the helminthomas that arise in *Oesophagostome apiostomum* lesions. The latter are small granulomas, but the two former may be significantly large granulomatous masses, producing intraluminal filling defects at barium enema examination with no specific signs to indicate their cause. As such they may be indistinguishable from neoplasm of the colon, from tuberculosis of the large bowel (a condition that still occurs with some frequency among the peoples of the developing countries where tuberculosis in all its forms is a major community problem) or from other rare granulomatous masses caused for example by a fungus infection like Histoplasmosis duboisii, which is being diagnosed with increasing frequency in tropical Africa.

Tissue reactions that may be caused by hypersensitivity have been shown to occur in the small bowel in *Schistosoma mansoni* infections, and roentgenologically these appear like Crohn's disease or regional enteritis. At present it is not known whether these appearances are caused by

Crohn's disease occurring by chance in individuals with schistosomiasis or whether they are caused by Crohn's disease occurring because of the schistosomiasis, or whether they are nonspecific changes caused by the passage of schistosome ova through that part of the bowel wall.

Finally, the last type of tissue reaction caused by the presence of parasites locally is cicatrization. This may produce strictures and stenoses at varying sites and of varying lengths. In *Strongyloides* infection stenosis of the third part of the duodenum may occur. This feature alone is nonspecific, though in endemic areas it would arouse suspicion of *Strongyloides* infection. Similarly, in chronic amebic dysentery stenoses may arise in the colon. These also are nonspecific. Stenoses of a similar character may occur after repeated acute episodes of bacillary dysentery, in long-standing ulcerative colitis, and in Crohn's disease of the colon; even neoplastic strictures may be difficult to differentiate. Amebic strictures are sometimes multiple, are often long, and commonly affect the proximal half of the colon. This perhaps helps to differentiate them from lymphogranuloma venereum in which there may also be skip areas but which almost always affects the distal third of the large bowel.

It can be seen thus that in dealing with the functional and structural changes that may occur in the alimentary tract because of gastrointestinal parasites there is little in the way of specific signs to incriminate or identify a particular etiologic factor. The corollary to this is that when they work in particular areas and deal with particular groups of peoples, radiologists will have a "clinical awareness" that will sometimes enable them to suggest a particular diagnosis that will still require laboratory confirmation. Apart from this, roentgenologic investigation is the only satisfactory method of demonstrating the extent of the involvement of the alimentary tract in many of the conditions that have been discussed here.

REFERENCES

1. Amini, F.: Giardiasis and steatorrhea, J. Trop. Med. Hyg. **66**:190, 1963.
2. Ardran, G. M.: Armillifer armillatus, Brit. J. Radiol. **21**:342, 1948.
3. Barker, E. M.: Colonic perforations in amoebiasis, S. Afr. Med. J. **32**:634, 1958.
4. Bras, G., Richards, R. C., Irvine, R. A., Milner, P.

F., and Ragbeer, M. M.: Infection with *Strongyloides* stercoralis in Jamaica, Lancet. 2:1257, 1964.

4a. Briers, P.: Personal communication, 1971.

5. Chait, A.: Schistosomiasis mansoni, Amer. J. Roentgen. **90**:688, 1963.

6. Ch'en, M. C., and Ch'en Wang, S. C.: Acute colonic obstruction in schistosomiasis japonica, Chin. Med. J. **75**:517, 1957.

7. Cortner, J. A.: Giardiasis, a cause of celiac syndrome, A.M.A. J. Dis. Child. **98**:311, 1959.

8. Cywes, S., and Krige, H.: Intravenous cholangiography and tomography in the diagnosis of biliary ascariasis, Clin. Radiol. **14**:271, 1963.

9. Dimmette, R. M., and Sproat, H. F.: Rectosigmoid polyps in schistosomiasis, Amer. J. Trop. Med. **4**:1057, 1955.

10. Ellman, B., McLeod, I. N., and Powell, S. J.: Diagnostic pneumoperitoneum in amoebic liver abscess, Brit. Med. J. **2**:1406, 1965.

11. Evans, S. S., Lubben, J. F., Jr., and Whigham, H. E.: Pancreatic pseudocyst of ascaris origin, Ann. Surg. **138**:801, 1953.

12. Facey, R. V., and Marsden, P. D.: Fascioliasis in man, Brit. Med. J. **2**:619, 1960.

13. Gilles, H. M., Watson Williams, E. J., and Ball, P. A.: Hookworm infection and anaemia, Quart. J. Med. **33**:1, 1964.

14. Hamilton, J. B.: Taenia saginata, Radiology **47**:64, 1946.

15. Ho, H. C.: Clonorchiasis. In Middlemiss, H., editor: Tropical radiology, London, 1961, Heinemann.

16. Hsu, F. H.: Clinical observation on 110 cases of Ascaris invasion into the biliary tract, Nagoya J. Med. Sci. **24**:215, 1962.

17. Jassinowsky, M. A.: Ueber die Anzahl der Parasiten bei der Lambliose der Kaninchen, Trop. Dis. Bull. **24**:871, 1927 (abstr.).

18. Krause, G. R., and Crilly, J. A.: Roentgenologic changes in small intestine in presence of hookworm, Amer. J. Roentgen. **49**:719, 1943.

19. Makidono, J.: Observations on Ascaris during fluoroscopy, Amer. J. Trop. Med. **5**:699, 1956.

20. Manson-Bahr, P. H.: Manson's tropical diseases, ed. 15, London, 1960, Cassell.

21. Medina, J. T., Seaman, W. B., Guzman-Acosta, C., and Diaz-Bonnet, R. B.: The roentgen appearance of schistosomiasis Mansoni involving the colon, Radiology **85**:682, 1965.

22. Middlemiss, H.: Tropical radiology, London, 1961, Heinemann.

23. Middlemiss, H.: Radiology in the tropics, Trans. Roy. Soc. Trop. Med. Hyg. **58**:197, 1964.

24. Milner, P. F., Irvine, R. A., Barton, C. J., Bras, G., and Richards, R.: Intestinal malabsorption in Strongyloides stercoralis infestation, Gut **6**:574, 1965.

25. Monroe, L. S., and Norton, R. A.: Roentgenographic signs produced by Taenia saginata, Amer. J. Dig. Dis. **7**:519, 1962.

26. Peterson, G. M.: Intestinal changes in giardia lamblia infestation, Amer. J. Roentgen. **77**:670, 1957.

27. Pinheiro, G. C., Pinheiro, R. M., and Dacorso Filho, P.: Strongyloidiasis as the cause of fatal intestinal subocclusion, Med. Cir. Farm. No. **280**:311, 1959.

28. Powell, E. D. U.: Giardiasis, Irish J. M. Sc. No. **371**:509, 1956.

29. Ragheb, M.: Radiological manifestations in bilharziasis, Brit. J. Radiol. **12**:21, 1939.

30. Rowland, H. A.: Radiological changes in amoebic liver abscess, J. Trop. Med. Hyg. **66**:113, 1963.

31. Salem, S. N., and Truelove, S. C.: Hookworm disease in immigrants, Brit. Med. J. **1**:1074, 1964.

32. Sheehy, T. W., Meroney, W. H., Cox, R. S., Jr., and Soler, J. E.: Hookworm disease and malabsorption, Gastroenterology **42**:148, 1962.

33. Sobrinho, J., and Kelsch, F.: Aspectos tumorais de esquistosomose do colon, Rev. Brasil. Radiol. **2**:1, 1959.

34. Tesluk, H.: Segmental ileitis due to schistosomiasis Mansoni, Henry Ford Hosp. Med. Bull. **1**:18, 1953.

35. Watson, J. M.: Medical helminthology, London, 1960, Baillière, Tindall & Cox, Ltd.

36. Welchman, J. M.: Helminithic abscess of the bowel, Brit. J. Radiol. **39**:372, 1966.

37. Zinneman, H. H., and Kaplan, A. P.: The association of giardiasis with reduced intestinal secretory immunoglobulin A, Dig. Dis. **17**:793, 1972.

Infections and infestations of the gastrointestinal tract | 60

Henry I. Goldberg
Maurice M. Reeder

GASTROINTESTINAL TUBERCULOSIS

Bovine *Mycobacterium tuberculosis* is virtually nonexistent in the United States, although it still accounts for much intestinal disease in countries where milk is not pasteurized. Those rare instances of gastrointestinal tuberculosis in the United States are usually secondary to coexisting pulmonary tuberculosis. Because of the effectiveness of chemotherapy in pulmonary tuberculosis, the incidence of gastrointestinal tuberculosis has fallen sharply in the past two decades.

The development of gastrointestinal tuberculosis without roentgenographic or clinical evidence of pulmonary involvement at some time in the patient's life is uncommon. Cases have been reported, however, in which there was no pulmonary involvement.[11] Roentgenograms of the chest may appear normal when the pulmonary lesions have healed. Tuberculous peritonitis, in particular, may not be associated with pulmonary tuberculosis.[11] Studies on many tuberculous patients in the 1930s and 1940s[8,14] revealed the incidence of gastrointestinal tuberculosis to be greater in patients with cavitating pulmonary lesions and positive sputum tests. Gastrointestinal involvement has been reported in 6% to 38% of patients with pulmonary tuberculosis.[1]

Swallowed sputum that contains tubercle bacilli is the most common means of spread of tuberculosis to the gastrointestinal tract. Swallowed bacilli are absorbed by phagocytosis by intestinal mucosal cells and may colonize in submucosal lymphoid tissue.[5]

Once the tubercle bacilli proliferate in submucosal lymphoid tissue, typical tubercles of epitheloid cells and lymphocytes are formed. Submucosal tubercles may expand toward the bowel lumen, resulting in mucosal ulceration, usually manifested as circumferential ulcers. Ex-

pansion of submucosal tubercles also involves serosa with formation of fistulas. Tuberculous involvement of the gastrointestinal tract is a transmural granulomatous process that thickens the bowel wall and eventually leads to fibrosis and stricture. Regional lymph nodes may become involved when submucosal tubercles undergo necrosis and caseation with the release of organisms into intramural lymphatics.

Tuberculous involvement of the gastrointestinal tract is often asymptomatic. In a series reported by Abrams and Holden, about one third of the patients with roentgenographic evidence of tuberculous enteritis had symptoms.[1] Nausea and vomiting are the most common symptoms, followed by anorexia and crampy, diffuse abdominal pain. Symptoms of gastric tuberculosis may resemble the typical symptoms of peptic ulcer. Tuberculous colitis occasionally produces diarrhea in those instances in which the colon is diffusely involved. Massive gastrointestinal hemorrhage after tuberculous involvement of the gastrointestinal tract has been described[16] but is rare.

Roentgenographic findings

Tuberculosis of the gastrointestinal tract is distributed according to the richness of gastrointestinal lymphoid tissue and according to areas of greatest stasis. Therefore, the most common site of involvement is the ileocecal region (80% to 90%), which contains the highest density of Peyer's patches and is the major site of stasis in the gastrointestinal tract.[5] Less likely involved sites include, in order of descending frequency, the ascending colon, jejunum, appendiceal, duodenum, stomach, and rectosigmoid.

Evidence of tuberculous peritonitis and of tuberculous mesenteric lymph nodes may be seen on plain roentgenograms of the abdomen. Tuberculous peritonitis may be manifested as ascites and small-bowel obstruction from underlying serosal tubercles that form adhesions. These findings on plain roentgenograms, however, are not specific for tuberculosis. The typical calcified tuberculous lymph nodes tend to cluster, with lobulated contours and spotty calcification throughout. These nodes vary in size from 0.5 to 10 cm. (Fig. 60-1). Calcification of mesenteric lymph nodes 1 to 2 years after the onset of intestinal infection has been reported.[13]

The classic roentgenographic appearance of ileocecal tuberculosis has been described on barium enema examination as a conical, shrunken, retracted cecum associated with a narrow ulcerated terminal ileum (Fig. 60-2).[2] The cecal deformity is the result of spasm early in the disease and transmural infiltrate with fibrosis in more advanced phases. Narrowing of the terminal ileum may be caused by persistent irritability with rapid emptying of the narrowed segment when filling retrograde or antegrade

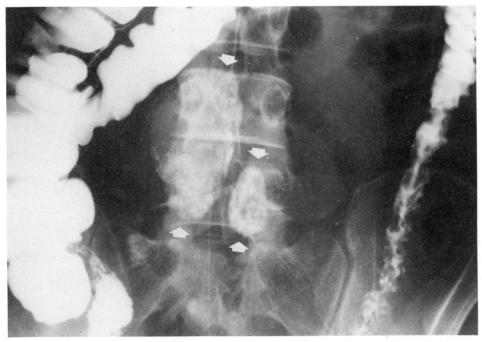

Fig. 60-1. Irregular patchy calcifications distributed throughout large tuberculous mesenteric lymph nodes (arrows). This patient had inactive pulmonary tuberculosis.

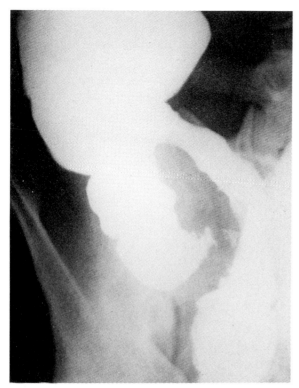

Fig. 60-2. The typical, narrowed, shrunken, conical cecum and narrowed ulcerated terminal ileum of ileocecal tuberculosis. Note the gaping ileocecal valve.

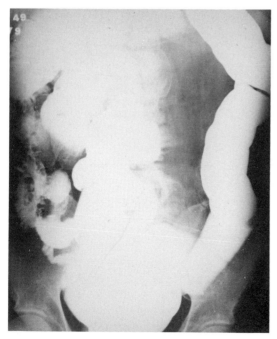

Fig. 60-3. Deep penetrating ulcers and fissures of the cecum and ascending colon cause extensive narrowing and deformity of the right portion of the colon in a patient with ileocecal tuberculosis.

(Stierlin's sign) from a barium enema. This narrowing corresponds to the acute inflammatory phase of the disease. It may be the result of stricture with thickening and ulceration of the bowel wall in advanced ileocecal tuberculosis. The ileocecal valve has been described as "gaping,"[7] similar to that in chronic ulcerative colitis (Fig. 60-2).[12] In the more advanced ileal lesions, deep fissures and ulcers develop, as well as enterocutaneous fistulas (Fig. 60-3).[9] Circumferential deep ileal ulcers may progress to perforation at those times when clinical and pulmonary response to antitubercular drugs is seen. Most perforations, however, are of the walled-off type rather than of the free intraperitoneal type.[18]

When tuberculosis organisms spread to the peritoneum, ascites, bulging flanks, an opaque granular appearance to the abdomen, and centrally located loops of small bowel may be present. Caseating nodules on the serosa may lead to serosal and mesenteric thickening. This is manifested on roentgenograms of the small bowel by retraction and nodularity of the mucosal contour, by fixation and separation of bowel loops, or by partial or complete small-bowel obstruction from adhesions.[4,11,17] Localized tuberculous abscesses representing walled-off perforations may efface and displace loops of bowel. Roentgenographic differentiation between tuberculous peritonitis and other causes of ascites, separation of bowel loops, spiking and retraction of mucosa, and fixation of loops is difficult. Nontuberculous peritonitis, lymphoma, Crohn's disease, metastasis to small bowel, and pseudomyxoma peritonei may all produce similar roentgenographic findings.

Tuberculous colitis, except for cecal involvement, is rare.[3] Involvement of the cecum and terminal ileum is usually in continuity with that of the rest of the colon (Fig. 60-4), but right-sided tuberculosis without involvement of the terminal ileum may be seen. Tuberculous colitis may also involve other areas of the colon either in continuity with cecal involvement or separately, as in isolated rectal tuberculosis (Fig. 60-5).[3,9] Extension of tuberculous salpingitis may involve the sigmoid colon secondarily. The roentgenographic findings of tuberculous colitis are similar to those of Crohn's disease. A diffuse ulcerating colitis with pseudopolyps may be present, but more often thickening, shortening,

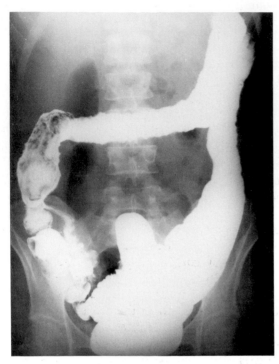

Fig. 60-4. Tuberculous ileocolitis manifested by narrowed ileum and cecum, narrowing of right and transverse portions of the colon with loss of haustra, and extensive ulceration. Left portion of the colon is normal. Crohn's disease and occasionally amebiasis may produce this roentgenographic pattern.

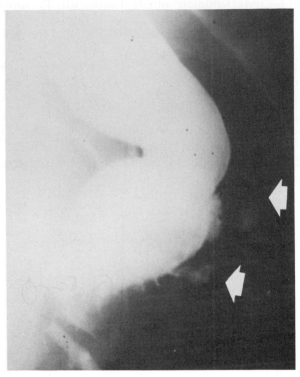

Fig. 60-5. Deep penetrating rectal ulcers and fissures with production of perirectal abscesses (arrows), the result of tuberculosis. This patient also had pulmonary tuberculosis.

and stricture of the colon are seen along with deep penetrating ulcers and fissures.

Gastroduodenal tuberculosis is rare.[15] In most of the patients reported the disease had caused multiple ulcerations of the lesser curvature of the stomach of an irregular and ragged appearance.[6,15] Tuberculous gastric ulcers may extend to form fistulas. Besides the ulcerative form, thickening of the gastric wall may lead to marked narrowing of the stomach and produce the appearance of linitis plastica. When the pylorus is involved, it may become stenotic. Large gastric folds have resulted from tuberculous infiltrate and solitary tuberculomas have also been noted. Gastric tuberculosis should be suspected when irregular ragged gastric ulcers or pyloric ulcers do not respond to medical treatment. Gastric tuberculosis should also be suspected when the stomach and duodenum are involved simultaneously with ulcer disease and fistulas tracts.[6,15] When the duodenum is involved its mucosal

folds are enlarged. If the wall of the duodenum is infiltrated its contour may be irregular and it may be dilated. Involvement of celiac lymph nodes may cause obstruction of the third portion of duodenum (Fig. 60-6).

Differential diagnosis

Gastric tuberculosis must be differentiated roentgenographically from gastric carcinoma, lymphoma, and syphilis.

Intestinal tuberculosis is a granulomatous disease that involves all layers of the bowel wall. As in other granulomatous processes, it produces deep ulcers and may progress to formation of fistula and stricture. Crohn's disease must be the first entity considered in the differential diagnosis particularly when the ileocecal region is involved. These two processes may be indistinguishable roentgenographically.[18] Definite apical pulmonary infiltrates seen on the chest roentgenogram in cases of typical ileocecal deformity

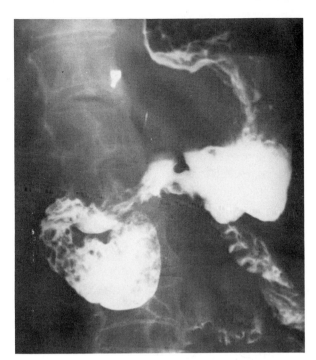

Fig. 60-6. Tuberculosis involving the stomach and duodenum. Infiltration along lesser curvature has narrowed the stomach. The duodenal bulb is deformed. A nodular mucosal contour is evident in the duodenum. Partial obstruction of the third portion of the duodenum is caused by tuberculous celiac lymph nodes.

suggest a tuberculous granulomatous process rather than Crohn's disease. Periappendiceal abscess may also produce the cecal deformities and narrowing of the terminal ileum that are suggestive of tuberculosis. Cecal diverticulitis has produced similar cecal and ileal narrowing. Although amebiasis may produce the typical shrunken cecum seen in tuberculosis, associated small-bowel involvement with this infestation is rare. Lymphoma and carcinoma of the cecum may produce a short truncated cecal tip. For cecal carcinoma to cross the ileocecal valve and involve the ileum is rare, however. Also, the margins of a carcinoma do not ordinarily taper but tend to be sharply demarcated.

More extensive tuberculosis that involves the colon must be differentiated from ulcerative colitis, Crohn's disease, the colitis of bacillary dysentery, amebic colitis, ischemic colitis, and pseudomembranous colitis. Idiopathic ulcerative colitis does not produce deep ulcerations and fistulas as does tuberculous colitis. However, the other forms of ulcerating colitis may be roentgenographically indistinguishable from tuberculous colitis.

SALMONELLA INFECTIONS

Many species of *Salmonella* organisms may be responsible for "food poisoning" that originates from the ingestion of contaminated foods.[20-22] Food poisoning caused by *Salmonella* infection, in which the salmonellae produce a thermostable endotoxin that irritates the mucosa of the stomach and small and large bowels, must be differentiated from that caused by enterotoxin-producing organisms such as staphylococci."[7]

Infected carrier animals or their by-products such as eggs, meat, and milk are a major source of *Salmonella* infections in man. Human chronic or temporary carriers, especially those engaged in the handling of food, can contribute significantly to the transmission of the disease as can flies, cockroaches, and other insects.[23]

Once ingested, salmonellae organisms incubate for 7 to 30 hours before they cause gastroenteritis. Infected persons may have headache, pyrexia, nausea, vomiting, and diarrhea with fluid stools that contain mucus and occasionally a small amount of blood. Patients with *Salmonella* food poisoning usually recover in about 5 days. Occasionally they may become extremely toxic and may advance into a typhoid state. Mortality from this fulminant form of the disease is 1% to 2%.[23]

On necropsy the mucosa of the stomach and of the small and large bowels may appear inflamed and hyperemic and covered with a slimy exudate, small hemorrhages, and superficial ulcers, especially in the colon.[20,23] Peyer's patches are usually swollen and the spleen may be enlarged and soft in patients with septicemia. In infants, complications such as osteomyelitis, purulent arthritis, intraperitoneal abscess, subacute bacterial endocarditis, and meningitis may result from septicemia.[23] Reports of roentgenologic evaluation of patients with *Salmonella* gastroenterocolitis are virtually nonexistent. Golden observed rapid transit of barium through the intestine with hypertonicity in one patient with probable "food poisoning."[19] The case illustrated here with diffuse ulcerations of the colon may be unique in the roentgenologic literature (Fig. 60-7).

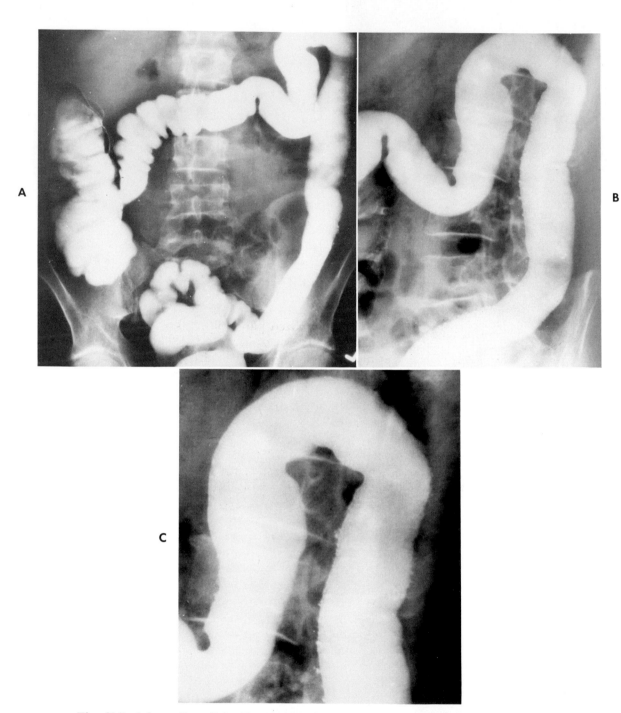

Fig. 60-7. *Salmonella* colitis. Numerous collar-button ulcerations are seen along both borders of the sigmoid, **A,** and along the descending and transverse colon, with diffuse loss of haustrations, **B** and **C.** The rectal valves and sigmoid haustra are enlarged and edematous, **A.** Sigmoidoscopy revealed friable, ulcerated mucosa. *Salmonella* organisms were cultured from the feces and from the scraping of rectal mucosa. The roentgenographic findings of this type of colitis are indistinguishable from those of idiopathic ulcerative colitis. (Courtesy Dr. Proper.)

TYPHOID FEVER

Typhoid fever, caused by *Salmonella typhi*, and the paratyphoid fevers, caused by the *para-typhi A, B,* and *C* bacilli of the *Salmonella* group, are specifically human diseases. They are transmitted by the excreta of one infected person to another, usually through polluted drinking water. Occasionally organisms are transmitted through dairy products or other food items that are contaminated by chronic carriers of the organism. Although flies and contaminated shellfish may also act as intermediaries, the enteric fevers are primarily water-borne diseases. This fact explains the explosive onset of epidemics in military or civilian populations.[29] After the bacilli enter the gastrointestinal tract, they invade the intestinal lymphatics and multiply, eventually entering the bloodstream. In the bloodstream they are phagocytized by reticuloendothelial cells, liver, and spleen. A second bacteremia develops when the bacilli are released from the liver and spleen. This release coincides with the beginning clinical manifestations of the disease.[29]

The incubation period for typhoid fever is usually 10 to 15 days. Characteristic lesions develop in the intestinal lymphatic tissues, especially in the terminal ileum. The colon is involved in only one third of patients, although not extensively.[29] The involvement includes hyperplasia of Peyer's patches, hyperemia and edema of the follicles, and mucosal inflammation. The inflammatory changes are maximal about the tenth day, after which they may resolve or, more commonly, progress to necrosis of the hyperplastic lymphoid tissue. This necrosis results in sloughing of overlying mucosa, leaving ulcers of various extent and depth.[24,29] The oval-shaped ulcers situated on the long axis of the intestinal lumen on the antimesenteric margin of the distal ileum coincide with the distribution of Peyer's patches.[24] Near the ileocecal valve, where perforation is most frequent, the ulcers are deepest. Toward the end of the second week or during the third week of illness further sloughing of necrotic ulcerating tissue may lead to intestinal perforation and hemorrhage.[24]

Roentgenographic findings

Because the pathologic anatomy and clinical course of typhoid and paratyphoid fevers are well known, roentgenographic examination is rarely indicated except when perforation of a typhoid ulcer is suspected. Such perforation in the distal ileum is a complication in 2% to 4% of all such ulcers and is the cause of 25% to 40% of deaths from typhoid.[24] Most investigators agree that perforation occurs between the end of the second week and the fourth week of clinical illness.[27,28] Others have noted perforation earlier, sometimes after only 3 to 7 days of clinical symptoms.[24,27] The clinical severity of the typhoid illness is apparently not related to the occurrence of perforation.[24]

The main roentgenographic finding in patients with typhoid fever but without intestinal perforation is accumulation of gas produced by a paralytic ileus in distended loops of bowel, especially in the small bowel.[24,26,27] Fluid levels are uncommon. By contrast, peritonitis resulting from other diseases typically produces a generalized paralytic ileus with gaseous distention of the entire intestine, with the colon more distended than the small bowel. In typhoid fever, distention of the small bowel primarily may be explained by paresis and functional obstruction before perforation. Mechanical obstruction from kinking, edema, and adhesions may further distend the small bowel.[24,27]

The presence of free intraperitoneal gas in typhoid patients with perforation is controversial. Held to be uncommon by some,[31] others have reported that up to 65% of patients with free perforation had evidence of free gas.[24] In Bohrer's study of twelve patients with perforation resulting from typhoid ulcers, clinical evidence in all suggested peritonitis. In ten of the patients roentgenographic findings also were suggestive. These findings consisted of loss of the properitoneal fat lines, free abdominal fluid, distention of gas-filled bowel, elevation of the diaphragm, and outlining of the outer wall of intestine by free intraperitoneal gas. Most roentgenograms showed fluid levels within the small bowel. In five instances segments of the distal portion of the small bowel were narrowed irregularly and fixed, as outlined by intraluminal gas (Fig. 60-8).[24] When combined with paralytic ileus from generalized peritonitis, inflammatory hyperplasia of the ileocecal valve may add to the roentgenographic appearance of a mixed paralytic-obstructive ileus.[24]

Large amounts of free intraperitoneal gas

Fig. 60-8. Typhoid fever with perforation. **A,** Note the multiple loops of distended, gas-filled small bowel on the supine view. **B,** In the upright projection, multiple resting fluid levels are seen. The properitoneal fat lines are lost and several of the small-bowel loops, especially those in the right lower quadrant, appear fixed on the two projections. Free gas can be seen below the liver margin on both views. A roentgenogram of the chest in the erect position showed free air beneath the right hemidiaphragm. (Courtesy Dr. Stanley Bohrer.)

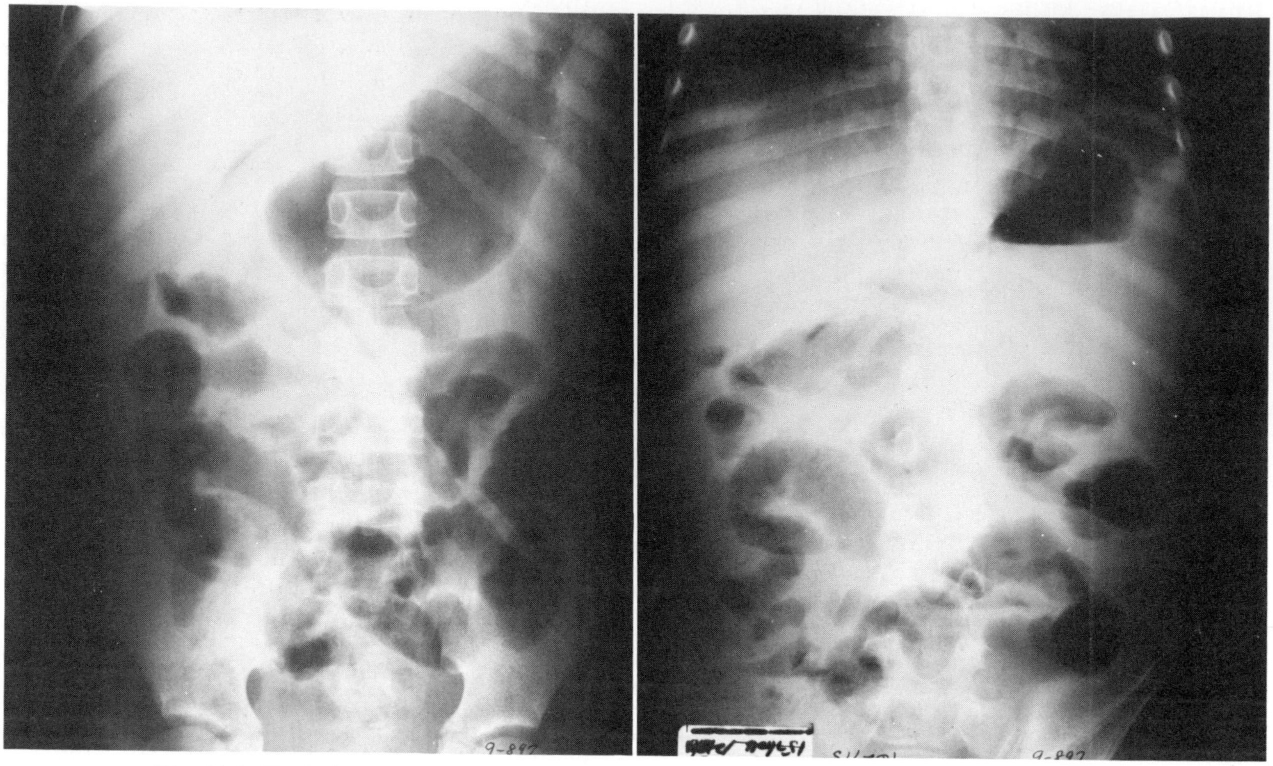

after perforation in some patients may be explained by excessive gas that distends the small bowel before perforation. The absence of free intraperitoneal gas in other instances may be the result of insidious perforations walled off by adhesions prior to roentgenographic examination.[24]

Reports of barium studies of the small intestine and colon in patients with typhoid fever are rare. Chérigié and associates reported the results of examinations of the small bowel in thirty-two patients studied during a typhoid epidemic in France in 1950.[25] They found the caliber of the jejunum to be dilated to two or three times its normal size, with enlargement and edema of the valves of Kerckring suggesting a stacked plate appearance. The barium in the ileum appeared segmented as a result of multiple areas of spasm. Small pea-sized mucosal nodules were found in the distal ileum, which

represented hypertrophy of the Peyer's patches. In only three of their patients were small ulcerations of the distal ileum demonstrated. The ileum, however, was the least well-opacified portion of the small bowel. Transit of barium through the small intestine required about 5 hours with delay noted in the dilated areas.

Schinz and co-workers have noted that, as in tuberculosis, typhoid bacilli tend to invade the lower ileum because of the greater abundance of lymphatic tissue in that location.[31] In the initial stages the dominant pathologic and roentgenographic appearances are those of mucosal edema with thickening of the folds, narrowing of the lumen, and mural rigidity. During the advanced stage of typhoid fever the extensively ulcerated intestinal surface appears as a ragged ill-defined contour on roentgenograms (Fig. 60-9). Because of the disturbed motility of the small bowel, aperistalsis may alternate with hyper-

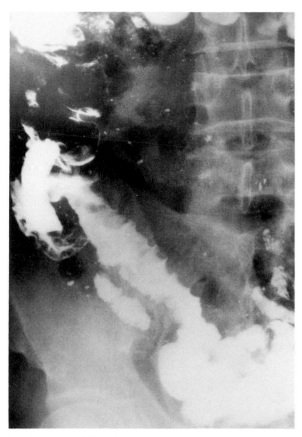

Fig. 60-9. Straightening and rigidity of the terminal ileum with pronounced edema and irregularity of the lumen—the result of typhoid fever. Numerous ulcers that project from both sides of the ileum produce a spiked, ragged bowel contour. There are several lucent areas near the ileocecal area that represent hypertrophied Peyer's patches. The cecum and ascending colon are incompletely filled.

peristalsis. In a still later stage, if perforation has not occurred, the ulcerations may disappear, indicating healing of the disease.[31] Healing of ulcers by granulation tissue may begin in about the fourth week of the disease. When healing is complete a slightly depressed, smooth scar remains, which does not cause stricture or intestinal obstruction.[29]

A chronic typhoid infection of the intestinal tract of 4 years' duration has been described.[30] The serial roentgenograms of the small bowel revealed extensive segmentation and puddling of barium throughout the ileum, with loss of normal mucosal folds and dilatation of loops of bowel. Hypermotility of the intestine was observed, and barium reached the cecum in 1 hour.

Similar findings have been reported as the result of paratyphoid fever caused by *Salmonella schottmülleri (paratyphi B).*[32] Usually, paratyphoid fevers do not produce extensive lymphatic invasion and ulceration, as does typhoid fever. More often on postmortem studies of intestinal specimens in paratyphoid fever little or no change is noted, although the entire intestines may be acutely inflamed.[28] In the paratyphoid fevers and some other forms of salmonellosis, ulceration of the large intestine is more frequent than in typhoid fever.

The differential diagnosis of terminal ileal spasticity and ulceration, and later luminal rigidity includes regional enteritis, tuberculous ileitis, histoplasmosis, lymphosarcoma, radiation vasculitis, ischemia, and periarteritis nodosa. Regional enteritis in particular may resemble the roentgenographic findings of typhoid fever.

BACILLARY DYSENTERY

Bacillary dysentery is an acute or chronic inflammatory disease that involves the colon and occasionally the distal ileum. The disease is worldwide in distribution and is caused by members of the genus *Shigella,* the dysentery bacilli. Members of this genus differ widely both in antigenicity and pathogenicity. *Shigella dysenteriae,* the Shiga bacillus, produces a potent endotoxin that accounts for epidemics of severe diarrhea in the tropics and subtropics.

Shigellosis occurs almost exclusively in man. Human carriers are common where the disease is prevalent and are the only important reservoir of shigellosis. Fecal pollution of water supply, contamination of food by infected food handlers, or transfer of the bacilli by flies are the principle means of transmission.[34,36] Epidemics commonly occur after mild cases are overlooked. In epidemics positive cultures may be obtained from up to 25% of apparently healthy contacts. About 3% of those who recover from an attack of shigellosis become carriers for various periods.[36]

Clinically, the incubation period may vary from 24 hours to a week or longer. The disease most commonly begins as a simple diarrhea but may vary in its severity, so that it is classified as one of the following clinical types: mild (catarrhal), acute, fulminant, relapsing, and chronic dysentery.

A swollen, diffusely inflamed rectal mucosa, often covered with mucus and pus, may be seen through the proctoscope. Underlying this exudate is a granular mucous membrane that oozes blood freely. Shallow ulcerations, irregular in size and shape and covered with pus, may be present.

Pathologically, bacillary dysentery is characterized by acute diffuse inflammation of the colon with initial hyperemia of the mucosa followed by edema, hemorrhage, and leukocytic infiltration. This process often extends into the submucosa and causes marked thickening of the intestinal wall. Epithelial necrosis and desquamation with formation of a diphtheritic membrane is followed by ulceration that may extend deep into the submucosa.[33,36] The inflammation is usually not distributed uniformly throughout the colon but is most severe in the distal portion. The terminal ileum is involved occasionally. Perforation is rare. Secondary bacterial infection occurs once ulcerative lesions have developed. The secondary infection may be important in the development of the chronic stage of the disease, in which adjacent ulcers may be joined by ulcerating channels beneath bridges of hyperplastic mucosa. Mucosal retention cysts may harbor *Shigella* bacilli, which are intermittently discharged in the chronic carrier state.[33,36]

In chronic bacillary dysentery extensive scarring and fibrosis of the colon, indolent ulceration, and a continued subacute or chronic inflammation that becomes acute periodically, are characteristic. The disease differs little from both clinically and pathologically chronic idiopathic ulcerative colitis, including a tendency to undergo exacerbation and remission. During periods of active disease fever may be present as well as diarrhea, with various amounts of blood, mucus, and characteristic cellular exudate in the stools.[36]

Roentgenographic findings

The roentgenographic findings are influenced by the severity and stage of the disease. Many roentgenographic features of bacillary dysentery are similar to those of other inflammatory diseases of the large and small bowels. A large

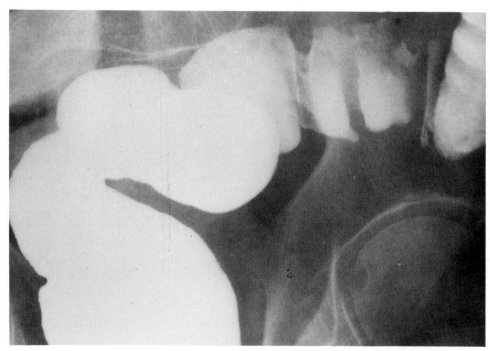

Fig. 60-10. Bacillary dysentery has produced a proctocolitis characterized by small superficial mucosal erosions that impart a finely serrated appearance to the rectal contour. Haustral folds in the sigmoid are edematous. (Courtesy Dr. Wylie Dodds.)

amount of gas may be seen in the small and large bowels. In the small intestine, mucosal edema, segmentation, loss of normal fold pattern, hypersecretion, and especially hypermotility may be noted.[35,37,38] Barium is often observed in the terminal ileum within an hour after ingestion and in some cases has reached the descending colon in that time.

In many instances no roentgenographic changes are observed in the colon on barium enema examination. Edema of the entire mucosa with spasm and irregularity of the bowel wall may be present in active, moderately advanced disease (Fig. 60-10).[39] Complete filling of the colon by barium enema is difficult because of pronounced spasmodic contractions and tenesmus. Postevacuation roentgenograms usually reveal complete elimination of the barium.[35]

In more severe *Shigella* dysentery, focal ulcerations may be present, which are usually not deep and rarely extend into the muscularis. These superficial ulcers may extend throughout the colon but are more common in the rectosigmoid area (Fig. 60-11). The ulcerative ap-

pearance of the colon in bacillary dysentery may resemble acute generalized ulcerative colitis, with irregular bowel contours, considerable spasm, and eventual partial cicatricial stenoses.[37,39]

In chronic cases transient spasmodic emptyings and reflux fillings may take place and the colon may be rigid and tubelike in some segments with lack of haustration. Postevacuation roentgenograms show segmental puddling of barium with lack of haustral markings.[35]

The roentgenographic differential diagnosis of bacillary dysentery includes acute and chronic idiopathic ulcerative colitis, *Salmonella* enterocolitis, pseudomembranous enterocolitis, and amebiasis. These are all inflammatory diseases that produce edema, spasm, and ulceration of the small bowel or colon. Crohn's disease and tuberculosis may produce similar roentgenographic findings, although these inflammatory diseases tend to be more segmental and eccentric in distribution.

PSEUDOMEMBRANOUS ENTEROCOLITIS

Necrotizing enterocolitis of the newborn and in Hirschsprung's disease are discussed in Chapter 56. Pseudomembranous enterocolitis is a disease that involves both the small and large bowels. It derives its name from the fact that a pseudomembrane composed of necrotic debris adherent to ulcerated mucosa follows necrosis of the intestinal mucosa. Of the many causes, the one most frequently associated with the name pseudomembranous enterocolitis is antibiotic-induced change in intestinal flora.[45] Penicillin,[47] lincomycin,[40] streptomycin,[43] chlortetracycline, and chloramphenicol[50] have been known to alter the normal *E. coli* and *Bacteroides* flora of the intestine. The result may be an overgrowth of pathogenic organisms, the most common being *Staphylococcus aureus*.[43,47,51] Mixed gram-positive and gram-negative rods have been reported, as well as *Proteus* infections.[40,43] Enterocolitis after antibiotics, however, has been associated with no definable bacterial overgrowth.[47] Intestinal vascular insufficiency,[41] sometimes associated with intestinal surgery, is thought to initiate acute pseudomembranous enterocolitis, either from hypoperfusion, arteriosclerotic disease, or bleeding disorders. Many cases of pseudomembranous enterocolitis have

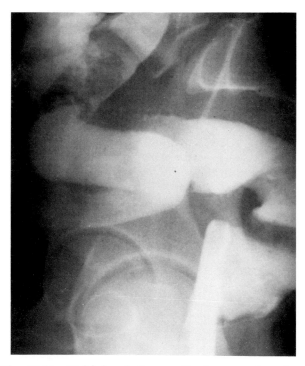

Fig. 60-11. Multiple, shallow, collar-button ulcerations are present in the sigmoid colon of this patient with bacillary dysentery *(Shigellosis)*. The presacral space is widened and the rectal valves thickened because of the inflammatory process in the rectosigmoid.

been reported in patients with debilitating diseases, such as lymphosarcoma and leukemia, or after irradiation for malignant disease.[41,45] Long-term steroid therapy has also been implicated.[42,46] A similar form of colitis has been noted in patients with intestinal obstruction proximal to the site of obstruction.[46,49]

The onset of pseudomembranous enterocolitis is usually heralded by severe diarrhea with or without blood.[43,47] In drug-induced *S. aureus* infections, the organism is capable of producing an enterotoxin that is itself diarrheagenic[43,51] Abdominal cramps and abdominal tenderness, and sometimes signs of peritonitis,[43,47,49] are associated with the diarrhea. Hypoproteinemia with peripheral edema and ascites has also been reported.[47]

Proctoscopic examination demonstrates a friable and erythematous mucosa with yellowish-green exudate or patchy, adherent, elevated yellow mucosal plaques, which may progress to become a confluent purulent pseudomembrane.[40,43,47,49]

In the gross specimen of bowel involved with pseudomembranous colitis the bowel wall is markedly thickened, a yellow-greenish patchy or confluent pseudomembrane is present, and the mucosa is ulcerated.[47,49] Histologically, the pseudomembrane is composed of mucus, fibrin, leukocytes, occasional gram-positive or gram-negative rods, and frequently identifiable *S. aureus*.[43,51] Shallow mucosal ulcerations are present although occasionally ulceration may extend into the submucosa. Goblet-cell hypertrophy of the mucosa may be seen. The lamina propria and submucosal areas are edematous and filled with cellular infiltrate. These histologic changes are nonspecific, however, and may be seen with many other forms of enteritis, such as typhoid fever, bacillary dysentery, septicemia, and uremia.[48]

Roentgenographic findings

Plain roentgenograms of the abdomen are usually the first obtained in patients with the sudden onset of severe diarrhea. An adynamic ileus pattern with distention of the small and large bowels may be seen.[43] The ileus may be caused by associated peritonitis, by electrolyte disturbances because of severe diarrhea, or possibly by release of enterotoxin by offending bacteria. Frequently, the colon is greatly distended,

and its contour is irregular. Thumbprint-like indentations in the gas-filled transverse colon may simulate the appearance of toxic megacolon of chronic ulcerative colitis[42,43] or ischemic colitis. In severe advanced colitis, air in the bowel wall may be seen.[43]

Because of these colonic findings extreme caution should be exercised before barium enema is performed. A markedly dilated colon with an irregular contour in a febrile patient with bloody diarrhea contraindicates a barium enema examination. The high pressure from the barium enema examination is conducive to perforation of the necrotic megacolon. With some resolution of the acute colonic dilatation, however, and a change in symptoms, barium enema examination may be performed with caution under low pressure. Thumbprint-like indentations in the contour of the colon may be seen, these are most prominent in the transverse colon. These indentations are believed to be the result of hematoma formation in the bowel wall from mesenteric and submucosal bleeding.[43] Extensive vascular involvement with occlusion of small vessels and lymphatics has been reported in pseudomembranous colitis and may be reversible.[43] An irregular, ragged, polypoid contour to the colon wall is seen on barium enema examination.[40,44] An alteration of the mucosal-barium interface is the cause of this irregularity. The pseudomembrane itself ordinarily covers a vast area of the mucosa and accounts for the irregular appearance on barium enema examination (Fig. 60-12).[40] Ulcerations, although present, are usually shallow and often are covered by pseudomembrane. These findings are similar, both histologically and roentgenographically, to ischemic colitis.

The small bowel may also be involved.[46,47] Its involvement is indicated by edema of the valvulae conniventes and of the bowel wall, with thickening and separation of loops. Ulceration and complete loss of the fold pattern may be seen in more severely involved areas.

Treatment by supportive measures, discontinuation of the offending antibiotic, and addition of *E. coli* to reestablish the bacterial flora may result in healing to such an extent that follow-up roentgenograms appear normal. Pseudomembranous enterocolitis may resolve so that a smooth atrophic appearing colon without haustra remains, which simulates inactive

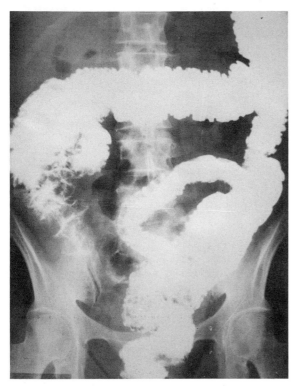

Fig. 60-12. Irregular, ragged contour of the entire colon with loss of haustra, and thumb-print–like indentations in the cecum, the result of extensive pseudomembranous colitis in a patient receiving antibiotics for suppurative otitis. *Staphylococcus aureus* organisms were cultured from stools.

chronic ulcerative colitis.[42] Stenosis and strictures of both the large and small bowels may also take place.

Differential diagnosis

Many other diseases may produce roentgenographic similarities. Ulcerative colitis, both in the active and healed phases, may resemble pseudomembranous enterocolitis on plain roentgenograms (toxic megacolon) and on barium enema examination.[46] The distribution of pseudomembranous enterocolitis may be more patchy than that of ulcerative colitis. Identifiable pseudopolyps as seen in some instances of ulcerative colitis are rarely produced by pseudomembranous enterocolitis. However, any form of ulcerating colitis may produce roentgenographic findings similar to those of pseudomembranous enterocolitis. These findings include Crohn's disease, amebiasis, *Salmonella-Shigella* colitis,

and particularly ischemic colitis. When the small bowel is involved, ischemia, radiation enteritis, regional enteritis, periarteritis nodosa, and lymphoma should be considered in the differential diagnoses.

HISTOPLASMOSIS

Gastrointestinal involvement by the fungus, *Histoplasma capsulatum,* produces clinical and roentgenographic findings similar to those of tuberculosis. As in tuberculosis, the lung is the main portal of entry and the site of primary infection.[58,61] Occasionally, primary intestinal infection has been reported.[52,61] More often, however, roentgenographic evidence of pulmonary histoplasmosis is present in patients with gastrointestinal involvement.[58,61]

The swallowing of organism-laden sputum results in mucosal involvement, whereas hematogenous spread involves the submucosa of bowel.[61] Dissemination to the gastrointestinal tract is accompanied with symptoms in only 20% of patients.[59] These symptoms consist of weight loss, anorexia, abdominal pain, and watery diarrhea with involvement of colon. Gastrointestinal hemorrhage with perforation, peritonitis, and intestinal obstruction have also been initial manifestations.[58]

Involvement by histoplasmosis has been reported in nearly all areas of the gastrointestinal tract. Ulcerating granulomatous lesions of the pharynx[61] and anus[62] have been noted, as well as lesions of more common areas of disease, such as the ileum, cecum, jejunum, and colon.[53,54,56-58] The esophagus may be involved secondary to spread from involved mediastinal lymph nodes.[55]

Roentgenographic findings

Plain roentgenograms of the abdomen in patients with gastrointestinal histoplasmosis may frequently show small, round, calcified granulomas in the spleen. Hepatosplenomegaly caused by frequent involvement of the reticuloendothelial system by histoplasmosis may also be present.[61]

Gastrointestinal histoplasmosis involves lymphoid aggregates in the submucosa and causes a granulomatous infiltrate with transmural involvement. A roentgenographic pattern is produced, similar to that of tuberculosis. Three types of roentgenographic findings are seen: (1) The mucosal pattern may be distorted either by

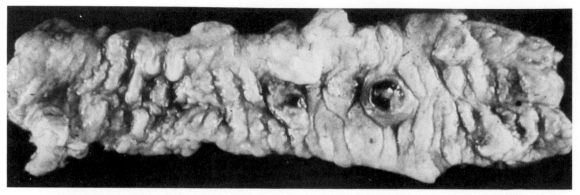

Fig. 60-13. Section of colon from a child with disseminated histoplasmosis, showing thickened indurated mucosal folds. The nodular lesions resulted from microabscesses in the colon wall, which were filled with fungi that had become necrotic and ulcerated. (From Silverman, F. N., Schwarz, J., Lahey, M., and Carson, R. P.: Histoplasmosis, Amer. J. Med. **19**:410, 1955.)

small nodules or ulcerations from underlying granulomatous reaction (Fig. 60-13).[53,54,57,58,60] The ulcers are generally shallow and difficult to demonstrate roentgenographically. (2) A mass in the area of the terminal ileum and cecum, the result of involvement of Peyer's patches and regional nodes, may indent the cecal tip.[54] In a later phase of the disease scarring and fibrosis may cause stricture and deformity.[54,55,58] (3) Generalized widening of mucosal folds of small bowel by edema of protein-losing enteropathy, with underlying intestinal histoplasmosis, has been reported.[52]

The differential diagnoses are identical to those of tuberculosis: Crohn's disease, tuberculosis, periappendiceal abscess, carcinoma, and lymphoma.

GASTROINTESTINAL CANDIDIASIS

Gastrointestinal candidiasis, termed "candidosis" in the European literature, is caused by the fungus, *Candida albicans.* This commensal organism is found in the gastrointestinal tract of many normal persons. It nearly always becomes pathogenic secondary to an underlying debilitating state. Such a state could be caused by prolonged antibiotic therapy[70,71] that alters gastrointestinal flora, malignancy, and chemotherapy for neoplastic disease (immunosuppressive agents, steroids, and antimetabolites). Blood dyscrasias, particularly leukemia,[64] advanced diabetes, and malnutrition, either dietary or resulting from abnormal intestinal absorption, are

other underlying causes. *Candida* infections of the gastrointestinal tract are frequently accompanied by oral thrush or ulcerations of the buccal mucosa, but this relationship is not absolute.[68] Although all sites in the gastrointestinal tract may be invaded by *Candida albicans,* the oral cavity, pharynx, and esophagus are most commonly involved. Dysphagia is therefore the most common presenting symptom. In children, vomiting and dehydration from esophagitis is common and may lead to aspiration and pulmonary infection.[72] Plaquelike white patches on the gums and pharyngeal mucosa indicate oral involvement. Esophagoscopy may reveal erythematous and ulcerated esophageal mucosa, sometimes with a visible pseudomembrane.

The diagnosis of candidal gastrointestinal lesions is more difficult. Identification of mycelia in the feces is important for the diagnosis. Mycelia are thought to be evidence of invasion of mucosa rather than of simple saprophytic activity, as may be the case when only yeast cells are found in the feces.[72] The ultimate diagnosis is established by demonstration of mycelia in material from the gastrointestinal ulcerations or on histologic section. Invasion of the gastrointestinal tract by *Candida* may be followed by septicemia.[70,72] The ulcerating gastrointestinal lesions provide a portal of entry for *Candida albicans* into the intestinal venules and thus into the circulation. Specific antibody titers have been found in the blood and are of diagnostic value.[67,70]

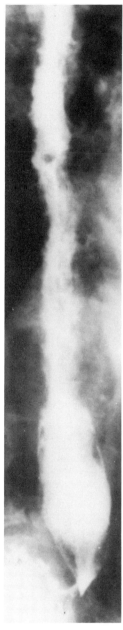

Fig. 60-14. Irregular, shaggy, esophageal contour, the result of ulcerating candidal esophagitis.

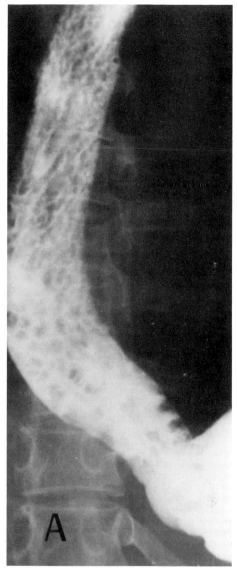

Fig. 60-15. Small nodular contour defects from candidal invasion without ulceration (cobblestone esophagus). (From Goldberg, H. I., and Dodds, W. J.: Cobblestone esophagus due to monilial infection, Amer. J. Roentgen. **104:**608, 1968.)

Roentgenographic findings

Roentgenographic abnormalities resulting from *Candida albicans* are most frequently seen in the esophagus. A long segment, particularly the lower half of the esophagus, is involved, although short, plaquelike lesions have been seen. The typical roentgenographic appearance is an irregular, ragged, shaggy contour of the barium-filled esophageal lumen (Fig. 60-14). This appearance is produced by mucosal ulceration and by pseudomembrane covering areas of ulceration.[65,66] Multiple, small, smooth, nodules, caused by edema and infiltrate without ulceration of the esophagus, may produce a cobblestone pattern (Fig. 60-15).[65] Esophageal spasm as well as atony has been noted in candidal esophagitis.[69] The roentgenographic findings reverse rapidly when antibiotics and steroids are stopped and antifungal drugs are administered.

Candida albicans esophagitis must be differentiated from esophagitis that results from other causes, such as caustic agents and reflux esophagitis. A history of ingestion of caustics or of long-standing heartburn is helpful in the differentiation. Reflux esophagitis is usually not as extensive nor are the ulcerations as prominent as in candidal esophagitis. At times, esophageal varices may be confused with candidal esophagitis, but the contour irregularity is smooth and not ragged. A varicoid carcinoma of the esophagus with ulceration and irregularity also may be confused with *Candida albicans* esophagitis.

Occasionally, in infants with oral or esophageal candidiasis the stomach is involved.[72] Candidiasis in the stomach and small bowel is usually revealed only at autopsy, without signs having been demonstrated roentgenographically. In one large series no specific gastrointestinal roentgenographic abnormality below the esophagus was reported.[63] Changes in the stomach and small bowel are secondary to extensive ulceration and invasion by the fungus. A secondary pseudomembranous formation results in a ragged, irregular-appearing ulcer with associated edema. The pseudomembrane may be proliferative and contain many mycelia that produce irregular intraluminal filling defects (Fig. 60-16).

ACUTE GASTROENTERITIS

Acute nonspecific gastroenteritis is the most frequent gastrointestinal disease and yet one in which a cause has rarely, if ever, been proved. So-called traveler's diarrhea, acute epidemic gastroenteritis, or "mal de turista" may be caused by enteropathic *E. coli* (EEC),[74] by intestinal viruses, such as enteric cytopathogenic human orphan (ECHO) and Coxsackie A and B, or by mixed flora.[73] The disease is a self-limiting pathophysiologic process of altered water and electrolyte absorption, increased intestinal motility, or, in some instances, ileus of small and large bowels.

Roentgenographic findings in acute gastroenteritis are nearly always confined to the plain roentgenograms of the abdomen. Air-fluid levels may be seen in dilated loops of small and large bowels (Fig. 60-17). Dilatation and fluid may

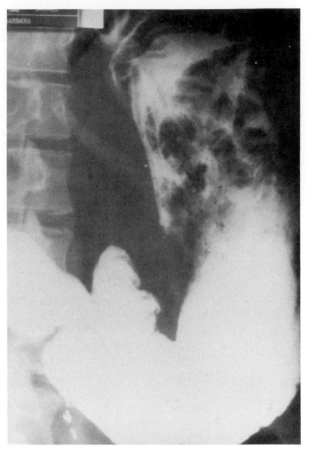

Fig. 60-16. Amorphous, irregular, filling defects in the body of the stomach, which persisted in location and appearance. These filling defects are the result of massive candidal invasion with ulceration and pseudomembranous formation. (Courtesy Dr. Harold Jacobson.)

become so prominent as to simulate mechanical obstruction of the large bowel. Outpouring of large amounts of water and electrolytes into the small bowel results in dilatation, air-fluid levels, and increased but often incoordinate motor activity. Electrolyte loss may also produce adynamic ileus pattern. Some experimental evidence exists that in EEC diarrhea a toxin may be produced, further potentiating the ileus.[73] Air-fluid levels in distended large and small bowels, coupled with the history of diarrhea of acute onset, permit differentiation from mechanical obstruction.

On those rare occasions when barium meals are administered or barium enema examination is performed on patients with acute diarrhea, no specific roentgenographic findings are noted.

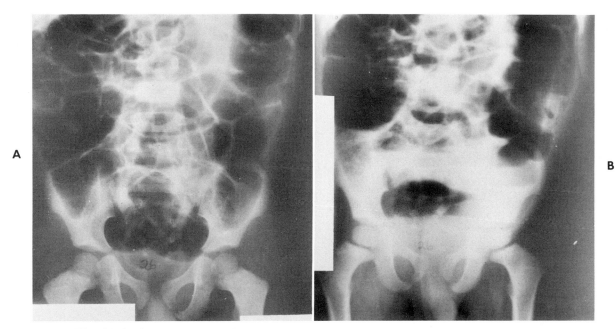

Fig. 60-17. Acute gastroenteritis in a child who had a sudden onset of diarrhea and abdominal cramps with one episode of vomiting. Although acute gastroenteritis was epidemic in the community, no specific etiologic agent was found in this child. Note dilatation, **A,** and air-fluid levels, **B,** in small and large bowels.

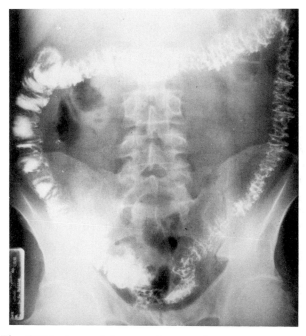

Fig. 60-18. Loss of haustra in an edematous, partially collapsed colon of an adult male with acute gastroenteritis, which resolved without treatment after 4 days.

The small bowel is dilated but the mucosal pattern is normal. Motility may be increased during fluoroscopic examination, producing rapid changes in the location and extent of air-fluid levels. When ileus is pronounced, little activity is noted. On barium enema examination mucosal edema is best demonstrated on the post-evacuation roentgenogram (Fig. 60-18). The mucosal pattern remains coarse in the partially collapsed colon and haustra, and septa are often not present. These changes may be seen in any cause of acute diarrhea, for example, food poisoning, bacillary dysentery, cholera, and ulcerative and amebic colitis.

LYMPHOGRANULOMA VENEREUM

Lymphogranuloma venereum, also referred to as lymphopathia venereum or lymphogranuloma inguinale, is a venereal disease caused by a filtrable virus of 200 to 300 microns in size, which may result in proctocolitis or rectosigmoid stricture. The disease has been reported in all races and in most countries. It is especially common in the tropics among Negro females.[76,77] Ulcers

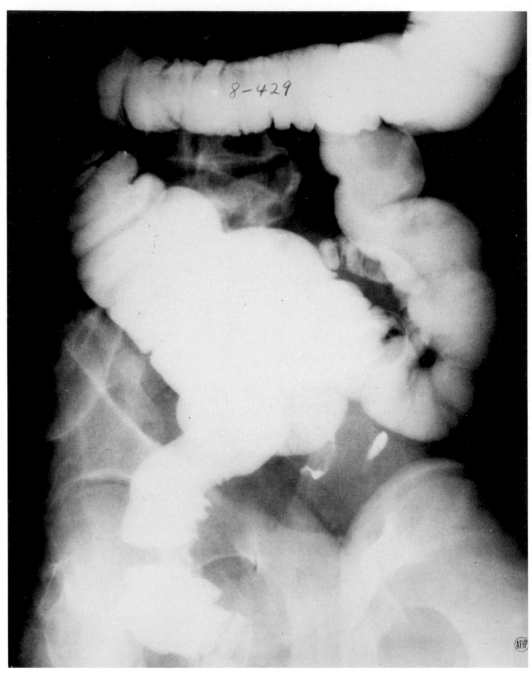

Fig. 60-19. Ulcerative proctitis, with localized rectal narrowing, deep ulcerations, and thickened rectal valves caused by lymphogranuloma venereum.

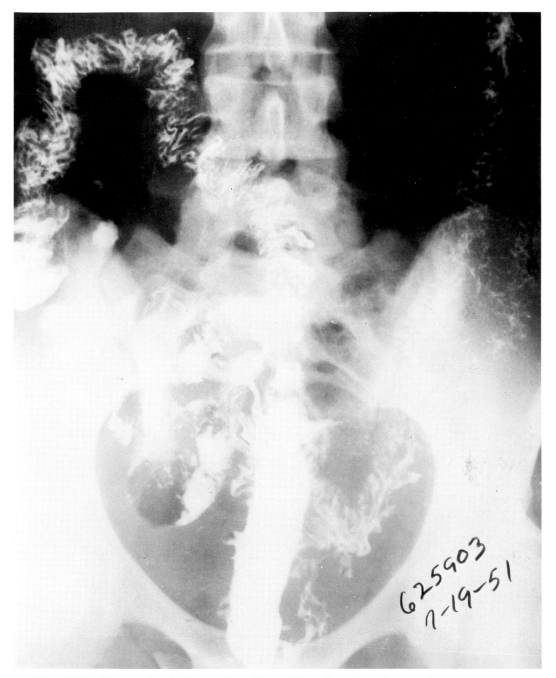

Fig. 60-20. Narrowed, rigid rectosigmoid resulting from lymphogranuloma venereum. The rectosigmoid junction is straightened because of a large perirectal abscess. Multiple deep and shallow perirectal sinuses extend laterally and downward to the perineum.

and strictures of the rectum and colon appear almost exclusively in females.[75,76] The virus invades the vulvar and vaginal lymphatics and produces a herpetiform mucosal lesion.

Rectal bleeding and rectal discharge of purulent material may be the first clinical symptoms.[75,82] These symptoms of proctocolitis may occur as early as 3 weeks after the sexual contact. As stricture forms, rectal pain, tenesmus, constipation, and narrow caliber of stool become prominent features. Rectovaginal fistula frequently develops[76] as may perianal abscesses and vulvar swelling. Systemic manifestations, such as a rash, arthralgias, fever, and leukocytosis may also be present.

On sigmoidoscopy, an acute proctitis may be seen in the early nonstenotic phase and a pseudomembrane noted on a bleeding friable mucosa. In the stenotic phase, the rectal ampulla is markedly narrowed by scarring. Frequently, a friable, bleeding, ulcerated mucosa overlies the stricture. Initially, invasion and blockage of the rectal lymphatics by the virus results in lymphangitis, rectal edema, cellular infiltrate in the submucosa and muscularis, some endarteritis and phlebitis, and subsequent mucosal destruction.[80,82,87] Rectal biopsy may show granulomas in the wall of the rectum with nuclear debris surrounded by macrophages and palisades of epitheloid cells.[86,87] On rectal biopsy later in the course, fibrosis is seen to have produced the rectal stricture, and thrombolymphangitis and vascularitis associated with mucosal destruction are evident.[80] The diagnosis is confirmed by an intradermal test—the Frei test—and by a complement fixation test, both said to show positive reactions in two thirds to three fourths of the patients.

Roentgenographic findings

Roentgenographic features of lymphogranuloma venereum have been thoroughly documented by Annamunthodo and Marryatt,[76] although several investigators have contributed to the literature.[79-81,83-85,88]

The findings on barium enema examination depend to some extent on the phase and activity of the disease. In the prestenotic phase the rectal ampulla is narrowed and spasm is present.[75,79,80,82] The contour of the narrowed rectal region is irregular and ulcerated (Fig. 60-19). Fistulous tracts and perirectal abscesses,

as well as widening of the presacral space may be seen (Fig. 60-20).[80,84] Fistulas may extend to the buttocks and occasionally upward to involve the paramentrium, peritoneum, sigmoid colon and, rarely, small bowel.[83]

As the disease progresses to fibrosis, strictures of varied lengths develop.[75] Short distal rectal strictures slightly above the anorectal junction may extend to narrow the entire rectal ampulla.[82] Strictures as long as 25 cm. have been noted to progress into the sigmoid (Fig. 60-21).[80,82] The contour of the narrow colon may be smooth, but frequently it is irregular, the result of mucosal ulceration and occasional fistulous tracts.[80] Usually the stricture of the rectum and colon are in continuity, but occasionally, separate skip lesions have been reported,[75,78] similar to those seen in Crohn's disease and tuberculous colitis.

The colon is often dilated proximal to a stricture, and sometimes mucosal edema and

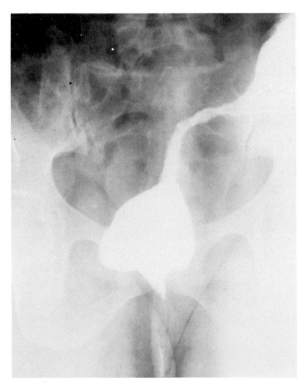

Fig. 60-21. Adult woman with rectosigmoid stricture caused by lymphogranuloma venereum. Note sparing of the distal rectum and the ulcerated appearance of the stricture lumen. Both proximal and distal margins taper smoothly. Dilatation and loss of haustration above the stricture impart a conical appearance to the cecum.

loss of haustra may be seen in the colon just proximal to a stricture. Oblique and lateral roentgenograms of the rectum are necessary to best demonstrate rectovaginal fistula and retrorectal sinuses when present.

Differential diagnosis

Many differential diagnoses must be considered in the interpretation of rectal stricture. Inflammatory diseases such as idiopathic, chronic ulcerative colitis, Crohn's disease, and tuberculous proctosigmoiditis all may produce roentgenographic findings similar to those of lymphogranuloma venereum. In these three diseases, rectal biopsies may also show granulomas similar to those of lymphogranuloma venereum. Actinomycosis, although a rare disease, is known to produce fistulous tracts and ulcers of the rectum and may be confused with lymphogranuloma venereum. Schistosomiasis of the rectum and sigmoid produces diffuse narrowing and ulceration similar to that seen in lymphogranuloma. The ulcerative pattern in schistosomiasis is much coarser, however, than in lymphogranuloma, and the typical mucosal pattern consists of large polypoid lesions. Posttraumatic strictures caused by foreign bodies or by sclerosing agents from hemorrhoid injection may produce smooth rectal strictures, which roentgenographically may appear similar to those of lymphogranuloma venereum. Colitis cystica profunda may cause nodular rectal lesions with narrowing of the rectum suggestive of lymphogranuloma, but the rectal narrowing is not extended. The appearance on sigmoidoscopy is different from that of lymphogranuloma: the nodular lesions are covered with mucosa, and on rectal biopsy the two diseases are differentiated easily. Perirectal abscess or tumor may cause narrowing of the rectum. Usually in these instances the mucosa overlying the narrow rectal wall is not ulcerated. A scirrhous infiltrating type of carcinoma may also produce considerable rectal stricture of a long segment. But, again, the mucosa does not appear ulcerated as it so often does in lymphogranuloma venereum, and sinus tracts and fistulas do not often develop in cancer.

CHAGAS' DISEASE

Chagas' disease is a systemic infection, either acute or chronic, caused by *Trypanosoma cruzi,* a protozoan that inhabits the blood and tissues of man or animals. The heart is the most commonly infected organ and the resultant myocarditis accounts for greater morbidity and mortality than does involvement of other organs. In addition to the cardiac involvement the ganglion cells in the peripheral autonomic nervous system may be destroyed in the chronic phase of the disease. In this event, pronounced dilatation of the esophagus, colon, and other hollow viscera result. Chronic Chagas' disease is now known to account for the thousands of cases of mega-esophagus, megacolon, and myocardiopathy seen in endemic areas of Central and South America, especially in the rural areas of eastern Brazil.[90,92,95] In 1960 a World Health Organization study estimated that seven million people are infected with *T. cruzi* and thirty-five million are exposed to the infection.[101]

T. cruzi was first described in 1909 in Brazil by Carlos Chagas. The organism is transmitted to man by the bite of reduviid bugs *(Triatoma),* which become infected after feeding on an armadillo or other animal host. These bloodsucking bugs inhabit mud huts in rural areas, where they may bite sleeping children about the face at night. Contamination of the punctured skin by the insect's feces, which contains trypanosomes, results in infection. The protozoa travel within the bloodstream in flagellar form, but, upon invading tissue cells, they undergo transformation to *Leishmania,* which divide by binary fission to fill and rupture the somatic cells.[94] Liberated organisms either invade adjacent cells or are destroyed by macrophages, releasing a neurotoxin that attacks and destroys the ganglion cells in the myenteric plexuses of the affected organ.[92,95] The heart, brain, esophagus, colon, spleen, liver, lymph nodes, bronchi, ureters, and salivary glands are the main sites of involvement. In the acute phase of the infection—most commonly in children—fever, edema, lymphadenitis, anemia, meningoencephalitis, and myocarditis may be present.[94]

Usually after a period of many years and probably after repeated infection with the organism systemic changes may develop. Several Brazilian investigators have established that aperistalsis and dilatation of the colon and esophagus are common late sequels to infection with *T. cruzi.*[91-93,95] The result of the complement fixation test for trypanosomiasis was posi-

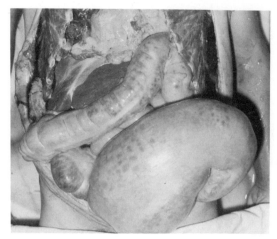

Fig. 60-22. Chronic Chagas' megacolon at necropsy. Note the massive distention and elongation of the rectosigmoid colon with less marked dilatation of the more proximal portion of the colon. (Courtesy Dr. Clovis Simão.)

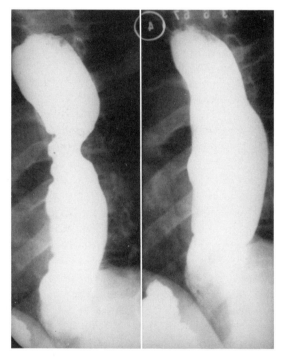

Fig. 60-23. Mega-esophagus in a Brazilian patient with chronic Chagas' disease. The considerable esophageal dilatation and altered peristalsis denote advanced disease. Local, incoordinate, nonpropulsive contractions are present. (From Reeder, M. M., and Hamilton, L. C.: Seminars Roentgen. 3:62, 1968.)

tive in 95% of a large group of patients with esophageal and colonic aperistalsis who were proved to have Chagas' disease at surgery or necropsy. The age range in these instances, reported by Ferreira-Santos, was 2 to 75 years, with an average age of 33 years.[92]

The term "aperistalsis" was applied to chronic Chagas' disease by Brasil to connote the pathophysiologic disturbances of motor incoordination, defective esophageal and colonic motility, and disturbed or absent peristalsis without propulsive efficiency.[91] Köberle demonstrated that the quantitative and qualitative reduction in the number of ganglia throughout the entire gastrointestinal tract, especially the colon and esophagus, is the primary cause of aperistalsis and atony, which in turn results in dilatation of these hollow viscera.[95,96]

Ganglia are deficient throughout the entire gastrointestinal tract in Chagas' disease. The esophagus and rectosigmoid, however, manifest the greatest distention roentgenographically and clinically, probably because they are subjected to greater mechanical pressure (Fig. 60-22).

Roentgenographic findings

The earliest roentgenographic manifestations of Chagas' disease in the esophagus relate only to motor dysfunction. Initially, tonicity is maintained and there is little or no dilatation. Hypercontractility, increased tonus, and hypertrophy of circular muscle layers are manifestations of motor dysfunction, often resulting in dysphagia. In early severe cases, however, or as denervation progresses, esophageal dilatation becomes extreme. The transverse diameter of the flaccid esophagus may be 7 cm. or more, tone may be lessened markedly, and contractions may be weak and uncoordinated (Fig. 60-23).[92] Food may become lodged in the esophagus and cause local irritation that may lead to inflammation, ulceration, bleeding, perforation, and fistulas. Carcinoma develops in 7% of patients with mega-esophagus.[92]

Usually, roentgenograms show no changes in the stomach or small bowel other than occasional instances of enlarged stomach, duodenum, or jejunum (Fig. 60-24). Transit time through the small bowel may be either accelerated or delayed in some patients.[98,100]

In patients with megacolon the outstanding symptom is chronic obstipation; the bowels

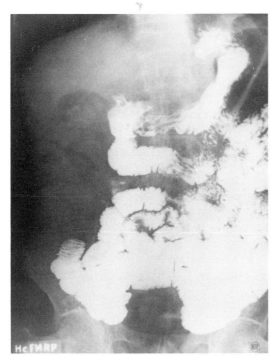

Fig. 60-24. Chagas' megaduodenum and megajejunum in a 57-year-old Brazilian man. At surgery the duodenum was dilated throughout its length. Neither ulcers nor obstruction by aortic mesenteric vessels were present. (Courtesy Dr. Clovis Simão.)

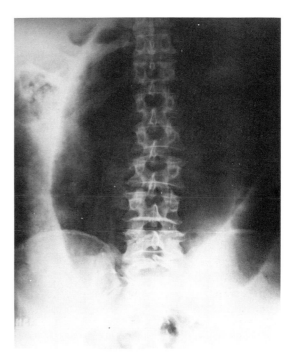

Fig. 60-25. Volvulus of the sigmoid colon in a 59-year-old Brazilian man with Chagas' disease who had abdominal colic, distention, and obstipation for 15 days. A 180-degree torsion of the mesosigmoid was discovered at surgery. (From Reeder, M. M., and Hamilton, L. C.: Seminars Roentgen. 3:62, 1968.)

move at intervals of 8 days to 5 months. Large boluses of desiccated feces may become impacted in the dilated, atonic rectosigmoid, leading to inflammation and stasis ulceration. Sigmoid volvulus, present in 10% of patients, is often the presenting manifestation of the disease (Fig. 60-25).[93]

On plain roentgenograms of the abdomen large fecaliths may be seen within a dilated often redundant colon (Fig. 60-26).[98] A dilated splenic flexure or elongated sigmoid colon may be seen at times beneath an elevated left hemidiaphragm. The striking elongation and dilatation of the rectosigmoid and descending colon are best demonstrated by barium enema (Fig. 60-27). The haustral markings of the colon are diminished or absent. Colonic contractility and evacuation are poor.[93] A cobblestone mucosal pattern is occasionally seen within a portion of the dilated distal colon or rectum, probably the result of stasis ulceration from chronic fecal impactions (Fig. 60-28).[97,98,100]

In advanced Chagas' disease a generalized enlargement of the heart is nearly always present and acute or chronic myocardiopathy results in secondary decreased pulsations (Fig. 60-29).[89,96,99] The bronchi and ureters may be dilated in rare instances.[98,100]

The roentgenographic differential diagnoses of advanced Chagas' disease, in which megaesophagus and megacolon are present, includes scleroderma and myotonia dystrophica.[100]

GIARDIASIS

Giardia lamblia is the most ubiquitous of the intestinal flagellates of man and is found in or infests 4% to 16% of inhabitants of tropical countries and in 3% to 20% of children in parts of the Southern United States.[109,116] The organisms are usually harmless protozoa attached to the mucosal surface of the duodenum and jejunum by their sucking disks. The organisms reproduce by formation of cysts, which are passed in the stool. Man acquires giardiasis by

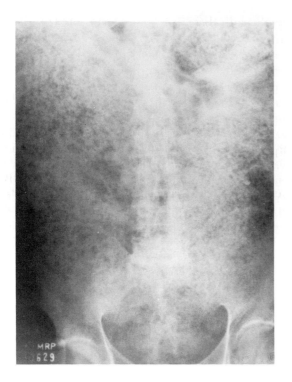

Fig. 60-26. Chronic Chagas' megacolon with a massive amount of retained feces throughout a grossly dilated colon, opacifying virtually the entire abdomen. This 51-year-old Brazilian man had progressive intestinal constipation for more than 14 years, despite two previous partial resections of the colon. Following this examination, the entire colon was removed after it was emptied of fecalomas. The colon measured 10 cm. in diameter and contained numerous small mucosal ulcers and secondary inflammation. The wall was not thickened uniformly; it was thin in some places and thick in others. (Courtesy Dr. Clovis Simão.)

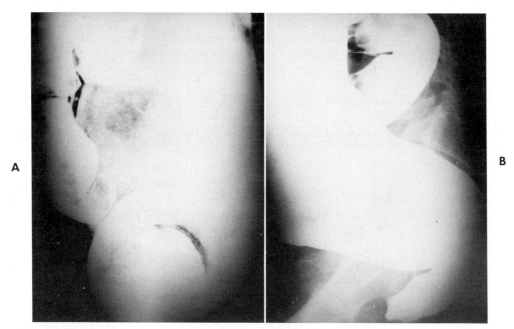

Fig. 60-27. Chagas' disease of the colon in a 56-year-old Brazilian woman with chronic trypanosomiasis. The anteroposterior, **A,** and lateral, **B,** views show massive dilatation of the entire left colon. Note the large fecaliths within the colon. The rectum is not dilated to the same degree as the sigmoid and descending colon because of the action of the pelvic musculature. A follow-up roentgenogram 47 days later showed marked retention of barium from this examination. (From Reeder, M. M., and Hamilton, L. C.: Seminars Roentgen. **3:**62, 1968.)

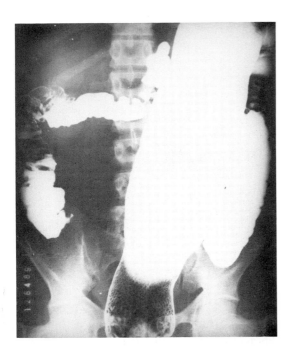

Fig. 60-28. Chagas' disease of the colon. Severe distention and elongation of the rectum, sigmoid, and descending colon with normal caliber of the proximal portion of the colon in a Brazilian man. A cobblestone or cantaloupe-rind appearance of the mucosal pattern is seen in the rectum, probably secondary to stasis ulcerations from chronic fecal impactions. (From Reeder, M. M., and Hamilton, L. C.: Seminars Roentgen. 3:62, 1968.)

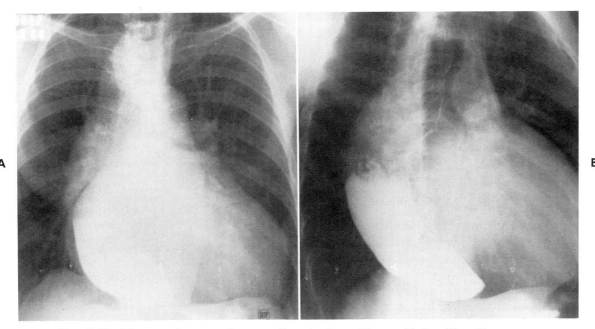

A   B

Fig. 60-29. Mega-esophagus and myocardiopathy in a 58-year-old Brazilian Negro man with Chagas' disease. **A,** The posteroanterior view shows a prominent soft-tissue density along the entire right mediastinal border caused by a greatly dilated esophagus partially filled with barium. The convexities of the right and left side of the heart are prominent because of enlargement of both sides of the heart. Left atrial enlargement produces a bulge along the left upper cardiac border and upward displacement of the left main bronchus. No pulmonary vascular congestion is noted. **B,** The right oblique view shows posterior displacement of the mega-esophagus by the grossly dilated left atrium. (From Reeder, M. M., and Simão, C.: Seminars Roentgen. 4:374, 1969.)

ingesting viable cysts, which pass unharmed through the gastric juices and undergo excystation to the trophozoite form in the upper portion of the small bowel. Though at times massive quantities of parasites may be present, only occasionally do they cause clinical symptoms, more often in children. These symptoms consist of abdominal colic, nausea, flatulence, and diarrhea, often with steatorrhea.[102,105,109] The stools and clinical manifestations in children may resemble those of sprue or celiac disease.[105,109] The individual response of a patient to infection with *Giardia* varies, depending on the number of organisms present, age, nutrition, associated bacterical infection, and immunoglobulin deficiency.[111,119]

Previously these organisms were thought not to invade tissue and thus no specific manifestations of inflammatory small-bowel disease were reported in patients with giardiasis.[106] Recent histopathologic studies, however, have shown that these flagellates can indeed invade the mucosa of the duodenum and jejunum and produce a mild inflammatory reaction.[104,113,117] Histologic examination of biopsy specimens of the small bowel may show acute and chronic inflammation, abnormal villus configuration, and damage to epithelial cells with increased mitoses.[108,119] The mechanism of malabsorption in giardiasis remains unproved, since there appears to be no direct correlation between malabsorption and the severity of underlying mucosal changes.[111] Defective intestinal absorption has been postulated to be caused by irritation and a mechanical barrier produced when an overwhelming number of parasites attach to the microvillar mucosal surface.[113]

Until recently, reports of roentgenographic changes in giardiasis have been rare. In 1944, Welch described irritability of the duodenal cap with coarsening of the mucosal pattern in twenty-two of twenty-nine patients with giardiasis.[118] Later, Peterson described a deficiency pattern in patients with *Giardia* infestation, which consisted of pronounced segmentation, a moderate degree of dilatation of small-bowel loops, coarsening of the mucosal folds in the midportion of small bowel, and prolonged transit time.[114] More recently, Marshak and co-workers,[110,111] Basu,[103] McLaughlin,[112] Reeder,[115] and Reeder and Hamilton[116] have reported roentgenographic changes of an inflammatory

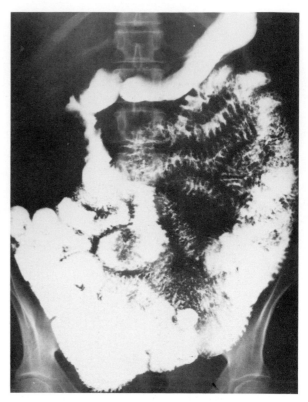

Fig. 60-30. Giardiasis. The second portion of the duodenum is markedly irregular and considerable spasm is noted within the duodenal sweep and proximal jejunum. These loops are poorly filled because of irritability and are separated from each other. The mucosal folds are thickened, and secretions are increased. The lumen of the bowel is slightly rigid and narrowed. The changes suggest actual inflammatory reaction rather than a malabsorption pattern. They disappeared after atebrine therapy for giardiasis. (Courtesy Dr. R. H. Marshak.)

nature usually localized to the duodenum and jejunum in patients with giardiasis. The ileum is rarely involved and the colon appears normal. The mucosal folds are thickened, blunted, and distorted, and there is associated spasm, irritability, and hypermotility (Fig. 60-30). Because of the resultant poor filling of the duodenum and jejunum with barium, fluoroscopic spot filming is difficult unless the patient is given large amounts of barium. Secretions are often increased, causing blurring of the mucosal folds, sometimes associated with fragmentation and segmentation. The bowel lumen may be narrow because of spasm. Cure or clinical improvement

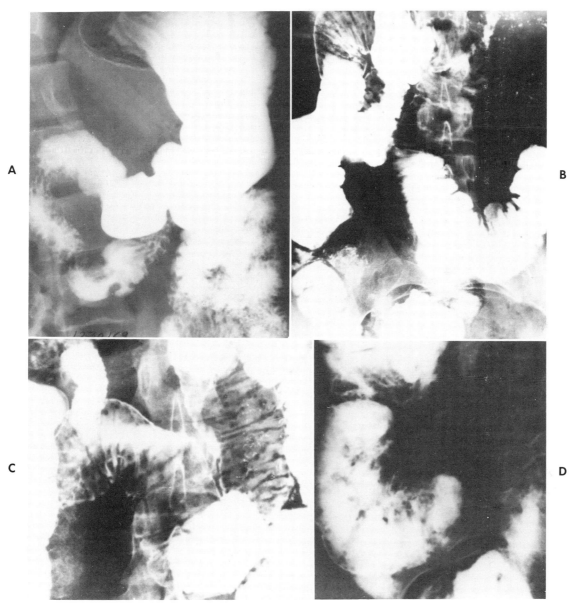

Fig. 60-31. Giardiasis and nodular lymphoid hyperplasia of the small intestine in a 24-year-old woman with dysgammaglobulinemia, recurrent respiratory infections, and constant spruelike diarrhea. **A,** The mucosal pattern within the duodenal bulb and C loop is coarse, with some edema of the folds. The duodenal sweep failed to fill out normally as seen on multiple spot films, indicating slight spasm. **B,** Abnormal motor activity with dilatation of multiple loops of jejunum and ileum, together with segmentation of the barium column and coarsening of the mucosal folds, is seen in some areas. **B** and **C,** The mucosa of the entire jejunum and ileum is uniformly studded with numerous, tiny, round polypoid lesions, 1 to 3 mm. in diameter. These nodules are especially well outlined in areas of air-barium contrast. **D,** Nodules are also present in the terminal ileum and right portion of the colon. (From Reeder, M. M.: Radiology **93:**427, 1969.

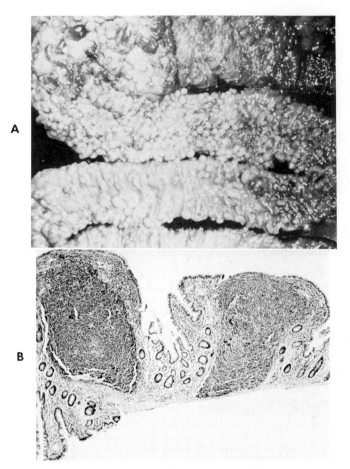

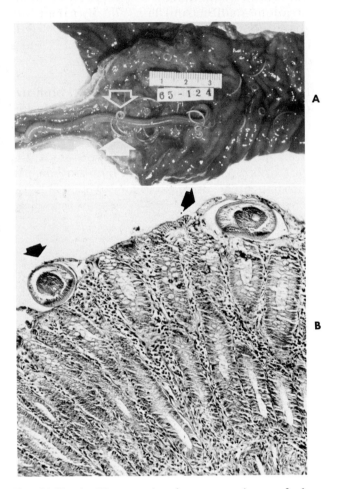

Fig. 60-32. A, Gross specimen of the small intestine from a patient with nodular lymphoid hyperplasia, in which innumerable small, uniform polypoid lesions studded the mucosal surface. These tiny nodules account for the multiple, round, filling defects noted on the roentgenograms of the small bowel. **B,** Photomicrograph from a jejunal biopsy of a patient with dysgammaglobulinemia and nodular lymphoid hyperplasia. The lymphoid follicles within the lamina propria are greatly enlarged, elevating the mucosal surface to produce a polypoid appearance. The overlying villi appear flattened. (Hemotoxylin and eosin; × 50.)

Fig. 60-33. A, Photograph of gross specimen of the cecum and appendix of a patient from San Salvador shows coexistent whipworm and *Ascaris* infection, a frequent combination. The glistening mucosal surface is not inflammed or ulcerated. It is coated with thick mucus secreted in the vicinity of the numerous whipworms, especially near the appendix. Note the typical coiled appearance of the male parasites (open arrow) and the curved semilunar configuration of the female worms (solid arrow), as their posterior portions protrude into the lumen of the bowel. **B,** The anterior portions of two whipworms are seen in cross section as they lie embedded in their typical location beneath the surface epithelium of the colonic mucosa (arrows). Note the lack of any significant inflammatory reaction in the vicinity of the worms. (Hemotoxylin and eosin; × 40.) (From Reeder, M. M., Astacio, J. E., and Theros, E. G.: Case of the month from AFID: an exercise in radiologic-pathologic correlation, Radiology **90**:382, 1968.)

of the patient is associated with return to a normal intestinal pattern after the organisms are eradicated by quinacrine (Atabrine) hydrochloride.[111]

Recently, Hermans and associates,[105] Hodgson and co-workers,[107] and Reeder[115] have reported dysgammaglobulinemia associated with nodular lymphoid hyperplasia of the small bowel and with recurrent respiratory and urinary tract infections (Fig. 60-31). These patients also have

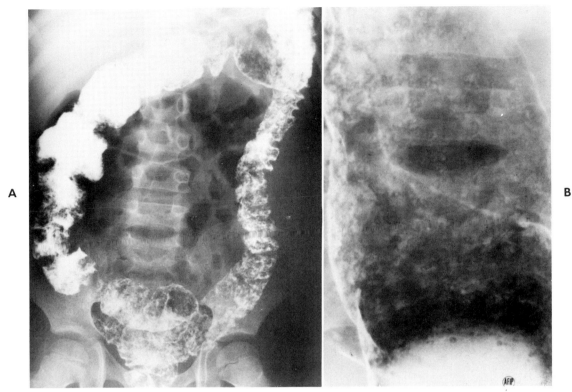

Fig. 60-34. A, Trichuriasis in a 7-year-old boy with profuse rectal bleeding. Innumerable whipworms were seen to be attached to the rectal mucosa at proctoscopy. A granular mucosal pattern was noted on a barium enema examination, similar in appearance to mucoviscidosis. The flocculation of barium and poor mucosal coating are produced by excessive mucous secretions surrounding numerous whipworms. **B,** A magnified view of the rectosigmoid on an air-contrast barium enema examination shows the outlines of many tiny whipworms attached to the mucosa with their posterior portions either tightly coiled or unfurled in whiplike configuration. (From Reeder, M. M., Astacio, J. E., and Theros, E. G.: Case of the month from AFID: an exercise in radiologic-pathologic correlation, Radiology **90:**382, 1968.)

a chronic spruelike diarrhea and other clinical and roentgenographic evidences of malabsorption. The numerous tiny polypoid defects in the small bowel are the result of nodular lymphoid hyperplasia and are not caused by giardiasis (Fig. 60-32). In most of these patients, *Giardia lamblia* cysts were present in the stools. The generally lowered resistance of the patients permits these usually innocuous sewage organisms to flourish in the small bowel.

TRICHURIASIS

Trichuriasis of the human colon is caused by the whipworm, *Trichuris trichiura*. This nematode is cosmopolitan in distribution but thrives chiefly in the warm moist tropics, where several

hundred worms may be present in a severely infested patient. These ubiquitous parasites usually inhabit the cecum, although in severe instances the entire colon, appendix, and even the terminal ileum may be infested. In 1947 more than 350 million persons were estimated to be infested with whipworms.[126] In the United States trichuriasis prevails chiefly in areas of the Southern Appalachian mountains and Louisiana, where dooryard pollution, dense shade near the house, and heavy rainfall favor the growth of whipworm.

Human beings become infested by ingesting contaminated vegetables or soil that contains infective ova passed in feces. The ova hatch into larvae, which attach briefly to the duodenal wall before they pass into the cecum to evolve into adult worms. The whipworms are 3 to 5 cm. long and possess a characteristic, long, whip-like anterior end, which contains a mouth and esophagus, and a broader posterior end for the reproductive organs. The worms are attached to the colon by means of their slender anterior ends, which transfix superficial folds of mucosa.[123] They lie embedded between the intestinal villi amid much mucus, with their blunt posterior portions either coiled or projecting freely into the bowel lumen as semilunar arcs (Fig. 60-33). Tissue reaction is absent or slight at the sites of attachment, although liquefaction of adjacent cells and bleeding may be noted.

Milder infections are usually asymptomatic and are discovered incidentally during evaluation of a patient concomitantly infected with *Ascaris,* hookworms, or amebas. A heavy infestation with *Trichuris,* however, especially in children, can cause severe chronic diarrhea or dysentery, with blood and mucus in the stool, tenesmus, abdominal pain, weakness, anorexia, dehydration, weight loss, rectal prolapse, eosinophilia, and anemia.[122] Occasional deaths from profuse hemorrhage or intussusception have been reported.[121,124]

The roentgenographic pattern in trichuriasis has recently been described by Reeder and co-workers,[124,125] who noted a granular mucosal pattern throughout the colon on routine barium examination of a severely infested Central American child (Fig. 60-34). The barium becomes flocculated because of mucus secretions surrounding the worms. The appearance is similar to that of mucoviscidosis of the colon. On air-contrast examination the wavy radiolucent outlines of innumerable tiny *Trichuris* organisms are clearly outlined against the air-barium background of the colon and rectum. The posterior portions of the male worms are coiled tightly in the mixed mucus and barium, whereas the female worms assume a typical crescentic or whip-like configuration, suggesting a pinwheel or target appearance of the mucosal pattern. Fisher and Cremin[120] recently reported on three patients from South Africa with similar findings on air-contrast barium enema examination.[120] They noted no clumping of barium on the standard barium enema examination, however. Roentgenographic examination should not be necessary for the diagnosis of trichuriasis, but the typical roentgenographic features should be kept in mind, especially in patients from areas of high prevalence and poor socioeconomic conditions.

REFERENCES
Gastrointestinal tuberculosis

1. Abrams, J. S., and Holden, W. D.: Tuberculosis of the gastrointestinal tract, Arch. Surg. **89**:282, 1964.
2. Anscombe, A. R., Keddie, N. C., and Schofield, P. F.: Caecal tuberculosis, Gut **8**:337, 1967.
3. Brenner, S. M., Annes, G., and Parker, J. G.: Tuberculous colitis simulating nonspecific granulomatous disease of the colon, Amer. J. Dig. Dis. **15**:85, 1970.
4. Burack, W. R., and Hollister, R. M.: Tuberculous peritonitis: a study of forty-seven proved cases encountered by a general medical unit in twenty-five years, Amer. J. Med. **28**:510, 1960.
5. Chazan, B. I., and Aitchison, J. D.: Gastric tuberculosis, Brit. Med. J. **2**:1288, 1960.
6. Gaines, W., Steinbach, H. L., and Lowenhaupt, E.: Tuberculosis of the stomach, Radiology **58**:808, 1952.
7. Gershon-Cohen, J., and Kremens, V.: X-ray studies of the ileocecal valve in ileocecal tuberculosis, Radiology **62**:251, 1954.
8. Granet, E.: Intestinal tuberculosis: a clinical, roentgenological and pathological study of 2086 patients affected with pulmonary tuberculosis, Amer. J. Dig. Dis. **2**:209, 1935.
9. Hancock, D. M.: Hyperplastic tuberculosis of the distal colon, Brit. J. Surg. **46**:63, 1958.
10. Hoon, J. R., Dockerty, M. G., and Pemberton, J. deJ.: Collective review; ileocecal tuberculosis including comparison of this disease with nonspecific regional enterocolitis and noncaseous tuberculated enterocolitis, Int. Abstr. Surg. **91**:417, 1950.
11. Hughes, H. J., Carr, D. T., and Geraci, J. E.: Tuberculous peritonitis: a review of 34 cases with emphasis on the diagnostic aspects, Dis. Chest **38**:42, 1960.
12. Margulis, A. R., Goldberg, H. I., Lawson, T. L., Montgomery, C. K., Rambo, O. N., Noonan, C. D., and Amberg, J. R.: The overlapping spectrum of ulcerative and granulomatous colitis: a roentgenographic-pathologic study, Amer. J. Roentgen. **113**:325, 1971.
13. Marshak, R. H., and Lindner, A. E.: Radiology of the small intestine, Philadelphia, 1970, W. B. Saunders Co.
14. Mitchell, R. S., and Bristol, L. J.: Intestinal tuberculosis: an analysis of 346 cases diagnosed by routine intestinal radiography on 5,529 admissions for pulmonary tuberculosis, 1924-1949, Amer. J. Med. Sci. **227**:241, 1954.
15. Pinto, R. S., Zausner, J., and Beranbaum, E. R.: Gastric tuberculosis. Report of a case with discussion of angiographic findings, Amer. J. Roentgen. **110**:808, 1970.

16. Schinz, H. R., Baensch, W. E., Friedl, E., and Uehlinger, E.: Roentgen-diagnostics, vol. 4, New York, 1954, Grune & Stratton, Inc., p. 3772.
17. Stassa, G.: Tuberculous peritonitis, Amer. J. Roentgen. 101:409, 1967.
18. Sweetman, W. R., and Wise, R. A.: Acute perforated tuberculous enteritis: surgical treatment, Ann. Surg. 149:143, 1959.

Salmonella infections

19. Felsenfeld, O.: Synopsis of clinical tropical medicine, St. Louis, 1965, The C. V. Mosby Co.
20. Golden, R.: Radiologic examination of the small intestine, ed. 2, Springfield, 1959, Charles C Thomas, Publisher.
21. Hunter, G. W., III, Frye, W. W., and Swartzwelder, J. C.: A manual of tropical medicine, ed. 4, Philadelphia, 1966, W. B. Saunders Co.
22. Manson-Bahr, P. H.: Manson's tropical diseases; a manual of diseases of warm climates, ed. 16, London, 1966, Baillière, Tindall & Cassell, Ltd.
23. Pontes, J. F.: Disorders of the small intestine, CIBA Clinical Symposia 12:107, 1960.

Typhoid fever

24. Bohrer, S. P.: Typhoid perforation of the ileum, Brit. J. Radiol. 39:37, 1966.
25. Chérigié, E., Laporte, A., and Verspyck, R.: Aspect radiologique du grêle chez les typhiques, J. Radiol. Électr. 34:522, 1953.
26. Frimann-Dahl, J.: Roentgen examinations in acute abdominal disorders, ed. 2, Springfield, 1960, Charles C Thomas, Publisher.
27. Huckstep, R. L.: Typhoid fever, and other *Salmonella* infections, Edinburgh, 1962, E. & S. Livingstone, Ltd.
28. Manson-Bahr, P. H.: Manson's tropical diseases; a manual of diseases of warm climates, ed. 16, London, 1966, Baillière, Tindall & Cassell, Ltd.
29. Pontes, J. F.: Disorders of the small intestine, CIBA Clinical Symposia 12:107, 1960.
30. Rappaport, E. M., and Rappaport, E. O.: Typhoid enterocolitis simulating chronic bacillary dysentery: report of a case with cure by chloromycetin, New Eng. J. Med. 242:698, 1950.
31. Schinz, H. R., Baensch, W. E., Friedl, E., and Uehlinger, E.: Roentgen-diagnostics, vol. 4, New York, 1954, Grune & Stratton, Inc.
32. Silverman, D. N., and Leslie, A.: Simulation of chronic bacterial dysentery by paratyphoid B infection, Gastroenterology 4:53, 1945.

Bacillary dysentery

33. Ash, J. E., and Spitz, S.: Pathology of tropical diseases, Philadelphia, 1945, W. B. Saunders Co.
34. Christie, A. B.: Bacillary dysentery, Brit. Med. J. 2:285, 1968.
35. de Lorimier, A. A., Moehring, H. G., and Hannan, J. R.: Clinical roentgenology, vol. 4, Springfield, 1956, Charles C Thomas, Publisher.
36. Hunter, G. W., III, Frye, W. W., and Swartzwelder,

J. C.: A manual of tropical medicine, ed. 4, Philadelphia, 1966, W. B. Saunders Co.
37. Schinz, H. R., Baensch, W. E., Friedl, E., and Uehlinger, E.: Roentgen-diagnostics, vol. 4, New York, 1954, Grune & Stratton, Inc.
38. Silverman, D. N., and Leslie, A.: Simulation of chronic bacterial dysentery by paratyphoid B. infection, Gastroenterology 4:53, 1945.
39. Teplick, J. G., Haskin, M. E., Schimert, A. P.: Roentgenologic diagnosis, vol. 1, Philadelphia, 1967, W. B. Saunders Co.

Pseudomembranous enterocolitis

40. Benner, E. J., and Tellman, W. H.: Pseudomembranous colitis as a sequel to oral lincomycin therapy, Amer. J. Gastroent. 54:55, 1970.
41. Birnbaum, D., Laufer, A., and Freund, M.: Pseudomembranous enterocolitis: a clinicopathologic study, Gastroenterology 41:345, 1961.
42. Brown, C. H., Ferrante, W. A., and Davis, W. D. Jr.: Toxic dilatation of the colon complicating pseudomembranous enterocolitis, Amer. J. Dig. Dis. 13:813, 1968.
43. Ecker, J. A., Williams, R. G., McKittrick, J. E., and Failing, R. M.: Pseudomembraneous enterocolitis—an unwelcome gastrointestinal complication of antibiotic therapy, Amer. J. Gastroent. 54:214, 1970.
44. Feinberg, S. B.: The roentgen findings in severe pseudomembranous enterocolitis, Radiology 74:778, 1960.
45. Gildenhorn, H. L., Springer, E. B., and Amromin, G. D.: Necrotizing enteropathy: roentgenographic features, Amer. J. Roentgen. 88:942, 1962.
46. Goulston, S. J., and McGovern, V. J.: Pseudo-membranous colitis, Gut 6:207, 1965.
47. Groll, A., Vlassembrouck, M. J., Ramchand, S., and Valberg, L. S.: Fulminating noninfective pseudomembranous colitis, Gastroenterology 58:88, 1970.
48. Hale, H. W., Jr., and Cosgriff, J. H., Jr.: Pseudomembranous enterocolitis, Amer. J. Surg. 94:710, 1957.
49. Pettet, J. D., Baggenstoss, A. H., Judd, E. S., Jr., and Dearing, W. H.: Generalized postoperative pseudomembranous enterocolitis, Proc. Staff Meet. Mayo Clin. 29:342, 1954.
50. Reiner, L., Schlesinger, M. J., and Miller, G. M.: Pseudomembranous colitis following aureomycin and chloramphenicol, A.M.A. Arch. Path. 54:39, 1952.
51. Speare, G. S.: Staphylococcus pseudomembranous enterocolitis, complication of antibiotic therapy, Amer. J. Surg. 88:523, 1954.

Histoplasmosis

52. Bank, S., Trey, C., Gans, I., Marks, I. N., and Groll, A.: Histoplasmosis of the small bowel with "giant" intestinal villi and secondary protein-losing enteropathy, Amer. J. Med. 39:492, 1965.
53. Brown, A. E., Havens, F. Z., and Magath, T. B.:

Histoplasmosis: report of case, Proc. Staff Meet. Mayo Clin. **15:**812, 1940.

54. Dietz, M. W.: Ileocecal histoplasmosis, Radiology **91:**285, 1968.

55. Felson, B.: Less familiar roentgen patterns of pulmonary granulomas, Amer. J. Roentgen. **81:**211, 1959.

56. Henderson, R. G., Pinkerton, H., and Moore, L. T.: Histoplasma capsulatum as cause of chronic ulcerative enteritis, J.A.M.A. **118:**885, 1942.

57. Negroni, P.: Histoplasmosis: diagnosis and treatment, rev. ed., Springfield, Ill., 1965, Charles C Thomas, Publisher, p. 28.

58. Perez, C. A., Sturim, H. S., Kouchoukos, N. T., and Kamberg, S.: Some clinical and radiographic features of gastrointestinal histoplasmosis, Radiology **86:**482, 1966.

59. Schwarz, E.: Radiologic contributions to the diagnosis of histoplasmosis, J.A.M.A. **170:**2171, 1959.

60. Shull, H. J.: Human histoplasmosis: disease with protean manifestations often with digestive system involvement, Gastroenterology **25:**582, 1953.

61. Silverman, F. N., Schwarz, J., Lahey, M., and Carson, R. P.: Histoplasmosis, Amer. J. Med. **19:**410, 1955.

62. Weiss, E. D., and Haskell, B. F.: Anorectal manifestations of histoplasmosis, Amer. J. Surg. **84:**541, 1952.

Gastrointestinal candidiasis

63. Brabander, J. O., Blank, F., and Butas, C. A.: Intestinal moniliasis in adults, Canad. Med. Ass. J. **77:**478, 1957.

64. Craig, J. M., and Farber, S.: The development of disseminated visceral mycosis during therapy for acute leukemia, Amer. J. Path. **29:**601, 1953.

65. Goldberg, H. I., and Dodds, W. J.: Cobblestone esophagus due to monilial infection, Amer. J. Roentgen. **104:**608, 1968.

66. Kaufman, S. A., Scheff, S., and Levene, G.: Esophageal moniliasis, Radiology **75:**726, 1960.

67. Murray, I. G., and Buckley, H. R.: Serological study of Candida species. In Winner, H. I., and Hurley, R., editors: Symposium on Candida infections, London, 1966, E. & S. Livingstone, Ltd.

68. Rogers, K. B.: Candida infections in paediatrics. In Winner, H. I., and Hurley, R., editors: Symposium on Candida infections, London, 1966, E. & S. Livingstone, Ltd.

69. Sanders, E., Levinthal, C., and Donner, M. W.: Monilial esophagitis in a patient with hemoglobin SC disease: demonstration of esophageal motor abnormality by cine-radiofluorography, Ann. Intern. Med. **57:**650, 1962.

70. Smith, J. M.: Mycoses of the alimentary tract, Gut **10:**1035, 1969.

71. Winner, H. I.: General features of Candida infections. In Winner, H. I., and Hurley, R., editors: Symposium on Candida infections, London, 1966, E. & S. Livingstone, Ltd.

72. Winner, H. I., and Hurley, R.: Candida albicans, London, 1964, J. & A. Churchill, Ltd.

Acute gastroenteritis

73. Dodd, K.: Gastroenteritis of viral origin, Med. Clin. N. Amer. **43:**1349, 1959.

74. Gorbach, S. L.: Acute diarrhea—a "toxin" disease? New Eng. J. Med. **283:**44, 1970.

Lymphogranuloma venereum

75. Annamunthodo, H.: Rectal lymphogranuloma venereum in Jamaica, Dis. Colon Rectum **4:**17, 1961.

76. Annamunthodo, H., and Marryatt, J.: Barium studies in intestinal lymphogranuloma venereum, Brit. J. Radiol. **34:**53, 1961.

77. Davey, W. W.: Companion to surgery in Africa, London, 1968, E. & S. Livingstone, Ltd.

78. David, V. C., and Loring, M.: Extragenital lesions of lymphogranuloma inguinale, J.A.M.A. **106:**1875, 1936.

79. de Lorimier, A. A., Moehring, H. G., and Hannan, J. R.: Clinical roentgenology, vol. 4, Springfield, 1956, Charles C Thomas, Publisher.

80. Helper, M., and Szilagyi, D. E.: Venereal lymphogranulomatous rectal stricture, Amer. J. Roentgen. **48:**179, 1942.

81. Klein, I.: Roentgen study of lymphogranuloma venereum: report of twenty-four cases, Amer. J. Roentgen. **51:**70, 1944.

82. Pessel, J. F.: Lymphogranuloma venereum. In Bockus, H. L., editor: Gastroenterology, ed. 2, vol. 2, Philadelphia, 1964, W. B. Saunders Co., pp. 1051-1063.

83. Rendich, R. A., and Poppel, M. H.: Lymphogranuloma of the colon, Radiology **33:**472, 1939.

84. Spiesman, M. G., Levy, R. C., and Brotman, D. M.: Lymphogranuloma inguinale: rectal stricture and pre-stricture, Amer. J. Dig. Dis. **3:**931, 1937.

85. Steinert, R.: Die Rectumverengerung bei Lymphopathia venerea und ihr röntgenologisches Bild, Acta Radiol. (Stockholm) **21:**368, 1940.

86. Valdes-Dapena, A. M., and Stein, G. N.: Morphologic pathology of the alimentary canal, Philadelphia, 1970, W. B. Saunders Co.

87. von Haam, E.: Venereal diseases and spirochetal infections. In Anderson, W. A. D., editor: Pathology, ed. 5, vol. 1, St. Louis, 1966, The C. V. Mosby Co., pp. 244-264.

88. Wright, L. T., Freeman, W. A., and Bolden, J. V.: Lymphogranulomatous strictures of rectum; résumé of 476 cases, Arch. Surg. **53:**499, 1946.

Chagas' disease

89. Anselmi, A., Pisani, F., Suárez, J. A., Gurdiel, O., and Lapco, L.: Cardiovascular radiology in acute and chronic Chagas' myocardiopathy: morphologic and dynamic study of the cardiac contour correlated with the histologic changes observed in myocardiopathies attributed to *Schizotrypanum cruzi*, Amer. Heart J. **73:**626, 1967.

90. Atías, A., Neghme, A., MacKay, L. A., and Jarpa, S.: Megaesophagus, megacolon, and Chagas' disease in Chile, Gastroenterology **44:**433, 1963.

91. Brasil, A.: Aperistalsis of the oesophagus, Rev. Brasil. Gastroent. **7:**21, 1955.

92. Ferreira-Santos, R.: Aperistalsis of the esophagus and colon (megaesophagus and megacolon) etiologically related to Chagas' disease, Amer. J. Dig. Dis. **6:**700, 1961.

93. Ferreira-Santos, R., and Carril, C. F.: Acquired megacolon in Chagas' disease, Dis. Colon Rectum **7:**353, 1964.

94. Johnson, C. M.: American trypanosomiasis, Med. Clin. N. Amer. **27:**822, 1943.

95. Köberle, F.: Megaesophagus, Gastroenterology **34:**460, 1958.

96. Köberle, F.: Enteromegaly and cardiomegaly in Chagas disease, Gut **4:**399, 1963.

97. Reeder, M. M., and Hamilton, L. C.: Tropical diseases of the colon, Seminars Roentgen. **3:**62, 1968.

98. Reeder, M. M., and Hamilton, L. C.: Radiologic diagnosis of tropical diseases of the gastrointestinal tract, Radiol. Clin. N. Amer. **7:**57, 1969.

99. Reeder, M. M., and Simão, C.: Chagas' myocardiopathy, Seminars Roentgen. **4:**374, 1969.

100. Simão, C.: Personal communication.

101. World Health Organization: Chagas' disease: report of a study group, WHO Techn. Rep. Ser. **202:**1, 1960.

Giardiasis

102. Antia, F. P., Desai, H. G., Jeejeebhoy, K. N., Kane, M. P., and Borkar, A. V.: Giardiasis in adults: incidence symptomatology and absorption studies, Indian J. Med. Sci. **20:**471, 1966.

103. Basu, S. P.: Radiological appearance of duodenal bulb in giardiasis, Bull. Calcutta School Trop. Med. **13:**64, 1965.

104. Brandborg, L. L., Tankersley, C. B., Gottlieb, S., Barancik, M., and Sartor, V. E.: Histological demonstration of mucosal invasion by Giardia lamblia in man, Gastroenterology **52:**143, 1967.

105. Cortner, J. A.: Giardiasis, a cause of celiac syndrome, A.M.A. Amer. J. Dis. Child. **98:**311, 1959.

106. Hermans, P. E., Huizenga, K. A., Hoffman, H. N., Brown, A. L., Jr., and Markowitz, H.: Dysgammaglobulinemia associated with nodular lymphoid hyperplasia of the small intestine, Amer. J. Med. **40:**78, 1966.

107. Hodgson, J. R., Hoffman, H. N., II, and Huizenga, K. A.: Roentgenologic features of lymphoid hyperplasia of the small intestine associated with dysgammaglobulinemia, Radiology **88:**883, 1967.

108. Hoskins, L. C., Winawer, S. J., Broitman, S. A., Gottlieb, L. S., and Zamcheck, N.: Clinical giardiasis and intestinal malabsorption, Gastroenterology **53:**265, 1967.

109. Manson-Bahr, P. H.: Manson's tropical diseases; a manual of diseases of warm climates, ed. 16, London, 1966, Baillière, Tindall & Cassell, Ltd.

110. Marshak, R. H., and Lindner, A. E.: Radiology of the small intestine, Philadelphia, 1970, W. B. Saunders Co.

111. Marshak, R. H., Ruoff, M., and Lindner, A. E.: Roentgen manifestations of giardiasis, Amer. J. Roentgen. **104:**557, 1968.

112. McLaughlin, L. A., Jr.: Giardial duodenitis: clinical manifestations of giardiasis in children (report of three cases), J. Louisiana Med. Soc. **115:**350, 1963.

113. Morecki, R., and Parker, J. G.: Ultrastructural studies of the human *Giardia lamblia* and subjacent jejunal mucosa in a subject with steatorrhea, Gastroenterology **52:**151, 1967.

114. Peterson, G. M.: Intestinal changes in *Giardia lamblia* infestation, Amer. J. Roentgen. **77:**670, 1957.

115. Reeder, M. M.: RPC of the month from the AFIP, Radiology **93:**427, 1969.

116. Reeder, M. M., and Hamilton, L. C.: Radiologic diagnosis of tropical diseases of the gastrointestinal tract, Radiol. Clin. N. Amer. **7:**57, 1969.

117. Takano, J., and Yardley, J. H.: Jejunal lesions in patients with giardiasis and malabsorption: an electron microscopic study, Bull. Johns Hopkins Hosp. **116:**413, 1965.

118. Welch, P. B.: Giardiasis with unusual findings, Gastroenterology **3:**98, 1944.

119. Yardley, J. H., and Bayless, T. M.: Giardiasis, Gastroenterology **52:**301, 1967.

Trichuriasis

120. Fisher, R. M., and Cremin, B. J.: Rectal bleeding due to Trichuris trichiura, Brit. J. Radiol. **43:**214, 1970.

121. Getz, L.: Massive infection with Trichuris trichiura in children; report of 4 cases with autopsy, Amer. J. Dis. Child. **70:**19, 1945.

122. Hunter, G. W., III, Frye, W. W., and Swartzwelder, J. C.: A manual of tropical medicine, ed. 4., Philadelphia, 1966, W. B. Saunders Co.

123. Manson-Bahr, P. H.: Manson's tropical diseases; a manual of diseases of warm climates, ed. 16, London, 1966, Baillière, Tindall & Cassell, Ltd.

124. Reeder, M. M., Astacio, J. E., and Theros, E. G.: Case of the month from the AFIP: an exercise in radiologic-pathologic correlation, Radiology **90:**382, 1968.

125. Reeder, M. M., and Hamilton, L. C.: Tropical diseases of the colon, Seminars Roentgen. **3:**62, 1968.

126. Stoll, N. R.: This wormy world, J. Parasit. **33:**1, 1947.

61 | Vascular disease

Richard H. Marshak
Arthur E. Lindner

ISCHEMIC JEJUNITIS, ILEITIS, AND COLITIS

Disturbances of the arterial or venous blood supply to the small bowel or colon may be responsible for a variety of clinical manifestations and roentgenographic findings.

The consequences of vascular occlusion depend upon the rapidity of onset, the length of intestine involved, and the efficiency of the collateral circulation.[9,10,13] Rapid occlusion of the major vessels supplying the intestine results in massive tissue necrosis and death from peritonitis and shock. Such catastrophic events usually allow little opportunity for roentgenographic study and are not reviewed in this chapter. When, however, the insult involves segmental rather than trunk vessels or when closure is slow enough to allow collateral flow to provide an adequate blood supply, total infarction of the intestine may not occur. In this case complete healing may subsequently take place.

Of great roentgenologic interest is an intermediate situation in which blood flow is sufficient to prevent death of the intestine yet not adequate for complete recovery of the damaged bowel wall. Such partial recovery may be associated with a variety of pathologic changes, including muscle atrophy or hypertrophy, fibrosis, and stricture formation. These changes may produce roentgenographic features that must be distinguished from inflammatory bowel disease and from tumor.

The layers of a segment of bowel are not equally sensitive to impairment of their blood supply. The mucosa appears to be most dependent on intact blood flow, and the initial change in vascular occlusion is superficial ulceration, often circumferential. The ulcer may subsequently heal or perforate or, with ensuing fibrosis, produce a stricture. The muscular layers are next involved, but the connective tissue layers of the submucosa and the subserosa may retain viability for considerable periods. Submucosal hemorrhage and edema cause localized nodularity or diffuse thickening of the mucosal folds. Ileus develops, either local or diffuse, and fluid accumulates within the lumen of the damaged intestine. After the vascular injury recovery may be complete, as the intramural blood and edema fluid are resorbed and the ulcerations heal without scars. On the other hand, fibrosis may result from the healing process, causing permanent stricture and proximal dilatation.

Clinically significant impairment of blood supply can occur even in the absence of gross changes in the bowel wall. When blood flow is sufficient to maintain function of the bowel at rest but inadequate to support the work of absorption and transit of a meal, the syndrome of intestinal angina may occur.[1] Characteristic clinical features are anorexia, weight loss, and postprandial abdominal pain. At times intestinal angina may be associated with a biochemically demonstrable malabsorption syndrome.

Mesenteric thromboses and emboli

Mesenteric arterial thrombosis is a complication of atherosclerosis. Gradual thrombosis, even if complete, may cause no changes in the intestine because collateral flow is adequate. Sudden occlusion, however, or gradual closure in the absence of collaterals leads to infarction of the bowel.

Venous thrombosis is less common than arterial occlusion and tends to occur in patients with abdominal neoplasms, polycythemia, venous impairment, or diseases associated with a hypercoagulable state.

Arterial emboli usually originate as mural thrombi in the heart after a myocardial infarction or as thrombi in a fibrillating atrium. These emboli tend to lodge in the branches of the superior mesenteric artery.

It is generally considered that all varieties of vascular accidents involve the branches of the superior mesenteric vessels more commonly than the inferior mesenteric. It has become apparent, however, that segmental vascular occlusion of the colon may be clinically mild, reversible, and difficult to diagnose[9,10] and may be more common than has been thought.

Nonocclusive mesenteric ischemia

With the advent of angiographic studies and early surgery in the management of acute mesenteric vascular disease, a surprising finding became apparent: in a large proportion of patients with mesenteric infarction neither thrombosis nor embolism can be demonstrated. In one study of 136 patients with mesenteric infarction, no vascular lesion could be found in half the cases.[12] This entity, which appears to be common, has been termed "nonocclusive mesenteric ischemia" and, although the mechanism remains to be established, it presumably represents a perfusion defect within the wall of the bowel.[14]

Ischemic disease

British workers have used the term "ischemic colitis" to designate the changes that occur in the colon after vascular occlusion.[10] The terms "ischemic ileitis" and "ischemic jejunitis" might

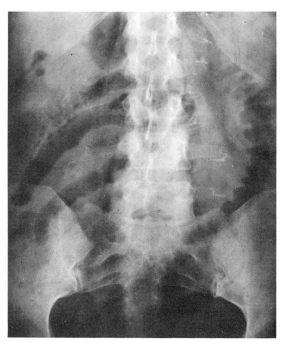

Fig. 61-1. Infarction of the small bowel. Two loops of jejunum in the right upper quadrant are moderately narrowed, rigid, and separated. The separation is the result of thickening of the walls, secondary to the venous congestion. The valvulae conniventes are absent. An additional loop of jejunum on the left side is involved to a lesser extent.

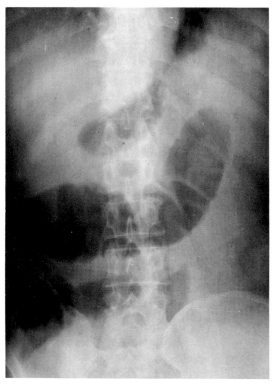

Fig. 61-2. Incomplete segmental infarction of the colon. Segmental dilatation of the right side of the colon is seen, and the haustral markings are still present.

be applied to similar processes in the small bowel. The roentgenologic findings in segmental ischemic disease in the small bowel and colon are remarkably similar except for differences in location. Any segment of the small bowel may be involved.[6] In the colon the most common locations appear to be the distal transverse colon, the splenic flexure, and the cecum; any segment of colon, however, including the rectum,[8] may be implicated.

The typical clinical presentation of mesenteric infarction is an acute episode of abdominal pain, first crampy and then continuous, sometimes associated with nausea, vomiting, diarrhea, abdominal distention, sweating, and apprehension. Gross blood usually is passed from the rectum. The color and the volume of the blood that is passed depend on the rapidity and severity of the hemorrhage and on the site of the infarction. The clinical manifestations vary greatly in severity. They may be so intense that they lead to peritonitis and shock, or they may be so mild that the episode is hardly noticed by the patient and is recalled only on direct questioning.

Characteristic roentgenographic features

A preliminary film of the abdomen is sometimes diagnostic. In the initial stages, no significant alterations may be identified. As the process continues, however, paralytic ileus occurs with edema of the valvulae or haustral markings and thickening of the wall (Fig. 61-1). As edema increases, the valvulae or haustra disappear. Segmental dilatation of the colon can be distinct (Fig. 61-2). Localized perforations may be identified; these occur more frequently in the colon, where they appear as pneumatosis coli.

Barium studies in the early stages reveal a marked degree of spasm associated with separation and uncoiling of the loops (Fig. 61-3). The involved segment may be difficult to fill because of the distinct spasm and irritability. The individual loops of bowel are separated from one another as if by thickening of the mesentery. The bowel lumen is narrowed, but there is no significant proximal dilatation at this stage. The folds are thickened and blunted, and in some segments a rigid picket fence, as seen in regional enteritis, is identified (Fig. 61-4). Multiple indentures, which have been described as "scalloping" or "thumb-printing," are seen along the contours of the bowel (Fig. 61-4). When seen face-on they appear as multiple polypoid filling defects. As edema progresses the folds become more thickened and hazy (Fig. 61-5). Although ulcerations are frequently seen in resected specimens of bowel with ischemic ileitis and colitis,

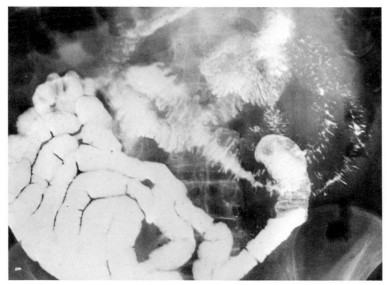

Fig. 61-3. Segmental infarction of the small bowel. There is marked spasm and irritability of several jejunal loops as well as separation and uncoiling.

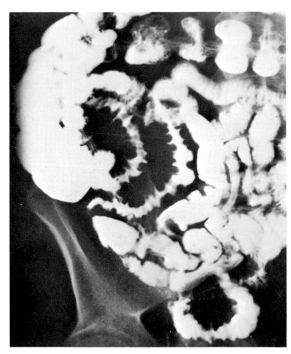

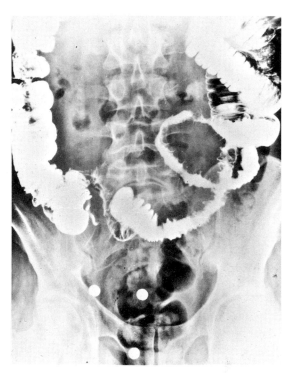

Fig. 61-4. Segmental infarction. Moderate narrowing and rigidity of the distal loops of ileum, associated with thickening and blunting of the folds, are demonstrated. The involved loops of bowel are moderately separated. These findings are similar to those of regional enteritis.

Fig. 61-5. Segmental infarction. Moderate narrowing and rigidity of the distal ileal loops is shown. The narrowing is most pronounced in the terminal ileum. The proximal loops are dilated. The mucosal folds are thickened and blurred, and there is increased secretion.

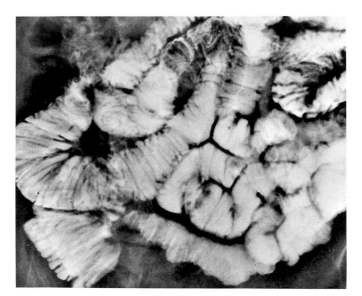

Fig. 61-6. Segmental infarction. A view during the healing stage of a loop of proximal ileum for a distance of 9 inches reveals slight narrowing, slight thickening of the folds, and rigidity. The inferior aspect of the loop is irregular as a result of early pseudodiverticula or sacculations.

the ulcerations are not always deep enough to be recognized as individual ulcers on roentgenographic studies. With diffuse ulceration the entire mucosa may be completely effaced, and the barium column presents a smooth, homogeneous configuration.

We have studied two unusual cases of ischemic disease of the colon in which deep ulcerations were found to involve the entire thickness of the bowel wall. In one, the lesion mimicked a large submucosal tumor with extensive ulceration. In the other, a large pocket of gas was seen adjacent to the sigmoid and was related to a deep ulcer in this segment.

As healing and fibrosis progress, flattening and rigidity of one border may ensue. The antimesenteric border then becomes pleated or plicated, forming multiple sacculations or pseudodiverticula (Fig. 61-6). As fibrosis continues, a long tubular segment with smooth contours and a concentric lumen is identified, and finally a stricture with proximal dilatation is seen (Figs. 61-7 and 61-8). The strictures may be short, but more commonly they are 3 or 4 inches long.

The sequence of findings just described is rapid. In a period of several weeks the lesion progresses from the initial stage of spasm and edema to stricture formation (Figs. 61-9 to 61-12). In the stages before fibrosis develops, partial or complete reversibility may occur (Figs. 61-13 and 61-14). The process may stop at any one of the stages, and the patient may be first seen at any stage. In some cases not only is the bowel dilated proximal to the stricture, but poststenotic dilatation is also seen. The fact that the stricture is usually shorter than the initial area of involvement suggests that at the onset there was probably more widespread impairment of the blood supply. Since ulcerations are rarely deep, sinus tracts and fistulas are unusual.

In the colon a similar sequence of roentgenographic findings is identified, but pleating and sacculation are more common. A toxic megacolon resembling that observed in the course of ulcerative colitis has been reported.[11] In these cases marked colonic distention occurred in association with large penetrating ulcers and pseudopolypoid changes.

It must be noted that ischemic colitis may develop proximal to a colonic carcinoma (Figs. 61-15 to 61-28), so it is important to rule out a neoplasm by appropriate clinical and roent-

Text continued on p. 1622.

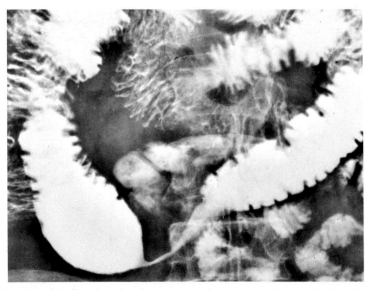

Fig. 61-7. Segmental infarction. In the same patient as was shown in Fig. 61-3, 4 weeks later there is a strictured segment of bowel with smooth contours. The stricture is concenric and joins the proximal and distal bowel in a fusiform tapering fashion. The proximal and distal bowel are dilated.

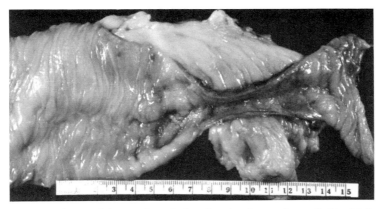

Fig. 61-8. Gross specimen of incomplete infarction in the patient of Fig. 61-7. A tubular fibrotic segment 7 cm. long with a conical transition to the adjacent bowel is shown. Microscopic examination revealed partial necrosis of all the walls of the bowel associated with the fibrosis.

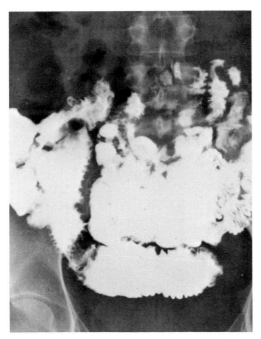

Fig. 61-9. Incomplete infarction. In a 22-year-old female patient 1 month following an uncomplicated pregnancy and delivery, the distal ileum is slightly spastic and irritable, with slight thickening of the folds.

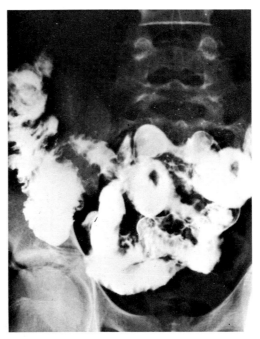

Fig. 61-10. Incomplete infarction. In the same patient as was shown in Fig. 61-9, 3 weeks later there is more narrowing and rigidity of the ileum. The folds are more thickened and polypoid defects are identified.

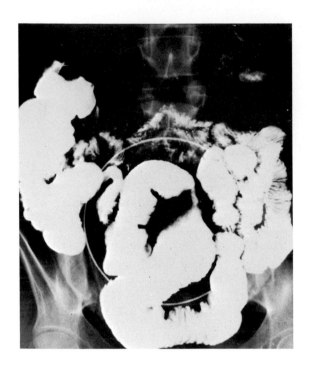

Fig. 61-11. In the same patient as in Fig. 61-9, 1 month after the initial study a short stricture is seen. The proximal portion of the bowel is dilated, and the terminal ileum reveals a moderate degree of narrowing.

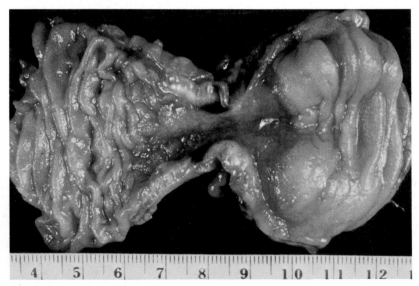

Fig. 61-12. Gross specimen demonstrating a short stricture secondary to incomplete infarction in the patient of Fig. 61-9.

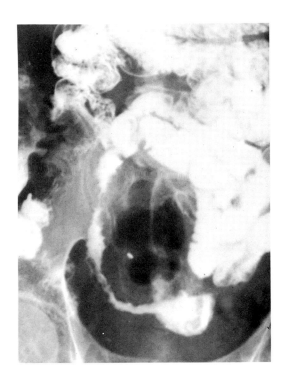

Fig. 61-13. Incomplete infarction. Considerable narrowing and moderate rigidity of the distal ileum is demonstrated. The proximal portion of the bowel is not dilated, indicating that some of the narrowing is secondary to spasm.

Fig. 61-14. In the patient of Fig. 61-13, reexamination 3 weeks later reveals only minimal narrowing and rigidity of the distal ileum, and slight blunting of the folds. The terminal ileum itself is normal except for slight dilatation. The patient was a 72-year-old man who experienced severe right lower quadrant pain associated with the passage of dark red stools. He made an uneventful recovery.

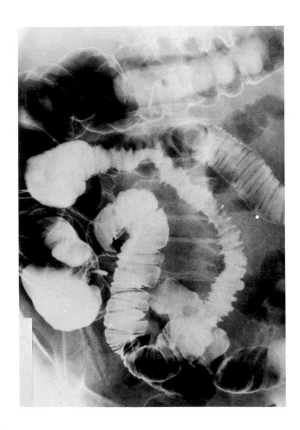

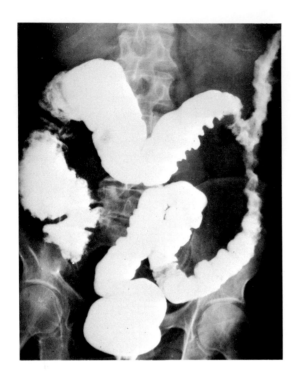

Fig. 61-15. Segmental infarction of the colon in a 67-year-old man who had had a coronary occlusion 4 years previously. There is a moderate degree of spasm and rigidity of the distal transverse and descending colon. The folds are thickened, associated with scalloping of the contours. No discrete ulcerations are identified. The segmental infarction was confirmed at autopsy.

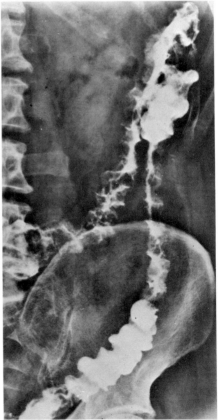

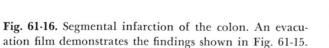

Fig. 61-16. Segmental infarction of the colon. An evacuation film demonstrates the findings shown in Fig. 61-15.

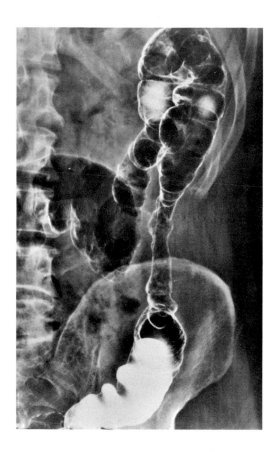

Fig. 61-17. Segmental infarction in the patient of Fig. 61-15, 1 month after the original examination. In the middescending colon there is a narrowed segment of bowel approximately 5 inches long with smooth contours.

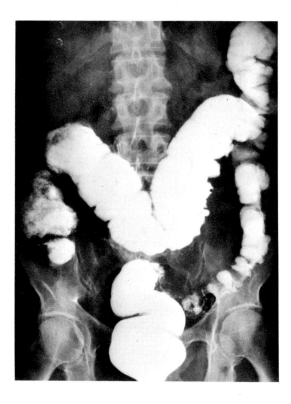

Fig. 61-18. In the patient of Fig. 61-15, 2 months after the original episode moderate reversibility of the lesion is demonstrated. At this time there is slight flattening of the inferior wall of the distal transverse colon. The descending colon reveals sacculation and a moderate number of pseudodiverticula.

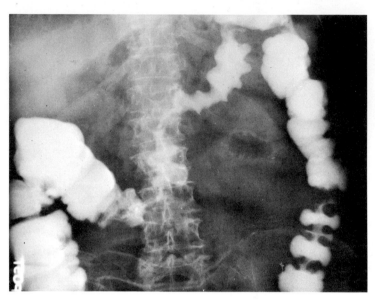

Fig. 61-19. Incomplete segmental infarction of the colon in a 70-year-old woman occurring with acute onset of abdominal pain and subsequent passage of bright red blood in the stool. Considerable spasm and irritability of the transverse colon took place, associated with thickening of the folds. Moderate degree of scalloping of the contours is noted.

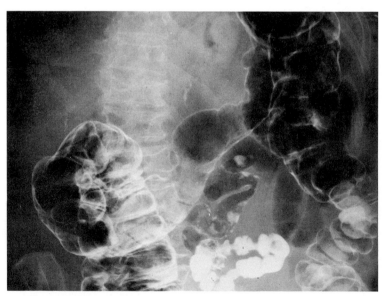

Fig. 61-20. In the patient of Fig. 61-19, 1 month later the transverse colon reveals only slight narrowing and rigidity with minimal irregularity of the superior contour. These findings persisted for 1 year after the onset of infarction.

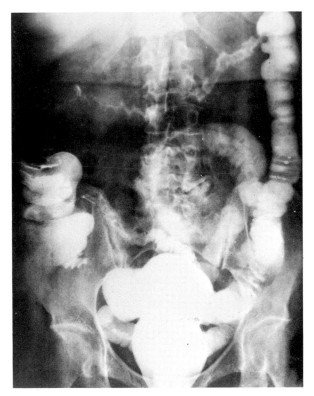

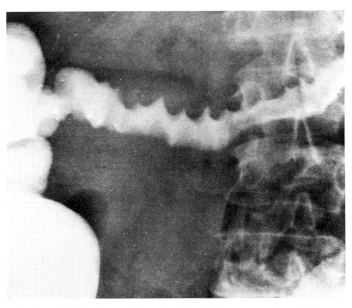

Fig. 61-22. In the patient of Fig. 61-21, a spot film of the transverse colon reveals narrowing, rigidity, and a moderate degree of scalloping. The barium enema examination returned to normal in 1 month.

Fig. 61-21. Incomplete segmental infarction with marked spasm and irritability of the transverse colon. A barium enema was performed 2 days after a severe abdominal episode associated with a moderate amount of rectal bleeding in a 70-year-old woman.

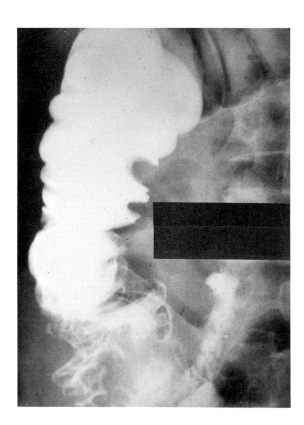

Fig. 61-23. Segmental incomplete infarction with reversibility in a 60-year-old woman. The cecum and ascending colon are slightly narrowed and rigid. There is a moderate degree of scalloping on the medial aspect of the colon.

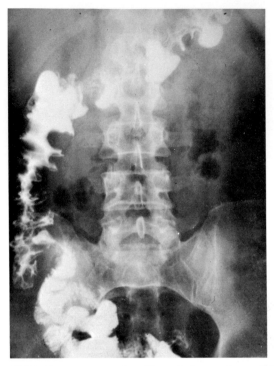

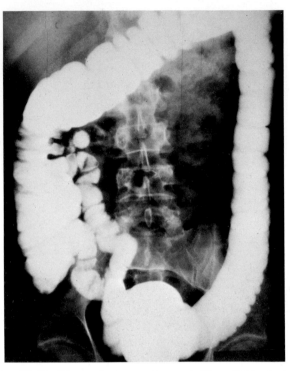

Fig. 61-24. In an evacuation film of the patient of Fig. 61-23, thickening of the folds is shown.

Fig. 61-25. View of the patient of Fig. 61-23 shows complete reversibility of the previous findings.

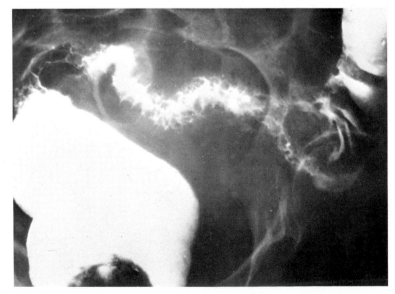

Fig. 61-26. Early stage of segmental infarction involving the sigmoid. The condition is characterized by a moderate degree of narrowing, rigidity, and thickening of the folds.

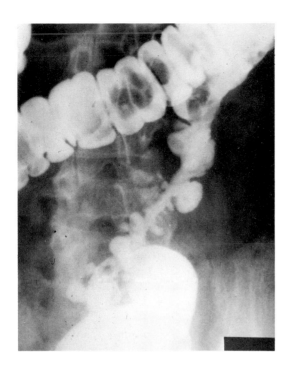

Fig. 61-27. Late stage of segmental incomplete infarction of the colon. Narrowing and rigidity of the colon are revealed, as well as multiple sacculations or pseudodiverticula of the descending colon.

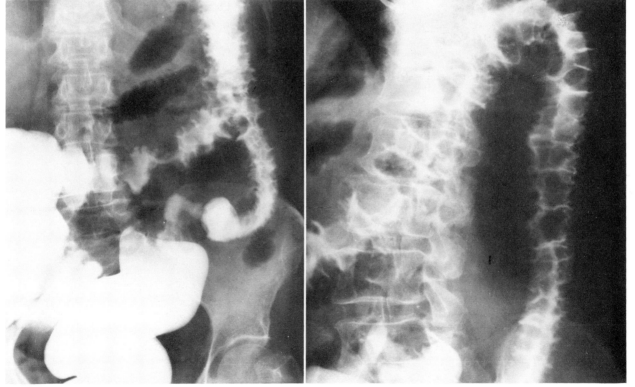

A

B

Fig. 61-28. A, Carcinoma with appearance of ischemic colitis proximal to a sigmoid carcinoma. Carcinoma obstructs the sigmoid. The changes proximal to the sigmoid and involving the entire descending colon and distal half of the transverse colon are typical of ischemic colitis. The roentgenographic findings were confirmed at necropsy. B, Same examination. Spot film of the splenic flexure. Marked edema of the folds (thumb-printing) is apparent.

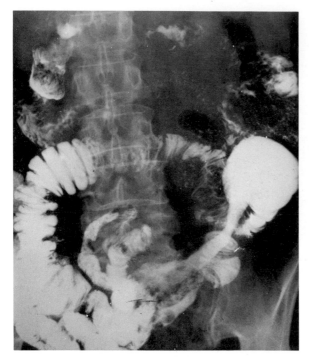

Fig. 61-29. Reduced strangulated hernia. In a 54-year-old woman with a right femoral hernia containing a loop of ileum a segment of ileum about 6 inches long shows tubular stenosis with effacement of the mucosal pattern and conical transition to the proximal dilated bowel. The surgeon thought the loop of bowel was viable despite the fact that it appeared discolored. The ileal loop was returned to the abdomen and the wound closed. Three weeks after operation symptoms of intestinal obstruction occurred.

genologic studies in all patients with vascular disease of the colon. The mechanism of development of colitis in association with colonic carcinoma is unclear, but experimental studies[5] suggest that large-bowel obstruction may be responsible for interference with the transmural blood supply to the colon proximal to the lesion.

In summary, then, the characteristic roentgenographic features of ischemic ileitis and colitis are thumb-printing, picket-fence thickening of the folds, sacculation, tubular narrowing, and stricture. The differential diagnosis includes carcinoma and granulomatous inflammatory disease. The stricture in infarction is smooth and tapering, with a concentric lumen and without overhanging margins or discrete ulcerations. Sacculations are common, especially in the colon. Skip lesions are unusual. In contrast to these findings, longitudinal ulcerations, fissuring, and skip lesions are frequent findings in granulomatous disease. Carcinoma is easily excluded by the lack of overhanging margins and the absence of an eccentric lumen.

Segmental vascular compromise

Segmental vascular compromise may occur from incarceration of bowel in a hernial sac (Figs. 61-29 to 61-31), from bands or adhesions, and from volvulus or intussusception.[16] When

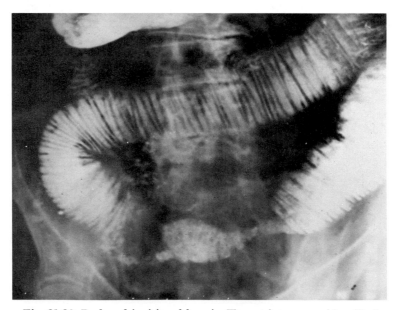

Fig. 61-30. Reduced incisional hernia. Two strictures are identified.

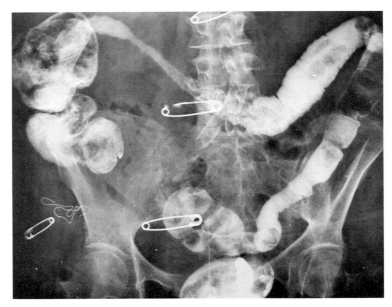

Fig. 61-31. Reduced incisional hernia. There is tubular narrowing of the proximal transverse colon.

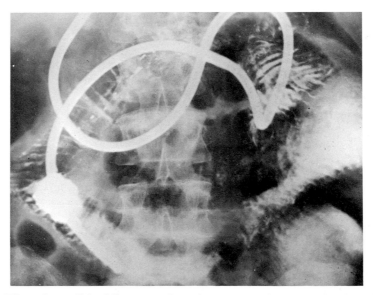

Fig. 61-32. Thromboangiitis obliterans. There is a narrowed segment in the midjejunum where the mucosa is effaced secondary to edema. There is probably diffuse superficial ulceration present in this segment.

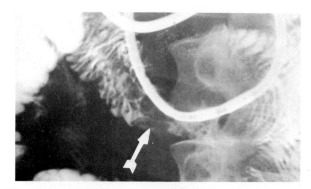

Fig. 61-33. In the patient of Fig. 61-32, the involved jejunal segment now reveals more narrowing and rigidity, with slight polypoid thickening of the folds.

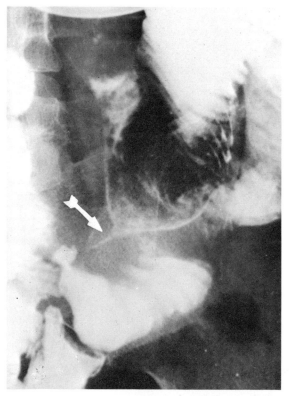

Fig. 61-34. In the patient of Fig. 61-32, 4 weeks later a stenotic segment measuring 2 cm. in length is identified. This patient passed a cast of the small intestine by way of his intestinal tract. Pathologic examination of this material confirmed the fact that it represented necrotic small intestinal wall, 18 cm. in length. At operation, two areas of stenosis and an obliterating endophlebitis of the mesenteric veins were revealed.

infarction is incomplete but the bowel is not resected, stricture formation may occur just as in segmental infarction of the bowel.

Vasculitis

Vasculitis, as in polyarteritis nodosa,[4] lupus erythematosus, or Buerger's disease (Figs. 61-32 to 61-34), may narrow the arterial lumen sufficiently to cause ischemic changes in the bowel. These alterations may be responsible for some of the obscure abdominal pain patterns in these diseases and also for mucosal ulceration and perforation.

The roentgenographic changes in vasculitis are remarkably similar to those in segmental infarction. In the early stages there is narrowing of the lumen associated with a mild degree of rigidity. The folds are thickened, hazy, and blunted. Increased secretions are prominent because of the inflammatory process. Discrete ulcerations are usually not deep enough to be identified on roentgenographic studies, but in more severe cases the entire mucosa appears effaced because of diffuse ulceration. Skip lesions are not unusual. Although perforations occur, sinus tracts and fistulas with walled-off abscesses are infrequent.

Schönlein-Henoch syndrome

Schönlein-Henoch syndrome is an acute arteritis characterized by purpura, nephritis, abdominal pain, and joint pain. The disease tends to be self-limited, often developing several weeks after a streptococcal infection. At times, however, it evolves into a syndrome indistinguishable from polyarteritis nodosa or glomerulonephritis. In the bowel Schönlein-Henoch changes are marked by submucosal edema. All portions of the gastrointestinal tract except the esophagus have been reported to be involved.[6] Pain and tenderness in the abdomen are the clinical features, and when fever is present an acute condition within the abdomen may be suspected. Either diarrhea or constipation may occur. At exploratory laparotomy the involved bowel has been described as appearing reddened and edematous, but unlike the findings in infarction, the mesenteric vessels pulsate normally. Histologic section shows an arteritis with extensive edema of the mucosa and submucosa. The disease process is reversible, and healing is complete without fibrosis or stenosis.

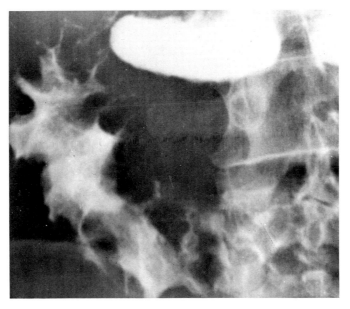

Fig. 61-35. Henoch's purpura. The folds in the second portion of duodenum are markedly exaggerated and have a hazy nodular appearance.

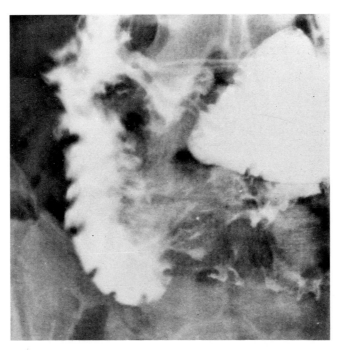

Fig. 61-36. In the patient of Fig. 61-35, 1 month later there is a marked improvement in the appearance of the folds.

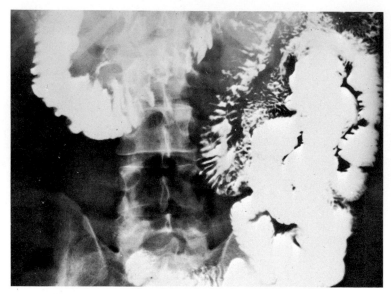

Fig. 61-37. Henoch's purpura. Exaggerated thickened folds accompanied by spasm and irritability are seen in the fourth portion of the duodenum and in the proximal jejunum.

In Schönlein-Henoch syndrome the most conspicuous roentgenographic alteration is the appearance of the fold pattern. The folds are thickened and blurred because of the marked edema and increased secretions (Figs. 61-35 to 61-38). The blurring and indistinctness of the folds may become so pronounced that complete effacement of the entire fold pattern may be seen (Figs. 61-39 and 61-40). As the edema and secretions increase, the barium column becomes segmented and fragmented. Occasionally, scalloping and marked thumb-printing resulting from excessive edema and hemorrhage may be identified. In the colon an appearance of carcinoma may be simulated (Figs. 61-41 and 61-42). Discrete ulcerations are not seen. Because of the increased secretions and the thickening of the folds, intestinal lymphangiectasia may be suggested in the differential diagnosis.

Ulceration with potassium ingestion

Another form of vasculitis appears to be responsible for the occasional development of ulcerations of the small bowel when enteric-coated potassium tablets are ingested. Patients may present with obstruction, perforation, or bleeding,[2] and at laparotomy the lesion is found to be a circumferential ulcer. Experimental data indicate

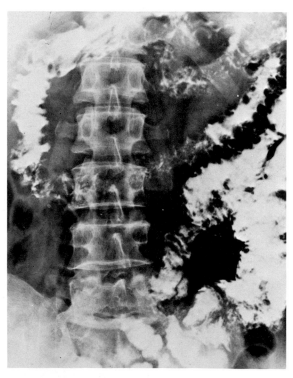

Fig. 61-38. Henoch's purpura. Almost the entire small intestine is involved. The condition is characterized by an irregular thickening of the mucosal folds, increased secretions, and minimal segmentation. The bowel lumen is of normal caliber.

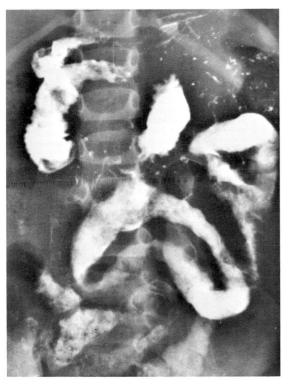

Fig. 61-39. Henoch's purpura. The small intestine is slightly dilated. The mucosal pattern is coarse and in some areas effaced, presumably because of increased secretions and mucosal edema.

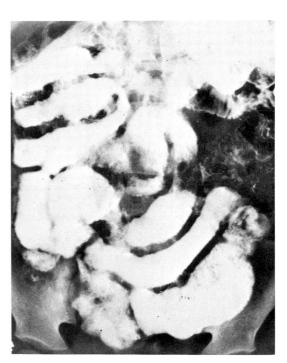

Fig. 61-40. Henoch's purpura. In the patient of Fig. 61-39, 3 days later the small bowel changes are slightly less pronounced.

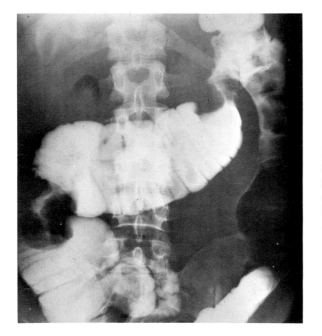

Fig. 61-41. Henoch's purpura. Two segmental areas of narrowing in the colon are characterized by sharply defined margins, a concentric lumen that contains some degree of flexibility, and irregular thickening of the folds without mucosal ulceration. The appearance is consistent with a circumferential submucosal lesion.

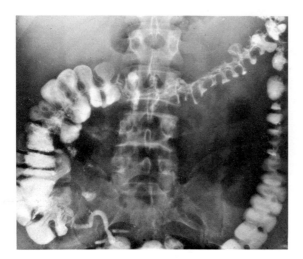

Fig. 61-42. In the patient of Fig. 61-41, 2 weeks later the colon appears normal.

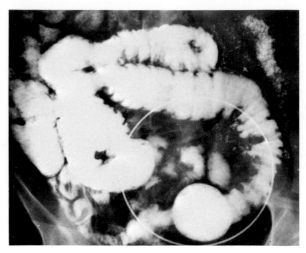

Fig. 61-44. In the patient of Fig. 61-43, 2 weeks later the jejunum and proximal ileum are more dilated; the distal ileum shows a normal configuration. A strictured segment is obscured by the round dilated segment in midileum (cobra-head deformity). At operation a moderate degree of fibrosis, and a small area of stenosis secondary to a tiny ulcer were revealed. All these changes are secondary to the local release of potassium.

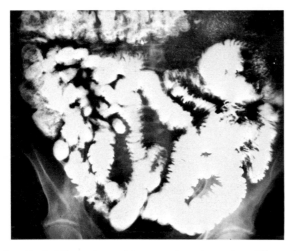

Fig. 61-43. Ulceration with potassium ingestion. There is marked hyperactivity of the jejunum and proximal ileum with minimal dilatation. The patient was a 54-year-old man who had been receiving enteric-coated potassium tablets for 4 weeks. The gastrointestinal series was performed for intermittent abdominal cramps.

that the precipitating factor is rapid release of potassium from enteric-coated tablets, with absorption over a short segment of bowel.[3] This high concentration is believed to cause spasm or paralysis of intramural and submucosal veins with venous stasis, edema, and local infarction. Circumferential ulceration ensues. With mild injury complete recovery may occur, but with greater degrees of damage, hemorrhage or perforation may result or subsequent fibrosis may lead to intestinal obstruction.

In the early stages of ulceration caused by enteric-coated potassium, there are no specific roentgenographic changes. Spasm with overactivity of the bowel and slight narrowing of the lumen may be seen (Fig. 61-43). After an interval, usually 2 to 4 weeks, a short segment of stenosis is identified. The bowel immediately proximal to the stenosis is dilated in a smooth, elliptical fashion. This has been termed a "cobra-head" deformity (Fig. 61-44). Because the segment proximal to the small stenotic area is dilated, it is frequently difficult to demonstrate the segment of stenosis. On rare occasions the ulceration in the stenotic segment can be visualized (Figs. 61-45 and 61-46). More often, however, the ulcer is so superficial that it fails to fill with contrast material. The lesions are usually single but may be multiple. The marked hyperactivity of the dilated proximal bowel should not be interpreted as the evidence of multiple ulcerations. Perforation can occur at the ulcer site.

INTRAMURAL BLEEDING

Bleeding into the intestinal wall may occur with trauma to the abdomen, with coagulation defects, and with the use of anticoagulant medi-

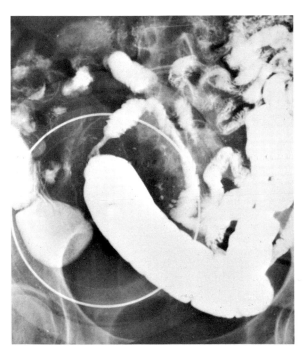

Fig. 61-45. Ulceration with potassium ingestion. A tiny ulcer crater with a short stricture and proximal dilatation is seen in midileum.

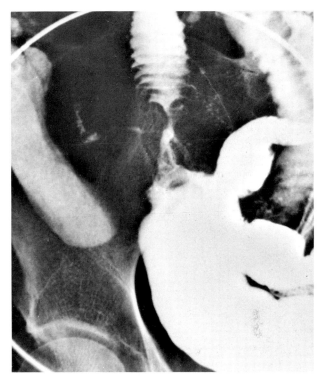

Fig. 61-46. In a 50-year-old woman who had received enteric-coated potassium tablets for 2 weeks the ulcer crater is well visualized with compression. Operation revealed the small ulcer and an area of stenosis. The patient made an uneventful recovery. Visualization of the ulcer crater on small-bowel examination is unusual.

cations. It may also occur in association with the coagulation defects of such neoplasms as leukemia, myeloma, lymphoma, or metastatic carcinoma. Thrombocytopenia, hypofibrinogenemia, circulating anticoagulants, activation of the fibrinolytic system, and dysproteinemia have been implicated in intramural bleeding.

In cases associated with trauma, an intramural mass develops, and the duodenum is commonly the area involved. This localization may occur because the bowel tends to fix the duodenum between its ligamentous supports and the spinc.[15] In spontaneously occurring hematomas there tends to be a diffuse infiltration of the bowel wall rather than a localized intramural mass, and any portion of the bowel may be involved without predilection for the duodenum.[7] With passage of time and correction of coagulation defects, if these are present, the intramural hematoma is resorbed and the bowel returns to its normal appearance.

Histologic examination of the bowel involved in intramural hemorrhage shows thickening of the intestinal wall with submucosal extravasation of blood.

Symptoms

Symptoms of intramural bleeding may range from mild abdominal discomfort to the clinical features of intestinal obstruction. Either gross or microscopic blood is often present in the stool, but it may be only a transitory finding, easy to overlook. Paralytic ileus commonly occurs, but if the lumen is narrowed the picture may be one of mechanical obstruction. Full clinical recovery following supportive medical treatment is the rule, and surgical intervention is rarely required if the diagnosis of intramural bleeding can be established from the clinical and roentgenologic features.

Roentgenographic findings

A preliminary roentgenogram of the abdomen may demonstrate significant findings. If there

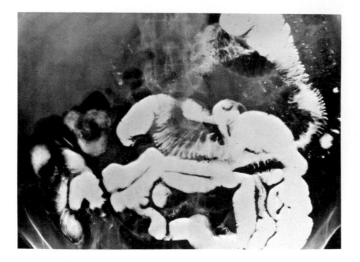

Fig. 61-47. Intramural bleeding secondary to anticoagulant therapy. For a distance of 9 inches the distal jejunum is slightly narrowed and shows some loss of flexibility. Marked alterations, characterized by sharp delineation, uniform thickening, a spikelike configuration, and symmetric regular spacing simulating a stack of coins, are present in the folds. There is no mucosal ulceration or nodularity suggestive of inflammatory or neoplastic process. The bowel immediately proximal to this segment is slightly dilated. All these changes are secondary to anticoagulant therapy.

Fig. 61-48. In the patient of Fig. 61-47, 2 days later there has been considerable resolution of the degree and extent of involvement. The folds are less thickened and the bowel lumen has become wider. Autopsy 9 months later showed no abnormality of the small bowel.

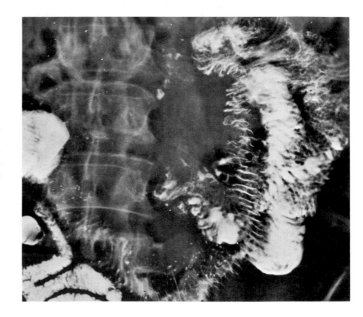

is a solitary hematoma of sufficient size, it may be recognized either by its increased density or by the displacement of loops of the small or large bowel. If the hemorrhage is confined to the bowel wall, varying degrees of paralytic ileus, narrowing of the bowel lumen, or localized filling defects producing marked scalloping of the bowel may be seen. Differentiation from infarction on the preliminary roentgenogram alone can be difficult.

With barium studies, the roentgenographic changes caused by intramural hemorrhage have many typical features. The variation in the roentgenographic appearance seems to be a reflection of the difference in the extent of intramural hemorrhage and the presence of mucosal edema and intestinal secretions. Changes in the small intestine have been reported more frequently than in the large bowel, and involvement of the esophagus and stomach has not been documented.

The roentgenographic alterations are usually segmental but may be diffuse. The involved segments of small bowel reveal varying degrees

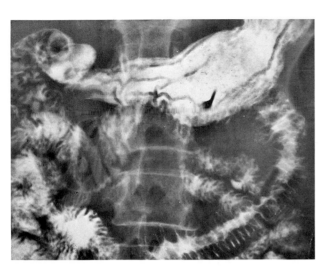

Fig. 61-49. Intramural bleeding secondary to anticoagulant therapy. The changes noted in hemorrhage into the bowel are again seen. On the antimesenteric side the irregularly thickened folds have a uniform appearance. On the mesenteric side the folds are irregularly flattened, not only by the intramural hematoma but by blood in the mesentery as well.

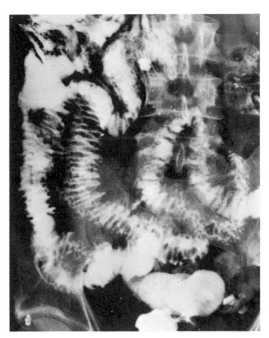

Fig. 61-50. Idiopathic thrombocytopenic purpura with hemorrhage into the small intestinal wall. The folds in the distal ileum are thickened and have a stacked coin appearance. The appearance is similar to that noted in intramural bleeding secondary to anticoagulant therapy. The findings in this patient were confirmed at surgery during splenectomy.

of rigidity and uncoiling of the loops, depending on the amount and extent of bleeding into the bowel wall and mesentery. Marked rigidity and separation of the loops of bowel are rarely observed. As a rule, mechanical or clinical obstruction is not prominent, although some degree of narrowing of the bowel lumen is frequent. We have observed transient intussusception proximal to the lesion in one case. When bleeding ceases, resorption of the hemorrhage and complete resolution appear to be the rule.

The small intestine fold pattern has a characteristic appearance. There is a uniform, regular thickening of the folds, sharp delineation of their margins, and a parallel arrangement producing a symmetric, spikelike configuration that resembles a stack of coins. This stacked-coin appearance is the most prominent alteration and is more striking in the jejunum than the ileum because of the better developed jejunal folds (Figs. 61-47 and 61-48). There is a conspicuous lack of spasm or changeability of folds. Bleeding into the mesentery is a frequent

finding, especially in patients receiving anticoagulants and in hemophiliac patients. Evidence of a mass, flattening of the folds on the mesenteric side of the bowel, and separation and uncoiling of the bowel loops is noted. If the mesenteric hemorrhage is large, hammock-like configuration of the bowel segments may result (Fig. 61-49). Resolution of these findings in a short period of time is observed on followup examinations (Figs. 61-50 to 61-53).

The changes in the colon are similar to those seen in the small bowel, except that the scalloped areas may be large (Figs. 61-54 to 61-56).

Differential diagnosis

Differentiation of the roentgenographic changes of mesenteric vascular occlusion from those caused by intramural bleeding may be difficult. This is especially true because a patient who is receiving anticoagulants may develop a mesenteric occlusion. In favor of anticoagulant-induced changes are the stacked-coin appearance, lack of spasm or irritability, presence of a

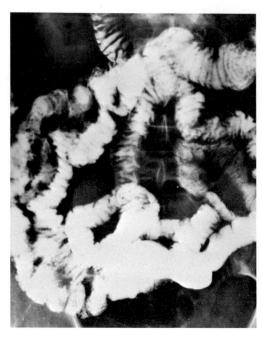

Fig. 61-51. In the patient of Fig. 61-50, 5 weeks later the abnormal findings have completely disappeared.

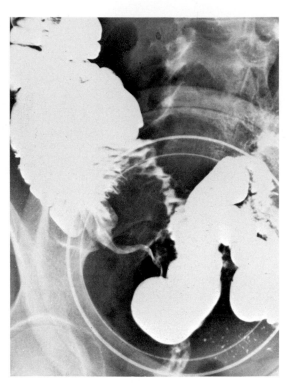

Fig. 61-52. Intramural bleeding with hemophilia. The terminal ileum is moderately narrowed and rigid with irregularity of the contours. The folds are thickened. There was no evidence of spasm or irritability.

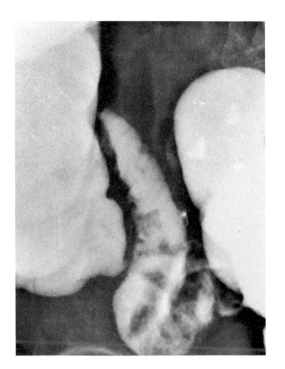

Fig. 61-53. In the patient of Fig. 61-52, 2 months later there is complete resolution of the changes.

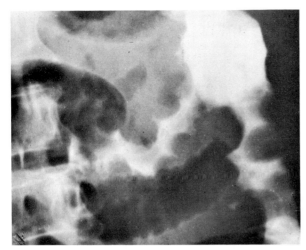

Fig. 61-54. Intramural bleeding in the colon. There is marked scalloping and thumb-printing of the distal transverse colon and proximal descending colon secondary to intramural hemorrhage following anticoagulant therapy.

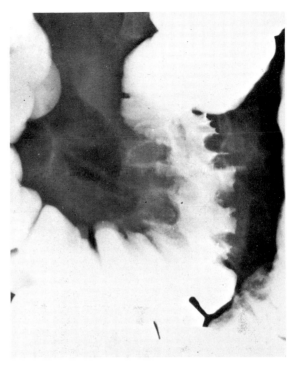

Fig. 61-56. Intramural bleeding with hemophilia. A short segment of the transverse colon is slightly narrowed and the contours are scalloped.

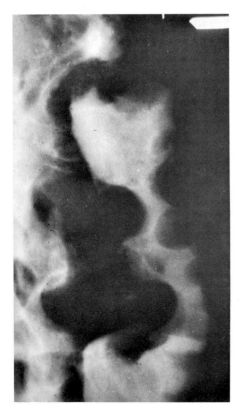

Fig. 61-55. In the patient of Fig. 61-54, a spot roentgenogram demonstrates the characteristic thumb-printing and scalloping in the colon. Except for the fact that the changes are more pronounced, the appearance is similar to that of infarction.

mesenteric mass, and complete resolution of the roentgenographic findings. In mesenteric vascular occlusion a localized mesenteric mass caused by bleeding is uncommon, and the folds exhibit varying degrees of edema, spasm, and irritability. The usual sequel of vascular occlusion is a stricture at the site of the maximally infarcted segment. In some cases, however, differential diagnosis is impossible since complete resolution of the roentgenographic changes has been noted in mesenteric vascular occlusion (Figs. 61-57 to 61-59).

Inflammatory lesions of the small bowel can readily be differentiated from intramural hemorrhage. In the early stages there is marked spasm and irritability; later, ulceration, inflammatory polyps, marked rigidity, and separation of the loops of bowel are evident. Neoplastic diseases of the small bowel, specifically lymphosarcoma, can be distinguished by ulceration, localized dilatation, tumor nodules, or multiple areas of involvement.

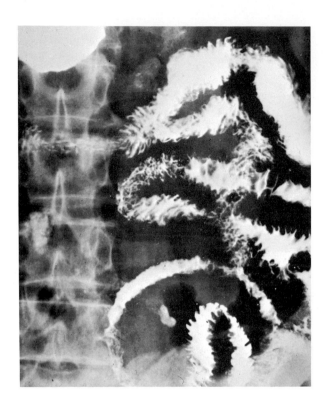

Fig. 61-57. Mesenteric venous thrombosis. The visualized portion of the bowel in this film reveals a moderate degree of narrowing, rigidity, separation of the loops of bowel, and thickening and blunting of the folds. In the proximal portion of the bowel the alterations are highly suggestive of intramural hemorrhage. Distally the folds appear to be effaced. The patient was an 80-year-old woman who died the day following the small-bowel examination. Study of the small bowel at autopsy revealed an extensive mesenteric venous thrombosis. The mucosal changes were caused by a combination of hemorrhage and edema.

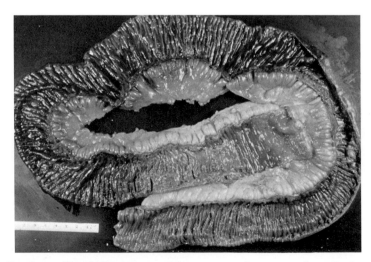

Fig. 61-58. Specimen illustrating an extensive mesenteric venous thrombosis, responsible for the roentgenographic changes described in Fig. 61-57.

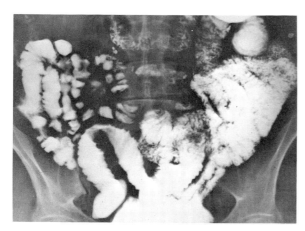

Fig. 61-59. This film shows an abnormal loop of jejunum characterized by thickening and flattening of the folds, without ulceration or nodularity. Some abnormal motor activity is identified. The patient, a 58-year-old woman on anticoagulation therapy, 3 months following a myocardial infarction developed midabdominal pain. She made an uneventful recovery and a follow-up study showed no abnormality of the small bowel. It was impossible to determine whether these changes were secondary to anticoagulant therapy or to a mesenteric infarction.

REFERENCES

1. Bircher, J., Bartholomew, L. G., Cain, J. C., and Adson, M. A.: Syndrome of intestinal arterial insufficiency ("abdominal angina"), Arch. Intern. Med. **117**:632, 1966.
2. Boley, S. J., Allen, A. C., Schultz, L., and Schwartz, S.: Potassium-induced lesions of the small bowel, I. Clinical aspects, J.A.M.A. **193**:997, 1965.
3. Boley, S. J., Schultz, L., Krieger, H., Schwartz, S., Elguezabal, A., and Allen, A. C.: Experimental evaluation of thiazides and potassium as a cause of small-bowel ulcer, J.A.M.A. **192**:763, 1965.
4. Ettinger, A., and Perez-Tamayo, R.: Ulcerative jejunitis in polyarteritis, Radiology **68**:669, 1957.
5. Glotzer, D. J., and Pihl, B. G.: Experimental obstructive colitis, Arch. Surg. (Chicago) **92**:1, 1966.
6. Handel, J., and Schwartz, S.: Gastrointestinal manifestations of the Schönlein-Henoch syndrome, Amer. J. Roentgen. **78**:643, 1957.
7. Khilnani, M. T., Marshak, R. H., Eliasoph, J., and Wolf, B. S.: Intramural intestinal hemorrhage, Amer. J. Roentgen. **92**:1061, 1964.
8. Kilpatrick, Z. M., Farman, J., Yesner, R., and Spiro, H. M.: Ischemic proctitis, J.A.M.A. **205**:71, 1960.
9. Marshak, R. H., Maklansky, D., and Calem, S. H.: Segmental infarction of the colon, Amer. J. Dig. Dis. **10**:86, 1965.
10. Marston, A., Pheils, M. T., Thomas, M. L., and Morson, B. C.: Ischemic colitis, Gut **7**:1, 1966.
11. Miller, W. T., Scott, J., Rosato, E. F., Rosato, F. E., and Crow, H.: Ischemic colitis with gangrene, Radiology **94**:291, 1970.
12. Ottinger, L. W., and Austin, W. G.: A study of 136 patients with mesenteric infarction, Surg. Gynec. Obstet. **124**:251, 1967.
13. Schwartz, S., Boley, S., Schultz, L., and Allen, A.: A survey of vascular diseases of the small intestine, Seminars Roentgenol. **1**:178, 1966.
14. Williams, L. F.: Vascular insufficiency of the bowels, Disease-a-Month, August, 1970, Chicago, 1970, Yearbook Medical Publishers.
15. Wiot, J. F.: Intramural small intestinal hemorrhage—a differential diagnosis, Seminars Roentgenol. **1**:219, 1966.
16. Wolf, B. S., and Marshak, R. H.: Segmental infarction of the small bowel, Radiology **66**:701, 1956.

Part XII

Combined roentgenologic and endoscopic procedures

Peroral retrograde cholangiography and pancreatography | 62

Jack A. Vennes

The biliary tree and the pancreas remain as difficult areas in which to evaluate disease precisely. The pancreas is particularly inaccessible, and improved diagnostic methods are badly needed. Available techniques for visualizing the biliary ductal system are more advanced and have provided a background of experience in this system. However, all cholangiographic methods operate with some limitation. Because of the inherently difficult diagnostic problems in both organ systems, any method of visualizing both the pancreatic and the biliary duct system in a diagnostic evaluation must receive serious consideration. Endoscopic cannulation and retrograde injection of one or both ductal systems is the most recent method to be evaluated.

Although the initial fiberoptic concepts of light transmission were developed in the United States and in Europe,[4] Japan has been a very important contributor to their further engineering and medical application.[11] Instrumentation developed both in the United States and Japan has been widely used and developed to make fiberoptic endoscopy available as a safe, precise technique in evaluation of the gastrointestinal tract. Extension of fiberoptic methods to evaluation of the biliary and pancreatic systems is a potentially important advance also developed in Japan.[6-10] Experience with the technique has now been reported from other centers.[1,3,12]

THE INSTRUMENT

The instrument used is a flexible fiberoptic side-viewing duodenoscope. My colleagues and I have used the Olympus JF instrument; it has a 10 mm. diameter and greater flexibility than fiberscopes designed for other uses (Figs. 62-1 and 62-2). A 70 degree angle, cold-lighted view of excellent detail can be seen with variable magnification. An auxiliary teaching attachment allows viewing by a second observer, and a 35 mm. camera may also be attached for photo-

graphic record. Biplane controls plus rotation of the device permit steering the tip in any plane or direction. Options of insufflating air or water or applying suction are provided. A 1.6 mm. Teflon cannula can be inserted through the instrument, and its distal tip can be precisely positioned in the visual field by a simple, hand-operated lever control. A.C.M.I.* has developed another side-viewing instrument, incorporating the same features, through which the cannulation procedure can be satisfactorily performed.

After suitable preparation of the patient, the ampulla of Vater can be visualized through these flexible fiberoptic instruments; contrast material can be injected through a cannula inserted into the ductal orifice, with subsequent roentgenography. With proper attention to detail a study of diagnostic quality can be quite predictably obtained. The procedure is well tolerated by patients, and morbidity is acceptably low.

TECHNIQUE OF EXAMINATION

The procedure is carried out in a radiology examining room equipped with high-resolution fluoroscopic monitoring. Fifteen minutes before

---

*American Cystoscope Makers, Inc.

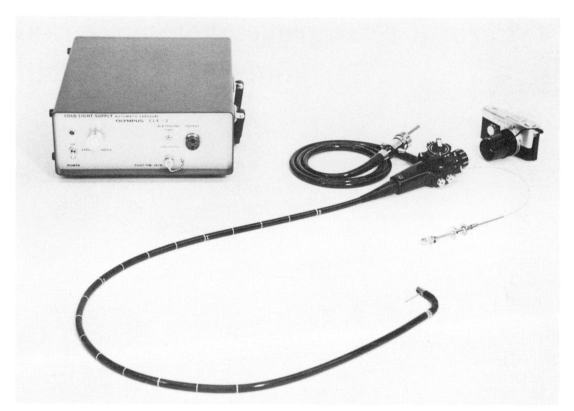

Fig. 62-1. Side-viewing duodenoscope used for cannulation (Olympus JF-B2). Cold light is transmitted to the instrument through one fiber bundle and to the distal tip through a light-carrying bundle in the instrument. A high resolution image is returned to the observer's magnified field of vision through another fiber bundle. Controls allow precise fourway manipulation of the tip and of the cannula. In this particular illustration a biopsy forceps is in place.

the procedure, duodenal atony and papillary smooth muscle relaxation are achieved by administration of anticholinergics, dicyclomine (Bentyl) hydrochloride or glucagon. Through an intravenous drip positioned in the right arm, diazepam (Valium), from 2 to 30 mg., is slowly administered to sedate the patient to a level of cooperative somnolence. Smooth muscle relaxants and diazepam may be added to the intravenous drip as needed during the procedure. The pharynx is lightly anesthetized with a topical agent of choice. The obvious may need stating at this point, namely that a thorough discussion of the procedure, and of any concerns the patient may have about it, is of fundamental importance for the success of the procedure.

The patient is placed in the left lateral position on the padded x-ray table. The instrument is introduced orally and gently passed through the stomach and duodenal bulb into the descending duodenum. Although other endoscopic observations may be made incidentally during the withdrawal of the scope, if the process is prolonged this is best done on another occasion as needed. When the instrument is in the descending duodenum it is usually most helpful to turn the patient into the prone position, which offers a more panoramic view of the descending duodenum. A minimal amount of insufflated air now remains trapped in the duodenum, offering a good field of view if the pharmacologic preparation has rendered the duodenum atonic. A brief spray of water containing a defoaming agent removes interfering bubbles of mucus. If at all indicated, the third portion of the duodenum can be quickly examined at this point in the procedure, as in a case in which pancreatic disease is suspected or suspected radiologic de-

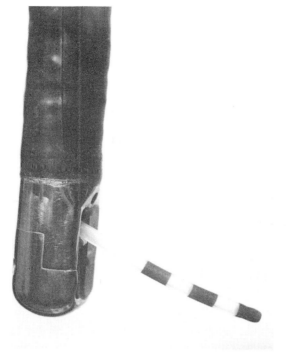

Fig. 62-2. Distal tip of endoscope. The diameter is 10 mm. A marked cannula, 1.6 mm in diameter, is protruding from the tip of the instrument.

fects require evaluation. The scope can then be retracted to search for the papilla of Vater. The search can begin downward from the junction of the bulb with the descending duodenum or upward from a point low in the descending duodenum. The tip of the instrument is rotated as the lumen is examined circumferentially on withdrawal.

Generally, the papilla is seen as a raised structure on the posterior medial wall about 6 or 8 cm. beyond the bulb. It is frequently found at the superior end of a serpiginous vertical fold that interrupts the continuity of the transverse plicae. It may usually be identified by color and shape, since it has a redder color than the surrounding tan duodenal mucosa and usually presents a profile protruding into the duodenal lumen. Its shape depends in some measure on the state of smooth muscle relaxation induced by the prior drug preparation and may change during the examination from a conical to hemispherical profile. Rarely, the papillary excrescence is absent and the ductal orifice may be recognized only as a discrete reddened area. In about 25% of patients a second papilla, smaller and paler, can be found where the duct of Santorini enters the duodenum, a few centimeters cephalad to the main papilla. This main papilla is the one through which the pancreatic duct of Wirsung and the common bile duct usually enter. The several varying relationships of these two ductal drainages of the pancreas are usually unimportant for purposes of this study. Visualization of the duct of Wirsung is much easier and on all but rare occasions provides a diagnostic study.

The correct papilla having been identified, it remains for the operator to position the cannula so that it is close to the ductal orifice and addresses it squarely. Search of the papilla will usually provide some indication of where the ductal orifice is emerging, although the orifice itself is not visible. Search for a small, more reddened, often slightly depressed area near the center of the papillary mass usually provides a needed clue as to location of the orifice. There may be converging folds, and occasionally an overlying fine, white, mucoid reticular network is seen. In some patients there are two ductal orifices on the same papillary mass; this poses a separate set of problems in terms of visualizing both ducts or, more specifically, the clinically desired ductal system.

The cannula is now advanced through the scope so that its tip emerges into the field of vision, having been previously filled with water soluble contrast agent. Our experience has been with meglumine diatrizoate and sodium diatrizoate (Renografin). The cannula must be occluded proximally by a short guide wire or by the contrast-filled syringe, so that air bubbles are precluded from entering the ductal system as filling artifacts.

With the ductal orifice centered close to the scope the cannula is now gently but confidently advanced. Further positioning and insinuation of the cannula into a ductal orifice require integrated manipulation of the biplane controls, elevating or depressing the cannula tip, rotation of the entire instrument, and occasionally changing the patient's position. If the papillary mass feels firm to the exploring cannula and if no tachycardia exists, the patient may be given an anticholinergic or glucagon intravenously for more complete smooth muscle relaxation. Once entry is achieved, the cannula depth is adjusted so that it remains just engaged during tidal respiration.

Contrast agent is now cautiously injected under close fluoroscopic control. If only the pancreatic duct is being opacified, from 2 to 5 ml. of 60% Renografin is injected slowly to avoid over distention. If the common bile duct is entered from 5 to 40 ml. of contrast agent is needed to fill all structures; the larger amounts are required if the gallbladder fills during the procedure. In visualizing the gallbladder or a dilated common bile duct, the use of a more dilute solution of contrast material is frequently advisable so that small filling defects are not overlooked. The dye having been injected, the instrument is temporarily withdrawn from the field of radiation while appropriate roentgenograms are taken. The instrument can be advanced and the cannula reinserted if the other ductal system is to be visualized or if the first attempt is inconclusive.

Selection of the clinically desired duct depends on a number of largely anatomic variables, such as the existence of a significant common channel or existence of two separate ductal orifices, separated only by a septum or at times by some relatively considerable distance on the papilla. To visualize the common bile duct it is often necessary to recall the very early cephalad course that it pursues even in its intramural portion.[5] Technical details will not be gone into further here; suffice it to state that most of them have been mastered. In our last 100 attempts the clinically desired duct was visualized in diagnostic detail on 92 occasions, probably approaching an irreducible minimum of failures. Ampullary infiltrations by tumor, failure to cannulate the very high-lying papilla, and incomplete understanding of the intramural ductal relationship all contribute to occasional failure.

INDICATIONS

Indications for endoscopic ductal visualization are still evolving. Cholangiographic indications are fairly definitive and similar to those of other established methods—intravenous, percutaneous, or surgical cholangiography. In our experience with 230 examinations about half were for possible extrahepatic biliary obstruction. In most of these patients a clinical diagnosis of obstructive jaundice had been made by all usual criteria, in-

cluding intravenous cholangiography when applicable. A preoperative study was requested to confirm the diagnosis and establish the site and etiology of obstruction. Another subgroup was studied with primary liver disease as the presumptive cause of jaundice, but because of persisting hyperbilirubinemia and some evidence suggesting possible extrahepatic obstruction a cholangiogram was requested. The list of primary liver diseases included alcoholic liver disease, biliary cirrhosis, chronic active hepatitis, as well as sclerosing cholangitis. Concern over possible coexisting extrahepatic obstruction in this group of patients is a familiar and nagging clinical problem.

During the developmental phase of this technique, most investigators have applied pancreatography to discovery of definable disease entities—carcinoma, chronic pancreatitis, pancreatic pseudocyst, and acute pancreatitis. In six instances we have successfully used the laterally viewed course of the pancreatic duct to evaluate suspicious retrogastric mass lesions.

CONTRAINDICATIONS

Contraindications to peroral retrograde ductal visualization are few. Pancreatography in the study of acute pancreatitis is arbitrarily delayed for four weeks after clinical remission. While not contraindicated, study of patients with probable common duct obstruction and of patients with suspected pancreatic pseudocyst should be deferred until the day prior to scheduled tentative surgery to avoid some of the complications listed later. Patients up to 88 years of age with various cardiopulmonary problems have been studied without difficulty except for transient respiratory depression in one patient due to premedication. The presence of pyloric stenosis, tumor infiltration, or extrinsic compression (as by a pseudocyst) will occasionally preclude adequate study.

COMPLICATIONS

Complications of the procedure have been thoroughly reviewed by Cotton.[2] Febrile reactions and acute pancreatitis are of most concern. In our experience with 230 examinations, pancreatitis, defined as amylase elevation with pain persisting longer than 2 hours, developed in 7 patients, most of whom were studied early in our experience. It is our impression that the

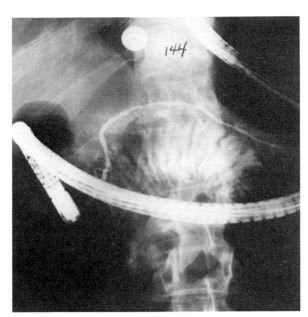

Fig. 62-3. Normal pancreatic duct. Note the normal lateral branching and tapering and one of the many variations in the normal course of the duct.

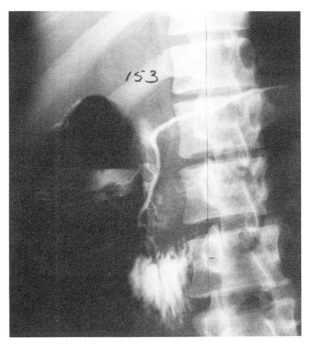

Fig. 62-4. Contrast material refluxing back through the duct of Santorini.

incidence has decreased as the pancreatic duct is filled more slowly and cautiously under better fluoroscopic control. Eight patients have developed febrile reactions 24 hours after the procedure. Two of these cases occurred after dye entered a pancreatic pseudocyst and the other six after visualization of an obstructed common bile duct. Three of this latter group had clinical evidence of cholangitis. All patients recovered. These serious reactions have been successfully avoided since we adopted a policy of early surgery when indicated. When obstruction of either ductal system is clinically suspected, the patient is tentatively scheduled for surgical management the day after endoscopic study. Since this practice has been observed, no further febrile reactions have occurred. Their etiology remains obscure, however, and is being investigated. One elderly patient developed transient respiratory depression after a small dose of premedication. Our experience is similar to that of others in that asymptomatic hyperamylasuria occurs after cannulation in over one third of patients; this occurs frequently although pancreatography may not have been included as part of the study.

ROENTGENOGRAPHIC FINDINGS

Our own experience to date has resulted in 230 successful cannulation studies in 260 attempts. Much more importantly, the clinically desired duct can now be visualized in nine of ten patients (Figs. 62-3 to 62-5).

Endoscopic cholangiography proves to be highly specific in determining the existence, site, and etiology of extrahepatic obstruction. Results of pancreatography (Figs. 62-6 to 62-9) are less definitive, and clear-cut diagnostic criteria must await attention to finer detail in a larger collective experience. The principal findings in pancreatic carcinoma have been ductal obstruction or stricture. Ductal disruption is usually part of the necrotizing process of pseudocyst formation, and the cystic space fills readily as contrast material enters the duct. However, on two occasions simple ductal obstruction by the cystic mass has been observed. Ductal obstruction is therefore not a specific finding. A group of patients with chronic pancreatitis is being systematically studied to determine whether ductal characteristics offer any pathognomonic clues. Tortuous dilatation, with or without obstruction,

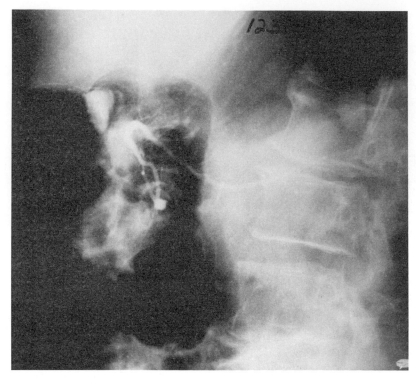

Fig. 62-5. Lateral view of normal pancreatic duct.

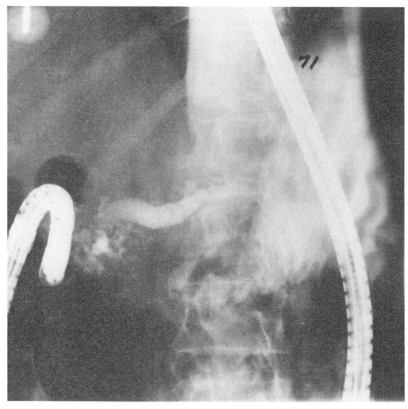

Fig. 62-6. For legend see opposite page.

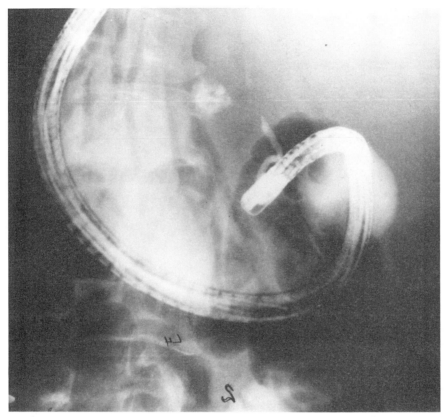

Fig. 62-7. Pancreatic adenocarcinoma. Seen laterally, the normal duct in the head of the gland is attenuated in the body and terminates in a small pool of contrast material. This proved to be a small cystic space within the center of an unresectable tumor mass. The smooth bolus of contrast material overlying the bend of the scope is in the duodenal bulb.

Fig. 62-6. Chronic pancreatitis. Typical findings include ductal dilatation (with or without obstruction), tortuosity, and dilated stubby lateral branches. Note tremendous dilatation of smaller ducts in the uncinate process, with dilated lateral branches. This particular duct is obstructed at about the point at which it blends with contrast material in the stomach.

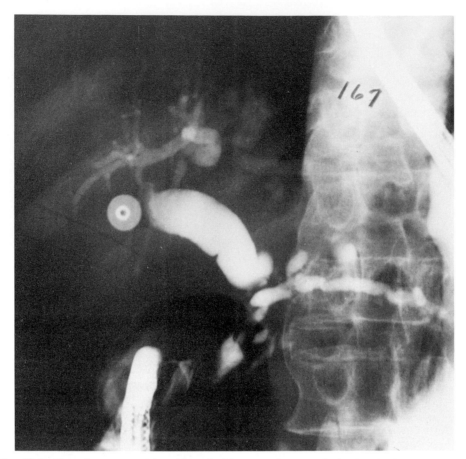

Fig. 62-8. Chronic pancreatitis with coincident carcinoma of the head of the pancreas. The somewhat dilated pancreatic duct with dilated sacular lateral branching is seen over the spine. Both the dilated common bile duct and the pancreatic duct, however, are attenuated for some distance between the papilla at the lower border of the picture and the medial edge of the duodenal shadow. The typical findings of chronic pancreatitis plus ductal stricture in the head have been present in four cases so far in our experience of coincident malignant disease.

and dilated, snubbed-off lateral branches are characteristic findings in the alcoholic patient who has greatly reduced exocrine pancreatic function and fibrotic glands when seen surgically. Several studies have revealed irregular cavernous spaces inside a fibrotic shell. Again, our diagnostic confidence is shaken by the coincident finding of adenocarcinoma in the head of an otherwise fibrotic gland with chronic pancreatitis on four occasions. The need for more critically analyzed experience is evident. Details of fine lateral ductal branches and the time required for ductal emptying are two of the variables as yet not systematically evaluated. The

routine study of patients after acute pancreatitis may prove to be worthwhile. Two unsuspected pseudocysts and several instances of calculi in the gallbladder or common duct or both have been discovered in study of eighteen patients thus far. Radiologically suggested retrogastric mass lesions have been evaluated by this means in a small number of patients. Endoscopic observations can be helpful at times whether or not cannulation studies are possible. Malignant infiltration can be recognized and biopsied when present. Impacted stones may present as smooth submucosal masses at the papilla; they usually disimpact as the cannula is advanced.

Text continued on p. 1652.

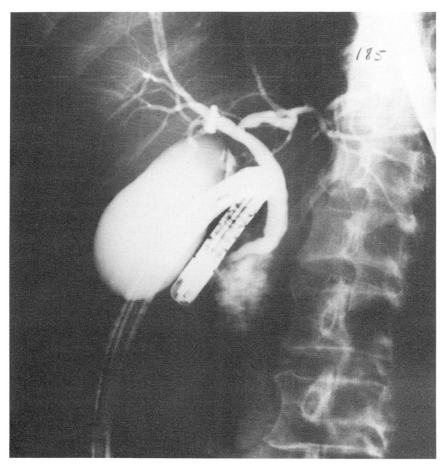

Fig. 62-9. Pancreatic pseudocyst, with normal biliary tree and cystic duct and gallbladder. As the pancreatic duct was entered, an immediate blush of dye was seen filling the space noted between the scope tip and the spine. No attempt was made to completely fill the cystic space, and the larger cyst was evident at surgery.

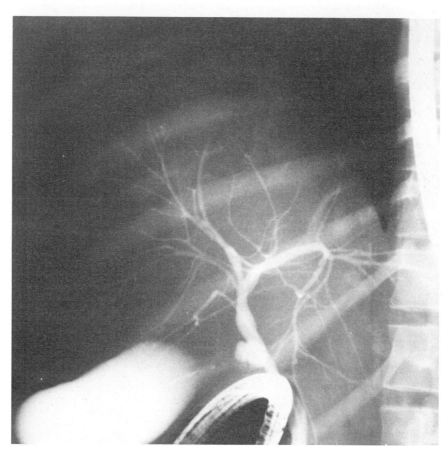

Fig. 62-10. Normal biliary tree. Note the normal contour, course, and caliber of the extra-hepatic bile duct. The scope (diameter of 10 mm.) is in approximately the same plane as the duct.

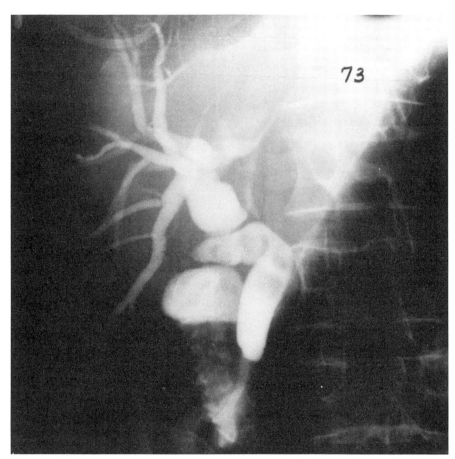

Fig. 62-11. Choledocholithiasis and benign common bile duct stricture. Painless jaundice occurred in an 88-year-old man, 19 years after a cholecystectomy. In the common duct and cystic duct remnant are four large calculi. A benign stricture is present. The intrahepatic branches are only partially filled.

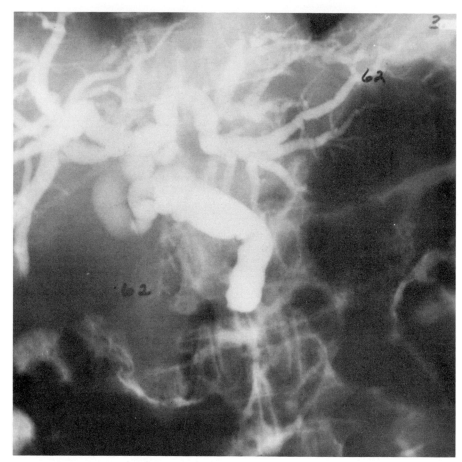

Fig. 62-12. Obstruction of the common bile duct secondary to pancreatic carcinoma. The patient had painless progressive jaundice. Tremendous dilatation of the biliary tree includes a cystic duct remnant. The pancreatic duct is completely occluded. Pancreatic calcifications of chronic pancreatitis are seen to the left of the spine.

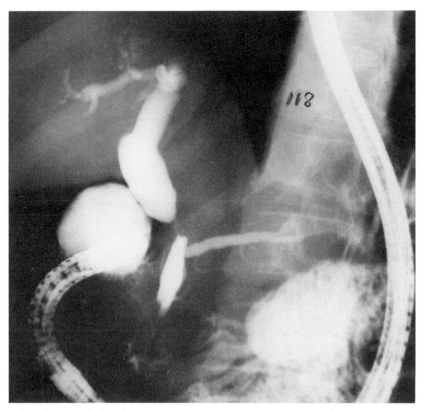

Fig. 62-13. Primary cholangiocarcinoma. Note a rather severe stricture of the common duct above an initially normal duct next to a partially drained normal pancreatic duct. The dilated common bile duct above is incompletely filled with dye. There is a bolus of contrast material in the duodenal bulb.

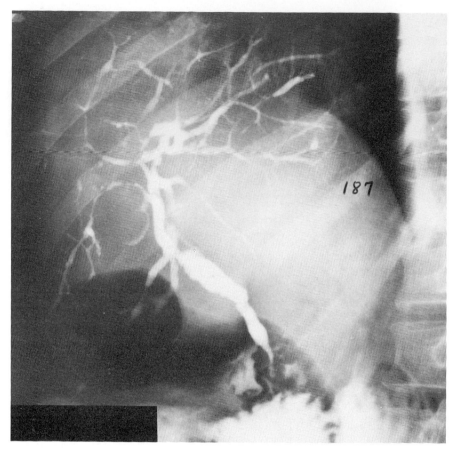

Fig. 62-14. Sclerosing cholangitis. The patient had mild jaundice and liver disease after 8 years of mild ulcerative colitis. The irregular caliber of both the common duct and the intrahepatic branches is consistent with this finding.

CONCLUSIONS

It is evident that ductal cannulation is a fairly sophisticated endoscopic procedure. Many of the technical details have been worked out during the developmental phase, however, so that it can be mastered by experienced endoscopists who have reasonable experience and give attention to detail. Visualization of the clinically desired system may be expected with acceptably high frequency, producing studies of diagnostic quality. A low morbidity can now be expected. Endoscopic cannulation studies have important diagnostic potential. This is more evident in the biliary tree at present (Figs. 62-10 to 62-15). Our results are more clear cut and can be evaluated against an already existing experience with other prior methods. Hopefully, diagnostic criteria for various disease states can be worked out successfully in the pancreatic ductal system, although at present caution is necessary in interpretation of findings.

REFERENCES

1. Classen, M.: Fibreendoscopy of the intestines, Gut **12:**330, 1971.
2. Cotton, P. B.: Cannulation of the papilla of Vater by endoscopy and retrograde cholangiopancreatography (ERCP), Gut **13:**1014, 1972.
3. Cotton, P. B., Salmon, P. R., Beales, J. S. M., and Burwood, R. J.: Endoscopic trans-papillary radiographs of pancreatic and bile ducts, Gastrointest. Endosc. **19:**60, 1972.
4. Goldman, J. A., Bereskin, S. and Shackney, C.: Fiber optics in medicine, New Eng. J. Med. **273:** 1425, 1965.
5. Hand, B. H.: An anatomical study of the choledochoduodenal area, Brit. J. Surg. **50:**486, 1962.

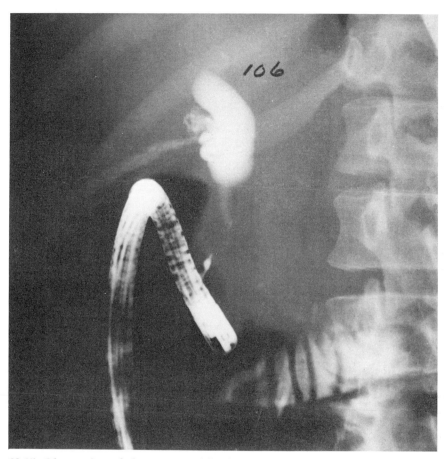

Fig. 62-15. Obstruction of the common bile duct caused by pancreatic fibrosis. The patient was studied for probable chronic pancreatitis, and was thought to have alcoholic liver disease as the cause of jaundice. The pancreatic duct, not shown here, was nearly completely occluded. The intrapancreatic common duct, attenuated and dilated above, is incompletely filled.

6. Kasugai, T., Kuno, N., Kizu, M., Kobayashi, S., and Hattori, K.: Endoscopic pancreatocholangiography. II. The pathological endosopic pancreatocholangiogram, Gastroenterology 63:227, 1972.

7. Ogoshi, K., Niwa, M., Hara, Y., et al: Endoscopic pancreatocholangiography in the evaluation of pancreatic and biliary disease, Gastroenterology 64:210, 1973.

8. Ogoshi, K., Tobita, Y., Hara, Y.: Endoscopic observations of the duodenum and pancreato-choledochography using duodenal fiberscope under direct vision, Gastrointest. Endosc. (Tokyo) 12:83, 1970.

9. Oi, I.: Fiberduodenoscopy and endoscopic pancreatocholangiography, Gastrointest. Endosc. 17:59, 1970.

10. Takagi, K., Ikeda, S., Nakagawa, Y., Sakaguchi, N., Takahashi, T., Kumakura, K., Maruyama, M., Someya, N., Nakano, H., Takada, T., Takekoshi, T., and Kin, T.: Retrograde pancreatography and cholangiography by fiber duodenoscope, Gastroenterology 59:445, 1970.

11. Takemoto, T., Nakao, K.: Progress in the structure of various fiber gastroscopes. In Proceedings of the First Congress of the International Society of Endoscopy, Tokyo, 1966, p. 89.

12. Vennes, J. A., and Silvis, S. E. Endoscopic visualization of bile and pancreatic ducts, Gastrointest. Endosc. 18:149, 1972.

Part XIII

Alimentary tract roentgenology from the viewpoint of the gastroenterologist

General gastroenterologic considerations | 63

Walter L. Palmer

EXAMINATION
Roentgenologic examination

In the 70 years since Cannon first proved the feasibility of the use of the roentgen ray for the study of the digestive tract[18] the procedure has advanced steadily. There has been progressive improvement in the clarity of the image, continued reduction in the radiation required, and decreasing risk of radiation injury. The early studies of Barclay,[5] Carman and Miller,[19] Cole,[22] and others with fluoroscopy and unaimed films progressed to the mucosal relief techniques using the spot films and aimed exposures of Åkerlund,[2] Berg,[10] and Templeton,[72] and now to image amplification and cinephotography. These procedures enable the clinician to see the films and thus to share responsibility for their interpretation.

The radiologist is entitled to know the pertinent facts of the patient's history. He should be informed as to the nature of the primary problem: Is it difficulty in swallowing, substernal pain, epigastric pain, or abdominal pain? Is it acute or chronic? Is it related to taking food or to bowel movements? Has there been nausea and vomiting, diarrhea or constipation, a gain or loss of weight? Is the patient anemic; has there been bleeding? The roentgenographic examination is not a substitute for a good history; the two go hand in hand.

In general terms, the roentgenographic study provides, with minimal discomfort to the patient, the most reliable objective evidence of gastrointestinal disease beyond the reach of the scope. Frequently the radiologist finds conditions unsuspected by the clinician. Partly because of these facts, physicians and patients have developed the habit of expecting the radiologist to be infallible. Certain roentgenographic pictures are pathognomonic, but the majority are subject to interpretation. The radioligist should not hesitate to request the privilege of a reexamination when the patient may be more relaxed, stronger, and easier to examine. The

clinician should readily grant this request, realizing that it will best serve the interest of the patient. Roentgenology should not be expected to give a tissue diagnosis. The radiologist should describe what he sees; if possible, show it on the film; and give a diagnostic impression concerning the nature of the lesion. It is not the responsibility of a radiologist to make a clinical diagnosis or to prescribe treatment.

The innumerable problems, the limitations, and the extraordinary possibilities of roentgenographic diagnosis have been presented in the preceding chapters of this book. The present discussion is an attempt to describe the more important clinical applications and implications.

Auxiliary diagnostic procedures

Additional methods used for the demonstration of organic disease may be mentioned briefly. *Esophagoscopy* with the old rigid esophagoscope was a hazardous procedure to be entrusted only to the skilled specialist. The more flexible instrument developed in recent years is much less dangerous but is still an instrument to be used only by experienced workers. Esophagoscopy enables the physician to observe the mucosa directly and to assess the presence or absence of a lesion. Biopsies may be taken only through the open tube.

Gastroscopy with the rigid instrument was equally hazardous, but after the development of the more flexible gastroscope by Schindler in 1932,[66] using a system of mirrors and lenses, the procedure in competent hands became safer. Biopsy is not possible with the usual instruments, but modifications to permit this have been devised. The more flexible gastroscopes have the great advantage of permitting inspection of most of the stomach and the antrum. The flexible fiberscope of Hirschowitz[36] gives visualization of the stomach and sometimes of the proximal duodenum, but opinions differ as to the clarity of the image and the reliability of the instrument; biopsy has been combined with it.

With newer instruments the duodenum can be routinely examined and the common bile duct and the pancreatic duct can be cannulated.

Gastric photography was first developed so that pictures were taken through the gastroscope, but in time cameras capable of taking pictures within the stomach itself were devised; they have been used with some degree of success. *Blind biopsy* tubes and capsules yield valuable information. The location of these instruments in the stomach or bowel can be assessed fairly well by reference to the roentgenogram or by fluoroscopy. *Proctosigmoidoscopy* is such a common and rewarding procedure that it should be almost routine. Biopsies may be taken through the standard instrument without difficulty. *Colonoscopy* is also becoming a routine procedure and smaller polyps can be removed during the examination. Larger lesions can be biopsied. *Peritoneoscopy* has not yet become a standard procedure, although some workers have found it highly useful. *Exfoliative cytology* enables the examiner to see the desquamated cells and to identify the malignant ones in a high percentage of cases. Table 63-1 gives the results of Raskin's study.[61]

Table 63-1. Accuracy of exfoliative cytology*

Area	Number of cancers	Cells found	Accuracy
Esophagus	110	105	95%
Stomach	226	203	90%
Duodenum	118	61	52%
Colon	108	98	91%

*Figures revised to 1962.

CLINICAL SYNOPSIS
Esophagus
Function and symptoms

The function of the esophagus is to conduct food and liquids from the mouth to the stomach. The first symptom of significant esophageal disease is usually difficulty in swallowing. The type of dysphagia, as will be shown later, is important. Substernal pain, heartburn, and discomfort are not necessarily attributable to esophageal disease, but if the symptoms persist for more than a few days they merit roentgenographic study. Hematemesis of esophageal origin comes chiefly from varices and occasionally from neoplasm or benign ulcer.

Esophagitis

Substernal pain, burning, and discomfort on swallowing are usually caused by esophageal irritation and are transitory phenomena. A positive diagnosis is made by means of esophagoscopy; a negative roentgenologic study is reassuring.

Peptic esophagitis is limited to the lower third of the esophagus and is much more persistent and troublesome than simple esophagitis. It may be associated with duodenal as well as esophageal ulcer, hiatal hernia, or prolonged gastric intubation resulting in stricture.[8] The discomfort may be produced by the regurgitation of acid gastric content into the esophagus or by esophageal spasm, as Jones has demonstrated.[41] The diagnosis may be suspected on the basis of the localized spasm noted by the radiologist and confirmed by the inflammation found by the esophagoscopist. The acid test has been utilized for the indirect diagnosis of esophagitis.[11,48]

Diverticula

The so-called pulsion diverticulum of Zenker is really a pharyngeal diverticulum, since it arises from the posterior wall of the pharynx, between the inferior constrictor muscle of the pharynx and the lower fibers of this muscle composing the cricopharyngeus or superior constrictor muscle of the esophagus. The sac may vary greatly in size; symptoms usually arise in the later decades of life when the sac is large.

The first symptom is often that of a foreign body in the throat. Dysphagia develops, and as it progresses, the patient may notice that the site of the obstruction behind the sternum seems to be lower than it was formerly. The difficulty is less noticeable for solid foods than for liquids, and it is less marked for the first few mouthfuls than later, when the sac is full. Regurgitation may be reduced by pressure on the side of the neck, usually the left. Slight swelling of the neck is noticeable in about one third of the cases. The diagnosis is easily established by roentgenography.

Traction diverticula occur in the midintrathoracic portion of the esophagus and apparently result from the tendency of the wall of the esophagus to adhere to a lymph node; as the esophagus falls away, a pouch of the wall is formed by means of traction. Such lesions are painless and of no clinical significance.

Traction-pulsion diverticula, or epiphrenic diverticula, are combinations of pulsion and traction diverticula occasionally found in the lower portion of the esophagus. If the pouch of the sac is lower than the neck, food and drink may be retained and, in time, as the bag increases in size symptoms may develop.

Pseudodiverticulosis of the esophagus, or curling of the esophagus, is an occasional roentgenographic finding in patients without esophageal symptoms and without anatomic lesions at autopsy.

Nonsphincteric spasm (Fig. 63-1) roentgenologically simulates curling but is usually accompanied by minor degrees of dysphagia. Anatomic abnormality is not demonstrable at autopsy.

Physiologic narrowing and foreign bodies

Physiologic narrowing of the esophagus occurs at three points of some clinical significance, particularly in patients who have ingested foreign objects. Coins are likely to stick above the level of the manubrium sterni. Other objects may lodge at the level of the aortic arch of the bifurcation of the trachea, where strictures also are particularly likely to form. The prune pit held at the aortic arch in Fig. 63-2 is above **a** minor lye stricture easily dilated with bougies. The third point of physiologic narrowing is located at the diaphragm, where large chunks of meat or other foods may stick and fail to pass— a form of "steak-eater's disease."

Stricture

Esophageal strictures may be either congenital or acquired. Acquired strictures usually follow the ingestion of corrosive objects, or esophagitis associated with a diaphragmatic hernia, or a peptic ulcer of the esophagus. Strictures are usually demonstrable by roentgenography, but a few may be missed, particularly when only a small amount of barium is used.

Cancer

Cancer of the esophagus, formerly common in the United States and presently endemic in the West Indies and in other areas of the world, occurs more frequently in males than in females. It is characterized by difficulty in swallowing meat, followed in a few weeks by difficulty in

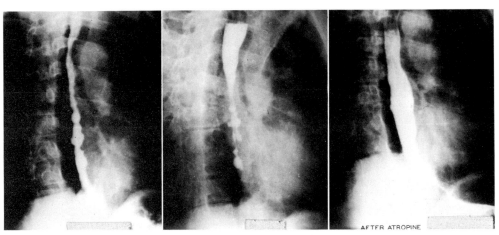

Fig. 63-1. Nonsphincteric spasm of the esophagus.

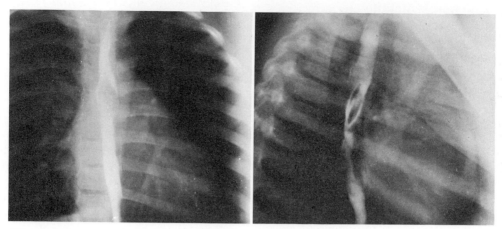

Fig. 63-2. Prune pit lodged above a minor lye stricture at the level of the second point of physiologic narrowing.

swallowing other foods; finally, in a few months, liquids may fail to pass. Bennett considers progressive dysphagia of this type in men over 40 to be pathognomonic of cancer.[9] Pain is the initial symptom in less than 2% of the victims. The majority of the lesions are composed of squamous cells, although basal cell and adenomatous types are frequent. Their locations, in order of frequency, are in the middle third, the upper third, and the lower third of the esophagus. Neoplasia may develop in strictures or may be associated with cardiospasm.

While the symptoms of esophageal cancer are alleged to occur early, because of obstruction produced in the narrow esophagus, the unfortunate fact is that metastases are usually present by the time therapy is undertaken.

Achalasia

The term "cardiospasm" does not accurately describe the condition under consideration, nor are "mega-esophagus" or "idiopathic dilatation" entirely satisfactory names; "achalasia"[39] is perhaps most suitable, but as a word it is clumsy. The disorder is caused by interruption of impulses from the vagus nerves to the esophagus, as a result of which the normal peristaltic waves do not occur and there is no relaxation of the cardia. The tonicity of the muscle is variable, and hence the height of the fluid column required to open the cardia by means of hydrostatic pressure is also variable. The disorder is usually of long duration; the degree of dilatation of the esophagus may be great. The relaxa-

tion of the cardia produced by the administration of amyl nitrite is quite dramatic when seen under the fluoroscope, but it is so transitory that it is not helpful as a method of therapy.

Symptomatically, achalasia is characterized by minimal pain under the lower sternum and by difficulty in eating, increasing with the continued ingestion of the meal. The symptoms can be bizarre; frequently they are of long duration and somewhat periodic. Some patients will eat part of a meal, vomit (or more correctly, regurgitate the contents of the esophagus), and then proceed with the meal. There is no nausea. The regurgitated food always contains thick, ropy mucus without acid or bile. Loss of weight is rare. Many patients describe a deposit of mucus on the pillow when they awaken. The roentgenologic examination demonstrates a dilated esophagus with a conical tip, lack of normal peristalsis, and failure of the cardia to relax. Aspiration pneumonitis may be detected first in the roentgenogram of the chest.

Ulcers

Esophageal ulcers are relatively uncommon and are found almost invariably in the lower third of the esophagus. They result from peptic digestion, and hence, in a sense, they are a complication of peptic esophagitis. The two conditions may result from ectopic parietal cells or from an abnormal regurgitation of gastric juice, occasionally in association with paraesophageal hernias or after operative procedures on the cardia. Barrett[6] described a pathologic syndrome

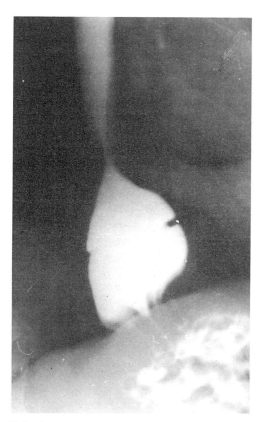

Fig. 63-3. Asymptomatic Schatzki ring. (Courtesy Dr. L. R. Donaldson.)

characterized by columnar epithelium lining the lower esophagus, esophageal stricture, esophageal ulcer, and hiatal hernia.[55] The symptoms include substernal pain and difficulty in the passage of food into the stomach.

Scleroderma

The esophagus is usually the first visceral organ to give symptoms in scleroderma and may do so months or years before the dermatologic diagnosis is evident. The symptoms of scleroderma often result from esophagitis. The roentgenologic diagnosis is based upon the flaccid appearance of the esophagus, almost complete lack of peristalsis, and some narrowing of the lumen. The disease is slowly progressive.

Hiatal hernia

A variety of abnormalities occur in the neighborhood of the diaphragmatic opening when the stomach crowds, or is pushed back into, the chest; however, symptoms are relatively uncommon. The hernias may slide in and out. They rarely become incarcerated.[70] The lower esophagus may be exposed to gastric juice for an abnormal time, resulting in esophagitis, peptic ulcer, and stricture formation. In

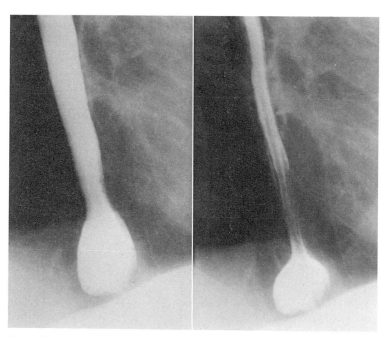

Fig. 63-4. Physiologic ampulla of the lower esophagus. (Courtesy Dr. L. R. Donaldson.)

some patients the angle of entry of the esophagus into the cardia becomes acute and is associated with some narrowing and difficulty in the emptying of solid foods into the stomach, a condition called "steak-eater's disease." A relatively frequent associated finding is a so-called Schatzki ring (Fig. 63-3), which is ordinarily of no significance, although in occasional instances such a ring has been found at autopsy and has been thought to be associated with symptoms.[64] Traumatic hernias usually involve the dome of the diaphragm. They are important because of the frequency with which one or more loops of bowel pass into the thorax, with a part or all of the stomach, and undergo volvulus.

A phrenic ampulla is a dilatation of the lower end of the esophagus, simulating a small diaphragmatic hernia (Fig. 63-4). It does not produce symptoms and is of no clinical significance.

Varices

Esophageal varices occur as a manifestation of portal hypertension because the short gastric veins are in direct communication with the esophageal veins and the superior vena cava through the azygos veins, unprotected by valves. Hepatic disease is usually responsible for the portal hypertension, although extrahepatic portal thrombosis may occur, particularly in children, secondary to neonatal omphalitis and thrombophlebitis of the umbilical vein. Splenomegaly is almost invariably present.

Roentgenologic evidence of the varices may be obtained following the Valsalva maneuver, although opinions differ as to the value of the procedure. Varices large enough to bleed are usually demonstrable by roentgenogram, although in the phase of active hemorrhage esophagoscopy may be a more acceptable procedure.

Stomach
Foreign bodies

The small coins and marbles swallowed by children usually pass through the stomach and the digestive tract without difficulty. Needles and pins, particularly open safety pins, are exceptions because they may perforate the wall of the stomach or intestine and lead to bizarre complications. Demented individuals may carry an assortment of metal objects in their stomachs without symptoms.

Bezoars are conglomerations of swallowed matted foreign material such as hair (trichobezoars), vegetable fiber (phytobezoars), gastroliths, or gallstones extruded through a spontaneous gastrocholecystic fistula. The opaque objects are identified easily by roentgenogram, but the nonopaque objects may simulate benign or malignant polyps. Gastric ulcers may be found on the lesser curvature opposite the bezoars.

Gastroptosis

Gastroptosis is neither a disease nor a cause of symptoms. It scarcely deserves mention.

Diverticulum

Diverticulum of the stomach occurs classically on the posterior wall just below the cardia. It does not cause symptoms.

Gastritis

Nonspecific gastritis, the most frequent inflammation of the stomach, has been thought to be the cause of peptic ulcer and gastric cancer.[32,43-45,80] The atrophic gastropathy of pernicious anemia seems to precede the anemia and to play a causal role.[20] The pathologists have been unable to agree on a satisfactory classification. Atrophy, gastritis, erosions, and erosive gastritis are recognizable anatomically. Schindler[67] divided gastrititis into three gastroscopic types: superficial, atrophic, and hypertrophic. The roentgenologic demonstration of unusually shallow or flat folds may suggest mucosal atrophy[46] and the diagnosis of pernicious anemia. Recent evidence indicates that plasma vitamin B_{12} levels correlate with parietal cell mass.[4] Mucosal atrophy, of itself, does not cause symptoms; indeed gastritis produces few if any symptoms, although Wood and Taft[80] provide a different point of view. Erosions or acute ulcers may be sought roentgenologically, but they are difficult to demonstrate; usually such lesions are best identified gastroscopically.

Giant hypertrophic gastritis is rare but of great importance to the radiologist, the clinician, and the patient.[50] In its pure form it probably produces few if any symptoms except for an occasional protein-losing gastropathy. There may be superimposed adenomatous sessile or pedunculated polyps. Roentgenologically, the folds resemble the convolutions of the brain.

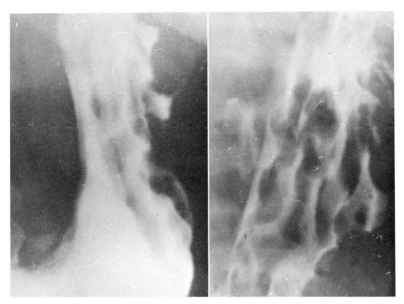

Fig. 63-5. Giant hypertrophic gastric folds.

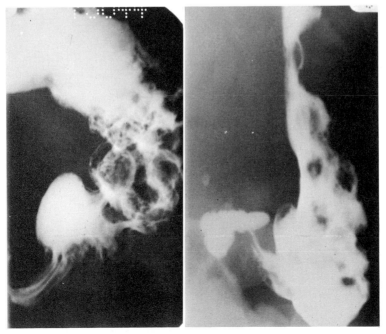

Fig. 63-6. Benign gastric polyposis.

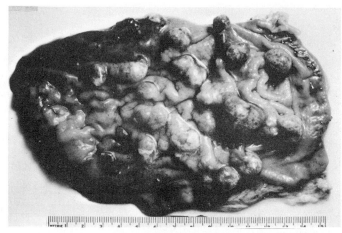

Fig. 63-7. Resected specimen of benign gastric polyposis; see Fig. 63-6.

The process is diffuse, but the greatest involvement is in the body of the stomach and along the greater curvature. The large, broad, soft, pliable folds (Fig. 63-5) may be difficult if not impossible to differentiate roentgenologically and gastroscopically from those of an infiltrating lymphoma or carcinoma. Exfoliative cytology or blind biopsy often gives the definitive diagnosis, but laparotomy with direct inspection and biopsy may be necessary.

Polyposis of the stomach may be superimposed upon giant hypertrophic gastritis or may simulate it roentgenologically. The adenomatous polyps are usually benign and asymptomatic, but they raise the question of neoplasm (Figs. 63-6 and 63-7).

Granuloma

Syphilis of the stomach may simulate roentgenologically either a benign ulcer or an infiltrative neoplasm[57] (Fig. 63-8). Neither the radiologist nor the gastroscopist should attempt the differential diagnosis. With a history of lues, positive results of serologic study, and a negative results of cytologic examination, antiluetic therapy may be undertaken. The lesions should be studied again carefully at the end of 3 weeks; resolution should occur promptly. A good axiom to remember is that in patients with proved syphilis, gastric cancer and benign peptic ulcer are each more common than is gastric lues.

Tuberculous ulcers are multiple, atypical, usually nearly terminal lesions in patients with advanced pulmonary tuberculosis.

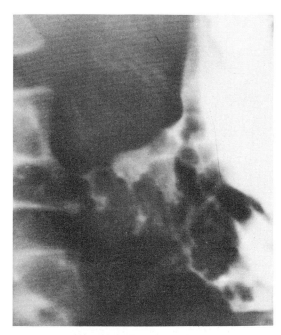

Fig. 63-8. Gastric syphilis.

Nonspecific granulomas are rarely encountered in studies of the stomach. They are diagnosed by the pathologist, not by the radiologist or the clinician.[40]

Abnormalities of the pylorus

Hypertrophic stenosis of the pylorus ordinarily is diagnosed clinically in the first 2 or 3 weeks of infancy. The roentgenographic findings are pyloric obstruction and gastric reten-

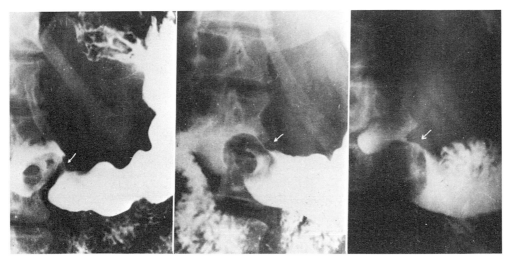

Fig. 63-9. Benign prepyloric polyp prolapsing through the pylorus into the base of the duodenal bulb.

tion. The lesion is rare in adults, and when it occurs it is frequently accompanied by a gastric ulcer; it is difficult to know which condition is antecedent. The chief roentgenographic sign, aside from the gastric retention, is the gap between the end of the antrum and the base of the bulb; it is often difficult to get barium through the pylorus and into the bulb.

The differential problems are simple pylorospasm, intrapyloric ulcer, and carcinoma of the pylorus—the carcinoma fibrosum of Konjetzny[45] —which may be almost indistinguishable pathologically from hypertrophic stenosis. Clinically, the neoplastic obstruction is characterized by the rather sudden onset and the severity of the symptoms. If the tumor extends back into the antrum, the deformity gives the clue to the diagnosis. The diagnosis of *pyloric ulcer* depends upon the demonstration of a crater.

Simple pylorospasm may be caused by reflux spasm from an adjacent ulcer, but more frequently the condition is simple failure of the pylorus to open. Radiologists learned years ago that for many patients the strategy of engaging them in pleasant conversation about choice foods frequently promoted gastric emptying. If this procedure failed, the patients were "benched" and allowed to wait for 30 to 45 minutes while other patients were examined; the pylorus usually was then found to have opened.

"Pyloric obstruction" technically and correctly means obstruction at the pylorus, but the term is frequently used to mean outlet obstruction of any kind, including a stenosing duodenal ulcer. True pyloric obstruction may be produced by a channel or intrapyloric ulcer, by a juxtapyloric ulcer with reflex spasm, by tumor, or by hypertrophic stenosis. True obstruction is characterized by abnormal retention of secretion, food, and barium.

Prolapsing polyp of the pylorus may cause intermittent obstruction of the outlet as the polyp is pushed backward and forward through the pylorus (Fig. 63-9). Such a polyp may produce intermittent obstruction, nausea, and vomiting; it rarely bleeds.

Prolapsing gastric mucosa may indent the base of the bulb sufficiently to simulate a polyp. Ordinarily the differentiation between polyp and prolapse is made without difficulty. Symptoms of various kinds, including bleeding, ascribed to prolapse have been controversial for over 50 years. White, Bargen, and Saghafi have reviewed the subject and presented excellent evidence of bleeding from prolapsed mucosa.[78]

Neoplasms

Carcinoma. In spite of the dramatic and unexplained decrease in deaths from gastric cancer in the past 50 years in the United States, the disease is still fairly common and must always be

Table 63-2. Accuracy of roentgenologic diagnosis of gastric cancer

	Number	Percentage
Correct diagnosis	219	78
Inability to differentiate	18	6
Incorrect diagnosis (called normal or benign)	45	16
Total patients with cancer	282	100

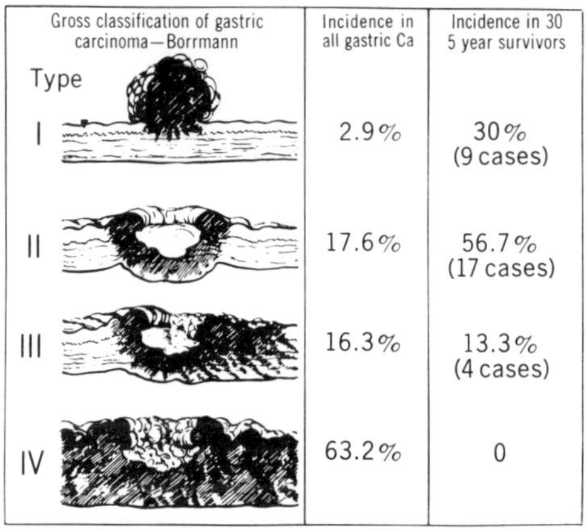

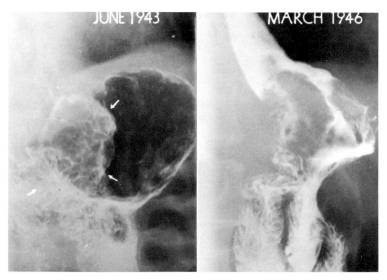

Gross classification of gastric carcinoma—Borrmann	Incidence in all gastric Ca	Incidence in 30 5 year survivors
Type I	2.9%	30% (9 cases)
II	17.6%	56.7% (17 cases)
III	16.3%	13.3% (4 cases)
IV	63.2%	0

Fig. 63-10. Distribution of gastric cancer according to Borrmann's classification and also the distribution of tumor by type in 30 patients surviving 5 years or longer.

borne in mind by radiologists and clinicians dealing with patients with abdominal distress. In other countries, such as Great Britain, Germany, and Japan, the incidence of carcinoma of the stomach has not decreased.

In the early stages, the history and the clinical findings may not be especially remarkable, and hence the radiologist may be the first to direct attention to the stomach. The clinician must utilize and correlate the various diagnostic procedures and bear final responsibility for the diagnosis. It is neither realistic nor fair to rely completely upon the roentgenographic examination, as is illustrated by the data provided in Table 63-2 by Strandjord, Moseley, and Schweinfus.[71]

Gastric cancers vary in type and in their rate of growth; some are acute fulminating tumors, others grow more slowly. Borrmann's classification[14a] is of some value to the radiologist and clinician. Type I tumors are localized, polypoid, relatively noninvasive, nonulcerated lesions. Type II cancers are ulcerated, well circumscribed, and minimally invasive. Type III tumors are ulcerated, invasive, and poorly circumscribed lesions. Type IV carcinomas are diffusely invasive, with or without ulceration. Fig. 63-10 shows the usual distribution of gastric cancer according to Borrmann's grouping and also

Fig. 63-11. Recurrent polypoid tumor, Type I of Borrmann, increasing slowly in size from 1943 to 1946.

the distribution by type of thirty 5-year survivors after resection.[51] (See also Figs. 63-11 to 63-16.)

While it is clear that there may be a considerable difference in the rate of growth in the various types of gastric cancers and even in those of one group, as in the Type IV infiltrative tumors, it is nevertheless true that the degree of malignancy and the rate of growth go together. The old dictum of the pathologist still holds: the larger the primary growth, the smaller the metastases, and vice versa. Surgeons press for earlier diagnosis in order to remove the cancer before it has spread. The goal is laudable, but it is well to bear in mind that rate of growth is not directly related to the size of the lesion but rather to the as yet unknown factors that control or fail to control the growth of cancers.

Lymphoma. Lymphoma may simulate infiltrating carcinoma. While the roentgenologic differentiation of the two tumors may be supported by gastroscopic or cytologic evidence, histologic examination (lymph node resection or gastric resection) is mandatory because many of these tumors are surprisingly sensitive to radiation. Some lymphomas are relatively benign, whereas others are highly malignant.[74]

Gastric ulcers

Malignant gastric ulcer. A primary problem for the radiologist and the clinician is the differentiation between benign and malignant ulcer. Frequently the clinician relies entirely upon the radiologist for the diagnosis. This is improper.

Peptic ulceration in neoplasm may heal and rarely simulate benign ulcer as shown in Fig. 63-17. The patient whose roentgenogram is shown had had ulcer symptoms for 18 months. She deferred operation. During this time the

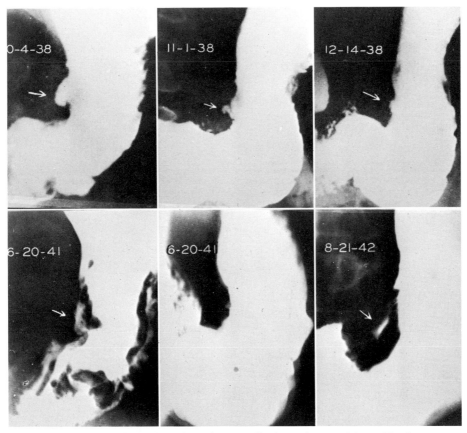

Fig. 63-12. Slowly growing ulcerating circumscribed carcinoma, Type II of Borrmann.

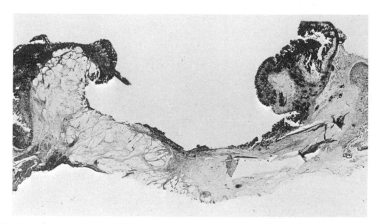

Fig. 63-13. Specimen removed 4 years after the original diagnosis was made. The patient survived more than 25 years (see Fig. 63-12).

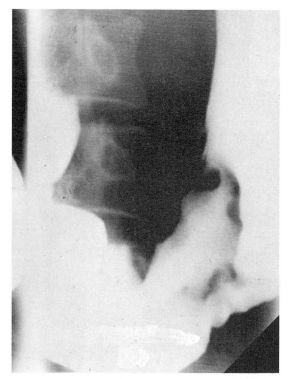

Fig. 63-14. Ulcerating infiltrative carcinoma. Type III of Borrmann. The patient survived resection for 21 years.

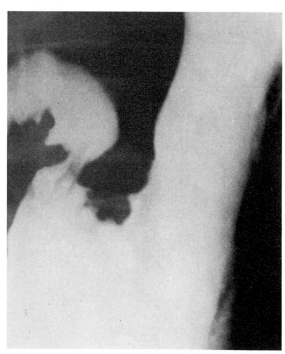

Fig. 63-15. Ulcerating carcinoma, Type IV of Borrmann, simulating benign ulcer with early widespread metastases and rapid downhill course.

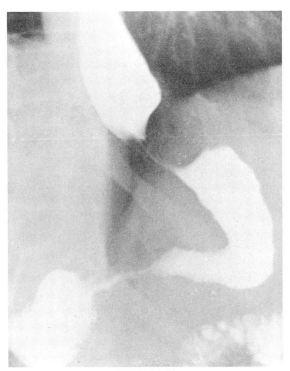

Fig. 63-16. Infiltrative carcinoma, Type IV of Borrmann, "leather bottle stomach" or "stomach in miniature."

roentgenologic crater disappeared, but the *infiltration of the gastric wall* persisted and gave convincing evidence of neoplasm; at no time was the lesion considered to be benign.[56a] The patient is still alive, 25 years postoperatively.

Strandjord, Moseley, and Schweinfus have analyzed the accuracy of the roentgenologic diagnosis in twenty-seven patients with proved neoplastic ulcers without a mass as follows:

Definite criteria of malignancy	14
No differentiation made	7
Interpreted as benign or missed	6
Total patients	27

When the roentgenologic and clinical evidence are combined, the discrimination is improved. Doll, Jones, Pygott, and Stubbe found that, of 266 ulcers confidently diagnosed as benign, 0.4% turned out to be neoplastic, whereas of nineteen reluctantly treated as benign, 21% were neoplastic.[29] Bolt, Wilson, and Pollard found that when all procedures indicated benignancy the incidence of cancer was 2.8%, whereas when the evidence was conflicting, the rate of cancer rose to 25%.[14] Dworken, Roth, and Duber, in a follow-up of 130 gastric lesions treated as benign, found cancer in 3%.[31] Paustian, Stein, Young, Roth, and Bockus in a study of 152 gastric ulcers concluded, at the end of a 2-week trial, that 4% were malignant; four

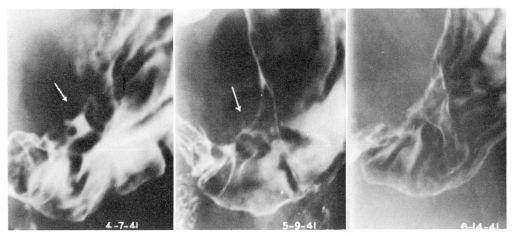

Fig. 63-17. Healing of peptic ulceration in ulcerating carcinoma. Note the persistence of mass, with deformity of the gastric wall.

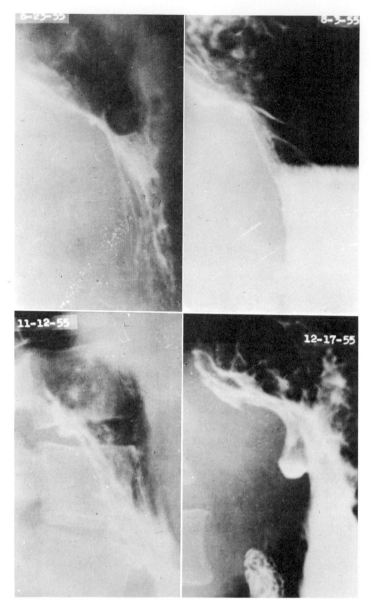

Fig. 63-18. Benign ulcer high on the lesser curvature, increasing in size from June to December 1955.

additional patients (2.6%) were considered failures (three patient failures and one physician failure).[59] Levin, Palmer, and Kirsner considered five of 121 cases (4%) to have been diagnostic errors.[47] In all of the studies cited, the diagnoses were made without the aid of exfoliative cytology, a procedure that should reduce further the incidence of error.

Benign gastric ulcer. Of the various roentgenologic criteria suggestive of benignancy, per-

haps the most important is the response to therapy. Some writers insist that the crater should disappear completely within 3 to 6 weeks. The exact period of time is less important than the behavior of the lesions, such as lack of infiltration and preservation of the fold pattern. The healing of the ulcer must be demonstrated roentgenologically (Figs. 63-18 to 63-21). There should be no residual infiltration of the gastric wall although there may be a slight pit and per-

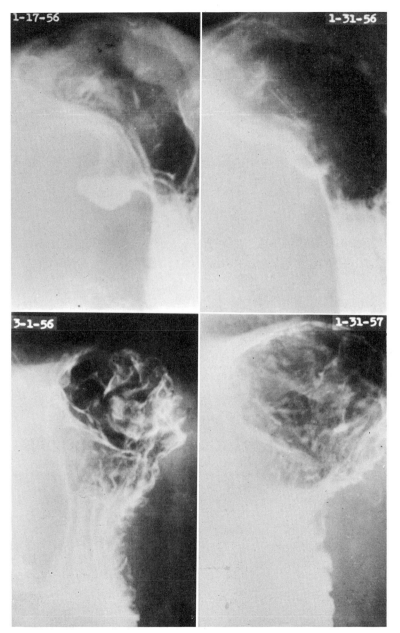

Fig. 63-19. Decrease in size from January to March 1956 of lesser curvature ulcer pictured in previous figure, followed by complete healing as shown in Fig. 63-21.

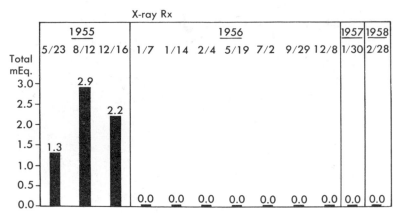

Fig. 63-20. Production of persistent achlorhydria to roentgen-ray irradiation in patient in Fig. 63-19.

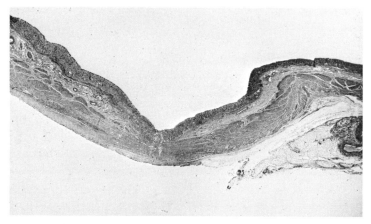

Fig. 63-21. Cross section of healed ulcer found at autopsy of patient in Fig. 63-20 in 1958 after cerebral hemorrhage.

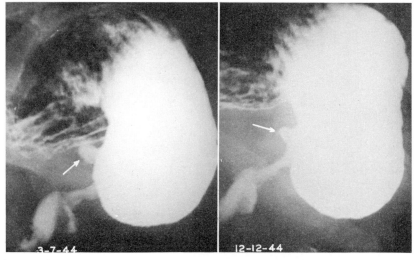

Fig. 63-22. Deformity of the antrum, secondary to a benign ulcer of the lesser curvature.

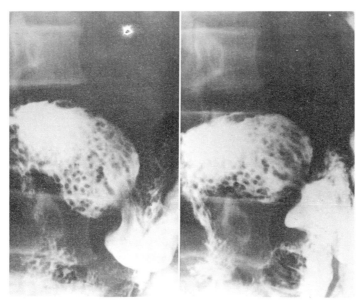

Fig. 63-23. Lymphoid hyperplasia of the duodenal bulb histologically confirmed. (Courtesy Dr. R. D. Moseley.)

haps a convergence of the fold pattern toward the healed ulcer.

Pyloric obstruction, a very frequent complication of peptic ulcer, is usually outlet obstruction caused by a stenosing postpyloric, duodenal, or even postbulbar ulcer; hence, strictly speaking, it is not pyloric in location. True pyloric obstruction results ordinarily from an active or healed pyloric or channel ulcer.

Deformity of the antrum is frequently seen in association with gastric ulcer, as shown in Fig. 63-22. It is variously ascribed to spasm, antral gastritis, and shortening of the lesser curvature by scar. The ulcer may be secondary to the antral process.

Hourglass deformity of the stomach is usually the result of contraction induced by a long-standing ulcer of the lesser curvature. Spasm has been alleged to play a role, but usually the deformity is caused by submucosal scar tissue contraction not visible from the serosal surface. Cancer can simulate a benign hourglass deformity.

Duodenum

The first portion of the duodenum is relatively devoid of pattern, but the folds of the second portion may extend back into the upper portion of the bulb. Barium may lodge between the folds and simulate an ulcer crater, just as a star-shaped collection of barium may remain on the duodenal side of the pylorus for a few moments—the "pyloric star"—and be mistaken for an ulcer crater. The pylorus frequently indents the base of the bulb, protruding into it almost in the manner the cervix uteri protrudes into the vaginal vault.

Hyperplasia of Brunner's glands may create a distinctive pattern; it does not give rise to symptoms. Similarly, lymphoid hyperplasia may produce extensive mottling (Fig. 63-23). It is important to recognize this change as benign and of no clinical significance; a similar pattern may be seen in the terminal ileum.

Duodenal stasis

Barium ordinarily progresses rapidly from the pylorus through the duodenum into the small intestine, but occasionally it delays in the second and third portions of the duodenum, and considerable churning motion seems to be required to force the barium up through the fourth portion into the jejunum. As a rule this finding is not significant; it occurs more frequently in tall, thin individuals than in short, stout ones and is simply an anatomic variation.

Occasionally the distal duodenum is involved in the inflammation of an ulcer in the bulb or other extrinsic disease. Some workers tend to attribute such stasis to the pressure of the superior mesenteric vessels anteriorly and the spine posteriorly. The temptation of such a diagnosis is particularly great when the patient is a young woman with nervous vomiting. The clinician and the radiologist must both be aware of the hazard involved in making a diagnosis of duodenal stasis as a disease sui generis. On the other hand, duodenal stasis may be present in the vicious cycle of the postoperative stomach with a gastroenterostomy or be involved in such generalized and yet intrinsic disease as scleroderma, Crohn's disease, and gluten-induced enteropathy.

Duodenitis

Duodenitis is a pathologic entity but not a clinical one, because there is no clear evidence that it produces symptoms in the absence of erosions or acute ulcers that may bleed or produce ulcer pain. Konjetzny and his associates were staunch advocates of the concept of duodenitis as a clinically significant disease.[44] Radiologists sometimes infer a diagnosis of duodenitis from indirect signs such as irritability and spasm of the bulb, but these are very unreliable criteria. Consequently, the term "duodenitis" is not acceptable as a roentgenologic or clinical diagnosis unless one intends to imply simply the existence of peptic ulcer disease of the duodenal bulb with erosions and acute ulcer or with ulcer pain or bleeding. The inference may be correct, but the roentgenologic diagnosis is hazardous.

Diverticula

True diverticula are common in the second and third portions of the duodenum, but they do not occur in the bulb. Diverticula of the duodenal bulb are acquired diverticula secondary to duodenal ulcer. The deformity is produced by the healing and recurrence of the ulcer; the crater, if present, is always located in or just proximal to the deformity. Diverticula rarely produce symptoms, although instances of ulcer in a diverticulum and of peridiverticular inflammation have been reported.

Duodenal ulcer

Peptic ulcers occur primarily in the duodenal bulb, occasionally in the upper second portion of the duodenum, and rarely as far down as the middle of the second portion. Peptic ulceration beyond that point is seen in the Zollinger-Ellison syndrome[81]; in patients who have had operations for ulcer, with a gastrointestinal anastomosis; and in association with ectopic gastric mucosa, usually located in a Meckel's diverticulum. It is rarely seen with duplication of the bowel (ileum)[65] and even more rarely with the simple ectopic location of gastric mucosa in the ileum.

The roentgenologic signs of duodenal ulcer are: (1) the classic crater, consisting of a circumscribed collection of barium surrounded by a halo, and (2) a sharp indentation of both curvatures of the bulb, producing the typical cloverleaf deformity; occasionally the deformity is unilateral, incomplete, or absent.[10] The crater heals with treatment, but the deformity persists, although it may decrease in magnitude; that is, there may be some increase in the lumen of the bulb at the site of the deformity. The presence or absence of crater is of importance to the clinician, because it is the only positive roentgenographic sign of active ulcer. It should be noted, however, that no radiologist has ever claimed to be able to identify craters in all active ulcers. Templeton's figures are among the highest, 65%.[72]

The diameter of the lumen is also of importance to the clinician, because it is a direct appraisal of the degree of stenosis produced by the deformity. The roentgenogram does not necessarily provide satisfactory information regarding the channel, but the fluoroscopist usually sees it and may catch it on the film. Considerable stenosis is required to produce significant interference with gastric emptying and hence gastric retention.

Complications of duodenal ulcer. The most frequent complication of duodenal ulcer is stenosis. The most acute and life-threatening complications are free perforation into the peritoneal cavity and massive hemorrhage. The positive roentgenographic sign of the former is free air under the diaphragm. As mentioned previously, roentgenographic studies may be carried out early if a modicum of care is used. Some patients faint when they try to stand and are in greater danger from a fall than they are from additional bleeding. Important information can be gained from an examination carried out care-

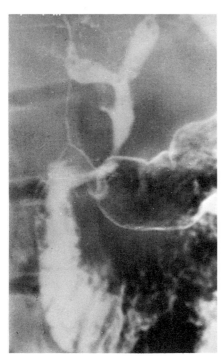

Fig. 63-24. Perforation of a duodenal ulcer into the common bile duct.

fully, with a minimum of manipulation. There is no evidence that barium itself is harmful.

Chronic perforation of a duodenal ulcer onto the capsule of the pancreas is fairly common. It does not in itself alter the pattern of pain, contrary to popular teaching. Extension of the ulcer into the pancreas may produce a chemical type of localized pancreatitis, usually with severe pain. In peptic ulcer there is no absolute relationship between the size and depth of the ulcer and the severity of the pain, although in general they increase together and decrease together, with the pain pattern leading the advance and the recession. Ulcers may perforate into other organs. As shown in Fig. 63-24, a duodenal ulcer may perforate into the common bile duct.

Neoplasms

Primary malignant tumors of the duodenal bulb are almost unknown; relatively few have been reported in the literature of the world. Carcinomas of the second, third, and fourth portions, however, are common; they produce ulcerating, bleeding, stenosing lesions easily differentiated from diverticula. Carcinomas of the pancreas may invade any portion of the duo-

denum or the stomach, ulcerate, and be roentgenologically indistinguishable from primary lesions of these organs. Crohn's disease of the duodenum may be indistinguishable roentgenologically.

Sequelae of gastric surgery

The various sequelae of gastric surgery may tax the diagnostic acumen of the radiologist and the clinician. A few simple rules may be helpful. Gastric ulcers removed by wedge resection are likely to recur at the site of excision. Jejunal ulcers almost never develop after gastrojejunostomy for simple gastric ulcer. Duodenal ulcers almost invariably heal after simple gastroenterostomy (anterior or posterior), but the incidence of recurrent jejunal or anastomotic ulcer is between 20% and 40%. Fig. 63-25, showing the presence of coexisting duodenal and jejunal ulcers, is an exception to the rule of healing of the duodenal ulcer after gastroenterostomy. Jejunal ulcers may be difficult to demonstrate roentgenologically; they are rarely seen gastroscopically.

The so-called dumping syndrome may be more debilitating than the ulcer itself. It consists of a variety of symptoms brought on by eating: palpitation, tachycardia, weakness, nausea, sweating, fear, and prostration. Diarrhea is not a necessary feature of the syndrome, but it is fairly common. Various degrees of steatorrhea are demonstrable.[24] Burhenne has provided roentgenographic confirmation of the role of intestinal hyperosmolarity and consequent circulatory hypovolemia in the pathogenesis of symptoms.[16] In general, the greater the resection, the more likely the development of the syndrome and the more severe the symptoms, but they may appear following gastroenterostomy alone. The symptoms may be relieved partially or completely by undoing the anastomosis or by conversion of a Polya or Billroth II anastomosis into a Billroth I. Usually the dumping syndrome may be controlled by minor dietary changes, anticholinergic drugs, and sedatives. A somewhat similar group of symptoms is seen at times in patients who have not undergone operation.

The postvagotomy syndrome may include diarrhea, a foul-smelling belch, and various portions of the dumping syndrome. The diarrhea ordinarily may be handled quite easily by simple manipulation of the diet and by medication.

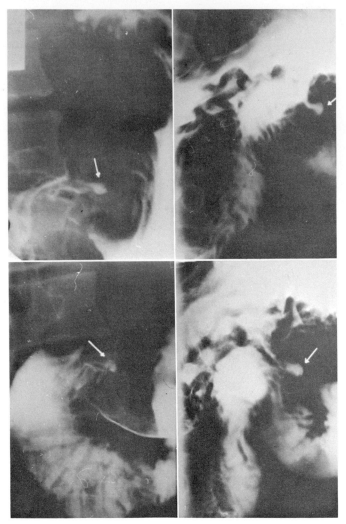

Fig. 63-25. Coexisting duodenal and jejunal ulcers, after gastroenterostomy.

The drainage procedures have eliminated the retention responsible for the foul belch.

Small intestine
Diverticula

Roentgenologically spectacular single or multiple diverticula may occur in the jejunum or ileum, usually in older adults. The existence of such diverticula was recognized early in the last century, but their clinical significance, except for acute diverticulitis and its complications and rare instances of tumor formation, was not appreciated until a few years ago. The clinical concept has been altered by the demonstration that duodenal and jejunal diverticulosis may be as-sociated with a megaloblastic anemia (Fig. 63-26), diarrhea caused by a malabsorption syndrome, and neuritis simulating the neuropathy of pernicious anemia.[23,28,68] The vitamin B_{12} levels are low and are raised by the administration of this vitamin. Apparently the anemia is caused by a vitamin B_{12} deficiency attributed to competitive uptake of the vitamin by certain strains of *Escherichia coli* found in the diverticula. The anemia and vitamin B_{12} levels respond to the administration of tetracycline, which lowers the bacterial count in the diverticula and alters the flora, specifically the strain of *E. coli* requiring histidine.[58] A blind loop of intestine may produce the same syndrome. The

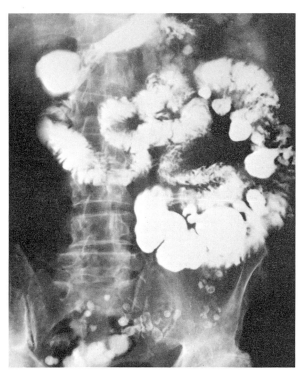

Fig. 63-26. Spectacular acquired jejunal diverticula in a male 84 years of age with steatorrhea and macrocytic anemia (B_{12} deficiency).

malabsorption apparently results from histologic changes in the mucosa of the jejunum similar to those found in other malabsorptive states.

Meckel's diverticulum

Meckel's diverticulum, resulting from incomplete closure of the vitelline duct, may occur at any point in the intestine; however, it classically occurs in the distal ileum, 30 to 40 cm. proximal to the ileocecal valve. It is common in children and young adults. The more typical manifestation is that of acute diverticulitis, simulating acute appendicitis—the "left-sided appendicitis." It may produce intestinal obstruction or intussusception. Ectopic gastric mucosa occurs frequently in such diverticula and secretes sufficient unneutralized hydrochloric acid and pepsin to produce peptic ulcers in the mouth of the diverticulum or in the adjacent intestine. Such ulcers may give rise to periumbilical pain, poorly related to food taking and not relieved thereby. Massive bleeding is fairly common;

acute perforation may occur. Roentgenologic demonstration of such diverticula is infrequent. Ectopic gastric mucosa has been reported in the distal small bowel, not associated with diverticula or with duplication of the intestine but producing pain and melena.

Potassium-induced ulcers

Following the introduction of drugs for maintaining diuresis, the frequency of electrolyte depletion was recognized. Emphasis was placed on the potassium ion, and hence it became more or less customary to prescribe potassium chloride to protect against hypokalemia and hypochloremia. Potassium chloride had long been recognized as an irritant to the bowel, but only recently was it discovered that the tablets may have a sufficiently corrosive effect to produce ulcers of the small bowel with acute and chronic inflammation. The clinical picture consists of cramplike abdominal pain with diarrhea or with obstipation and the classic findings of acute intestinal obstruction. Laparotomy reveals a localized resectable ulcer,[3,13] as in Fig. 63-27.

Acute intestinal obstruction

The classic clinical picture of acute intestinal obstruction consists of (1) rhythmic, intermittent peristaltic pain; (2) nausea and vomiting, at first gastric, then duodenal, and finally intestinal (fecal); and (3) obstipatient. In high obstruction there is less pain; vomiting appears earlier, and the emesis consists only of gastric and duodenal content. Dilated loops of small bowel are almost invariably demonstrable roentgenologically, except in some patients with volvulus. In paralytic ileus the pain is less, even absent, and the abdomen is more distended, tympanitic, and tender. The dilated loops of small bowel are present in an abdomen "silent as the grave." Intussusception of the small bowel into the colon may be identified by a barium enema and often may be reduced thereby. Volvulus of the small bowel may not be evident on the plain film, whereas volvulus of the sigmoid colon may be identified easily. It must be remembered that loops of bowel filled with fluid do not yield gas shadows on the roentgenogram.

In many instances the use of the Miller-Abbott tube may be of diagnostic and therapeutic value. The radiologist helps greatly in checking the transit of the tube. In earlier years this was

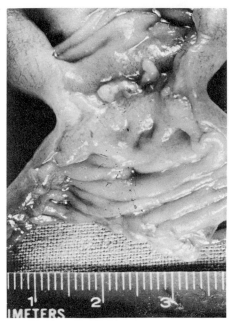

Fig. 63-27. Localized ulceration and stricture presumably produced by oral administration of diuretics and potassium chloride. (Courtesy Dr. E. M. Goldberg.)

done fluoroscopically, but roentgenograms involve less work and less irradiation and provide a permanent record. Effective use of the Miller-Abbott tube requires trained personnel and careful attention to the procedure. One of the dangers of the method is the failure to recognize volvulus and gangrene of the bowel. In short, the procedure may be of great value when properly carried out in appropriate cases.

Chronic intestinal obstruction

Chronic intestinal obstruction may be produced by a number of lesions. The diagnostic problem primarily involves localization and, if possible, identification of the obstructive process. Clinically it is hazardous to diagnose chronic or intermittent intestinal obstruction unless the radiologist is able to demonstrate a lesion, a point of obstruction, or at least abnormal loops of small bowel. Admittedly, the small bowel gives the radiologist his greatest difficulties, and it may do the same for the clinician. Perhaps the most frequent clinical error is the vague diagnosis of "adhesions." Certainly, adhesive bands can and do produce intestinal obstruction, but the clinical picture is not that of recurring day-to-day abdominal distress for

months or years. Almost any abdomen opened by the surgeon contains some adhesions; the greater the number of previous operations, the greater the number of adhesions, but such findings rarely are responsible for the symptoms. To be sure, the easiest thing to do is to ascribe the pain to the adhesions, break them up, and then with satisfaction tell the patient what has been accomplished. The procedure may be helpful mechanically or psychotherapeutically to both the doctor and the patient, but too often it accomplishes nothing of permanent value.

Polyposis

Polyposis of the small intestine is relatively rare and occurs primarily as part of the Peutz-Jeghers syndrome, a hereditary disorder characterized not only by polyposis but also by spotty melanin pigmentation of the skin and mucous membranes. There is agreement that the polyps are benign and devoid of any malignant potential.[15,17] However, Warren, Kune, and Poulantzas have described a patient with the Peutz-Jeghers syndrome and a carcinoma of the duodenum. These authors point out that "in the only recorded case of a metastasizing small bowel tumor of the Peutz-Jeghers type, the malignant polyp also arose in the duodenum."[76]

Specific infections

Aside from typhoid fever, which rarely comes into roentgenologic consideration, the only important specific infection of the small intestine is tuberculosis. It occurs almost exclusively in patients with advanced pulmonary tuberculosis. The motility disturbances it creates in the intestine simulate those of the malabsorption syndrome and of regional enteritis (Crohn's disease). Sarcoidosis rarely affects the bowel. The reported cases of localized sarcoidosis of the intestine are almost surely Crohn's disease.

Granulomatous enteritis (Crohn's disease)

In 1932, Crohn, Ginzburg, and Oppenheimer presented a paper[25] on regional enteritis, a disease of unknown etiology not previously recognized as an entity, although occasional cases had been described under varying titles in the previous century. Since then the diagnosis has been made with increasing frequency, so that the patients known to be afflicted with it now number many hundreds, possibly thousands, and are no longer reported as curiosities.[26]

While the process most frequently involves the ileum, any portion of the small bowel may be affected, even the stomach and duodenum, frequently with so-called skip areas. Disease of the terminal ileum and the proximal colon has been termed "ileocolitis." The recognition of granulomatous colitis is relatively recent and will be discussed later. Typically, Crohn's disease is a chronic, progressive, ulcerative, sclerosing process producing abdominal cramps, diarrhea, and loss of appetite and of weight, with secondary anemia. Fistulas are fairly common in advanced cases. The disease is one of the recognized causes of fever of unknown origin. Rheumatoid-like arthritis, erythema nodosum, and pyoderma gangrenosum may occur; they constitute one of the reasons for the suggestion that the disorder is one of the autoimmune diseases. Acute and chronic forms occur, but even the chronic form may produce only acute symptoms, such as acute intestinal obstruction or profuse bleeding. The disease may occasionally run a rapidly progressive and fatal course, but usually it is slowly progressive with exacerbations and remissions. More or less spontaneous recovery may occur.

Fistula formation may occur spontaneously, producing internal fistulas to other loops of small intestine, the cecum, the sigmoid, or the urinary bladder. External fistulas may develop spontaneously through the anterior abdominal wall, posteriorly, or even through the chest wall. Enterocutaneous fistulas may follow abscess formation and external drainage, but more frequently they appear after surgery. The roentgenologic examination gives the best information available prior to surgery concerning the extent of the disease and its location. Injection methods for the identification of fistulous communications have been disappointing; barium solutions given orally or by enema are generally more instructive.

Malabsorption syndrome

Malabsorption of variable degree is observed in many conditions, including nearly all short-circuiting operations on the gut and the various inflammatory diseases of the small intestine and even of the colon.[75] The roentgenologic diagnosis of malabsorption is less precise than is that of specific intestinal lesions.

The identification of Whipple's disease on roentgenologic grounds is hazardous. Fortunately the various biopsy and biochemical techniques developed in the past 20 years have helped greatly to clarify the diagnostic and therapeutic problems of the malabsorption syndrome.

Scleroderma

Visceral scleroderma, while usually affecting the esophagus first may also involve other organs, including the small intestine and the colon, producing more or less inability to eat, nausea, vomiting, diarrhea, or alternating diarrhea and constipation.[35,63] The roentgenologic picture may simulate that of the malabsorption syndrome, but there is more stagnation and partial obstruction in various loops of bowel.[34]

Tumors

Malignant tumors of the small bowel may be carcinomas, carcinoids, or lymphomas of various types. The presenting symptoms are those of obstruction or bleeding unless metastases have occurred. In this case, more unusual features, such as the carcinoid flush, may dominate the clinical picture. Benign tumors may ulcerate and bleed. Any tumor may play a leading role in intussusception.

Colon
Megacolon

One of the more common congenital anomalies is Hirschsprung's disease, or idiopathic megacolon, resulting in severe constipation from birth, with an enormous colon containing impacted feces.[73] This can be seen in a plain roentgenogram of the abdomen or by means of barium enema. There is great validity in the dictum, "A baby's first enema should be a barium enema." Congenital megacolon is caused by an aganglionic segment of the rectum or rectosigmoid.

In the adult, redundant colons are common and bear no resemblance to Hirschsprung's disease. Fecal impactions may occur on the basis of bad habits. In Brazil, Chagas' disease (trypanosomiasis) produces destruction of the myenteric ganglia in the esophagus and the colon, resulting in an aganglionic mega-esophagus and megacolon.

Appendicitis

Acute appendicitis is still, in a sense, the most frequent disease of the colon. Roentgenologic examination with its attendant procedures is contraindicated, but when it is done, an appendiceal mass may be found to indent the cecum in a fairly characteristic fashion. Chronic appendicitis is not an acceptable clinical or roentgenologic diagnosis.

A postappendectomy deformity of the cecum is occasionally troublesome in that it suggests the presence of a tumor. The history of operation, absence of symptoms, absence of a palpable mass in the right lower quadrant, and the absence of anemia and of occult blood in the feces are all helpful.

Diverticula

Diverticula of the colon are extremely common, increasing in incidence with each decade of life. They are found least frequently in the cecum and ascending colon, most frequently in the sigmoid colon, and commonly in the transverse and descending colons.

Although diverticulosis rarely causes symptoms and may be ignored clinically, diverticulitis presents a variety of problems.[55a] The most serious of these is perforation, either free into the peritoneal cavity or walled off with abscess for-

mation. Acute diverticulitis produces a fairly characteristic clinical syndrome, with localized pain, rigidity, fever, and leukocytosis. Chronic diverticulitis may be relatively painless; the deformity of the bowel, as shown in Fig. 63-28, is usually quite different from that of cancer.

The possibility of neoplasm in a patient with diverticulosis must always be borne in mind, since the two diseases are so common and rather

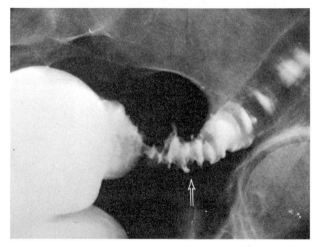

Fig. 63-28. Chronic obstructing diverticulitis of the sigmoid.

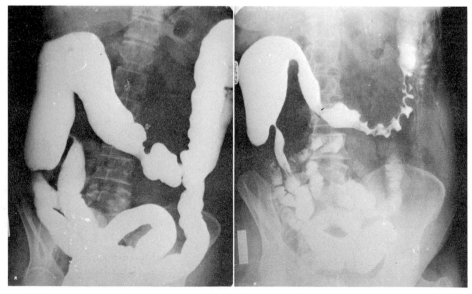

Fig. 63-29. Roentgenographic abnormality of the bowel produced by chronic catharsis.

frequently occur together. Carcinomas usually ooze blood and hence give anemia and occult blood in the feces, whereas diverticulosis rarely bleeds; if it does, the bleeding tends to be profuse, at times almost exsanguinating.

Irritable colon syndrome

The irritable colon syndrome, commonly called "colitis," with adjectives such as "spastic," "mucous," or "cathartic," and with variants such as "hepatic" and "splenic" flexure syndromes, should not be diagnosed roentgenologically, although frequently the examiner may be struck by the excessive irritability and activity of the colon. The small bowel may participate in the hypermotility, as is evident from the rapid transit time from the stomach to the ileocecal valve and to the rectum. The enema may reproduce the patient's typical distress, a consideration of considerable significance, and the radiologist may even note some correlation between bowel spasm and pain. Such information is helpful to the clinician, but it does not have the objective validity of the demonstration of a napkin ring deformity or a polypoid tumor. Occasionally patients with a long history of chronic catharsis will be found to have colons devoid of haustral pattern, simulating chronic ulcerative colitis (Fig. 63-29), or visceral sclerodermal involving the colon. The diagnosis of irritable colon is based on the history, the absence of pus and blood in the feces, and the negative proctoscopic examination except for the frequent demonstration of melanosis coli.

Postdysenteric enteritis

Postdysenteric enteritis is a painful hypermotility of the bowel that, as the name implies, may follow any type of acute enteritis, bacterial, viral, or amebic, and may persist for a number of months. The radiologist may detect the spasm and hyperactivity of an "angry" or irritated bowel, but there is nothing pathognomonic about the picture.

Specific granulomas

In the earlier years, and even now in some areas, the most important specific intestinal lesion was and is tuberculosis secondary to pulmonary tuberculosis.

Typically the lesions are found in the ileum and in the proximal colon of patients with active pulmonary tuberculosis; they constitute a form if ileocolitis, as illustrated in Fig. 63-30. Healing can occur if the tuberculosis is treated properly. Bovine tuberculosis, now extinct in North America, may produce a hyperplastic type of disease in the cecum and ascending colon.

Actinomycosis may also result in a mass in the proximal colon that is hard and fixed and tending toward fistulization. Amebic granulomas of the colon may simulate tuberculosis or

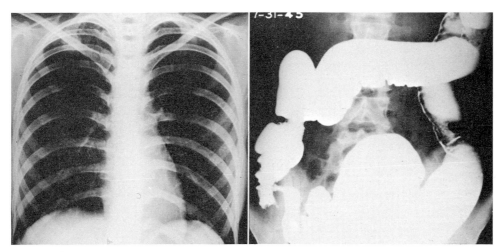

Fig. 63-30. Tuberculous ileocolitis (clinically and surgically controlled); the soft infiltration in the apex of the right lung is poorly reproduced.

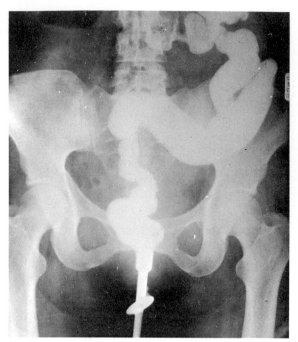

Fig. 63-31. Glove and finger stricture of the rectosigmoid caused by lymphopathia venereum.

Crohn's disease, although the ileum is very rarely involved. Amebic colitis is roentgenologically indistinguishable from the other forms of granulomatous colitis. The diagnosis depends upon the history, the proctoscopic picture, and above all the demonstration by direct examination or by culture of *Entamoeba histolytica* in the feces or in swabs obtained at proctoscopy.[69,79] Lymphopathia venereum may produce a "glove and finger" stricture of the rectum or rectosigmoid (Fig. 63-31).

Granulomatous colitis (Crohn's disease)

The frequency of granulomatous colitis or Crohn's disease of the colon has not been appreciated until recent years. When the process involves the entire colon it simulates chronic nonspecific ulcerative colitis. In some patients the anus, rectum, and sigmoid seem to be the primary site of the disease, producing rectal bleeding, more or less diarrhea, anal fistulas, and dense anal strictures interfering with defecation.[33]

Ulcerative colitis

Chronic nonspecific ulcerative colitis is a disease of considerable antiquity and, like Crohn's

disease, one of increasing frequency. Both are of unknown etiology and pathogenesis; they seem at times to merge into each other and are sometimes difficult to differentiate. Pathologically they are quite different.[49,77]

Crohn's disease is a chronic inflammatory disease of the entire wall of the bowel, with fibrosis and ulceration. Granulomas are frequently, but not invariably, present in the intestine as well as in the enlarged lymph nodes. Nonspecific ulcerative colitis starts as a mucosal disease, with thickening of the mucosa, edema, and friability; ulceration is a later manifestation, characteristically producing longitudinal ulceration above the rectosigmoid and eventually denuding the wall of the bowel completely in areas of variable size. Tags of old mucosa may be seen proctoscopically; on the roentgenogram they appear as pseudopolyposis.

Proctoscopic differentiation of the two diseases is difficult, if not impossible, although the granular, friable, edematous mucosa is much more typical of ulcerative colitis. It has been customary to consider this process as beginning in the rectum in 90% to 95% of the cases. The diagnosis of regional colitis was made in the 5% to 10% of patients in whom there was no proctoscopic evidence of disease although there were clinical and roentgenologic signs of involvement higher in the colon. In retrospect it seems to me probable that these were cases of Crohn's disease of the colon.[26] If more than a few centimeters of terminal ileum are involved, the disease is almost invariably Crohn's disease; backwash ileitis is limited and not progressive. On the other hand, recurring proctitis involving only the lower part of the ampulla or the rectosigmoid may come and go for years and apparently be related to ulcerative colitis rather than to Crohn's disease. Granulomas may be found in the wall of the bowel in ulcerative colitis.

In both ulcerative colitis and Crohn's disease chronic, inflammatory, ulcerative lesions, more or less granulomatous in nature, are found. One distinction between the two has been alleged to be that ulcerative colitis is curable by colectomy, whereas Crohn's disease is incurable; in terms of prognosis and therapy the distinction is important, but the statement is not entirely acceptable, for Crohn's disease may heal, regress, or be controlled by therapy.

The two most urgent acute complications of ulcerative colitis are free perforation and massive hemorrhage, either of which is an indication for immediate colectomy. Of almost equal urgency is so-called toxic megacolon, or paralytic ileus of a portion of the colon, usually the transverse.

The incidence of carcinoma in patients with long-standing ulcerative colitis is at least 3 times higher than it is in patients with otherwise normal colons; some authors set the figure at tenfold.

Polyposis

The Peutz-Jeghers syndrome may involve the colon, but the tumors are benign. Gardner's syndrome[27] is another familial disease, inherited as an autosomal dominant trait, with polyposis of the colon, multiple sebaceous cysts, and osteomas; the tendency toward neoplasm is high. In this respect it resembles multiple polyposis (Fig. 63-32), which also is a mendelian dominant almost invariably resulting in carcinoma, and frequently at an early age. Early colectomy is the only effective treatment. Adenomatous polyps are almost invariably benign, but they are usually subjected to surgical excision or biopsy because of the difficulty in their roentgenologic differentiation. Pedunculated polyps may appear neoplastic in cross section, but they

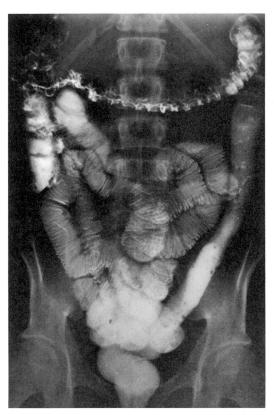

Fig. 63-32. Familial polyposis of the colon in an 18-year-old white male. (Courtesy Dr. R. D. Moseley.)

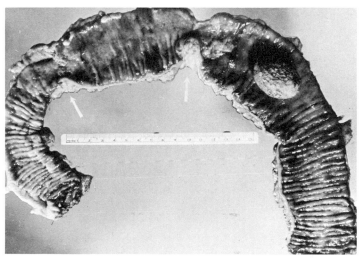

Fig. 63-33. Radiation-induced stricture of small intestine with fecalith.

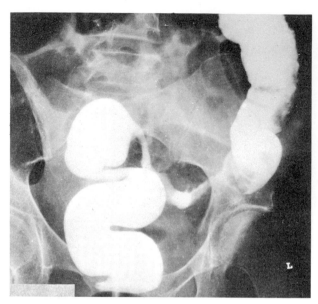

Fig. 63-34. Stenosis of the sigmoid 3 months after irradiation of an endometrial carcinoma with the linear accelerator.

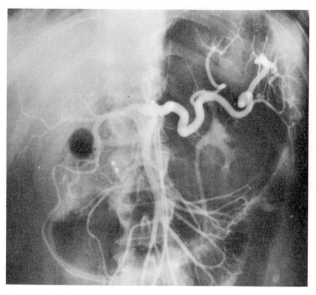

Fig. 63-35. Transfemoral aortography of a normal individual with one catheter in the celiac axis and the other in the superior mesenteric artery. The various branches of both arteries are clearly shown, together with contrast material in the pelvis of the left kidney. (Courtesy Dr. K. Ranniger.)

rarely invade the stalk or the wall of the bowel and still more rarely do they metastasize.

Cancer

Cancers of the colon are almost all adenocarcinomas. Colonic cancer has become one of the most common neoplasms of civilized man. In one study, the 5-year survival for all patients treated surgically was 50%; in the patients with localized tumor the 5-year survival was 70%.[21]

Typically, cancers of the proximal colon bleed early, producing secondary anemia, whereas those of the distal colon obstruct early. The outlook for patients with cancer of the rectum, when it is surgically resected, is essentially the same as that for cancer of the colon. The first symptom almost invariably is rectal bleeding. In patients with abdominal distress or rectal bleeding, digital examination, proctoscopy, and the barium enema constitute a triad. Omission by the physician of any one of these three procedures carries great risk to the patient.

Radiation reaction

Radiation reaction of the bowel is usually encountered in women subjected to external and internal radiation for carcinoma of the cervix. The lesions in the anterior rectal wall, in the

sigmoid, or even in the small bowel may occur early or late. Fig. 63-33 shows two such points of stricture in a loop of small intestine; a large fecalith proximal to the first stricture is responsible for the acute obstruction. Fig. 63-34 illustrates the roentgenographic appearance of the sigmoid in a 48-year-old woman treated approximately 3 months earlier for endometrial carcinoma by means of the linear accelerator. At autopsy, 25 days after the film was made, multiple strictures of the ileum and sigmoid were found, with necrosis of the bowel, fistulas, and generalized peritonitis.

Vascular disease

Arterial occlusion of the celiac axis, superior mesenteric, and inferior mesenteric vessels may produce different clinical syndromes.[12,52,56] Sudden occlusion of the superior mesenteric artery produces gangrene of the small bowel from the duodenum to the proximal colon. Occlusion of smaller vessels may result in partial infarction, with spontaneous recovery if the artery is small; if a larger vessel is affected, surgery may be life-saving.[42]

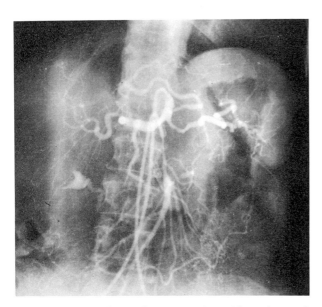

Fig. 63-36. Transfemoral aortography with catheters in the celiac axis and superior mesenteric arteries; narrowing of the artery leading to the splenic and short gastric arteries is well shown, as is narrowing of the superior mesenteric artery. (Courtesy Dr. K. Ranniger.)

Gradual narrowing and occlusion of the blood supply to the intestine may produce the picture of abdominal angina—an angina of digestive effort—with pain induced by eating and not relieved by anything. Robb coined an appropriate phrase for the clinical picture, namely, the "small meal syndrome"[62]; it is quite different from any other abdominal pain. As Maynard has pointed out, its course is progressive, inexorably leading to infarction of the bowel.[54]

Recent developments in arteriography have provided valuable tools for the demonstration of such vascular lesions.[60] Fig. 63-35 shows a visualization of the normal celiac axis and superior mesenteric arteries, whereas Fig. 63-36 demonstrates the narrowing found in the superior mesenteric artery and in the branch of the celiac axis leading to the short gastric and splenic vessels. The patient underwent an endarterectomy of the superior mesenteric artery with symptomatic relief.[60]

Mesenteric venous occlusions may arise spontaneously and be completely reversible, as in the case reported by Mayer and Poore.[53] The symptoms are slower in onset and in their evolution than is the case with arterial occlusion.

REFERENCES

1. Adams, W. E., and Phemister, D. B.: Carcinoma of the lower thoracic esophagus, J. Thorac. Surg. **7**:621, 1938.
2. Åkerlund, A.: Röntgenologische Studien uber den Bulbus duodeni mit besonderer Berucksichtigung des Ulcus duodoni, Acta Radiol. **1** (Supp.): 1, 1921.
3. Allen, A. C., Boley, S. J., Schultz, L., and Schwartz, S.: Potassium-induced lesions of the small bowel, II. Pathology and pathogenesis, J.A.M.A. **193**:1001, 1965.
4. Ardeman, S., and Chanarin, I.: Intrinsic factor secretion in gastric atrophy, Gut **7**:1, 1966.
5. Barclay, A. E.: The normal and pathological stomach as seen by x-rays, Brit. Med. J. **2**:537, 1910.
6. Barrett, N. R.: Chronic peptic ulcer of the oesophagus and "oesophagitis," Brit. J. Surg. **38**:175, 1950.
7. Benedict, E. B.: An extraordinary body in the esophagus, New Eng. J. Med. **269**:146, 1963.
8. Benedict, E. B.: Esophageal stenosis caused by peptic esophagitis or ulceration, Surg. Gynec. Obstet. **122**:613, 1966.
9. Bennett, T. I.: The stomach and upper alimentary canal in health and disease, London, 1925, Wm. Wood and Company.
10. Berg, H. H.: Roentgenuntersuchungen am Innerrelief des Verdauungskanals, Leipzig, 1930, Georg Thieme.
11. Bernot, R., and Norton, R.: The esophageal acid perfusion test, Lahey Clin. Found. Bull. **14**:2, 1965.
12. Bircher, J., Bartholomew, L. G., Cain, J. C., and Adson, M. A.: Syndrome of intestinal arterial insufficiency, Arch. Intern. Med. **117**:5, 1966.
13. Boley, S. J., Allen, A. C., Schultz, L., and Schwartz, S.: Potassium-induced lesions of the small bowel, I. Clinical aspects, J.A.M.A. **193**:997, 1965.
14. Bolt, R. J., Wilson, W. S., and Pollard, H. M.: Gastric ulcer; evaluation of methods of treatment, Univ. Michigan Med. Cent. J. **23**:126, 1957.
14a. Borrmann, R.: Magenkarcinom. In Henke, F., and Lubarsch, O.: Handbuch der speziellen pathologischen Anatomie und Histologie, Berlin, 1926, Julius Springer.
15. Burdick, D., Prior, J. T., and Scanlon, G. T.: Peutz-Jeghers syndrome; a clinical-pathological study of a large family with a 10-year follow-up, Cancer **16**:854, 1963.
16. Burhenne, H. J.: Radiographic confirmation of the hyperosmolar-hypovolemic concept of the dumping syndrome. In II World Congress of Gastroenterology, vol. 2, Munich, 1962, S. Karger.
17. Calabro, J. J.: Heritable multiple polyposis syndromes of the gastrointestinal tract, Amer. J. Med. **33**:276, 1962.
18. Cannon, W. B., and Moser, A.: The movements of food in the oesophagus, Amer. J. Physiol. **1**:435, 1898.
19. Carman, R. D., and Miller, A.: Roentgenologic diagnosis of diseases of the alimentary canal, Philadelphia, 1920, W. B. Saunders Co.
20. Castle, W. B.: Treatment of pernicious anemia;

clinical aspects, Clin. Pharmacol. Ther. 7:2, 1966.

21. Clayman, C. B., Webber, W. W., and Palmer, W. L.: The measurement of cancer survival by a hospital registry, Surg. Gynec. Obstet. 112:173, 1961.

22. Cole, L. G.: The value of serial radiography in gastro-intestinal diagnosis, J.A.M.A. 59:1947, 1912.

23. Cooke, W. T., Cox, E. V., Fone, D. J., Meynell, M. J., and Gaddie, R.: The clinical and metabolic significance of jejunal diverticula, Gut 4:115, 1963.

24. Corsini, G., Gandolfi, E., Bonechi, I., and Cerri, B.: Postgastrectomy malabsorption, Gastroenterology 50:3, 1966.

25. Crohn, B. B., Ginzburg, L., and Oppenheimer, G. D.: Regional ileitis; a pathologic and clinical entity, J.A.M.A. 99:1323, 1932.

26. Crohn, B. B., and Yarnis, H.: Regional ileitis, ed. 2, New York, 1958, Grune & Stratton, Inc.

26a. Dashiell, G. F., and Palmer, W. L.: Carcinoma of the pancreas; diagnostic criteria, Arch. Intern. Med. 81:173, 1948.

27. Dawborn, J. K., Ferguson, J., and Sanistreet, R. H.: Familial polyposis coli with multiple sebaceous cysts and osteomata; Gardner's syndrome, Aust. Ann. Med. 11:3, 1962.

28. Delaney, W. E., and Hedges, R. C.: Acquired ileal diverticulosis and hemorrhagic diverticulitis, Gastroenterology 42:56, 1962.

29. Doll, R., Jones, F. A., Pygott, F., and Stubbe, J. L.: The risk of gastric cancer after medical treatment for gastric ulcer, Gastroenterologia 88:1, 1957.

30. Dragstedt, L. R., and Woodward, E. R.: Appraisal of vagotomy for peptic ulcer after seven years. J.A.M.A. 145:795, 1951.

31. Dworken, H. J., Roth, H. P., and Duber, H. A.: The efficacy of medical criteria in differentiating benign from malignant gastric ulcers, Ann Intern. Med. 47:711, 1957.

32. Faber, K.: Gastritis and its consequences, New York, 1935, Oxford University Press, Inc.

33. Gray, B. K., Lockhart-Mummery, H. E., and Morson, B. C.: Crohn's disease of the anal region, Gut 6:515, 1965.

34. Hale, C. H., and Schatzki, R.: The visceral manifestations of scleroderma; a review of the recent literature, Amer. J. Roentgen. 51:407, 1944.

35. Heinz, E. R., Steinberg, A. J., and Sackner, M. A.: Roentgenographic and pathologic aspects of intestinal scleroderma, Ann. Intern. Med. 822, 1963.

36. Hirschowitz, B. I.: Endoscopic examination of the stomach and duodenal cap with the fiberscope, Lancet 1:1074, 1961.

37. Hodges, P. C.: Personal communication.

38. Howell, J. S., and Knapton, P. J.: Ileal cecal tuberculosis, Gut 5:524, 1964.

39. Hurst, A. F.: Treatment of achalasia of the cardia, Lancet 1:667, 1927.

40. Johnson, O. A., Hoskins, D. W., Todd, J., and Thorbjarnarson, B.: Crohn's disease of the stomach, Gastroenterology 50:571, 1966.

41. Jones, C. M.: Digestive tract pain, New York, 1938, The Macmillan Company.

42. Joske, R. A., Shamma'a, M. H., and Drummey, G.

D.: Intestinal malabsorption following temporary occlusion of the superior mesenteric artery, Amer. J. Med. 25:449, 1958.

43. Kirsner, J. B., and Palmer, W. L.: Gastritis. In The cyclopedia of medicine, surgery, specialties, vol. 13, Philadelphia, 1951, F. A. Davis Co.

44. Konjetzny, G. E.: Die entzündliche Grundlage der typischen Geschwürsbildung im Magen und Duodenum, Berlin, 1930, Julius Springer.

45. Konjetzny, G. E.: Der Magenkrebs, Stuttgart, 1939, Ferdinand Enke.

46. Laws, J. W., Mollin, D. L., and Coghill, N. F.: Relation of radiological appearance to gastric function in simple atrophic gastritis, Lancet 1:510, 1966.

47. Levin, E., Palmer, W. L., and Kirsner, J. B.: Observations on the diagnosis, treatment, and course of gastric ulcer, J.A.M.A. 156:1383, 1954.

48. Littman, A., and Bernstein, L. M.: Clinical diagnosis in peptic ulcer and esophagitis, Med. Clin. N. Amer. 46:747, 1962.

49. Lockhart-Mummery, H. E., and Morson, B. C.: Crohn's disease of the large intestine, Gut 5:492, 1964.

50. Maimon, S. N., Bartlett, J. P., Humphreys, E. M., and Palmer, W. L.: Giant hypertrophic gastritis, Gastroenterol. 8:4, 1947.

51. Maimon, S. N., Palmer, W. L., and Kirsner, J. B.: Prognosis in gastric cancer; a study of five-year survivors, Amer. J. Med. 5:230, 1948.

52. Marston, A., Pheils, M. T., Thomas, M. L., and Morson, B. C.: Ischaemic colitis, Gut 7:1, 1966.

53. Mayer, H., and Poore, T. B.: Reversible mesenteric venous thrombosis, Arch. Intern. Med. 114:359, 1964.

54. Maynard, E. P., III: Intestinal angina. In McHardy, G., editor: Current gastroenterology, New York, 1962, Paul B. Hoeber, Inc.

55. Mossberg, S. M.: The columnar-lined esophagus (Barrett syndrome)—an acquired condition? Gastroenterol. 50:671, 1966.

55a. Nash, E. C., and Palmer, W. L.: The clinical significance of diverticulosis, including diverticulitis of the gastrointestinal tract, Ann. Intern. Med. 27:41, 1947.

56. Palmer, W. L.: Clinical features of mesenteric artery insufficiency, J. Tenn. Med. Ass. 59:152, 1966.

56a. Palmer, W. L., and Humphreys, E. M.: Gastric carcinoma; observations on peptic ulceration and healing, Gastroenterol. 3:266, 1944.

57. Palmer, W. L., Schindler, R., Templeton, F., and Humphreys, E. M.: Syphilis of the stomach; a case report, Ann. Intern. Med. 18:3, 1943.

58. Paulk, E. A., Jr., and Farrar, W. E., Jr.: Diverticulosis of the small intestine and megaloblastic anemia, Amer. J. Med. 37:473, 1964.

59. Paustian, F. F., Stein, G. N., Young, J. F., Roth, J. L. A., and Bockus, H. L.: The importance of the brief trial of rigid medical management in the diagnosis of benign versus malignant gastric ulcer, Gastroenterol. 38:155, 1960.

60. Ranniger, K.: Personal communication.

61. Raskin, H. F., Kirsner, J. B., and Palmer, W. L.:

Role of exfoliative cytology in the diagnosis of cancer of the digestive tract, J.A.M.A. **169**:789, 1959.

62. Robb, G. P.: Discussion of revascularization of the celiac and superior mesenteric arteries, Arch. Surg. (Chicago) **84**:107, 1962.

63. Salen, G., Goldstein, F., and Wirts, C. W.: Malabsorption in intestinal scleroderma; relation to bacterial flora and treatment with antibiotics, Ann. Intern. Med. **64**:4, 1966.

64. Schatzki, R., MacMahon, H. E., and Gary, J. E.: Pathology of a lower esophageal ring; report of a case with autopsy, observed for nine years, New Eng. J. Med. **259** (1):1, 1958.

65. Schatzki, R., and Castleman, B.: Lower abdominal pain, fever and melena in a nineteen-year-old girl, New Eng. J. Med. **274**:10, 1966.

66. Schindler, R.: Gastroscopy; the endoscopic study of gastric pathology, Chicago, 1937, The University of Chicago Press.

67. Schindler, R.: Gastroscopy; the endoscopic study of gastric pathology, ed. 2, Chicago, 1950, The University of Chicago Press.

68. Schiffer, L. M., Faloon, W. W., Chodos, R. E., and Lozner, E. L.: Malabsorption syndrome associated with intestinal diverticulosis, Gastroenterol. **42**:63, 1962.

69. Shaffer, J. G., Shlaes, W. H., and Radke, R. A.: Amebiasis; a biomedical problem, Springfield, Ill., 1965, Charles C Thomas, Publisher.

70. Shocket, E., Neber, J., and Drosd, R. E.: The acutely obstructed incarcerated paraesophageal hiatal hernia, Amer. J. Surg. **108**:805, 1964.

71. Strandjord, N. M., Moseley, R. D., Jr., and Schweinfus, R. L.: Gastric carcinoma; accuracy of radiologic diagnosis, Radiology **74**:442, 1960.

72. Templeton, F. E.: X-ray examination of the stomach, Chicago, 1944, The University of Chicago Press.

73. Truelove, S. C., and Reynell, P. C.: Diseases of the digestive system, Philadelphia, 1963, F. A. Davis Co.

74. Valdes-Dapena, A., Affolter, H., and Vilardell, F.: The gradient of malignancy in lymphoid lesions of the stomach, Gastroenterology **50**:382, 1966.

75. Waldman, T. A.: Protein-losing enteropathy, Gastroenterol. **50**:3, 1966.

76. Warren, K. W., Kune, G. A., and Poulantzas, J. K.: Peutz-Jeghers syndrome with carcinoma of the duodenum and jejunum, Lahey Clin. Found. Bull. **4**:97, 1965.

77. Warren, S., and Sommers, S. C.: Pathology of regional ileitis and ulcerative colitis, J.A.M.A. **154** (3): 189, 1954.

78. White, R. R., Bargen, J. A., and Saghafi, M. M.: Prolapse of gastric mucosa into the duodenum, Postgrad. Med. **39**:512, 1966.

79. Wilmot, A. J.: Clinical amoebiasis, Philadelphia, 1962, F. A. Davis Company.

80. Wood, I. J., and Taft, L. I.: Diffuse lesions of the stomach, London, 1958, Edward Arnold, Ltd.

81. Zollinger, R. M., and Craig, T.: Endocrine tumors and peptic ulcer, Amer. J. Med. **29**:761, 1960.

I wish to acknowledge permission to reproduce illustrations from the following sources:

Cecil, R. L., and Loeb, R. F., editors: A textbook of medicine, ed. 9, Philadelphia, 1955, W. B. Saunders Co.

Maimon, S. N., Bartlett, J. P., Humphreys, E. M., and Palmer, W. L.: Gastroenterology **8**:397, 1947.

Nash, E. C., and Palmer, W. L.: Ann. Intern. Med. **27**:41, 1947.

Palmer, W. L.: Ann. Intern. Med. **13**:317, 1939.

Palmer, W. L.: Gastroenterology **1**:723, 1943.

Palmer, W. L.: Postgrad. Med. **39**:123, 1966.

Palmer, W. L., and Humphreys, E. M.: Gastroenterology **3**:257, 1944.

Palmer, W. L., Schindler, R., Templeton, F. E., and Humphreys, E. M.: Ann. Intern. Med. **13**:317, 1939.

64 | Communication between the radiologist and the clinician

John V. Carbone

The patient with gastrointestinal disease represents a unique challenge to the physician. For the most part, the gastrointestinal tract is inaccessible except by endoscopic and roentgenographic techniques.

The clinician dealing with gastrointestinal tract disease must decide whether he would serve his patients most effectively by limiting himself strictly to diseases of the intestinal tract and knowing all the necessary techniques of gastrointestinal examination. The alternative is an emphasis on the clinical aspects of all branches of gastroenterology and specialized support by an appropriately trained radiologist.

Ideally, a physician should be able to perform most studies on his patients. Realistically, this is no longer true. The breadth and complexity of modern medicine have channeled and will continue to channel physicians into specialized areas. Because the physician will no longer be able to perform all procedures on his patients, he can provide the best patient service by calling upon those most highly skilled in the techniques involved. Roentgenology of the intestinal tract should be done by the person best qualified, in some instances the gastroenterologist, in most the radiologist. It is then the responsibility of the gastroenterologist to be familiar with techniques of the radiologist, and the radiologist doing gastrointestinal roentgenology must be informed on advances in clinical gastroenterology.

The radiologist is a colleague and collaborator in the practice of gastroenterology. In order to have a good working relationship, effective communication between physicians must be established. Communication, by definition, is an exchange of information. Both the clinician and the radiologist must participate. The remainder of this discussion will be devoted to this topic.

Communication begins with the patient. The clinician is confronted with the problem of defining the disease entity that has caused the patient's complaint of: (1) pain, and/or (2) gastrointestinal dysfunction (such as diarrhea, constipation, dysphagia), and/or (3) change in appearance of body or excrement (weight loss, jaundice, pallor, melena). The clinician formulates the history and physical examination into concepts relating to the disease process. This material should be available to all physicians participating in the patient's diagnosis and treatment. If the clinician has failed to provide information, the radiologist should seek the necessary data himself prior to examination. Effective roentgenologic consultation requires an adequate history. There is no excuse for withholding information from a consultant. Whether it be deliberate or inadvertent, it detracts from the value of the consultation. The radiologist's final opinion should reflect a careful analysis of the clinical as well as the roentgenologic observations.

Effective communication prior to the procedure enables the radiologist to individualize his approach in problem cases. Variations in contrast media, intensity of examination, and techniques employed may be indicated and should be determined by the best roentgenologic approach to a problem rather than by the referring clinician's inclination.

The clinician is often concerned about whether or not he should be present during the roentgenologic examination of his patient. Ideally, the best roentgenologic observations are those made with the least distraction. However, when the patient's state is precarious, the clinician should be present to evaluate the patient and assist the radiologist, should the need arise.

There are also occasions when the radiologist and clinician collaborate to position intraluminal tubes for biopsy and aspiration.

The radiologist's opinion is formalized in a written report. The information most useful to the clinician includes the following: (1) technical factors (preparation, type of barium); (2) observations in terms of structure and function of the organ system under study, with description of these findings in the body of the report; (3) conclusions and diagnosis (where applicable, a differential diagnosis may prove helpful to the clinician); and (4) suggestions for further roentgenologic study and follow-up when appropriate.

In instances in which the gastroenterologist may be working with a general radiologist who has no particular interest in gastrointestinal roentgenology, it is helpful to discuss the information desired prior to the roentgenographic study. It makes the radiologist more aware of the data necessary for the clinician's diagnosis and treatment. This attention by the clinician will be appreciated by the radiologist and may foster his special interest in gastrointestinal tract examination.

The radiologist should be on guard not to extend his conclusions beyond the bounds of his technique. There are instances in which histologic diagnoses such as gastritis, duodenitis, or colitis are made by the radiologist, when the roentgenologic observations are those of altered tone and motility of the intestine. When the radiologist or clinician suspects mucosal disease, it may be appropriate for one or the other to suggest colonoscopy or fiberoptic endoscopy of the upper gastrointestinal tract. These new techniques complement the roentgenologic examination rather than compete with it. The radiologist is uniquely able to describe and document many anatomic and physiologic functions of the gastrointestinal tract. The finer details of mucosal disease that do not alter structure, tone, or motility may escape him. In this instance, the endoscopist is uniquely qualified by direct visualization and biopsy to substantiate mucosal disease. It is essential that the radiologist and clinician appreciate the advantages and limitations of each technique.

Retrospective diagnoses are inappropriate. If the data are inadequate for a diagnosis, the radiologist should so state and advise repeat studies. Prompt reporting to the clinician is mandatory; personal reporting is gratifying and may prove useful in preventing delay of appropriate studies or treatment.

The relationship between the radiologist and the clinician should not end with the roentgenologic report. Follow-up studies and conclusions are necessary for continuing education and for substantiation of their observations. Referral to other data, such as manometric motility studies, biopsy, or necropsy, should serve in this regard. The radiologist must maintain an active interest in clinical medicine.

In summary, the radiologist functions as a consultant, with specialized techniques and knowledge in the investigation of the alimentary tract. The relationship between the clinician and the radiologist is based upon effective communication. It is the responsibility of both physicians. The needs of patients will be served best by mutually well-informed radiologists and clinicians.

Index

1

Syndromes—cont'd
body cast, 628, 731, 747
Boerhaave's, 750
Budd-Chiari, 1214-1215
hepatocarcinoma and, 1238, 1241
suprahepatic obstruction and, 1374
chiliaditis, 1501, 1502
Courvoisier's, 1304
Cronkhite-Canada, 914, 1055-1056, 1061-1062, 1063
diffuse esophageal spasm, 421, 472-473, 527, 537, 539-542
Down's, 43, 710, 1542-1543
dumping, 773-774, 1675
Gardner's, 914, 1055-1056, 1057-1060, 1063
carcinoma and, 1068, 1096
clinical synopsis of, 1683
gastric polyposis and, 700
mesenteric fibromatosis and, 796
hypertensive esophagogastric sphincter as, 539
inspissated bile, 1523
irritable colon
clinical synopsis of, 1681
diverticular disease and, 1027-1032
MacMahon-Tannhauser, 1507
malabsorption; *see* Malabsorption
Mallory-Weiss, 341, 457-459, 749, 756
meconium plug, 1485-1487, 1533
Milkman's, 774
Mirizzi, 1304
mucosal neuroma, in children, 1548
oculopharyngeal, 326
Paterson-Kelly, 332-333
Peutz-Jeghers; *see* Peutz-Jeghers syndrome
Plummer-Vinson, 332-334
polyposis; *see* Polyposis and syndromes
postcholecystectomy, 1275, 1322-1326
postgastrectomy, 585, 772-775
postvagotomy, 476-477, 481, 1675
proximal loop, 764, 765, 774-775
Rendu-Osler-Weber, 879-880
Riley-Day, 326, 1544
Sandifer's, 1544
Schatzki's, 447, 451, 452, 453; *see also* Schatzki's ring
Schönlein-Henoch, 1499, 1542, 1624-1626, 1627, 1628
small meal, 1685
superior mesenteric artery, 731
trisomy, 1542-1544
Turcot, 914, 1055-1056, 1061, 1063, 1068, 1096
watery diarrhea hypokalemia achlorhydria, 1121
Wilkie's, 628
Zollinger-Ellison; *see* Zollinger-Ellison syndrome
Syphilis
colonic malignancy and, 1095
of stomach, 557, 614-615, 1664
tuberculosis and, 1578
Systemic diseases in children, 1531-1553
cystic fibrosis of pancreas in, 1531-1537
exocrine pancreatic insufficiency, blood disorders, and metaphyseal dysostosis in, 1537, 1538

Systemic diseases in children—cont'd
hematologic disease and, 1537-1542
mucosal neuroma syndrome in, 1547, 1548
neurofibromatosis and, 1548
pharyngeal and esophageal abnormalities in, 1544-1545
psychogenic disorders in, 1545-1548
renal tubular ectasia and hepatic fibrosis in, 1549, 1550
trisomy syndromes and, 1542-1544
Zollinger-Ellison syndrome in, 1548-1550
Systemic sclerosis, progressive; *see* Progressive systemic sclerosis

T

T tube cholangiography, 1303, 1327; *see also* Biliary system, operative and postoperative study of
Taenia saginata and *taenia solium*, 1566-1567
Tannic acid, 933-934
in barium sulfate suspension, 936
and bisacodyl, 933, 937, 948, 1038-1039
in enemas, 1038
Tapered nipple configuration, 1348, 1349, 1350
Tapeworms, 1566-1567
Tartaric acid, duodenal receptors and, 67
Tears; *see* Lacerations
Telangiectasia, hereditary hemorrhagic, 1400, 1429, 1444, 1445
Telepaque; *see* Iopanoic acid
Television
equipment for, 26-28
in fluoroscopic images, magnetic recording and, 31-32
test equipment for, 28
Tensilon; *see* Edrophonium chloride
Tenting of wall and mucosa of small bowel, 900
Teratomas
duodenal metastasis and, 734, 736
of stomach, cystic, 555
Teridax; *see* Propionic acid
Tertiary contractions of esophagus, 418-420, 421, 469, 473, 477, 542, 543
Tests
Casoni's, 1228
complement fixation, 1594, 1595
four-day iopanoic acid, 1309
Frei, 1594
histamine, familial dysautonomia and, 1544
Kveim, 614
methacholine, 367, 427, 428, 469, 470-471, 479
serum amylase, 258-260
sniff, 498
turning, for esophageal reflux, 505
Valsalva, esophagogastric ring and, 454; *see also* Valsalva maneuver
Tetracycline, 1676
Tetraethylammonium chloride, small-bowel examinations and, 805
Thalassemia with extramedullary hematopoiesis in liver, 1210

Thallium intoxication, 1218
Thiazides, small-bowel ulcers and, 790
Thiokinase, 110
Thixotrophy, 117
Thoracic duct, compression of, 484, 485
Thorax, amebiasis and changes in, 1570-1571
Thorium, liver density and, 1218-1220
Thorium compounds as contrast medium, 7, 15
Thorium dioxide, 1219, 1220
Thorotrast; *see* Thorium dioxide
Thrombocytopenia, intramural bleeding and, 1629
Thromboembolism, gastric surgery and, 747
Thrombosis
of abdominal veins, 1441
acute pancreatitis and, 220
arteriography and, 1400
gastric surgery and, 747
mesenteric, 173, 211-213, 1608-1609
Thumb-printing defects, 968, 969, 1499
of bowel wall, 286, 287
of colon, 1586, 1587, 1610
in hemophilia, 1541
submucosal hemorrhage and, 1542
Thymoma, 380
Thyrohyoid membrane, anatomic weak area of, 309, 312
Thyroid
carcinoma of, stomach metastasis and, 564
hypertrophy of, 398, 399, 400, 401, 402
lingual, 37
myopathy and, 328
Thyrotoxicosis, 477
Tiered spasms in esophagus, 469
Tilting table, invention of, 9
Time-density-retention concept in cholangiography, 1296-1297, 1298-1299
Tissue-paper folds of stomach, 612
Tissue staining, arteriography and, 1400
Tolazoline hydrochloride, 1363
Tomography
of kidneys, 175
pancreatic size and, 729
of pharynx, 302, 303
retropneumoperitoneum with, 1122
Tongue, phonation and, 301
Tongue worms, 1567-1568
Torsion
diaphragmatic hernias and, 201
of omentum, 565
in volvulus, 207, 209, 210
Tortuosity of descending aorta, 417, 418, 419
Torus hyperplasia, 605-607
Tracheoesophageal fistula, 38-39, 339, 473-474
in children, 1470, 1471-1472
contrast media and, 277
differential diagnosis in, 480
Traction diverticula of esophagus, 340, 352, 393
Transduodenal pancreatography, 1123-1125
Transfusional hemosiderosis, 1218